Health, United States, 1998

With Socioeconomic Status and Health Chartbook

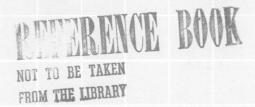
U.S. DEPARTMENT OF HEALTH AND HUMAN SERVICES
Centers for Disease Control and Prevention
National Center for Health Statistics
6525 Belcrest Road
Hyattsville, Maryland 20782

DHHS Publication number (PHS) 98-1232

D1299787

U.S. Department of Health and Human Services

Donna E. Shalala
Secretary

Office of Public Health and Science

David Satcher, M.D., Ph.D.
Assistant Secretary for Health

Centers for Disease Control and Prevention (CDC)

Claire V. Broome, M.D.
Acting Director

National Center for Health Statistics

Edward J. Sondik, Ph.D.
Director

For sale by the U.S. Government Printing Office
Superintendent of Documents, Mail Stop: SSOP, Washington, DC 20402-9328
ISBN 0-16-049631-4

Health, United States, 1998 is the 22d report on the health status of the Nation submitted by the Secretary of Health and Human Services to the President and Congress of the United States in compliance with Section 308 of the Public Health Service Act. This report was compiled by the Centers for Disease Control and Prevention (CDC), National Center for Health Statistics (NCHS). The National Committee on Vital and Health Statistics served in a review capacity.

Health, United States presents national trends in health statistics. Major findings are presented in the Highlights. The report includes a chartbook and detailed tables. In each edition of *Health, United States*, the chartbook focuses on a major health topic. This year socioeconomic status and health was selected as the subject of the chartbook. The chartbook consists of 49 figures and accompanying text divided into sections on the population, children's health, and adults' health. The sections on children's and adults' health include subsections on health status, risk factors, and health care access and utilization.

The chartbook is followed by 149 detailed tables organized around four major subject areas: health status and determinants, utilization of health resources, health care resources, and health care expenditures. A major criterion used in selecting the detailed tables is the availability of comparable national data over a period of several years. The detailed tables report data for selected years to highlight major trends in health statistics. Similar tables appear in each volume of *Health, United States* to enhance the use of this publication as a standard reference source. For tables that show extended trends, earlier editions of *Health, United States* may present data for intervening years that are not included in the current printed report. Where possible, intervening years in an extended trend are retained in the Lotus 1–2–3 spreadsheet files (described below).

Several tables in *Health, United States* present data according to race and Hispanic origin consistent with Department-wide emphasis on expanding racial and ethnic detail in the presentation of health data. The presentation of data on race and ethnicity in the

detailed tables is usually in the greatest detail possible, after taking into account the quality of data, the amount of missing data, and the number of observations. The large differences in health status according to race and Hispanic origin that are documented in this report may be explained by several factors including socioeconomic status, health practices, psychosocial stress and resources, environmental exposures, discrimination, and access to health care.

Each year new tables are added to *Health, United States* to reflect emerging topics in public health and new variables are added to existing tables to enhance their usefulness. *Health, United States, 1998* includes the following four new tables. For the first time vaccination rates for children 19–35 months of age are provided for States and selected urban areas (table 53); access to health care according to poverty status and health insurance status is measured by no physican contact in the past year for children under 6 years of age and by no usual source of care for children under 18 years of age (tables 78 and 79); and data on medical care benefits for employees of private companies are presented (table 136). The following enhancements were made to existing tables. Data for racial and ethnic groups were expanded in tables showing years of potential life lost rates (table 32) and maternal mortality rates (table 45). Data by race were added to other tables as follows: the poverty rate in 1990 among the American Indian population (NOTE, table 2); vaccination rates for children by race and poverty status (table 52); and functional status of nursing home residents by race, sex, and age (table 96). Data on health care coverage were expanded to include employer-sponsored private insurance and additional race, age, and poverty status subgroups (tables 133 and 134). To address heightened interest in persons 55–64 years of age approaching Medicare eligibility, data by age were expanded for ambulatory care visits (tables 81 and 82). The percent of Medicare enrollees in managed care and the percent of Medicaid recipients in managed care in each State were added to tables 146 and 147.

Preface

To use *Health, United States* most effectively, the reader should become familiar with two appendixes at the end of the report. Appendix I describes each data source used in the report and provides references for further information about the sources. Appendix II is an alphabetical listing of terms used in the report. It also contains standard populations used for age adjustment and *International Classification of Diseases* codes for cause of death and diagnostic and procedure categories.

Health, United States can be accessed electronically in several formats. First, the entire *Health, United States, 1998* is available, along with other NCHS reports, on a CD-ROM entitled "Publications from the National Center for Health Statistics, featuring *Health, United States, 1998*," vol 1 no 4, 1998. These publications can be viewed, searched, printed, and saved using the Adobe Acrobat software on the CD-ROM. The CD-ROM may be purchased from the Government Printing Office or the National Technical Information Service.

Second, the complete *Health, United States, 1998* is available as an Acrobat .pdf file on the Internet through the NCHS home page on the World Wide Web. The direct Uniform Locator Code (URL) address is:

www.cdc.gov/nchswww/products/pubs/pubd/hus/hus.htm.

Third, the 149 detailed tables in *Health, United States, 1998* are available on the FTP server as Lotus 1–2–3 spreadsheet files that can be downloaded. An electronic index is included that enables the user to search the tables by topic. The URL address for the FTP server is:

www.cdc.gov/nchswww/datawh/ftpserv/ftpserv.htm.

The detailed tables and electronic index are also included as Lotus 1–2–3 spreadsheet files on the CD-ROM mentioned above.

Fourth, for users who do not have access to the Internet or to a CD-ROM reader, the 149 detailed tables can be made available on diskette as Lotus 1–2–3 spreadsheet files for use with IBM compatible personal computers. To obtain a copy of the diskette, contact the NCHS Data Dissemination Branch.

For answers to questions about this report, contact:

Data Dissemination Branch
National Center for Health Statistics
Centers for Disease Control and Prevention
6525 Belcrest Road, Room 1064
Hyattsville, Maryland 20782-2003

phone: 301-436-8500

E-mail: nchsquery@cdc.gov

Overall responsibility for planning and coordinating the content of this volume rested with the Office of Analysis, Epidemiology, and Health Promotion, National Center for Health Statistics (NCHS), under the supervision of Kate Prager, Diane M. Makuc, and Jacob J. Feldman. Highlights of the detailed tables were written by Margaret A. Cooke, Virginia M. Freid, Michael E. Mussolino, and Kate Prager. Detailed tables were prepared by Alan J. Cohen, Margaret A. Cooke, Virginia M. Freid, Michael E. Mussolino, Mitchell B. Pierre, Jr., Rebecca A. Placek, and Kate Prager with assistance from La-Tonya Curl, Catherine Duran, Deborah D. Ingram, Patricia A. Knapp, Jaleh Mousavi, Mark F. Pioli, Anita L. Powell, Ronica N. Rooks, Kenneth C. Schoendorf, Fred Seitz, and Jean F. Williams. The appendixes, index to detailed tables, and pocket edition were prepared by Anita L. Powell. Production planning and coordination were managed by Rebecca A. Placek with typing assistance from Carole J. Hunt.

The chartbook was prepared by Elsie R. Pamuk, Diane M. Makuc, Katherine E. Heck, Cynthia Reuben, and Kimberly Lochner in the Office of Analysis, Epidemiology, and Health Promotion under the general direction of Jacob J. Feldman. Data for specific charts were provided by Sylvia A. Ellison (figure 23) and Lois A. Fingerhut (figures 30–31) of NCHS; Joseph Gfroerer of the Substance Abuse and Mental Health Administration (figure 37); and Paul Sorlie of the National Heart, Lung, and Blood Institute (figure 25). Technical help was provided by Alan J. Cohen and Catherine Duran of TRW, Information Services Division; Laura Porter, Joyce Abma, Debra Brody, Catherine W. Burt, Margaret Carroll, Margaret A. Cooke, Virginia M. Freid, Wilbur C. Hadden, Tamy Hickman, Meena Khare, John L. Kiely, Patricia A. Knapp, Lola Jean Kozak, Jeffrey D. Maurer, Laura E. Montgomery, Cynthia Ogden, Linda W. Pickle, Mitchell B. Pierre, Jr., Ronica N. Rooks, Kenneth C. Schoendorf, Richard P. Troiano, Kathleen M. Turczyn, and Clemencia M. Vargas of NCHS; Edmond F. Maes

of the National Immunization Program, CDC; and Deborah Dawson of the National Institute on Alcohol Abuse and Alcoholism.

Dr. Philip R. Lee, former Assistant Secretary for Health and currently at the University of California at San Francisco, was instrumental in the development of the chartbook. Dr. Lee has long been committed to the study of the relationship between socioeconomic status and health and to applying the knowledge gained to improving the health of disadvantaged populations. Advice and encouragement was also graciously provided by the following individuals: Dr. Norman Anderson of the National Institutes of Health; Dr. A. John Fox of the Office for National Statistics, England; Dr. George Kaplan of the University of Michigan; Dr. Roz Lasker of the New York Academy of Medicine; Dr. Paul Newacheck of the University of California at San Francisco; and Dr. David Williams of the University of Michigan.

Publications management and editorial review were provided by Thelma W. Sanders and Rolfe W. Larson. The designer was Sarah M. Hinkle. Graphics were supervised by Stephen L. Sloan. Production was done by Jacqueline M. Davis and Annette F. Holman. Printing was managed by Patricia L. Wilson and Joan D. Burton.

Publication of *Health, United States* would not have been possible without the contributions of numerous staff members throughout the National Center for Health Statistics and several other agencies. These people gave generously of their time and knowledge, providing data from their surveys and programs; their cooperation and assistance are gratefully acknowledged.

Contents

Preface _____ iii

Acknowledgments _____ v

List of Figures on Socioeconomic Status and Health _____ ix

Geographic Regions and Divisions of the United States _____ xi

Highlights
Socioeconomic Status and Health Chartbook _____ 3
Detailed Tables _____ 9

Socioeconomic Status and Health Chartbook

Introduction _____ 23

Population _____ 29
    Income _____ 32
    Poverty _____ 36
    Education _____ 40
    Occupation _____ 44
Children's Health _____ 46
    Health Status
        Infant Mortality _____ 50
        Low Birthweight _____ 54
        Activity Limitation _____ 56
    Risk Factors
        Teenage Childbearing _____ 58
        Smoking in Pregnancy _____ 60
        Blood Lead _____ 62
        Cigarette Smoking _____ 64
        Overweight _____ 66
        Sedentary Lifestyle _____ 68
    Health Care Access and Utilization
        Prenatal Care _____ 70
        Health Insurance _____ 74
        Vaccinations _____ 76
        No Physician Contact _____ 78
        Ambulatory Care _____ 80
        Asthma Hospitalization _____ 82
Adults' Health _____ 84
    Health Status
        Life Expectancy _____ 88
        Cause of Death _____ 90
        Heart Disease Mortality _____ 92
        Lung Cancer Mortality _____ 94
        Diabetes Mortality _____ 96
        Homicide _____ 98
        Suicide _____ 100
        Fair or Poor Health _____ 102
        Activity Limitation _____ 104
        Activities of Daily Living _____ 106

Contents

Risk Factors
    Cigarette Smoking ___ 108
    Alcohol Use ___ 112
    Overweight ___ 114
    Sedentary Lifestyle ___ 118
    Hypertension ___ 120
    Blood Lead ___ 122
Health Care Access and Utilization
    Health Insurance ___ 124
    No Physician Contact ___ 126
    Mammography ___ 128
    Unmet Need for Care ___ 130
    Avoidable Hospitalization ___ 134
    Dental Care ___ 136

Technical Notes ___ 138
Data Tables for Figures 1–49 ___ 144

Detailed Tables

List of Detailed Tables ___ 163

Health Status and Determinants ___ 169
    Population ___ 169
    Fertility and Natality ___ 172
    Mortality ___ 190
    Determinants and Measures of Health ___ 261
Utilization of Health Resources ___ 287
    Ambulatory Care ___ 287
    Inpatient Care ___ 302
Health Care Resources ___ 321
    Personnel ___ 321
    Facilities ___ 334
Health Care Expenditures ___ 341
    National Health Expenditures ___ 341
    Health Care Coverage and Major Federal Programs ___ 361
    State Health Expenditures ___ 372

Appendixes

Contents ___ 383
I. Sources and Limitations of Data ___ 386
II. Glossary ___ 419

Index to Detailed Tables ___ 446

Population

1. Household income at selected percentiles of the household income distribution: United States, 1970–96__ **33**

2. Median household income by race and Hispanic origin: United States, 1980–96_____ **35**

3. Percent of persons poor and near poor by race and Hispanic origin: United States, 1996_____ **37**

4. Percent of persons in poverty by State: United States, average annual 1994–96_____ **39**

5. Educational attainment among persons 25 years of age and over by age, race, and Hispanic origin: United States, 1996_____ **41**

6. Median household income among persons 25 years of age and over by education, sex, race, and Hispanic origin: United States, 1996_____ **43**

7. Current occupation for persons 25–64 years of age by sex, race, and Hispanic origin: United States, 1996_____ **45**

Children's Health

Health Status

8. Infant mortality rates among infants of mothers 20 years of age and over by mother's education and race: United States, 1983–95_____ **51**

9. Infant mortality rates among infants of mothers 20 years of age and over by mother's education, race, and Hispanic origin: United States, 1995_____ **53**

10. Low-birthweight live births among mothers 20 years of age and over by mother's education, race, and Hispanic origin: United States, 1996_____ **55**

11. Activity limitation among children under 18 years of age by family income, race, and Hispanic origin: United States, average annual, 1984–87, 1988–91, and 1992–95_____ **56**

Risk Factors

12. Percent of women 20–29 years of age who had a teenage birth, by respondent's mother's education and respondent's race and Hispanic origin: United States, 1995_____ **59**

13. Cigarette smoking during pregnancy among mothers 20 years of age and over by mother's education, race, and Hispanic origin: United States, 1996_____ **61**

14. Elevated blood lead among children 1–5 years of age by family income, race, and Hispanic origin: United States, average annual 1988–94_____ **62**

15. Cigarette smoking among adolescents 12–17 years of age by family income, race, and Hispanic origin: United States, 1992_____ **65**

16. Overweight among adolescents 12–17 years of age by family income, race, and Hispanic origin: United States, average annual 1988–94_____ **67**

17. Sedentary lifestyle among adolescents 12–17 years of age by family income and sex: United States, 1992__ **69**

Health Care Access and Utilization

18. Prenatal care use in the first trimester among mothers 20 years of age and over by mother's education and race: United States, 1980–96_____ **71**

19. Prenatal care use in the first trimester among mothers 20 years of age and over by mother's education, race, and Hispanic origin: United States, 1996_____ **73**

20. Percent of children under 18 years of age with no health insurance coverage by family income, race, and Hispanic origin: United States, average annual 1994–95_ **75**

21. Vaccinations among children 19–35 months of age by poverty status, race, and Hispanic origin: United States, 1996_____ **77**

22. Percent of children under 6 years of age with no physician contact during the past year by family income, health insurance status, race, and Hispanic origin: United States, average annual 1994–95_____ **78**

23. Ambulatory care visits among children under 18 years of age by median household income in ZIP Code of residence and place of visit: United States, 1995_____ **81**

24. Asthma hospitalization rates among children 1–14 years of age by median household income in ZIP Code of residence and race: United States, average annual 1989–91_____ **83**

Adults' Health

Health Status

25. Life expectancy among adults 45 and 65 years of age by family income, sex, and race: United States, average annual 1979–89_____ **89**

26. Death rates for selected causes for adults 25–64 years of age, by education level and sex: Selected States, 1995_____ **91**

27. Heart disease death rates among adults 25–64 years of age and 65 years of age and over by family income, sex, race, and Hispanic origin: United States, average annual 1979–89_____ **92**

List of Figures ....

28. Lung cancer death rates among adults 25–64 years of age and 65 years of age and over by family income and sex: United States, average annual 1979–89_____ 95

29. Diabetes death rates among adults 45 years of age and over by family income and sex: United States, average annual 1979–89_____ 97

30. Homicide rates among adults 25–44 years of age by education, sex, race, and Hispanic origin: Selected States, average annual 1994–95_____ 99

31. Suicide rates among adults 25–64 years of age by education, sex, race and Hispanic origin: Selected States, average annual 1994–95_____ 101

32. Fair or poor health among adults 18 years of age and over by family income, sex, race, and Hispanic origin: United States, 1995_____ 103

33. Activity limitation among adults 18–64 years of age by family income, race, and Hispanic origin: United States average annual, 1984–87, 1988–91, and 1992–95_____ 104

34. Difficulties with one or more activities of daily living among adults 70 years of age and over by family income and sex: United States, 1995_____ 107

Risk Factors

35. Cigarette smoking among adults 25 years of age and over by education and sex: United States, 1974–95_____ 109

36. Cigarette smoking among adults 18 years of age and over, by family income, sex, race, and Hispanic origin: United States, 1995_____ 110

37. Heavy alcohol use during the past month among adults 25–49 years of age by education, sex, race, and Hispanic origin: United States, average annual 1994–96_____ 112

38. Overweight among adults 25–74 years of age by sex and education: United States, average annual 1971–74, 1976–80, and 1988–94_____ 115

39. Overweight among adults 20 years of age and over by family income, sex, race, and Hispanic origin: United States, average annual 1988–94_____ 116

40. Sedentary lifestyle among adults 18 years of age and over by family income, sex, race, and Hispanic origin: United States, 1991_____ 119

41. Hypertension among adults 20 years of age and over by family income, sex, race, and Hispanic origin: United States, average annual 1988–94_____ 120

42. Elevated blood lead among men 20 years of age and over, by family income, race, and Hispanic origin: United States, average annual 1988–94_____ 122

Health Care Access and Utilization

43. No health insurance coverage among adults 18–64 years of age by family income, race, and Hispanic origin, United States, average annual 1994–95_____ 125

44. No physician contact within the past year among adults 18–64 years of age with a health problem by family income, race, and Hispanic origin: United States, average annual 1994–95_____ 127

45. Mammography within the past 2 years among women 50 years of age and over by family income, race, and Hispanic origin: United States, average annual 1993–94_____ 128

46. Unmet need for health care during the past year among adults 18–64 years of age, by family income, age, and sex: United States, average annual 1994–95____ 131

47. Unmet need for health care during the past year among adults 65 years of age and over by family income, race, and Hispanic origin: United States, average annual 1994–95_____ 132

48. Avoidable hospitalizations among adults 18–64 years of age by median household income in ZIP Code of residence and race: United States, average annual 1989–91_____ 135

49. Dental visit within the past year among adults 18–64 years of age by family income, race, and Hispanic origin: United States, 1993_____ 136

Geographic Regions and Divisions of the United States

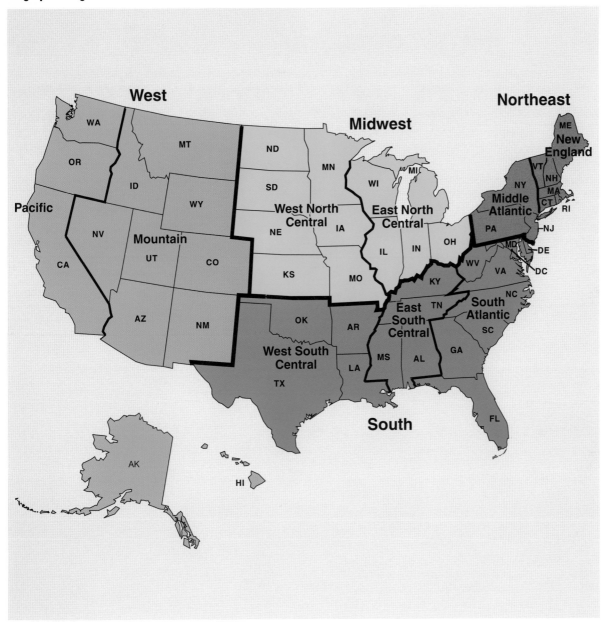

Population

■   **Income inequality** in the United States increased between 1970 and 1996. The growth in inequality was due primarily to larger increases in income among high-income than low-income households. While income increased by 5–7 percent in constant dollars for households in the 20th and the 50th percentiles of income, those at the 80th percentile experienced a 22 percent increase in their earnings, and the income of those in the 95th percentile increased by 36 percent (figure 1).

■   Children under 18 years of age were 40 percent more likely to live in **poverty** than was the population as a whole in 1996 (20 compared with 14 percent). Children in female-headed households were particularly unlikely to have adequate incomes. One-half of children in female-headed households were poor in 1996 and an additional 27 percent were near poor. Black and Hispanic children and adults were more likely than non-Hispanic white or Asian persons to be poor or near poor. On the whole, black persons and Hispanic persons had a poverty rate about 3.3 times that of non-Hispanic white persons (figure 3).

■   State **poverty** rates in 1994–96 varied more than threefold from 7 to 24 percent. Higher rates of poverty tended to be found in Southern and Southwestern States, while lower rates were found among New England and North Central States (figure 4).

■   Between 1980 and 1996 **median household incomes** increased about 5 percent in constant dollars. Non-Hispanic white households saw a 7 percent rise in their median incomes and black households a 14 percent rise, while Hispanic incomes declined by 4 percent. In 1996 Asian or Pacific Islander households had the highest median income, around $43,300, with non-Hispanic white incomes slightly less, at about $38,800; incomes of black and Hispanic households were similar and substantially lower: $23,500 and $24,900, respectively (figure 2).

■   In 1996 median **family incomes** rose with each higher level of **education** for men and women in each race and ethnic group. Among non-Hispanic white, non-Hispanic black, and Hispanic persons the ratio of median family income of college graduates to median income of those with less than a high school education ranged from 2.4–2.7 for men and from 2.9–3.6 for women. This ratio was 1.8–2.0 for Asian women and men (figure 6).

■   Asian or Pacific Islander adults had the most **education** as well as the largest proportion of men whose **occupation** was white collar. Fully 45 percent of Asian or Pacific Islander persons 25–64 years of age had 16 or more years of education in 1996, compared with 29 percent of non-Hispanic white persons, 15 percent of non-Hispanic black persons, and 10 percent of Hispanic persons. Conversely, 44 percent of Hispanic adults 25–64 years of age had less than 12 years of education, compared with 20 percent of non-Hispanic black adults, 14 percent of Asian or Pacific Islander adults, and 10 percent of non-Hispanic white adults. Education levels were lower among adults 65 and over; in each race and ethnic group, 6 to 20 percent of adults in this age group had 16 or more years of education. The distribution of occupational categories by race and ethnicity reflected the educational patterns in race and ethnic groups. A majority of Asian or Pacific Islander and non-Hispanic white men worked in white collar occupations, while a plurality (almost one-half) of non-Hispanic black and Hispanic men were classified as blue collar. A majority (52 to 78 percent) of women in every race and ethnic group were classified as white collar. Non-Hispanic black and Hispanic men and women were about twice as likely as their non-Hispanic white counterparts to be in service occupations. More than one-quarter of Hispanic and black women were in service jobs as were 15–18 percent of non-Hispanic black and Hispanic men (figures 5 and 7).

Children's Health

■ **Infant mortality** declined between 1983 and 1995 for infants of black and white mothers at all educational levels, but substantial socioeconomic disparities remained in 1995. **Low birthweight** and infant mortality were more common among the children of less educated mothers than among children of more educated mothers; for example, in 1995, infants born to non-Hispanic white mothers with less than 12 years of education were 2.4 times as likely to die in the first year of life as those whose mothers had at least 16 years of education. However, not all race and ethnic groups demonstrated identical patterns; a relationship between maternal education and these infant health outcomes was more apparent for non-Hispanic white, non-Hispanic black, and American Indian or Alaska Native infants than for Asian or Pacific Islander and Hispanic infants (figures 8, 9, and 10).

■ Mothers with more education are more likely to have received early **prenatal care** than less educated mothers; in 1996 mothers with 16 or more years of education were 40 percent more likely to obtain first-trimester prenatal care than those with fewer than 12 years of education. Mothers with fewer than 12 years of education were almost 10 times as likely to **smoke during pregnancy** as mothers with 16 or more years of education in 1996. These maternal risk factors are likely contributors to the higher incidence of low birthweight and infant mortality among the infants of less-educated mothers (figures 8–10, 13, 18, and 19).

■ The relationship between maternal education and health differed for **Hispanic** mothers and their infants compared with non-Hispanic mothers and infants. Non-Hispanic white mothers with fewer than 12 years of education were 80 percent more likely to have a low birthweight infant than those with a college degree. However, the incidence of **low birthweight** among Hispanic infants did not vary by mother's education. The relationship between mother's education and both low birthweight and **smoking during pregnancy**

varied according to Hispanic subgroup; for example, Puerto Rican and Cuban American mothers were less likely to smoke during pregnancy if they had higher education levels, but there was no relationship with education for Mexican American and Central and South American mothers, all of whom were unlikely to smoke during pregnancy. Although an inverse educational gradient was found for Hispanic infant mortality, the relationship was weaker for Hispanic infants (40 percent higher mortality in infants of the least educated compared with the most educated mothers) than for non-Hispanic white infants (140 percent higher) (figures 9, 10, and 13).

■ Young children who are exposed to environmental lead may be at risk for a range of mental and physical problems. **Elevated blood lead levels** were more common among poor children and among black children than among children of other groups. Children 1–5 years of age living in poor families in 1988–94 were over seven times as likely to have an elevated blood lead level as children in high-income families. Over one in five non-Hispanic black children who were poor had an elevated level of blood lead, compared with 8 percent of poor non-Hispanic white children and 6 percent of poor Mexican American children (figure 14).

■ Early childbearing is more common among girls from lower socioeconomic-status families. According to a 1995 survey, women in their twenties whose mothers did not finish high school were about five times as likely to have had a **teenage birth** as those whose mothers had 4 years of college education. The adolescent mothers, now in their twenties, had lower family incomes than women the same age who had not had a teenage birth (figure 12).

■ In 1992 non-Hispanic white girls and boys 12–17 years of age from poor families were 45 percent more likely to **smoke** cigarettes than similar adolescents from middle- or high-income families, while poor non-Hispanic black teen boys were almost 3 times as likely to smoke as those from middle- or high-income families. There was no relationship between family income and smoking for non-Hispanic black girls, while for Hispanic girls the pattern was reversed: those from middle- or high-income families were 60 percent more likely to smoke than those from poor families. However, smoking prevalence tended to differ more by race and ethnicity than by family income: smoking was most common among non-Hispanic white teens, somewhat less common among Hispanic teens, and least common among non-Hispanic black teens. For example, in 1992 among poor adolescents, the proportion who smoked was 33 percent for non-Hispanic white males, 23 percent for Hispanic males, and 12 percent for non-Hispanic black males (figure 15).

■ **Overweight** was inversely related to family income among non-Hispanic white adolescents, but not among Mexican American or non-Hispanic black adolescents. The percent of poor non-Hispanic white adolescents who were overweight during 1988–94 (19 percent) was about 2.6 times that for middle- or high-income adolescents (7 percent). **Sedentary lifestyle** was inversely related to family income among teenage girls and to a lesser extent among teenage boys. Poor female adolescents were more than twice as likely as those with high incomes to be sedentary. Girls were more likely than boys to be sedentary, and this difference was most pronounced among lower income youths. Among the poor and near poor, girls were 70–80 percent more likely than boys to be sedentary (figures 16 and 17).

■ Children from higher income families are more likely to have **health insurance** coverage than those from lower income families. More than one in five poor and near-poor children had no health insurance in 1994–95, while 9 percent of middle-income children and 4 percent of high-income children were uninsured. These differences were reflected in less use of health care for low-income children. During 1994–95, poor and near-poor children under 6 years of age were only about one-half as likely to have seen a physician in the

prior year as middle- or high-income children. Uninsured children were particularly unlikely to have seen a doctor, especially if they were poor: almost one-quarter of poor uninsured young children had not seen a doctor in the past year, compared with about 1 in 12 poor children with health insurance. Poor uninsured children were almost twice as likely to have had **no recent physician contacts** as middle or upper income uninsured children. When children in lower income areas received **ambulatory care** in 1995, it was less likely to be at a physician's office and more likely to be at a hospital emergency room: 22 percent of visits among children living in areas where the median income was less than $20,000 took place in emergency rooms, while only 8 percent of visits were in emergency rooms for children living in areas where the median income was at least $40,000 (figures 20, 22, and 23 and table 78).

■ Children in lower income families are less likely to receive needed health care. In 1996 two-thirds of poor children 19–35 months of age had been fully **vaccinated**, compared with more than three-quarters of those above the poverty level. Children 1–14 years of age living in low-income areas were more than twice as likely to be **hospitalized for asthma** as those in high-income areas during 1989–91, suggesting they may have been unable to receive outpatient care that could prevent such a hospitalization (figures 21 and 24).

Adults' Health

■ **Life expectancy** is related to family income; people with lower family income tend to die at younger ages than those with higher income. During 1979–89 white men who were 45 years of age and who had a family income of at least $25,000 could expect to live 6.6 years longer than men with family income less than $10,000 (33.9 years compared with 27.3 years). Among black men, the difference in life expectancy at age 45 between those with low and high incomes was 7.4 years; among white women, 2.7

years, and among black women, 3.8 years. At age 65, when life expectancy was shorter, the income disparities were somewhat less: the disparity in life expectancy between the lowest and highest income persons was 1.0 to 3.1 years, depending on sex and race (figure 25).

■ Among persons 25–64 years of age **death rates for chronic diseases, communicable diseases, and injuries** are all inversely related to education for men and women. In 1995 the death rate for chronic diseases among men with less than 12 years of education was 2.5 times that for men with more than 12 years education and among women the comparable ratio was 2.1. For men and women non-HIV communicable disease mortality among the least educated was three times that of the most educated. The education gradient in HIV mortality was much stronger among women than men. The ratio of the death rate for injuries for the least educated to the rate for most educated was 3.4 for men and 2.3 for women in 1995 (figure 26).

■ Less educated men and women have higher rates of **homicide** and **suicide** than those with more education. In 1994–95 homicide rates for adults 25–44 years of age were between three (for Hispanic women) and nine (for non-Hispanic white men) times as high among those with less than 12 years of education as among those with 13 or more years of education. In 1994–95 suicide rates for 25–44 year old men and women with less than 13 years of education were generally about twice the rates for those with more education. For non-Hispanic white men, however, suicide rates for the less educated were close to 4 times the rates for those with 13 or more years of education. (figures 30 and 31).

■ Adults with low incomes are far more likely than those with higher incomes to report **fair or poor health** status. In 1995 poor adults 18 years of age and over were about four to seven times as likely (depending on race, ethnicity, and sex) as high-income adults to report that their health status was fair or poor.

Poor persons 18–64 years of age were about three times as likely as middle- or high-income persons to report **limitations in activities** due to chronic conditions (34 percent compared with 11 percent in 1992–95). The gap between poor and middle- or high-income persons widened slightly between 1984–87 and 1992–95, primarily due to a 17 percent increase in the percent reporting limitations among poor non-Hispanic white adults. In addition, adults 70 years of age and over with low incomes were more likely than higher income older persons to report difficulty with **activities of daily living** (the ability to perform routine personal care); in 1995, 36 percent of poor men and 43 percent of poor women reported difficulty with activities of daily living while 20 percent of middle- or high-income men and 28 percent of middle- or high-income women reported such limitations (figures 32, 33, and 34).

■ Cigarette **smoking** among adults 25 years of age and over declined between 1974 and 1995, but rates of decline were steeper among more educated adults. While smoking rates declined 51 percent among men with 16 or more years of education, they declined 24 percent among those with less than a high school education. Declines for women were similar (down 49 percent for the college educated, compared with a drop of 13 percent among those who did not finish high school). In 1995 the least educated men and women were more than twice as likely to smoke as the most educated. Smoking also varies inversely with income. In 1995 poor non-Hispanic white, non-Hispanic black, and Hispanic persons 18 years of age and over were 1.2–2.0 times as likely to smoke as those with middle or high income (figures 35 and 36).

■ Higher prevalence of cigarette smoking among those of lower socioeconomic status was manifested in elevated **lung cancer and heart disease** death rates for lower income adults during 1979–89. Men with family incomes less than $10,000 were more than twice as likely to die of lung cancer as those earning at least $25,000. Among women, whose smoking and mortality rates were lower, there was no clear income gradient in lung cancer mortality during 1979–89. However, heart disease mortality was higher among those with lower incomes, regardless of sex, age, or race (figures 27 and 28).

■ Between 1971–74 and 1988–94 the prevalence of **overweight** increased by 20 to 80 percent, depending on sex and education level. By 1988–94, overweight prevalence was similar among men with less than 12, 12, or 13 to 15 years of education (37–40 percent), but men with 16 or more years of education were less likely to be overweight (28 percent). There were significant educational differences in the prevalence of overweight for women during 1988–94; each increase in education level was associated with a decline in the percent of women who were overweight, from 46 percent among women with less than 12 years of education, down to 26 percent among women with 16 or more years of education. Prevalence of overweight was similar for men of different income levels but it varied inversely with income among women. Non-Hispanic white and Mexican American (but not non-Hispanic black) women with lower income were more likely to be overweight than their higher income counterparts. **Hypertension** was also more common among lower income women in 1988–94. Poor women were 1.6 times as likely as high-income women to be hypertensive. **Sedentary lifestyle** is more common among lower income persons as well; in 1991 poor persons were 1.6 to 3.1 times as likely to be sedentary as high-income persons, depending on sex, race, and ethnicity. Overweight and sedentary persons are more likely to develop **diabetes**; in 1979–89 the death rate for diabetes among low–income women was three times that for high income women and the income gradient in diabetes mortality was only slightly less steep for men (figures 29, 38, 39, 40, and 41).

■ Heavy and chronic alcohol use can cause cirrhosis, poor pregnancy outcomes, and motor vehicle crashes as well as other health problems. In 1994–96 the percent of men and women 25–49 years of age

reporting **heavy alcohol use** (five or more drinks on at least one occasion in the past month) was 30 percent higher among those with less than a high school education than among college graduates and men were almost three times as likely as women to report heavy drinking during the past month. The percent of heavy alcohol use varied by education and sex from 9 percent among college-educated women to 32 percent among men with less than a high school education (figure 37).

■ Adults under age 65 with low family incomes are less likely to have **health insurance coverage** than higher income adults. In 1994–95 poor men were six to seven times as likely to be uninsured as high-income men, depending on race and ethnicity, while poor women were four to eight times as likely as high-income women to be uninsured. Among the poor and the near poor, coverage for women was somewhat higher than among men, due primarily to higher proportions of women than men with Medicaid coverage. In most income groups, non-Hispanic white and non-Hispanic black adults were more likely to be insured than Hispanic adults (figure 43).

■ The use of sick care, preventive care, and dental care by adults varies with income. Among adults 18–64 years of age who report a health problem there is a strong inverse income gradient in the percent with **no recent physician contact**, and the gradient is similar across race and ethnic groups. In 1994–95 poor women with a health problem were almost three times as likely, and poor men with a health problem almost twice as likely, not to have seen a doctor within the past year as high-income men and women. There is a strong direct relationship between income and use of recent **mammography**. During 1993–94, high-income women 50 years of age and over were about 70 percent more likely than poor women to have received a mammogram in the past 2 years. In 1993 the percent of adults 18–64 years of age with a **dental visit** within the past 12 months rose sharply with income from 41 percent among the poor to 77 percent among those with high family income (figures 44, 45, and 49).

■   Poor persons were far more likely than middle- or high-income persons to report an **unmet need for health care**. Among adults 18–64 years of age, about one-third of poor persons reported an unmet need for care in 1994–95, compared with about 7 percent of high-income persons; among adults 65 years of age and over, about one-fifth of the poor reported an unmet need, compared with 2 percent of high-income persons. Although the elderly have more health care needs than younger persons, almost universal Medicare coverage among the elderly assisted older adults in obtaining needed care (figures 46 and 47).

■   **Avoidable hospitalizations** are hospital stays for conditions that may be preventable with appropriate outpatient care. In 1989–91 the rate of **avoidable hospitalizations** among adults 18–64 years of age living in areas where median incomes were lowest (less than $20,000) was 2.4 times the rate among those living in areas where incomes were highest ($40,000 or more) (figure 48).

Health Status and Determinants

Population

■ In 1996 some 58 million children under the age of 15 years comprised the U.S. population, which totaled 265 million persons. Populations of **Asian or Pacific Islander children and Hispanic children** in the United States are increasing more rapidly than children in the U.S. population as a whole. Between 1990 and 1996 the average annual rate of increase was 4.5 percent for Asian or Pacific Islander children and 4.1 percent for Hispanic children compared with 1.2 percent for all U.S. children (table 1).

Fertility and Natality

■ In 1996 the **birth rate** for teenagers declined for the fifth consecutive year to 54.4 births per 1,000 women aged 15–19 years. Between 1991 and 1996 the teen birth rate declined 12 percent, with larger reductions for 15–17 year-olds than for 18–19 year-olds (13 percent compared with 9 percent) and larger reductions for black than for white teens (21 percent compared with 9 percent). In 1996 the overall fertility rate declined slightly from 65.6 to 65.3 births per 1,000 women 15–44 years of age, after declining at an average annual rate of 1.5 percent between 1990 and 1995 (table 3).

■ Between 1994 and 1996 the percent of **births to unmarried mothers** remained essentially level at about 32–33 percent following a threefold increase between 1970 and 1994. Between 1994 and 1996 the birth rate for unmarried black women declined 9 percent to 74 births per 1,000 unmarried black women aged 15–44 years and the birth rate for unmarried Hispanic women declined 8 percent to 93 per 1,000 while the birth rate for unmarried non-Hispanic white women remained stable at about 28 per 1,000 (table 8).

■ A trend toward **delayed childbearing** in the United States that began in the mid- to late-1960's has been relatively stable since 1985. The percent of women 25–29 years of age who had not had at least one live birth increased from 20 percent in 1965 to 42 percent in 1985 and 44 percent in 1990–96. Among women 30–34 years of age, the percent who had not had at least one live birth increased from 12 percent in 1970 to 25 percent in 1985 and 26 percent in 1987–96 (table 4).

■ **Low birthweight** is associated with elevated risk of death and disability in infants. In 1996 the incidence of low birthweight (less than 2,500 grams) among live-born infants was 7.4 percent. Between 1991 and 1996 low birthweight increased among white infants from 5.8 to 6.3 percent and decreased among black infants from 13.6 to 13.0 percent. Between 1991 and 1996 the incidence of very low birthweight (less than 1,500 grams) rose slightly for white infants from 1.0 to 1.1 percent and was stable at 3.0 percent for black infants (table 11).

■ In 1995 **mortality for low-birthweight infants** (weighing less than 2,500 grams at birth) was 22 times that for infants of normal weight (2,500 grams or more) (65.3 compared with 3.0 deaths per 1,000 live births). In 1995 mortality for very low birthweight infants (weighing less than 1,500 grams at birth) was 90 times that for infants of normal weight (table 22).

Mortality

■ In 1996 the **infant mortality rate** fell to a record low of 7.3 deaths per 1,000 live births, continuing the longterm downward trend in infant mortality. In 1996 mortality also reached record low rates for black infants (14.7) and white infants (6.1) (table 23).

■ In 1995 **infant mortality** for Puerto Rican and American Indian infants (8.9 and 9.0 deaths per 1,000 live births) was about 40 percent higher than mortality for non-Hispanic white infants. Compared with mortality for non-Hispanic white babies, Puerto Rican neonatal mortality (death before 28 days of age) was about 50 percent higher and postneonatal mortality (death in the 1st through 11th month of life) was nearly 30 percent higher. For American Indian babies the race differential in infant mortality was due entirely to a postneonatal mortality rate that was more than double that for white postneonates (table 20).

■ In 1996 **life expectancy** at birth reached an all-time high of 76.1 years. Life expectancy for black males increased for the third consecutive year to a record high of 66.1 years in 1996, following a period between 1984 and 1993 generally characterized by year-to-year declines in life expectancy. Life expectancy for white females rose slightly to 79.7 years but was still below the record high attained in 1992. In 1996 the gender gap in life expectancy narrowed to 6.0 years and the race differential between the white and black populations narrowed to 6.6 years (table 29).

■ Substantial **geographic differences** persist in the death rates for States and geographic divisions in the United States. In 1994–96 the age-adjusted death rate for the East South Central Division (575.5 deaths per 100,000 population) was 15 percent higher than for the United States as a whole whereas age-adjusted death rates for the Mountain, Pacific, West North Central, and New England Divisions were 7–10 percent lower than the U.S. average (table 30).

■ **Years of potential life lost** (YPLL) per 100,000 population under 75 years of age is a measure of premature mortality. In 1996 unintentional injuries were the leading cause of YPLL under 75 years of age among Hispanic males and American Indian females and males, accounting for 20–29 percent of all YPLL in each group. Heart disease was the leading cause of YPLL among black males and non–Hispanic white males, accounting for 14–21 percent of all YPLL. Cancer was the leading cause of YPLL among black, Hispanic, Asian American, and non-Hispanic white females, accounting for 18–32 percent of all YPLL in each group (table 32).

■ Although the first three leading causes of death, heart disease, cancer, and stroke, are the same for **males and females** in the United States, other leading causes of death differ for males and females. In 1996 unintentional injuries ranked higher for males (4th)

than for females (7th) and HIV infection and suicide, which ranked 8th and 9th for males, were not among the 10 leading causes for females. For males the age-adjusted death rate for unintentional injuries (43.3 deaths per 100,000 population) was 2.4 times the rate for females and the rates for HIV infection (18.1) and suicide (18.0) were 4–5 times the rates for females (tables 31 and 33).

■ Although the first two leading causes of death, heart disease and cancer, are the same for the **American Indian** and white populations in the United States, other leading causes of death differ for the two populations. In 1996 unintentional injuries and diabetes ranked higher for American Indians (3d and 4th) than for white persons (5th and 7th), and cirrhosis, which ranked 6th for American Indians, ranked 9th for white persons. For American Indians the age-adjusted death rates for unintentional injuries (57.6 deaths per 100,000 population) and diabetes (27.8) were about double the rates for white persons, and the rate for cirrhosis (20.7) was nearly 3 times the rate for white persons (table 31 and 33).

■ In 1996 overall mortality for **Hispanic Americans** was 22 percent lower than for non-Hispanic white Americans. However for males 15–44 years of age death rates were higher for Hispanics than for non-Hispanic white persons, primarily due to elevated death rates for homicide and HIV infection among young Hispanic males. In 1996 homicide rates for Hispanic males 15–24 and 25–44 years of age were 8 times and 4 times the rates for non-Hispanic white males of similar ages and the death rate for HIV infection for Hispanic males 25–44 years of age was about double the rate for non-Hispanic white males (tables 31, 37, 44, and 47).

■ In 1996 the age-adjusted death rate for **black Americans** declined 4 percent to 738 deaths per 100,000 population. Between 1995 and 1996 mortality due to HIV infection, the fourth leading cause of death among black persons, declined 20 percent, following an average increase of 15 percent per year between

1990 and 1995. Mortality among black persons continued to decline for heart disease and injuries. In 1996 age-adjusted death rates declined 4 percent for heart disease, 2 percent for unintentional injuries, and 8 percent for homicide, and homicide dropped from sixth to seventh in the ranking of leading causes of death for black persons (tables 31 and 33).

■ Between 1992 and 1996 the age-adjusted death rate for **stroke**, the third leading cause of death overall, was stable following a long downward trend. Between 1980 and 1992 stroke mortality declined at an average rate of 3.6 percent per year. Stroke mortality is higher for the black population than for other racial groups. In 1996 the age-adjusted death rate for stroke for the black population was 80 percent higher than for the white population (tables 31, 33, and 39).

■ In 1996 age-adjusted death rates for cancer and heart disease for the **Asian-American** population were 39 percent and 45 percent lower than the rates for the white population, while death rates for stroke were similar for the two populations. Death rates for stroke for Asian-American males 55–64 and 65–74 years of age were 14–28 percent higher than for white males of those ages, while death rates for Asian males age 75 years and over were 12–14 percent lower than for elderly white males (tables 31 and 39).

■ Between 1990 and 1996 the age-adjusted death rate for **cancer,** the second leading cause of death, decreased 5 percent, after increasing slowly but steadily over the 20-year period, 1970 to 1990 (tables 31 and 33).

■ In 1996 the age-adjusted death rate for **chronic obstructive pulmonary diseases (COPD)**, the fourth leading cause of death overall, was 47 percent higher for males than females (25.9 and 17.6 deaths per 100,000 population). Between 1980 and 1996 age-adjusted death rates for males were relatively stable while death rates for females nearly doubled. COPD death rates are highest for the elderly and have been increasing most rapidly among females age 75 years and over (tables 33 and 43).

■ In 1996 the age-adjusted death rate for **HIV infection** declined 29 percent to 11.1 deaths per 100,000 population. Between 1994 and 1995 HIV mortality increased by only 1 percent following a period between 1987 and 1994 in which mortality had increased at an average rate of 16 percent per year. In 1996 the death rate for HIV infection for persons 25–44 years of age declined 30 percent and HIV infection dropped from first to third in the ranking of leading causes of death for this age group (tables 31, 34, and 44).

■ Between 1980 and 1996 the age-adjusted **maternal mortality** rate declined by nearly one-third, to 6.4 maternal deaths per 100,000 live births. In 1996, 294 women died of maternal causes compared with 334 women in 1980. In 1996 age-adjusted maternal mortality for black women (19.9 per 100,000 live births) was 5 times the rate for non-Hispanic white women. Maternal mortality for Hispanic women (4.8) was 23 percent higher than the rate for non-Hispanic white women (table 45).

■ Between 1993 and 1996 the age-adjusted death rate for **firearm-related injuries** declined by about 6 percent annually on average to 12.9 deaths per 100,000 population, after increasing almost every year since the late 1980's. Two-thirds of the decline in the firearm-related death rate resulted from the decline in the homicide rate associated with firearms. Between 1993 and 1996 the firearm-related death rate for young black males 15–24 years of age declined at an average annual rate of nearly 10 percent to 131.6 deaths per 100,000. Despite the decline, the firearm-related death rate for young black males was still 6.5 times the rate for young non-Hispanic white males (table 49).

■ In general the workplace is safer today than it was over a decade ago. Between 1980 and 1993 the overall **occupational injury death rate** declined 45 percent to 4.2 deaths per 100,000 workers and decreases occurred in all industries. Of the industries with the highest occupational injury mortality, declines of 52 percent occurred in transportation, communication, and public utilities; 45 percent in construction; 42 percent in mining; and 24 percent in agriculture, forestry, and fishing. Although occupational injury mortality in 1993 for wholesale and retail trade was lower than in 1980, rates have increased since 1989. In 1993 the occupational injury death rate was 3.6 deaths per 100,000 workers for wholesale trade and 2.9 for retail trade (table 51).

Determinants and Measures of Health

■   In 1996, 77 percent of children 19–35 months of age received the combined **vaccination** series of 4 doses of DTP (diphtheria-tetanus-pertussis) vaccine, 3 doses of polio vaccine, 1 dose of measles-containing vaccine, and 3 doses of Hib (Haemophilus influenzae type b) vaccine, up from 69 percent in 1994. Substantial differences exist among the States in the percent of children 19–35 months of age who received the combined vaccination series, ranging from a high of 87 percent in Connecticut to a low of 63 percent in Utah (tables 52 and 53).

■   In 1996 **tuberculosis** incidence declined to 8 cases per 100,000 population. This, the fourth consecutive year of decline, is the lowest rate ever reported and reflects improvements in TB-prevention and TB-control programs. Between 1990 and 1996 the case rate for primary and secondary syphilis declined nearly 80 percent to 4 cases per 100,000 and gonorrhea incidence declined 55 percent to 124 per 100,000 (table 54).

■   Between 1995 and 1996 the number of reported **AIDS cases** decreased 6 percent overall. However the decrease was not observed for all population groups. In contrast to other groups, incident AIDS cases for non-Hispanic black females 13 years of age and over increased 6 percent. In 1996 incident AIDS cases decreased for all exposure categories except for the undetermined category, which increased 24 percent overall, and for persons infected through heterosexual contact, which increased 14 percent for non-Hispanic black persons (tables 55 and 56).

■   In 1997 the first leveling off of drug use was found in eighth graders since 1992, with **marijuana** use in the past month declining to 10 percent. The percent of eighth graders who drank alcohol (25) or smoked cigarettes (19) also decreased slightly in 1997. Among high school seniors, 37 percent reported smoking cigarettes in the past month; 1997 marked the fifth consecutive year of increase. Marijuana use among high school seniors in 1997 was 24 percent, double that in 1992 (table 65).

■   In 1996, 51 percent of the population 12 years of age and over reported using **alcohol** in the past month and 15 percent reported having five or more drinks on at least one occasion in the past month. Young people 18–25 years of age were more likely to drink heavily than were other age groups. Among 18–25 year olds, heavy drinking was more than twice as likely for males as females (44 and 21 percent) and about twice as likely for non-Hispanic white persons as for non-Hispanic black persons (37 and 19 percent) (table 64).

■   In 1994 and 1995 there were more than 142,000 **cocaine-related emergency room episodes** per year, the highest number ever reported since these events were tracked starting in 1978. Between 1988 and 1995 cocaine-related episodes among persons 35 years of age and over have almost tripled, reflecting an aging population of drug abusers being treated in emergency departments (table 66).

■   An **environmental health** objective for the year 2000 is that at least 85 percent of the U.S. population should be living in counties that meet the Environmental Protection Agency's National Ambient Air Quality Standards (NAAQS). In 1996, 81 percent of Americans lived in counties that met the NAAQS for all pollutants, up from 68 percent in 1995. In 1995, one of the hottest summers on record, a 7-percentage point decline in compliance with air quality standards occurred, following 3 years of higher levels of compliance (table 72).

■ Between 1990 and 1996 the **injuries with lost workdays** rate decreased 21 percent to 3.1 per 100 full-time equivalents (FTE's) in the private sector. The industries reporting the largest declines during this period (33–35 percent) were mining; agriculture, fishing, and forestry; and construction. The 1996 rate for the manufacturing industry (4.3 per 100 FTE's) was 19 percent lower than in 1990 and the rate for the transportation, communication, and public utilities industry (5.0 per 100 FTE's) was 7 percent lower than in 1990 (table 73).

Utilization of Health Resources

Ambulatory Care

■ In 1994–95, 4 percent of children under 6 years of age had no **usual source of health care**. Being without a usual source of care was more likely for Hispanic children than for non-Hispanic white and non-Hispanic black children (8 percent compared with 3–4 percent); more likely for poor and near poor children (in families whose income was below 200 percent of the poverty threshhold) than for nonpoor children (6 percent compared with 2 percent); and more likely for children without health insurance than for children with insurance (16 percent compared with 2 percent). Among poor children under 6 years of age, 21 percent of uninsured children had no usual source of care compared with 4 percent of insured children (table 79).

■ In 1996 there were 892 million **ambulatory care visits,** 82 percent occurring in physician offices, 8 percent in hospital outpatient departments, and 10 percent in hospital emergency departments. Compared with older persons, a larger proportion of the ambulatory care visits by younger persons are to hospital emergency departments. In 1996 hospital emergency department visits accounted for 12–14 percent of ambulatory care visits among persons under 45 years of age and 8 percent of visits among persons 75 years of age and over (table 81).

■ In 1996, 60 percent of all **surgical operations** in community hospitals were performed on an outpatient basis, almost 4 times the percent in 1980. The upward trend in the proportion of surgery performed on outpatients is slowing. During the 1980's the proportion of surgery that was outpatient increased 12 percent per year on the average whereas by the 1990's that growth had slowed to 3 percent per year (table 94).

■ In 1995 there were 457 **clients in specialty substance abuse treatment** per 100,000 population 12 years of age and over, 5 percent higher than in 1992. Nearly one-half (46 percent) of the clients were enrolled in simultaneous treatment for alcohol and drug abuse in 1995, up from 38 percent in 1992. In 1995 30 percent of clients were enrolled in alcohol-only treatment and 23 percent in drug abuse-only treatment. The total number of substance abuse clients in all specialty treatment units per 100,000 population was lowest in the West South Central (258) and West North Central divisions (279) and highest in the Pacific (618) and Middle Atlantic divisions (596) (table 84).

■ In 1996 **home health agencies** provided care to about 2.4 million persons on an average day. Two-thirds of users of home health services were female. Home health services are provided mainly to the elderly. In 1996 one-third of those being served were 75–84 years of age at the time of admission and one-sixth were 85 years of age and over. In 1996 the most common primary admission diagnoses were heart disease (11 percent of patients), diseases of the musculoskeletal system and diabetes (9 percent each), and cerebrovascular diseases and diseases of the respiratory system (8 percent each) (table 86).

Inpatient Care

■ Utilization of **inpatient short-stay hospital care** is greater for persons with low family income (less than $15,000) than for persons with high family income ($50,000 or more). In 1995 the age-adjusted days of care rate for low income persons was almost 3 times the rate for high income persons (880 and 300 days of care per 1,000 population) (table 87).

■ Between 1988 and 1995 the age-adjusted **hospital discharge rate** for non-Federal short-stay hospitals declined 11 percent to 105 discharges per 1,000 population. The decline was greater for persons under 64 years of age (14–17 percent) than for persons 65–74 years of age (3 percent). By contrast the hospital discharge rate increased 5 percent for persons 75 years of age and over. Between 1988 and 1995 the **average length of stay** decreased for persons of all ages with larger declines for elderly than for younger persons. The average length of stay declined by more than 2 days for persons 65 years of age and over, 1.3 days for persons 45–64 years of age, and by less than 1 day for persons under 45 years of age (table 88).

■ In 1995 among elderly persons with a first-listed diagnosis of **ischemic heart disease**, the hospital discharge rate for non-Federal short-stay hospitals was higher for men than for women, but the difference diminished with increasing age. In 1995 among persons 65–74 years of age the rate of ischemic heart disease discharges for men was 1.8 times the rate for women (43.7 and 24.0 per 1,000 population). Among persons 75 years of age and over, the rate for men was 1.4 times the rate for women (51.6 and 36.8) (table 90).

■ In 1995 for persons 65 years of age and over, the hospital discharge rate for **coronary bypass surgery** for men was 3 times the rate for women and this difference did not diminish with increasing age. For persons 65–74 years of age, the discharge rate for men was 11.2 per 1,000 population compared with 3.8 for women. For persons 75 years of age and over, the rate for men was 8.9 compared with 3.0 for women (table 92).

■ Between 1990 and 1994, overall **additions to mental health inpatient and residential treatment organizations** (admissions and readmissions) remained stable at 830–840 per 100,000 civilian population.

However, trends differed for different types of mental health organizations. Additions declined 19–24 percent in State and county mental health organizations and the Department of Veterans Affairs while additions increased 5–11 percent in non-Federal general hospitals and private psychiatric hospitals (table 85).

■ Between 1985 and 1995 the number of **nursing home residents** 85 years of age and over per 1,000 population decreased 10 percent to 199. During this 10-year period the number of nursing home residents 85 years of age and over increased 21 percent while this age group in the population increased 36 percent. In 1995 the nursing home residency rate among persons 85 years and over was about 70 percent higher for women than men and 20 percent higher for white persons than for black persons (tables 1 and 95).

■ Functional dependencies most commonly afflicting **nursing home residents** are in mobility, incontinence, and eating. In 1995, 79 percent of nursing home residents 65 years of age and over were dependent in mobility, 64 percent were incontinent, 45 percent were dependent in eating, and 37 percent were dependent in all three functionalities. Compared with 1985 a larger proportion of nursing home residents were functionally dependent in 1995. In 1995 a larger proportion of black than white residents had functional dependencies (table 96).

Health Care Resources

Personnel

■ In 1996 the number of active **doctors of medicine in patient care** per 10,000 civilian population was 22 for the United States as a whole, an increase of 61 percent since 1975. In 1996 the divisions with the highest ratios were New England and Middle Atlantic (28–29) and the divisions with the lowest ratios were East South Central, West South Central, and Mountain (18), a pattern similar to that in 1975 (table 100).

■ Between 1980 and 1995 the **supply of active registered nurses** increased 42 percent to 798 per

100,000 population. Registered nurses are generally more educated today than they were 15 years ago. In 1995, 58 percent of active registered nurses were prepared at the associate and diploma level, 32 percent at the baccalaureate level, and 10 percent at the masters and doctoral level. By contrast in 1980, the mix was 71 percent associate and diploma, 23 percent baccalaureate, and 5 percent masters and doctoral nurses (table 103).

■ In 1993 through 1996 the annual number of **graduates from dentistry school** was stable at 3,700–3,800 after declining steadily from 5,400 in 1985. Between 1985 and 1996 the number of professional schools of dentistry declined from 60 to 53 (table 106).

■ In academic year 1995–96, women comprised 42 percent of total student enrollment in **allopathic schools of medicine** compared with 27 percent in academic year 1980–81. In academic year 1995–96 women comprised 40–45 percent of the non-Hispanic white, Asian, Hispanic, and American Indian students compared with 60 percent of the non-Hispanic black students (table 108).

Facilities

■ In 1996 **occupancy rates in community hospitals** averaged 62 percent. Community hospital occupancy varied inversely by bed size ranging from 33 percent for hospitals with 6–24 beds to 70 percent for hospitals with 500 beds or more (table 109).

■ Between 1990 and 1994 the number of **mental health inpatient and residential treatment beds** per 100,000 population declined 13 percent to 98 after remaining relatively stable between 1984 and 1990. Between 1990 and 1994, the bed to population ratio declined 24 percent for State and county mental hospitals to 31 per 100,000 and declined 14 percent for private psychiatric hospitals to 16. By contrast, the mental health bed to population ratio remained relatively stable for non-Federal general hospitals, Department of Veterans Affairs hospitals, and

residential treatment centers for emotionally disturbed children (table 110).

■ Between 1992 and 1996 the number of **nursing home beds** in the United States increased by 9 percent to 1.8 million beds. During the same period, occupancy rates in nursing homes declined by 3 percentage points from 86 percent to 83 percent. In 1996 occupancy rates varied among the geographic divisions from a low of 72 percent in the West South Central division to a high of 90–93 percent in the East South Central, New England, and Middle Atlantic divisions (table 114).

Health Care Expenditures

National Health Expenditures

■ In 1996 **national health care expenditures** in the United States totaled $1,035 billion, an average of $3,759 per person. In 1996 the 4-percent increase in national health expenditures continued the steady slowdown in growth of the 1990's. During the 1980's national health expenditures grew at an average annual rate of 11 percent compared with 7 percent between 1990 and 1995 (tables 115 and 119).

■ **Health expenditures as a percent of the gross domestic product** remained stable at 13.6 percent between 1993 and 1996, after increasing steadily from 8.9 percent in 1980 (table 115).

■ In 1995 health spending in the United States continued to account for a larger **share of gross domestic product** (GDP) than in any other major industrialized country. The United States devoted 13.6 percent of GDP to health in 1995. The countries with the next highest share of GDP devoted to health in 1995 were Germany with 10.4 percent and Canada, Switzerland, and France with 9.7 to 9.9 percent each. In the United Kingdom the percent of GDP devoted to health care has been stable at 6.9 percent during 1992–95 while in Japan the percent has been steadily rising during the 1990's to 7.2 percent in 1995 (table 116).

■ During the 1990's the rate of increase in the medical care component of the **Consumer Price Index** (CPI) has declined every year from 9.0 percent in 1990 to 2.8 percent in 1997. From 1990 to 1995 the inflation rate for the medical care component of CPI (6.3 percent) averaged more than double the overall inflation rate of 3.1 percent. However for the last two years medical care inflation averaged 20 percent higher than the overall rate of inflation. In 1997 inflation for dental services (4.7 percent) and outpatient services (4.6 percent) outpaced inflation for all other types of medical care services and commodities (tables 117 and 118).

■ During the 1990's the percent of **national health expenditures that were publicly funded** increased steadily to 47 percent in 1996. Between 1990 and 1996 public funds for national health expenditures grew at an average annual rate of 9.2 percent compared with 4.9 percent for private funds (table 119).

■ Expenditures for hospital care continued to decline as a percent of **national health expenditures** from 42 percent in 1980 to 35 percent in 1996. Physician services accounted for 20 percent of the total in 1996 and drugs and nursing home care each for 8–9 percent (table 120).

■ In 1995, 34 percent of **expenditures for health services and supplies** was paid by households, 26 percent by private business, and 38 percent by the Federal and State and local governments. Between 1990 and 1995 the share of expenditures from out-of-pocket health spending by individuals declined from 22 percent to 19 percent and the share of expenditures paid by private business declined from 28 percent to 26 percent (table 121).

■ Between 1994 and 1997 **private employers' health insurance costs** per employee-hour worked declined from $1.14 to $.99 per hour after increasing by 24 percent between 1991 and 1994. In 1997 private employers with 500 or more employees paid 2.2 times as much for health insurance per employee-hour worked ($1.57) as did the employers with fewer than

100 employees ($.72), and 2.4 times as much for health insurance per employee-hour worked for union workers ($2.01) as for nonunion workers ($.85). Among private employers the share of total compensation devoted to health insurance declined from 6.7 percent in 1994 to 5.5 percent in 1997 (table 122).

■ In 1996, 19 percent of **personal health care expenditures** were paid out-of-pocket; private health insurance paid 32 percent, the Federal Government paid 36 percent, and State and local government paid 10 percent. Between 1990 and 1996 the share paid by the Federal Government increased nearly 7 percentage points, while the share paid out-of-pocket decreased by nearly 5 percentage points (table 124).

■ In 1996 the major **sources of funds** for hospital care were Medicare (33 percent) and private health insurance (32 percent). In 1996 physician services were also primarily funded by private health insurance (50 percent) and Medicare (21 percent). In contrast, in 1996 nursing home care was financed primarily by Medicaid (48 percent) and out-of-pocket payments (31 percent). In 1996 out-of-pocket payments financed only 3 percent of hospital care and 15 percent of physician services (table 125).

■ Between 1990 and 1996 the proportion of **health expenditures** paid by Medicaid increased from 12 to 15 percent for hospital care and from 5 to 8 percent for physician services. Over the same period Medicare funding for hospital care increased from 27 to 33 percent and for nursing home care increased from 3 to 11 percent (table 125).

■ Between 1993 and 1996 the average annual increase in **total expenses in community hospitals** was 3.4 percent, following a period of higher growth that averaged 9.3 percent per year from 1985 to 1993. Between 1993 and 1996 expenses per inpatient day increased by 5.1 percent per year in nonprofit hospitals and by 1.1 percent per year in proprietary hospitals, while expenses per inpatient stay increased by 0.9 percent per year in nonprofit community hospitals and decreased by 2.6 percent per year in proprietary hospitals. In 1996 employee costs accounted for 53 percent of total hospital costs in nonprofit community hospitals compared with 48 percent in proprietary hospitals (table 126).

■ In 1995 the **average monthly charge in a nursing home** was $3,135 per resident. The monthly charge varied widely by geographic region from about $2,700 in the Midwest and South to $3,700 and $3,900 in the West and Northeast. In 1995 nearly one-half of the nursing home residents were 85 years of age or older and nearly three-quarters were women (table 127).

■ The **average monthly nursing home charge** varies according to the primary source of payment. In 1995 the average monthly charge for patients funded by Medicaid (60 percent of residents) was $2,769 per resident, one-half of the charge of $5,546 for Medicare patients (10 percent of residents). Medicare funds nursing home patients who have been discharged directly from the hospital to the nursing home and who are likely to be sicker than nursing home patients funded by Medicaid. Residents paying for nursing home care with their own income, family support, or private health insurance paid $3,081 per month (28 percent of residents) (table 128).

■ **Expenditures by mental health organizations** increased between 1990 and 1994 from $28 to $33 billion. Spending on mental health was $128 per capita in 1994, up from $117 per capita in 1990 and 1992. Private psychiatric hospitals continued to account for about one-fifth of the mental health dollar. State and county mental hospitals continued to decrease their share of mental health expenditures from 27 percent in 1990 to 24 percent in 1994 (table 129).

■ In 1995 **funding for health research and development** increased by 7 percent to $36 billion. The average annual rate of increase in health research funding during 1992–95 (7 percent) was less rapid than during 1990–92 (12.5 percent). Between 1990 and 1995 industry's share of funding for health research

increased from 46 to 52 percent while the Federal Government's share decreased from 42 to 37 percent (table 130).

■ Between 1995 and 1997 **Federal expenditures for HIV-related activities** increased at an average annual rate of 11 percent to $8.5 billion compared with an average annual increase of 17 percent between 1990 and 1995. Of the total Federal spending in 1997, 56 percent was for medical care, 21 percent for research, 15 percent for cash assistance (Disability Insurance, Supplemental Security Income, and Housing and Urban Development assistance), and 8 percent for education and prevention. Between 1996 and 1997 expenditures for medical care increased by 17 percent, cash assistance by 10 percent, education and prevention expenditures by 7 percent, and research by 5 percent (table 132).

Health Care Coverage and Major Federal Programs

■ Between 1993 and 1996 the age-adjusted proportion of the population under 65 years of age with **private health insurance** has remained stable at 70–71 percent after declining from 76 percent in 1989. More than 90 percent of private coverage was obtained through the workplace (a current or former employer or union) in 1996. Compared with persons living in the South, those living in the Northeast and Midwest geographic regions were about 14–19 percent more likely to have private health insurance in 1996. Persons living in the South and West were about equally likely to have private health insurance (table 133).

■ Expansions in the **Medicaid** program have resulted in an increase in the percentage of poor children under 18 years of age with Medicaid or other public assistance from 48 percent in 1989 to 66 percent in 1996. During this period the percentage of near poor children with Medicaid doubled from 12 to 25 percent for children at 100–149 percent of the poverty threshold and from 6 to 11 percent for children at 150–199 percent of the poverty threshold (table 133).

■ Nearly all persons 65 years of age or older are eligible for **Medicare**, the Federal health program for the elderly, but most of the elderly have additional health care coverage. In 1996, 72 percent of the elderly had private health insurance and 38 percent had private health insurance obtained through the workplace (a current or former employer or union). In 1996, 9 percent of the elderly had Medicaid or other public assistance and 18 percent had Medicare only, with no other health plan (table 134).

■ In 1997, one-quarter of the U.S. population was enrolled in **health maintenance organizations (HMO's)**, ranging from only 18 percent in the South to 36 percent in the West. HMO enrollment is steadily increasing. Enrollment in 1997 was 67 million persons, double the enrollment in 1991. The distribution of enrollees among model types is also changing. Between 1991 and 1997 the percent of HMO members enrolled in group HMO's declined from 50 to 17 percent while the percent enrolled in mixed HMO's increased from 10 to 43 percent. During the same period the percent of HMO members enrolled in individual practice associations was relatively unchanged at about 40 percent (table 135).

■ Employee participation in **medical care benefits** is related to the size of the company. In 1995, 77 percent of full-time and 19 percent of part-time employees in medium and large private establishments (100 or more employees) participated in the medical care benefits offered by their company. In 1994, 66 percent of full-time and only 7 percent of part-time employees in small private establishments (less than 100 employees) participated in the company's medical care benefits (table 136).

■ In private companies with 100 or more employees the percent of full-time **employees participating in health care benefits** declined between 1991 and 1995 from 83 to 77 percent. The decline among blue collar and service employees was 9 percentage points compared with a 5-percentage point decline among employees in other occupational groups (table 136).

■ During the 1990's the use of **traditional fee-for-service** medical care benefits by employees in private companies declined sharply. In 1994 in small companies, 55 percent of full-time employees who participated in medical care benefits were in traditional fee-for-service medical care, down from 74 percent in 1990. In 1995 in medium and large companies, only 37 percent of participating full-time employees were in traditional fee-for-service medical care, down from 67 percent in 1991 (table 136).

■ During the 1990's **full financing of medical care coverage** became less common. In 1994, 47 percent of full-time participating employees in small companies received full financing of individual medical coverage compared with 58 percent in 1990. In 1995, 33 percent of full-time participating employees in larger companies received full financing of individual medical coverage compared with 49 percent in 1991. Similar declines in full financing of family medical coverage were also seen in small and larger companies (table 136).

■ The average **monthly contribution** by full-time employees for family **medical care benefits** was 36 percent higher in small companies ($160 in 1994) than in medium and large companies ($118 in 1995). Average monthly contributions by full-time employees for individual medical care benefits were more than 20 percent higher in small than in medium and large companies ($41 in 1994 compared with $34 in 1995). Average employee contributions for HMO medical care benefits were higher than for non-HMO fee arrangements, regardless of company size (table 136).

■ In 1996 the **Medicare** program had 38.1 million enrollees and expenditures of $200 billion. The total number of enrollees increased less than 2 percent over the previous year while expenditures increased nearly 9 percent. In 1996 supplementary medical insurance (SMI) accounted for 35 percent of Medicare expenditures. Expenditures for home health agency care increased to 13.5 percent of hospital insurance (HI) expenditures in 1996 up from 5.5 percent in 1990.

Expenditures for skilled nursing facilities more than doubled to 9 percent of the HI expenditures over the same period. Group practice prepayment increased from 6 percent of the SMI expenditures in 1990 to 13 percent in 1996 (table 137).

■ Of the 33.1 million elderly **Medicare** enrollees in 1995, 11 percent were 85 years of age and over. In 1995 the average payment per Medicare enrollee for those 85 years of age and over ($6,356) was 2.5 times that for those aged 65–66 years ($2,546). In every age group for those 65 years of age and over, Medicare payments per person served and payments per enrollee were higher for men than for women. In 1995 in the West there were 663 persons served per 1,000 enrollees compared with 865 or more in the other three regions of the country (table 138).

■ In 1996 **Medicaid** vendor payments totaled $122 billion for 36.1 million recipients, showing little change from the previous year. Between 1993 and 1995 the average annual increase slowed to 9 percent for payments and 4 percent for recipients, about one-half the growth during the period 1990 to 1993. In 1996 children under the age of 21 years comprised 46 percent of recipients but accounted for only 14 percent of expenditures. The aged, blind, and disabled accounted for 29 percent of recipients and 73 percent of expenditures (table 139).

■ In 1996 nearly one-quarter of **Medicaid** payments went to nursing facilities and 21 percent to general hospitals. Home health care accounted for 9 percent of Medicaid payments in 1996, up from 1 percent in 1980. In 1996, 5 percent of Medicaid recipients received home health care at a cost averaging $6,293 per recipient. Early and periodic screening, rural health clinics, and family planning services combined received less than 2 percent of Medicaid funds in 1996, with the cost per recipient averaging between $200 and $215 (table 140).

■ Between 1995 and 1996 spending on health care by the **Department of Veterans Affairs** increased by less than 2 percent to $16.4 billion. In 1996, 46 percent

of the total was for inpatient hospital care, down from 58 percent in 1990, one-third for outpatient care, up from one-quarter in 1990, and 10 percent for nursing home care. The number of inpatient stays decreased by 8 percent between 1995 and 1996 and the number of outpatient visits increased by 6 percent. In 1996 veterans with service-connected disabilities accounted for 40 percent of inpatients and 38 percent of outpatients. Low-income veterans with no service-connected disability were the largest group served accounting for 56 percent of inpatients and 42 percent of outpatients (table 141).

State Health Expenditures

■ In 1995 **Medicare payments per enrollee** averaged $4,750 in the United States, ranging from $3,300 in Nebraska, Iowa, and Idaho to more than $6,000 in Massachusetts and Louisiana. In 1995 utilization of short-stay hospitals by Medicare enrollees varied among the States from 250 discharges per 1,000 enrollees in Utah to 432 in Mississippi. The length of stay in short-stay hospitals by Medicare enrollees averaged 5.6 and 5.7 days in the Mountain and Pacific geographic divisions compared with 9.0 days in the Middle Atlantic division in 1995 (table 146).

■ In 1996 **Medicaid payments per recipient** averaged $3,369 and ranged from $2,049 in Tennessee to $6,811 in New York. For the United States as a whole, the ratio of Medicaid recipients to persons below the poverty level increased from 75 per 100 in 1989–90 to 99 per 100 in 1995–96. For 1995–96 the ratio of Medicaid recipients to persons below the poverty level was above the average in all States in the New England geographic division and below the average in all States in the West South Central and Mountain divisions (table 147).

■ In 1997 the percent of the population enrolled in a **health maintenance organization (HMO)** varied among the States from 0 in Alaska and Vermont to 47 percent in Oregon. In seven other States more than one-third of the population was enrolled in an HMO in

1997 including Massachusetts (45 percent), New York (36 percent), Connecticut (35 percent), Maryland and Delaware (38–39 percent), Utah (41 percent), and California (44 percent) (table 148).

■ In 1996 the proportion of the population without **health care coverage** was 15.6 percent, compared with 15.4 percent the previous year and 12.9 percent in 1987. In 1996 the proportion of the population without health care coverage varied from less than 9 percent in Wisconsin, Michigan, and Hawaii to more than 20 percent in Arkansas, Louisiana, Texas, New Mexico, Arizona, and California (table 149).

Socioeconomic Status and Health Chartbook

One of the three overarching goals of *Healthy People 2000*, the Public Health Service's national health objectives for the year 2000, is to reduce health disparities among Americans (1). *Healthy People 2000*, the Nation's prevention agenda, seeks to reduce such disparities by encouraging preventive efforts targeted for "special population" groups: low-income persons, racial and ethnic minorities, and persons with disabilities. In the United States health disparities among racial and ethnic subgroups of the population, especially between white persons and black persons, have received much of the attention. However, individuals' access to social and economic resources, as indicated by income, level of education, or type of occupation, is a major source of disparities in health in this country, and many others (2–4). *Healthy People 2000* implicitly recognizes the strength and persistence of disparities in health outcomes and access to health services by setting separate targets for special population groups that represent a more rapid rate of improvement and thus a narrowing of the gap. In 1997, goals for *Healthy People 2010* were proposed that seek to eliminate, rather than reduce, health disparities.

The first section of this chartbook documents the strong relationship between race, ethnicity, and various measures of socioeconomic status: household or family income (figures 2 and 6), poverty status (figure 3), level of education (figure 5), and type of occupation (figure 7). Racial and ethnic minorities are disproportionately represented among the poor in the United States. In 1996 African Americans comprised 13 percent of the overall U.S. population and 26 percent of the poor population; persons of Hispanic origin comprised 11 percent of the overall population and 22 percent of the poor; while non-Hispanic white persons made up 72 percent of the overall population and 45 percent of the poor. By contrast, the high-income population was considerably more homogeneous with respect to race and Hispanic origin; 87 percent of individuals with incomes of $50,000 or more in 1996 were non-Hispanic white persons. This chartbook addresses the overlap between race, ethnicity, and socioeconomic status by documenting

health disparities across levels of socioeconomic status for as many race and ethnic subgroups as possible, given the limitations of the data.

The chartbook includes separate sections on the health of children under 18 years of age (figures 8–24) and adults 18 years of age and over (figures 25–49). Each of these sections is divided into subsections on health status, health risk factors, and health care access and utilization. Many of the charts in each section present data by gender where appropriate and feasible. The charts are followed by Technical Notes that describe data sources, definitions, and methods and a Data Table that includes data points presented in the charts and standard errors. Appendixes I and II present additional information on data sources and definitions.

Data Issues

With the exception of data derived from the Census and from the vital registration system (birth and death certificates), the existing sources of health data do not permit examination of socioeconomic differences for any but the three largest race and ethnic categories: non-Hispanic white persons, non-Hispanic black persons, and persons of Hispanic or Mexican origin. Much of the data used in this chartbook was collected by surveys that may provide reliable estimates for entire race and ethnic subgroups, but usually have insufficient numbers to make good estimates for detailed subcategories within these populations. This problem is particularly acute when the subcategories reflect socioeconomic levels, because of the tendency for race and ethnic groups to be disproportionately concentrated at either the low or high ends of the socioeconomic distribution (as shown in the Population section). The reader will notice that, even for the three largest race and ethnic groups, sample sizes often require collapsing socioeconomic variables into fewer categories than reported for the population as a whole.

Combining into larger groups is an expedient solution to problems of small numbers, but it is not without cost. Readers should be aware that the broad groupings presented in this chartbook may mask differences among subgroups. For example, "Asian or Pacific Islander" includes persons with ancestry in such countries as China, Vietnam, the Phillippines, Japan, and Samoa, while "Hispanic" combines persons whose origins were in Cuba, Puerto Rico, Mexico, or any of the countries of Central or South America. These subgroups often have very diverse socioeconomic profiles and may also have very different health status and risk behaviors.

This problem of hidden heterogeneity also affects the socioeconomic categories. For example, in many of the charts that follow, "high income" persons may have a family income for the year ranging from $50,000 to $500,000 or more; the category of 16 or more years of education combines persons with baccalaureate degrees with those with graduate and professional degrees, such as lawyers and doctors. There are likely to be differences within each of these categories that are not discernable in the charts. In addition, race and ethnic groups are likely to have different "mixes" of persons within a uniformly named category. In 1996, in an income category labeled "$50,000 or more," 25 percent of the non-Hispanic white households in this group would have incomes of $100,000 or more, compared with only 17 percent of Hispanic households and 14 percent of black households (5). The reader should also bear in mind that race and ethnic groups are distributed very differently across socioeconomic strata, although the categories are depicted equally in the charts. Thus, in the charts for children under the age of 18, the category "poor" usually represents around 11 percent of non-Hispanic white children, but 40 percent or more of Hispanic or black children (figure 3).

Another difficulty in presenting health data by socioeconomic status is that each indicator used to stratify the population into levels of SES has certain conceptual and practical limitations.

Income is the most common measure of socioeconomic status, and is probably the most relevant to health policy formulation. Current income provides a direct measure of the quality of food, housing, leisure-time amenities, and health care an

individual is able to acquire, as well as reflecting their relative position in society. However, income may fluctuate over time so that income received in a given year may not accurately reflect one's lifetime income stream, the measure of resources more relevant to health. Among the elderly, persons who have low incomes may also have accumulated assets that offset their need for a high annual income. Of particular importance in considering the relationship between income and health is the fact that income may be low because illness has limited the amount of income earned or prevented earning income entirely.

The use of income as a measure of SES also involves more practical difficulties. A fairly high percent of persons either do not know or refuse to report their incomes. In the income-based charts shown in this report, the proportion of the population excluded because of missing data on family income generally varied between 10 and 16 percent, although it was as high as 24 percent for persons 70 years of age and older (figure 34). To reduce nonresponse, income is most often collected in categories. The categorization of income, however, introduces a certain amount of error into calculation of poverty status (family income as a percent of the Federal poverty level), although the error is likely to be small when the number of categories is large. Since low-income populations are of particular interest to health researchers, income data has traditionally been collected at a finer level of detail at the lower end of the income distribution. In most of the surveys used in this report, less detailed income categories were collected at higher income levels; in particular, all persons with family incomes of $50,000 or more were grouped together (see Technical Notes).

Converting family income into percent of the Federal poverty level is generally desirable because family size is taken into account and poverty definitions are adjusted each year to account for inflation (See Technical Notes and Appendix II). Since the calculation of poverty status was not feasible for the full range of incomes, trend data are generally presented by level of education. Education is frequently used as the measure of SES in presentations of health data. There are several reasons for this preference. Education is generally better reported than income; usually 95 percent or more of respondents report their attained level of education. Unlike occupation, all adults may be characterized by their education level. Education, unlike income, remains fixed for most people after the age of 25 and usually is not influenced by health. In addition, education is highly related to income as shown in figure 6. However, education cannot be used to characterize the socioeconomic position of children (except through parental education), and the average education level of the U.S. population has increased dramatically over time, complicating comparisons across age groups.

This chartbook relies most heavily on poverty, income, and education as measures of socioeconomic status. We have included average income level in the individual's area of residence as a measure of SES where an individual-level indicator was not available (figures 23, 24, and 48). Occupation is another indicator of SES that reflects education and income. However, occupation as usually collected is not relevant to children, retired persons, or women not currently employed, which characterizes a significant portion of women during childbearing. Since these stages of the life cycle are of great interest to health researchers and policymakers, we have not included in this report charts showing health variables by occupation.

Socioeconomic Disparities in Health

This chartbook is intended to document the extent to which socioeconomic disparities continue to exist in indicators of health status, health behaviors and other risk factors, and health care access and utilization within the United States. This demonstration provides a cautionary note when examining progress toward the *Healthy People 2000* objectives for the population as a whole. Although progress is occurring toward most targets, data presented in this chartbook demonstrate that, for many objectives, only the higher socioeconomic groups have achieved or are close to achieving the target, while lower socioeconomic

groups lag farther behind. For a broad cross section of indicators where substantial progress toward the year 2000 objectives has already occurred—mortality from heart disease (figure 27) and lung cancer (figure 28), infant mortality (figures 8 and 9), cigarette smoking (figures 35 and 36) and smoking during pregnancy (figure 13), receipt of early prenatal care (figure 19), and having regular mammograms (figure 45)—further improvement clearly depends on achieving greater gains among persons of lower socioeconomic status. This chartbook does not attempt to present a complete examination of differential progress toward all of the Year 2000 objectives since this is routinely presented in the *Healthy People 2000 Progress Reviews* (6). We have however tried to include a broad cross-section of indicators reflecting different aspects of health and health care and applicable to several age groups, that demonstrate both the magnitude and complexity of the effects of socioeconomic status.

Often examinations of the relationship between SES and health have focused on the lowest end of the SES distribution, comparing poor persons to those above the poverty threshold or persons with less than a high school education to everyone else (7). Although poverty is a powerful determinant and consequence of ill health, focus on the extreme end of the SES distribution implies uniformity among persons above the thresholds of poverty or high school graduation. Evidence from previous studies in Europe and the United States have indicated that the association between SES and health generally takes the form of a gradient; that is, while persons of lowest SES have the worst health outcomes, persons of middle SES have worse health than persons of high SES (8,9).

The data presented in this chartbook support the existence of a socioeconomic gradient in most of the health indicators examined; each increase in social position, measured either by income or education, improves the likelihood of being in good health. For most of the health indicators, this SES gradient was observed for persons in every race and ethnic group examined. In general, the SES gradient was strongest for non-Hispanic white persons and weakest for Mexican American or all Hispanic persons or, in the few instances where data were available, for Asians and Pacific Islanders. In addition, lower SES Hispanic persons tend to have better health status than non-Hispanic persons at a similar social position. The different pattern of SES and health among persons of Hispanic origin characterizes Mexican Americans, who make up the largest share of the U.S. Hispanic population. Evidence suggests that this pattern may be due, in part, to protective effects of traditional culture, which is likely to be more prevalent among recent immigrants who are also most likely to have lower incomes and educational attainment (10–12).

Although documenting socioeconomic disparities in health is not new, identifying and understanding the causes still remain a challenge. The sections of this chartbook on risk factors and health care access demonstrate the likely contributions of these two broad areas toward disparities seen in health outcomes. The socioeconomic differences apparent in risk factors, such as smoking (figures 13, 15, 35, and 36), overweight (figures 16, 38, and 39), elevated blood lead (figures 14 and 42), and sedentary lifestyle (figures 17 and 40), as well as differential access to and utilization of health care, such as seen in health insurance coverage (figures 20 and 43), physician visits (figures 22, 23, 44, 46, and 47), and avoidable hospitalizations (figures 24 and 48), influence the rates of health outcomes such as low birthweight (figure 10), heart disease mortality (figure 27), fair or poor health (figure 32), diabetes mortality (figure 29), and activity limitation (figures 11 and 33).

Given the ubiquity of SES differences in health risk factors, we need to address the question of why these behaviors are disproportionately concentrated among persons with fewer socioeconomic resources. Differences in the life circumstances of high- and low-SES persons in the United States are substantial. Higher socioeconomic position may directly influence health through income- and education-related differences including having knowledge and time to pursue healthy behaviors, having sufficient income to assure access to comfortable housing, healthy food, and appropriate health care, access to safe and

affordable locations to exercise and relax, and living and working in a safe, healthy environment (13,14). In addition, a more direct connection may exist in that persons whose attention and energy are focused on attaining economic security, or dealing with the lack of it, may have few resources, financial and emotional, for pursuing healthy lifestyles and obtaining preventive health care. It has also been suggested that simply being at a lower position on the economic distribution exacts an emotional or psychological cost that translates into poorer health practices, or simply poorer health (15,16). This latter explanation may also apply to the effects of racial and ethnic discrimination, proposed by some as a contributor to the poorer health outcomes experienced by many minorities even after adjusting for differences in their socioeconomic profile (17,18).

References

1. U.S. Department of Health and Human Services. Healthy people 2000: National health promotion and disease prevention objectives. Washington: Public Health Service. 1990.

2. Department of Health (U.K.). Variations in health: What can the Department of Health and the N.H.S. do? London. 1996.

3. Williams DR. Socioeconomic differentials in health: A review and redirection. Social Psychology Quarterly 53:81–99. 1990.

4. Townsend P, Davidson N. Inequalities in health: The Black report. Penguin: London. 1982.

5. U.S. Bureau of the Census. Current Population Survey, 1996.

6. Department of Health and Human Services. Office of Disease Prevention and Health Promotion. <http://odphp.osophs.dhhs.gov/pubs/hp2000>.

7. Haan MN, Kaplan GA, Syme SL. Socioeconomic status and health: Old observations and new thoughts, in Bunker DS, Gomby DS, Kehrer BH (eds.) Pathways to health: The role of social factors. Menlo Park, CA: Henry Kaiser Family Foundation. 1989.

8. Marmot M, Smith GD, Stansfeld S et al. Health inequalities among British civil servants: The Whitehall Study II. Lancet 337:1387–93. 1991.

9. Adler N, Boyce T, Chesney M, et al. Socioeconomic status and health: The challenge of the gradient. Am Psychol 49:15–24. 1994.

10. Marin G, Perez-Stable EJ, Marin BV. Cigarette smoking among San Francisco Hispanics: The role of acculturation and gender. Am J Public Health 79:196–8. 1989.

11. Council on Scientific Affairs. Hispanic health in the United States. JAMA 265:248–52. 1991.

12. Molina CW, Aguirre-Molina M (eds.). Latino Health in the US: A growing challenge. American Public Health Association. 1994.

13. Lundberg O. Causal explanations for class inequality in health an empirical analysis. Soc Sci Med 32:385–93. 1991.

14. Link BG, Phelan J. Social conditions as fundamental causes of disease. J Health Soc Behav (extra issue):80–94. 1995.

15. Wilkinson RG. The epidemiologic transition: From material scarcity to social disadvantage. Daedalus 123:61–77. 1994.

16. Wilkinson RG. Health inequalities: Relative or absolute material standards? BMJ 314:1427–28. 1997.

17. Krieger N, Rowley D, Herman AA, et al. Racism, sexism, and social class: Implications for studies of health disease and well-being. Am J Prev Med 9:82–122. 1993.

18. Williams DR. Racism and health: A research agenda. Ethn Dis 6:1–6. 1996.

This section presents current patterns and recent trends in measures of socioeconomic status (SES) in the United States population. To the extent possible, distributions and trends in measures of SES are shown for major race and ethnic subgroups of the population, and for gender and age groups where appropriate.

Figure 1 shows household income at selected percentiles of the household income distribution for the years 1970 to 1996 and demonstrates increasing income inequality in recent years in the United States. In 1996 the bottom 20 percent of U.S. households had incomes below $14,770; adjusted for inflation, this represents an increase of less than $800 since 1970. In contrast, the top 20 percent of households had incomes above $68,000 in 1996, $12,300 more than in 1970. A major contributor to the increase in income inequality has been increasing inequality in wages. The increase in earnings inequality over the last 25 years was primarily produced by technological change that increased returns to highly skilled labor at the same time that less skilled workers saw their real wages stagnate or decline. This trend was exacerbated to some degree by "globalization" of the economy, declines in the real minimum wage and in unionization, and an increase in immigration. Household income, however, is also a product of household composition and income from sources other than earnings. A significant part of the increase in income inequality can be attributed to changes in family composition and an increase in female labor-force participation. Because individuals tend to marry individuals with similar earnings profiles, increasing the number of families with both husband and wife working increases income inequality. In addition, an increase in families headed by women (from 10 percent of families in 1970 to 18 percent in 1996) has acted to increase income inequality since these households generally have lower incomes (1–5).

Income may be related to health because it increases access to medical care, enables one to live in better neighborhoods and afford better housing, and increases the opportunity to engage in health-promoting behaviors. Income may also be affected by poor health, by restricting type or amount of employment, or preventing an individual from

working entirely. Figure 2 shows median household income by race and Hispanic origin for the years 1980 to 1996. Throughout this period, the median income of non-Hispanic white households has been much higher than that of black or Hispanic households, but the income gap between white and Hispanic households widened, whereas the gap between white and black households narrowed slightly. In 1996 Asian or Pacific Islander households had the highest median income, with the median income of these households showing no significant change between 1991 and 1996. Trends in median income for Hispanic and Asian or Pacific Islander households are likely to have been affected by increasing immigration into the United States in recent years since recent immigrants have a lower median income than natives or longer term residents (6).

As mentioned above, household income is affected by household composition. The poverty index takes household size and composition into account (see Technical Notes). Figure 3 shows the proportion of persons poor and near poor by race and Hispanic origin for 1996. Overall, almost 14 percent of the population lived in poverty in 1996 and 20 percent more had incomes that were near poverty.

There are distinct demographic differences in poverty by age, race, ethnicity and household composition. In accordance with differences in median household income, black persons and persons of Hispanic origin are disproportionately represented among the poor and near poor. Poverty rates also vary across age groups. In 1996 over one-fifth of all children lived in poverty. Between 1970 and 1980 the poverty rate among children rose from around 15 percent to more than 20 percent and it has remained at or above 20 percent for the last 16 years. In contrast, nearly one-quarter of persons 65 years of age and over were poor in 1970, but by 1980 the proportion in poverty had decreased to 16 percent. Between 1980 and 1996 poverty among the elderly continued to decline to 10.8 percent, slightly below the rate for working-age adults (18–64 years of age) (7).

Race and ethnic differences in the poverty rate are as pronounced among children as among adults; in 1996, 11 percent of non-Hispanic white children were poor compared with 40 percent of black and Hispanic children. Children in female-headed households had the highest rates of poverty; nearly one-half of the children living in female-headed households in 1996 were below the poverty line. Even among female-headed households, however, poverty rates for children were higher in black and Hispanic households than white households.

Figure 4 demonstrates that there are substantial geographic differences in poverty rates in the United States. The average State poverty levels for the years 1994–96 ranged from 7–8 percent in New Hampshire and Utah to 22 percent and more in New Mexico, the District of Columbia, and Louisiana with the South and West having disproportionately larger shares of the Nation's poor population. Geographic differences in health outcomes may be related to these variations in poverty.

Education is a widely used indicator of socioeconomic status in the United States. Educational attainment is a major determinant of earnings. In addition, education is also likely to influence health through a variety of cultural, social, and psychological mechanisms (8). For example, higher levels of education may increase exposure to health-related information as well as equip individuals with the skills to adopt health promoting behaviors. Education may also influence health-related values such as a belief in prevention.

Figure 5 shows the distribution of educational attainment for persons 25 years and over by age, race, and Hispanic origin in 1996. Educational attainment is presented for persons 25–64 years and 65 years or over because educational attainment varies by age cohort, with persons 65 years and over much less likely to have completed high school. Educational attainment also differs substantially by race and ethnicity. The race and ethnic patterns in household income (figure 2) are mirrored in the educational distributions of these groups. Among persons 25 to 64 years of age in 1996, 45 percent of Asian or Pacific Islanders and nearly 30 percent of non-Hispanic white persons have college degrees, compared with 15 percent of non-Hispanic black persons and 10 percent of Hispanic persons. This pattern is essentially reversed at the low end of educational

attainment; 10 percent of non-Hispanic white persons and 14 percent of Asian or Pacific Islander persons have not completed high school, compared with 20 percent of non-Hispanic black persons and 44 percent of Hispanic persons.

Figures 2 and 5 show that income and education vary by race and ethnicity, but even within the same category of educational attainment, median family income varies by race and ethnicity and also gender (figure 6). For men and women across all race and ethnic groups, the higher the level of education, the higher the median family income. However, within education level categories, men have higher median family incomes than women, and median family incomes of Asian or Pacific Islander and white persons were higher than median family incomes of black or Hispanic men and women. Some of these differences, especially differences between men and women, may be attributed to the number of family members who are employed and to whether employed family members work full-time or part-time.

Type of occupation can also significantly impact health, largely because occupation and income are intrinsically connected. However, occupation may additionally influence health directly by determining exposure to hazards in the work environment, as well as exposure to job-associated stress (9). Figure 7 shows the distribution of men and women by racial and ethnic groups across occupational categories (see Technical Notes for a description of each occupational category). The majority of persons 25–64 years of age are employed in white collar occupations. However, a greater proportion of Asian or Pacific Islander and non-Hispanic white men are employed in white collar jobs while more black and Hispanic men are employed in blue collar jobs. Women were twice as likely to be employed in service occupations than men, with black and Hispanic women more likely to be employed in service occupations than Asian or Pacific Islander or white women.

As these charts briefly demonstrate, the most common measures of socioeconomic status (income, education, and occupation) can vary substantially by race, ethnicity, and sex. The two following sections of the chartbook will demonstrate how measures of socioeconomic status—particularly income and education—are strongly associated with health outcomes, health-related behaviors and other risk factors, and measures of health care access and utilization.

References

1. Ryscavage P, Henle P. Earnings inequality accelerates in the 1980's. Monthly Labor Review 113:3–16. 1990.

2. Danziger S, Gottschalk (eds.). Uneven tides: Rising inequality in America. New York: Russell Sage Foundation. 1993.

3. Karoly LA, Burtless G. Demographic change, rising earnings inequality, and the distribution of personal well-being, 1959–89. Demography 32(3):379–405. 1995.

4. U.S. Council of Economic Advisors. Economic report of the President. Washington: U.S. Government Printing Office. Chapter 4. 1992.

5. U.S. Council of Economic Advisors. Economic report of the President Washington: U.S. Government Printing Office. Chapter 5. 1995.

6. Hansen KA, Faber CS. The foreign-born population, 1996. U.S. Bureau of the Census. Current Population Survey, P20–494. 1997.

7. U.S. Council of Economic Advisors. Economic report of the President. Washington: U.S. Government Printing Office. Chapter 5. 1997.

8. Liberatos P. Link BG. Kelsey JL. The measurement of social class in epidemiology. Epidemiologic Reviews.10:87–121. 1988.

9. Karasek R, Theorell T. Healthy work: Stress, productivity, and the reconstruction of working life. New York: Basic Books. 1990.

Population

Income

■ In 1996, 20 percent of U.S. households had incomes above $68,015 and 20 percent had incomes below $14,768, so that household income at the 80th percentile of the household income distribution was 4.6 times household income at the 20th percentile.

■ The ratio of income at the 80th percentile to that at the 20th percentile increased over the past 26 years; in 1970 this ratio was 4.0. The increase in the ratio of income at the 95th percentile to that at the 20th percentile has been even greater, from 6.3 in 1970 to 8.1 in 1996. By contrast, income at the 50th percentile remained approximately 2.4 times income at the 20th percentile over the 26 year period.

■ Measured in 1996 dollars, household income at the 20th and 50th percentiles changed little between 1970 and 1996. Between 1970 and 1990, income at the 20th percentile increased slightly, then fell by a small amount between 1990 and 1996, yielding an average annual increase of 0.20 percent over the 26-year period. Income at the 50th percentile followed a similar pattern with an average annual increase of 0.26 percent between 1970 and 1996. Income at the 80th percentile increased consistently over the period at an average annual rate of 0.77 percent, while the top 5 percent of the income distribution showed the greatest increase at 1.18 percent per year.

Figure 1. Household income at selected percentiles of the household income distribution: United States, 1970–96

Household income (in thousands of 1996 dollars)

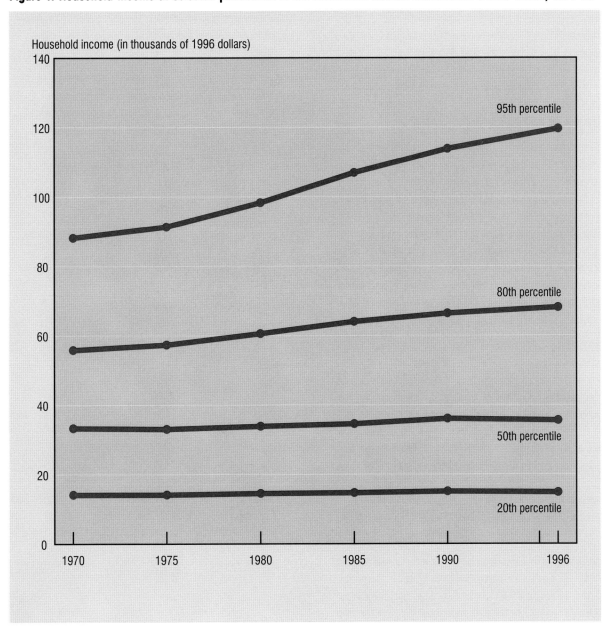

NOTES: See Technical Notes for the definition of income. In 1995, the 1990 Census adjusted population controls and sample redesign were implemented: there was a change in data collection method from paper-pencil to computer-assisted interviewing, and income reporting limits changed. In 1980, the 1980 Census population controls were implemented. In 1975, the 1970 population controls were implemented.

SOURCE: U.S. Census Bureau. Money Income in the United States: 1996. Current Population Reports, Series P60-197, Washington: U.S. Government Printing Office. September 1997.

Population

Income

- In 1996 median household income in the United States was $35,492. Asian or Pacific Islander households had the highest median income ($43,276), followed by non-Hispanic white households ($38,787). Median incomes for black and Hispanic households ($23,482 and $24,906) were less than 65 percent of the median for non-Hispanic white households.

- Between 1982 and 1989, median income increased for black, non-Hispanic white, and Hispanic households (by 17 percent, 12 percent and 11 percent, respectively), then declined for all race and ethnic groups between 1989 and 1992. Between 1992 and 1996 median incomes rose for black, Asian or Pacific Islander, and non-Hispanic white households, but not for Hispanic households. In 1996 median income for black households was slightly higher than it had been in 1989, but median income for white households was still slightly lower than in 1989.

- Between 1980 and 1996 the difference in income between non-Hispanic white households and black households decreased slightly, but the difference between Hispanic households and non-Hispanic white households widened. In 1980 the median income for white households was 39 percent higher than for Hispanic households; in 1990, 43 percent higher; and in 1996, 56 percent higher. In contrast, median income for non-Hispanic white households in 1980 was 77 percent higher than for black households; it was 71 percent higher in 1990, and 65 percent higher in 1996.

- Similarly, the income difference between Hispanic and black households decreased considerably between 1980 and 1996. In 1980 median income for Hispanic households was 27 percent higher than median income

for black households; in 1990 it was 20 percent higher, but by 1996 it was only 6 percent higher.

- Household income is influenced by number of earners per household and comparison across race and ethnic groups is affected by differences in average household size. In 1996, the total money income per household member was $20,216 for non-Hispanic white persons, $17,928 for persons of Asian or Pacific Islander origin, $11,543 for black persons, and $9,545 for persons of Hispanic origin (1).

Reference

1. U.S. Census Bureau. "Historical Income Tables, Household Table H-15. Total Money Income Per Household Member, by Race and Hispanic Origin of Householder: 1980 to 1996." Published 29 September, 1997.<www.census.gov/hhes/income/histinc/h15.html>

Figure 2. Median household income by race and Hispanic origin: United States, 1980–96

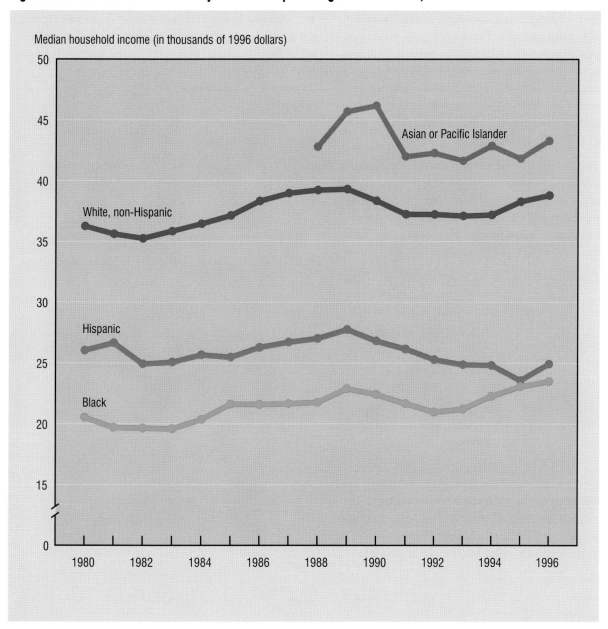

Median household income (in thousands of 1996 dollars)

NOTES: See Technical Notes for the definition of income. In 1995 the 1990 census adjusted population controls and sample redesign were implemented: there was a change in data collection method from paper-pencil to computer-assisted interviewing, and income reporting limits changed. In 1980, the 1980 Census population controls were implemented. In 1975, the 1970 population controls were implemented.

SOURCE: U.S. Census Bureau. "Historical Income Tables, Household Table H-5. Race and Hispanic Origin of Householder—Households by Median and Mean Income: 1967 to 1996." Published 29 September 1997. <www.census.gov/hhes/income/histic/h05.html>

Poverty

■ In 1996, 36.5 million residents of the United States (14 percent) were living in poverty. Forty-five percent (16.5 million) of persons living below the poverty line were non-Hispanic white persons, 27 percent (9.7 million) were black persons, 24 percent (8.7 million) were persons of Hispanic origin, and 4 percent (1.5 million) were persons of Asian or Pacific Islander origin.

■ The poverty rate was lowest among non-Hispanic white persons (9 percent) followed by persons of Asian or Pacific Islander origin (15 percent). Poverty rates for black persons and persons of Hispanic origin were more than three times the rate for non-Hispanic white persons.

■ Over one-third of the U.S. population was living in or near poverty in 1996. The majority of black persons (55 percent) and persons of Hispanic origin (60 percent) lived in families classified as poor or near poor.

■ In 1996, one out of every five children in the United States (14.5 million) lived in poverty. Poverty rates for black and Hispanic children were much higher (40 percent in each group) than the overall rate, and almost 4 times the poverty rate for non-Hispanic white children.

■ Over two-thirds of black children and nearly three-quarters of Hispanic children were living in or near poverty in 1996; 31 percent of non-Hispanic white children and 36 percent of children of Asian or Pacific Islander origin were classified as poor or near poor.

■ Children living in female-headed households had the highest rates of poverty. In 1996 nearly one-half of all children in female-headed households (8 million) were living below the poverty line and another 27 percent were near poor. Poverty rates for black and Hispanic children in female-headed households were considerably higher than the rates for non-Hispanic white children or children of Asian or Pacific Islander origin.

Figure 3. Percent of persons poor and near poor by race and Hispanic origin: United States, 1996

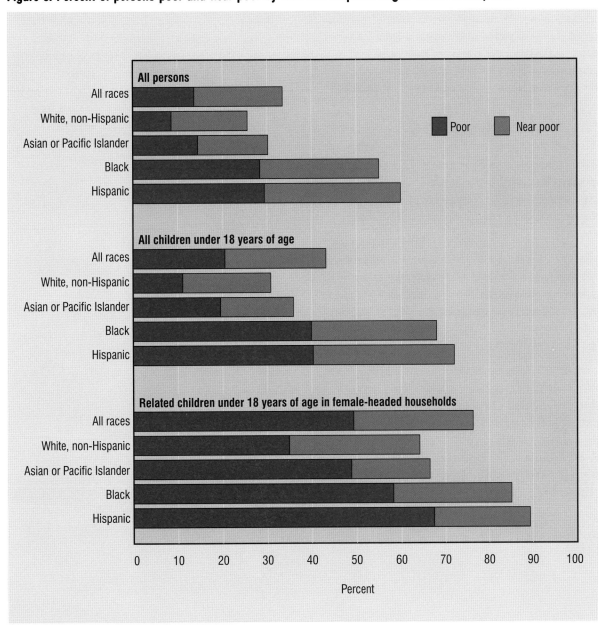

NOTES: All figures refer to persons. "All children under 18 years of age" includes unrelated children. "Female-headed households" above are families with female householder and no spouse present. See Technical Notes for a description of poverty status.

SOURCE: U.S. Census Bureau. "Detailed Poverty Tables, Table 2. Age, Sex, Household Relationship, Race and Hispanic origin, and Selected Statuses-Ratio of Income to Poverty level in 1996." Last revised: October 3, 1997. <http://ferret.bls.census.gov/macro/031997/pov/2_001-3.htm>. See related *Health, United States, 1998*, table 2.

Poverty

■ Across States the average annual poverty rates for the years 1994–96 varied over threefold from 7 to 24 percent. Poverty rates were lowest in New Hampshire and Utah (7–8 percent) and highest in Louisiana, New Mexico, and the District of Columbia (22–24 percent).

■ The South has a disproportionately large share of the Nation's poor population. In 1996, 35 percent of the U.S. population, but 38 percent of persons below the poverty line, lived in the South. One-quarter of poor persons lived in the West, while the Midwest and Northeast each contained 18 percent of the Nation's poor.

■ Before 1994 the South had the highest poverty rate of any region. In 1996 the poverty rate in the West was not significantly different from that in the South; both were 15 percent. Thirteen percent of persons living in the Northeast were poor in 1996, as were 11 percent of persons living in the Midwest.

■ Within the West, the States with the highest poverty rates during 1994–96 include New Mexico (24 percent), Arizona (18 percent), and California (17 percent). Within the South the following eight States had poverty rates of 16 percent or higher during 1994–96: Louisiana, the District of Columbia, Mississippi, West Virginia, Alabama, Texas, Oklahoma, and Kentucky.

Figure 4. Percent of persons in poverty by State: United States, average annual 1994–96

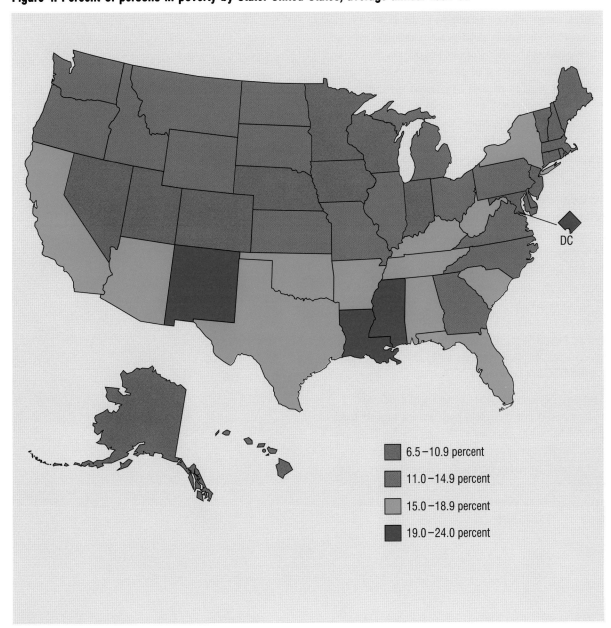

DC

6.5–10.9 percent
11.0–14.9 percent
15.0–18.9 percent
19.0–24.0 percent

NOTE: See Technical Notes for a description of poverty status.

SOURCE: U.S. Bureau of the Census. Poverty in the United States: 1996. Current Population Reports, Series P60-194. Washington: U.S. Government Printing Office. September 1997.

Education

■ The average level of education in the U.S. population has increased steadily since this information was first collected by the Current Population Survey in 1947. In 1996, 35 percent of persons 65 years of age and over, but only 14 percent of persons ages 25–64 years, had not completed high school. In contrast, more than one-half of persons 25–64 years of age had some education beyond high school, whereas only 31 percent of persons 65 years of age and over had more than a high school diploma.

■ Educational levels vary considerably among race and ethnic subgroups. Among persons 25–64 years of age, the proportion who had not completed high school in 1996 ranged from 10 percent for white persons to 44 percent for Hispanic persons. In this age group, one out of every five black persons and one out of every eight Asian or Pacific Islander persons had less than a high school education. The percent with a college degree or higher level of education ranged from 10 percent for Hispanic persons to 45 percent for Asian or Pacific Islander persons.

■ Among persons 65 years of age and older, the percent who did not complete high school ranged from 31 percent for white persons to 70 percent for Hispanic persons. In this age group, one-third of white persons and 35 percent of Asian or Pacific Islander persons had some education beyond high school, compared with 18 percent of black persons and 14 percent of Hispanic persons.

Figure 5. Educational attainment among persons 25 years and over by age, race, and Hispanic origin: United States, 1996

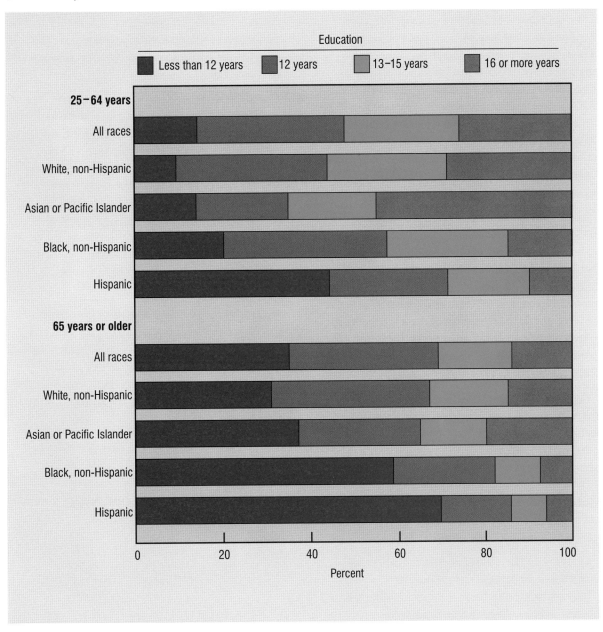

NOTES: Less than 12 years includes persons with 12 years of schooling but no high school diploma. Twelve years includes persons with a high school diploma or G.E.D. Thirteen to fifteen years includes persons without a degree and persons with associate's degrees. Sixteen years or more includes all persons with a baccalaurate degree or higher.

SOURCE: U.S. Bureau of the Census. Current Population Survey, March 1996.

Education

■ Median household income increases with each higher level of education. Men 25 years of age and over with at least a college degree had a median family income of $66,690 in 1996, 2.7 times the median for men who did not complete high school ($24,386). The income gradient with increasing education was similar for women; median family income for women with a college degree or higher level of education was 3.4 times as high as the median for women without a high school diploma ($62,050 compared with $18,200).

■ At each level of attained education, women generally lived in households with less income than men, but the gender disparity tended to decrease at higher levels of education. Median household income for men who had not finished high school was 34 percent higher than the median for women with the same level of education; median household income for men with at least a college degree was 7 percent higher than the median for women at the same education level.

■ The disparity between the median household incomes of men and women at the same level of education was greatest for black persons; median income for men exceeded that for women by 52 percent for persons with less than a high school education, and by 16 percent for college graduates. Among Asian or Pacific Islander persons, there was essentially no gender disparity in median household income within levels of education.

■ Among men, the education-related gradient in median household income was greatest for non-Hispanic white and black men; in 1996 black and white men with a college degree had median household incomes 2.7 times higher than the median income for those with no high school diploma. This ratio was 2.4 for Hispanic men and 2.0 for Asian or Pacific Islander men.

■ The education-related gradient in median household income was similar for black and white women; those with at least a college degree lived in households where the median family income was approximately 3.5 times greater than that for women who had not finished high school. Among Hispanic women, this ratio was 2.9. There was less of an education-related gradient in income for Asian or Pacific Islander women; those with a college degree or higher lived in households with a median income less than twice that of women with no high school diploma.

■ At each level of education, median household incomes for women varied more across the race and ethnic subgroups than did those for men. Within each education level, median household income in 1996 was similar for Hispanic and black men, but the median for black women was lower than that for Hispanic women.

Figure 6. Median household income among persons 25 years of age and over by education, sex, race, and Hispanic origin: United States, 1996

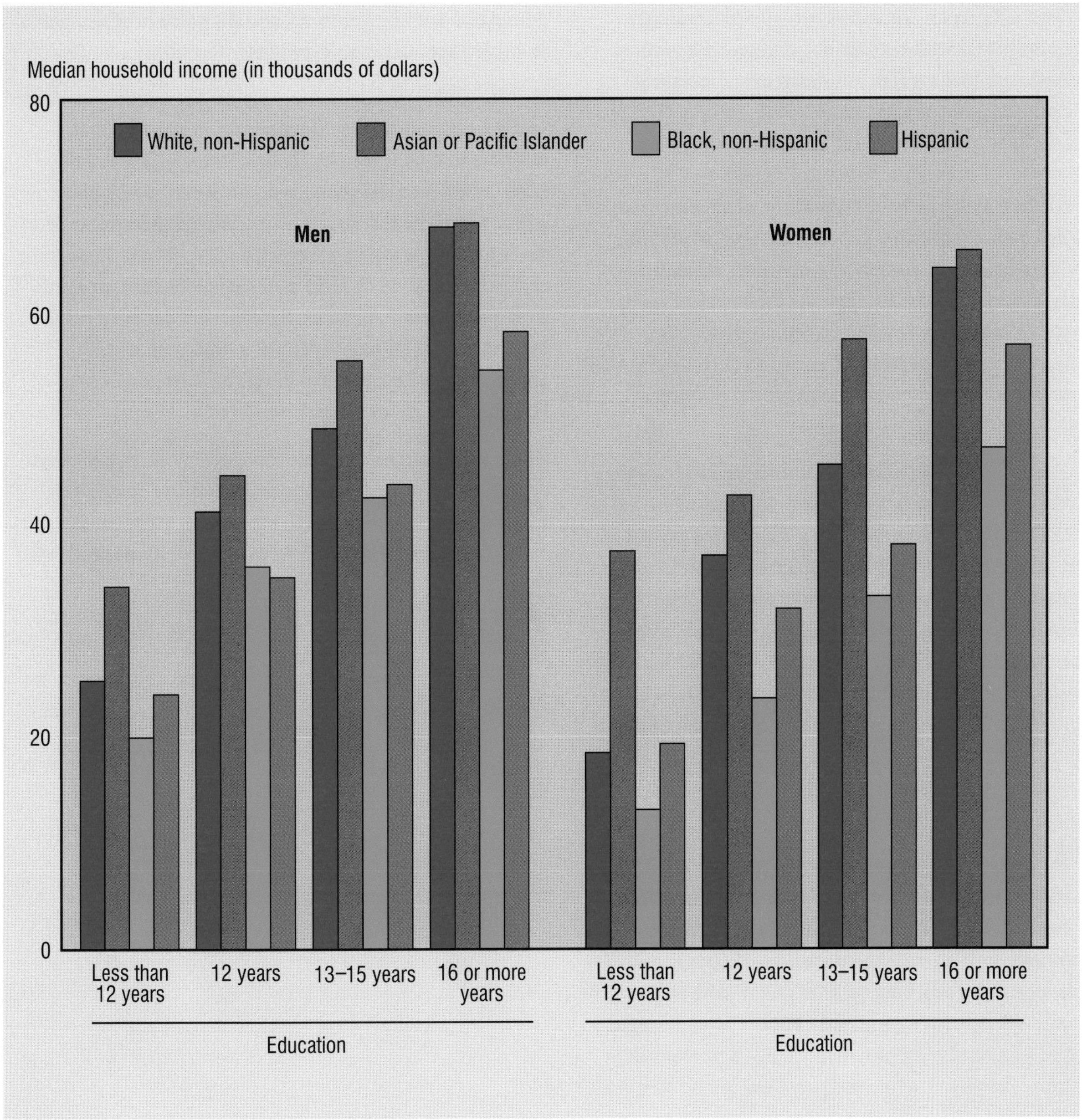

Median household income (in thousands of dollars)

Legend: White, non-Hispanic | Asian or Pacific Islander | Black, non-Hispanic | Hispanic

Men / Women

Education: Less than 12 years, 12 years, 13–15 years, 16 or more years

NOTES: Median income is based on total household income (earnings and other income) and is not adjusted for work status or number of hours worked by household members. Median is calculated using actual reported household income, not grouped data. Educational attainment is as of March 1997. Less than 12 years includes persons with 12 years of schooling but no high school diploma. Twelve years includes persons with a high school diploma or G.E.D. Thirteen to fifteen years includes persons without a degree and persons with Associate's degrees. Sixteen years or more includes all persons with a baccalaurate degree or higher.

SOURCE: U.S. Bureau of the Census. Current Population Survey: March 1997.

Occupation

■ The U.S. labor force has become increasingly concentrated in white collar occupations: executive, professional, managerial, administrative, technical, clerical, and sales positions. In 1996, among civilians 25–64 years of age reporting a current occupation, 48 percent of men and 73 percent of women held white collar positions. Thirty–nine percent of civilian men in this age range held blue collar jobs, compared with only 10 percent of women. By contrast, women were nearly twice as likely as men to be employed in service occupations (16 percent compared with 9 percent). Only 4 percent of men and just 1 percent of women reported their major occupation as farm related.

■ Asian or Pacific Islander men and non-Hispanic white men were much more likely to hold white collar positions than black or Hispanic men; three out of every five Asian or Pacific Islander men and over one-half of white men were employed in white collar occupations, compared with one out of every three black men and about one-quarter of Hispanic men. For each race and ethnic group examined, the majority of employed civilian women between 25 and 64 years of age held white collar positions, from 52 percent of Hispanic women to over three-quarters of white women.

■ In 1996 average compensation for persons holding blue-collar jobs was 81 percent of that for white collar workers (see *Health, United States, 1998*, table 122). Nearly one-half of employed civilian Hispanic and black men were working in blue collar jobs in 1996, but only 28 percent of Asian or Pacific Islander men were in blue collar employment. Only 8 percent of currently employed white women held blue collar jobs, compared with between 15 and 18 percent of women in other race and ethnic groups.

■ In 1996 average compensation for service workers was 41 percent of that for persons in white collar employment (see *Health, United States, 1998*, table 122). Black and Hispanic women were nearly twice as likely as white and Asian or Pacific Islander women to be employed in service occupations (26 and 27 percent compared with 13 and 15 percent, respectively) in 1996. White and Asian or Pacific Islander men were least likely to be employed in service occupations, 7 and 9 percent compared with 15 and 18 percent for Hispanic and black men, respectively.

■ Hispanic men and women were more likely to be employed in farm occupations than those in other race and ethnic groups. In 1996, 9 percent of Hispanic men and 3 percent of Hispanic women reported farm-related work as their major occupation.

Figure 7. Current occupation for persons 25–64 years of age by sex, race, and Hispanic origin: United States, 1996

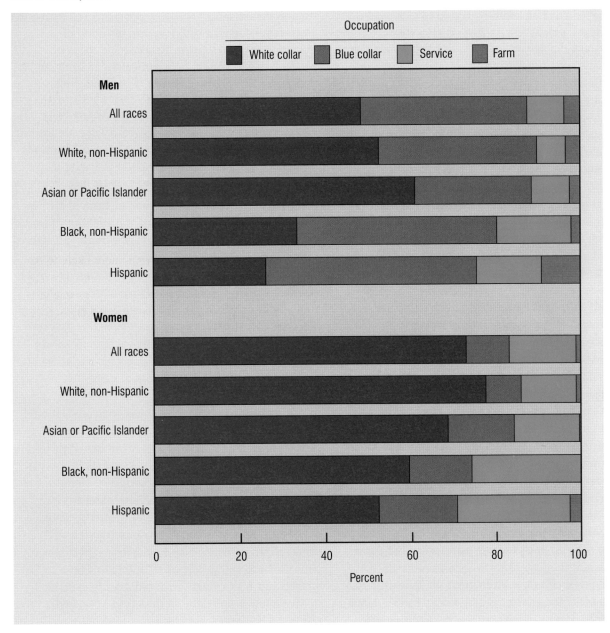

NOTES: Within the occupational categories there is a great deal of occupational diversity. See Technical Notes for description of each occupational category. Persons in the military are excluded.

SOURCE: U.S. Bureau of the Census. Current Population Survey: March 1996.

A healthy childhood is a foundation of success and health in later life. This section of the chartbook shows the relationship between socioeconomic status (SES) of a child's family and indicators of health status in childhood, risk factors for poor health during pregnancy through adolescence, and health care access and utilization for children.

Receiving prenatal care and maintaining good health behaviors during pregnancy are the first steps toward having a healthy child. Early and consistent prenatal care reduces the risk of poor birth outcomes. Figures 18 and 19 present data on prenatal care utilization. During the 1990's early initiation of prenatal care increased for mothers at every level of education. This improvement may have been due partly to expansions in Medicaid coverage for pregnant women (1). However, data indicated that in 1996 more educated mothers were still more likely than less educated mothers to obtain prenatal care in the first trimester, regardless of race or ethnicity. The *Healthy People 2000* goal for prenatal care is for 90 percent of live births to have received prenatal care in the first trimester. While mothers with 16 or more years of education were close to the goal or achieved it in most race and ethnic groups, fewer than three-quarters of mothers who had not completed high school obtained early prenatal care in any race and ethnic group; in some groups the percent with early prenatal care was closer to one-half. In addition to lack of insurance or other financial problems, other factors, such as lack of transportation, scheduling difficulties, or lack of knowledge about the pregnancy, may act as barriers to receiving early care (2,3).

Maternal behaviors also influence the health of the infant at birth. Infants whose mothers smoked during pregnancy are more likely to experience health problems, such as low birthweight, abruptio placentae (4), intrauterine growth retardation (5), Sudden Infant Death Syndrome (6), and asthma in childhood (7). Figure 13 demonstrates that in 1996 less educated women were more likely to smoke during pregnancy, but there were significant differences by race and ethnicity; less educated non-Hispanic white women were far more likely to smoke than women of other backgrounds. Almost one-half of non-Hispanic white women without a high school diploma smoked during pregnancy, compared with less than one-third of women in any other group. Hispanic and Asian or Pacific Islander women were particularly unlikely to smoke, yet even in these groups, an education-related gradient was apparent.

Adolescent childbearing, another risk factor for poor health in childhood, was more common among mothers of lower socioeconomic status (figure 12). Women whose own mothers were less educated were more likely to become teenage parents. The low education levels of the respondents' mothers likely reflected lower household incomes, on average, when the teenage mothers were young, and perhaps different expectations for educational attainment or childbearing than were found among the daughters of more educated women (8). Early childbearing is associated with a wide range of poor health and economic outcomes (9), and the teenage mothers in this data set had much lower incomes in adulthood than those who delayed their first birth. Lower socioeconomic status was a predictor and a consequence of early childbearing.

Infants born to mothers of lower socioeconomic status tended to have poorer health, as measured by their rates of low birthweight and infant mortality. In addition to the importance of infant survival in its own right, the infant mortality rate is correlated strongly with a variety of other health measures, and is considered to be a good measure of overall community health (10). Low birthweight is associated with an increased risk of health and developmental problems during infancy and childhood (11). Infants whose mothers had fewer years of education were more likely to have a low weight at birth (less than 5.5 pounds) and to die before reaching their first birthday (figures 8, 9, and 10). These two measures are closely associated as low birthweight is a frequent antecedent to infant mortality. Among white and black infants, each increase in maternal education was associated with a decline in low birthweight and infant mortality rates. This pattern was evident among Hispanic children for infant mortality but not for low birthweight. Neither infant mortality nor low birthweight was clearly associated with maternal education among American Indian or Alaska Native children or among Asian or Pacific Islander children, although the infants of the least educated American Indian or Alaska Native women had higher rates of both measures. Analysis of data for Hispanic and Asian or Pacific Islander subgroups found the association with socioeconomic status to be evident among some groups and less so among others. Analysis of trends in infant mortality (figure 8) indicated that the health gaps between children of higher and lower socioeconomic status have been fairly wide throughout the 1980's and early 1990's, and that declines in infant mortality during 1983–95 were fairly consistent across maternal education groups.

Health insurance may be a contributing factor in health disparities. Children without health insurance coverage are likely to have difficulties obtaining medical care (12,13). The parents of children with public (usually Medicaid) coverage may also have trouble finding a physician since many do not accept Medicaid patients, often because Medicaid reimburses at a lower rate than does private insurance (14). Children who have no insurance may be forced to bypass well-child and preventive visits. Those without adequate access may procure services at an emergency room as a last-resort location for health care (13).

Children from low-income families were much less likely to be insured (figure 20), although there were few differences between poor and near-poor children. Among black and Hispanic children, the near-poor had lower coverage rates, probably because many of the poor were insured through the Medicaid program, for which most of the near-poor children were not eligible. Very few children in high-income families were uninsured (from 4 to 7 percent), while

up to one-third of children in low-income families had no health insurance.

Several measures of health status and health care utilization indicated that children from lower SES families had worse health status and more risk factors for poor health while having less adequate access to and utilization of health services. Health care utilization reflected the disparities evident in insurance coverage. Children under age 6 who were from poor and near-poor families were less likely than those from middle- or high-income families to have seen a physician in the past year, and uninsured children from every income group were substantially less likely than insured children to have seen a doctor (figure 22). Children living in lower income areas had lower rates of outpatient visits than those living in higher income areas, and were more likely to have received care in hospital emergency or outpatient departments than at a physician's office (figure 23).

Children from poor families were less likely to be fully vaccinated on schedule than children from higher income families (figure 21). Prompt vaccination is important to protect children's health, and may be a marker of the quality of children's health care early in life. Insufficient vaccine levels may indicate that the child has not had timely use of well-child visits.

Another indicator of adequacy of preventive care is hospitalization for asthma. Asthma is one of the most common chronic diseases in childhood, and is generally managed via outpatient care and, occasionally, emergency room visits. Hospitalization for asthma indicates severe disease and may suggest that the child has not had adequate care from a physician who can help them control their asthma (15). Children who lived in poorer neighborhoods had higher rates of hospitalization for asthma (figure 24) and black children had higher rates than those of white children at every level of neighborhood socioeconomic status during 1989–91.

Disparity in environmental quality is another factor contributing to the influence of socioeconomic status on health. Figure 14 shows that children in lower income households were more likely to have elevated levels of blood lead, which is associated with less than optimal developmental outcome, such as lower intelligence (16). Poorer children may be more subject to environmental degradation, such as substandard housing, putting them at greater risk of lead intake (17).

Activity limitation due to a chronic health condition is a broad measure of health and functioning. In contrast to the declines in infant mortality, rates of reported activity limitation among children increased slightly between 1984–87 and 1992–95. This increase appeared to be greater among children in lower income than higher income families, resulting in a slight widening of the disparity by income (figure 11). Hispanic children had lower rates of reported activity limitation in each income group and a less marked income gradient than white or black children. The increase in reported rates of activity limitation may have been a result of a true increase in limitation, but also may have been influenced if there was an increase in diagnosis of existing limitations (such as the diagnosis of learning disability) or a change in awareness of such limitations.

Many risk factors for poor health in later life develop in adolescence. Smoking is most frequently begun in adolescence (18), and obesity in youth may remain into adulthood (19). Although smoking rates among pregnant women were inversely related to level of education, there was no clear gradient in smoking rates for adolescents by family income group overall (figures 13 and 15). However, when adolescent smoking data were broken down by race and ethnic group, results appeared more similar to those of childbearing women: the proportion smoking was highest and the income gradient strongest among white adolescents. However, smoking was more common among Hispanic adolescents and less common among black adolescents than among pregnant women of the same race or ethnicity.

Overall, adolescents from lower income families were more likely to be overweight than those from higher income families. However, within the race and ethnic subgroups examined, the negative relationship of income and overweight was true only for non-Hispanic white adolescents (figure 16). Black adolescents had no clear pattern of overweight in relation to family socioeconomic status, while Mexican American teenagers from higher income families were more likely to be overweight. Since sedentary behavior is a strong risk factor for overweight, one might expect the two to have a similar socioeconomic profile, and sedentariness was associated with socioeconomic status (figure 17), with the association more marked for girls than for boys. The overall relationship between income and sedentary behavior may obscure substantial differences among race and ethnic groups, which could not be examined here due to insufficient sample size.

Data suggested that health status of children has improved in some areas since the early 1980's and worsened in others. However, the health gap between children of higher and lower socioeconomic status parents was constant through the time period and remained in the mid-1990's. Children who had well-educated or high-income parents had a better chance of being born healthy and continuing to remain healthy throughout childhood. Access to appropriate health care, health behaviors of parents and children, and exposure to environmental risks are among the factors contributing to the socioeconomic disparities in children's health.

References

1. Ray WA, Mitchel EF, Piper JM. Effect of Medicaid expansions on preterm birth. Am J Prev Med 13(4): 292–7. 1997.

2. Lewis CT, Mathews TJ, Heuser RL. Prenatal care in the United States, 1980–94. Vital Health Stat 21(54):1–17. 1996.

3. Rogers C, Schiff M. Early versus late prenatal care in New Mexico: Barriers and motivators. Birth 23(1):26–30. 1996.

4. Kramer MS, Usher RH, Pollack R, Boyd M, Usher S. Etiologic determinants of abruptio placentae. Obstet Gynecol 89:221–6. 1997.

5. Nordentoft M, Lou HC, Hansen D, et al. Intrauterine growth retardation and premature delivery: The influence of maternal smoking and psychosocial factors. Am J Public Health 86: 1996.

6. Hoffman HJ, Damus K, Hillman L, Krongrad E. Risk factors for SIDS: Results of the National Institute of Child Health and Human Development SIDS Cooperative Epidemiological Study. Ann NY Acad Sci1 8: 113–20. 1988.

7. Ehrlich RI, Du-Toit D, Jordaan E, et al. Risk factors for childhood asthma and wheezing: Importance of maternal and household smoking. Am J Respir Crit Care Med 154: 681–8. 1996.

8. Nord CW, Moore KA, Morrison DR, et al. Consequences of teenage parenting. J School Health 62:310–8. 1992.

9. Hoffman SD, Foster EM, Furstenberg FF Jr. Reevaluating the costs of teenage childbearing. Demography 30(1):1–13. 1993.

10. Freedman MA. Health status indicators for the year 2000. Healthy People 2000 Statistical Notes 1(1): 1–4. National Center for Health Statistics. 1991.

11. Hack M, Klein NK, Taylor HG. Long-term developmental outcomes of low birth weight infants. In: The Future of Children. Low Birth Weight. Shiano PH and Berhman RE, eds. David and Lucille Packard Foundation. 176–96. 1995.

12. Newacheck PW, Hughes DC, Stoddard JJ. Children's access to primary care: Differences by race, income, and insurance status. Pediatrics 97(1):26–32. 1996.

13. Weissman JS, Epstein AM. Falling through the safety net. Baltimore, Maryland: The Johns Hopkins University Press. 1994.

14. Cykert S, Kissling G, Layson R, Hansen C. Health insurance does not guarantee access to primary care: A national study of physicians' acceptance of publicly insured patients. J Gen Intern Med 10(6):345–8. 1995.

15. Lieu TA, Quesenberry CP Jr, Capra AM, et al. Outpatient management practices associated with reduced risk of pediatric asthma hospitalization and emergency department visits. Pediatrics 100(3 Pt 1): 334–41. 1997.

16. Pocock SJ, Smith M, Baghurst P. Environmental lead and children's intelligence: A systematic review of the epidemiological evidence. BMJ 309:1189–97. 1994.

17. Lanphear BP, Weitzman M, Eberly S. Racial differences in urban children's environmental exposures to lead. Am J Public Health 86:1460–63. 1996.

18. Centers for Disease Control and Prevention. Trends in smoking initiation among adolescents and young adults - United States, 1980–1989. MMWR 44(28): 521–5. 1995.

19. Serdula MK, Ivery D, Coates RJ, et al. Do obese children become obese adults? A review of the literature. Prev Med 22:167–77. 1993.

Children's Health ....

Infant Mortality

■ Infant mortality is comprised of deaths that occur before an infant's first birthday. Infant mortality is an important indicator of the health of infants and pregnant women because it is closely related to factors such as maternal health, quality of and access to medical care, socioeconomic conditions, and public health practices. About two-thirds of infant deaths are associated with problems of the infant or the pregnancy, while one-third result from conditions arising after the delivery, often reflecting social or environmental factors (1). The *Healthy People 2000* target is for no more than 7 deaths per 1,000 infants in the United States as a whole, and no more than 11 deaths per 1,000 black infants.

■ Between 1983 and 1995, the infant mortality rate in the United States among infants born to mothers 20 years of age and over declined from 10.3 to 7.1 deaths per 1,000 live births. Reductions in infant mortality were seen in all race and education groups examined, though the decline occurred more steadily in some groups than in others.

■ The infant mortality gap across education levels remained approximately constant during the time period among white and black infants. In every year, infants born to less educated mothers had higher rates of mortality than infants born to more educated mothers, but the disparity was constant or decreased slightly over time. Between 1983 and 1995, among infants born to white mothers, the relative decline in infant mortality was greatest among infants born to women with less than 12 years of education (39 percent) and least among infants of mothers with 12 years of education (26 percent). Among infants born to black women the relative decline in infant mortality ranged from 16 percent among those born to the most

educated mothers to 27 percent among those born to the least educated mothers.

■ In every year black infants remained at higher risk of dying than white infants at every level of mother's education. By 1995 rates among infants born to more educated black mothers were approaching rates seen in the mid-1980's among infants of less educated white mothers.

■ White infants' mortality rates declined more rapidly than those of black infants at each level of mother's education. In 1983, the ratio of black to white infant mortality rates ranged from 1.9 for infants born to the least educated mothers to 2.1 among infants born to the most educated mothers. In 1995 the black-white infant mortality ratio increased to 2.2 for infants born to the least educated mothers to 2.7 among infants born to the most educated mothers.

Reference

1. Centers for Disease Control and Prevention. Poverty and infant mortality. United States, 1988. MMWR 44(49): 922–27. 1995.

Figure 8. Infant mortality rates among infants of mothers 20 years of age and over by mother's education and race: United States, 1983–95

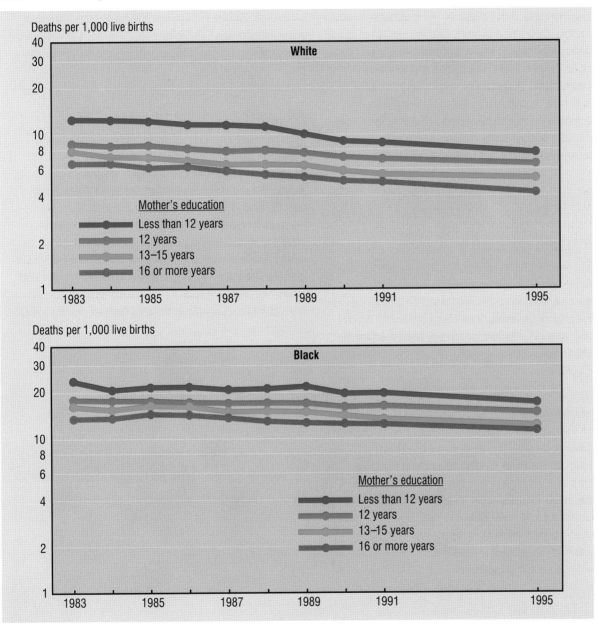

Deaths per 1,000 live births

White

Mother's education
- Less than 12 years
- 12 years
- 13–15 years
- 16 or more years

Deaths per 1,000 live births

Black

Mother's education
- Less than 12 years
- 12 years
- 13–15 years
- 16 or more years

NOTES: 1995 data were calculated on a period basis, while prior years were calculated on a cohort basis; 1995 data used weighting for the first time. See *Health, United States, 1998* Appendix I for an explanation of the differences in the methods.

SOURCE: Centers for Disease Control and Prevention, National Center for Health Statistics, National Linked Files of Live Births and Infant Deaths. See related *Health, United States, 1998*, table 21.

Children's Health ....

Health Status

Infant Mortality

■ During 1995 about seven in every thousand infants died before their first birthday. The likelihood of death in infancy was related to the mother's education; each higher level of maternal education was associated with an improvement in the infant mortality rate. Among live births to mothers 20 years of age and over in 1995, babies born to mothers who did not finish high school were almost 1.9 times as likely to die as those whose mothers graduated from college.

■ Infant mortality rates varied significantly among racial and ethnic groups. Hispanic and Asian or Pacific Islander infants tended to have similar infant mortality rates. Black infants had higher rates. Non-Hispanic white and American Indian or Alaska Native infants had intermediate rates at lower education levels, but rates among non-Hispanic white infants approached Hispanic and Asian or Pacific Islander rates at the highest education levels. The *Healthy People 2000* goal for American Indian or Alaska Native infants is 8.5 deaths per 1,000.

■ Although apparent for all race and ethnic groups, the educational gradient in infant mortality was stronger for white and American Indian or Alaska Native infants than for black, Asian or Pacific Islander, or Hispanic infants. White infants had the steepest gradient; infants born to mothers with fewer than 12 years of education were 2.4 times as likely to die as those born to mothers with 16 or more years of education. Among both Hispanic and Asian or Pacific Islander infants, babies born to the least educated mothers were 1.4 times as likely to die as those born to the most educated mothers.

■ There was diversity in the educational disparities among Hispanic and Asian or Pacific Islander

subgroups. When Hispanic subgroups were examined separately for the 3-year period 1989–91, Cuban and Puerto Rican infants had stronger maternal educational gradients in mortality (the infants of the least educated women were 1.8 or 1.9 times as likely to die as infants of the most educated women) than did Mexican or Central and South American infants (where the disparity was 1.1–1.3). *Healthy People 2000* sets a target for Puerto Rican infants of 8 deaths per 1,000 by the year 2000. During the same time period, among Asian or Pacific Islander infants, Filipino American and Chinese American infants had a relatively lower gradient (infants born to the least educated women were 1.2 to 1.4 times as likely to die as infants of the most educated), while Japanese American (infants of the least educated were 1.7 times as likely to die) and Hawaiian infants (infants of the least educated were over three times as likely to die) had steeper maternal educational gradients.

Figure 9. Infant mortality rates among infants of mothers 20 years of age and over by mother's education, race, and Hispanic origin: United States, 1995

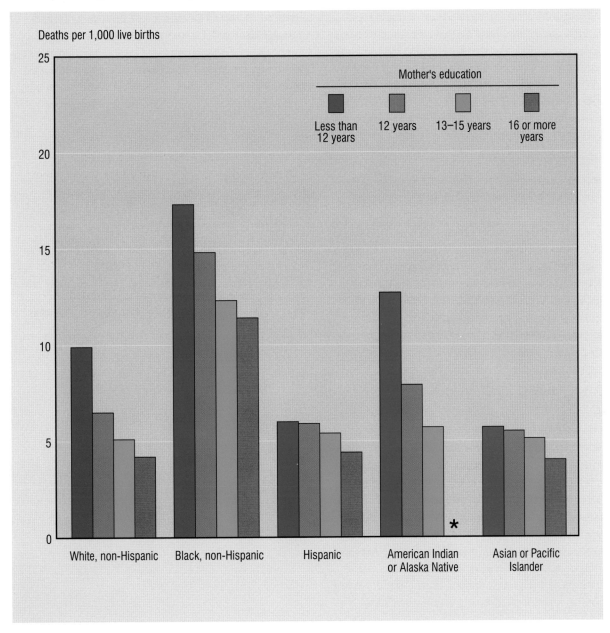

Deaths per 1,000 live births

Mother's education

Less than 12 years | 12 years | 13–15 years | 16 or more years

White, non-Hispanic | Black, non-Hispanic | Hispanic | American Indian or Alaska Native | Asian or Pacific Islander

*The number of infant deaths among American Indian or Alaska Native mothers with 16 or more years of education was too small for stable rate calculation.

SOURCE: Centers for Disease Control and Prevention, National Center for Health Statistics, National Linked File of Live Births and Infant Deaths. See related *Health, United States, 1998*, table 21.

Low Birthweight

■ Low-birthweight infants are born weighing less than 2,500 grams, or about 5.5 pounds. Infants of low birthweight are less likely to survive and have a higher risk of disability if they live. Low birthweight may result from premature birth and/or from insufficient growth for the gestational age. *Healthy People 2000* sets a low-birthweight goal of 5 percent overall, and 9 percent for black infants.

■ Among births to non-Hispanic white, black, and American Indian or Alaska Native mothers 20 years of age and over, greater maternal education was associated with a decreased likelihood of low birthweight. In 1996 the prevalence of low birthweight among births to white mothers with less than 12 years of education was 1.8 times as high as among mothers with at least 16 years of education; among black mothers, the least educated had low birthweight rates 1.5 times those of their counterparts who had 16 or more years of education. For American Indian or Alaska Native infants, low birthweight was 1.2 times as high among births to mothers with less than a high school education as among births to mothers who had at least some college.

■ Overall, births to Hispanic and Asian or Pacific Islander mothers did not show the same kind of trend; no matter what the mother's education level, the infants were equally likely to be low birthweight, and the rates were uniformly low (on average, 6 percent of Hispanic infants and 7 percent of Asian or Pacific Islander infants). When Asian or Pacific Islander subgroups were examined, only Hawaiian mothers had a strong relationship between education and birthweight; other groups did not show a trend. Among Hispanics, less educated Puerto Rican and Cuban

American mothers had higher low birthweight rates, while Mexican and Central and South American mothers had no such gradient. The *Healthy People 2000* target for Puerto Rican infants is 6 percent with low birthweight.

■ There was a greater disparity in low birthweight across race and ethnic groups than by maternal education. Black women were much more likely to have a low-birthweight infant than women of any other background. Over 13 percent of black infants were low birthweight, compared with between 6 and 7 percent of infants for the four other groups. The reasons for this disparity are unclear, but socioeconomic status could not fully account for it; the most educated black women were more likely to have a low-birthweight infant than the least educated women of any other race or ethnic group.

Figure 10. Low-birthweight live births among mothers 20 years of age and over by mother's education, race, and Hispanic origin: United States, 1996

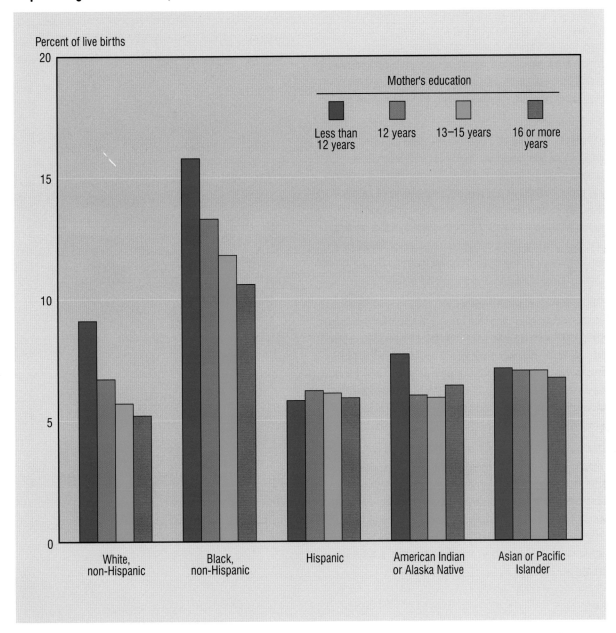

NOTE: Low birthweight refers to an infant weighing less than 2,500 grams at birth.

SOURCES: Centers for Disease Control and Prevention, National Center for Health Statistics, National Vital Statistics System. See related *Health, United States, 1998*, table 12.

Activity Limitation

■ This chart refers to the proportion of children whose usual activities, such as playing and going to school, are limited due to chronic health conditions. Conditions included here have persisted at least 3 months and may include illnesses, such as asthma or diabetes, injuries, or impairments affecting abilities such as vision, hearing, or speech.

■ Overall, the rate of children who are reported to have some kind of limitation in their everyday activities increased slightly between 1984–87 and 1992–95. There was a clear pattern of socioeconomic disparity in each time period, such that children from lower income families were more likely to have some kind of activity limitation. During 1992–95 children in poor families were about 1.9 times as likely to have an activity limitation as children living in higher income households.

■ In every race and ethnic group for every time period, limitation of activity rates increased as income declined. In 1992–95, poor non-Hispanic white children were about 2.2 times as likely, and poor black children twice as likely, to have an activity limitation as white and black children in higher income households. Hispanic children, however, had less of a gradient; the lower income children were only 1.4 times as likely as upper income children to have a limitation.

■ Data suggested that the disparity between the lowest and highest income groups may have increased over time. During 1984–87 children living in poor families were 1.7 times as likely to have a limitation of activity as those in the highest income families, while in 1992–95 poor children were almost twice as likely to have a limitation as wealthier children.

Figure 11. Activity limitation among children under 18 years of age by family income, race, and Hispanic origin: United States, average annual, 1984–87, 1988–91, and 1992–95

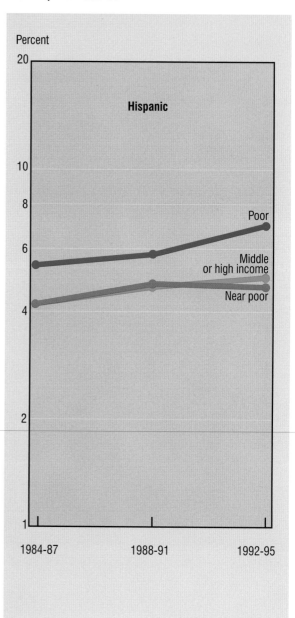

Figure 11. Activity limitation among children under 18 years of age by family income, race, and Hispanic origin: United States, average annual, 1984–87, 1988–91, and 1992–95—Continued

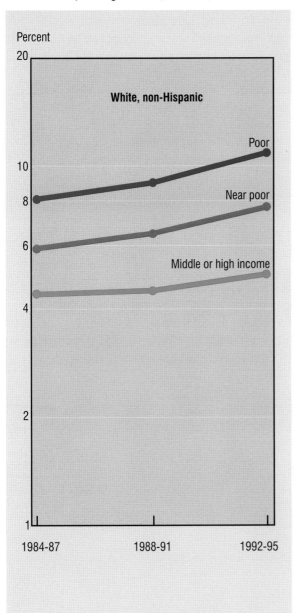

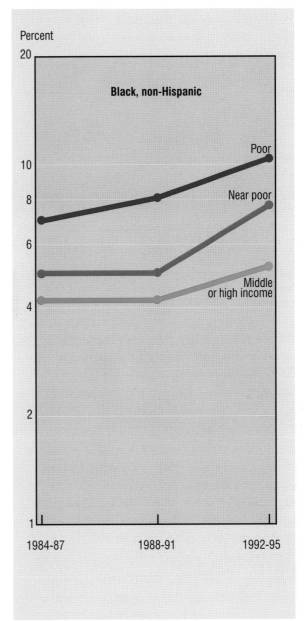

NOTE: See Technical Notes for definitions of activity limitation and family income categories.

SOURCE: Centers for Disease Control and Prevention, National Center for Health Statistics, National Health Interview Survey. See related *Health, United States, 1998*, table 60.

Teenage Childbearing

■ Teenage childbearing often leads to poor economic and social outcomes for teenage parents and their children. Adolescent mothers are unlikely to attain a high level of education, their relationships with the father are highly unstable, and they are far more likely than other women to live in poverty. Children born to teenagers have higher infant mortality rates, and sequelae continue throughout childhood, including higher rates of abuse and neglect and poorer rates of high school completion.

■ Almost one out of five women aged 20–29 in 1995 had a first birth before the age of 20. The likelihood of having had a child as a teenager was much higher among women whose own mothers were less educated. Nearly one out of every three women whose mothers had not completed high school began childbearing as an adolescent. The proportion dropped to fewer than one in five among those whose mothers had completed only high school, to 13 percent of women whose mothers had some college, and to 7 percent of women whose mothers had completed college.

■ In every race and ethnic group analyzed, there was an inverse relationship between the respondent's mother's education level and the proportion of women who had a teenage birth. Women whose mothers had more education were less likely to have become a teenage parent, no matter what their race or ethnic background, although the magnitude of this disparity differed among the race and ethnic groups.

■ The proportion of non-Hispanic white women in their twenties who had their first birth as a teenager declined from more than 1 in 4 among those whose mothers had less than a high school education to less than 1 in 20 among those whose mothers completed college. Among black women, almost one-half of women with the least educated mothers had a teenage birth while about one in seven of those with college-educated mothers had a teenage birth. Hispanic women showed the least disparity; about one-third of women whose mothers were the least educated had a teen birth while one in five daughters of college-educated mothers were teen parents.

■ The family income of women in their twenties at the time of the survey suggested that those who had been teen mothers were much worse off economically than those who were not (data not shown). Forty-three percent of women who began childbearing in adolescence were poor in their twenties, while only 16 percent had high incomes in their twenties. Among women in their twenties who had not been teenage mothers, these figures were almost reversed; 13 percent were below the poverty line at the time of the survey and 40 percent were in high-income families.

Figure 12. Percent of women 20–29 years of age who had a teenage birth, by respondent's mother's education and respondent's race and Hispanic origin: United States, 1995

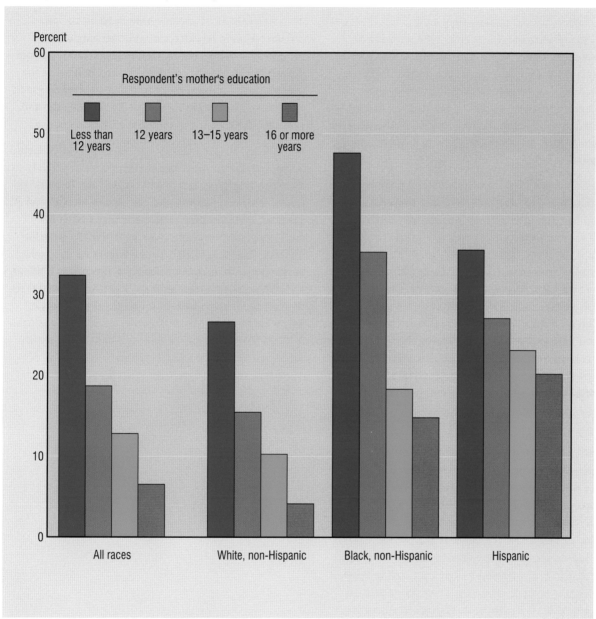

NOTES: Education level is for the infant's maternal grandmother. See Technical Notes for further information.

SOURCE: Centers for Disease Control and Prevention, National Center for Health Statistics, 1995 National Survey of Family Growth.

Risk Factors

Smoking in Pregnancy

■ Infants whose mothers smoke cigarettes during pregnancy are more likely to be born with low birthweight. Other health outcomes associated with maternal smoking include Sudden Infant Death Syndrome (1), pregnancy complications such as placenta previa and abruptio placentae (2), and asthma in childhood (3). The *Healthy People 2000* goal is for no more than 10 percent of mothers to smoke during pregnancy.

■ Data from 1996 birth certificates for mothers 20 years of age and older indicated that smoking cigarettes during pregnancy was strongly associated with socioeconomic status among all racial and ethnic groups. In every race and ethnic group, the more education women had, the less likely they were to report smoking during their pregnancy. Overall, non-Hispanic white mothers (16 percent) and American Indian or Alaska Native mothers (21 percent) were most likely to report smoking during their pregnancies, while black mothers had a somewhat lower rate (12 percent), and Hispanic (4 percent) and Asian or Pacific Islander mothers (3 percent) had the lowest rates of smoking.

■ Non-Hispanic white mothers with less than a high school education were the most likely of any group to smoke during pregnancy. In 1996 nearly one-half of these women reported smoking during pregnancy, compared with only 3 percent of white mothers with 16 or more years of education. Among American Indian or Alaska Native mothers, the percent who smoked during pregnancy decreased from 32 percent among the least educated to 7 percent among those at the highest level of education. Over one-quarter of black mothers with less than 12 years of education smoked, compared with 3 percent among those with 16

or more years of education. Among Hispanic and Asian or Pacific Islander mothers, smoking during pregnancy was rare but an education gradient was still apparent. The proportion varied from 5 percent at the lowest education level to 1 percent at the highest education level for both Asian or Pacific Islander and Hispanic mothers.

■ Among Hispanic subgroups, more educated Puerto Rican and Cuban American mothers were less likely to smoke during pregnancy, but Mexican and Central and South American mothers did not show a strong gradient; their smoking rates were very low at all levels of education. Among Asian or Pacific Islander mothers, data suggested a strong negative relationship between education and smoking for Hawaiian, Filipino, and Japanese American mothers, but Chinese American mothers were very unlikely to smoke at all levels of education.

References

1. Golding J. Sudden infant death syndrome and parental smoking—a literature review. Paediatr Perinat Epidemiol 11(1): 67–77. 1997.

2. Andres RL. The association of cigarette smoking with placenta previa and abruptio placentae. Semin Perinatol 20(2): 154–159. 1996.

3. Oliveti JF. Pre- and perinatal risk factors for asthma in inner city African-American children. Am J Epidemiol 143(6): 570–577. 1996.

Figure 13. Cigarette smoking during pregnancy among mothers 20 years of age and over by mother's education, race, and Hispanic origin: United States, 1996

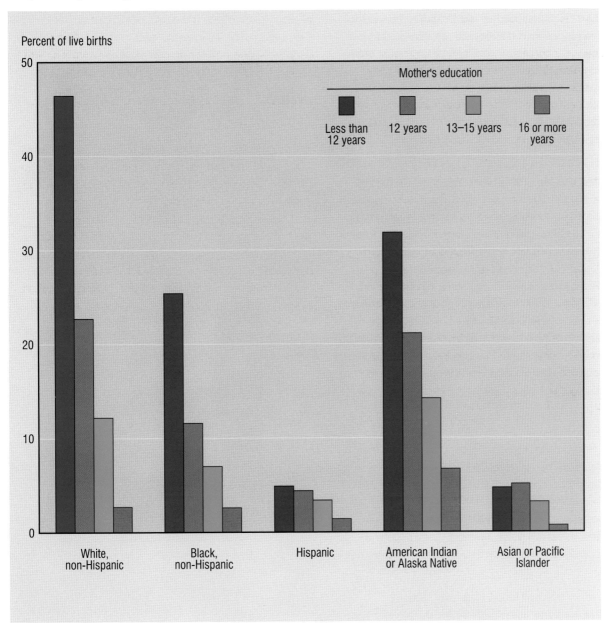

Percent of live births

SOURCE: Centers for Disease Control and Prevention, National Center for Health Statistics, National Vital Statistics System. See related *Health, United States, 1998*, table 10.

Blood Lead

■ Lead is dangerous for small children because it can lead to lowered intelligence (1). Elevated blood lead among children in the United States most often results from residence in an older house that has lead paint, which may flake or peel, causing lead dust to be distributed in the house. Young children may eat paint chips or inadvertently take in lead by tasting dusty objects.

■ Data presented here are drawn from the Third National Health and Nutrition Examination Survey. In general, children 1 to 5 years of age who lived in families with lower socioeconomic status had a greater likelihood of having a high blood lead level (defined as a level of blood lead at or above 10 μg/dL). About 12 percent of children living in poor families had an elevated lead level, compared with about 2 percent of children in high-income families. There was a clear income-related gradient in the prevalence of high blood lead levels; each increase in family income level was associated with a decline in the proportion of children with elevated blood lead.

■ The income-associated gradient in the prevalence of high blood lead levels was seen in each of the race and ethnic groups examined. The gradient was strongest for non-Hispanic black children; 22 percent of black children in families below poverty had an elevated blood lead level, compared with only 6 percent in high-income families.

■ In each income group, black children were more likely than children of other race and ethnic groups to have an elevated blood lead level. Among children living in households below the poverty line, black children were 2.7 times as likely as non-Hispanic white children and 3.4 times as likely as Mexican American children to have an elevated blood lead level.

Reference

1. Pocock SJ, Smith M, Baghurst P. Environmental lead and children's intelligence: A systematic review of the epidemiological evidence. BMJ 309:1189–97. 1994.

Figure 14. Elevated blood lead among children 1–5 years of age by family income, race, and Hispanic origin: United States, average annual 1988–94

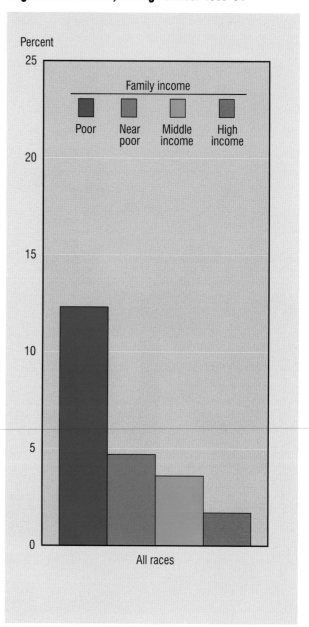

Figure 14. Elevated blood lead among children 1–5 years of age by family income, race, and Hispanic origin: United States, average annual 1988–94—Continued

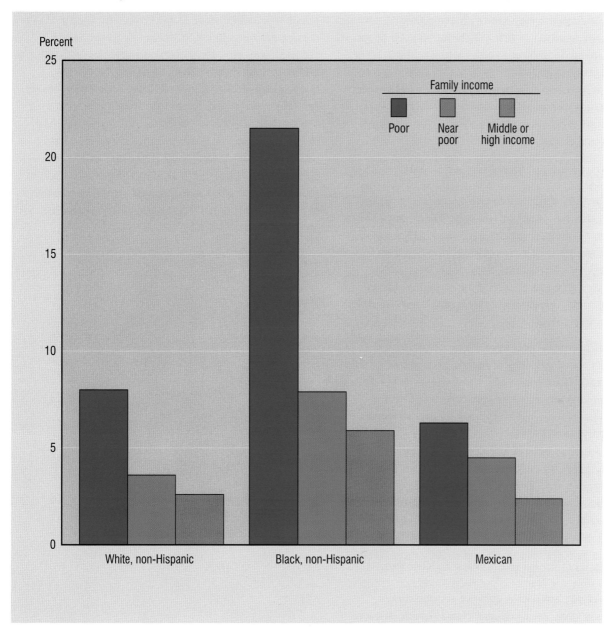

NOTES: Elevated blood lead was defined as having at least 10 micrograms of lead per deciliter of blood. See Technical Notes for definition of family income categories.

SOURCE: Centers for Disease Control and Prevention, National Center for Health Statistics, Third National Health and Nutrition Examination Survey.

Cigarette Smoking

■ Adolescence is the most common time to take up cigarette smoking, which kills about 400,000 people in the United States every year. Each day, about 3,000 teenagers become daily smokers (1). Smoking may lead to heart disease, lung or other forms of cancer, bronchitis and emphysema (also known as chronic obstructive pulmonary disease), and other health problems. The *Healthy People 2000* goal is for no more than 6 percent of adolescents 12–17 to have smoked in the past month.

■ In 1992 about one in five adolescents age 12–17 years said they were current cigarette smokers. When all race and ethnic groups were examined together, there was no clear socioeconomic trend in smoking: teenagers in low-income households were about equally likely to smoke as those in higher income households. Boys and girls were also about equally likely to smoke.

■ However, a breakdown by race and ethnicity demonstrated that socioeconomic gradients in smoking did exist. In each race and ethnic group, the prevalence of smoking among adolescent boys was lower in households with higher incomes. In every income category, non-Hispanic white boys had higher rates of smoking than boys of any other race or ethnic background. Among teenagers in poor families, white teen boys were 2.8 times as likely as black teen boys to smoke and 1.5 times as likely as Hispanic teen boys. Among adolescents in higher income households, white teen males were over five times as likely to smoke as black teen males and slightly more likely than Hispanic teen males.

■ Among adolescent girls the socioeconomic patterns were less consistent. Non-Hispanic white teen girls had a similar trend to the boys, with higher income girls less likely to smoke. However, in Hispanic teen girls the pattern was reversed with higher income girls more likely to smoke. Among black teen girls there appeared to be little difference in smoking rates by income group. Smoking rates among black adolescents were uniformly lower than the rates in any other race or ethnic group. Almost 1 in 3 poor white, but fewer than 1 in 12 poor black adolescent girls, was a smoker in 1992. About one in five middle- or high-income white and Hispanic teen girls smoked, but only 8 percent of black teen girls in this income group smoked.

Reference

1. Centers for Disease Control and Prevention. The great American smokeout–November 21, 1996. MMWR 45(44): 961. 1996.

Figure 15. Cigarette smoking among adolescents 12–17 years of age by family income, race, and Hispanic origin: United States, 1992

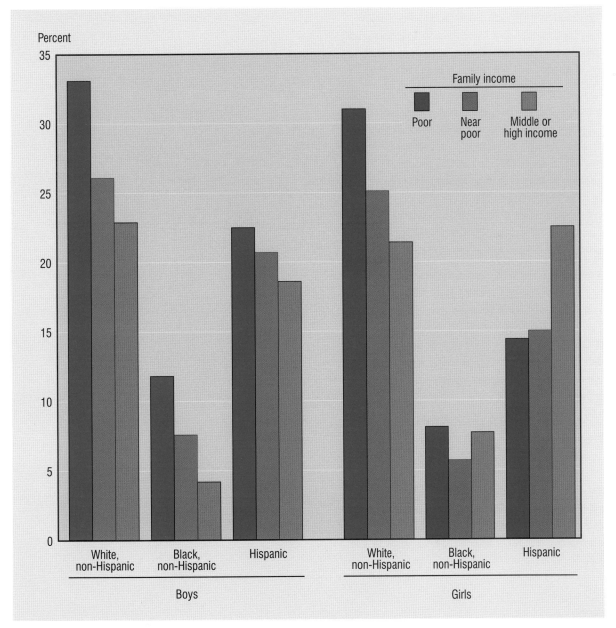

NOTES: Smoking is defined as any smoking in the past month. Percents are age adjusted. See Technical notes for definition of family income categories and age adjustment procedure.

SOURCE: Centers for Disease Control and Prevention, National Center for Health Statistics, National Health Interview Survey, Youth Risk Behavior Survey, 1992.

Overweight

■ Overweight in adolescence is associated with overweight in adulthood. Excessive weight for height is a risk factor for heart disease, several forms of cancer, diabetes, and other health problems (1).

■ Data from the third National Health and Nutrition Examination Survey suggested that among adolescents 12–17 years of age during 1988–94, socioeconomic status was closely related to the prevalence of overweight in some race and ethnic groups. Overall, adolescents in higher income households were less likely to be overweight than those in poorer households. Among adolescents in middle- or high-income households, 9 percent were overweight, compared with 17 percent in poor households.

■ Despite the apparent socioeconomic gradient in overweight, only non-Hispanic white adolescents exhibited an association between overweight and socioeconomic status. Poor white adolescents were about 2.6 times as likely to be overweight as those in middle- or high-income families, and adolescents with near-poor family income had an intermediate prevalence.

■ Among black and Mexican-origin adolescents, there was no such trend. Adolescents in these groups had lower rates of overweight if they were poor than if they were in middle- or high-income households. The highest rates of overweight were found among Mexican American adolescents whose families were middle- or high-income; about one in five of these teens were overweight. The lowest rates were in middle- or high-income white teens, 7 percent of whom were overweight.

Reference

1. Troiano RP, Flegal KM, Kuczmarski RJ, Campbell SM, Johnson CL. Overweight prevalence and trends for children and adolescents. The National Health and Nutrition Examination Surveys, 1963 to 1991. Arch Pediatr Adolesc Med 149(10):1085–91. 1995.

Figure 16. Overweight among adolescents 12–17 years of age by family income, race, and Hispanic origin: United States, average annual 1988–94

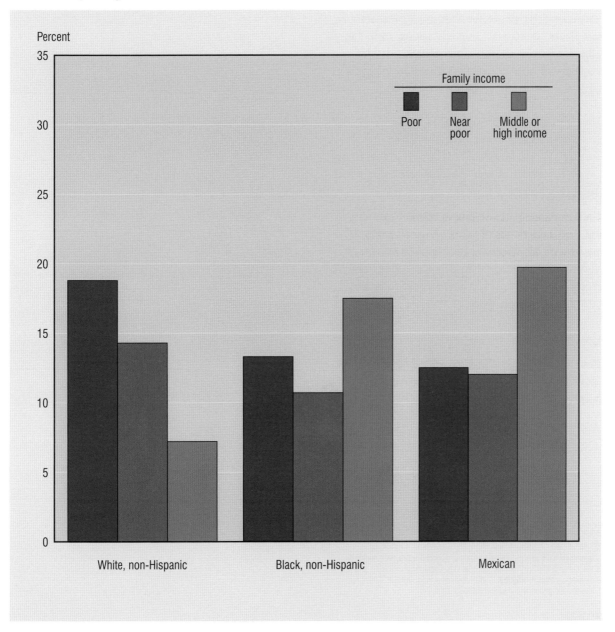

NOTES: Overweight was defined for adolescents by the sex-specific 95th percentile of weight for height and age in the National Health Examination Survey, 1966–70. Percents are age adjusted. See Technical Notes for definition of family income categories, age adjustment, and for more information on classifying overweight.

SOURCE: Centers for Disease Control and Prevention, National Center for Health Statistics, Third National Health and Nutrition Examination Survey. See related *Health, United States, 1998*, table 71.

Sedentary Lifestyle

■   Sedentary lifestyle, or the lack of physical activity, is a risk factor for several chronic diseases, including heart disease, stroke, diabetes, and certain forms of cancer. Physical activity has been shown to improve mental health and is important for the health of muscles, bones and joints. Lack of physical activity contributes to obesity. Participation in all forms of physical activity declines dramatically during adolescence (1). *Healthy People 2000* sets a goal of no more than 15 percent of individuals 6 years of age and over to have a sedentary lifestyle.

■   Data from the Youth Risk Behavioral Survey showed that females 12–17 years of age in lower income households were more likely to be sedentary than those in higher-income households. Among male adolescents, there was less socioeconomic variation. Poor females were over twice as likely as high-income females to be sedentary, while poor males were 1.4 times as likely as high-income males to be sedentary.

■   In every income group, girls were more likely than boys to say they were sedentary during the past week. However, the differences between boys and girls also varied with socioeconomic status. The sex differential appeared primarily among lower income youth; poor and near-poor girls were 1.7–1.8 times as likely to be sedentary as poor or near-poor boys, while girls and boys in high-income families had nearly equal rates of inactivity.

Reference

1. U.S. Department of Health and Human Services. Physical activity and health: A report of the Surgeon General. Atlanta, Georgia: U.S. Department of Health and Human Services, Centers for Disease Control and Prevention, National Center for Chronic Disease Prevention and Health Promotion. 1996.

Figure 17. Sedentary lifestyle among adolescents 12–17 years of age by family income and sex: United States, 1992

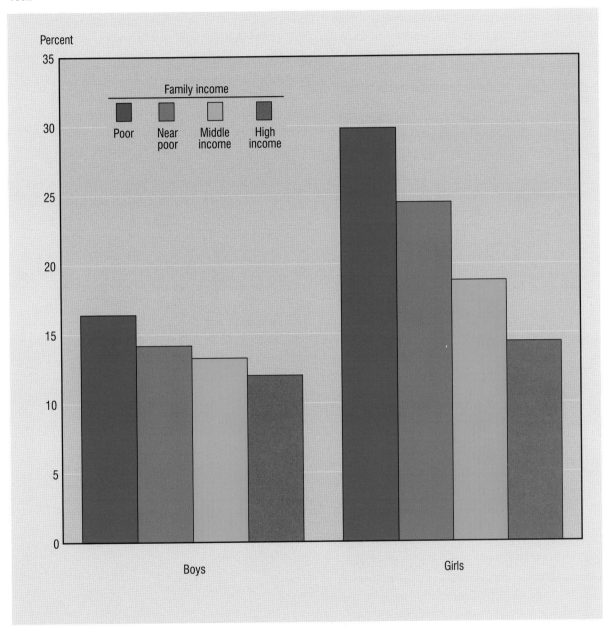

NOTES: Percents are age adjusted. See Technical Notes for definition of family income categories, sedentary lifestyle, and age adjustment procedure.

SOURCE: Centers for Disease Control and Prevention, National Center for Health Statistics, National Health Interview Survey, Youth Risk Behavior Survey, 1992.

Prenatal Care

■ Pregnant women are encouraged to obtain regular prenatal care beginning in the first trimester of pregnancy to help ensure a healthy pregnancy and birth. The *Healthy People 2000* goal is for 90 percent of pregnant women to obtain first-trimester prenatal care. Expansion of the Medicaid program to cover pregnant women with incomes up to 185 percent of poverty improved access to prenatal care in some States (1).

■ After declining slightly during the 1980's, prenatal care attendance rates increased steadily if slowly during the 1990's.

■ Prenatal care utilization is directly associated with education level. Pregnant women who have more education are more likely to start prenatal care early and to have more visits. Throughout the period 1980–96, rates of early prenatal care use among mothers at least 20 years of age were higher among those with more education.

■ Among white mothers, there was little change in rates of prenatal care use between 1980 and 1996 except among mothers with fewer than 13 years of education; prenatal care use among white mothers who had not finished high school declined until 1990, when it began to rise again and in 1994 attained the level achieved in 1980. White mothers with 12 years of education evidenced a similar though more moderate pattern. Those with 16 or more years of education had rates that rose throughout the period, resulting in a 3-percent increase in prenatal care use by 1995; among mothers with some college, rates changed relatively little during the time period with less than a 2 percent increase in usage overall. In both 1980 and 1996 white mothers with at least 16 years of education were 1.4 times as likely to have early prenatal care as those with fewer than 12 years of education.

■ Black mothers' rates in each education group tended to be lower than the rates among white mothers, but their early prenatal attendance rates increased more rapidly in the 1990's than white mothers' rates. Particularly among those without any college education, rates declined until 1990 and then increased again to surpass the 1980 levels. By 1989 only about one-half of black mothers with fewer than 12 years of education received first-trimester prenatal care. However, between 1990 and 1996 these mothers' rates rose rapidly, so that about 61 percent received early prenatal care in 1996. Similar changes were seen among mothers with 12 years of education, while those with 13–15 and 16 or more years of education experienced slower increases. In 1996 black mothers with 16 or more years of education were about 1.4 times as likely to receive early prenatal care as those with fewer than 12 years of education.

Reference

1. Ray WA. Effect of Medicaid expansions on preterm birth. Am J Prev Med 13(4): 292–7. 1997.

Figure 18. Prenatal care use in the first trimester among mothers 20 years of age and over by mother's education and race: United States, 1980–96

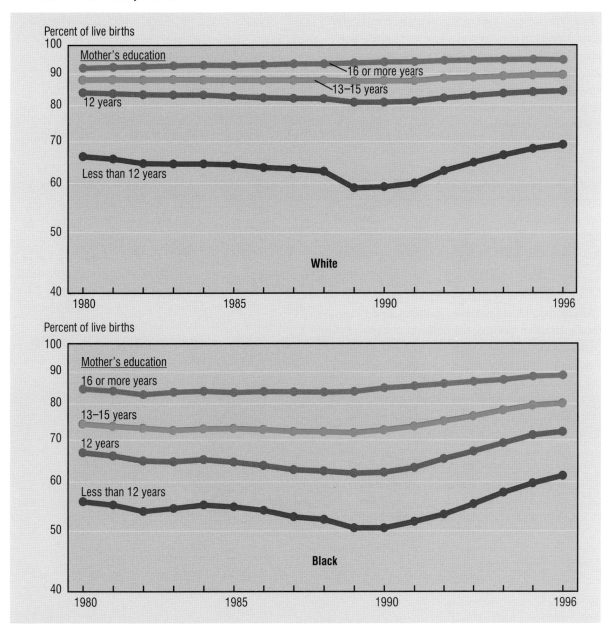

SOURCES: Centers for Disease Control and Prevention, National Center for Health Statistics, National Vital Statistics System. See related *Health, United States, 1998*, table 6.

Health Care

Prenatal Care

■ In 1996, 82 percent of mothers received early (first trimester) prenatal care, though there was substantial variation among racial and ethnic groups. Japanese and Cuban American mothers were the most likely to obtain early prenatal care in 1996 (89 percent), while American Indian or Alaska Native mothers were the least likely (68 percent).

■ In 1996 there was a clear socioeconomic gradient among mothers 20 years of age and over in use of early prenatal care. In every race and ethnic group, mothers with more education were more likely to receive early prenatal care; overall, the most educated mothers (those with at least 16 years of education) were 1.4 times as likely to receive early prenatal care as the least educated mothers (those with fewer than 12 years of education).

■ Among non-Hispanic white, Hispanic, and Asian or Pacific Islander mothers, the most educated were 1.3 times as likely to have early prenatal care as the least educated. The most educated black and American Indian or Alaska Native mothers were 1.5 times as likely to receive early care as the least educated. White mothers with at least 13 years of education have achieved the *Healthy People 2000* goal of 90 percent or more first trimester prenatal care attendance; rates were above 87 percent among the most educated mothers of all other racial and ethnic groups, but substantially lower among less educated mothers.

Figure 19. Prenatal care use in the first trimester among mothers 20 years of age and over by mother's education, race, and Hispanic origin: United States, 1996

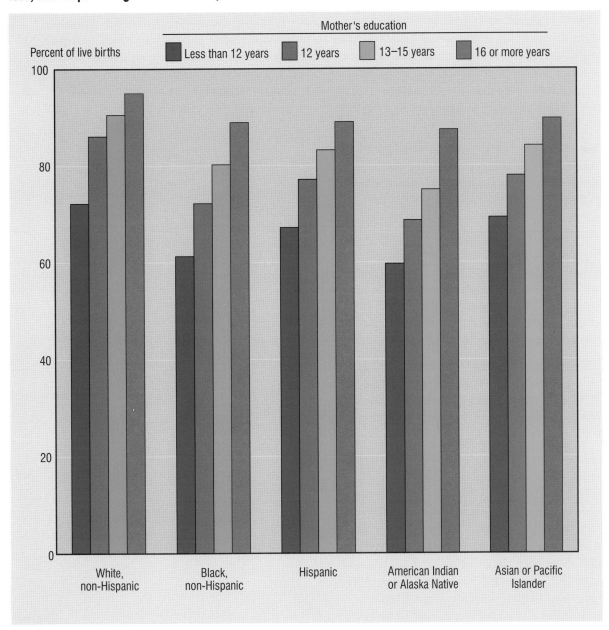

SOURCE: Centers for Disease Control and Prevention, National Center for Health Statistics, National Vital Statistics System. See related *Health, United States, 1998*, table 6.

Children's Health ....

Health Insurance

■ Health insurance coverage is an important component of financial access to health care. Children without health insurance coverage are less likely to have a usual source of health care and are more likely to delay or not receive care when it is needed (1). The *Healthy People 2000* goal is for no one to be without health insurance.

■ In 1995, 14 percent of children under age 18 had no health insurance coverage during the month prior to interview in the National Health Interview Survey, while 21 percent had Medicaid or public assistance coverage, and 66 percent had private coverage (see *Health, United States, 1998*, table 133). Between 1989 and 1995 the proportion of children covered by Medicaid increased by more than 60 percent, primarily due to State expansions in Medicaid eligibility for children, while the proportion of children with private coverage declined by 8 percent, and the percent with no coverage remained fairly stable.

■ The percent of children who are uninsured is strongly associated with family income. Overall, in 1994–95 poor and near-poor children were more than five times as likely as those with high family income to be uninsured.

■ Family income is a strong predictor of insurance coverage, regardless of race and ethnicity. Poor white children were six times as likely as those with high incomes to be uninsured. Among black and Hispanic children those with near-poor family income were somewhat more likely to be uninsured than poor children. Near-poor black children were 3.2 times as likely as high- income black children to be uninsured and near-poor Hispanic children were 4.5 times as likely as high-income Hispanic children to be uninsured.

■ Poor Hispanic children were twice as likely as poor black children to be uninsured and near-poor Hispanic children were almost 80 percent more likely than near-poor black children to be uninsured, due in large part to lower rates of Medicaid coverage among Hispanic than black children.

Reference

1. Simpson G, Bloom B, Cohen RA, Parsons PE. Access to health care. Part 1: Children. National Center for Health Statistics. Vital Health Stat 10(196). 1997.

Figure 20. Percent of children under 18 years of age with no health insurance coverage by family income, race, and Hispanic origin: United States, average annual 1994–95

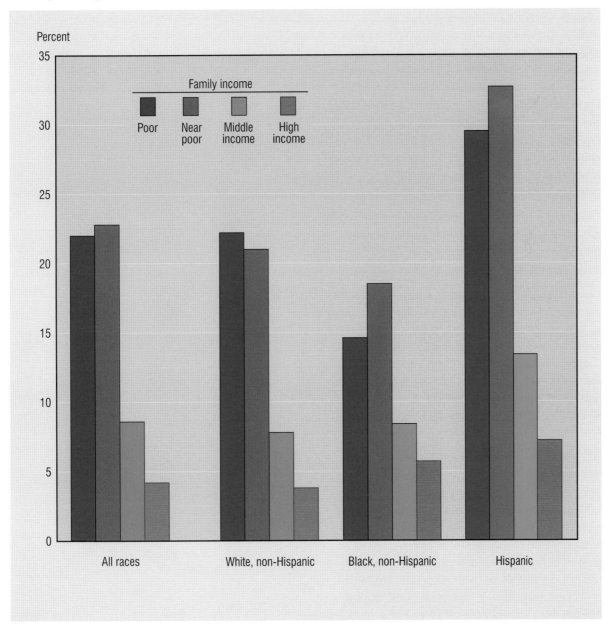

Percent

Family income

Poor　Near poor　Middle income　High income

All races　White, non-Hispanic　Black, non-Hispanic　Hispanic

NOTE: See Technical Notes for definitions of the uninsured and family income categories.

SOURCE: Centers for Disease Control and Prevention, National Center for Health Statistics, National Health Interview Survey. See related *Health, United States, 1998*, table 133.

Children's Health

Vaccinations

■ Timely vaccination protects children from life-threatening and disabling diseases. In 1996 over three-quarters (77 percent) of children ages 19–35 months received the combined series of recommended vaccines consisting of 4 doses of diphtheria, tetanus, and pertussis (DTP) vaccine, 3 doses of polio vaccine, 1 dose of measles-containing vaccine, and 3 doses of *Haemophilus influenzae* type b (Hib) vaccine. The *Healthy People 2000* goal is for 90 percent of children under 2 years of age to have received the recommended immunization series.

■ Children with family incomes below the poverty level were less likely to receive the combined series than children with family incomes at or above the poverty level (69 percent compared with 80 percent).

■ Non-Hispanic white, black, and Hispanic children whose families were not poor were slightly more likely to be fully vaccinated than those in poor families. Poor white, black, and Hispanic children had similar levels of vaccine coverage, with 68–70 percent having a full series of vaccines. Among those in families above the poverty line, non-Hispanic white children were slightly more likely to be fully vaccinated than Hispanic children; black children had an intermediate level of vaccination.

■ In 1996 about 92 percent of children living in families at or above the poverty level were fully vaccinated with polio, Hib, and a measles-containing vaccine (data not shown). About 88 percent of poor children were vaccinated for these diseases. About 84 percent of children in nonpoor families were fully vaccinated for DTP (4 or more doses) and Hepatitis B (3 or more doses). Among children in poor families, 73 percent were vaccinated for DTP and 78 percent for Hepatitis B.

Figure 21. Vaccinations among children 19–35 months of age by poverty status, race, and Hispanic origin: United States, 1996

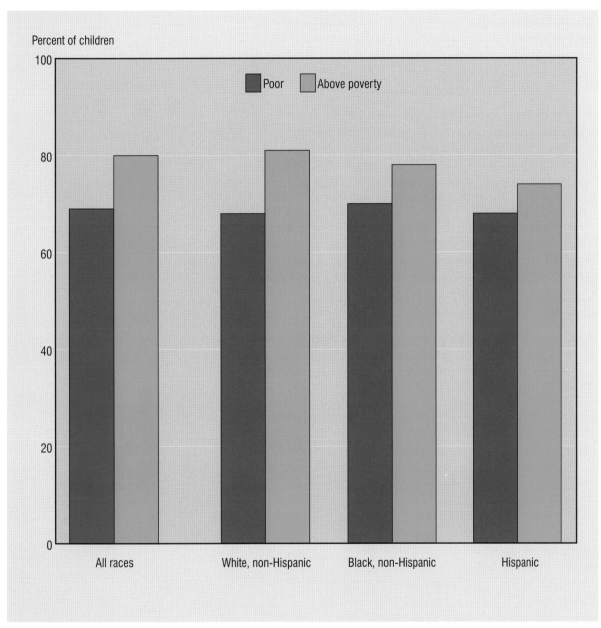

Percent of children

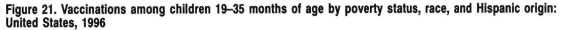

■ Poor ■ Above poverty

All races | White, non-Hispanic | Black, non-Hispanic | Hispanic

NOTES: Vaccinations included in the full series are 4 doses of diphtheria-tetanus-pertussis (DTP) vaccine, 3 doses of polio vaccine, 1 dose of a measles-containing vaccine, and 3 doses of *Haemophilus influenzae* type b (Hib) vaccine. See Technical Notes for definition of poverty status.

SOURCE: Centers for Disease Control and Prevention, National Center for Health Statistics and National Immunization Program, National Immunization Survey. See related *Health, United States, 1998*, table 52.

No Physician Contact

■ All children under age 6 should have at least one physician visit each year to assess the child's growth and development and to ensure that vaccinations are up to date. The proportion of young children who have visited a physician at least once in the previous year varies with family income and health insurance coverage.

■ In 1994–95 the percent of young children without a recent physician visit declined with increasing income. Near poor and poor children were 2.5–2.7 times as likely to lack a recent physician visit as high-income children. Eleven percent of poor children and 10 percent of near-poor children lacked a physician visit within the past year compared with 4 percent of high-income children.

■ Within each income group the percent of young children without a recent physician visit did not vary by race and ethnicity. In each of the three race and ethnic groups shown, the percent of young children without a recent physician visit declined with increasing income and 11 percent of poor children within each group did not have a recent physician visit.

■ Within each income group the percent without a recent visit was greater for uninsured than insured children. Poor children without health insurance coverage were 2.8 times as likely to lack a recent physician visit as poor children with health insurance.

■ Among uninsured children the percent without a recent visit ranged from 12 percent for those with middle or high incomes to 23 percent for poor children. Lacking a recent physician visit was less common among insured children at each income level and ranged from 5 percent of those with middle or high incomes to 8–9 percent of the poor and near poor.

Figure 22. Percent of children under 6 years of age with no physician contact during the past year by family income, health insurance status, race, and Hispanic origin: United States, average annual 1994–95

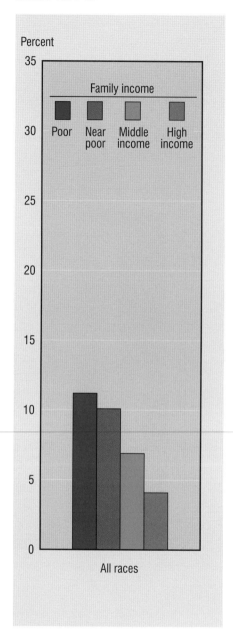

Figure 22. Percent of children under 6 years of age with no physician contact during the past year by family income, health insurance status, race, and Hispanic origin: United States, average annual 1994–95—Continued

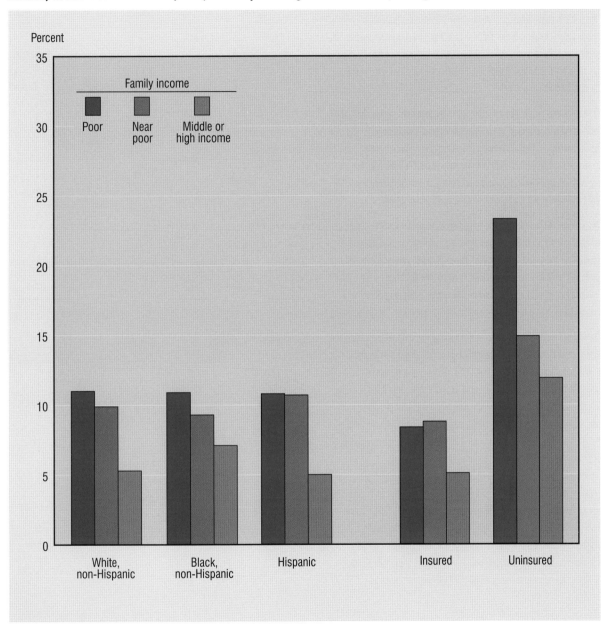

NOTES: See Technical Notes for definitions of the uninsured and family income categories.
SOURCE: Centers for Disease Control and Prevention, National Center for Health Statistics, National Health Interview Survey. See related *Health, United States, 1998*, table 78.

Ambulatory Care

■ In 1995 ambulatory care utilization among children who resided in areas with a median income of $40,000 or more was 65–75 percent higher than for children who resided in areas with a median income below $30,000.

■ There was a particularly strong income gradient in the use of ambulatory care in physician offices. Children who resided in the highest-income areas had more than twice as many visits as those residing in areas with a median income of less than $20,000 (339 and 145 visits per 100 children, respectively).

■ In contrast to physician offices, the use of ambulatory care in hospital settings (emergency departments and outpatient departments) was almost 50 percent higher for children residing in the lowest-income areas (median income below $20,000) than for those in the highest income areas (79 and 54 visits per 100 children, respectively).

■ The distribution of the place of ambulatory care visits for children varies substantially by median income of the patient's area of residence. In 1995, 22 percent of visits by children residing in the lowest income areas were to hospital emergency departments, compared with only 8 percent of visits by children in the highest income areas. Hospital outpatient departments accounted for 13 percent of visits by children residing in the lowest income areas and only 6 percent of visits by children in the highest income areas. In contrast, 86 percent of visits by children in the highest income areas took place in physician offices while 65 percent of visits by children residing in the lowest income areas occurred in physician offices.

Figure 23. Ambulatory care visits among children under 18 years of age by median household income in ZIP Code of residence and place of visit: United States, 1995

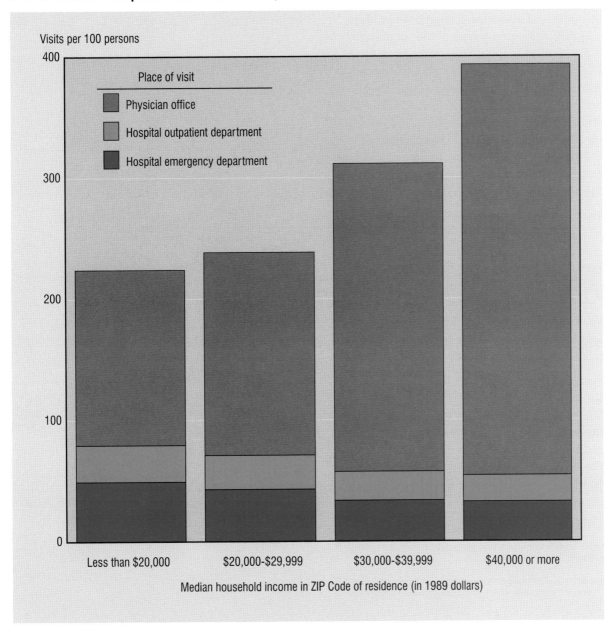

NOTES: Median income is for persons who resided in the ZIP Code area in 1990. See Technical Notes for methods.

SOURCE: Centers for Disease Control and Prevention, National Center for Health Statistics, 1995 National Ambulatory Medical Care Survey and 1995 National Hospital Ambulatory Medical Care Survey. Bureau of the Census, 1990 decennial Census.

Children's Health

Asthma Hospitalization

■   Access to and utilization of appropriate medical care can prevent severe episodes of asthma in many cases. Hospitalization for asthma may indicate that the child has not had adequate outpatient management for the disease. Research suggests that asthma, which is the most common chronic disease in childhood, may be increasing in the United States (1,2). The *Healthy People 2000* goal is for no more than 2.25 asthma hospitalizations per 1,000 population for children 0–14 years of age. White, but not black, children in each socioeconomic group attained the goal by 1989–91.

■   Data presented here were for hospitalizations in 1989–91 and were categorized by the median family income in the child's ZIP Code in 1990. There was an inverse relationship between median income and hospital admission rates for asthma among children 1–14 years of age. Children living in communities with a median family income below $20,000 were 2.4 times as likely to be hospitalized with asthma as those living in neighborhoods with an income of at least $40,000.

■   Asthma hospitalization rates were higher among black children than among white children. Black children had a rate 3.3 times that of white children, and the hospitalization rates of black children were higher than those of white children in each neighborhood income group. Racial disparities were similar within neighborhood income groups.

References

1. Farber HJ. Trends in asthma prevalence: The Bogalusa heart study. Ann Allergy Asthma Immunol 78(3): 265–69. 1997.

2. Centers for Disease Control and Prevention. Asthma mortality and hospitalization among children and young adults—United States, 1980–1993. MMWR 45(17): 350–3. 1996.

Figure 24. Asthma hospitalization rates among children 1–14 years of age by median household income in ZIP Code of residence and race: United States, average annual 1989–91

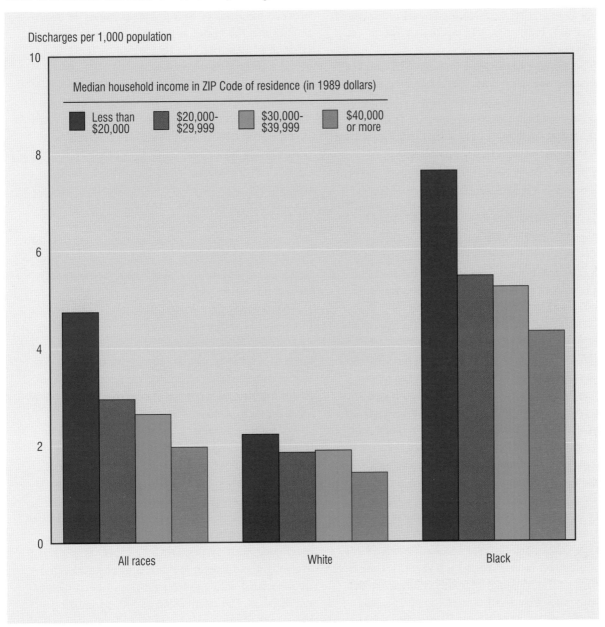

Discharges per 1,000 population

Median household income in ZIP Code of residence (in 1989 dollars)

- Less than $20,000
- $20,000–$29,999
- $30,000–$39,999
- $40,000 or more

All races   White   Black

NOTE: See Technical Notes for methods.

SOURCE: Centers for Disease Control and Prevention, National Center for Health Statistics, National Hospital Discharge Survey; Bureau of the Census, 1990 decennial Census.

Adults' Health

This section describes the relationship between socioeconomic status (SES) and adult health. Using national data from several sources, the figures in this section show this relationship for several indicators of health status, health risk, and health care access and utilization.

The negative relationship between SES and health is perhaps made most evident by examining differences in death rates and life expectancy. As far back as the mid-19th century, vital records from Great Britain indicated that death rates were higher and average age at death lower for men in trade and laboring occupations than for men in the professional class (1). Several of the factors, such as grossly inadequate housing, poor sanitation, and insufficient nutrition, that contributed to SES differences in health a century ago no longer contribute substantially to mortality today; and yet, persons of lower SES still experience higher death rates and lower life expectancy. Furthermore, there is evidence that socioeconomic disparities in death rates have widened since 1960 (2).

Throughout this century, average life expectancy for all persons in the United States has been increasing (*Health, United States, 1998*, table 29), but data show that during 1979–89, 45-year-olds with the highest incomes could expect to live 3 to 7 years longer than those with the lowest incomes (figure 25). Figure 26 shows that the advantage experienced by those with higher social position is evident in death rates for the major categories of natural causes (chronic and communicable diseases) and injuries.

Deaths due to chronic disease now account for nearly three-fourths of all deaths to persons 25–64 years of age. Considered together, cardiovascular diseases, cancer, and diabetes account for over $300 billion in direct medical costs each year (3). Data from the National Longitudinal Mortality Study show that mortality rates from heart disease (figure 27), lung cancer (figure 28), and diabetes (figure 29) increased as family income decreased, indicating that much of the burden of chronic disease is disproportionately concentrated among persons with fewer resources.

These discrepancies tended to be larger for young and middle-aged adults than for the elderly.

The consistency of the inverse relationship between measures of SES and most causes of death implies that the health of persons of lower social position is more likely to be affected by these same diseases or injuries while they remain alive. In addition, the greater susceptibility associated with lower SES implies a greater likelihood of having multiple health conditions adversely affecting overall health status. Global health assessments, such as a person rating his or her health as "poor," "fair," "good," or "excellent," have been shown to be reliable indicators of a person's health status as well as being an independent risk factor for mortality (4,5). Figure 32 shows the strong relationship between self-reported health and family income; regardless of gender, race, or ethnicity, the percent reporting their health as only "fair" or "poor" increases as family income decreases.

Chronically poor health often results in a decline in a person's ability to perform their usual activities; it may prevent them from holding a job or limit the kinds of work they can do, affect their ability to do routine chores inside or outside the home, or, when health impairment is severe, render them incapable of handling their personal care needs (6,7). Figure 33 shows a strong inverse association between income level and health-related activity limitation among working-age adults, while figure 34 demonstrates a similar association for difficulty performing personal care activities among the elderly.

Many chronic diseases have common risk factors. For example, smoking increases a person's risk of developing heart disease and lung cancer while being overweight and having low levels of physical activity are associated with an increased risk of heart disease and diabetes. The relationship of SES to smoking, prevalence of overweight, and lack of physical activity are described in figures 35–36 and 38–40. The decline in cigarette smoking among U.S. adults since the publication of the first Surgeon General's report on smoking in 1964 has been one of the major success stories of public health (8). However, figure 35 shows that the decline in smoking has been disproportionately concentrated among the more educated, and figure 36 shows the prevalence of smoking among lower income persons remains higher than among middle- and high-income persons regardless of gender, race, or ethnicity.

In contrast to smoking, the prevalence of overweight in the United States is increasing among adults and children (9,10). A consistent inverse relationship between overweight and SES exists for women, but not for men, and the gradient is strongest for non-Hispanic white women (figures 38–39). Overweight contributes to diabetes (11) and to hypertension (12), health conditions that are also major risk factors for heart disease and stroke. Like overweight, hypertension is strongly related to SES among women, but not men (figure 41). Lack of physical activity, however, increases sharply as family income decreases within each sex, race, and ethnic group examined (figure 40).

The reasons why lower SES groups experience higher morbidity and mortality are complex. Established risk factors for chronic diseases, such as smoking, being overweight, and low physical activity levels that tend to increase as SES declines account for part of the observed relationship between SES and health. However, many studies have found that an elevated risk of heart disease among lower SES groups remains even after adjustment for the known major behavioral risk factors, such as smoking, obesity, and hypertension (13). This suggests that the relationship between SES and chronic disease mortality may not be fully explained by the differential distribution of health-related behaviors. In addition, as figure 26 demonstrates, the SES gradients in mortality from communicable diseases and injuries are larger, relatively, than that for chronic disease mortality, indicating that environmental and social exposures may be even more unequally distributed than the behavioral risk factors for chronic diseases. For example,

figure 42 shows a strong income gradient in elevated blood lead level among adult men that likely results from differential occupational and environmental exposures.

The association between socioeconomic status and the health status of adults may also be explained in part by reduced access to health care among those with lower socioeconomic status. Figures 43–48 provide national data on the relationship between income and a selected set of indicators of access to health care and health care utilization. Access to health care may be defined as "the attainment of timely, sufficient, and appropriate health care of adequate quality such that health outcomes are maximized" (14). Having adequate health insurance coverage is key to assuring access to health care. However, nonfinancial factors such as race, ethnicity, language, culture, education, geographic isolation, and provider availability also have been shown to affect access to care (14).

Almost all U.S. adults age 65 and over have Medicare coverage. About three-quarters of adults 18–64 years of age have private health insurance coverage, most commonly through an employer-sponsored health insurance plan. However, in 1994–95 almost one-fifth of adults under age 65 lacked coverage and the proportion uninsured rose sharply as income declined (figure 43). Reasons for lacking employer-sponsored coverage include not being offered health insurance through work or not being able to afford the coverage offered, losing a job or changing employers, or losing coverage through divorce or the death of a spouse. Persons employed in small firms are less likely to be offered coverage than those in large firms and part-time workers are less likely to be offered coverage than full-time workers. Establishments with predominantly low-wage workers are also less likely to offer coverage than establishments where a majority of employees earn at least $10,000 per year (15). Even those with health insurance may have problems accessing health care for financial reasons. Insurance plans may exclude coverage for certain types of care or require substantial out-of-pocket spending through deductibles and copayments.

Medicaid provides coverage to eligible needy persons, but eligibility varies from State to State and is undergoing major changes with the implementation of welfare reform. Those eligible for Medicaid have included families with children receiving Aid to Families with Dependent Children (AFDC), pregnant women and young children in low-income families, the aged, blind, and disabled receiving assistance under Supplemental Security Income (SSI), and the medically needy (persons who become poor due to illness). The Medicaid eligibility criteria have resulted in greater Medicaid coverage and lower proportions uninsured among poor women than poor men (figure 43). In addition to meeting Medicaid eligibility requirements, individuals must know about the program, complete necessary forms, and provide required documentation to gain access to benefits. These requirements may present difficult barriers to some persons who are eligible for Medicaid. Among the poor and near poor, Hispanic adults are more likely to be uninsured than non-Hispanic white or black adults (figure 43). Immigration status and language and cultural barriers as well as their greater likelihood of employment in service and farm occupations may contribute to the lower proportions with coverage among the Hispanic population.

Low-income adults are more likely to experience financial barriers to health care use than those with higher incomes. They are less able to afford out-of-pocket expenses for health care, but are also more likely to lack health insurance coverage and incur high out-of-pocket expenses when they use health care. Results from the RAND Health Insurance Experiment indicate that cost sharing reduces the use of appropriate and inappropriate services (16). Cost sharing also reduces the use of preventive care (16). While financial barriers may discourage the use of health care among the low-income population, adults with low incomes are more likely to be sick than those

with higher incomes and therefore could be expected to need more health care (figures 32–33).

The use of sick care, preventive care, and dental care by adults varies with income. Among adults 18–64 years of age who report a health problem there is a strong inverse income gradient in the percent without a recent physician contact (figure 44), and the gradient is similar across race and ethnic groups. Similarly, the percent of adults 18–64 years of age with a recent dental visit rises sharply with income (figure 49). Women 50 years of age and older from higher income families are more likely to have recently used mammography (figure 45). This relationship is particularly pronounced among non-Hispanic white women. Poor and near-poor black women were more likely than poor and near-poor non-Hispanic white women to have received recent mammography, perhaps as a result of targeted screening programs (17).

Perceived unmet need for health care provides another indicator of access to health care (18,19). Data from the National Health Interview Survey show a strong inverse income gradient in the percent of adults who perceive that they have unmet needs for health care (figures 46–47). This measure incorporates needs for services that may not be covered by health insurance plans (prescription drugs, mental health care, and dental care) as well as delaying or not receiving needed medical care. Although the percent who report unmet need for care is lower among the elderly (who have Medicare coverage) than among those 18–64 years of age, there was a strong inverse relationship between income and unmet need for the elderly as well as for younger adults.

Persons who delay or do not receive needed ambulatory care may become more seriously ill and require hospitalization. Avoidable hospitalizations have been defined as those that could potentially be avoided in the presence of appropriate and timely ambulatory care (20,21). Among adults 18–64 years of age the rate of avoidable hospitalizations during 1989–91 was inversely associated with the median household income of ZIP Code of residence (figure 48). In addition, among residents of low-income areas the avoidable hospitalization rate for black persons was substantially greater than that for white persons. The higher rate of avoidable hospitalizations among black persons than white persons in low income-areas could be due in part to lower family income among black persons than white persons who reside in low income ZIP Code areas.

The direct provision and financing of personal health care services is an area where government has played an important role in the United States (22). Programs such as Medicaid, community health centers, and the National Health Service Corps have had an important effect on improving access to health care for disadvantaged groups. Recent legislative efforts to further extend health insurance coverage to the uninsured have focused on expanding coverage for uninsured children. However, the data in figures 43–48 as well as other published literature demonstrate that low-income adults also clearly face difficulties in accessing the health care system (23).

References

1. Macintyre S. The Black report and beyond: What are the issues? Soc Sci Med 44(6):723–45. 1997.

2. Feldman JJ, Makuc DM, Kleinman JC, Cornoni-Huntley J. National trends in educational differentials in mortality. AJE 129: 919–33. 1989.

3. Institute of Medicine. Disability in America. 1991.

4. Tissue T. Another look at self-rated health among the elderly. J Geront 27:91–4. 1972.

5. Idler EL, Benyamini Y. Self-rated health and mortality: A review of twenty-seven community studies. J Hlth Soc Beh 38:21–37. 1997.

6. Centers for Disease Control and Prevention. Prevalence of work disability—United States, 1990. MMWR 42:757–9. 1993.

7. Centers for Disease Control and Prevention. Prevalence of mobility and self-care disability—United States, 1990. MMWR 42:760–7. 1993.

8. Centers for Disease Control and Prevention. Reducing the health consequences of smoking: 25 years of progress—a report of the Surgeon General. Rockville, Maryland: Department of Health and Human Services. Public Health Service. 1989.

9. Kuczmarski RJ, Flegal KM, Campbell SM, Johnson CL. Increasing prevalence of overweight among U.S. adults: The National Health and Nutrition Examination surveys, 1960 to 1991. JAMA 272:205–11. 1994.

10. Centers for Disease Control and Prevention. Update: Prevalence of overweight among children, adolescents, and adults—United States, 1988–94. MMWR 46:199—202. 1997.

11. Pi-Sunyer FX. Medical hazards of obesity. Ann Intern Med 119:655–60. 1993.

12. Joint National Committee on Detection, Evaluation, and Treatment of High Blood Pressure. The fifth report on the Joint National Committee on Detection, Evaluation, and Treatment of High Blood Pressure. Arch Intern Med 153:154–83. 1993.

13. Davey Smith G, Shipley R, Rose G. Magnitude and causes of socioeconomic differentials in mortality: Further evidence from the Whitehall Study. J Epid Comm Hlth 44:265–70. 1990.

14. Weissman JS, Epstein AM. Falling through the safety net. Insurance and access to health care. The Johns Hopkins University Press: Baltimore. 1994.

15. National Center for Health Statistics. Employer-sponsored health insurance: State and national estimates. Hyattsville, Maryland. 1997.

16. Newhouse JP and the Insurance Experiment Group. Free for all? Lessons from the RAND Health Insurance Experiment. Harvard University Press: Cambridge. 1993.

17. Henson RM, Wyatt SW, Lee NC. The National Breast and Cervical Cancer Early Detection Program: a comprehensive public health response to two major health issues for women. J Public Health Management Practice 2(2): 36–47. 1996.

18. Bloom B, Simpson G, Cohen RA, Parsons PE. Access to health care. Part 2: Working-age adults. National Center for Health Statistics. Vital Health Stat 10(197). 1997.

19. Cohen RA, Bloom B, Simpson G. Parsons PE. Access to heath care. Part 3: Older adults. National Center for Health Statistics. Vital Health Stat 10(198). 1997.

20. Weissman JS, Gatsonis C, Epstein AM. Rates of avoidable hospitalization by insurance status in Massachusetts and Maryland. JAMA 268: 2388–94. 1992.

21. Pappas G, Hadden WC, Kozak LF, Fisher GF. Potentially avoidable hospitalizations: Inequalities in rates between U.S. socioeconomic groups. AJPH 87(5):811–16. 1997.

22. Shonick W. Government and health services. Oxford University Press: New York. 1995.

23. Schoen C, Lyons B, Rowland D, et al.. Insurance matters for low income adults: results from a five-State survey. Health Affairs 16 (5), 163–71. 1997.

Life Expectancy

■   U.S. vital statistics data show that average life expectancy of all persons in the United States has been increasing. Life expectancy from birth has increased from 70.8 years in 1970 to 75.8 years in 1995. Life expectancy varies by race and sex. Women have a longer life expectancy than men and black persons have a shorter life expectancy than white persons (see *Health, United States, 1998*, table 29). Data from the National Longitudinal Mortality Study for 1979–89 indicate that, among the noninstitutionalized population of the United States, life expectancy also varies by family income level.

■   During 1979–89 life expectancy at age 45 increased with each increase in family income, regardless of sex or race. Black men 45 years of age in families earning at least $25,000 could expect to live 7.4 years longer than black men in families earning less than $10,000; among white men the difference was 6.6 years. The differences between the highest and the lowest income groups tended to be smaller for women than for men. At 45 years of age, black women in the highest income group could expect to live 3.8 years longer than those in the lowest income group; among white women the difference was 2.7 years.

■   At age 65, white men in the highest income families could expect to live 3.1 years longer than white men in the lowest income families; the difference was 2.5 years for black men, 1.3 years for black women, and 1 year for white women.

■   Race differences in life expectancy were larger at age 45 than at age 65. The life expectancy of white persons at age 45 exceeded that of black persons at every income level. Differences between black and white persons in life expectancy at age 45 were larger for women than for men, and larger for persons with family incomes below $15,000 than for persons with higher incomes.

Figure 25. Life expectancy among adults 45 and 65 years of age by family income, sex, and race: United States, average annual 1979–89

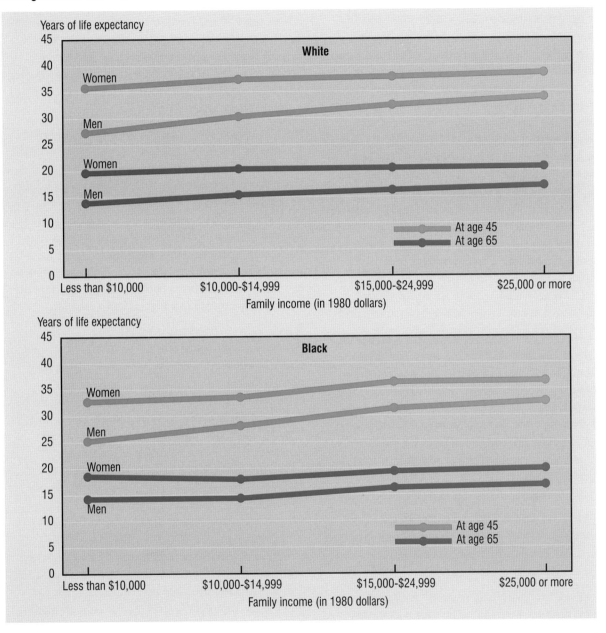

NOTE: See Appendix II for definition of life expectancy.
SOURCE: U.S. Bureau of the Census and National Institutes of Health, National Heart, Lung, and Blood Institute, National Longitudinal Mortality Study.

Adults' Health

Cause of Death

■ Although socioeconomic (SES) differences in mortality have been persistent over time, the nature of the SES relationship for specific causes of death has changed. In earlier times when communicable diseases were the primary causes of death, the higher death rate among persons of lower SES was due to their poor nutrition and unsanitary living conditions. Today chronic diseases, such as heart disease, are the major contributors to death, and although heart disease currently fits the pattern of higher rates among lower SES, this represents a change from the pattern in the past. As recently as the 1950's, heart disease mortality rates were greater among higher SES groups (1). As the factors that influence chronic diseases, such as smoking, high-fat diet, and preventive care, have diffused throughout society, there has been a shift to lower SES groups being more adversely affected, presumably because higher SES groups more quickly adopt practices to reduce their risk of chronic diseases.

■ In 1995 nearly three out of every four deaths to persons 25–64 years of age was due to a chronic disease, intentional and unintentional injuries accounted for 15 percent of deaths in this age range, and communicable diseases accounted for 11 percent. Communicable diseases and injuries were responsible for a larger proportion of deaths to men (13 and 18 percent, respectively) than to women (7 and 10 percent, respectively).

■ Men and women with more than a high school education had lower age-adjusted death rates than their less educated counterparts within each of these major cause groupings.

■ Education gradients in mortality attributed to chronic diseases were similar for men and women

25–64 years of age. In 1995 the chronic disease death rate for men with a high school education or less was 2.3–2.5 times that for men with more than a high school education; less educated women had death rates 1.9–2.2 times the rate of women with education beyond high school.

■ The overall death rate and the education gradient for injuries was higher for men than women. In 1995 the death rate from injuries for men was over three times that for women. Men with 12 years of education or less had age-adjusted injury death rates approximately three times that for men with more than 12 years of education. Among women, the education gradient in injury mortality was similar to that for mortality from chronic diseases; less educated women had injury mortality rates approximately twice that of women with more than a high school education.

■ At ages 25–64 years, mortality from communicable diseases was 3.5 times higher for men than women, and the education gradient was much stronger for women than for men. The discrepancy between men and women in the education gradient for communicable diseases was due entirely to mortality from HIV infection (see data table). For men and women, non-HIV communicable disease mortality among the least educated was three times that of the most educated, and those with 12 years of education had mortality rates twice as high as persons with more than 12 years. In contrast, mortality from HIV infection among men with 12 or fewer years of education was 60–70 percent higher than among those with more than 12 years. By contrast, women with less than 12 years of education were almost six times as likely to die from HIV infection as those with more than 12 years.

Reference

1. Marmot MG, Shipley MJ, Rose G. Inequalities in death: Specific explanations of a general pattern? Lancet 1:1003–6. 1984.

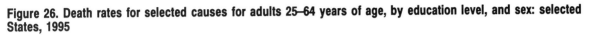

Figure 26. Death rates for selected causes for adults 25–64 years of age, by education level, and sex: selected States, 1995

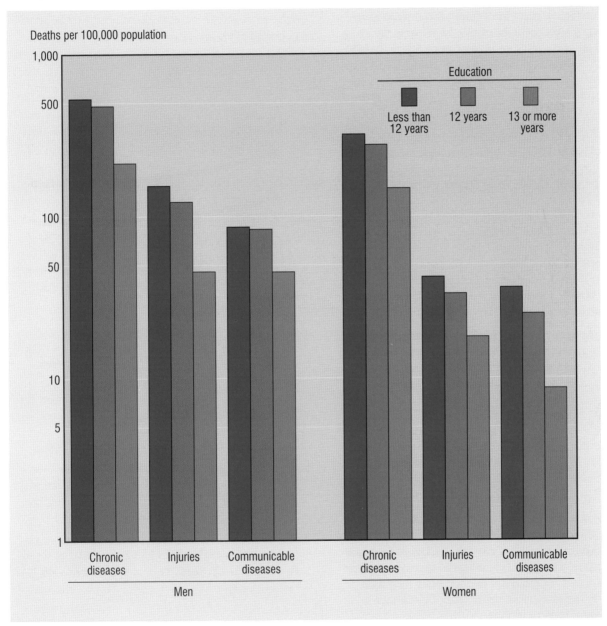

NOTES: Death rates are age adjusted; see Technical Notes. For a description of International Classification of Diseases code numbers for causes of death, see Appendix II. "Injuries" includes homicide, suicide, unintentional injuries, and deaths from adverse effects of medical procedures. See Appendix I, National Vital Statistics System, for a discussion of reporting of education of decedent on death certificates. Rates are plotted on a log scale.

SOURCE: Centers for Disease Control and Prevention, National Center for Health Statistics, National Vital Statistics System.

Heart Disease Mortality

■ Although death rates from heart disease have dropped since 1970, heart disease remains the leading cause of death in the United States. In 1995 heart disease accounted for an estimated $79 billion in direct medical expenditures (1). Risk factors for heart disease include diabetes, hypertension, high serum cholesterol, smoking, obesity, and lack of physical activity (2).

■ During 1979–89 death rates from heart disease declined as family income increased. Among men 25–64 years of age, heart disease mortality for those with incomes less than $10,000 was 2.5 times that for those with incomes of $25,000 or more. The poorest women in this age range were 3.4 times as likely to die from heart disease as those with the highest incomes. For persons 65 years of age and over, the income gradient in heart disease mortality was similar for men and women and flatter than at younger ages.

■ At ages 25–64, income-related gradients in heart disease mortality were similar across sex, race, and ethnic groups; persons with incomes under $10,000 were 2.4–2.9 times as likely to die from heart disease as those with incomes of $15,000 or more. Among persons 65 years of age and older, income gradients were less steep. Ratios of the heart disease death rate in the lowest income group to that in the highest income group ranged from 1.3 for black women to 1.7 for black men.

■ Within each income level, non-Hispanic black women had higher mortality from heart disease than non-Hispanic white women. At 25–64 years of age the death rate for heart disease was higher for black men than white men, regardless of income; at older ages, however, the death rate for white men was nearly the same or exceeded that of black men at the same level of income.

■ Heart disease mortality varied by sex. The poorest women had death rates similar to those of the highest income men.

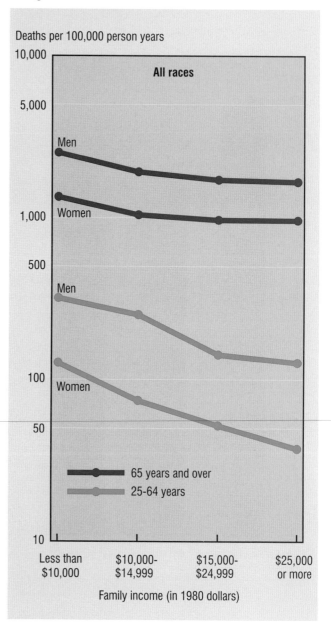

Figure 27. Heart disease death rates among adults 25–64 years of age and 65 years of age and over by family income, sex, race, and Hispanic origin: United States, average annual 1979–89

References

1. Hodgson TA. National Center for Health Statistics, Centers for Disease Control and Prevention. Unpublished estimates. 1997.

2. White CC, Tolsma DD, Haynes SG, McGee D. Cardiovascular disease. In: Amler RW, Dull HB, eds. Closing the gap: The burden of unnecessary illness. New York: Oxford University Press. 1987.

Figure 27. Heart disease death rates among adults 25–64 years of age and 65 years of age and over by family income, sex, race, and Hispanic origin: United States, average annual 1979–89—Continued

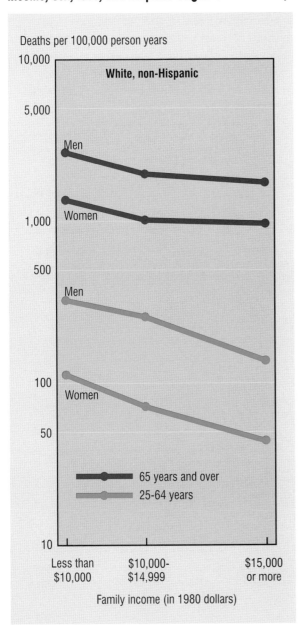

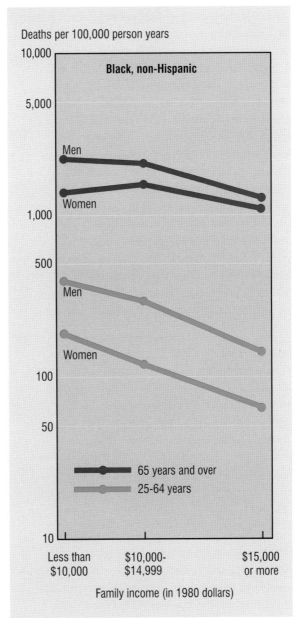

NOTES: Death rates are age adjusted; see Technical Notes. For a description of International Classification of Diseases code numbers for causes of death, see Appendix II. Rates are plotted on a log scale.

SOURCE: U.S. Bureau of the Census and National Institutes of Health, National Heart, Lung, and Blood Institute, National Longitudinal Mortality Study.

Health Status

Lung Cancer Mortality

■ Cancer is the second leading cause of death in the United States, and lung cancer accounted for approximately 28 percent of all cancer deaths in 1996 (1,2). Since 1987 lung cancer has been the leading cause of cancer deaths for men and women. Death rates for lung cancer have been consistently higher for men than women. Between 1950 and 1990 the overall age-adjusted death rate for lung cancer increased. However, among men, the rate of increase began to slow during the early 1980's while the rate for women continued to increase sharply. Between 1990 and 1995 the age-adjusted death rate for lung cancer for males decreased 9 percent while the corresponding rate for females increased 5 percent. In 1995 medical expenditures for lung cancer were estimated to be nearly $4 billion (3). Tobacco is the leading contributor to lung cancer incidence, and the majority of lung cancer cases could be prevented by refraining from smoking (4).

■ Data from the National Longitudinal Mortality Study for 1979–89 show that, among men, lung cancer mortality rates declined as family income increased. The relationship between family income and lung cancer mortality was somewhat stronger for younger than for older men. Men 25–64 years of age in families earning less than $10,000 had a mortality rate 2.4 times the rate among men in families with an income of at least $25,000. Among men 65 years and over, the lowest income group had a rate twice as high as that of the highest.

■ Among women the relationship between family income and lung cancer mortality was weaker and less consistent than among men. Women 25–64 years of age in families earning less than $15,000 had lung cancer death rates 40–60 percent higher than the rates

for women with incomes of $15,000 and more. For women ages 65 years and over, there was some indication that mortality from lung cancer increased with income, although differences were small. Lung cancer mortality among elderly women with incomes of $25,000 and more was 25–30 percent higher than among those with incomes below $15,000.

References

1. Ventura SJ, Peters KD, Martin JA, Maurer JD. Births and deaths: United States, 1996. Monthly vital statistics report; vol 46 no 1, supp 2. Hyattsville, Maryland: National Center for Health Statistics. 1997.

2. Ries LAG, Miller BA, Hankey BF, eds. SEER Cancer Statistics Review, 1973–1993. National Cancer Institute. NIH Pub. No. 94-2789. 1996.

3. Hodgson TA. National Center for Health Statistics, Centers for Disease Control and Prevention. Unpublished estimates. 1997.

4. National Cancer Institute. Cancer control objectives for the nation: 1985–2000. National Cancer Institute Monographs 2. Bethesda, Maryland: U.S. Department of Health and Human Services. 1986.

Figure 28. Lung cancer death rates among adults 25–64 years of age and 65 years of age and over by family income and sex: United States, average annual 1979–89

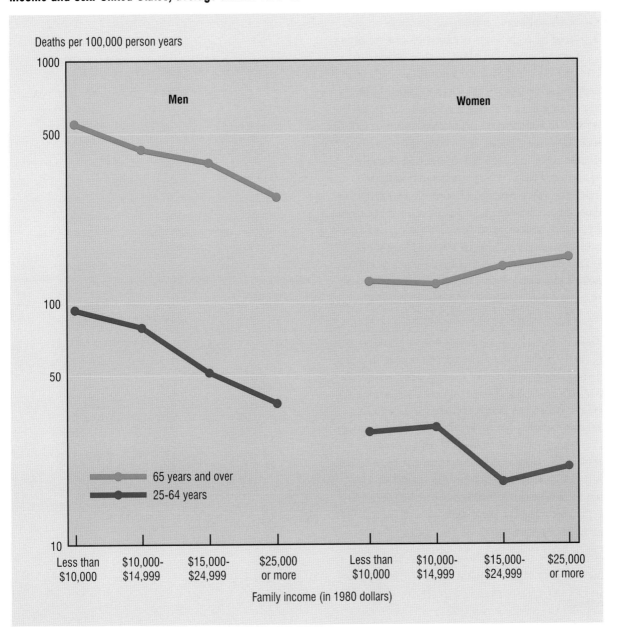

Deaths per 100,000 person years

NOTES: Death rates are age adjusted; see Technical Notes. For a description of International Classification of Diseases code numbers for causes of death, see Appendix II. Rates are plotted on a log scale.

SOURCE: U.S. Bureau of the Census and National Institutes of Health, National Heart, Lung, and Blood Institute, National Longitudinal Mortality Study.

Diabetes Mortality

■   Diabetes mellitus is a group of diseases characterized by high levels of blood glucose resulting from defects in insulin secretion, insulin action, or both. In 1995 diabetes was the seventh leading cause of death for all persons in the United States. In recent years mortality from diabetes has been increasing; between 1990 and 1995, the age-adjusted death rate for diabetes increased 17 percent for men and 12 percent for women. Diabetes death rates vary considerably across race and ethnic groups; compared with non-Hispanic white persons, diabetes death rates were 2.5 times higher among black persons, 2.4 times higher among American Indians or Alaska Natives, and 1.7 times higher among persons of Hispanic origin in 1995. Diabetes was responsible for nearly $48 billion in medical expenditures in 1995 (1). The primary risk factor for noninsulin dependent diabetes mellitus is obesity (2).

■   Data from the National Longitudinal Mortality Study for 1979–89 show a strong relationship between diabetes mortality and family income. For persons 45 years of age and over, the age-adjusted death rate from diabetes decreased as family income increased. The relationship between family income and death from diabetes was similar for men and women; for both sexes mortality from diabetes decreased at each higher level of family income. The diabetes death rate for women in families with incomes below $10,000 was 3 times the death rate for those with incomes of $25,000 or more; among men, the death rate for the lowest income group was 2.6 times that of the highest income group.

References

1. Hodgson TA. National Center for Health Statistics, Centers for Disease Control and Prevention. Unpublished estimates. 1997.

2. Herman WH, Teutsch SM, Geiss LS. Diabetes mellitus. In: Amler RW, Dull HB, eds. Closing the gap: The burden of unnecessary illness. New York: Oxford University Press. 1987.

Figure 29. Diabetes death rates among adults 45 years of age and over by family income and sex: United States, average annual 1979–89

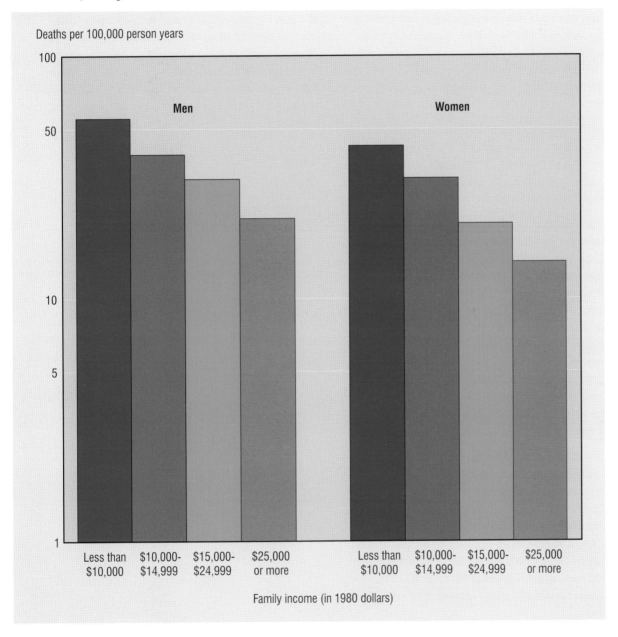

Deaths per 100,000 person years

Men

Women

Family income (in 1980 dollars)

NOTES: Death rates are age adjusted; See Technical Notes. For a description of International Classification of Diseases code numbers for causes of death, see Appendix II. Rates are plotted on a log scale.

SOURCE: U.S. Bureau of the Census and National Institutes of Health, National Heart, Lung, and Blood Institute, National Longitudinal Mortality Study.

Homicide

■ The homicide rate in the United States increased sharply between 1985 and 1991 and then began to decline in 1992 (1). In 1995 homicide ranked as the 11th leading cause of death in the United States overall and the 6th leading cause among persons 25–44 years of age.

■ In 1994–95 homicide rates decreased as years of education increased for persons 25–44 years of age. For those with less than 12 years of education, the rate was more than 7 times the rate for persons who had 13 or more years of education.

■ The education gradient in homicide rates was strongest for non-Hispanic white men. The homicide rate for white men with less than 12 years of education was 8.6 times the rate for those with 13 or more years; for black and Hispanic men, those with the least education were about 5 times as likely to be the victim of homicide as those with the most education. Among women the education gradient for homicide was also strongest for non-Hispanic whites; the rate of the least educated women was 6.4 times the rate for the most educated. Homicide rates for Hispanic and black women with less than 12 years of education were 3–4 times that of those with 13 or more years.

■ For all levels of education combined, the homicide rates for black and Hispanic men were 12 and 4 times the rate for non-Hispanic white men. For those with less than a high school education, the relative difference in homicide rates among the race and ethnic groups was much smaller than for those with more education. By contrast, homicide rates for black women were about 4–6 times the rates for non-Hispanic white women, regardless of educational attainment.

■ Among white, black, and Hispanic men 25–44 years of age, firearms were the cause of about 70–80 percent of homicides; among women 50–60 percent of homicides were caused by firearms. The proportion of homicides caused by firearms did not vary by education level for any sex, race, or ethnic group.

Reference

1. Centers for Disease Control and Prevention. Trends in rates of homicide-United States, 1985–94. MMWR 45:460–64. 1996.

Figure 30. Homicide rates among adults 25–44 years of age by education, sex, race, and Hispanic origin: Selected States, average annual 1994–95

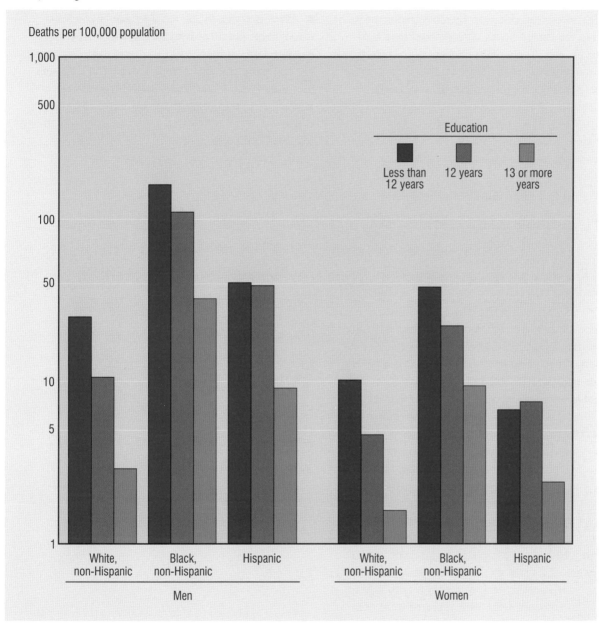

Deaths per 100,000 population

NOTES: Death rates are age adjusted; see Technical Notes. For a description of International Classification of Diseases code numbers for causes of death, see Appendix II. See Appendix I, National Vital Statistics System, for a discussion of reporting of education of decedent on death certificates. Rates are plotted on a log scale.

SOURCE: Centers for Disease Control and Prevention, National Center for Health Statistics, National Vital Statistics System.

Suicide

■ In 1994–95 suicide was the ninth leading cause of death in the United States. Suicide rates tend to be higher for men than women, higher for the elderly than for younger persons, and higher among American Indian or Alaska Native and non-Hispanic white persons than other race and ethnic groups (see *Health, United States, 1998*, table 48). Suicide rates vary by geographic region; for 1990–94, suicide rates were higher in the West and lower in the Northeast, after adjustment for differences in the age, sex, race, and ethnic distributions of regional populations(1).

■ In 1994–95 suicide rates at ages 25–44 were highest for non-Hispanic white persons, and slightly higher for non-Hispanic black persons than for persons of Hispanic origin. In this age group, suicide rates among men were 4–6 times higher than among women for each race and ethnic group examined.

■ For 1994–95, the relationship between education and suicide at ages 25–44 differed by race and ethnicity. The strongest education-related gradient in suicide rates was observed for non-Hispanic white men; the rate for those with less than a high school education was 3.7 times the rate for men with at least some college. Suicide rates for black men who had not gone to college were twice that of those who had, but there was little evidence of a gradient among Hispanic men. Among women 25–44 years of age, the education-related patterns in suicide were similar to those of men in the same race and ethnic group, although not as pronounced. Non-Hispanic white women who had not completed high school had a suicide rate 2.2 times that of those with some college; among non-Hispanic black women this ratio was 1.8. Similar to Hispanic men, there appeared to be no education-related gradient in suicide for Hispanic women.

■ Firearms caused about 55 percent of suicides among men and 40 percent among women. Firearm use in suicide did not vary by education among men, but was more common among less educated women than among more-educated women. Poisoning as a method was more common among those of higher education, while suffocation was more common among less educated persons.

Reference

1. Centers for Disease Control and Prevention. Regional variations in suicide rates, United States, 1990–94. MMWR 46:789–93. 1997.

Figure 31. Suicide rates among adults 25–44 years of age by education, sex, race, and Hispanic origin: Selected States, average annual 1994–95

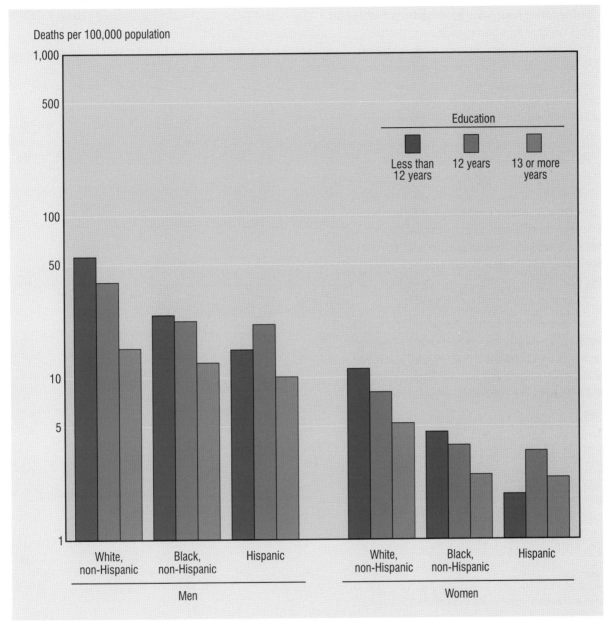

NOTES: Death rates are age adjusted; see Technical Notes. For a description of International Classification of Diseases code numbers for causes of death, see Appendix II. See Appendix I, National Vital Statistics System, for a discussion of reporting of education of decedent on death certificates. Rates are plotted on a log scale.

SOURCE: Centers for Disease Control and Prevention, National Center for Health Statistics, National Vital Statistics System.

Fair or Poor Health

■ Self-assessed health is a broad indicator of health and well being, which incorporates a variety of physical, emotional, and personal components of health. Several studies have shown self-assessed health to be a valid and reliable indicator of a person's overall health status (1) and a powerful predictor of mortality (2) and changes in physical functioning (3).

■ In 1995, one in eight persons 18 years of age and over classified themselves as being in fair or poor health, while seven in eight said they were in good to excellent health. Black and Hispanic persons were more likely to consider themselves in fair or poor health than non-Hispanic white persons. However, within each race and gender group there was a strong income gradient in self-assessed health.

■ Men in poor households were 1.5 times as likely to be in fair or poor health as men near the poverty line, and over 7 times as likely to report their health as fair or poor as men in the highest-income households. Only 4–5 percent of high-income white, black, and Hispanic men were in fair or poor health, compared with 27–37 percent of those below the poverty line.

■ Similar to men, poor women were 1.6 times as likely to say their health was fair or poor as women near the poverty line and over 5 times as likely as high-income women to report their health as less than good. Income disparities in self-assessed health were similar across race and ethnic groups; poor women were four to five times as likely to be in fair or poor health as high-income women.

References

1. Tissue T. Another look at self-rated health among the elderly. J Gerontol (27):91–4. 1972.

2. Idler EL, Benyamini Y. Self-rated health and mortality: A review of twenty-seven community studies. J Health Soc Behav (38):21–37. 1997.

3. Idler EL, Kasl SV. Self-ratings of health: Do they also predict change in functional ability? J Gerontol 50B(6):S344–53. 1995.

Figure 32. Fair or poor health among adults 18 years of age and over by family income, sex, race, and Hispanic origin: United States, 1995

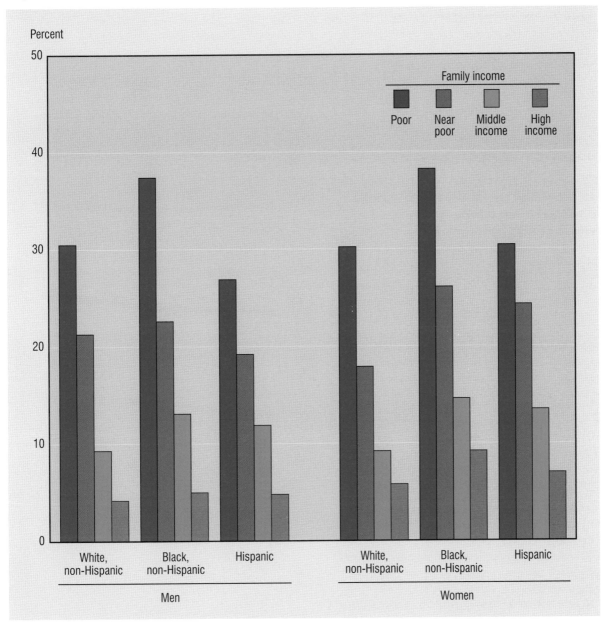

NOTE: Percents are age adjusted. See Technical Notes for definition of family income categories and age adjustment procedure.

SOURCE: Centers for Disease Control and Prevention, National Center for Health Statistics, National Health Interview Survey. See related *Health, United States, 1998*, table 61.

Activity Limitation

■ Chronic conditions and injuries can have long term health consequences, sometimes resulting in limiting individuals in the performance of their usual activities, such as work, household tasks, or other routine activities. In 1995, 22.5 million Americans 18 to 64 years of age experienced some limitation in normal activities because of a chronic health problem. The conditions responsible for most activity limitation in nonelderly adults include back, spine, and lower extremity injuries and impairments, heart disease, arthritis, and visual problems (1,2).

■ In 1992–95 the age-adjusted percent reporting activity limitation was slightly higher among black persons (19 percent) than among white or Hispanic persons (14 percent). However, at each level of income, white persons had the highest rates of activity limitation.

■ At each period and within each race and ethnic group, a larger proportion of poor persons reported activity limitation. In 1992–95 one-third of poor persons, 22 percent of near-poor persons, and 11 percent of middle- and high-income persons had activity limitation.

■ In 1992–95 the income gradient was larger for non-Hispanic black and non-Hispanic white persons than for Hispanic persons; white and black persons in poor families were nearly 3.5 times as likely to be limited as their middle- and high-income counterparts. Poor Hispanic persons were 2.6 times as likely to be limited as those with middle or high incomes.

■ Between 1984–87 and 1992–95 the prevalence of activity limitations among poor white persons increased by 17 percent while the prevalence among those with middle and high incomes increased by only 3 percent. Among black persons increases in the percent with a limitation were similar across income levels (11–15 percent), while among Hispanic persons there was some evidence of an increase in activity limitation for those with incomes above poverty (9–11 percent), but there was no change for those below poverty.

References

1. Verbrugge LM, Patrick DL. Seven chronic conditions and their impact on U.S. adult activity levels and use of medical services. Am J Public Health 85(2):173–82. 1995.

2. Stoto MA, Durch JS. National health objectives for the year 2000: The demographic impact of health promotion and disease prevention. Am J Public Health 1991 81(11):1456–65. 1995.

Figure 33. Activity limitation among adults 18–64 years of age by family income, race, and Hispanic origin: United States, average annual, 1984–87, 1988–91, and 1992–95

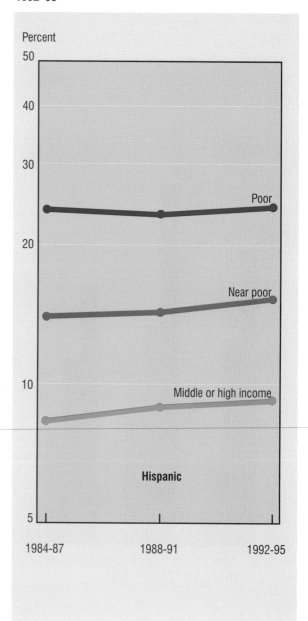

Figure 33. Activity limitation among adults 18–64 years of age by family income, race, and Hispanic origin: United States, average annual, 1984–87, 1988–91, and 1992–95—Continued

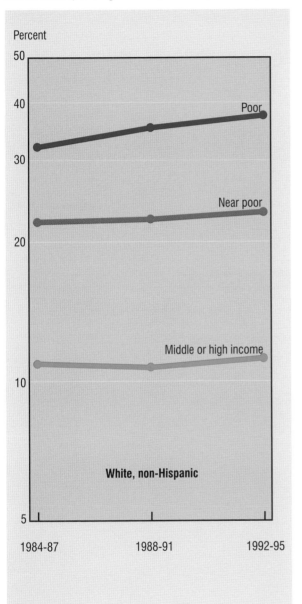

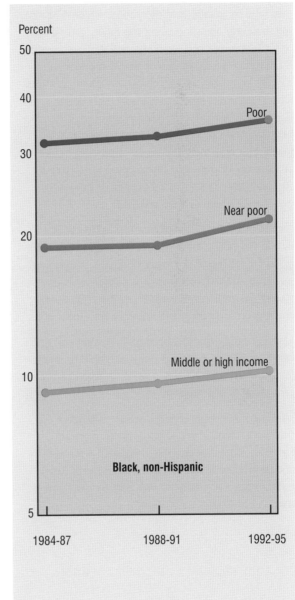

NOTES: Percents are age adjusted and plotted on a log scale. See Technical Notes for definition of family income categories and age adjustment procedure.

SOURCE: Centers for Disease Control and Prevention, National Center for Health Statistics, National Health Interview Survey. See related *Health, United States, 1998*, table 60.

Activities of Daily Living

■ The ability to take care of routine personal needs (eating, bathing, dressing, using the toilet, getting in and out of chairs or bed, walking, and getting outside), is an important aspect of health status, particularly for the elderly population. Needing the assistance of other persons to perform these activities of daily living (ADL) constitutes a physical and psychological burden to the individual affected. The inability to function independently may also impose an additional burden, either in terms of time and foregone opportunities to family members, or a financial burden, if help is obtained from a paid service provider.

■ In 1995, 24 percent of men and 32 percent of women in the noninstitutionalized population 70 years of age and over reported having difficulty performing one or more ADL. Twelve percent of men and 15 percent of women received assistance from another person with at least one of these daily activities.

■ Among noninstitutionalized men 70 years of age and over, poor men were 1.8 times as likely to report having difficulty and 2.5 times as likely to receive help as were middle- and high-income men.

■ Among noninstitutionalized women 70 years of age and over, income gradients in the proportions experiencing difficulty and receiving help were similar. Poor women were about 1.5 times as likely to have difficulty and to receive help with routine care as were middle- and high-income women.

Figure 34. Difficulty with one or more activities of daily living among adults 70 years of age and over by family income and sex: United States, 1995

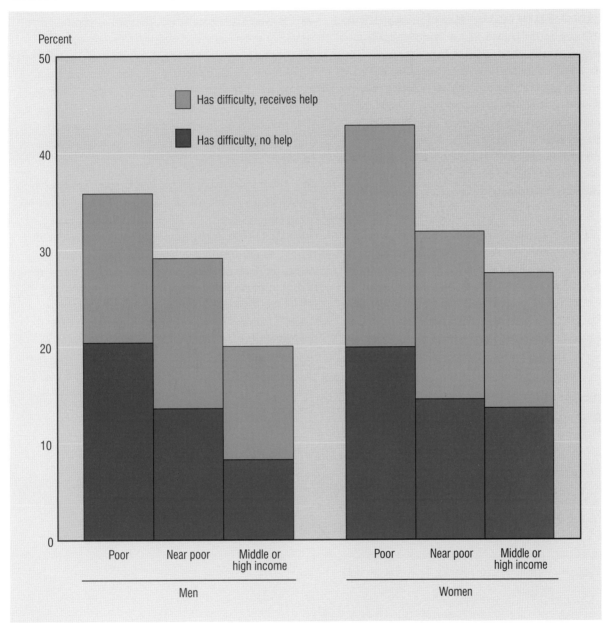

NOTES: Based on interviews conducted between October 1994 and March 1996 with noninstitutionalized persons. Percents are age adjusted. See Technical Notes for definitions of activities of daily living, family income categories, and age adjustment procedure.

SOURCE: Centers for Disease Control and Prevention, National Center for Health Statistics, National Health Interview Survey.

Risk Factors

Cigarette Smoking

■ Smoking is the leading cause of preventable death and disease in the United States. Smoking leads to an increased risk for heart disease, lung cancer, emphysema, and other respiratory diseases. Each year approximately 400,000 deaths in the United States are attributed to smoking (1) and smoking results annually in more than $50 billion in direct medical costs (1). Although there have been recent declines in the prevalence of smoking, the public health burden of smoking-related illness is expected to continue over the next several decades.

■ Between 1974 and 1990, cigarette smoking in the United States declined substantially for persons 25 years of age and over. Among men, the age adjusted prevalence of smoking decreased from 43 percent in 1974 to 28 percent in 1990; among women, smoking declined from 32 percent to 23 percent over the same period. Between 1990 and 1995, however, there was little change in smoking prevalence; in 1995, the age adjusted smoking prevalence was 26 percent for men and 23 percent for women.

■ Between 1974 and 1990, cigarette smoking declined at all levels of education for both men and women. The rate of decline, however, was greater among persons with more education. Among men, smoking declined at an average annual rate of about 1.5 percent among those with a high school diploma or less education and 2.9 percent per year among those with some college. Average annual declines ranged from 0.9 to 2.2 percent for women with less than a college degree. Among college graduates, cigarette smoking declined by approximately 4 percent per year for men and women.

■ Between 1990 and 1995, the rate of decline in smoking prevalence was considerably less than occurred during 1974 to 1990. In addition, declines showed no education-related gradient, ranging from 0.4 percent per year among high school graduates to 1.5 percent per year among men with some college. For women at all levels of education, the age-adjusted prevalence of smoking in 1995 was nearly the same as in 1990.

■ Differential declines across education groups have produced a widening in the socioeconomic gradient in smoking prevalence. In 1974, men with less than a high school education were nearly twice as likely to smoke as those with a college degree or more; by 1995, the least educated men were nearly 3 times as likely to smoke as the most educated. Likewise, in 1974, the least educated women were 1.4 times as likely to smoke as women with 16 or more years of education; by 1995 they were 2.4 times as likely to smoke.

Reference

1. Centers for Disease Control and Prevention. Cigarette smoking-attributable mortality and years of potential life lost—United States, 1990. MMWR 42:654–9. 1993.

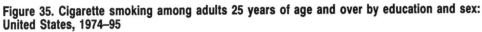

Figure 35. Cigarette smoking among adults 25 years of age and over by education and sex: United States, 1974–95

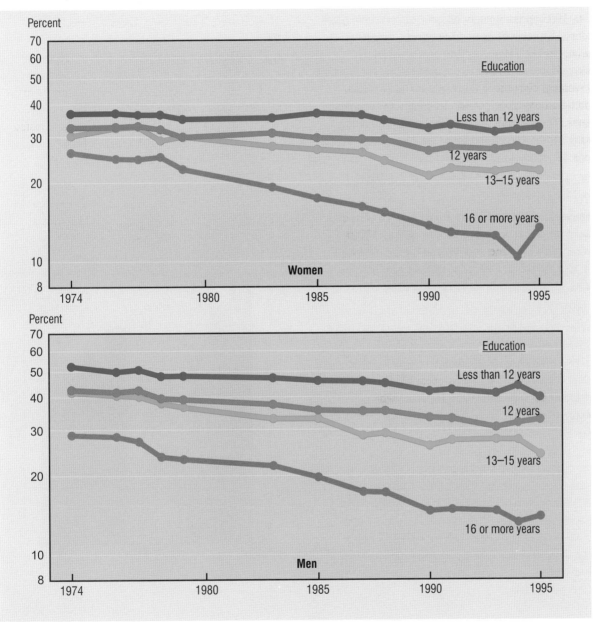

NOTES: Percents are age adjusted (see Technical Notes) and plotted on a log scale. The definition of current smoker was revised in 1992 and 1993. See Appendix II for definition of "current smoker."

SOURCE: Centers for Disease Control and Prevention, National Center for Health Statistics, National Health Interview Survey. See related *Health, United States, 1998*, table 63.

Risk Factors

Cigarette Smoking

■ In 1995 approximately one out of every four U.S. residents 18 years of age and over was a current cigarette smoker. However, the percent currently smoking decreased as family income increased. For men and women, cigarette smoking was about twice as common among poor persons as among high-income persons. The *Healthy People 2000* goal is to reduce smoking prevalence to no more than 15 percent among persons 18 years of age and older.

■ Non-Hispanic white and black persons living below poverty were more likely to smoke than persons with higher incomes. Poor black men and women were twice as likely to smoke as those with middle and high incomes; for white men and women the ratio was 1.7. There appeared to be less of an income gradient in smoking prevalence among Hispanic persons.

■ At all income levels, the prevalence of cigarette smoking was similar for non-Hispanic white and black men, whereas non-Hispanic white women were more likely to smoke than black women regardless of income Hispanic men and women in or near poverty were less likely to smoke than their non-Hispanic white or black counterparts.

Figure 36. Cigarette smoking among adults 18 years of age and over, by family income, sex, race, and Hispanic origin: United States, 1995

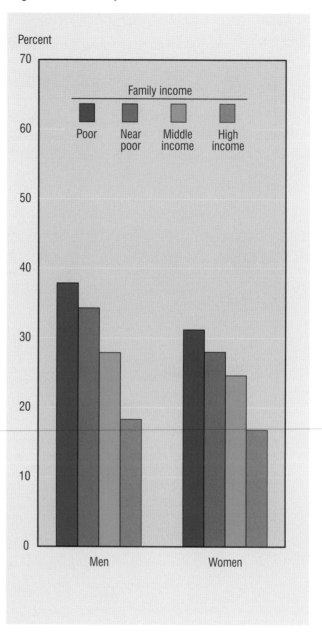

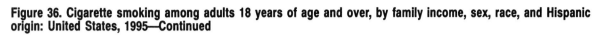

Figure 36. Cigarette smoking among adults 18 years of age and over, by family income, sex, race, and Hispanic origin: United States, 1995—Continued

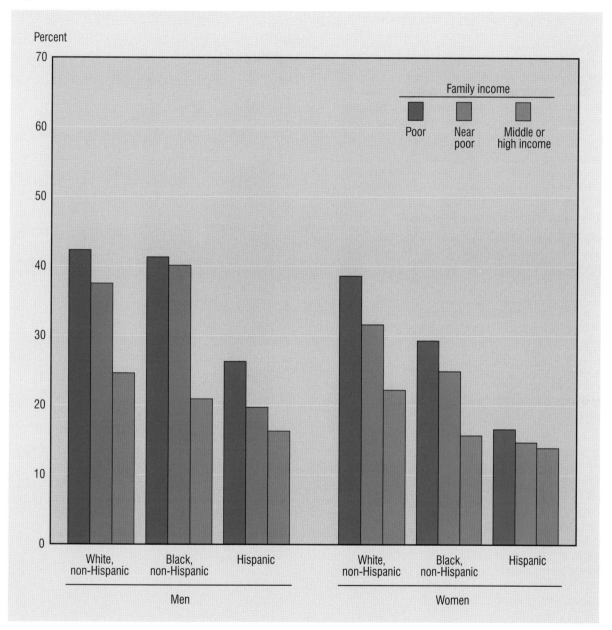

NOTES: Percents are age adjusted. See Technical Notes for definition of family income categories and age adjustment procedure. See Appendix II for definition of "current smoker."

SOURCE: Centers for Disease Control and Prevention, National Center for Health Statistics, National Health Interview Survey.

Alcohol Use

■ Heavy and chronic alcohol use has numerous harmful effects on the body (1). For example, alcohol use and abuse can cause cirrhosis, poor pregnancy outcomes, and motor vehicle crashes (1). The relationship between socioeconomic status and alcohol differs for moderate and heavy use of alcohol. Heavy drinking decreases with more education, whereas moderate alcohol use increases with educational level (2).

■ In 1994–96, 19 percent of persons 25–49 years of age reported heavy alcohol use, defined as having five or more drinks on at least one occasion in the past month. Men were 2.8 times as likely as women to report heavy drinking during the past month.

■ The relationship between education and heavy drinking in the past month differed by race, ethnicity, and gender. In 1994–96 black men and women with less than a high school education were almost twice as likely to report heavy alcohol use in the past month as those with more than a high school education. White men with a high school degree were 20 percent more likely to report heavy alcohol use than those with more education and white women with less than a high school degree were 40 percent more likely to report heavy drinking than women with more education. Heavy drinking in the past month did not differ by education among Hispanic women.

■ Another measure of heavy alcohol use, drinking five or more drinks on five or more occasions in the past month, shows an even stronger inverse relationship with educational attainment (see data table for figure 37). In 1994–96, 7 percent of persons 25–49 years reported this measure of heavy alcohol use. Those with less than a high school education were 2.7 times as likely to report frequent heavy alcohol use during the past month as college graduates. Except for Hispanic women, all race, ethnicity, and gender groups showed a strong inverse relationship between education and frequent heavy alcohol use.

References

1. U.S. Department of Health and Human Services. Eighth special report to Congress on alcohol and health. National Institutes of Health, National Institute on Alcohol Abuse and Alcoholism. Public Health Service. 1993.

2. Substance Abuse and Mental Health Services Administration. Race/ethnicity, socioeconomic status, and drug abuse. U.S. Department of Health and Human Services. No. (SMA) 93–2062. 1993.

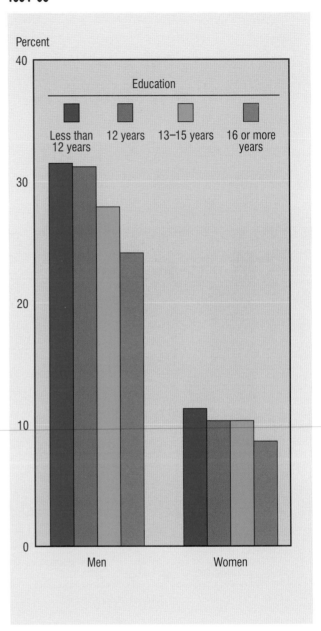

Figure 37. Heavy alcohol use during the past month among adults 25–49 years of age by education, sex, race, and Hispanic origin: United States, average annual 1994–96

Figure 37. Heavy alcohol use during the past month among adults 25–49 years of age by education, sex, race, and Hispanic origin: United States, average annual 1994–96—Continued

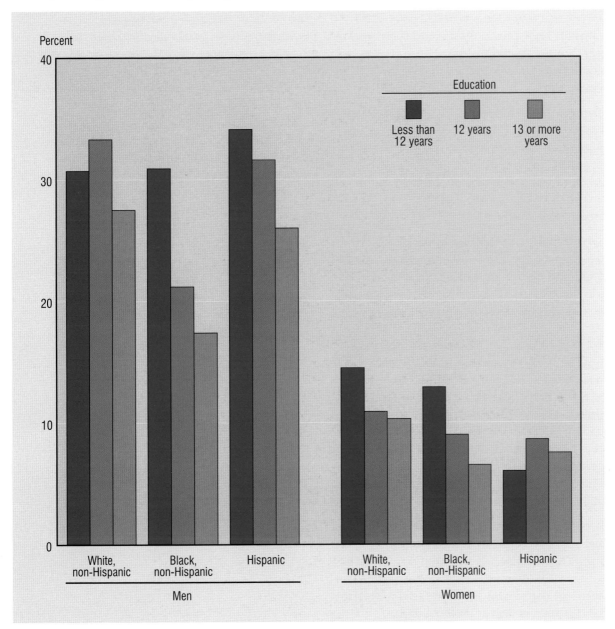

NOTE: Heavy alcohol use during the past month is defined as drinking five or more drinks on the same occasion at least once in the past month.

SOURCE: Substance Abuse and Mental Health Services Administration, Office of Applied Studies, National Household Survey on Drug Abuse, 1994B–96.

Risk Factors

Overweight

■ Overweight adults are at increased risk for hypertension, heart disease, diabetes and some types of cancer (1). A healthy diet and engaging in regular physical activity are important for maintaining a healthy weight.

■ Between 1971–1974 and 1976–80 the prevalence of overweight among U.S. adults 25–74 years of age remained nearly constant at around 26 percent for men and 29 percent for women. By 1988–94, however, 36 percent of men and 39 percent of women in this age range were overweight, an increase of 38 and 33 percent, respectively.

■ Over the three time periods, the prevalence of overweight among men has risen continuously only for those with less than 12 years of education, increasing from 25 percent in 1971–74 to 40 percent in 1988–94. For men at all higher levels of education, the prevalence of overweight remained stable between 1971–74 and 1976–80 and then increased between 1976–80 and 1988–94. Among women the trends were different. Between 1971–74 and 1976–80 the prevalence of overweight was stable for women with less than 12 years of education and increased most among women with higher levels of education. Between 1976–80 and 1988–94 overweight increased among women at all levels of education. The increases were greatest for women with 13–15 years of education.

■ Among men the greatest educational differences in prevalence of overweight are between men with 16 or more years of education and men with fewer than 16 years. Overweight prevalences among men with less than a college degree were similar at each time period and 1.3–1.5 times as high as those of college

graduates. However, among women, overweight prevalence declined as education increased. In 1971–74, overweight prevalence among women with less than 12 years of education was nearly 2.5 times the prevalence among those with 16 or more years. By 1988–94 overweight prevalence among women with less than 12 years of education was only 1.7 times as high as the prevalence among college graduates, due to increases in overweight among college graduates between 1971–74 and 1988–94.

Reference

1. Pi-Sunyer FX. Medical hazards of obesity. Annals of Internal Medicine 119:655–60. 1993.

Figure 38. Overweight among adults 25–74 years of age by sex and education: United States, average annual 1971–74, 1976–80, and 1988–94

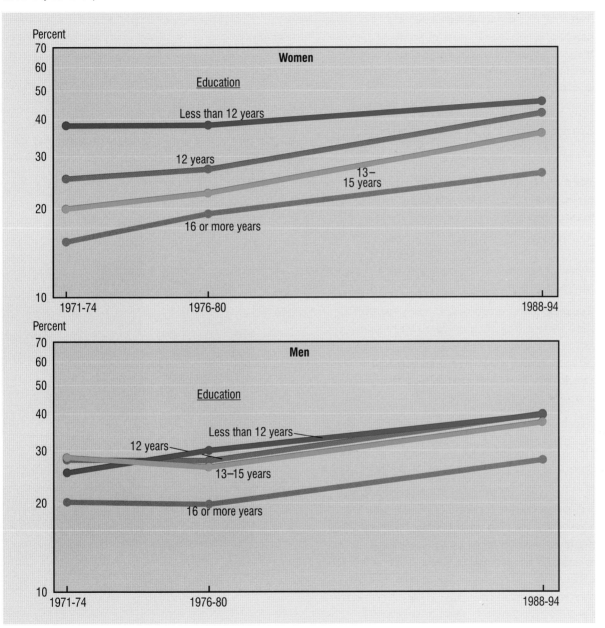

NOTES: Percents are age adjusted and plotted on a log scale. See Technical Notes for definition of overweight and age adjustment procedure.

SOURCE: Centers for Disease Control and Prevention, National Center for Health Statistics, National Health and Nutrition Examination Surveys. See related *Health, United States, 1998*, table 70.

Risk Factors

Overweight

■ The *Healthy People 2000* goal is for no more than 20 percent of adults 20–74 years of age to be overweight; the target for low-income women is 25 percent. During 1988–94, approximately one-third of adults in the United States were overweight. The prevalence of overweight was similar for men and women, except for persons living below the poverty line. Among the poor, 46 percent of women and 31 percent of men were overweight.

■ For men of all races there was little evidence of an income-related gradient in the prevalence of overweight. In contrast, there was a clear income gradient in overweight prevalence among women, with overweight prevalence for poor women 1.4 times that of women with middle incomes and 1.6 times that for women with high incomes.

■ The prevalence of overweight was 58 percent higher for black women than for black men. Mexican American women were also more likely than Mexican American men to be overweight, while the prevalence of overweight was the same for white women and men.

■ For Mexican American and non-Hispanic white women, there was an income-related gradient in the prevalence of overweight. In 1988–94, 42 percent of poor white women were overweight, 1.4 times the proportion overweight among middle- or high-income white women. Among Mexican American women, overweight prevalence for those in poverty was 1.2 times that for those with middle or high incomes. Among black women, however, the prevalence of overweight did not vary much across the income categories.

Figure 39. Overweight among adults 20 years of age and over by family income, sex, race, and Hispanic origin: United States, average annual 1988–94

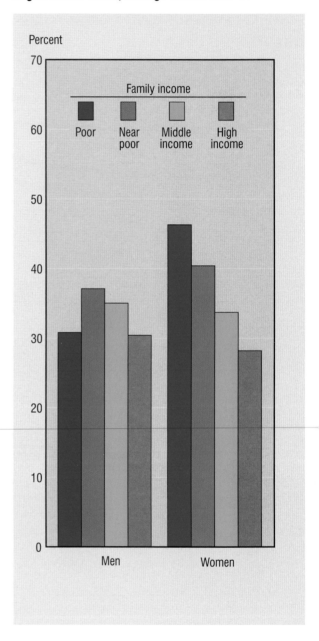

Figure 39. Overweight among adults 20 years of age and over by family income, sex, race, and Hispanic origin: United States, average annual 1988–94—Continued

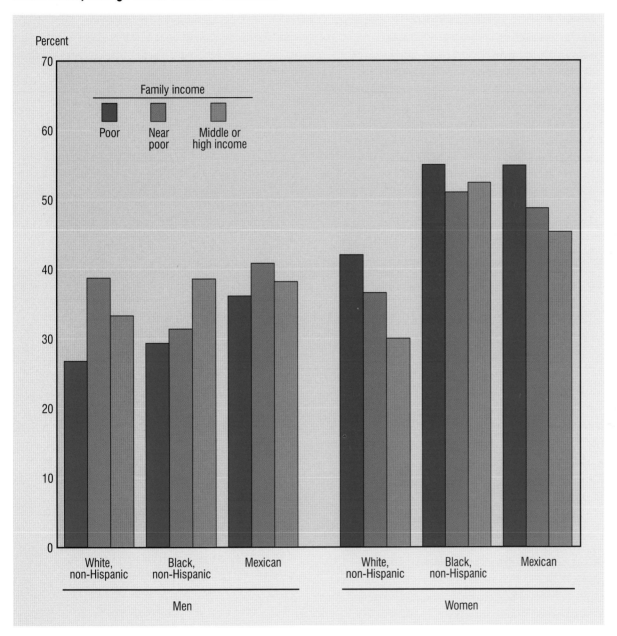

NOTES: Percents are age adjusted. See Technical Notes for definition of family income categories, overweight, and age adjustment procedure.

SOURCE: Centers for Disease Control and Prevention, National Center for Health Statistics, National Health and Nutrition Examination Survey. See related *Health, United States, 1998*, table 70.

Sedentary Lifestyle

■ Regular physical activity can reduce the risk of developing coronary heart disease, noninsulin-dependent diabetes, hypertension, and colon cancer, and thus lower the risk of premature death and disability. Physical activity also helps to control and maintain weight as well as reduce anxiety and depression. Recent research has shown that adults and children do not have to engage in strenuous physical activity to gain health benefits, but rather Americans can improve their health and quality of life by incorporating moderate amounts of physical activity (for example, walking, dancing, or yard work) in their daily lives (1). No more than 15 percent of adults 18 years of age and over should lead a sedentary lifestyle, according to the *Healthy People 2000* goal.

■ In 1991 one out of every five men and one out of every four women 18 years of age and over were not physically active during their leisure time. Although sedentary lifestyle was more common for Hispanic and black persons than for white persons, sedentary lifestyle showed a strong relationship to income in every sex, race, and ethnic group. The percent who were sedentary in their leisure time declined at each higher income level.

■ Black men living in poverty were three times as likely to have a sedentary lifestyle as those with high family incomes. For Hispanic and non-Hispanic white men, the prevalence of sedentary lifestyle for the poor was around 2.5 times the prevalence among those with high family incomes.

■ Women had similar income-related gradients in sedentary lifestyle, with higher income groups having lower prevalences. Poor Hispanic women and poor white women were more than twice as likely to be sedentary as their high income counterparts. The percent sedentary among poor black women was 1.6 times the percent sedentary among black women with high incomes.

Reference

1. U.S. Department of Health and Human Services. Physical activity and health: A report of the Surgeon General. Atlanta, Georgia: Public Health Service. Centers for Disease Control and Prevention, National Center for Chronic Disease Prevention and Health Promotion. 1996.

Figure 40. Sedentary lifestyle among adults 18 years of age and over by family income, sex, race, and Hispanic origin: United States, 1991

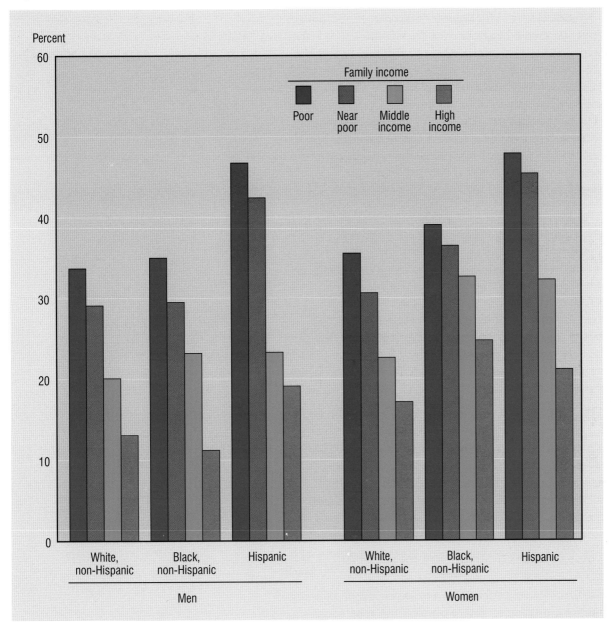

NOTES: Percents are age adjusted. See Technical Notes for definitions of sedentary lifestyle, family income categories, and age adjustment procedure.

SOURCE: Centers for Disease Control and Prevention, National Center for Health Statistics, National Health Interview Survey.

Hypertension

■ Hypertension is a risk factor for heart disease and stroke, the first and third leading causes of death in the United States. During 1988–94 hypertension affected nearly one in four U.S. adults 20 years of age and over, 25 percent of men and 23 percent of women. Twenty percent of men and 17 percent of women had uncontrolled high blood pressure while 18 percent of hypertensive men and 28 percent of hypertensive women were controlling their blood pressure with medication. The *Healthy People 2000* goal is for 50 percent of hypertensives (40 percent of hypertensive men) to be controlling their hypertension.

■ For men of all races, there was little evidence of an income-related gradient in hypertension prevalence in 1988–94. The prevalence of hypertension was 26–27 percent for poor, near poor, and middle income men. Men with high family incomes, however, had a somewhat lower prevalence of hypertension (22 percent). In contrast, there was a clear income-related gradient in hypertension prevalence among women. The prevalence of hypertension ranged from 31 percent for poor women to 19 percent for high-income women and poor women were 1.8 times as likely as high-income women to have uncontrolled hypertension.

■ The income-associated prevalences of hypertension for all men and women mask considerable differences across race and ethnic groups. Among non-Hispanic white men, hypertension prevalence was similar across income groups. Hypertension prevalence was higher for black men than for white and Mexican American men, and also varied little across income categories (33–34 percent). However, poor black men were less likely than those with higher incomes to control their hypertension with medication. Among Mexican American men, uncontrolled hypertension increased at higher levels of income.

■ In 1988–94 total hypertension prevalence and uncontrolled hypertension declined as income increased for white and black women. Forty percent of poor black women had hypertension, compared with 30 percent of middle- and high-income women. Among white women the prevalence of hypertension ranged from 30 percent for those in poverty to 20 percent for those with middle or high incomes. Among Mexican American women there was no association between income and hypertension.

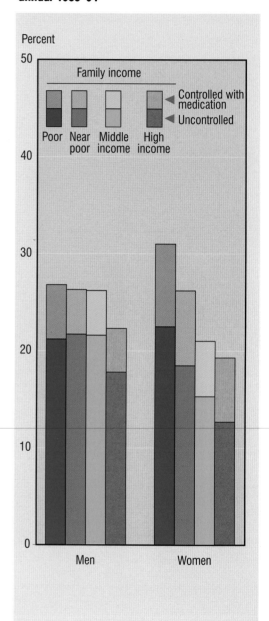

Figure 41. Hypertension among adults 20 years of age and over by family income, sex, race, and Hispanic origin: United States, average annual 1988–94

Figure 41. Hypertension among adults 20 years of age and over by family income, sex, race, and Hispanic origin: United States, average annual 1988–94—Continued

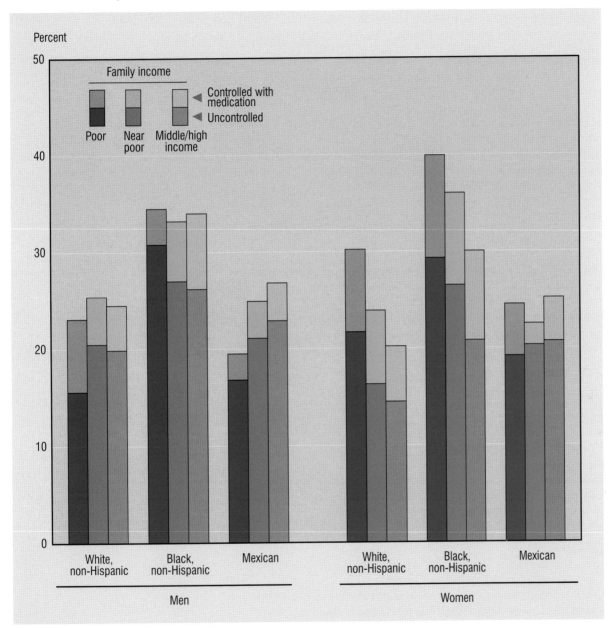

NOTES: Percents are age adjusted. See Technical Notes for definition of family income categories and age adjustment procedure. A person with hypertension is defined as either having elevated blood pressure (systolic pressure of at least 140 mmHg or diastolic pressure of at least 90 mmHg) or taking antihypertensive medication. Percents are based on an average of up to six measurements of blood pressure.

SOURCE: Centers for Disease Control and Prevention, National Center for Health Statistics, Third National Health and Nutrition Examination Survey. See related *Health, United States, 1998*, table 68.

Risk Factors

Blood Lead

■ Lead can be absorbed by breathing air that is contaminated with lead particles, drinking water that comes from lead pipes or lead-soldered fittings, or eating foods that have been grown in soil containing lead. Adults may be exposed to lead in the environment, but the most common high-dose exposures for men come from the workplace. There are a wide variety of occupations in which a worker may be exposed to lead including smelting and refining industries, battery manufacturing plants, gasoline stations, construction, and residential painting. Elevated levels of lead in adults may have a variety of adverse effects on health including decreased reaction time, possible memory loss, anemia, kidney damage, as well as damaging male and female reproductive functions (1).

■ There is a clear gradient between income and prevalence of high blood lead in men. (Rates for women were very low and are not presented here.) In 1988–94 poor men had a greater likelihood of having high levels of lead in their blood (defined as blood lead at or above 10 μg/dL) than men with higher incomes. Over 13 percent of poor men had an elevated blood lead level, a prevalence that was 1.8 times that for near-poor men, 2.8 times that for middle-income men, and almost six times that for men with high incomes.

■ Across all race and ethnic groups, poor men had higher prevalences of elevated blood lead than men with high incomes. Non-Hispanic white men living in poverty were over three times as likely to have high blood lead as white men with middle and high incomes. Poor black and Mexican American men had a prevalence of elevated blood lead that was over twice as high as those of black and Mexican American men with middle and high incomes.

■ Non-Hispanic white and Mexican American men had similar prevalences of high blood lead levels at each income category; however, the data suggest that black men were more likely to have high blood lead levels than white or Mexican American men at each income level.

Reference

1. U.S. Department of Health and Human Services. Toxicological profile for lead. Atlanta, Georgia: Agency for Toxic Substances and Disease Registry (ATSDR). Public Health Service. 1993.

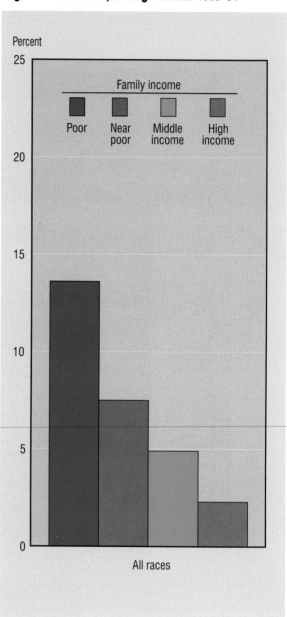

Figure 42. Elevated blood lead among men 20 years of age and over, by family income, race, and Hispanic origin: United States, average annual 1988–94

Figure 42. Elevated blood lead among men 20 years of age and over, by family income, race, and Hispanic origin: United States, average annual 1988–94—Continued

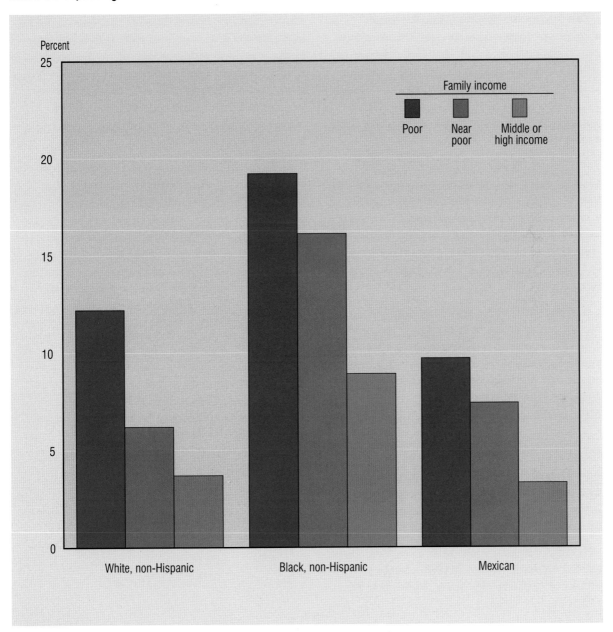

NOTES: Percents are age adjusted. See Technical Notes for definition of family income categories and age adjustment procedure. An elevated blood lead level is defined as blood lead at or above 10 µg/dL.

SOURCE: Centers for Disease Control and Prevention, National Center for Health Statistics, Third National Health and Nutrition Examination Survey.

Health Care

Health Insurance

■ Health insurance coverage is an important determinant of access to health care. Persons without either private or public health insurance coverage are less likely to have a usual source of health care, are more likely to report an unmet need for health care, and are less likely to receive preventive health care services (1,2). The *Healthy People 2000* goal is for no one to be without health insurance.

■ In 1994–95, 18 percent of adults 18–64 years of age had no health insurance coverage, 73 percent had private coverage, 7 percent had Medicaid or public assistance coverage, and 2 percent had other coverage (Medicare or military). Among adults age 65 and over, the proportion who were uninsured was very low (less than 1 percent) due to Medicare coverage of older persons.

■ Hispanic adults under age 65 are substantially more likely to be uninsured than white or black adults. In 1994–95, 34 percent of Hispanic adults 18–64 years of age lacked health care coverage, more than twice the percent of non-Hispanic white persons without coverage and about 60 percent more than the percent of black persons without coverage.

■ The percent of adults under 65 years of age who are uninsured is strongly associated with family income. Overall, in 1994–95 poor adults were seven times as likely to be uninsured as those with high incomes and near-poor adults were six times as likely to be uninsured.

■ Poor and near-poor adults were much more likely to be uninsured than those with high incomes regardless of race, ethnicity, or sex. Poor white, black, and Hispanic men were six–seven times as likely to be uninsured as their high-income counterparts. Among

white women the poor were more than eight times as likely and the near poor were more than seven times as likely as those with high incomes to be uninsured. Among Hispanic women the poor and near poor were about five-six times as likely as those with high incomes to be uninsured; poor and near-poor black women were about four times as likely as those with high incomes to be uninsured.

■ At each level of income Hispanic men and women were more likely to be uninsured than either their black or white counterparts. Within most income groups the percent of black men and women without coverage was somewhat higher or similar to the percent of white men and women without coverage. However, poor and near-poor black women were less likely to be uninsured than white women at those income levels due to greater Medicaid coverage among black women.

■ Men were more likely than women to be uninsured and the difference was greatest among black adults. Poor black men were about 70 percent more likely than poor black women to be uninsured, primarily due to the fact that poor black women were more than twice as likely as poor black men to have Medicaid coverage (55 percent compared with 27 percent).

References

1. Bloom B, Simpson G, Cohen RA, Parsons PE. Access to health care. Part 2: Working-age adults. National Center for Health Statistics. Vital Heath Stat 10(197). 1997.

2. Makuc DM, Freid VM, Parsons PE. Health insurance and cancer screening among women. Advance data from vital and health statistics; no 254. National Center for Health Statistics. 1994.

Figure 43. No health insurance coverage among persons 18–64 years of age by family income, race, and Hispanic origin: United States, average annual 1994–95

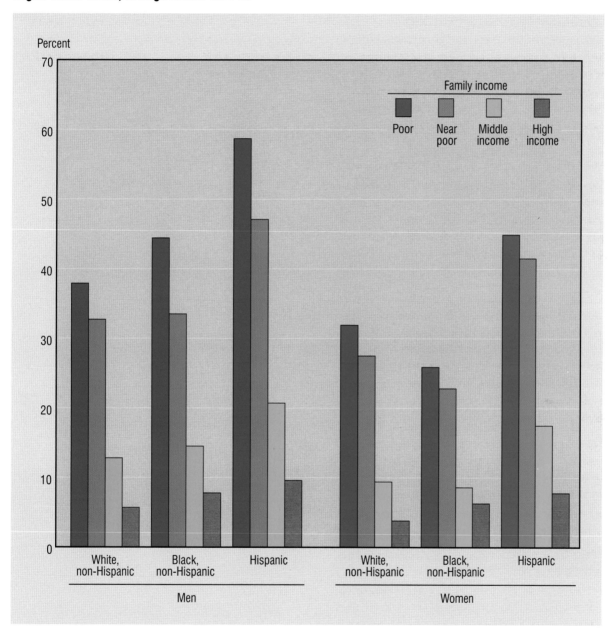

NOTES: Percents are age adjusted. See Technical Notes for definitions of the uninsured, family income categories, and age adjustment procedure.

SOURCE: Centers for Disease Control and Prevention, National Center for Health Statistics, National Health Interview Survey. See related *Health, United States, 1998*, table 133.

No Physician Contact

■　Those who do not receive timely and appropriate ambulatory care when ill may suffer adverse health consequences that require more intensive care in the future. The proportion of adults without a physician visit within the past year among those with health problems is one measure of access to care for those who are ill and may have a need for health care.

■　In 1993–95, 22 percent of persons 18–64 years of age reported a health problem, defined as reporting any one of the following: fair or poor health, a limitation in activity due to a chronic condition, or 10 or more bed-days in the past year. The percent of persons who had not visited a physician in the past year was 12 percent among those with a health problem and 31 percent among those without a health problem.

■　Among adults with a health problem the percent who had not visited a physician in the past year was inversely related to family income, regardless of race, ethnicity, or sex. Poor women were almost three times as likely to be without a recent physician visit as women with high incomes and poor men were almost two times as likely to lack a recent physician visit as men with high incomes.

■　Men with a health problem were more likely than women with a health problem to lack a recent physician contact, regardless of income, race, and ethnicity. Among the poor and near-poor, men were almost twice as likely as women to lack a recent physician contact, and among middle- and high-income persons men were about 2.5 times as likely as women to lack a recent physician contact.

Figure 44. No physician contact within the past year among adults 18–64 years of age with a health problem by family income, race, and Hispanic origin: United States, average annual 1994–95

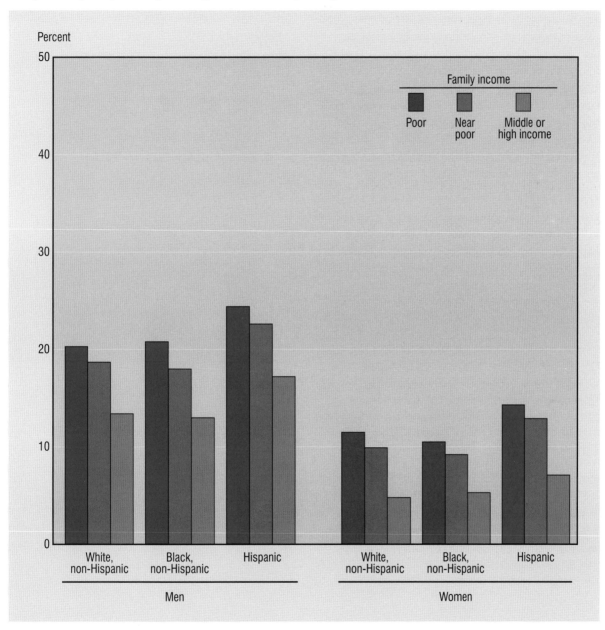

NOTES: Percents are age adjusted. See Technical Notes for definitions of persons with a health problem, family income categories, and age adjustment procedure.

SOURCES: Centers for Disease Control and Prevention, National Center for Health Statistics, National Health Interview Survey. See related *Health, United States, 1998*, table 77.

Mammography

■ Breast cancer is the most common site of new cancers among women and second to lung cancer as a leading cause of cancer deaths among women. Regular mammography screening has been shown to be effective in reducing breast cancer mortality. For women ages 50 years and over the National Cancer Institute recommends screening with mammography every 1 to 2 years. The *Healthy People 2000* goal is for 60 percent of women 50 years and older to have received a breast examination and mammogram within the past 2 years.

■ Overall in 1993–94, 60 percent of women 50 years of age and over reported having a mammogram in the last 2 years. Women with high incomes were about 60–70 percent more likely than poor or near-poor women to have had a recent mammogram. The income gradient in the percent with recent mammography holds for middle-aged women 50–64 years of age as well as for older women 65 years of age and over (data not shown).

■ Within each race and ethnic group women with middle and high incomes were more likely than poor or near-poor women to have recent mammography. This relationship was strongest among white women; the proportion of middle- and high-income white women with a recent mammogram was almost twice that for poor white women.

■ After controlling for income, black women were as likely or more likely than white women to report having a recent mammogram. Among the poor, black women were about 60 percent more likely than white women to have a recent mammogram. Among near-poor women, Hispanic women were less likely than either white women or black women to have recent mammography screening.

Figure 45. Mammography within the past 2 years among women 50 years of age and over by family income, race, and Hispanic origin: United States, average annual 1993–94

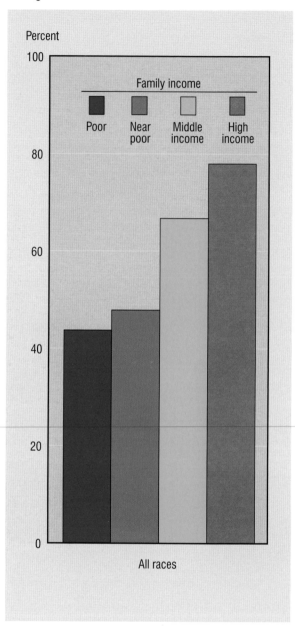

Figure 45. Mammography within the past 2 years among women 50 years of age and over by family income, race, and Hispanic origin: United States, average annual 1993–94—Continued

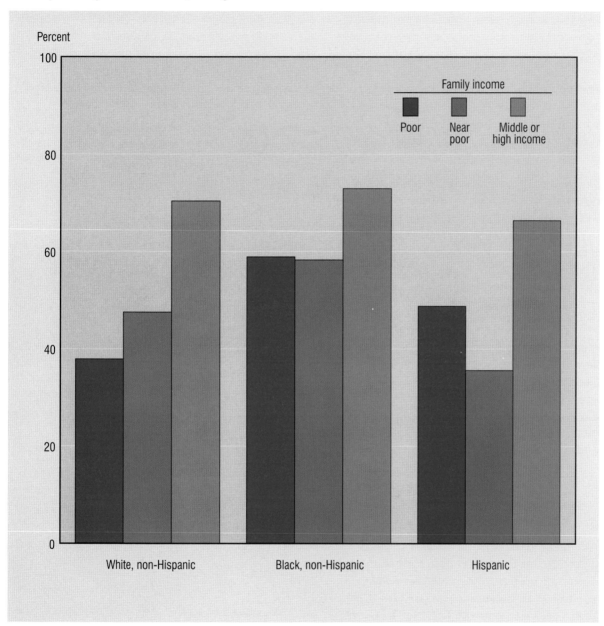

NOTES: Percents are age adjusted. See Technical Notes for definition of family income categories and age adjustment procedure.

SOURCE: Centers for Disease Control and Prevention, National Center for Health Statistics, National Health Interview Survey. See related *Health, United States, 1998*, table 80.

Unmet Need for Care

■ Delaying or not receiving needed health care can have adverse health consequences and may eventually result in the need for more intensive care if health status worsens. One approach to measuring the extent of unmet need for health care is to ask respondents whether they delayed or received care that they needed. This approach relies on the ability of respondents to accurately determine whether care was needed.

■ The proportion of persons who report unmet need for health care increases sharply as income declines. In 1994–95 the age-adjusted percent of poor persons 18–64 years of age who reported unmet need for health care was almost five times that for adults with high family income, and near-poor persons were four times as likely as those with high incomes to report unmet need for health care.

■ The inverse relationship between unmet need for health care and family income held true for young and middle-aged adults and for men and women. The relationship between income and having an unmet need was even stronger for middle-aged persons 45–64 years of age than for younger adults 18–44 years. Poor middle-aged men and women were almost seven times as likely as high-income men and women to report unmet need for care. Poor and near-poor men and women 18–44 years of age were almost four times as likely as their high-income counterparts to report unmet need for care.

■ Among the poor the percent of persons with unmet need for health care was higher among those 45–64 years of age than younger adults, whereas among middle- and high-income persons the percent with unmet need was somewhat lower for 45–64 year

olds than for younger adults. Poor men 45–64 years of age were 40 percent more likely than poor men 18–44 years of age to report unmet need for health care. Poor women 45–64 years of age were about one–third more likely than younger adult women to report unmet need for health care.

■ The proportion of adult women who report unmet need for health care tended to be somewhat higher than for adult men, regardless of income or age.

Figure 46. Unmet need for health care during the past year among adults 18–64 years of age, by family income, age, and sex: United States, average annual 1994–95

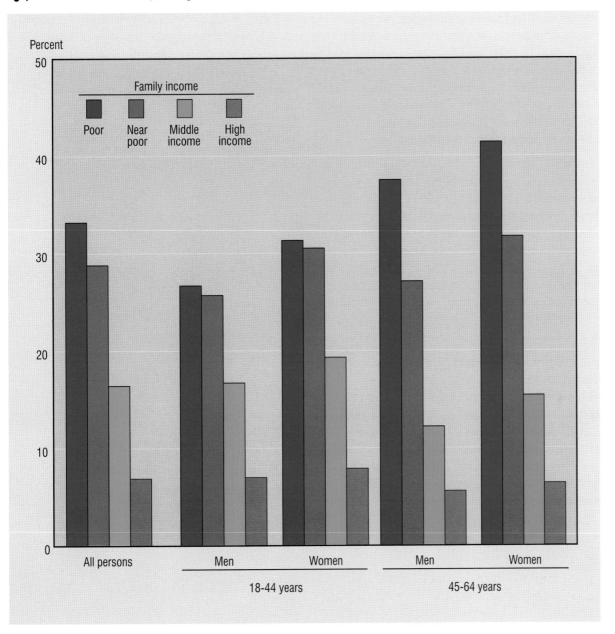

NOTE: See Technical Notes for definitions of unmet need for health care and family income categories.

SOURCE: Centers for Disease Control and Prevention, National Center for Health Statistics, National Health Interview Survey.

Health Care

Unmet Need for Care

■ Unmet need for health care increases sharply as income declines among the elderly as well as among younger adults. In 1994–95, 22 percent of persons 65 years and over who were poor reported unmet need for health care, 10 times the percent for older persons with high incomes. Twelve percent of near-poor older persons reported unmet need for health care, five times the percent for those with high incomes.

■ Compared with middle-aged persons 45–64 years of age, older persons are substantially less likely to report unmet need for care, due in large part to the fact that Medicare coverage comes into effect at age 65. The drop in unmet need between middle-aged and older persons occurs in every income group. Poor persons 45–64 years of age were 1.8 times as likely to report unmet need for care as poor persons 65 years and over. Among the near-poor the percent of those 65 years and over reporting unmet need was less than one–half that for middle-aged persons.

■ Among poor elderly persons and among near-poor elderly persons the percent with unmet need for health care did not differ significantly by race and Hispanic origin. However, in the middle- or high-income group, black and Hispanic older persons were about twice as likely to report unmet need as non-Hispanic white older persons. As a result the income gradient in unmet need was greater for white older persons than for black or Hispanic older persons.

Figure 47. Unmet need for health care during the past year among adults 65 years of age and over by family income, race, and Hispanic origin: United States, average annual 1994–95

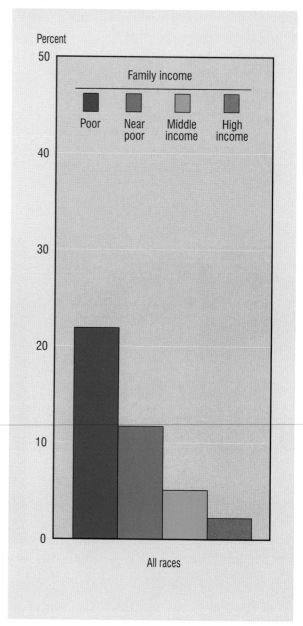

Figure 47. Unmet need for health care during the past year among adults 65 years of age and over by family income, race, and Hispanic origin: United States, average annual 1994–95—Continued

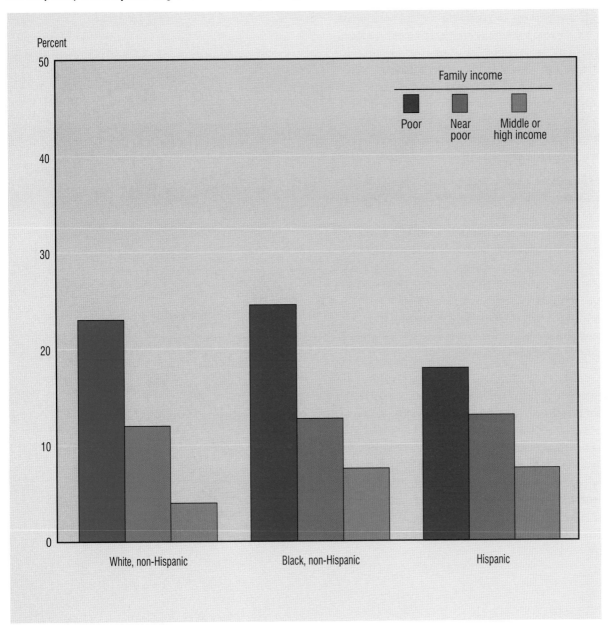

NOTE: See Technical Notes for definitions of unmet need for health care and family income categories.

SOURCE: Centers for Disease Control and Prevention, National Center for Health Statistics, National Health Interview Survey.

Avoidable Hospitalization

■ Delaying or not receiving timely and appropriate care for chronic conditions and other health problems may lead to the development of more serious health conditions that require hospitalization. Hospital stays for specific conditions have been identified as potentially avoidable in the presence of appropriate and timely ambulatory care. Hospitalization rates for these conditions provide a measure of access to ambulatory medical care.

■ The rate of avoidable hospitalizations is inversely associated with the median income of the patient's area of residence. In 1989–91 the avoidable hospitalization rate among residents of low-income areas with median household income less than $20,000 was 2.4 times that for residents of high-income areas with median income $40,000 and over. There was an income gradient in avoidable hospitalization rates for white persons and black persons. The ratio of low-income to high-income rates was 1.7 for white persons and 2.2 for black persons.

■ At each level of median area income, the avoidable hospitalization rate for black persons was higher than for white persons. This racial difference was largest for residents of the lowest income areas. The rate of avoidable hospitalizations for black persons living in the lowest income areas was 2.7 times that of white persons residing in areas with the lowest median income. In areas with higher median incomes black persons had about twice the rate of avoidable hospitalizations as white persons.

Figure 48. Avoidable hospitalizations among adults 18–64 years of age by median household income in ZIP Code of residence and race: United States, average annual 1989–91

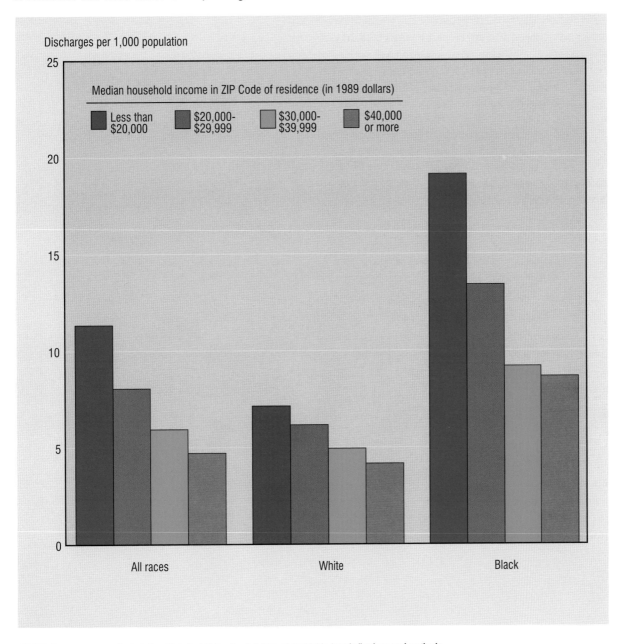

Discharges per 1,000 population

Median household income in ZIP Code of residence (in 1989 dollars)

- Less than $20,000
- $20,000–$29,999
- $30,000–$39,999
- $40,000 or more

NOTES: Rates are age adjusted. See Technical Notes for definition of avoidable hospitalizations and methods.

SOURCE: Centers for Disease Control and Prevention, National Center for Health Statistics, National Hospital Discharge Survey. U.S. Bureau of the Census, 1990 decennial Census.

Dental Care

■ Regular dental visits are important for preventing and treating oral diseases. Having at least one dental visit per year is an indicator of appropriate use of dental care services. The *Healthy People 2000* objective is for 70 percent of adults 35 years and over to use the oral health care system during each year.

■ In 1993, 63 percent of adults 18–64 years of age had a dental visit during the previous 12 months. The percent of adults with a recent dental visit rose sharply with income from 41 percent among the poor to 77 percent among those with high family income.

■ The strength of the association between family income and dental care utilization was similar for white, black, and Hispanic persons. The percent of middle- or high-income adults with a dental visit during the past 12 months was 60–65 percent higher than the percent of poor adults with a recent dental visit within each of these three race and ethnic groups.

■ Among poor adults non-Hispanic white persons were more likely to have had a dental visit in the past 12 months than black or Hispanic persons (45 percent compared with 38 and 36 percent). Among middle or high income adults a similar pattern was found with non-Hispanic white persons more likely than black or Hispanic persons to have had a recent dental visit.

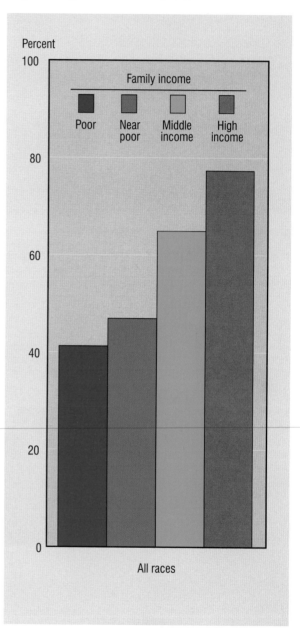

Figure 49. Dental visit within the past year among adults 18–64 years of age by family income, race, and Hispanic origin: United States, 1993

Figure 49. Dental visit within the past year among adults 18–64 years of age by family income, race, and Hispanic origin: United States, 1993—Continued

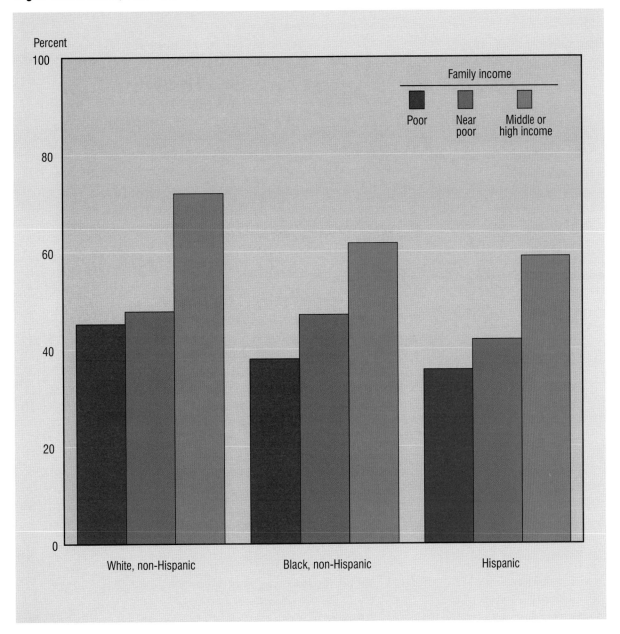

NOTES: Percents are age adjusted. See Technical Notes for definition of family income categories and age adjustment procedure.

SOURCE: Centers for Disease Control and Prevention, National Center for Health Statistics, National Health Interview Survey. See related *Health, United States, 1998*, table 83.

Technical Notes

Data Sources

Appendix I describes the data sources used in the chartbook except for the two surveys described below.

National Longitudinal Mortality Study (figures 25 and 27–29)

The National Longitudinal Mortality Study (NLMS) is a long-term prospective study of mortality in the United States. The study is funded and directed by the National Heart, Lung, and Blood Institute and is carried out with the help of the Census Bureau and the National Center for Health Statistics.

The study population for NLMS consists of samples drawn from the Current Population Survey (CPS). The primary purpose of CPS is to provide estimates of employment, unemployment, and other characteristics of the labor force, but it also includes data needed for the record linkage with the National Death Index.

The CPS sample includes persons of all ages, both sexes, and all races. Each sample is designated as a "cohort" for mortality follow up; that is, the persons in the sample were known to be alive on the survey date, and therefore are eligible for follow up for survivorship from that date forward. The CPS surveys used for the full NLMS were conducted in February 1978, March 1979, April 1980, August 1980, December 1980, March 1981, March 1982, March 1983, and March 1985. Data for figures 27–29 were obtained from the NLMS Public Use File, Release 2, which includes 9 years of follow up for the five CPS surveys conducted over the period 1979–81 (1).

Youth Risk Behavior Survey (figures 15 and 17)

The 1992 Youth Risk Behavior Survey is a followback survey of children 12–21 years of age, drawn from families who were interviewed in the 1992 National Health Interview Survey (NHIS). Interviews were completed for 10,645 children. The questionnaire focused on selected types of health behaviors that could lead to a greater risk for disease and injuries among youths.

Measures of Socioeconomic Status

Income refers solely to money income before taxes and does not include the value of noncash benefits such as food stamps, Medicare, Medicaid, public housing, and employer-provided fringe benefits.

Poverty status (figures 3, 4, 21) is based on family income and family size using the poverty thresholds developed by the U.S. Bureau of the Census (see Appendix II). Poor persons are defined as having incomes below the poverty threshold. Near poor persons have incomes of 100 percent to 199 percent of the poverty threshold.

Poverty rates by State (figure 4) are grouped into the following intervals according to the percent below the poverty threshold: 6.5–10.9 percent (19 States); 11.0–14.9 percent (16 States); 15.0–18.9 percent (12 States); and 19.0–24.0 (3 States and the District of Columbia).

Occupational category (figure 7) is based on current occupation and excludes persons on full-time active duty in the military. The category "white collar" includes executive, administrative, and managerial occupations, professional specialty occupations, technicians and related support occupations, sales occupations, and administrative support occupations. The category "blue collar" includes precision production, craft and repair occupations, machine operators, assemblers and inspectors, transportation and material moving occupations, handlers, equipment cleaners, helpers, and laborers. The category "service" includes private household occupations, protective and other service occupations. The category "farm" includes farming, forestry, and fishing occupations.

Family income categories (figures 11, 14–17, 20, 22, 32–34, 36, 39–47, and 49) were defined as follows:

■ **Poor** persons have family incomes below the Federal poverty level (See Appendix II). For a family of four, the Federal poverty level was $15,569 in 1995.

■ **Near poor** persons have family incomes between 100 and 199 percent of the Federal poverty level.

■ **Middle income** persons have family incomes at least 200 percent of the Federal poverty level but less than $50,000.

■ **High income** persons have family incomes at least 200 percent of the Federal poverty level and at least $50,000.

■ **Middle or high income** persons have family income at least 200 percent of the Federal poverty level.

Three or four family income categories were used in each chart, depending on whether there were sufficient numbers of observations to subdivide those persons with family incomes above twice the poverty level into two groups. Limitations in data collection required the subdivision of the group with incomes at least 200 percent of poverty to be based on family income rather than on percent of poverty level (the National Health Interview Survey and National Health and Nutrition Examination Survey had an upper income category of $50,000 or more for the survey years analyzed).

Median household income in ZIP Code of residence (figures 23, 24, and 48) based on the 1990 decennial Census was used as a measure of socioeconomic status for charts based on data sources that did not include a measure of socioeconomic status at the individual level. Four categories of median household income were used: under $20,000 (13 percent of the U.S. population), $20,000–$29,999 (39 percent of the U.S. population), $30,000–$39,999 (27 percent of the U.S. population), $40,000 and over (21 percent of the U.S. population) (2).

Race and Ethnicity

This chartbook presents data by race and ethnicity as well as socioeconomic status. In many charts, data are presented by both race and ethnicity (e.g., presenting information for Hispanic as well as non-Hispanic white and non-Hispanic black persons).

The chart labels provide a complete description of the data that are presented. In the text that accompanies the charts, in some places, shorthand terms ("white" and "black") were used for the sake of brevity. For example, where a chart presents data for black, non-Hispanic persons, the term "black" in the text refers to only non-Hispanic black persons.

Data throughout the chartbook were generally presented for each race and ethnic subgroup where data were available and numbers were sufficient to allow calculation of reliable estimates. Many charts present data only for the largest race and ethnic groups: non-Hispanic white, non-Hispanic black, and Hispanic (or Mexican-American) persons. National health data sources that permit tabulation by socioeconomic status are limited for smaller groups such as American Indians or Alaska Natives and Asians or Pacific Islanders. Figures 8 and 18 do not present trends for Hispanic births because the number of states reporting Hispanic origin on birth certificates has changed over the time period 1980–95 (See Appendix I, National Vital Statistics System). Figures 14, 16, 39, 41, and 42 present data for Mexican Americans, rather than all Hispanic persons, because Mexican Americans were oversampled in the National Health and Nutrition Examination Survey III. Figures 24 and 48, based on the National Hospital Discharge Survey, do not present data by Hispanic origin because ethnicity is not well reported in that survey.

Data are generally presented by both race and ethnicity so that data are shown for non-Hispanic white and non-Hispanic black persons rather than all white persons and all black persons. However, figures 2 and 3 present data for non-Hispanic white persons and all black persons because the data sources for these figures did not include tabulations for non-Hispanic black persons. Failing to separate black Hispanics from all black persons should not have a large effect on results for black persons, however. While 12.4 percent of the white population is Hispanic, only 2.4 percent of the black population is Hispanic.

Technical Notes ....

The proportion of the black population that is of Hispanic origin by sex and age is shown in the following table.

Percent of black persons who are of Hispanic origin, United States, 1996

Age	Male	Female
0–17 years.	2.7	2.6
18–64 years.	2.4	2.4
65 years and over	0.8	1.7

SOURCE: Current Population Survey, 1996.

The method of collection of race or ethnicity varies with the data source. Most of the data sources used in the chartbook collect race and ethnicity through self-report or the report of a household member. However, in medical records-based data sources such as the National Hospital Discharge Survey these data may be obtained through some self-reports and some observer reports. Race and ethnicity on death certificates are reported by the funeral director based on information provided by an informant such as next of kin, while birth certificates may combine some self-reports and some observer reports.

Age Adjustment

The age adjustment section of Appendix II explains age adjustment procedures and defines standard populations. The standard populations used in the chartbook are consistent with those used in the detailed tables section of Health, United States and vary with the data source.

- Figures 15, 16, and 17: data were age adjusted to the 1980 U.S. resident population using two age groups: 12–14 years and 15–17 years (see Appendix II, table III).

- Figures 26–31: data were age adjusted to the 1940 U.S. standard million age distribution (see Appendix II, table I) using 10-year age groups.

- Figures 32–36, 40, 44, 45, 46, 48: data were age adjusted to the 1970 U.S. civilian noninstitutionalized population (see Appendix II, table III) using the following age groups: 18–44, 45–64, 65–74, 75 and over (figure 32); 18–24, 25–34, 35–44, 45–64, and 65 and over (figures 36, 40); 18–24, 25–34, 35–44, 45–64 (figure 33); 70–74, 75–84, 85 and over (figure 34); 25–34, 35–44, 45–64, 65 and over (figure 35); 18–44, 45–64 (figures 44, 46); 50–64, 65 and over (figure 45); 18–24, 25–34, 35–44, 45–54, 55–64 (figure 48).

- Figures 38, 39, 41, and 42: data were age-adjusted to the 1980 U.S. resident population using the following age groups: 25–34, 35–44, 45–54, 55–64, 65–74 (figure 38); 20–34, 35–44, 45–54, 55–64, 65–74, 75 and over (figures 39, 41, 42).

Other Measures and Methods

Activity limitation among children (figure 11) refers to limitation in ability to perform activities usual for children of the same age. For children under 5 years of age, the National Health Interview Survey (NHIS) asked about "the usual kinds of play activities done by most children his/her age." For children ages 5 to 17, the NHIS asked whether "any impairment or health problem" limits school attendance, or requires the child "to attend a special school or special classes." In addition, respondents are asked whether the child is "limited in any way in any activities because of an impairment or health problem."

Teenage childbearing (figure 12) estimates are based on the 1995 National Survey of Family Growth (NSFG). Women were asked their age at first birth and some information about their family of origin. The education level shown is education of the respondent's mother, to provide information about the socioeconomic status of the respondent's family of origin. This chart included only women 20–29 years of age at the time of the survey in order to reduce recall bias and reduce age-related variability in respondents' current income.

Blood lead (figures 14 and 42) levels are based on data from the third National Health and Nutrition Examination Survey. Blood was drawn from most survey participants and the level of lead in the blood was assessed. These charts present the proportion of the population who were determined to have a high level of blood lead. An elevated blood lead level was defined as having at least 10 micrograms of lead per deciliter of blood. Data for adults are shown only for men; values for women were very low in every socioeconomic category.

Overweight among adolescents (figure 16) is measured by the body mass index (BMI), a measure of weight for height (kg/m^2). The lower boundaries for overweight in adolescents were defined by the sex-specific 95th percentile of BMI for every 6 months of age among respondents 12–17 years of age in the 1966–70 National Health Examination Survey (NHES). Adolescents in NHANES III (the third National Health and Nutrition Examination Survey) whose BMI's were greater than the 95th percentiles for NHES were defined as being overweight. Pregnant girls were excluded.

Sedentary lifestyle among adolescents (figure 17) is defined as having no heavy physical activity that resulted in sweating or heavy breathing during the past week.

Health insurance coverage (figures 20, 22, and 43) is defined as coverage during the month prior to interview in the National Health Interview Survey. The uninsured are defined as those who reported that they did not have the following types of health insurance coverage: private coverage, Medicaid, public assistance, Medicare, and military coverage. Persons who reported that they had any of these types of coverage during the month prior to interview are categorized as insured in figure 22. In the data table for figures 20 and 43 persons who had Medicaid and private coverage are classified as having Medicaid coverage.

Ambulatory care visits among children (figure 23) by median household income of ZIP Code

of residence were estimated by linking records from the 1995 National Ambulatory Medical Care Survey (NAMCS) and the National Hospital Ambulatory Medical Care Survey (NHAMCS) with 1990 Census data on median household income of ZIP Code of residence. Ratios of the number of ambulatory care visits during 1995 to Census population estimates in 1990 by median household income of ZIP Code of residence were estimated. The 1995 data on numbers of visits were used because 1995 was the first year with ZIP Code of residence available on NAMCS and NHAMCS. The only year for which information on median household income by ZIP Code is readily available from the Bureau of the Census is 1990.

Asthma hospitalizations among children (figure 24) include inpatient hospital stays; emergency room visits that did not result in a hospital stay are excluded. The data are based on the National Hospital Discharge Survey (NHDS). ZIP Code of the patient's place of residence from NHDS was linked with 1990 Census data on median household income by ZIP Code to produce hospitalization rates by median household income in the ZIP Code of residence. Census population estimates in 1990 by median household income of ZIP Code of residence, age, and race were used as the denominators of rates. These estimates were based on data for 1989–91 because 1990 is the only year for which information on median household income by ZIP Code is readily available from the Bureau of the Census.

Activity limitation among adults (figure 33) refers to a long-term reduction in a person's capacity to perform the usual kind or amount of activities associated with his or her age group.

Activities of daily living among persons 70 years and over (figure 34) are based on the activities of daily living scale (ADL) that is used to measure functional limitation, primarily in community dwelling populations. The ADL scale is comprised of a set of self-maintenance activities specifically designed to measure the ability to perform routine personal care functions. The activities included in the measure are:

Technical Notes

bathing or showering, dressing, eating, getting in and out of bed or chairs, walking, using the toilet, and getting outside. Questions about these activities ask whether, because of a health or physical problem, an individual has any difficulty performing the activity without personal assistance or the assistance of special equipment. If the individual has difficulty then the degree of difficulty is obtained, including whether he or she receives help from another person.

Overweight among adults (figures 38 and 39) is measured by the body mass index (BMI), a measure of weight for height (kg/m^2). Overweight is defined for men as a BMI greater than or equal to 27.8 kg/m^2, and for women as a BMI greater than or equal to 27.3 kg/m^2. These cut points were used because they represent the sex-specific 85th percentiles for persons 20–29 years of age in the 1976–80 National Health and Nutrition Examination Survey. Height was measured without shoes. Pregnant women were excluded.

Sedentary lifestyle among adults (figure 40) is defined as no self-reported leisure time physical activity during the past 2 weeks. Individuals with disabilities were asked if they had done any exercises, sports, or physically active hobbies in the past 2 weeks. All other persons were asked about the following specific activities: walking for exercise, gardening or yard work, stretching exercises, lifting weights, jogging or running, aerobics or aerobic dancing, bicycle riding, stair climbing, swimming for exercise, bowling, golfing, or playing the following sports: softball, baseball, tennis, handball/racquetball/squash, basketball, volleyball, soccer, or football. A final question was asked about doing any other sport, exercise, or physically active hobbies.

Physician contacts among adults (figure 44) are based on data from the 1993, 1994, and 1995 National Health Interview Survey. This figure presents the average annual age-adjusted proportion of adults 18–64 years of age who have not had a physician visit during the past 12 months among those who reported a health problem. Persons with a health problem are defined as those who met at least one of the following criteria: (a) respondent reported fair or poor health status, (b) a limitation in activity due to a chronic condition, or (c) 10 or more bed days within the past 12 months where a bed day is defined as staying in bed for at least half a day due to a health condition.

Mammography (figure 45) estimates are based on data from the 1993 and 1994 Healthy People Year 2000 Supplements to the National Health Interview Survey. These 1993 and 1994 supplements asked about selected topic areas related to the Department of Health and Human Service's year 2000 health objectives. These supplements were administered to one adult per family in one-half of the sampled households each year. During the 2-year period 1993–94 about 9,400 women age 50 and over responded to questions on mammography.

Unmet need for health care (figures 46 and 47) is based on data from the 1994 and 1995 Access to Care Supplements of the National Health Interview Survey. Persons who responded "yes" to at least one of the following series of questions on unmet need for care during the 12 months prior to being interviewed were categorized as having unmet need for health care: needed medical care or surgery, but did not get it; delayed medical care because of the cost; needed dental care, prescription medicine, eyeglasses, or mental health care but could not get it.

Avoidable hospitalizations (figure 48) were defined as hospital stays with a principal or first-listed diagnosis for which hospitalization may potentially be avoided if ambulatory care is provided in a timely and effective manner. Avoidable hospitalizations were defined as those with the following first-listed diagnoses based on *International Classification of Diseases, 9th Revision, Clinical Modifications* (ICD–9–CM) codes: pneumonia (481–483, 485–486); congestive heart failure (402.01, 402.11, 402.91, 428); asthma (493); cellulitis (681, 682); perforated or bleeding ulcer (531.0, 531.2, 531.4, 531.6, 532.0, 532.2, 532.4, 532.6, 533.0–533.2, 533.4–533.6);

pyelonephritis (590.0, 590.1, 590.8); diabetes with ketoacidosis or coma (250.1–250.3, 251.0); ruptured appendix (540.0–540.1), malignant hypertension (401.0, 402.0, 403.0, 404.0, 405.0, 437.2); hypokalemia (276.8); immunizable conditions (032, 033, 037, 045, 055, 072); and gangrene (785.4) (2, 3). ZIP Code of the patient's place of residence from NHDS was linked with 1990 Census data on median family income by ZIP Code to produce avoidable hospitalization rates by median family income in the ZIP Code of residence. Population estimates for denominators were based on the 1990 Census.

Dental visit estimates (figure 49) are based on data from the 1993 Healthy People 2000 Supplement to the National Health Interview Survey. This supplement was administered to one adult sample person per family during the last half of 1993. Adults defined as having a dental visit within the past year responded that they had one or more dental visits when asked the number of visits that they had made to a dentist during the past 12 months.

References

1. Rogot E, Sorlie PD, Johnson NJ, Schmitt C. NIH Publication No 92–3297. National Institutes of Health, PHS, DHHS. 1992.

2. Pappas G, Hadden WG, Kozak LJ, Fisher G. Potentially avoidable hospitalizations: Inequalities in rates between U.S. socioeconomic groups. AJPH 87(5), 811–6. 1997.

3. Weissman JS, Gatsonis C, Epstein AM. Rates of avoidable hospitalization by insurance status in Massachusetts and Maryland. JAMA 268:2388–94. 1992.

Data Tables for Figures 1–49 ....

Figure 1. Household income at selected percentiles of the household income distribution

Year	Percentiles of income distribution			
	20th percentile	50th percentile	80th percentile	95th percentile
1970	$14,007	$33,181	$55,698	$ 88,054
1975	14,029	32,943	57,221	91,239
1980	14,405	33,763	60,434	98,182
1985	14,582	34,439	63,881	106,830
1990	15,006	35,945	66,271	113,741
1996	14,768	35,492	68,015	119,540

Figure 2. Median household income

Year	All races	White, non-Hispanic	Black[1]	Hispanic	Asian or Pacific Islander
1980	$33,763	$36,251	$20,521	$26,025	---
1981	33,215	35,601	19,693	26,643	---
1982	33,105	35,238	19,642	24,910	---
1983	32,900	---	19,579	25,057	---
1984	33,849	36,451	20,343	25,660	---
1985	34,439	37,137	21,609	25,467	---
1986	35,642	38,323	21,588	26,272	---
1987	35,994	38,967	21,646	26,706	---
1988	36,108	39,224	21,760	27,002	$42,795
1989	36,575	39,301	22,881	27,737	45,681
1990	35,945	38,349	22,420	26,806	46,158
1991	34,705	37,236	21,665	26,140	41,989
1992	34,261	37,229	20,974	25,271	42,274
1993	33,922	37,105	21,209	24,850	41,638
1994	34,158	37,188	22,261	24,796	42,858
1995	35,082	38,276	23,054	23,535	41,813
1996	35,492	38,787	23,482	24,906	43,276

--- Data not available.
[1]Includes persons of Hispanic origin.

Figure 3. Percent of persons poor and near poor

Race and Hispanic origin	All persons		Children under 18 in families		Related children under 18 in female-headed households	
	Poor	Near poor	Poor	Near poor	Poor	Near poor
All races	13.7	19.8	20.5	22.7	49.3	27.0
White, non-Hispanic	8.6	17.0	11.1	19.7	34.9	29.2
Asian or Pacific Islander	14.5	15.7	19.5	16.4	48.8	17.6
Black[1]	28.4	26.7	39.9	28.1	58.2	26.8
Hispanic	29.4	30.5	40.3	31.7	67.4	21.9

[1]Includes persons of Hispanic origin.

Figure 4. Percent of persons in poverty

State	Percent	SE	State	Percent	SE	State	Percent	SE
Alabama	16.8	1.4	Kentucky	16.7	1.4	North Dakota	11.1	1.2
Alaska.	8.5	1.0	Louisiana.	22.0	1.5	Ohio	12.8	0.7
Arizona	17.5	1.3	Maine	10.6	1.3	Oklahoma	16.8	1.3
Arkansas.	15.8	1.3	Maryland	10.4	1.2	Oregon	11.6	1.2
California.	17.2	0.6	Massachusetts	10.3	0.8	Pennsylvania	12.1	0.7
Colorado	9.5	1.1	Michigan	12.5	0.7	Rhode Island	10.6	1.3
Connecticut	10.7	1.3	Minnesota	10.2	1.1	South Carolina	15.6	1.4
Delaware.	9.1	1.2	Mississippi.	21.3	1.5	South Dakota.	13.6	1.2
District of Columbia . . .	22.5	1.7	Missouri.	11.5	1.2	Tennessee.	15.3	1.3
Florida.	15.1	0.7	Montana	14.6	1.3	Texas	17.7	0.7
Georgia.	13.6	1.1	Nebraska.	9.5	1.1	Utah	8.0	0.9
Hawaii.	10.4	1.2	Nevada	10.1	1.1	Vermont.	10.2	1.2
Idaho	12.8	1.2	New Hampshire	6.5	1.1	Virginia	11.1	1.1
Illinois	12.3	0.7	New Jersey	8.7	0.6	Washington	12.0	1.2
Indiana	10.3	1.1	New Mexico.	24.0	1.5	West Virginia	17.9	1.4
Iowa	10.8	1.2	New York.	16.7	0.6	Wisconsin	8.8	1.0
Kansas	12.3	1.2	North Carolina	13.0	0.8	Wyoming.	11.1	1.2

SE Standard error.

Figure 5. Educational attainment among persons 25 years of age and over

Age, race, and Hispanic origin	Education			
	Less than 12 years	12 years	13–15 years	16 or more years
25–64 years				
All races	14.3	33.5	26.3	25.8
White, non-Hispanic	9.5	34.4	27.3	28.8
Asian or Pacific Islander	14.0	21.0	20.0	45.1
Black, non-Hispanic	20.3	37.1	27.9	14.8
Hispanic	44.3	27.1	18.9	9.7
65 years and over				
All races	35.1	34.0	17.0	13.9
White, non-Hispanic	31.0	36.1	18.1	14.8
Asian or Pacific Islander	37.2	27.7	15.3	19.8
Black, non-Hispanic	58.6	23.5	10.5	7.4
Hispanic	69.6	16.2	8.2	6.0

Data Tables for Figures 1–49

Figure 6. Median family income among persons 25 years of age and over

Sex, race, and Hispanic origin	Education			
	Less than 12 years	12 years	13–15 years	16 or more years
Men				
All races	$24,386	$40,000	$47,944	$66,690
White, non-Hispanic	$25,274	$41,200	$49,000	$67,952
Asian or Pacific Islander	$34,146	$44,612	$55,392	$68,327
Black, non-Hispanic	$19,957	$36,020	$42,500	$54,500
Hispanic	$24,000	$35,000	$43,734	$58,079
Women				
All races	$18,200	$35,300	$43,628	$62,050
White, non-Hispanic	$18,471	$37,000	$45,510	$64,007
Asian or Pacific Islander	$37,420	$42,658	$57,300	$65,675
Black, non-Hispanic	$13,100	$23,556	$33,162	$47,100
Hispanic	$19,310	$32,000	$38,000	$56,765

Figure 7. Current occupation for persons 25–64 years of age

Race and Hispanic origin	Men				Women			
	White collar	Blue collar	Service	Farm	White collar	Blue collar	Service	Farm
All races	48.4	39.2	8.7	3.8	72.9	10.2	15.8	1.1
White, non-Hispanic	52.6	37.4	6.7	3.4	77.6	8.3	13.0	1.1
Asian or Pacific Islander	60.9	27.7	8.9	2.5	68.5	15.7	15.4	0.4
Black, non-Hispanic	33.5	46.9	17.6	2.0	59.3	14.8	25.7	0.1
Hispanic	26.1	49.4	15.4	9.0	52.3	18.4	26.7	2.7

Figure 8. Infant mortality rates among infants of mothers 20 years of age and over

Maternal education and race	1983	1984	1985	1986	1987	1988	1989	1990	1991	1995
White[1]										
Less than 12 years..............	12.5	12.4	12.2	11.6	11.5	11.2	10.0	9.0	8.8	7.6
12 years	8.7	8.4	8.5	8.1	7.8	7.9	7.6	7.1	6.9	6.4
13–15 years...................	7.8	7.2	7.1	6.8	6.4	6.4	6.3	5.8	5.5	5.2
16 or more years	6.5	6.5	6.1	6.2	5.8	5.5	5.3	5.0	4.9	4.2
Black[1]										
Less than 12 years..............	23.4	20.6	21.5	21.6	20.7	21.0	21.7	19.5	19.6	17.0
12 years	17.8	17.6	17.6	17.2	17.0	17.0	16.9	16.0	16.2	14.7
13–15 years...................	16.1	15.4	16.4	16.2	15.0	15.1	14.9	14.1	13.4	12.2
16 or more years	13.5	13.6	14.5	14.3	13.7	13.0	12.7	12.5	12.4	11.3

[1]Includes persons of Hispanic origin. Method of rate calculation changed in 1995. See Technical Notes.

Figure 9. Infant mortality rates among infants of mothers 20 years of age and over

Maternal education	White, non-Hispanic	Black, non-Hispanic	Hispanic	American Indian or Alaska Native	Asian or Pacific Islander
Less than 12 years...............	9.9	17.3	6.0	12.7	5.7
12 years	6.5	14.8	5.9	7.9	5.5
13–15 years...................	5.1	12.3	5.4	5.7	5.1
16 or more years	4.2	11.4	4.4	*	4.0

* Number in this category is too small for stable rate calculation.

Figure 10. Low birthweight live births among mothers 20 years of age and over

Maternal education	All races	White, non-Hispanic	Black, non-Hispanic	Hispanic	American Indian or Alaska Native	Asian or Pacific Islander
Less than 12 years...............	8.4	9.1	15.8	5.8	7.7	7.1
12 years	7.7	6.7	13.3	6.2	6.0	7.0
13–15 years...................	6.7	5.7	11.8	6.1	5.9	7.0
16 or more years	5.7	5.2	10.6	5.9	6.4	6.7

Figure 11. Activity limitation among children under 18 years of age

Race, Hispanic origin, and family income	1984–87 Percent	1984–87 SE	1988–91 Percent	1988–91 SE	1992–95 Percent	1992–95 SE
All races						
Poor.........................	7.1	0.2	7.8	0.3	9.4	0.2
Near poor	5.5	0.2	5.9	0.2	7.1	0.2
Middle/high income................	4.3	0.1	4.4	0.1	5.0	0.1
White, non-Hispanic						
Poor.........................	8.1	0.4	9.0	0.5	10.9	0.4
Near poor	5.9	0.2	6.5	0.3	7.7	0.2
Middle/high income................	4.4	0.1	4.5	0.1	5.0	0.1
Black, non-Hispanic						
Poor.........................	7.0	0.3	8.1	0.4	10.4	0.5
Near poor	5.0	0.4	5.0	0.4	7.7	0.5
Middle/high income................	4.2	0.3	4.2	0.3	5.2	0.4
Hispanic						
Poor.........................	5.4	0.5	5.8	0.4	7.0	0.4
Near poor	4.2	0.4	4.8	0.4	4.7	0.3
Middle/high income................	4.2	0.4	4.7	0.3	5.0	0.3

SE Standard error.

Figure 12. Percent of women 20–29 years of age who had a teenage birth

Respondent's mother's education	All races Percent	All races SE	White, non-Hispanic Percent	White, non-Hispanic SE	Black, non-Hispanic Percent	Black, non-Hispanic SE	Hispanic Percent	Hispanic SE
Less than 12 years....................	32.4	1.6	26.7	2.6	47.6	3.5	35.6	2.8
12 years	18.7	1.2	15.5	1.3	35.3	3.2	27.1	4.1
13–15 years........................	12.8	1.6	10.3	1.8	18.4	4.2	23.2	5.5
16 or more years	6.5	1.1	4.2	1.1	14.9	3.5	20.3	8.0

SE Standard error.

Data Tables for Figures 1–49 ....

Figure 13. Cigarette smoking during pregnancy among mothers 20 years of age and over

Maternal education	All races	White, non-Hispanic	Black, non-Hispanic	Hispanic	American Indian or Alaska Native	Asian or Pacific Islander
Less than 12 years...............	25.3	46.4	25.4	4.9	31.8	4.7
12 years	18.0	22.7	11.6	4.4	21.1	5.1
13–15 years....................	10.4	12.2	7.0	3.4	14.2	3.2
16 or more years	2.6	2.7	2.6	1.4	6.7	0.7

Figure 14. Elevated blood lead among children 1–5 years of age

Family income	All races		White, non-Hispanic		Black, non-Hispanic		Mexican	
	Percent	SE	Percent	SE	Percent	SE	Percent	SE
Poor	12.3	1.7	8.0	1.7	21.5	3.2	6.3	1.6
Near poor	4.7	1.3	3.6	1.5	7.9	2.2	4.5	1.3
Middle income	3.6	0.9 }	2.6	0.8	5.9	1.5	2.4	1.3
High income.........	1.7	0.8 }						

SE Standard error.

Figure 15. Cigarette smoking among adolescents 12–17 years of age

Family income	Total		Boys		Girls	
	Percent	SE	Percent	SE	Percent	SE
Poor	20.3	1.7	22.0	2.1	18.5	2.4
Near poor	21.5	1.4	22.5	2.0	20.4	1.9
Middle income	21.0	1.2	19.5	1.7	22.6	1.8
High income................................	20.3	1.1	22.6	1.8	18.0	1.3

Sex and family income	White, non-Hispanic		Black, non-Hispanic		Hispanic	
	Percent	SE	Percent	SE	Percent	SE
Boys						
Poor	33.1	4.0	11.8	3.2	22.5	3.0
Near poor	26.1	2.5	7.6	2.7	20.7	4.3
Middle/high income..........................	22.9	1.6	4.2	1.6	18.6	3.6
Girls						
Poor	31.0	4.3	8.1	2.8	14.4	3.4
Near poor	25.1	2.6	5.7	1.9	15.0	2.9
Middle/high income..........................	21.4	1.3	7.7	3.4	22.5	4.2

SE Standard error.

Figure 16. Overweight among adolescents 12–17 years of age

Family income	All races		White, non-Hispanic		Black, non-Hispanic		Mexican	
	Percent	SE	Percent	SE	Percent	SE	Percent	SE
Poor	16.6	3.0	18.8	5.1	13.3	2.0	12.5	2.7
Near poor	12.6	2.0	14.3	3.0	10.7	2.1	12.0	2.4
Middle/high income.....	8.5	1.4	7.2	1.6	17.5	3.4	19.7	5.3

SE Standard error.

Figure 17. Sedentary lifestyle among adolescents 12–17 years of age

Family income	Boys		Girls	
	Percent	SE	Percent	SE
Poor	16.4	1.8	29.8	2.3
Near poor	14.2	1.8	24.4	2.0
Middle income	13.3	1.5	18.8	1.6
High income.	12.0	1.5	14.4	1.4

SE Standard error.

Figure 18. Prenatal care use in the first trimester among mothers 20 years of age and over

Year	Race and maternal education							
	White[1]				Black[1]			
	Less than 12 years	12 years	13–15 years	16 or more years	Less than 12 years	12 years	13–15 years	16 or more years
1980	66.3	83.9	87.9	91.9	55.8	66.8	74.2	84.5
1981	65.7	83.6	88.0	92.2	55.1	66.0	73.6	83.9
1982	64.6	83.3	87.9	92.4	53.8	64.8	73.1	82.8
1983	64.5	83.2	88.0	92.7	54.4	64.6	72.5	83.5
1984	64.5	83.2	87.9	92.9	55.1	65.1	72.9	83.8
1985	64.3	82.7	87.8	92.8	54.7	64.5	73.0	83.4
1986	63.6	82.3	87.8	93.0	54.0	63.7	72.7	83.7
1987	63.3	82.1	87.8	93.3	52.7	62.7	72.2	83.6
1988	62.7	82.0	87.8	93.3	52.2	62.4	72.1	83.5
1989	59.0	80.9	87.5	93.6	50.6	61.9	71.9	83.7
1990	59.2	80.9	87.6	93.9	50.6	62.1	72.6	84.8
1991	60.0	81.2	87.6	94.0	51.8	63.2	73.6	85.4
1992	62.8	82.2	88.4	94.4	53.2	65.3	75.0	86.1
1993	64.8	82.9	88.7	94.5	55.3	67.1	76.4	86.8
1994	66.6	83.6	89.1	94.7	57.7	69.2	78.1	87.4
1995	68.2	84.1	89.4	94.8	59.7	71.3	79.5	88.5
1996	69.2	84.4	89.6	94.7	61.4	72.2	80.1	88.9

[1]Includes persons of Hispanic origin.

Figure 19. Prenatal care use in the first trimester among mothers 20 years of age and over

Maternal education	All races	White, non-Hispanic	Black, non-Hispanic	Hispanic	American Indian or Alaska Native	Asian or Pacific Islander
Less than 12 years.	68.0	72.2	61.3	67.2	59.7	69.3
12 years	82.0	86.1	72.2	77.1	68.7	77.9
13–15 years.	87.8	90.5	80.2	83.2	75.0	84.1
16 or more years	93.9	95.0	88.9	89.0	87.4	89.7

Data Tables for Figures 1–49

Figure 20. Percent of children under 18 years of age with no health insurance coverage

| Race, Hispanic origin, and family income | Type of health insurance coverage | | | | | |
| | Uninsured | | Medicaid | | Private | |
	Percent	SE	Percent	SE	Percent	SE
All races						
Poor	22.0	0.7	64.5	0.8	12.7	0.6
Near poor	22.8	0.6	18.1	0.5	55.5	0.8
Middle income	8.6	0.4	3.5	0.2	85.4	0.5
High income	4.2	0.2	1.4	0.2	93.4	0.3
White, non-Hispanic						
Poor	22.2	1.2	60.0	1.4	16.5	1.0
Near poor	21.0	0.7	14.5	0.6	60.8	1.0
Middle income	7.8	0.4	2.8	0.2	87.2	0.6
High income	3.8	0.3	1.1	0.2	94.3	0.3
Black, non-Hispanic						
Poor	14.6	1.1	74.3	1.3	10.5	1.0
Near poor	18.5	1.4	30.7	1.6	46.4	1.8
Middle income	8.4	1.0	7.7	1.0	79.2	1.6
High income	5.7	1.1	4.9	1.0	88.6	1.5
Hispanic						
Poor	29.5	1.3	60.4	1.4	9.7	0.8
Near poor	32.7	1.4	21.6	1.2	43.4	1.5
Middle income	13.4	1.3	5.8	0.8	78.3	1.6
High income	7.2	1.0	3.0	0.7	88.2	1.3

SE Standard error.

Figure 21. Vaccinations among children 19–35 months of age

| Race and Hispanic origin | Poor | | Above poverty level | |
	Percent	SE	Percent	SE
All races	69	1.5	80	0.7
White, non-Hispanic	68	2.4	81	0.8
Black, non-Hispanic	70	2.7	78	2.3
Hispanic	68	2.9	74	2.6

SE Standard error.

Figure 22. Percent of children under 6 years of age with no physician contact during the past year

Family income	All races		White, non-Hispanic		Black non-Hispanic		Hispanic		Insured		Uninsured	
	Percent	SE	Percent	SE	Percent	SE	Percent	SE	Percent	SE	Percent	SE
Poor	11.2	0.6	11.0	1.1	10.9	1.0	10.8	0.9	8.4	0.6	23.3	1.9
Near poor	10.1	0.5	9.9	0.6	9.3	1.3	10.7	1.0	8.7	0.6	14.9	1.3
Middle income	6.9	0.5 }	5.3	0.3	7.1	1.2	5.0	0.7	5.1	0.3	11.8	1.6
High income.	4.1	0.4 }										

SE Standard error.

Figure 23. Ambulatory care visits among children under 18 years of age

Median income in ZIP Code of residence	Place of visit							
	All places		Emergency department		Outpatient department		Physician office	
	Ratio	SE	Ratio	SE	Ratio	SE	Ratio	SE
Less than $20,000	224.1	29.0	49.3	6.2	30.2	5.5	144.6	26.9
$20,000–29,999	238.5	19.1	43.1	3.2	28.1	5.1	167.3	16.3
$30,000–39,999	311.7	25.8	33.7	2.4	23.8	3.4	254.2	24.1
$40,000 or more.	393.0	40.8	32.6	3.0	21.7	4.6	338.8	39.9

SE Standard error.

Figure 24. Asthma hospitalization rates among children 1–14 years of age

Race	Median income in ZIP Code of residence									
	All incomes		Less than $20,000		$20,000–29,999		$30,000–39,999		$40,000 or more	
	Rate	SE	Rate	SE	Rate	SE	Rate	SE	Rate	SE
All races	3.1	0.4	4.7	1.0	3.0	0.4	2.6	0.5	2.0	0.2
White[1]	1.9	0.3	2.2	0.6	1.8	0.3	1.9	0.4	1.4	0.2
Black[1]	6.3	1.0	7.6	1.6	5.5	0.8	5.2	1.1	4.3	1.0

SE Standard error.
[1] Includes persons of Hispanic origin.

Data Tables for Figures 1–49 ....

Figure 25. Life expectancy among adults 45 and 65 years of age

Family income	White men[1]		Black men[1]		White women[1]		Black women[1]	
	45 years	65 years	45 years	65 years	45 years	65 years	45 years	65 years
Less than $10,000	27.3	14.0	25.2	14.3	35.8	19.7	32.7	18.6
$10,000–14,999	30.3	15.5	28.1	14.4	37.4	20.4	33.5	18.0
$15,000–24,999	32.4	16.3	31.3	16.3	37.8	20.5	36.3	19.4
$25,000 or more.	33.9	17.1	32.6	16.8	38.5	20.7	36.5	19.9

[1]Includes persons of Hispanic origin.

Figure 26. Death rates for selected causes among adults 25–64 years of age

Education	Chronic diseases	Injuries	Communicable diseases		
			Total	HIV	Other
Men					
Less than 12 years..............	530.8	154.0	85.7	58.9	26.8
12 years	479.2	122.7	82.8	63.5	19.3
13 years or more	212.3	45.6	45.3	36.9	8.4
Women					
Less than 12 years..............	317.9	41.9	36.0	19.8	16.2
12 years	273.8	33.1	24.8	13.8	11.0
13 years or more	147.6	17.9	8.6	3.4	5.2

HIV Human immunodeficiency virus.

Figure 27. Heart disease death rates among adults 25–64 years of age and 65 years of age and over

Race, Hispanic origin, and family income	Men		Women	
	25–64 years	65 or more years	25–64 years	65 or more years
All races				
Less than $10,000	318.7	2524.6	126.9	1346.0
$10,000–$14,999	251.4	1920.6	74.1	1043.6
$15,000–$24,999	142.3	1715.3	51.9	969.7
$25,000 or more.	126.8	1666.6	37.3	963.4
White, non-Hispanic				
Less than $10,000	324.1	2658.3	112.2	1352.6
$10,000-$14,999	255.4	1951.1	71.3	1016.2
$15,000 or more.	136.9	1723.1	43.7	961.4
Black, non-Hispanic				
Less than $10,000	390.8	2216.2	184.7	1374.2
$10,000-$14,999	292.8	2079.8	119.2	1542.0
$15,000 or more.	142.2	1272.5	64.8	1088.1

Figure 28. Lung cancer death rates among adults 25–64 years of age and 65 years of age and over

	Men		Women	
Family income	25–64 years	65 or more years	25–64 years	65 or more years
Less than $10,000	93.3	547.9	29.1	122.1
$10,000–$14,999	79.3	428.9	30.6	118.8
$15,000–$24,999	51.5	379.0	18.1	140.7
$25,000 or more.	38.5	273.6	20.9	153.4

Figure 29. Diabetes death rates among adults 45 years of age and over

Family income	Men	Women
Less than $10,000	55.3	42.6
$10,000–$14,999	39.3	31.3
$15,000–$24,999	31.1	20.3
$25,000 or more.	21.4	14.1

Figure 30. Homicide rates among adults 25–44 years of age

	Education		
Sex, race and Hispanic origin	Less than 12 years	12 years	13 or more years
Men			
White, non-Hispanic	25.0	10.6	2.9
Black, non-Hispanic	163.3	110.7	32.4
Hispanic	40.6	39.0	9.1
Women			
White, non-Hispanic	10.2	4.7	1.6
Black, non-Hispanic	38.2	22.0	9.4
Hispanic	6.7	7.5	2.4

Figure 31. Suicide rates among adults 25–44 years of age

	Education		
Sex, race, and Hispanic origin	Less than 12 years	12 years	13 or more years
Men			
White, non-Hispanic	56.0	38.9	15.2
Black, non-Hispanic	24.4	22.4	12.4
Hispanic	14.9	21.3	10.1
Women			
White, non-Hispanic	11.3	8.1	5.2
Black, non-Hispanic	4.6	3.8	2.5
Hispanic	1.9	3.5	2.4

Data Tables for Figures 1–49

Figure 32. Fair or poor health among adults 18 years of age and over

Sex and family income	All races		White, non-Hispanic		Black, non-Hispanic		Hispanic	
	Percent	SE	Percent	SE	Percent	SE	Percent	SE
Men								
Poor	31.1	1.1	30.5	1.5	37.4	2.3	26.9	2.0
Near poor	21.1	0.7	21.3	0.8	22.6	1.7	19.2	1.3
Middle income	9.8	0.3	9.3	0.3	13.1	1.1	11.9	1.2
High income	4.3	0.3	4.2	0.3	5.0	1.0	4.8	1.4
Women								
Poor	32.4	0.8	30.2	1.2	38.2	1.6	30.4	1.4
Near poor	19.8	0.6	17.9	0.7	26.1	1.6	24.3	1.4
Middle income	9.9	0.3	9.2	0.3	14.6	1.1	13.5	1.2
High income	6.0	0.3	5.8	0.3	9.2	1.7	7.0	1.2

SE Standard error.

Figure 33. Activity limitation among adults 18–64 years of age

Race and Hispanic origin, and year	Poor		Near poor		Middle/high income	
	Percent	SE	Percent	SE	Percent	SE
All races						
1984–87	30.4	0.4	20.6	0.3	10.5	0.2
1988–91	31.9	0.4	20.7	0.3	10.4	0.1
1992–95	33.6	0.4	21.5	0.3	10.9	0.1
White, non-Hispanic						
1984–87	32.1	0.6	22.1	0.4	10.9	0.2
1988–91	35.3	0.5	22.4	0.4	10.7	0.1
1992–95	37.5	0.5	23.2	0.3	11.2	0.1
Black, non-Hispanic						
1984–87	31.8	0.7	18.9	0.6	9.2	0.4
1988–91	32.8	0.7	19.1	0.6	9.6	0.3
1992–95	35.5	0.7	21.7	0.6	10.2	0.3
Hispanic						
1984–87	23.9	1.1	14.0	0.8	8.3	0.5
1988–91	23.3	0.7	14.3	0.6	8.9	0.3
1992–95	24.2	0.8	15.3	0.6	9.2	0.3

SE Standard error.

Figure 34. Difficulty with one or more activities of daily living among adults 70 years of age and over

Family income	Men						Women					
	Any difficulty		Receives help		No help		Any difficulty		Receives help		No help	
	Percent	SE	Percent	SE	Percent	SE	Percent	SE	Percent	SE	Percent	SE
Poor	35.8	2.8	20.4	2.7	15.4	2.3	42.8	1.9	19.9	1.5	22.9	1.7
Near poor	29.1	1.6	13.6	1.2	15.5	1.4	31.8	1.3	14.5	1.1	17.3	1.1
Middle/high income	20.0	1.1	8.3	0.7	11.7	0.9	27.5	1.1	13.6	0.9	13.9	0.9

SE Standard error.

Figure 35. Cigarette smoking among adults 25 years of age and over

Sex and year	Education							
	Less than 12 years		12 years		13–15 years		16 or more years	
	Percent	SE	Percent	SE	Percent	SE	Percent	SE
Men								
1974	52.4	0.9	42.6	1.9	41.6	1.4	28.6	1.3
1976	49.9	1.0	41.7	1.0	40.5	1.6	28.2	1.3
1977	50.8	1.1	42.4	1.2	40.1	1.6	27.0	1.2
1978	48.0	1.6	39.5	1.4	37.8	2.2	23.6	1.5
1979	48.1	1.0	39.1	0.9	36.5	1.3	23.1	1.1
1983	47.2	1.3	37.4	0.9	33.0	1.4	21.8	1.1
1985	46.0	1.2	35.5	0.9	33.0	1.2	19.7	0.9
1987	45.7	1.1	35.2	0.8	28.4	1.0	17.3	0.7
1988	44.9	0.8	35.2	0.7	29.0	1.0	17.2	0.7
1990	41.8	1.2	33.2	0.7	25.9	0.8	14.6	0.6
1991	42.4	1.1	32.9	0.7	27.2	1.0	14.8	0.7
1993	41.0	1.6	30.5	1.1	27.4	1.4	14.6	0.9
1994	43.9	1.5	31.7	1.1	27.3	1.3	13.2	0.8
1995	39.7	1.7	32.6	1.1	24.0	1.3	13.9	0.9
Women								
1974	36.8	0.8	32.5	0.8	30.2	1.4	26.1	1.4
1976	36.9	0.9	32.7	0.7	32.4	1.3	24.7	1.3
1977	36.4	0.9	33.0	0.7	32.7	1.2	24.6	1.4
1978	36.4	1.3	32.0	0.9	29.0	1.9	25.1	2.0
1979	35.0	0.9	29.9	0.7	30.0	1.2	22.5	1.1
1983	35.3	1.1	30.9	0.7	27.5	1.2	19.2	1.1
1985	36.7	1.0	29.6	0.6	26.7	1.0	17.4	1.0
1987	36.1	0.9	29.2	0.6	26.0	0.8	16.1	0.8
1988	34.5	0.9	29.1	0.6	24.1	0.7	15.3	0.8
1990	32.1	1.0	26.3	0.5	21.1	0.8	13.6	0.8
1991	33.0	0.9	27.1	0.6	22.5	0.8	12.8	0.7
1993	31.0	1.5	26.6	0.7	21.9	1.0	12.4	0.9
1994	31.6	1.4	27.3	0.9	22.5	1.1	10.3	0.7
1995	32.1	1.4	26.3	0.9	22.0	1.1	13.3	0.9

SE Standard error.

Figure 36. Cigarette smoking among adults 18 years of age and over

Family income	All races				White, non-Hispanic				Black, non-Hispanic				Hispanic			
	Men		Women		Men		Women		Men		Women		Men		Women	
	Percent	SE	Percent	SE	Percent	SE	Percent	SE	Percent	SE	Percent	SE	Percent	SE	Percent	SE
Poor	37.9	2.3	31.2	1.7	42.3	3.5	38.6	2.5	41.3	4.4	29.3	2.7	26.3	3.3	16.6	2.4
Near poor	34.3	1.6	28.0	1.3	37.5	2.0	31.6	1.7	40.1	4.5	24.9	3.0	19.7	2.5	14.7	1.9
Middle income	27.9	1.1	24.6	1.0	24.6	0.9	22.2	0.8	20.9	2.6	15.7	2.0	16.3	2.0	13.9	1.8
High income.	18.3	1.2	16.8	1.2												

SE Standard error.

Data Tables for Figures 1–49

Figure 37. Heavy alcohol use during the past month among adults 25–49 years of age

	Heavy alcohol use during the past month							
	On 1 or more occasions				On 5 or more occasions			
	Men		Women		Men		Women	
Race, Hispanic origin, and education	Percent	SE	Percent	SE	Percent	SE	Percent	SE
All races								
Less than 12 years.....................	31.5	1.5	11.3	0.8	16.3	1.1	3.9	0.5
12 years	31.2	1.2	10.3	0.7	14.0	0.8	2.6	0.3
13–15 years..........................	27.9	1.4	10.3	0.6	9.0	0.7	2.4	0.3
16 or more years	24.1	1.2	8.6	0.6	6.1	06	1.4	0.3
White, non-Hispanic								
Less than 12 years.....................	30.7	2.5	14.5	1.6	17.7	1.9	4.9	0.9
12 years	33.3	1.6	10.9	0.8	14.8	1.0	2.7	0.4
13 or more years	27.5	1.2	10.3	0.6	7.7	0.5	2.0	0.2
Black, non-Hispanic								
Less than 12 years.....................	30.9	3.1	12.9	1.4	17.6	2.6	5.0	0.8
12 years	21.2	1.7	9.0	0.9	10.6	1.3	2.9	0.4
13 or more years	17.4	1.5	6.5	0.9	5.7	0.8	1.9	0.5
Hispanic								
Less than 12 years.....................	34.1	1.9	6.0	0.7	13.6	1.3	1.8	0.4
12 years	31.6	1.9	8.6	1.1	13.5	1.6	3.2	0.9
13 or more years	26.0	1.9	7.5	1.1	8.4	1.3	1.7	0.5

SE Standard error.

Figure 38. Overweight among adults 25–74 years of age

| | Men | | | | | | Women | | | | | |
| | 1971–74 | | 1976–80 | | 1988–94 | | 1971–74 | | 1976–80 | | 1988–94 | |
Education	Percent	SE	Percent	SE	Percent	SE	Percent	SE	Percent	SE	Percent	SE
Less than 12 years....	25.2	1.3	30.0	1.5	39.5	1.7	38.0	1.4	38.1	1.3	45.8	1.8
12 years	27.9	2.0	27.7	1.3	39.8	1.8	25.1	1.0	27.1	1.4	41.8	1.6
13–15 years.........	28.4	2.7	26.4	1.9	37.3	2.3	19.9	2.2	22.5	1.3	35.9	2.0
16 or more years	20.1	2.2	19.8	1.5	27.9	2.3	15.4	2.1	19.2	1.8	26.3	2.1

SE Standard error.

Figure 39. Overweight among adults 20 years of age and over

| | All races | | | | White, non-Hispanic | | | | Black, non-Hispanic | | | | Mexican | | | |
| | Men | | Women | | Men | | Women | | Men | | Women | | Men | | Women | |
Family income	Percent	SE	Percent	SE	Percent	SE	Percent	SE	Percent	SE	Percent	SE	Percent	SE	Percent	SE
Poor	30.8	2.4	46.3	1.9	26.8	3.2	42.0	3.2	29.4	1.8	55.0	2.3	36.2	1.8	54.9	2.4
Near poor	37.1	1.8	40.4	1.8	38.7	2.7	36.6	2.4	31.4	2.1	51.0	1.9	40.8	2.0	48.7	2.2
Middle	35.0	1.5	33.7	1.3 }	33.3	1.3	30.0	1.2	38.6	1.7	52.4	2.4	38.2	2.2	45.3	2.2
High	30.4	2.3	28.2	1.7 }												

SE Standard error.

Figure 40. Sedentary lifestyle among adults 18 years of age and over

Sex, race, and Hispanic origin	Poor		Near poor		Middle income		High income	
	Percent	SE	Percent	SE	Percent	SE	Percent	SE
Men								
White, non-Hispanic	33.7	2.1	29.1	1.7	20.1	0.8	13.1	0.9
Black, non-Hispanic	35.0	3.4	29.5	3.2	23.2	2.3	11.2	3.0
Hispanic	46.7	5.0	42.4	3.9	23.3	3.2	19.1	5.3
Women								
White, non-Hispanic	35.5	1.7	30.6	1.2	22.6	0.8	17.1	1.0
Black, non-Hispanic	39.0	2.5	36.4	2.6	32.6	2.1	24.7	4.0
Hispanic	47.8	2.8	45.3	4.5	32.2	3.0	21.1	4.3

SE Standard error.

Figure 41. Hypertension among adults 20 years of age and over

Race, Hispanic origin, and family income	Men						Women					
	Hypertension		Uncontrolled		Controlled with medication		Hypertension		Uncontrolled		Controlled with medication	
	Percent	SE	Percent	SE	Percent	SE	Percent	SE	Percent	SE	Percent	SE
All races												
Poor	26.7	1.6	21.2	1.7	5.6	1.1	31.0	1.8	22.5	1.7	8.5	1.2
Near poor	26.3	1.7	21.7	1.5	4.6	1.5	26.1	1.3	18.5	1.2	7.7	0.7
Middle income	26.2	1.2	21.6	1.2	4.6	0.5	21.0	0.7	15.3	0.6	5.7	0.5
High income.	22.4	1.7	17.8	1.7	4.5	0.8	19.3	1.1	12.7	1.0	6.6	1.1
White, non-Hispanic												
Poor	23.2	2.6	15.6	2.5	7.5	1.7	30.2	3.1	21.7	2.6	8.5	2.2
Near poor	25.3	2.3	20.5	2.1	4.9	0.8	23.9	1.7	16.3	1.6	7.6	0.9
Middle/high income. . . .	24.5	1.1	19.9	1.1	4.6	0.5	20.2	0.7	14.5	0.5	4.6	0.5
Black, non-Hispanic												
Poor	34.4	1.6	30.8	1.6	3.7	0.7	39.9	1.6	29.3	2.5	10.6	1.8
Near poor	33.3	1.6	27.0	1.8	6.2	1.0	35.9	2.2	26.5	2.1	9.5	1.0
Middle/high income. . . .	34.0	1.7	26.2	1.4	7.8	0.9	30.0	1.5	20.8	1.4	9.2	1.3
Mexican												
Poor	19.5	1.6	16.8	1.4	2.7	0.6	24.5	1.4	19.2	1.3	5.3	0.8
Near poor	24.9	2.1	21.1	1.9	2.8	0.9	22.4	1.4	20.3	1.1	2.2	0.5
Middle/high income. . . .	26.8	1.1	22.9	1.1	3.9	0.8	25.2	2.1	20.7	2.3	4.5	1.2

SE Standard error.

Figure 42. Elevated blood lead among men 18 years of age and over

Family income	All races		White, non-Hispanic		Black, non-Hispanic		Mexican	
	Percent	SE	Percent	SE	Percent	SE	Percent	SE
Poor	13.6	1.6	12.2	2.7	19.2	2.2	9.7	1.5
Near poor	7.5	0.7	6.2	1.1	16.1	1.9	7.4	1.1
Middle income	4.9	0.7 ⎫	3.7	0.7	8.9	1.2	3.3	0.7
High income.	2.3	0.7 ⎬						

SE Standard error.

Data Tables for Figures 1–49

Figure 43. Health insurance coverage among adults 18–64 years of age

Race, Hispanic origin, and family income	Men						Women					
	Uninsured		Medicaid		Private		Uninsured		Medicaid		Private	
	Percent	SE	Percent	SE	Percent	SE	Percent	SE	Percent	SE	Percent	SE
All races												
Poor	44.1	1.0	23.0	0.8	26.9	1.0	33.3	0.7	42.6	0.8	21.6	0.8
Near Poor	35.3	0.6	5.8	0.3	52.9	0.6	28.6	0.5	11.2	0.4	56.4	0.6
Middle income	13.8	0.3	0.9	0.1	83.1	0.3	10.2	0.2	1.6	0.1	86.2	0.3
High income.	6.1	0.2	0.3	0.1	92.7	0.2	4.4	0.2	0.6	0.1	93.9	0.2
White, non-Hispanic												
Poor	37.9	1.4	22.3	1.0	32.7	1.6	31.9	1.0	37.1	1.1	28.2	1.3
Near poor	32.7	0.7	5.3	0.4	55.5	0.8	27.5	0.6	9.2	0.4	59.6	0.7
Middle income	12.8	0.3	0.8	0.1	84.3	0.3	9.4	0.3	1.3	0.1	87.4	0.3
High income.	5.7	0.2	0.3	0.1	93.2	0.3	3.8	0.2	0.5	0.1	94.7	0.2
Black, non-Hispanic												
Poor	44.4	2.0	26.5	1.7	22.4	1.9	25.9	1.2	55.4	1.4	16.4	1.0
Near poor	33.5	1.6	8.6	1.1	50.6	1.8	22.8	1.2	18.8	1.1	54.2	1.4
Middle income	14.5	0.9	1.7	0.3	80.1	1.1	8.6	0.7	2.4	0.4	86.4	0.9
High income.	7.8	1.0	1.1	0.4	90.0	1.1	6.3	0.9	1.4	0.4	91.4	1.0
Hispanic												
Poor	58.7	1.6	22.0	1.6	16.6	1.1	44.9	1.5	41.9	1.7	12.0	0.9
Near poor	47.1	1.4	5.6	0.7	44.6	1.4	41.5	1.3	12.3	0.9	43.4	1.3
Middle income	20.7	1.2	1.1	0.3	76.5	1.2	17.5	1.1	3.3	0.5	77.1	1.2
High income.	9.6	1.0	–	. . .	89.6	1.1	7.8	0.9	1.3	0.4	89.7	1.0

– Quantity zero.
. . . Not applicable
SE Standard error.

Figure 44. No physician contact within the past year among adults 18–64 years of age with a health problem

Race, Hispanic origin, and family income	Men		Women	
	Percent	SE	Percent	SE
All races				
Poor	21.2	0.8	11.7	0.5
Near poor	19.1	0.7	10.3	0.5
Middle income	14.9	0.6	5.7	0.3
High income.	11.4	0.7	4.0	0.3
White, non-Hispanic				
Poor	20.3	1.1	11.5	0.8
Near poor	18.7	0.8	9.9	0.5
Middle/high income.	13.4	0.5	4.8	0.2
Black, non-Hispanic				
Poor	20.8	1.6	10.5	0.8
Near poor	18.0	2.0	9.2	1.2
Middle/high income.	13.0	1.5	5.3	0.7
Hispanic				
Poor	24.4	1.8	14.3	1.2
Near poor	22.6	1.8	12.9	1.3
Middle/high income.	17.2	1.9	7.1	1.0

SE Standard error.

Figure 45. Mammography within the past 2 years among women 50 years of age and over

Family income	All races		White, non-Hispanic		Black, non-Hispanic		Hispanic	
	Percent	SE	Percent	SE	Percent	SE	Percent	SE
Poor	44.7	2.2	37.5	2.5	60.0	3.7	49.3	6.8
Near poor	48.2	1.5	47.9	1.8	57.4	3.7	38.2	5.1
Middle income	67.2	1.0 }	70.4	0.9	72.2	3.4	64.7	4.8
High income.	76.3	1.8 }						

SE Standard error.

Figure 46. Unmet need for health care during the past year among adults 18–64 years of age

Family income	18–64 years		18–44 years				45–64 years			
	Percent	SE	Percent	SE	Percent	SE	Percent	SE	Percent	SE
Poor	33.2	0.6	26.7	0.9	31.3	0.7	37.5	1.6	41.4	1.3
Near poor	28.8	0.	25.7	0.6	30.5	0.6	27.1	1.0	31.7	0.9
Middle income	16.4	0.3	16.7	0.4	19.3	0.4	12.2	0.4	15.4	0.5
High income.	6.9	0.2	7.0	0.3	7.9	0.3	5.6	0.3	6.4	0.3

SE Standard error.

Figure 47. Unmet need for health care during the past year among adults 65 years of age and over

Family income	All races		White, non-Hispanic		Black, non-Hispanic		Hispanic	
	Percent	SE	Percent	SE	Percent	SE	Percent	SE
Poor	21.9	0.9	22.6	1.2	24.5	1.8	17.9	2.2
Near poor	11.7	0.5	11.6	0.6	12.7	1.5	13.0	2.1
Middle income	5.1	0.3 }	4.2	0.2	7.9	1.5	7.5	1.5
High income.	2.2	0.4 }						

SE Standard error.

Figure 48. Avoidable hospitalizations among adults 18–64 years of age

Median income in ZIP code of residence	All races		White[1]		Black[1]	
	Rate	SE	Rate	SE	Rate	SE
Less than $20,000	11.3	1.0	7.1	0.8	19.1	2.4
$20,000–29,999	8.1	0.4	6.2	0.4	13.4	1.0
$30,000–39,999	5.9	0.3	4.9	0.4	9.2	0.8
$40,000 or more.	4.7	0.3	4.2	0.2	8.6	0.9

SE Standard error.
[1]Includes persons of Hispanic origin.

Figure 49. Dental visit within the past year among adults 18–64 years of age

Family income	All races		White, non-Hispanic		Black, non-Hispanic		Hispanic	
	Percent	SE	Percent	SE	Percent	SE	Percent	SE
Poor	41.3	1.4	45.2	2.0	38.0	2.4	35.7	3.3
Near poor	46.9	1.1	47.7	1.3	47.0	3.1	41.9	3.2
Middle income	64.9	0.8 }	72.0	0.7	61.7	2.3	58.9	2.4
High income.	77.3	1.1 }						

SE Standard error.

Health Status and Determinants

Population

1. **Resident population,** according to age, sex, detailed race, and Hispanic origin: United States, selected years 1950–96_____ 169

2. Persons and families below **poverty** level, according to selected characteristics, race, and Hispanic origin: United States, selected years 1973–96_____ 171

Fertility and Natality

3. Crude birth rates, **fertility rates, and birth rates** by age of mother, according to detailed race and Hispanic origin: United States, selected years 1950–96_____ 172

4. **Women** 15–44 years of age **who have not had at least one live birth,** by age: United States, selected years 1960–96_____ 174

5. **Live births,** according to detailed race of mother and Hispanic origin of mother: United States, selected years 1970–96_____ 175

6. **Prenatal care** for live births, according to detailed race of mother and Hispanic origin of mother: United States, selected years 1970–96_____ 176

7. **Teenage childbearing,** according to detailed race of mother and Hispanic origin of mother: United States, selected years 1970–96_____ 177

8. **Nonmarital childbearing** according to detailed race of mother, Hispanic origin of mother, and maternal age and birth rates for unmarried women by race of mother and Hispanic origin of mother: United States, selected years 1970–96_____ 178

9. **Maternal education** for live births, according to detailed race of mother and Hispanic origin of mother: United States, selected years 1970–96_____ 179

10. **Mothers who smoked cigarettes** during pregnancy, according to mother's detailed race, Hispanic origin, age, and educational attainment: Selected States, 1989–96_____ 180

11. **Low-birthweight** live births, according to mother's detailed race, Hispanic origin, and smoking status: United States, selected years 1970–96_____ 181

12. **Low-birthweight** live births among mothers 20 years of age and over, by mother's detailed race, Hispanic origin, and educational attainment: Selected States, 1989–96_____ 182

13. **Low-birthweight** live births, according to race of mother, geographic division, and State: United States, average annual 1984–86, 1989–91, and 1994–96_____ 183

14. **Very low-birthweight** live births, according to race of mother, geographic division, and State: United States, average annual 1984–86, 1989–91, and 1994–96_____ 184

15. Legal **abortion ratios,** according to selected patient characteristics: United States, selected years 1973–95_____ 185

16. Legal **abortions,** according to selected characteristics: United States, selected years 1973–95_____ 186

17. Legal abortions, **abortion-related deaths,** and abortion-related death rates, according to period of gestation: United States, 1974–76 through 1989–91_____ 187

18. Methods of **contraception** for women 15–44 years of age, according to race and age: United States, 1982, 1988, and 1995_____ 188

19. **Breastfeeding** by mothers 15–44 years of age by year of baby's birth, according to selected characteristics of mother: United States, 1972–74 to 1993–94_____ 189

Mortality

20. **Infant, neonatal, and postneonatal mortality rates,** according to detailed race of mother and Hispanic origin of mother: United States, selected birth cohorts 1983–95_____ 190

21. **Infant mortality rates** for mothers 20 years of age and over, according to educational attainment, detailed race of mother, and Hispanic origin of mother: United States, selected birth cohorts 1983–95_____ 191

22. **Infant mortality rates** according to birthweight: United States, selected birth cohorts 1983–95_____ 192

23. **Infant mortality rates,** fetal mortality rates, and perinatal mortality rates, according to race: United States, selected years 1950–96_____ 193

24. **Infant mortality rates,** according to race, geographic division, and State: United States, average annual 1984–86, 1989–91, and 1994–96____ 194

25. **Neonatal mortality rates,** according to race, geographic division, and State: United States, average annual 1984–86, 1989–91, and 1994–96____ 195

26. **Postneonatal mortality rates,** according to race, geographic division, and State: United States, average annual 1984–86, 1989–91, and 1994–96____ 196

27. **Infant mortality rates,** feto-infant mortality rates, and postneonatal mortality rates, and average annual percent change: Selected countries, 1989 and 1994_____ 197

List of Detailed Tables

28. **Life expectancy** at birth and at 65 years of age, according to sex: Selected countries, 1989 and 1994____ 198

29. **Life expectancy** at birth, at 65 years of age, and at 75 years of age, according to race and sex: United States, selected years 1900–96____ 200

30. **Age-adjusted death rates,** according to detailed race, Hispanic origin, geographic division, and State: United States, average annual 1984–86, 1989–91, and 1994–96____ 201

31. **Age-adjusted death rates** for selected causes of death, according to sex, detailed race, and Hispanic origin: United States, selected years 1950–96____ 203

32. **Years of potential life lost** before age 75 for selected causes of death, according to sex, detailed race, and Hispanic origin: United States, selected years 1980–96____ 207

33. **Leading causes of death** and numbers of deaths, according to sex, detailed race, and Hispanic origin: United States, 1980 and 1996____ 212

34. **Leading causes of death** and numbers of deaths, according to age: United States, 1980 and 1996____ 216

35. Age-adjusted death rates, according to race, sex, region, and **urbanization:** United States, average annual 1984–86, 1989–91, and 1993–95____ 218

36. Death rates for persons 25–64 years of age, for all races and the white population, according to sex, age, and **educational attainment:** Selected States, 1994–96____ 220

37. **Death rates** for all causes, according to sex, detailed race, Hispanic origin, and age: United States, selected years 1950–96____ 221

38. Death rates for **diseases of heart,** according to sex, detailed race, Hispanic origin, and age: United States, selected years 1950–96____ 225

39. Death rates for **cerebrovascular diseases,** according to sex, detailed race, Hispanic origin, and age: United States, selected years 1950–96____ 228

40. Death rates for **malignant neoplasms,** according to sex, detailed race, Hispanic origin, and age: United States, selected years 1950–96____ 231

41. Death rates for **malignant neoplasms of respiratory system,** according to sex, detailed race, Hispanic origin, and age: United States, selected years 1950–96____ 235

42. Death rates for **malignant neoplasm of breast** for females, according to detailed race, Hispanic origin, and age: United States, selected years 1950–96____ 238

43. Death rates for **chronic obstructive pulmonary diseases,** according to sex, detailed race, Hispanic origin, and age: United States, selected years 1980–96____ 240

44. Death rates for **human immunodeficiency virus (HIV) infection,** according to sex, detailed race, Hispanic origin, and age: United States, 1987–96____ 243

45. **Maternal mortality** for complications of pregnancy, childbirth, and the puerperium, according to race, Hispanic origin, and age: United States, selected years 1950–96____ 245

46. Death rates for **motor vehicle-related injuries,** according to sex, detailed race, Hispanic origin, and age: United States, selected years 1950–96____ 246

47. Death rates for **homicide** and legal intervention, according to sex, detailed race, Hispanic origin, and age: United States, selected years 1950–96____ 250

48. Death rates for **suicide,** according to sex, detailed race, Hispanic origin, and age: United States, selected years 1950–96____ 253

49. Death rates for **firearm-related injuries,** according to sex, detailed race, Hispanic origin, and age: United States, selected years 1970–96____ 256

50. Deaths from selected **occupational diseases** for males, according to age: United States, selected years 1970–96____ 259

51. **Occupational injury deaths,** according to industry: United States, selected years 1980–93____ 260

Determinants and Measures of Health

52. **Vaccinations** of children 19–35 months of age for selected diseases, according to race, Hispanic origin, poverty status, and residence in metropolitan statistical area (MSA): United States, 1994–96____ 261

53. **Vaccination coverage** among children 19–35 months of age according to geographic division, State, and selected urban areas: United States, 1994–96____ 262

54. Selected **notifiable disease rates,** according to disease: United States, selected years 1950–96____ 264

55. Acquired immunodeficiency syndrome (**AIDS**) cases, according to age at diagnosis, sex, detailed race, and Hispanic origin: United States, selected years 1985–97____ 265

56. Acquired immunodeficiency syndrome (AIDS) cases, according to race, Hispanic origin, sex, and transmission category for persons 13 years of age and over at diagnosis: United States, selected years 1985–97_____ 266

57. Acquired immunodeficiency syndrome (AIDS) cases, according to geographic division and State: United States, selected years 1985–97_____ 268

58. Age-adjusted cancer incidence rates for selected cancer sites, according to sex and race: Selected geographic areas, selected years 1973–95__ 269

59. Five-year relative cancer survival rates for selected cancer sites, according to race and sex: Selected geographic areas, 1974–79, 1980–82, 1983–85, 1986–88, and 1989–94_____ 270

60. Limitation of activity caused by chronic conditions, according to selected characteristics: United States, 1990 and 1995_____ 271

61. Respondent-assessed health status, according to selected characteristics: United States, 1987–95__ 272

62. Current cigarette smoking by persons 18 years of age and over, according to sex, race, and age: United States, selected years 1965–95_____ 273

63. Age-adjusted prevalence of current cigarette smoking by persons 25 years of age and over, according to sex, race, and education: United States, selected years 1974–95_____ 274

64. Use of selected substances in the past month by persons 12 years of age and over, according to age, sex, race, and Hispanic origin: United States, selected years 1979–96_____ 275

65. Use of selected substances in the past month and heavy alcohol use in the past 2 weeks by high school seniors and eighth-graders, according to sex and race: United States, selected years 1980–97____ 277

66. Cocaine-related emergency room episodes, according to age, sex, race, and Hispanic origin: United States, selected years 1985–95_____ 279

67. Alcohol consumption by persons 18 years of age and over, according to sex, race, Hispanic origin, and age: United States, 1985 and 1990_____ 280

68. Hypertension among persons 20 years of age and over, according to sex, age, race, and Hispanic origin: United States, 1960–62, 1971–74, 1976–80, and 1988–94_____ 281

69. Serum cholesterol levels among persons 20 years of age and over, according to sex, age, race, and Hispanic origin: United States, 1960–62, 1971–74, 1976–80, and 1988–94_____ 282

70. Overweight persons 20 years of age and over, according to sex, age, race, and Hispanic origin: United States, 1960–62, 1971–74, 1976–80, and 1988–94_____ 283

71. Overweight children and adolescents 6–17 years of age, according to sex, age, race, and Hispanic origin: United States, selected years 1963–65 through 1988–94_____ 284

72. Persons residing in counties that met national ambient air quality standards throughout the year, by race and Hispanic origin: United States, selected years 1988–96_____ 285

73. Occupational injuries with lost workdays in the private sector, according to industry: United States, selected years 1980–96_____ 286

Utilization of Health Resources

Ambulatory Care

74. Physician contacts, according to selected patient characteristics: United States, 1987–95_____ 287

75. Physician contacts, according to place of contact and selected patient characteristics: United States, 1990 and 1995_____ 288

76. Physician contacts, according to respondent-assessed health status, age, sex, and poverty status: United States, 1987–89 and 1993–95_____ 289

77. Interval since last physician contact, according to selected patient characteristics: United States, 1964, 1990, and 1995_____ 290

78. No physician contact within the past 12 months among children under 6 years of age according to selected characteristics: United States, average annual 1993–94 and 1994–95_____ 291

79. No usual source of health care among children under 18 years of age according to selected characteristics: United States, average annual 1993–94 and 1994–95_____ 292

80. Use of mammography for women 40 years of age and over according to selected characteristics: United States, selected years 1987–94_____ 293

81. Ambulatory care visits to physician offices and hospital outpatient and emergency departments by selected patient characteristics: United States, 1993–96_____ 295

List of Detailed Tables

82. **Ambulatory care visits** to physician offices, percent distribution according to selected patient characteristics and physician specialty: United States, 1975, 1985, and 1996_____ 297

83. Persons with a **dental visit** within the past year among persons 25 years of age and over, according to selected patient characteristics: United States, selected years 1983–93_____ 298

84. **Substance abuse clients** in specialty treatment units according to substance abused, geographic division, and State: United States, 1992 and 1995___ 299

85. **Additions to mental health organizations** according to type of service and organization: United States, selected years 1983–94_____ 300

86. **Home health care and hospice patients,** according to selected characteristics: United States, 1992–96_____ 301

Inpatient Care

87. **Discharges,** days of care, and average length of stay in short-stay hospitals, according to selected characteristics: United States, 1964, 1990, and 1995_____ 302

88. **Discharges,** days of care, and average length of stay in non-Federal short-stay hospitals, according to selected characteristics: United States, selected years 1980–95_____ 303

89. **Discharges,** days of care, and average length of stay in non-Federal short-stay hospitals for discharges with the diagnosis of human immunodeficiency virus (HIV) and for all discharges: United States, 1986–95_____ 304

90. **Rates of discharges** and days of care in non-Federal short-stay hospitals, according to sex, age, and selected first-listed diagnosis: United States, 1985, 1990, 1994, and 1995_____ 305

91. **Discharges** and average length of stay in non-Federal short-stay hospitals, according to sex, age, and selected first-listed diagnosis: United States, 1985, 1990, 1994, and 1995_____ 308

92. **Operations** for inpatients discharged from non-Federal short-stay hospitals, according to sex, age, and surgical category: United States, 1985, 1990, 1994, and 1995_____ 311

93. Diagnostic and other **nonsurgical procedures** for inpatients discharged from non-Federal short-stay hospitals, according to sex, age, and procedure category: United States, 1985, 1990, 1994, and 1995_____ 314

94. Hospital admissions, average length of stay, and outpatient visits, according to type of ownership and size of hospital, and percent **outpatient surgery:** United States, selected years 1975–96_____ 316

95. **Nursing home** and personal care home residents 65 years of age and over according to age, sex, and race: United States, 1963, 1973–74, 1985, and 1995_____ 317

96. **Nursing home residents** 65 years of age and over, according to selected functional status and age, sex, and race: United States, 1985 and 1995___ 318

97. **Additions** to selected inpatient **psychiatric organizations** according to sex, age, and race: United States, 1975, 1980, and 1986_____ 319

98. **Additions** to selected inpatient **psychiatric organizations,** according to selected primary diagnoses and age: United States, 1975, 1980, and 1986_____ 320

Health Care Resources

Personnel

99. **Persons employed** in health service sites: United States, selected years 1970–96_____ 321

100. Active non-Federal **physicians** and doctors of medicine in patient care, according to geographic division and State: United States, 1975, 1985, 1990, and 1996_____ 322

101. **Physicians,** according to activity and place of medical education: United States and outlying U.S. areas, selected years 1975–96_____ 324

102. **Primary care doctors of medicine,** according to specialty: United States and outlying U.S. areas, selected years 1949–96_____ 325

103. Active **health personnel** according to occupation and geographic region: United States, 1980, 1990, and 1995_____ 326

104. Full-time equivalent **employment in** selected occupations for **community hospitals:** United States, selected years 1983–93_____ 327

105. Full-time equivalent patient care **staff in mental health organizations,** according to type of organization and staff discipline: United States, selected years 1984–94_____ 328

106. First-year enrollment and **graduates of health professions schools** and number of schools, according to profession: United States, selected years 1950–96 and projections for year 2000_____ 330

107. Total **enrollment of minorities** in schools for selected health occupations, according to detailed race and Hispanic origin: United States, academic years 1970–71, 1980–81, 1990–91, and 1995–96___ 331

108. First-year and total **enrollment of women** in schools for selected health occupations, according to detailed race and Hispanic origin: United States, academic years 1971–72, 1980–81, 1990–91, and 1995–96___ 333

Facilities

109. **Hospitals,** beds, and occupancy rates, according to type of ownership and size of hospital: United States, selected years 1975–96___ 334

110. Inpatient and residential **mental health organizations** and beds, according to type of organization: United States, selected years 1984–94_ 335

111. **Community hospital beds** and average annual percent change, according to geographic division and State: United States, selected years 1940–96___ 336

112. **Occupancy rates** in community hospitals and average annual percent change, according to geographic division and State: United States, selected years 1940–96___ 337

113. **Nursing homes** with 3 or more beds, beds, and bed rates, according to geographic division and State: United States, 1976, 1986, and 1991___ 338

114. **Nursing homes,** beds, occupancy, and residents, according to geographic division and State: United States, 1992 and 1996___ 339

Health Care Expenditures

National Health Expenditures

115. Gross domestic product, **national health expenditures,** and Federal and State and local government expenditures and average annual percent change: United States, selected years 1960–96___ 341

116. **Total health expenditures** as a percent of gross domestic product and per capita health expenditures in dollars: Selected countries and years 1960–95___ 342

117. **Consumer Price Index** and average annual percent change for all items and selected items: United States, selected years 1960–97___ 343

118. **Consumer Price Index** and average annual percent change for all items and medical care components: United States, selected years 1960–97___ 344

119. **National health expenditures** and average annual percent change, according to source of funds: United States, selected years 1929–96___ 345

120. **National health expenditures,** percent distribution, and average annual percent change, according to type of expenditure: United States, selected years 1960–96___ 346

121. **Expenditures for health services** and supplies and percent distribution, by type of payer: United States, selected calendar years 1965–95___ 348

122. **Employers' costs** per employee hour worked for total compensation, wages and salaries, and **health insurance,** according to selected characteristics: United States, selected years 1991–97___ 350

123. **Personal health care expenditures** average annual percent increase and percent distribution of factors affecting growth: United States, 1960–96___ 351

124. **Personal health care expenditures** and percent distribution, according to source of funds: United States, selected years 1929–96___ 352

125. **Expenditures on hospital care,** nursing home care, physician services, and all other personal health care expenditures and percent distribution, according to source of funds: United States, selected years 1960–96___ 353

126. **Hospital expenses,** according to type of ownership and size of hospital: United States, selected years 1975–96___ 354

127. **Nursing home average monthly charges** per resident and percent of residents, according to selected facility and resident characteristics: United States, 1964, 1973–74, 1977, and 1985___ 355

128. **Nursing home average monthly charges** per resident and percent of residents, according to primary source of payments and selected facility characteristics: United States, 1977 and 1985___ 356

129. **Mental health expenditures,** percent distribution, and per capita expenditures, according to type of mental health organization: United States, selected years 1975–94___ 357

130. National **funding for health research** and development and average annual percent change, according to source of funds: United States, selected years 1960–95___ 358

List of Detailed Tables ....

131. Federal **funding for health research** and development and percent distribution, according to agency: United States, selected fiscal years 1970–95_____ 359

132. Federal **spending for human immunodeficiency virus (HIV)-related activities,** according to agency and type of activity: United States, selected fiscal years 1985–97_____ 360

Health Care Coverage and Major Federal Programs

133. **Health care coverage** for persons under 65 years of age, according to type of coverage and selected characteristics: United States, selected years 1984–96_____ 361

134. **Health care coverage** for persons 65 years of age and over, according to type of coverage and selected characteristics: United States, selected years 1984–96_____ 363

135. **Health maintenance organizations** (HMO's) and enrollment, according to model type, geographic region, and Federal program: United States, selected years 1976–97_____ 365

136. **Medical care benefits** for employees of private establishments by size of establishment and occupation: United States, selected years 1990–95__ 366

137. **Medicare** enrollees and expenditures and percent distribution, according to type of service: United States and other areas, selected years 1967–96_____ 367

138. **Medicare** enrollment, persons served, and payments for Medicare enrollees 65 years of age and over, according to selected characteristics: United States and other areas, selected years 1977–95_____ 368

139. **Medicaid** recipients and medical vendor payments, according to basis of eligibility: United States, selected fiscal years 1972–96_____ 369

140. **Medicaid** recipients and medical vendor payments, according to type of service: United States, selected fiscal years 1972–96_____ 370

141. **Department of Veterans Affairs** health care expenditures and use, and persons treated according to selected characteristics: United States, selected fiscal years 1970–96_____ 371

State Health Expenditures

142. **Hospital care expenditures** by geographic division and State and average annual percent change: United States, selected years 1980–93_____ 372

143. **Physician service expenditures** by geographic division and State and average annual percent change: United States, selected years 1980–93_____ 373

144. **Expenditures for purchases of prescription drugs** by geographic division and State and average annual percent change: United States, selected years 1980–93_____ 374

145. State mental health agency per capita **expenditures for mental health services** and average annual percent change by geographic division and State: United States, selected fiscal years 1981–93_____ 375

146. **Medicare** enrollees, enrollees in managed care, payments per enrollee, and short-stay hospital utilization by geographic division and State: United States, 1990 and 1995_____ 376

147. **Medicaid** recipients, recipients in managed care, payments per recipient, and recipients per 100 persons below the poverty level by geographic division and State: United States, selected fiscal years 1980–96_____ 377

148. Persons enrolled in **health maintenance organizations** (HMO's) by geographic division and State: United States, selected years 1980–97_____ 378

149. **Persons without health care coverage** by geographic division and State: United States, selected years 1987–96_____ 379

Table 1 (page 1 of 2). Resident population, according to age, sex, detailed race, and Hispanic origin: United States, selected years 1950–96

[Data are based on decennial census updated by data from multiple sources]

Sex, race, Hispanic origin, and year	Total resident population	Under 1 year	1–4 years	5–14 years	15–24 years	25–34 years	35–44 years	45–54 years	55–64 years	65–74 years	75–84 years	85 years and over
All persons						Number in thousands						
1950	150,697	3,147	13,017	24,319	22,098	23,759	21,450	17,343	13,370	8,340	3,278	577
1960	179,323	4,112	16,209	35,465	24,020	22,818	24,081	20,485	15,572	10,997	4,633	929
1970	203,212	3,485	13,669	40,746	35,441	24,907	23,088	23,220	18,590	12,435	6,119	1,511
1980	226,546	3,534	12,815	34,942	42,487	37,082	25,634	22,800	21,703	15,580	7,729	2,240
1990	248,710	3,946	14,812	35,095	37,013	43,161	37,435	25,057	21,113	18,045	10,012	3,021
1995	262,755	3,848	15,743	38,134	35,947	40,873	42,468	31,079	21,131	18,759	11,145	3,628
1996	265,284	3,769	15,516	38,422	36,221	40,368	43,393	32,370	21,361	18,669	11,430	3,762
Male												
1950	74,833	1,602	6,634	12,375	10,918	11,597	10,588	8,655	6,697	4,024	1,507	237
1960	88,331	2,090	8,240	18,029	11,906	11,179	11,755	10,093	7,537	5,116	2,025	362
1970	98,912	1,778	6,968	20,759	17,551	12,217	11,231	11,199	8,793	5,437	2,436	542
1980	110,053	1,806	6,556	17,855	21,418	18,382	12,570	11,009	10,152	6,757	2,867	682
1990	121,239	2,018	7,581	17,971	18,915	21,564	18,510	12,232	9,955	7,907	3,745	841
1995	128,314	1,970	8,055	19,529	18,352	20,432	21,062	15,182	10,044	8,342	4,330	1,017
1996	129,810	1,928	7,940	19,681	18,618	20,191	21,569	15,837	10,166	8,325	4,486	1,070
Female												
1950	75,864	1,545	6,383	11,944	11,181	12,162	10,863	8,688	6,672	4,316	1,771	340
1960	90,992	2,022	7,969	17,437	12,114	11,639	12,326	10,393	8,036	5,881	2,609	567
1970	104,300	1,707	6,701	19,986	17,890	12,690	11,857	12,021	9,797	6,998	3,683	969
1980	116,493	1,727	6,259	17,087	21,068	18,700	13,065	11,791	11,551	8,825	4,862	1,559
1990	127,471	1,928	7,231	17,124	18,098	21,596	18,925	12,824	11,158	10,139	6,267	2,180
1995	134,441	1,878	7,688	18,606	17,595	20,441	21,406	15,897	11,087	10,417	6,815	2,611
1996	135,474	1,841	7,577	18,741	17,604	20,177	21,825	16,533	11,195	10,345	6,944	2,692
White male												
1950	67,129	1,400	5,845	10,860	9,689	10,430	9,529	7,836	6,180	3,736	1,406	218
1960	78,367	1,784	7,065	15,659	10,483	9,940	10,564	9,114	6,850	4,702	1,875	331
1970	86,721	1,501	5,873	17,667	15,232	10,775	9,979	10,090	7,958	4,916	2,243	487
1980	94,924	1,485	5,397	14,764	18,110	15,928	11,005	9,771	9,149	6,095	2,600	621
1990	102,143	1,604	6,071	14,467	15,389	18,071	15,819	10,624	8,813	7,127	3,397	760
1995	106,994	1,547	6,377	15,539	14,714	16,858	17,743	13,125	8,778	7,455	3,940	919
1996	108,052	1,546	6,294	15,622	14,910	16,587	18,128	13,649	8,864	7,419	4,076	959
White female												
1950	67,813	1,341	5,599	10,431	9,821	10,851	9,719	7,868	6,168	4,031	1,669	314
1960	80,465	1,714	6,795	15,068	10,596	10,204	11,000	9,364	7,327	5,428	2,441	527
1970	91,028	1,434	5,615	16,912	15,420	11,004	10,349	10,756	8,853	6,366	3,429	890
1980	99,788	1,410	5,121	14,048	17,643	15,887	11,227	10,282	10,324	7,950	4,457	1,440
1990	106,561	1,524	5,762	13,706	14,599	17,757	15,834	10,946	9,698	9,048	5,687	2,001
1995	111,092	1,467	6,060	14,737	13,965	16,529	17,645	13,459	9,487	9,189	6,168	2,385
1996	111,696	1,469	5,980	14,816	13,937	16,230	17,953	13,946	9,551	9,093	6,273	2,447
Black male												
1950	7,300	- - -	- - -	1,442	1,162	1,105	1,003	772	460	299	- - -	- - -
1960	9,114	281	1,082	2,185	1,305	1,120	1,086	891	617	382	137	29
1970	10,748	245	975	2,784	2,041	1,226	1,084	979	739	461	169	46
1980	12,612	270	970	2,618	2,813	1,974	1,238	1,026	855	568	228	53
1990	14,420	322	1,164	2,700	2,669	2,592	1,962	1,175	878	614	277	66
1995	15,721	314	1,256	2,994	2,730	2,565	2,416	1,466	925	674	302	79
1996	15,903	277	1,218	3,044	2,756	2,565	2,485	1,545	937	682	311	83
Black female												
1950	7,745	- - -	- - -	1,446	1,300	1,260	1,112	796	443	322	- - -	- - -
1960	9,758	283	1,085	2,191	1,404	1,300	1,229	974	663	430	160	38
1970	11,832	243	970	2,773	2,196	1,456	1,309	1,134	868	582	230	71
1980	14,071	267	953	2,583	2,942	2,272	1,490	1,260	1,061	777	360	106
1990	16,063	316	1,137	2,641	2,700	2,905	2,279	1,416	1,135	884	495	156
1995	17,420	307	1,223	2,908	2,730	2,855	2,762	1,770	1,201	943	526	195
1996	17,600	270	1,185	2,953	2,741	2,847	2,830	1,864	1,221	951	535	203

See notes at end of table.

Table 1 (page 2 of 2). Resident population, according to age, sex, detailed race, and Hispanic origin: United States, selected years 1950–96

[Data are based on decennial census updated by data from multiple sources]

Sex, race, Hispanic origin, and year	Total resident population	Under 1 year	1–4 years	5–14 years	15–24 years	25–34 years	35–44 years	45–54 years	55–64 years	65–74 years	75–84 years	85 years and over
American Indian or Alaska Native male						Number in thousands						
1980	702	17	60	153	164	114	75	53	37	22	9	2
1990	1,024	24	88	206	192	183	140	86	55	32	13	3
1995	1,110	21	84	234	196	186	163	106	61	38	17	5
1996	1,136	20	82	236	203	192	168	110	63	39	18	5
American Indian or Alaska Native female												
1980	718	16	57	149	158	118	79	57	41	26	12	4
1990	1,041	24	85	200	178	186	148	92	61	41	21	6
1995	1,132	21	82	227	190	180	170	113	69	46	25	10
1996	1,152	20	80	228	195	182	174	118	71	47	26	11
Asian or Pacific Islander male												
1980	1,814	35	129	321	334	367	252	159	110	72	29	6
1990	3,652	68	258	598	665	718	588	347	208	133	57	12
1995	4,489	87	340	761	713	823	740	485	280	176	72	14
1996	4,719	86	346	779	749	849	788	532	302	185	82	22
Asian or Pacific Islander female												
1980	1,915	34	127	307	325	423	269	193	126	70	33	9
1990	3,805	65	247	578	621	749	664	371	264	166	65	17
1995	4,797	83	323	734	710	877	828	556	330	238	96	22
1996	5,024	83	332	743	731	918	867	605	352	254	110	31
Hispanic male												
1980	7,280	187	661	1,530	1,646	1,255	761	570	364	201	86	19
1990	11,388	279	980	2,128	2,376	2,310	1,471	818	551	312	131	32
1995	13,676	338	1,306	2,600	2,397	2,674	1,978	1,105	652	419	164	43
1996	14,519	343	1,334	2,658	2,677	2,779	2,164	1,212	683	439	179	51
Hispanic female												
1980	7,329	181	634	1,482	1,547	1,249	805	615	411	257	116	30
1990	10,966	268	939	2,039	2,028	2,073	1,448	868	632	403	209	59
1995	13,318	321	1,246	2,488	2,214	2,359	1,903	1,167	744	528	260	87
1996	13,750	326	1,269	2,534	2,298	2,373	2,016	1,242	769	549	275	99
Non-Hispanic White male												
1980	88,035	1,308	4,773	13,318	16,555	14,739	10,285	9,229	8,802	5,906	2,519	603
1990	91,743	1,351	5,181	12,525	13,219	15,967	14,481	9,875	8,303	6,837	3,275	729
1995	94,540	1,239	5,184	13,186	12,529	14,426	15,949	12,117	8,179	7,067	3,786	878
1996	94,799	1,232	5,075	13,216	12,455	14,049	16,160	12,542	8,237	7,012	3,909	911
Non-Hispanic White female												
1980	92,872	1,240	4,522	12,647	16,185	14,711	10,468	9,700	9,935	7,708	4,345	1,411
1990	96,557	1,280	4,909	11,846	12,749	15,872	14,520	10,153	9,116	8,674	5,491	1,945
1995	98,983	1,174	4,921	12,485	11,955	14,393	15,921	12,397	8,806	8,703	5,926	2,302
1996	99,179	1,171	4,821	12,521	11,843	14,075	16,125	12,817	8,848	8,587	6,017	2,353

- - - Data not available.

NOTES: The race groups, white, black, American Indian or Alaska Native, and Asian or Pacific Islander, include persons of Hispanic and non-Hispanic origin. Conversely, persons of Hispanic origin may be of any race. Population figures are census counts as of April 1 for 1950, 1960, 1970, 1980, and 1990 and estimates as of July 1 for other years. See Appendix I, Department of Commerce. Populations for age groups may not sum to the total due to rounding. Although population figures are shown rounded to the nearest 1,000, calculations of birth rates and death rates shown in this volume are based on unrounded population figures for decennial years and starting with data year 1992. See Appendix II, Rate. Some numbers have been revised and differ from the previous edition of *Health, United States*.

SOURCES: U.S. Bureau of the Census: 1950 Nonwhite Population by Race. Special Report P-E, No. 3B. Washington. U.S. Government Printing Office, 1951; U.S. Census of Population: 1960, Number of Inhabitants, PC(1)-A1, United States Summary, 1964; 1970, Number of Inhabitants, Final Report PC(1)-A1, United States Summary, 1971; U.S. population estimates, by age, sex, race, and Hispanic origin: 1980 to 1991. Current Population Reports. Series P–25, No. 1095. Washington. U.S. Government Printing Office, Feb. 1993; U.S. resident population—estimates by age, sex, race, and Hispanic origin (consistent with the 1990 Census, as enumerated): 1992. Census files RESP0792 in PPL–21, series 1294. 1993; July 1, 1993. RES0793. 1994; July 1, 1994. RESD0794. 1995; July 1, 1995. RESD0795. 1996; July 1, 1996. NESTV96 in PPL-S7. 1997.

Table 2. Persons and families below poverty level, according to selected characteristics, race, and Hispanic origin: United States, selected years 1973–96

[Data are based on household interviews of the civilian noninstitutionalized population]

Selected characteristics	1973	1980	1985	1989	1990	1991	1992	1993	1994	1995	1996
All persons					Percent below poverty						
All races.................	11.1	13.0	14.0	12.8	13.5	14.2	14.8	15.1	14.5	13.8	13.7
White...................	8.4	10.2	11.4	10.0	10.7	11.3	11.9	12.2	11.7	11.2	11.2
Black...................	31.4	32.5	31.3	30.7	31.9	32.7	33.4	33.1	30.6	29.3	28.4
Asian or Pacific Islander.......	- - -	- - -	- - -	14.1	12.2	13.8	12.7	15.3	14.6	14.6	14.5
Hispanic origin	21.9	25.7	29.0	26.2	28.1	28.7	29.6	30.6	30.7	30.3	29.4
Mexican.............	- - -	- - -	28.8	28.4	28.1	29.5	30.1	31.6	32.3	31.2	31.0
Puerto Rican...........	- - -	- - -	43.3	33.0	40.6	39.4	36.5	38.4	36.0	38.1	35.7
White, non-Hispanic..........	- - -	- - -	- - -	8.3	8.8	9.4	9.6	9.9	9.4	8.5	8.6
Related children under 18 years of age in families											
All races.................	14.2	17.9	20.1	19.0	19.9	21.1	21.6	22.0	21.2	20.2	19.8
White...................	9.7	13.4	15.6	14.1	15.1	16.1	16.5	17.0	16.3	15.5	15.5
Black...................	40.6	42.1	43.1	43.2	44.2	45.6	46.3	45.9	43.3	41.5	39.5
Asian or Pacific Islander.......	- - -	- - -	- - -	18.9	17.0	17.1	16.0	17.6	17.9	18.6	19.1
Hispanic origin	27.8	33.0	39.6	35.5	37.7	39.8	39.0	39.9	41.1	39.3	39.9
Mexican.............	- - -	- - -	37.4	36.3	35.5	38.9	38.2	39.5	41.8	39.3	40.7
Puerto Rican...........	- - -	- - -	58.6	48.0	56.7	57.7	52.2	53.8	50.5	53.2	49.4
White, non-Hispanic..........	- - -	- - -	- - -	10.9	11.6	12.4	12.4	12.8	11.8	10.6	10.4
Related children under 18 years of age in families with female householder and no spouse present											
All races.................	- - -	50.8	53.6	51.1	53.4	55.5	54.3	53.7	52.9	50.3	49.3
White...................	- - -	41.6	45.2	42.5	45.9	47.1	45.3	45.6	45.7	42.5	43.1
Black...................	- - -	64.8	66.9	63.1	64.7	68.2	67.1	65.9	63.2	61.6	58.2
Asian or Pacific Islander.......	- - -	- - -	- - -	63.7	32.2	31.9	43.5	32.2	36.8	42.4	48.8
Hispanic origin	- - -	65.0	72.4	64.3	68.4	68.6	65.7	66.1	68.3	65.7	67.4
Mexican.............	- - -	- - -	64.4	64.5	62.4	66.6	63.5	64.6	69.5	65.9	68.1
Puerto Rican...........	- - -	- - -	85.4	74.4	82.7	83.3	74.1	73.4	73.6	79.6	76.6
White, non-Hispanic..........	- - -	- - -	- - -	36.2	39.6	41.0	39.6	39.0	38.0	33.5	34.9
All persons					Number below poverty in thousands						
All races.................	22,973	29,272	33,064	31,528	33,585	35,708	38,014	39,265	38,059	36,425	36,529
White...................	15,142	19,699	22,860	20,785	22,326	23,747	25,259	26,226	25,379	24,423	24,650
Black...................	7,388	8,579	8,926	9,302	9,837	10,242	10,827	10,877	10,196	9,872	9,694
Asian or Pacific Islander.......	- - -	- - -	- - -	939	858	996	985	1,134	974	1,411	1,454
Hispanic origin	2,366	3,491	5,236	5,430	6,006	6,339	7,592	8,126	8,416	8,574	8,697
Mexican.............	- - -	- - -	3,220	3,777	3,764	4,149	4,404	5,373	5,781	5,608	5,815
Puerto Rican...........	- - -	- - -	1,011	720	966	924	874	1,061	981	1,183	1,116
White, non-Hispanic..........	- - -	- - -	- - -	15,599	16,622	17,741	18,202	18,882	18,110	16,267	16,462
Related children under 18 years of age in families											
All races.................	9,453	11,114	12,483	12,001	12,715	13,658	14,521	14,961	14,610	13,999	13,764
White...................	5,462	6,817	7,838	7,164	7,696	8,316	8,752	9,123	8,826	8,474	8,488
Black...................	3,822	3,906	4,057	4,257	4,412	4,637	5,015	5,030	4,787	4,644	4,411
Asian or Pacific Islander.......	- - -	- - -	- - -	368	356	348	352	358	308	532	553
Hispanic origin	1,364	1,718	2,512	2,496	2,750	2,977	3,440	3,666	3,956	3,938	4,090
Mexican.............	- - -	- - -	1,589	1,785	1,733	2,004	2,019	2,520	2,805	2,655	2,853
Puerto Rican...........	- - -	- - -	535	354	490	475	457	537	485	610	545
White, non-Hispanic..........	- - -	- - -	- - -	4,779	5,106	5,497	5,558	5,819	5,404	4,745	4,656
Related children under 18 years of age in families with female householder and no spouse present											
All races.................	- - -	5,866	6,716	6,808	7,363	8,065	8,032	8,503	8,427	8,364	7,990
White...................	- - -	2,813	3,372	3,255	3,597	3,941	3,783	4,102	4,099	4,051	4,029
Black...................	- - -	2,944	3,181	3,326	3,543	3,853	3,967	4,104	3,935	3,954	3,619
Asian or Pacific Islander.......	- - -	- - -	- - -	115	80	81	103	72	59	145	167
Hispanic origin	- - -	809	1,247	1,158	1,314	1,398	1,289	1,673	1,804	1,872	1,779
Mexican.............	- - -	- - -	553	677	615	785	679	890	1,054	1,056	948
Puerto Rican...........	- - -	- - -	449	281	382	369	363	430	394	459	444
White, non-Hispanic..........	- - -	- - -	- - -	2,160	2,411	2,661	2,588	2,636	2,563	2,299	2,419

- - - Data not available.

NOTES: The race groups, white and black, include persons of both Hispanic and non-Hispanic origin. Conversely, persons of Hispanic origin may be of any race. Poverty status is based on family income and family size using Bureau of the Census poverty thresholds. See Appendix II. In 1989, 31.2 percent of the American Indian population in the United States, or 585,000 persons, were below the poverty threshhold, based on 1989 income data from the 1990 decennial census (U.S. Bureau of the Census, 1990 Census of Population, *Characteristics of American Indians by Tribe and Language*, 1990 CP–3–7).

SOURCE: U.S. Bureau of the Census. Lamison-White L. Poverty in the United States: 1996. Current population reports, series P–60, no 198. Washington: U.S. Government Printing Office. 1997; unpublished data.

Table 3 (page 1 of 2). Crude birth rates, fertility rates, and birth rates by age of mother, according to detailed race and Hispanic origin: United States, selected years 1950–96

[Data are based on the National Vital Statistics System]

Race of mother, Hispanic origin of mother, and year	Crude birth rate[1]	Fertility rate[2]	10–14 years	15–19 years Total	15–17 years	18–19 years	20–24 years	25–29 years	30–34 years	35–39 years	40–44 years	45–49 years
All races						Live births per 1,000 women						
1950	24.1	106.2	1.0	81.6	40.7	132.7	196.6	166.1	103.7	52.9	15.1	1.2
1960	23.7	118.0	0.8	89.1	43.9	166.7	258.1	197.4	112.7	56.2	15.5	0.9
1970	18.4	87.9	1.2	68.3	38.8	114.7	167.8	145.1	73.3	31.7	8.1	0.5
1980	15.9	68.4	1.1	53.0	32.5	82.1	115.1	112.9	61.9	19.8	3.9	0.2
1985	15.8	66.3	1.2	51.0	31.0	79.6	108.3	111.0	69.1	24.0	4.0	0.2
1990	16.7	70.9	1.4	59.9	37.5	88.6	116.5	120.2	80.8	31.7	5.5	0.2
1991	16.3	69.6	1.4	62.1	38.7	94.4	115.7	118.2	79.5	32.0	5.5	0.2
1992	15.9	68.9	1.4	60.7	37.8	94.5	114.6	117.4	80.2	32.5	5.9	0.3
1993	15.5	67.6	1.4	59.6	37.8	92.1	112.6	115.5	80.8	32.9	6.1	0.3
1994	15.2	66.7	1.4	58.9	37.6	91.5	111.1	113.9	81.5	33.7	6.4	0.3
1995	14.8	65.6	1.3	56.8	36.0	89.1	109.8	112.2	82.5	34.3	6.6	0.3
1996	14.7	65.3	1.2	54.4	33.8	86.0	110.4	113.1	83.9	35.3	6.8	0.3
Race of child:[3] White												
1950	23.0	102.3	0.4	70.0	31.3	120.5	190.4	165.1	102.6	51.4	14.5	1.0
1960	22.7	113.2	0.4	79.4	35.5	154.6	252.8	194.9	109.6	54.0	14.7	0.8
1970	17.4	84.1	0.5	57.4	29.2	101.5	163.4	145.9	71.9	30.0	7.5	0.4
1980	14.9	64.7	0.6	44.7	25.2	72.1	109.5	112.4	60.4	18.5	3.4	0.2
Race of mother:[4] White												
1980	15.1	65.6	0.6	45.4	25.5	73.2	111.1	113.8	61.2	18.8	3.5	0.2
1985	15.0	64.1	0.6	43.3	24.4	70.4	104.1	112.3	69.9	23.3	3.7	0.2
1990	15.8	68.3	0.7	50.8	29.5	78.0	109.8	120.7	81.7	31.5	5.2	0.2
1991	15.4	67.0	0.8	52.8	30.7	83.5	109.0	118.8	80.5	31.8	5.2	0.2
1992	15.0	66.5	0.8	51.8	30.1	83.8	108.2	118.4	81.4	32.2	5.7	0.2
1993	14.7	65.4	0.8	51.1	30.3	82.1	106.9	116.6	82.1	32.7	5.9	0.3
1994	14.4	64.9	0.8	51.1	30.7	82.1	106.2	115.5	83.2	33.7	6.2	0.3
1995	14.2	64.4	0.8	50.1	30.0	81.2	106.3	114.8	84.6	34.5	6.4	0.3
1996	14.1	64.3	0.8	48.1	28.4	78.4	107.2	116.1	86.3	35.6	6.7	0.3
Race of child:[3] Black												
1960	31.9	153.5	4.3	156.1	- - -	- - -	295.4	218.6	137.1	73.9	21.9	1.1
1970	25.3	115.4	5.2	140.7	101.4	204.9	202.7	136.3	79.6	41.9	12.5	1.0
1980	22.1	88.1	4.3	100.0	73.6	138.8	146.3	109.1	62.9	24.5	5.8	0.3
Race of mother:[4] Black												
1980	21.3	84.9	4.3	97.8	72.5	135.1	140.0	103.9	59.9	23.5	5.6	0.3
1985	20.4	78.8	4.5	95.4	69.3	132.4	135.0	100.2	57.9	23.9	4.6	0.3
1990	22.4	86.8	4.9	112.8	82.3	152.9	160.2	115.5	68.7	28.1	5.5	0.3
1991	21.9	85.2	4.8	115.5	84.1	158.6	160.9	113.1	67.7	28.3	5.5	0.2
1992	21.3	83.2	4.7	112.4	81.3	157.9	158.0	111.1	67.5	28.8	5.6	0.2
1993	20.5	80.5	4.6	108.6	79.8	151.9	152.6	108.4	67.3	29.2	5.9	0.3
1994	19.5	76.9	4.6	104.5	76.3	148.3	146.0	104.0	65.8	28.9	5.9	0.3
1995	18.2	72.3	4.2	96.1	69.7	137.1	137.1	98.6	64.0	28.7	6.0	0.3
1996	17.8	70.7	3.6	91.4	64.7	132.5	136.8	98.2	63.3	29.1	6.1	0.3
American Indian or Alaska Native mothers[4]												
1980	20.7	82.7	1.9	82.2	51.5	129.5	143.7	106.6	61.8	28.1	8.2	*
1985	19.8	78.6	1.7	79.2	47.7	124.1	139.1	109.6	62.6	27.4	6.0	*
1990	18.9	76.2	1.6	81.1	48.5	129.3	148.7	110.3	61.5	27.5	5.9	*
1991	18.3	75.1	1.6	85.0	52.7	134.3	144.9	106.9	61.9	27.2	5.9	0.4
1992	18.4	75.4	1.6	84.4	53.8	132.6	145.5	109.4	63.0	28.0	6.1	*
1993	17.8	73.4	1.4	83.1	53.7	130.7	139.8	107.6	62.8	27.6	5.9	*
1994	17.1	70.9	1.9	80.8	51.3	130.3	134.2	104.1	61.2	27.5	5.9	0.4
1995	16.6	69.1	1.8	78.0	47.8	130.7	132.5	98.4	62.2	27.7	6.1	*
1996	16.6	68.7	1.7	73.9	46.4	122.3	133.9	98.5	63.2	28.5	6.3	*

See footnotes at end of table.

Table 3 (page 2 of 2). Crude birth rates, fertility rates, and birth rates by age of mother, according to detailed race and Hispanic origin: United States, selected years 1950–96

[Data are based on the National Vital Statistics System]

Race of mother, Hispanic origin of mother, and year	Crude birth rate[1]	Fertility rate[2]	10–14 years	15–19 years Total	15–17 years	18–19 years	20–24 years	25–29 years	30–34 years	35–39 years	40–44 years	45–49 years
Asian or Pacific Islander mothers[4]				Live births per 1,000 women								
1980	19.9	73.2	0.3	26.2	12.0	46.2	93.3	127.4	96.0	38.3	8.5	0.7
1985	18.7	68.4	0.4	23.8	12.5	40.8	83.6	123.0	93.6	42.7	8.7	1.2
1990	19.0	69.6	0.7	26.4	16.0	40.2	79.2	126.3	106.5	49.6	10.7	1.1
1991	18.2	67.6	0.8	27.4	16.1	43.1	75.2	123.2	103.3	49.0	11.2	1.1
1992	18.0	67.2	0.7	26.6	15.2	43.1	74.6	121.0	103.0	50.6	11.0	0.9
1993	17.7	66.7	0.6	27.0	16.0	43.3	73.3	119.9	103.9	50.2	11.3	0.9
1994	17.5	66.8	0.7	27.1	16.1	44.1	73.1	118.6	105.2	51.3	11.6	1.0
1995	17.3	66.4	0.7	26.1	15.4	43.4	72.4	113.4	106.9	52.4	12.1	0.8
1996	17.0	65.9	0.6	24.6	14.9	40.4	70.7	111.2	109.2	52.2	12.2	0.8
Hispanic mothers[4,5,6]												
1980	23.5	95.4	1.7	82.2	52.1	126.9	156.4	132.1	83.2	39.9	10.6	0.7
1990	26.7	107.7	2.4	100.3	65.9	147.7	181.0	153.0	98.3	45.3	10.9	0.7
1991	26.7	108.1	2.4	106.7	70.6	158.5	186.3	152.8	96.1	44.9	10.7	0.6
1992	26.5	108.6	2.6	107.1	71.4	159.7	190.6	154.4	96.8	45.6	10.9	0.6
1993	26.0	106.9	2.7	106.8	71.7	159.1	188.3	154.0	96.4	44.7	10.6	0.6
1994	25.5	105.6	2.7	107.7	74.0	158.0	188.2	153.2	95.4	44.3	10.7	0.6
1995	25.2	105.0	2.7	106.7	72.9	157.9	188.5	153.8	95.9	44.9	10.8	0.6
1996	24.8	104.9	2.6	101.8	69.0	151.1	189.5	161.0	98.1	45.1	10.8	0.6
White, non-Hispanic mothers[4,5,6]												
1980	14.2	62.4	0.4	41.2	22.4	67.7	105.5	110.6	59.9	17.7	3.0	0.1
1990	14.4	62.8	0.5	42.5	23.2	66.6	97.5	115.3	79.4	30.0	4.7	0.2
1991	13.9	61.0	0.5	43.4	23.6	70.5	94.2	110.9	76.5	29.6	4.6	0.2
1992	13.5	60.2	0.5	41.7	22.7	69.8	93.9	111.5	78.7	30.5	5.1	0.2
1993	13.1	59.0	0.5	40.7	22.7	67.7	90.8	107.6	78.0	30.4	5.2	0.2
1994	12.8	58.3	0.5	40.4	22.8	67.4	90.9	107.9	80.7	32.1	5.7	0.2
1995	12.6	57.6	0.4	39.3	22.0	66.1	90.0	106.5	82.0	32.9	5.9	0.3
1996	12.4	57.3	0.4	37.6	20.6	63.7	90.1	107.0	83.5	34.0	6.2	0.3

- - - Data not available.
* Based on fewer than 20 births.
[1]Live births per 1,000 population.
[2]Total number of live births regardless of age of mother per 1,000 women 15–44 years of age.
[3]Live births are tabulated by race of child.
[4]Live births are tabulated by race and/or Hispanic origin of mother.
[5]Trend data for Hispanics and non-Hispanics are affected by expansion of the reporting area for an Hispanic-origin item on the birth certificate and by immigration. These two factors affect numbers of events, composition of the Hispanic population, and maternal and infant health characteristics. The number of States in the reporting area increased from 22 in 1980, to 23 and the District of Columbia (DC) in 1983–87, 30 and DC in 1988, 47 and DC in 1989, 48 and DC in 1990, 49 and DC in 1991–92, and 50 and DC in 1993 (see Appendix I, National Vital Statistics System).
[6]Rates in 1985 were not calculated because estimates for the Hispanic and non-Hispanic populations were not available.

NOTES: Data are based on births adjusted for underregistration for 1950 and on registered births for all other years. Beginning in 1970, births to persons who were not residents of the 50 States and the District of Columbia are excluded. The race groups, white, black, American Indian or Alaska Native, and Asian or Pacific Islander, include persons of Hispanic and non-Hispanic origin. Conversely, persons of Hispanic origin may be of any race.

SOURCES: Centers for Disease Control and Prevention, National Center for Health Statistics: Ventura SJ, Martin JA, Curtin SC, Mathews TJ. Report of final natality statistics, 1996. Monthly vital statistics report; vol 46. Hyattsville, Maryland: 1998; Advance report of final natality statistics, 1990, 1991, 1992, 1993, 1994, and 1995. Monthly vital statistics report; vol 41 no 9, vol 42 no 3, vol 43 no 5, vol 44 no 3, suppl., vol 44 no 11, suppl., vol 45 no 11, suppl. Hyattsville, Maryland. 1992, 1993, 1994, 1995, 1996, 1997; Ventura SJ. Births of Hispanic parentage, 1980 and 1985. Monthly vital statistics report; vol 32 no 6 and vol 36 no 11, suppl. Public Health Service. Hyattsville, Maryland. 1983 and 1988; Vital statistics of the United States, 1992, vol I, natality, Washington: Public Health Service. 1996.

Table 4. Women 15–44 years of age who have not had at least one live birth, by age: United States, selected years 1960–96

[Data are based on the National Vital Statistics System]

Year[1]	15–19 years	20–24 years	25–29 years	30–34 years	35–39 years	40–44 years
	Percent of women					
1960	91.4	47.5	20.0	14.2	12.0	15.1
1965	92.7	51.4	19.7	11.7	11.4	11.0
1970	93.0	57.0	24.4	11.8	9.4	10.6
1975	92.6	62.5	31.1	15.2	9.6	8.8
1980	93.4	66.2	38.9	19.7	12.5	9.0
1985	93.7	67.7	41.5	24.6	15.4	11.7
1986	93.8	68.0	42.0	25.1	16.1	12.2
1987	93.8	68.2	42.5	25.5	16.9	12.6
1988	93.8	68.4	43.0	25.7	17.7	13.0
1989	93.7	68.4	43.3	25.9	18.2	13.5
1990	93.3	68.3	43.5	25.9	18.5	13.9
1991	93.0	67.9	43.6	26.0	18.7	14.5
1992	92.7	67.3	43.7	26.0	18.8	15.2
1993	92.6	66.7	43.8	26.1	18.8	15.8
1994	92.6	66.1	43.9	26.2	18.7	16.2
1995	92.5	65.5	44.0	26.2	18.6	16.5
1996	92.5	65.0	43.8	26.2	18.5	16.6

[1]As of January 1.

NOTES: Data are based on cohort fertility. See Appendix II, Cohort fertility. Percents are derived from the cumulative childbearing experience of cohorts of women, up to the ages specified. Data on births are adjusted for underregistration and population estimates are corrected for underregistration and misstatement of age. Beginning in 1970 births to persons who were not residents of the 50 States and the District of Columbia are excluded.

SOURCE: Centers for Disease Control and Prevention, National Center for Health Statistics. Vital statistics of the United States, vol I, 1995 natality, table 1–17. Washington, in preparation.

Table 5. Live births, according to detailed race of mother and Hispanic origin of mother: United States, selected years 1970–96

[Data are based on the National Vital Statistics System]

Race of mother and Hispanic origin of mother	1970	1975	1980	1985	1990	1993	1994	1995	1996
	Total number of live births								
All races.	3,731,386	3,144,198	3,612,258	3,760,561	4,158,212	4,000,240	3,952,767	3,899,589	3,891,494
White.	3,109,956	2,576,818	2,936,351	3,037,913	3,290,273	3,149,833	3,121,004	3,098,885	3,093,057
Black.	561,992	496,829	568,080	581,824	684,336	658,875	636,391	603,139	594,781
American Indian or Alaska Native	22,264	22,690	29,389	34,037	39,051	38,732	37,740	37,278	37,880
Asian or Pacific Islander	- - -	- - -	74,355	104,606	141,635	152,800	157,632	160,287	165,776
Chinese	7,044	7,778	11,671	16,405	22,737	25,530	26,578	27,380	28,500
Japanese	7,744	6,725	7,482	8,035	8,674	8,699	9,230	8,901	8,902
Filipino	8,066	10,359	13,968	20,058	25,770	29,643	30,495	30,551	31,106
Hawaiian and part Hawaiian	- - -	- - -	- - -	- - -	6,099	5,810	5,955	5,787	5,907
Other Asian or Pacific Islander	- - -	- - -	- - -	- - -	78,355	83,118	85,374	87,668	91,361
Hispanic origin (selected States)[1,2]	- - -	- - -	307,163	372,814	595,073	654,418	665,026	679,768	701,339
Mexican	- - -	- - -	215,439	242,976	385,640	443,733	454,536	469,615	489,666
Puerto Rican	- - -	- - -	33,671	35,147	58,807	58,102	57,240	54,824	54,863
Cuban.	- - -	- - -	7,163	10,024	11,311	11,916	11,889	12,473	12,613
Central and South American	- - -	- - -	21,268	40,985	83,008	92,371	93,485	94,996	97,888
Other and unknown Hispanic	- - -	- - -	29,622	43,682	56,307	48,296	47,876	47,860	46,309
White, non-Hispanic (selected States)[1] . .	- - -	- - -	1,245,221	1,394,729	2,626,500	2,472,031	2,438,855	2,382,638	2,358,989
Black, non-Hispanic (selected States)[1] . .	- - -	- - -	299,646	336,029	661,701	641,273	619,198	587,781	578,099

- - - Data not available.

[1]Trend data for Hispanics and non-Hispanics are affected by expansion of the reporting area for an Hispanic-origin item on the birth certificate and by immigration. These two factors affect numbers of events, composition of the Hispanic population, and maternal and infant health characteristics. The number of States in the reporting area increased from 22 in 1980, to 23 and the District of Columbia (DC) in 1983–87, 30 and DC in 1988, 47 and DC in 1989, 48 and DC in 1990, 49 and DC in 1991–92, and 50 and DC in 1993 and later years (see Appendix I, National Vital Statistics System).
[2]Includes mothers of all races.

NOTES: The race groups, white, black, American Indian or Alaska Native, and Asian or Pacific Islander, include persons of Hispanic and non-Hispanic origin. Conversely, persons of Hispanic origin may be of any race.

SOURCES: Centers for Disease Control and Prevention, National Center for Health Statistics. Data computed by the Division of Health and Utilization Analysis from data compiled by the Division of Vital Statistics; Ventura SJ, Martin JA, Curtin SC, Mathews TJ. Report of final natality statistics, 1996. Monthly vital statistics report; vol 46. Hyattsville, Maryland: 1998; Report of final natality statistics, for each data year 1970–95. Monthly vital statistics report. Hyattsville, Maryland.

Table 6. Prenatal care for live births, according to detailed race of mother and Hispanic origin of mother: United States, selected years 1970–96

[Data are based on the National Vital Statistics System]

Prenatal care, race of mother, and Hispanic origin of mother	1970	1975	1980	1985	1988	1989	1990	1991	1992	1993	1994	1995	1996
Prenatal care began during 1st trimester					Percent of live births[1]								
All races	68.0	72.4	76.3	76.2	75.9	75.5	75.8	76.2	77.7	78.9	80.2	81.3	81.9
White	72.3	75.8	79.2	79.3	79.3	78.9	79.2	79.5	80.8	81.8	82.8	83.6	84.0
Black	44.2	55.5	62.4	61.5	60.7	60.0	60.6	61.9	63.9	66.0	68.3	70.4	71.4
American Indian or Alaska Native	38.2	45.4	55.8	57.5	58.1	57.9	57.9	59.9	62.1	63.4	65.2	66.7	67.7
Asian or Pacific Islander	- - -	- - -	73.7	74.1	75.5	74.8	75.1	75.3	76.6	77.6	79.7	79.9	81.2
Chinese	71.8	76.7	82.6	82.0	82.3	81.5	81.3	82.3	83.8	84.6	86.2	85.7	86.8
Japanese	78.1	82.7	86.1	84.7	86.3	86.2	87.0	87.7	88.2	87.2	89.2	89.7	89.3
Filipino	60.6	70.6	77.3	76.5	78.4	77.6	77.1	77.1	78.7	79.3	81.3	80.9	82.5
Hawaiian and part Hawaiian	- - -	- - -	- - -	- - -	- - -	66.8	65.8	68.1	69.9	70.6	77.0	75.9	78.5
Other Asian or Pacific Islander	- - -	- - -	- - -	- - -	- - -	71.1	71.9	71.9	72.8	74.4	76.2	77.0	78.4
Hispanic origin (selected States)[2,3]	- - -	- - -	60.2	61.2	61.3	59.5	60.2	61.0	64.2	66.6	68.9	70.8	72.2
Mexican	- - -	- - -	59.6	60.0	58.3	56.7	57.8	58.7	62.1	64.8	67.3	69.1	70.7
Puerto Rican	- - -	- - -	55.1	58.3	63.2	62.7	63.5	65.0	67.8	70.0	71.7	74.0	75.0
Cuban	- - -	- - -	82.7	82.5	83.4	83.2	84.8	85.4	86.8	88.9	90.1	89.2	89.2
Central and South American	- - -	- - -	58.8	60.6	62.8	60.8	61.5	63.4	66.8	68.7	71.2	73.2	75.0
Other and unknown Hispanic	- - -	- - -	66.4	65.8	67.3	66.0	66.4	65.6	68.0	70.0	72.1	74.3	74.6
White, non-Hispanic (selected States)[2]	- - -	- - -	81.2	81.4	81.8	82.7	83.3	83.7	84.9	85.6	86.5	87.1	87.4
Black, non-Hispanic (selected States)[2]	- - -	- - -	60.7	60.1	60.4	59.9	60.7	61.9	64.0	66.1	68.3	70.4	71.5
Prenatal care began during 3d trimester or no prenatal care													
All races	7.9	6.0	5.1	5.7	6.1	6.4	6.1	5.8	5.2	4.8	4.4	4.2	4.0
White	6.3	5.0	4.3	4.8	5.0	5.2	4.9	4.7	4.2	3.9	3.6	3.5	3.3
Black	16.6	10.5	8.9	10.2	11.0	11.9	11.3	10.7	9.9	9.0	8.2	7.6	7.3
American Indian or Alaska Native	28.9	22.4	15.2	12.9	13.2	13.4	12.9	12.2	11.0	10.3	9.8	9.5	8.6
Asian or Pacific Islander	- - -	- - -	6.5	6.5	5.9	6.1	5.8	5.7	4.9	4.6	4.1	4.3	3.9
Chinese	6.5	4.4	3.7	4.4	3.4	3.6	3.4	3.4	2.9	2.9	2.7	3.0	2.5
Japanese	4.1	2.7	2.1	3.1	3.3	2.7	2.9	2.5	2.4	2.8	1.9	2.3	2.2
Filipino	7.2	4.1	4.0	4.8	4.8	4.7	4.5	5.0	4.3	4.0	3.6	4.1	3.3
Hawaiian and part Hawaiian	- - -	- - -	- - -	- - -	- - -	8.7	8.7	7.5	7.0	6.7	4.7	5.1	5.0
Other Asian or Pacific Islander	- - -	- - -	- - -	- - -	- - -	7.5	7.1	6.8	5.9	5.4	4.8	5.0	4.6
Hispanic origin (selected States)[2,3]	- - -	- - -	12.0	12.4	12.1	13.0	12.0	11.0	9.5	8.8	7.6	7.4	6.7
Mexican	- - -	- - -	11.8	12.9	13.9	14.6	13.2	12.2	10.5	9.7	8.3	8.1	7.2
Puerto Rican	- - -	- - -	16.2	15.5	10.2	11.3	10.6	9.1	8.0	7.1	6.5	5.5	5.7
Cuban	- - -	- - -	3.9	3.7	3.6	4.0	2.8	2.4	2.1	1.8	1.6	2.1	1.6
Central and South American	- - -	- - -	13.1	12.5	9.9	11.9	10.9	9.5	7.9	7.3	6.5	6.1	5.5
Other and unknown Hispanic	- - -	- - -	9.2	9.4	8.8	9.3	8.5	8.2	7.5	7.0	6.2	6.0	5.9
White, non-Hispanic (selected States)[2]	- - -	- - -	3.5	4.0	4.1	3.7	3.4	3.2	2.8	2.7	2.5	2.5	2.4
Black, non-Hispanic (selected States)[2]	- - -	- - -	9.7	10.9	11.0	12.0	11.2	10.7	9.8	9.0	8.2	7.6	7.3

- - - Data not available.

[1]Excludes live births for whom trimester when prenatal care began is unknown.

[2]Trend data for Hispanics and non-Hispanics are affected by expansion of the reporting area for an Hispanic-origin item on the birth certificate and by immigration. These two factors affect numbers of events, composition of the Hispanic population, and maternal and infant health characteristics. The number of States in the reporting area increased from 22 in 1980, to 23 and the District of Columbia (DC) in 1983–87, 30 and DC in 1988, 47 and DC in 1989, 48 and DC in 1990, 49 and DC in 1991–92, and 50 and DC in 1993 and later years (see Appendix I, National Vital Statistics System).

[3]Includes mothers of all races.

NOTES: Data for 1970 and 1975 exclude births that occurred in States not reporting prenatal care (see Appendix I). The race groups, white, black, American Indian or Alaska Native, and Asian or Pacific Islander, include persons of Hispanic and non-Hispanic origin. Conversely, persons of Hispanic origin may be of any race.

SOURCES: Centers for Disease Control and Prevention, National Center for Health Statistics. Data computed by the Division of Health and Utilization Analysis from data compiled by the Division of Vital Statistics; Ventura SJ, Martin JA, Curtin SC, Mathews TJ. Report of final natality statistics, 1996. Monthly vital statistics report; vol 46. Hyattsville, Maryland: 1998. Report of final natality statistics, for each data year 1970–95. Monthly vital statistics report. Hyattsville, Maryland.

Table 7. Teenage childbearing, according to detailed race of mother and Hispanic origin of mother: United States, selected years 1970–96

[Data are based on the National Vital Statistics System]

Maternal age, race of mother, and Hispanic origin of mother	1970	1975	1980	1985	1988	1989	1990	1991	1992	1993	1994	1995	1996
Age of mother under 18 years						Percent of live births							
All races	6.3	7.6	5.8	4.7	4.8	4.8	4.7	4.9	4.9	5.1	5.3	5.3	5.1
White	4.8	6.0	4.5	3.7	3.7	3.6	3.6	3.8	3.9	4.0	4.2	4.3	4.2
Black	14.8	16.3	12.5	10.6	10.6	10.5	10.1	10.3	10.3	10.6	10.8	10.8	10.3
American Indian or Alaska Native	7.5	11.2	9.4	7.6	7.8	7.5	7.2	7.9	8.0	8.4	8.7	8.7	8.7
Asian or Pacific Islander	- - -	- - -	1.5	1.6	1.8	2.0	2.1	2.1	2.0	2.1	2.2	2.2	2.1
Chinese	1.1	0.4	0.3	0.3	0.3	0.3	0.4	0.3	0.3	0.3	0.3	0.3	0.3
Japanese	2.0	1.7	1.0	0.9	0.8	0.9	0.8	1.0	0.9	0.9	0.9	0.8	0.9
Filipino	3.7	2.4	1.6	1.6	1.7	1.9	2.0	2.0	1.9	2.0	2.2	2.2	2.1
Hawaiian and part Hawaiian	- - -	- - -	- - -	- - -	- - -	5.9	6.5	6.8	7.0	7.1	8.0	7.6	6.8
Other Asian or Pacific Islander	- - -	- - -	- - -	- - -	- - -	2.4	2.4	2.4	2.3	2.5	2.5	2.5	2.5
Hispanic origin (selected States)[1,2]	- - -	- - -	7.4	6.4	6.6	6.7	6.6	6.9	7.1	7.2	7.6	7.6	7.3
Mexican	- - -	- - -	7.7	6.9	7.0	6.9	6.9	7.2	7.3	7.5	7.9	8.0	7.7
Puerto Rican	- - -	- - -	10.0	8.5	9.2	9.4	9.1	9.5	9.6	10.2	10.8	10.8	10.2
Cuban	- - -	- - -	3.8	2.2	2.2	2.7	2.7	2.6	2.5	2.5	3.0	2.8	2.8
Central and South American	- - -	- - -	2.4	2.4	2.7	3.0	3.2	3.5	3.6	3.8	4.0	4.1	4.0
Other and unknown Hispanic	- - -	- - -	6.5	7.0	7.6	8.0	8.0	8.3	8.9	9.4	9.4	9.0	8.8
White, non-Hispanic (selected States)[1]	- - -	- - -	4.0	3.2	3.2	3.0	3.0	3.1	3.1	3.2	3.4	3.4	3.3
Black, non-Hispanic (selected States)[1]	- - -	- - -	12.7	10.7	10.8	10.5	10.2	10.3	10.4	10.6	10.9	10.8	10.4
Age of mother 18–19 years													
All races	11.3	11.3	9.8	8.0	7.7	8.1	8.1	8.1	7.8	7.8	7.9	7.9	7.9
White	10.4	10.3	9.0	7.1	6.9	7.2	7.3	7.2	7.0	7.0	7.1	7.2	7.2
Black	16.6	16.9	14.5	12.9	12.3	12.9	13.0	12.8	12.4	12.1	12.3	12.4	12.5
American Indian or Alaska Native	12.8	15.2	14.6	12.4	11.4	12.1	12.3	12.4	11.9	11.9	12.3	12.7	12.3
Asian or Pacific Islander	- - -	- - -	3.9	3.4	3.4	3.7	3.7	3.7	3.6	3.6	3.5	3.5	3.2
Chinese	3.9	1.7	1.0	0.6	0.5	0.7	0.8	0.8	0.7	0.7	0.7	0.6	0.6
Japanese	4.1	3.3	2.3	1.9	1.8	1.8	2.0	1.7	1.7	1.8	1.9	1.7	1.6
Filipino	7.1	5.0	4.0	3.7	3.8	4.0	4.1	4.0	3.7	3.8	3.8	4.1	4.0
Hawaiian and part Hawaiian	- - -	- - -	- - -	- - -	- - -	11.3	11.9	11.3	11.4	11.3	11.6	11.5	11.6
Other Asian or Pacific Islander	- - -	- - -	- - -	- - -	- - -	4.1	3.9	4.1	4.1	4.0	3.9	3.8	3.4
Hispanic origin (selected States)[1,2]	- - -	- - -	11.6	10.1	9.8	10.0	10.2	10.3	10.1	10.1	10.2	10.3	10.1
Mexican	- - -	- - -	12.0	10.6	10.3	10.5	10.7	10.9	10.7	10.7	10.7	10.8	10.5
Puerto Rican	- - -	- - -	13.3	12.4	12.2	12.6	12.6	12.2	11.8	12.1	12.4	12.7	13.0
Cuban	- - -	- - -	9.2	4.9	3.9	4.3	5.0	4.5	4.6	4.3	4.3	4.9	4.9
Central and South American	- - -	- - -	6.0	5.8	5.4	5.6	5.9	6.0	5.9	6.1	6.4	6.5	6.5
Other and unknown Hispanic	- - -	- - -	10.8	10.5	10.8	11.2	11.1	11.4	11.1	11.6	11.4	11.1	11.1
White, non-Hispanic (selected States)[1]	- - -	- - -	8.5	6.6	6.6	6.5	6.6	6.5	6.3	6.2	6.3	6.4	6.4
Black, non-Hispanic (selected States)[1]	- - -	- - -	14.7	12.9	12.4	13.0	13.0	12.9	12.5	12.2	12.4	12.4	12.6

- - - Data not available.

[1]Trend data for Hispanics and non-Hispanics are affected by expansion of the reporting area for an Hispanic-origin item on the birth certificate and by immigration. These two factors affect numbers of events, composition of the Hispanic population, and maternal and infant health characteristics. The number of States in the reporting area increased from 22 in 1980, to 23 and the District of Columbia (DC) in 1983–87, 30 and DC in 1988, 47 and DC in 1989, 48 and DC in 1990, 49 and DC in 1991–92, and 50 and DC in 1993 and later years (see Appendix I, National Vital Statistics System).
[2]Includes mothers of all races.

NOTES: The race groups, white, black, American Indian or Alaska Native, and Asian or Pacific Islander, include persons of Hispanic and non-Hispanic origin. Conversely, persons of Hispanic origin may be of any race.

SOURCES: Centers for Disease Control and Prevention, National Center for Health Statistics. Data computed by the Division of Health and Utilization Analysis from data compiled by the Division of Vital Statistics; Ventura SJ, Martin JA, Curtin SC, Mathews TJ. Report of final natality statistics, 1996. Monthly vital statistics report; vol 46. Hyattsville, Maryland: 1998; Report of final natality statistics, for each data year 1970–95. Monthly vital statistics report. Hyattsville, Maryland.

Table 8. Nonmarital childbearing according to detailed race of mother, Hispanic origin of mother, and maternal age and birth rates for unmarried women by race of mother and Hispanic origin of mother: United States, selected years 1970–96

[Data are based on the National Vital Statistics System]

Race of mother, Hispanic origin of mother, and maternal age	1970	1975	1980	1985	1988	1989	1990	1991	1992	1993	1994	1995	1996
	Percent of live births to unmarried mothers												
All races	10.7	14.3	18.4	22.0	25.7	27.1	28.0	29.5	30.1	31.0	32.6	32.2	32.4
White	5.5	7.1	11.2	14.7	18.0	19.2	20.4	21.8	22.6	23.6	25.4	25.3	25.7
Black	37.5	49.5	56.1	61.2	64.7	65.7	66.5	67.9	68.1	68.7	70.4	69.9	69.8
American Indian or Alaska Native	22.4	32.7	39.2	46.8	51.7	52.7	53.6	55.3	55.3	55.8	57.0	57.2	58.0
Asian or Pacific Islander	- - -	- - -	7.3	9.5	11.5	12.4	13.2	13.9	14.7	15.7	16.2	16.3	16.7
Chinese	3.0	1.6	2.7	3.0	3.9	4.2	5.0	5.5	6.1	6.7	7.2	7.9	9.2
Japanese	4.6	4.6	5.2	7.9	8.8	9.4	9.6	9.8	9.8	10.0	11.2	10.8	11.4
Filipino	9.1	6.9	8.6	11.4	13.6	14.8	15.9	16.8	16.8	17.7	18.5	19.5	19.4
Hawaiian and part Hawaiian	- - -	- - -	- - -	- - -	- - -	42.7	45.0	45.0	45.7	47.8	48.6	49.0	49.9
Other Asian or Pacific Islander	- - -	- - -	- - -	- - -	- - -	12.0	12.6	13.5	14.9	16.1	16.4	16.2	16.5
Hispanic origin (selected States)[1,2]	- - -	- - -	23.6	29.5	34.0	35.5	36.7	38.5	39.1	40.0	43.1	40.8	40.7
Mexican	- - -	- - -	20.3	25.7	30.6	31.7	33.3	35.3	36.3	37.0	40.8	38.1	37.9
Puerto Rican	- - -	- - -	46.3	51.1	53.3	55.2	55.9	57.5	57.5	59.4	60.2	60.0	60.7
Cuban	- - -	- - -	10.0	16.1	16.3	17.5	18.2	19.5	20.2	21.0	22.9	23.8	24.7
Central and South American	- - -	- - -	27.1	34.9	36.4	38.9	41.2	43.1	43.9	45.2	45.9	44.1	44.1
Other and unknown Hispanic	- - -	- - -	22.4	31.1	35.5	37.0	37.2	37.9	37.6	38.7	43.5	44.0	43.5
White, non-Hispanic (selected States)[1]	- - -	- - -	9.6	12.4	15.2	16.1	16.9	18.0	18.5	19.5	20.8	21.2	21.5
Black, non-Hispanic (selected States)[1]	- - -	- - -	57.3	62.1	64.8	66.0	66.7	68.2	68.3	68.9	70.7	70.0	70.0
	Number of live births, in thousands												
Live births to unmarried mothers	399	448	666	828	1,005	1,094	1,165	1,214	1,225	1,240	1,290	1,254	1,260
Maternal age	Percent distribution of live births to unmarried mothers												
Under 20 years	50.1	52.1	40.8	33.8	32.1	31.8	30.9	30.4	29.8	29.7	30.5	30.9	30.4
20–24 years	31.8	29.9	35.6	36.3	34.9	34.6	34.7	35.4	35.6	35.4	34.8	34.5	34.2
25 years and over	18.1	18.0	23.5	29.9	33.0	33.6	34.4	34.3	34.6	34.9	34.6	34.7	35.3
	Live births per 1,000 unmarried women 15–44 years of age[3]												
All races and origins	26.4	24.5	29.4	32.8	38.5	41.6	43.8	45.2	45.2	45.3	46.9	45.1	44.8
White[4]	13.9	12.4	18.1	22.5	27.4	30.2	32.9	34.6	35.2	35.9	38.3	37.5	37.6
Black[4]	95.5	84.2	81.1	77.0	86.5	90.7	90.5	89.5	86.5	84.0	82.1	75.9	74.4
Hispanic origin (selected States)[1,2]	- - -	- - -	- - -	- - -	- - -	- - -	89.6	93.7	95.3	95.2	101.2	95.0	93.2
White, non-Hispanic	- - -	- - -	- - -	- - -	- - -	- - -	- - -	- - -	- - -	- - -	28.5	28.2	28.3

- - - Data not available.

[1]Trend data for Hispanics and non-Hispanics are affected by expansion of the reporting area for an Hispanic-origin item on the birth certificate and by immigration. These two factors affect numbers of events, composition of the Hispanic population, and maternal and infant health characteristics. The number of States in the reporting area increased from 22 in 1980, to 23 and the District of Columbia (DC) in 1983–87, 30 and DC in 1988, 47 and DC in 1989, 48 and DC in 1990, 49 and DC in 1991–92, and 50 and DC in 1993 and later years (see Appendix I, National Vital Statistics System).

[2]Includes mothers of all races.

[3]Rates computed by relating births to unmarried mothers, regardless of age of mother, to unmarried women 15–44 years of age.

[4]For 1970 and 1975, birth rates are by race of child.

NOTES: National estimates for 1970 and 1975 for unmarried mothers based on births occurring in States reporting marital status of mother (see Appendix I, National Vital Statistics System). The race groups, white, black, American Indian or Alaska Native, and Asian or Pacific Islander, include persons of Hispanic and non-Hispanic origin. Conversely, persons of Hispanic origin may be of any race. In 1995 procedures implemented in California to more accurately identify the marital status of Hispanic mothers account for some of the decline in measures of nonmarital childbearing for women of all races, white women, and Hispanic women between 1994 and 1995.

SOURCES: Centers for Disease Control and Prevention, National Center for Health Statistics. Ventura SJ. Births to unmarried mothers: United States, 1980–92. Vital Health Stat 21(53). 1995; Report of final natality statistics, for each data year 1993–95. Monthly vital statistics report. Hyattsville, Maryland; Ventura SJ, Martin JA, Curtin SC, Mathews TJ. Report of final natality statistics, 1996. Monthly vital statistics report; vol 46. Hyattsville, Maryland: 1998; and data computed by the Division of Health and Utilization Analysis from data compiled by the Division of Vital Statistics.

Table 9. Maternal education for live births, according to detailed race of mother and Hispanic origin of mother: United States, selected years 1970–96

[Data are based on the National Vital Statistics System]

Mother's education, race of mother, and Hispanic origin of mother	1970	1975	1980	1985	1988	1989	1990	1991	1992	1993	1994	1995	1996
Less than 12 years of education						Percent of live births[1]							
All races	30.8	28.6	23.7	20.6	20.4	23.2	23.8	23.9	23.6	23.3	22.9	22.6	22.4
White.	27.1	25.1	20.8	17.8	17.6	21.6	22.4	22.5	22.3	22.0	21.7	21.6	21.6
Black.	51.2	45.3	36.4	32.6	31.4	30.4	30.2	30.4	30.0	29.8	29.3	28.7	28.2
American Indian or Alaska Native.	60.5	52.7	44.2	39.0	37.9	37.2	36.4	36.3	35.9	34.8	34.0	33.0	33.0
Asian or Pacific Islander	- - -	- - -	21.0	19.4	17.9	19.5	20.0	19.7	19.0	18.1	17.4	16.1	15.0
Chinese	23.0	16.5	15.2	15.5	14.2	14.9	15.8	15.7	15.2	14.3	13.7	12.9	12.8
Japanese	11.8	9.1	5.0	4.8	3.5	3.3	3.5	3.0	2.4	2.6	2.8	2.6	2.7
Filipino	26.4	22.3	16.4	13.9	11.8	10.2	10.3	10.1	9.3	8.8	8.9	8.0	7.4
Hawaiian and part Hawaiian	- - -	- - -	- - -	- - -	- - -	17.3	19.3	19.4	18.6	17.3	18.5	17.6	16.9
Other Asian or Pacific Islander	- - -	- - -	- - -	- - -	- - -	26.8	26.8	26.0	25.7	24.6	23.3	21.2	19.4
Hispanic origin (selected States)[2,3]	- - -	- - -	51.1	44.5	42.5	52.8	53.9	54.3	54.1	53.4	52.7	52.1	51.4
Mexican	- - -	- - -	62.8	59.0	56.9	61.3	61.4	61.7	61.3	60.4	59.5	58.6	57.7
Puerto Rican.	- - -	- - -	55.3	46.6	45.2	43.7	42.7	41.9	41.0	40.3	39.6	38.6	38.1
Cuban	- - -	- - -	24.1	21.1	18.1	17.9	17.8	16.7	15.6	14.6	15.0	14.4	14.5
Central and South American.	- - -	- - -	41.2	37.0	31.8	43.6	44.2	44.5	43.6	43.0	42.0	41.7	40.8
Other and unknown Hispanic	- - -	- - -	40.1	36.5	34.1	34.5	33.3	34.4	34.7	33.9	33.9	33.8	33.0
White, non-Hispanic (selected States)[2]	- - -	- - -	18.3	15.8	16.7	15.3	15.2	15.0	14.5	14.0	13.5	13.3	13.0
Black, non-Hispanic (selected States)[2]	- - -	- - -	37.4	33.5	31.8	29.9	30.0	30.3	29.8	29.6	29.1	28.6	28.0
16 years or more of education													
All races	8.6	11.4	14.0	16.7	17.7	17.4	17.5	18.1	18.9	19.5	20.4	21.4	22.1
White.	9.6	12.7	15.5	18.6	20.1	19.2	19.3	19.9	20.7	21.4	22.2	23.1	23.9
Black.	2.8	4.3	6.2	7.0	7.1	7.2	7.2	7.3	7.8	8.2	8.7	9.5	10.0
American Indian or Alaska Native.	2.7	2.2	3.5	3.7	3.7	4.3	4.4	4.0	4.7	5.5	5.7	6.2	6.3
Asian or Pacific Islander	- - -	- - -	30.8	30.3	31.7	31.2	31.0	31.8	32.5	33.0	33.9	35.0	36.2
Chinese	34.0	37.8	41.5	35.2	36.4	40.5	40.3	41.7	44.0	45.7	46.6	49.0	49.1
Japanese	20.7	30.6	36.8	38.1	42.3	43.6	44.1	45.0	46.6	46.3	45.2	46.2	46.8
Filipino	28.1	36.6	37.1	35.2	35.5	36.0	34.5	34.1	35.8	36.1	36.6	36.7	38.0
Hawaiian and part Hawaiian	- - -	- - -	- - -	- - -	- - -	6.6	6.8	6.7	8.0	8.5	8.9	9.7	11.3
Other Asian or Pacific Islander	- - -	- - -	- - -	- - -	- - -	26.9	27.3	28.6	28.0	28.1	29.4	30.5	32.2
Hispanic origin (selected States)[2,3]	- - -	- - -	4.2	6.0	7.0	5.1	5.1	5.2	5.4	5.5	5.8	6.1	6.4
Mexican	- - -	- - -	2.2	3.0	3.7	3.2	3.3	3.3	3.5	3.5	3.8	4.0	4.2
Puerto Rican.	- - -	- - -	3.0	4.6	5.3	6.3	6.5	6.8	7.3	7.5	8.1	8.7	8.9
Cuban	- - -	- - -	11.6	15.0	18.2	19.2	20.4	21.9	22.5	24.3	24.8	26.5	27.0
Central and South American.	- - -	- - -	6.1	8.1	10.1	8.2	8.6	9.1	9.2	9.4	9.8	10.3	11.2
Other and unknown Hispanic	- - -	- - -	5.5	7.2	8.0	7.7	8.5	8.2	8.5	9.2	9.8	10.5	11.1
White, non-Hispanic (selected States)[2]	- - -	- - -	16.4	19.3	20.4	22.0	22.6	23.3	24.4	25.3	26.5	27.7	28.8
Black, non-Hispanic (selected States)[2]	- - -	- - -	5.7	6.7	6.9	7.2	7.3	7.3	7.8	8.2	8.7	9.5	10.0

- - - Data not available.

[1]Excludes live births for whom education of mother is unknown.

[2]Trend data for Hispanics and non-Hispanics are affected by expansion of the reporting area for an Hispanic-origin item on the birth certificate and by immigration. These two factors affect numbers of events, composition of the Hispanic population, and maternal and infant health characteristics. Data shown only for States with an Hispanic-origin item and education of mother item on their birth certificates. The number of States reporting both items increased from 20 in 1980, to 21 and the District of Columbia (DC) in 1983–87, 26 and DC in 1988, 45 and DC in 1989, 47 and DC in 1990–91, 49 and DC in 1992, and 50 and DC in 1993 (see Appendix I, National Vital Statistics System).

[3]Includes mothers of all races.

NOTES: Excludes births that occurred in States not reporting education (see Appendix I). The race groups, white, black, American Indian or Alaska Native, and Asian or Pacific Islander, include persons of Hispanic and non-Hispanic origin. Conversely, persons of Hispanic origin may be of any race. Maternal education groups shown in this table generally represent the group at highest risk for unfavorable birth outcomes (less than 12 years of education) and the group at lowest risk (16 years or more of education.)

SOURCE: Centers for Disease Control and Prevention, National Center for Health Statistics. Data computed by the Division of Health and Utilization Analysis from data compiled by the Division of Vital Statistics.

Table 10. Mothers who smoked cigarettes during pregnancy, according to mother's detailed race, Hispanic origin, age, and educational attainment: Selected States, 1989–96

[Data are based on the National Vital Statistics System]

Characteristic of mother	1989	1990	1991	1992	1993	1994	1995	1996
Race of mother[1]	Percent of mothers who smoked[2]							
All races	19.5	18.4	17.8	16.9	15.8	14.6	13.9	13.6
White	20.4	19.4	18.8	17.9	16.8	15.6	15.0	14.7
Black	17.1	15.9	14.6	13.8	12.7	11.4	10.6	10.2
American Indian or Alaska Native	23.0	22.4	22.6	22.5	21.6	21.0	20.9	21.3
Asian or Pacific Islander[3]	5.7	5.5	5.2	4.8	4.3	3.6	3.4	3.3
Chinese	2.7	2.0	1.9	1.7	1.1	0.9	0.8	0.7
Japanese	8.2	8.0	7.5	6.6	6.7	5.4	5.2	4.8
Filipino	5.1	5.3	5.3	4.8	4.3	3.7	3.4	3.5
Hawaiian and part Hawaiian	19.3	21.0	19.4	18.5	17.2	16.0	15.9	15.3
Other Asian or Pacific Islander	4.2	3.8	3.8	3.6	3.2	2.9	2.7	2.7
Hispanic origin and race of mother[4]								
Hispanic origin	8.0	6.7	6.3	5.8	5.0	4.6	4.3	4.3
Mexican	6.3	5.3	4.8	4.3	3.7	3.4	3.1	3.1
Puerto Rican	14.5	13.6	13.2	12.7	11.2	10.9	10.4	11.0
Cuban	6.9	6.4	6.2	5.9	5.0	4.8	4.1	4.7
Central and South American	3.6	3.0	2.8	2.6	2.3	1.8	1.8	1.8
Other and unknown Hispanic	12.1	10.8	10.7	10.1	9.3	8.1	8.2	9.1
White, non-Hispanic	21.7	21.0	20.5	19.7	18.6	17.7	17.1	16.9
Black, non-Hispanic	17.2	15.9	14.6	13.8	12.7	11.5	10.6	10.3
Age of mother[1]								
Under 15 years	7.7	7.5	7.6	6.9	7.0	6.7	7.3	7.7
15–19 years	22.2	20.8	19.7	18.6	17.5	16.7	16.8	17.2
15–17 years	19.0	17.6	16.6	15.6	14.8	14.4	14.6	15.4
18–19 years	23.9	22.5	21.5	20.3	19.1	18.1	18.1	18.3
20–24 years	23.5	22.1	21.2	20.3	19.2	17.8	17.1	16.8
25–29 years	19.0	18.0	17.2	16.1	14.8	13.5	12.8	12.3
30–34 years	15.7	15.3	15.1	14.5	13.4	12.3	11.4	10.9
35–39 years	13.6	13.3	13.3	13.4	12.8	12.2	12.0	11.7
40–49 years	13.2	12.3	11.9	11.6	11.0	10.3	10.1	10.1
Education of mother[5]	Percent of mothers 20 years of age and over who smoked[2]							
0–8 years	18.9	17.5	16.8	15.5	13.9	12.1	11.0	10.3
9–11 years	42.2	40.5	39.1	37.8	36.1	33.6	32.0	31.1
12 years	22.8	21.9	21.2	20.7	19.9	18.7	18.3	18.0
13–15 years	13.7	12.8	12.5	12.1	11.4	10.8	10.6	10.4
16 years or more	5.0	4.5	4.2	3.9	3.1	2.8	2.7	2.6

[1]Includes data for 43 States and the District of Columbia (DC) in 1989, 45 States and DC in 1990, 46 States and DC in 1991–93, and 46 States, DC, and New York City (NYC) in 1994–96. Excludes data for California, Indiana, New York (but includes NYC in 1994–96), and South Dakota (1989–96), Oklahoma (1989–90), and Louisiana and Nebraska (1989), which did not require the reporting of mother's tobacco use during pregnancy on the birth certificate (see Appendix I).
[2]Excludes live births for whom smoking status of mother is unknown.
[3]Maternal tobacco use during pregnancy was not reported on the birth certificates of California and New York, which during 1989–91 together accounted for 43–66 percent of the births in each Asian subgroup (except Hawaiian).
[4]Includes data for 42 States and DC in 1989, 44 States and DC in 1990, 45 States and DC in 1991–92, 46 States and DC in 1993, and 46 States, DC, and NYC in 1994–96. Excludes data for California, Indiana, New York (but includes NYC in 1994–96), and South Dakota (1989–96), New Hampshire (1989–92), Oklahoma (1989–90), and Louisiana and Nebraska (1989), which did not require the reporting of either Hispanic origin of mother or tobacco use during pregnancy on the birth certificate (see Appendix I).
[5]Includes data for 42 States and DC in 1989, 44 States and DC in 1990, 45 States and DC in 1991, 46 States and DC in 1992–93, and 46 States, DC, and NYC in 1994–96. Excludes data for California, Indiana, New York (but includes NYC in 1994–96), and South Dakota (1989–96), Washington (1989–91), Oklahoma (1989–90), and Louisiana and Nebraska (1989), which did not require the reporting of either mother's education or tobacco use during pregnancy on the birth certificate (see Appendix I).

NOTES: The race groups, white, black, American Indian or Alaska Native, and Asian or Pacific Islander, include persons of Hispanic and non-Hispanic origin. Conversely, persons of Hispanic origin may be of any race.

SOURCES: Centers for Disease Control and Prevention, National Center for Health Statistics. Data computed by the Division of Health and Utilization Analysis from data compiled by the Division of Vital Statistics; Ventura SJ, Martin JA, Curtin SC, Mathews TJ. Report of final natality statistics, 1996. Monthly vital statistics report; vol 46. Hyattsville, Maryland: 1998; Report of final natality statistics, for each data year 1989–95. Monthly vital statistics report. Hyattsville, Maryland.

Table 11. Low-birthweight live births, according to mother's detailed race, Hispanic origin, and smoking status: United States, selected years 1970–96

[Data are based on the National Vital Statistics System]

Birthweight, race of mother, Hispanic origin of mother, and smoking status of mother	1970	1975	1980	1985	1988	1989	1990	1991	1992	1993	1994	1995	1996
Low birthweight (less than 2,500 grams)					Percent of live births[1]								
All races	7.93	7.38	6.84	6.75	6.93	7.05	6.97	7.12	7.08	7.22	7.28	7.32	7.39
White	6.85	6.27	5.72	5.65	5.67	5.72	5.70	5.80	5.80	5.98	6.11	6.22	6.34
Black	13.90	13.19	12.69	12.65	13.26	13.51	13.25	13.55	13.31	13.34	13.24	13.13	13.01
American Indian or Alaska Native	7.97	6.41	6.44	5.86	6.00	6.26	6.11	6.15	6.22	6.42	6.45	6.61	6.49
Asian or Pacific Islander	- - -	- - -	6.68	6.16	6.31	6.51	6.45	6.54	6.57	6.55	6.81	6.90	7.07
Chinese	6.67	5.29	5.21	4.98	4.63	4.89	4.69	5.10	4.98	4.91	4.76	5.29	5.03
Japanese	9.03	7.47	6.60	6.21	6.69	6.67	6.16	5.90	7.00	6.53	6.91	7.26	7.27
Filipino	10.02	8.08	7.40	6.95	7.15	7.35	7.30	7.31	7.43	6.99	7.77	7.83	7.92
Hawaiian and part Hawaiian	- - -	- - -	- - -	- - -	- - -	7.29	7.24	6.73	6.89	6.76	7.20	6.84	6.77
Other Asian or Pacific Islander	- - -	- - -	- - -	- - -	- - -	6.61	6.65	6.74	6.68	6.89	7.06	7.05	7.42
Hispanic origin (selected States)[2,3]	- - -	- - -	6.12	6.16	6.17	6.18	6.06	6.15	6.10	6.24	6.25	6.29	6.28
Mexican	- - -	- - -	5.62	5.77	5.60	5.60	5.55	5.60	5.61	5.77	5.80	5.81	5.86
Puerto Rican	- - -	- - -	8.95	8.69	9.42	9.50	8.99	9.42	9.19	9.23	9.13	9.41	9.24
Cuban	- - -	- - -	5.62	6.02	5.94	5.77	5.67	5.57	6.10	6.18	6.27	6.50	6.46
Central and South American	- - -	- - -	5.76	5.68	5.58	5.81	5.84	5.87	5.77	5.94	6.02	6.20	6.03
Other and unknown Hispanic	- - -	- - -	6.96	6.83	6.85	6.74	6.87	7.25	7.24	7.51	7.54	7.55	7.68
White, non-Hispanic (selected States)[2]	- - -	- - -	5.67	5.60	5.62	5.62	5.61	5.72	5.73	5.92	6.06	6.20	6.36
Black, non-Hispanic (selected States)[2]	- - -	- - -	12.71	12.61	13.28	13.61	13.32	13.62	13.40	13.43	13.34	13.21	13.12
Cigarette smoker[4]	- - -	- - -	- - -	- - -	- - -	11.36	11.25	11.41	11.49	11.84	12.28	12.18	12.13
Nonsmoker[4]	- - -	- - -	- - -	- - -	- - -	6.02	6.14	6.36	6.35	6.56	6.71	6.79	6.91
Very low birthweight (less than 1,500 grams)													
All races	1.17	1.16	1.15	1.21	1.24	1.28	1.27	1.29	1.29	1.33	1.33	1.35	1.37
White	0.95	0.92	0.90	0.94	0.93	0.95	0.95	0.96	0.96	1.01	1.02	1.06	1.09
Black	2.40	2.40	2.48	2.71	2.86	2.95	2.92	2.96	2.96	2.96	2.96	2.97	2.99
American Indian or Alaska Native	0.98	0.95	0.92	1.01	1.00	1.00	1.01	1.07	0.95	1.05	1.10	1.10	1.21
Asian or Pacific Islander	- - -	- - -	0.92	0.85	0.84	0.90	0.87	0.85	0.91	0.86	0.93	0.91	0.99
Chinese	0.80	0.52	0.66	0.57	0.57	0.61	0.51	0.65	0.67	0.63	0.58	0.67	0.64
Japanese	1.48	0.89	0.94	0.84	0.92	0.86	0.73	0.62	0.85	0.74	0.92	0.87	0.81
Filipino	1.08	0.93	0.99	0.86	0.91	1.12	1.05	0.97	1.05	0.95	1.19	1.13	1.20
Hawaiian and part Hawaiian	- - -	- - -	- - -	- - -	- - -	1.13	0.97	1.02	1.02	1.14	1.20	0.94	0.97
Other Asian or Pacific Islander	- - -	- - -	- - -	- - -	- - -	0.89	0.92	0.87	0.93	0.89	0.93	0.91	1.04
Hispanic origin (selected States)[2,3]	- - -	- - -	0.98	1.01	1.01	1.05	1.03	1.02	1.04	1.06	1.08	1.11	1.12
Mexican	- - -	- - -	0.92	0.97	0.89	0.94	0.92	0.92	0.94	0.97	0.99	1.01	1.01
Puerto Rican	- - -	- - -	1.29	1.30	1.61	1.71	1.62	1.66	1.70	1.66	1.63	1.79	1.70
Cuban	- - -	- - -	1.02	1.18	1.17	1.13	1.20	1.15	1.24	1.23	1.31	1.19	1.35
Central and South American	- - -	- - -	0.99	1.01	0.97	1.05	1.05	1.02	1.02	1.02	1.06	1.13	1.14
Other and unknown Hispanic	- - -	- - -	1.01	0.96	1.11	1.04	1.09	1.09	1.10	1.23	1.29	1.28	1.48
White, non-Hispanic (selected States)[2]	- - -	- - -	0.86	0.90	0.89	0.93	0.93	0.94	0.94	1.00	1.01	1.04	1.08
Black, non-Hispanic (selected States)[2]	- - -	- - -	2.46	2.66	2.82	2.97	2.93	2.97	2.97	2.99	2.99	2.98	3.02
Cigarette smoker[4]	- - -	- - -	- - -	- - -	- - -	1.75	1.73	1.73	1.74	1.77	1.81	1.85	1.85
Nonsmoker[4]	- - -	- - -	- - -	- - -	- - -	1.16	1.18	1.21	1.22	1.28	1.30	1.31	1.35

- - - Data not available.

[1]Excludes live births with unknown birthweight. Percent based on live births with known birthweight.

[2]Trend data for Hispanics and non-Hispanics are affected by expansion of the reporting area for an Hispanic-origin item on the birth certificate and by immigration. These two factors affect numbers of events, composition of the Hispanic population, and maternal and infant health characteristics. The number of States in the reporting area increased from 22 in 1980, to 23 and the District of Columbia (DC) in 1983–87, 30 and DC in 1988, 47 and DC in 1989, 48 and DC in 1990, 49 and DC in 1991–92, and 50 and DC in 1993 and later years (see Appendix I, National Vital Statistics System).

[3]Includes mothers of all races.

[4]Percent based on live births with known smoking status of mother and known birthweight. Includes data for 43 States and the District of Columbia (DC) in 1989, 45 States and DC in 1990, 46 States and DC in 1991–93, and 46 States, DC, and New York City (NYC) in 1994–96. Excludes data for California, Indiana, New York (but includes NYC in 1994–96), and South Dakota (1989–96), Oklahoma (1989–90), and Louisiana and Nebraska (1989), which did not require the reporting of mother's tobacco use during pregnancy on the birth certificate (see Appendix I).

NOTES: The race groups, white, black, American Indian or Alaska Native, and Asian or Pacific Islander, include persons of Hispanic and non-Hispanic origin. Conversely, persons of Hispanic origin may be of any race.

SOURCES: Centers for Disease Control and Prevention, National Center for Health Statistics. Data computed by the Division of Health and Utilization Analysis from data compiled by the Division of Vital Statistics; Ventura SJ, Martin JA, Curtin SC, Mathews TJ. Report of final natality statistics, 1996. Monthly vital statistics report; vol 46. Hyattsville, Maryland: 1998; Report of final natality statistics, for each data year 1970–95. Monthly vital statistics report. Hyattsville, Maryland.

Table 12. Low-birthweight live births among mothers 20 years of age and over, by mother's detailed race, Hispanic origin, and educational attainment: Selected States, 1989–96

[Data are based on the National Vital Statistics System]

Mother's education, race of mother, and Hispanic origin of mother	1989	1990	1991	1992	1993	1994	1995	1996
Less than 12 years of education	\multicolumn{8}{c}{Percent of live births weighing less than 2,500 grams[1]}							
All races	9.0	8.6	8.7	8.4	8.6	8.5	8.4	8.3
White	7.3	7.0	7.1	6.9	7.1	7.1	7.1	7.1
Black	17.0	16.5	17.0	16.5	16.4	16.2	16.0	15.5
American Indian or Alaska Native	7.3	7.4	7.4	7.1	7.6	7.0	8.0	7.7
Asian or Pacific Islander	6.6	6.4	6.5	6.2	6.4	6.6	6.7	7.1
Chinese	5.4	5.2	5.0	4.4	4.6	4.6	5.3	5.0
Japanese	4.0	10.6	7.5	7.0	9.4	7.4	11.0	8.3
Filipino	6.9	7.2	7.4	6.8	6.2	8.2	7.5	8.0
Hawaiian and part Hawaiian	11.0	10.7	7.1	9.5	9.1	8.0	9.8	10.1
Other Asian or Pacific Islander	6.8	6.4	6.7	6.4	6.6	6.8	6.7	7.5
Hispanic origin (selected States)[2,3]	6.0	5.7	5.8	5.8	5.8	5.8	5.8	5.8
Mexican	5.3	5.2	5.3	5.3	5.4	5.4	5.4	5.4
Puerto Rican	11.3	10.3	11.2	10.4	10.3	10.7	10.5	10.4
Cuban	9.4	7.9	7.1	7.8	6.5	8.2	9.2	8.0
Central and South American	5.8	5.8	5.7	5.8	5.8	6.0	6.2	6.0
Other and unknown Hispanic	8.2	8.0	8.1	7.8	8.1	7.6	7.7	8.0
White, non-Hispanic (selected States)[2]	8.4	8.3	8.4	8.3	8.7	8.8	8.9	9.1
Black, non-Hispanic (selected States)[2]	17.6	16.7	17.2	16.7	16.7	16.6	16.2	15.8
12 years of education								
All races	7.1	7.1	7.3	7.2	7.4	7.5	7.6	7.7
White	5.7	5.8	5.9	5.9	6.1	6.3	6.4	6.6
Black	13.4	13.1	13.5	13.3	13.4	13.3	13.3	13.2
American Indian or Alaska Native	5.6	6.1	5.9	6.0	6.1	6.3	6.5	6.0
Asian or Pacific Islander	6.4	6.5	6.5	6.8	6.6	6.7	7.0	7.0
Chinese	5.1	4.9	5.5	5.7	4.9	5.3	5.7	4.9
Japanese	7.4	6.2	6.4	7.4	7.2	7.6	7.4	7.2
Filipino	6.8	7.6	6.9	7.4	6.5	7.5	7.7	7.8
Hawaiian and part Hawaiian	7.0	6.7	6.7	7.0	7.1	6.9	6.6	6.5
Other Asian or Pacific Islander	6.5	6.7	6.7	6.8	7.0	6.8	7.1	7.4
Hispanic origin (selected States)[2,3]	5.9	6.0	6.0	6.0	6.2	6.2	6.1	6.2
Mexican	5.2	5.5	5.4	5.5	5.7	5.8	5.6	5.8
Puerto Rican	8.8	8.3	8.4	8.3	8.5	8.1	8.7	8.8
Cuban	5.3	5.2	6.1	6.6	6.6	6.6	6.7	6.0
Central and South American	5.7	5.8	5.6	5.7	6.1	5.8	5.9	5.9
Other and unknown Hispanic	6.1	6.6	6.8	7.1	7.4	7.3	7.1	7.5
White, non-Hispanic (selected States)[2]	5.7	5.7	5.9	5.9	6.1	6.3	6.5	6.7
Black, non-Hispanic (selected States)[2]	13.6	13.2	13.6	13.4	13.5	13.4	13.4	13.3
13 years or more of education								
All races	5.5	5.4	5.6	5.6	5.8	5.9	6.0	6.2
White	4.6	4.6	4.7	4.8	5.0	5.1	5.3	5.5
Black	11.2	11.1	11.4	11.2	11.3	11.5	11.4	11.4
American Indian or Alaska Native	5.6	4.7	4.9	5.6	5.8	5.9	5.7	6.0
Asian or Pacific Islander	6.1	6.0	6.2	6.2	6.3	6.6	6.6	6.8
Chinese	4.5	4.4	4.9	4.7	4.9	4.6	5.1	5.0
Japanese	6.6	6.0	5.6	6.9	6.3	6.8	7.1	7.2
Filipino	7.2	7.0	7.1	7.3	6.9	7.5	7.6	7.8
Hawaiian and part Hawaiian	6.3	4.7	4.9	5.4	5.2	5.9	5.0	5.4
Other Asian or Pacific Islander	6.1	6.2	6.4	6.2	6.5	6.9	6.7	7.0
Hispanic origin (selected States)[2,3]	5.5	5.5	5.5	5.5	5.7	5.8	5.9	6.0
Mexican	5.1	5.2	5.0	5.1	5.5	5.5	5.6	5.6
Puerto Rican	7.4	7.4	7.5	7.5	7.4	7.3	7.9	7.8
Cuban	4.9	5.0	4.8	5.1	5.4	5.7	5.6	6.4
Central and South American	5.2	5.6	5.7	5.1	5.4	5.5	5.8	5.7
Other and unknown Hispanic	5.4	5.2	5.7	5.4	5.6	6.5	6.1	6.6
White, non-Hispanic (selected States)[2]	4.6	4.5	4.7	4.7	4.9	5.1	5.2	5.4
Black, non-Hispanic (selected States)[2]	11.2	11.1	11.4	11.2	11.4	11.5	11.5	11.4

[1]Excludes live births with unknown birthweight. Percent based on live births with known birthweight.

[2]Data shown only for States with an Hispanic-origin item and education of mother on their birth certificates. The number of States reporting both items increased from 45, the District of Columbia (DC), and New York City (NYC) in 1989, to 47, DC, and NYC in 1990–91, 49 and DC in 1992, and 50 and DC in 1993 and later years (see Appendix I, National Vital Statistics System).

[3]Includes mothers of all races.

NOTES: Includes data for 48 States, the District of Columbia (DC), and New York City (NYC) in 1989–91 and all 50 States and DC starting in 1992. Excludes data for births to residents of upstate New York and Washington (1989–91), which did not require the reporting of education of mother on the birth certificate (see Appendix I). The race groups, white, black, American Indian or Alaska Native, and Asian or Pacific Islander, include persons of Hispanic and non-Hispanic origin. Conversely, persons of Hispanic origin may be of any race.

SOURCE: Centers for Disease Control and Prevention, National Center for Health Statistics. Data computed by the Division of Health and Utilization Analysis from data compiled by the Division of Vital Statistics.

Table 13. Low-birthweight live births, according to race of mother, geographic division, and State: United States, average annual 1984–86, 1989–91, and 1994–96

[Data are based on the National Vital Statistics System]

Geographic division and State	All races 1984–86	All races 1989–91	All races 1994–96	White 1984–86	White 1989–91	White 1994–96	Black 1984–86	Black 1989–91	Black 1994–96
	Percent of live births weighing less than 2,500 grams								
United States	6.76	7.04	7.33	5.64	5.74	6.22	12.67	13.44	13.13
New England	5.92	5.97	6.41	5.46	5.39	5.92	12.23	11.91	11.47
Maine	5.24	5.14	5.89	5.19	5.13	5.87	*	*	*
New Hampshire	5.06	4.97	5.15	5.04	4.93	5.10	*	*	*
Vermont	5.74	5.47	5.85	5.73	5.45	5.83	*	*	*
Massachusetts	5.83	5.88	6.37	5.42	5.34	5.88	11.18	10.58	10.64
Rhode Island	6.26	6.14	6.71	5.85	5.58	6.27	*11.95	*11.41	*11.63
Connecticut	6.59	6.80	7.07	5.67	5.70	6.21	13.49	13.96	12.75
Middle Atlantic	6.94	7.45	7.57	5.65	5.88	6.30	12.73	13.92	12.92
New York	7.11	7.71	7.63	5.73	6.08	6.35	12.26	13.60	12.31
New Jersey	6.88	7.21	7.60	5.54	5.63	6.23	12.69	13.55	13.24
Pennsylvania	6.71	7.17	7.44	5.60	5.74	6.28	14.03	15.07	14.21
East North Central	6.65	7.23	7.52	5.44	5.69	6.23	13.40	14.38	14.02
Ohio	6.57	7.21	7.54	5.66	5.99	6.48	12.33	13.81	13.56
Indiana	6.37	6.61	7.32	5.74	5.87	6.64	11.92	12.49	13.08
Illinois	7.24	7.68	7.92	5.44	5.63	6.11	14.03	14.63	14.61
Michigan	6.88	7.65	7.72	5.46	5.68	6.25	14.10	15.12	14.00
Wisconsin	5.26	5.92	6.22	4.66	4.99	5.40	12.58	14.18	13.58
West North Central	5.69	5.97	6.49	5.14	5.31	5.91	12.68	13.11	12.99
Minnesota	4.94	5.09	5.78	4.69	4.66	5.38	*12.28	13.88	12.17
Iowa	5.08	5.50	6.06	4.91	5.30	5.81	*11.84	*11.65	*13.04
Missouri	6.73	7.18	7.57	5.62	5.91	6.48	12.93	13.39	13.45
North Dakota	4.85	5.11	5.48	4.69	5.00	5.30	*	*	*
South Dakota	5.29	5.27	5.75	4.99	5.12	5.64	*	*	*
Nebraska	5.39	5.56	6.25	5.03	5.12	5.93	*12.05	*12.50	*11.88
Kansas	6.13	6.19	6.61	5.56	5.60	6.08	12.59	12.33	12.69
South Atlantic	7.77	8.02	8.32	5.94	5.93	6.49	12.47	13.10	13.06
Delaware	7.38	7.67	8.09	5.92	5.75	6.58	12.42	13.68	12.87
Maryland	7.60	7.97	8.53	5.49	5.59	6.23	12.58	13.14	13.30
District of Columbia	12.65	15.45	13.94	5.33	6.47	6.12	14.57	17.94	16.25
Virginia	7.06	7.18	7.62	5.62	5.54	6.11	11.75	12.34	12.53
West Virginia	6.93	6.86	7.78	6.71	6.61	7.56	*12.62	*13.43	*13.70
North Carolina	7.88	8.17	8.69	6.08	6.10	6.78	12.43	12.98	13.75
South Carolina	8.64	9.03	9.22	6.09	6.33	6.84	12.73	13.29	13.37
Georgia	8.15	8.53	8.63	6.02	6.04	6.42	12.22	12.92	12.86
Florida	7.52	7.51	7.76	5.99	5.92	6.42	12.45	12.61	12.27
East South Central	7.88	8.32	8.82	6.26	6.50	7.16	12.26	13.06	13.43
Kentucky	7.02	7.03	7.71	6.48	6.50	7.23	12.47	12.09	12.64
Tennessee	7.91	8.41	8.78	6.46	6.66	7.22	12.95	14.07	14.26
Alabama	8.00	8.46	9.11	5.89	6.27	7.05	12.06	12.64	13.29
Mississippi	8.72	9.56	9.85	5.99	6.53	7.01	11.91	12.87	13.07
West South Central	7.14	7.39	7.57	5.96	6.05	6.44	12.61	13.30	13.11
Arkansas	7.71	8.22	8.29	6.28	6.57	6.90	12.33	13.59	13.16
Louisiana	8.62	9.24	9.73	5.81	6.08	6.65	13.08	13.70	14.11
Oklahoma	6.42	6.54	7.12	5.89	5.98	6.59	11.94	11.68	12.61
Texas	6.82	7.00	7.11	5.96	6.00	6.35	12.39	13.15	12.46
Mountain	6.56	6.76	7.16	6.36	6.50	6.94	13.30	14.08	13.71
Montana	5.79	5.76	6.16	5.73	5.77	6.12	*	*	*
Idaho	5.27	5.66	5.72	5.22	5.61	5.67	*	*	*
Wyoming	6.99	7.23	8.21	6.99	7.13	8.15	*	*	*
Colorado	7.69	7.99	8.59	7.34	7.53	8.20	14.43	15.18	15.44
New Mexico	7.25	7.14	7.46	7.41	7.18	7.57	*11.64	*12.14	*10.96
Arizona	6.18	6.38	6.75	5.97	6.13	6.56	12.83	12.74	12.75
Utah	5.56	5.81	6.28	5.48	5.77	6.23	*	*	*
Nevada	7.01	7.22	7.49	6.30	6.40	6.81	*12.89	15.05	13.94
Pacific	5.81	5.81	6.01	5.14	5.13	5.44	12.38	12.78	11.96
Washington	5.18	5.33	5.45	4.83	4.99	5.16	11.74	11.76	10.65
Oregon	5.13	5.04	5.37	4.99	4.83	5.24	*12.14	*11.75	*10.56
California	5.95	5.90	6.11	5.23	5.18	5.51	12.50	12.92	12.11
Alaska	4.77	4.80	5.45	4.27	4.34	5.03	*8.89	*9.10	*11.67
Hawaii	6.86	6.99	7.17	5.56	5.62	5.35	*9.85	*11.52	*10.61

* Data for States with fewer than 5,000 live births for the 3-year period are considered unreliable. Data for States with fewer than 1,000 live births are considered highly unreliable and are not shown.

SOURCE: Centers for Disease Control and Prevention, National Center for Health Statistics. Data computed by the Division of Health and Utilization Analysis from data compiled by the Division of Vital Statistics.

Table 14. Very low-birthweight live births, according to race of mother, geographic division, and State: United States, average annual 1984–86, 1989–91, and 1994–96

[Data are based on the National Vital Statistics System]

Geographic division and State	All races 1984–86	All races 1989–91	All races 1994–96	White 1984–86	White 1989–91	White 1994–96	Black 1984–86	Black 1989–91	Black 1994–96
	Percent of live births weighing less than 1,500 grams								
United States	1.20	1.28	1.35	0.93	0.96	1.06	2.68	2.94	2.97
New England	1.04	1.12	1.17	0.92	0.97	1.02	2.83	2.87	2.92
Maine	0.93	0.85	1.12	0.93	0.85	1.12	*	*	*
New Hampshire	0.86	0.93	0.83	0.86	0.91	0.82	*	*	*
Vermont	0.89	0.79	0.88	0.90	0.79	0.88	*	*	*
Massachusetts	0.99	1.10	1.15	0.88	0.97	1.00	2.46	2.37	2.66
Rhode Island	1.10	1.16	1.07	1.00	1.03	0.97	*2.56	*2.76	*2.37
Connecticut	1.25	1.37	1.41	0.97	1.03	1.12	3.33	3.61	3.44
Middle Atlantic	1.26	1.42	1.46	0.94	1.01	1.10	2.72	3.19	3.06
New York	1.29	1.44	1.47	0.94	1.01	1.10	2.59	3.06	2.93
New Jersey	1.26	1.41	1.54	0.95	1.03	1.15	2.65	3.04	3.28
Pennsylvania	1.23	1.38	1.38	0.94	0.99	1.08	3.14	3.64	3.17
East North Central	1.23	1.36	1.42	0.94	0.98	1.10	2.91	3.14	3.09
Ohio	1.20	1.32	1.40	0.98	1.02	1.12	2.61	2.98	3.04
Indiana	1.07	1.18	1.31	0.92	1.00	1.13	2.43	2.68	2.85
Illinois	1.37	1.46	1.52	0.94	0.98	1.10	3.02	3.10	3.13
Michigan	1.32	1.50	1.50	0.95	0.98	1.11	3.24	3.48	3.20
Wisconsin	0.97	1.08	1.17	0.82	0.87	0.98	2.82	3.03	2.94
West North Central	0.98	1.04	1.17	0.86	0.88	1.03	2.58	2.72	2.78
Minnesota	0.88	0.90	1.08	0.84	0.82	1.00	*2.15	2.81	2.64
Iowa	0.83	0.91	1.11	0.81	0.86	1.06	*1.84	*2.51	*2.98
Missouri	1.18	1.26	1.29	0.92	0.93	1.03	2.71	2.82	2.75
North Dakota	0.80	0.84	0.97	0.75	0.83	0.89	*	*	*
South Dakota	0.98	0.90	1.00	0.91	0.86	0.89	*	*	*
Nebraska	0.87	0.95	1.11	0.78	0.85	1.06	*2.45	*2.47	*2.19
Kansas	1.02	1.09	1.24	0.89	0.96	1.08	2.62	2.50	3.20
South Atlantic	1.50	1.59	1.65	1.02	1.02	1.11	2.73	2.98	3.07
Delaware	1.52	1.63	1.62	1.13	1.07	1.24	2.87	3.41	2.87
Maryland	1.64	1.67	1.80	1.06	0.99	1.08	3.08	3.18	3.33
District of Columbia	3.15	3.79	3.48	1.18	1.28	0.86	3.70	4.48	4.27
Virginia	1.30	1.41	1.50	0.93	0.95	1.05	2.51	2.88	3.03
West Virginia	1.16	1.15	1.26	1.10	1.08	1.22	*3.09	*2.97	*2.26
North Carolina	1.49	1.65	1.79	1.03	1.09	1.22	2.67	2.99	3.28
South Carolina	1.65	1.72	1.81	1.04	1.06	1.16	2.64	2.77	2.94
Georgia	1.58	1.67	1.71	1.02	1.00	1.06	2.64	2.85	2.95
Florida	1.39	1.43	1.47	1.02	1.01	1.09	2.59	2.79	2.81
East South Central	1.38	1.52	1.65	1.01	1.06	1.17	2.41	2.71	2.97
Kentucky	1.21	1.21	1.32	1.07	1.07	1.19	2.57	2.53	2.67
Tennessee	1.36	1.56	1.63	1.01	1.10	1.18	2.59	3.07	3.22
Alabama	1.42	1.61	1.84	0.93	1.06	1.21	2.38	2.66	3.10
Mississippi	1.57	1.70	1.81	0.98	0.94	1.03	2.26	2.52	2.70
West South Central	1.22	1.26	1.34	0.94	0.94	1.05	2.51	2.70	2.80
Arkansas	1.30	1.33	1.56	1.01	0.98	1.24	2.28	2.46	2.69
Louisiana	1.58	1.73	1.91	0.95	0.96	1.08	2.58	2.83	3.10
Oklahoma	1.04	1.08	1.16	0.90	0.97	1.01	2.40	2.21	2.68
Texas	1.14	1.17	1.23	0.94	0.92	1.04	2.52	2.73	2.62
Mountain	0.95	1.01	1.09	0.89	0.95	1.04	2.44	2.70	2.71
Montana	0.81	0.87	0.99	0.77	0.84	0.99	*	*	*
Idaho	0.83	0.90	0.85	0.81	0.88	0.82	*	*	*
Wyoming	1.02	0.90	1.06	1.02	0.91	1.07	*	*	*
Colorado	0.99	1.08	1.24	0.91	0.97	1.15	2.56	2.71	3.05
New Mexico	1.00	0.94	1.09	1.00	0.93	1.10	*2.19	*2.39	*2.02
Arizona	1.05	1.08	1.09	0.98	1.02	1.05	2.57	2.84	2.68
Utah	0.75	0.86	0.97	0.74	0.85	0.94	*	*	*
Nevada	0.98	1.14	1.13	0.87	0.97	1.01	*2.30	2.76	2.51
Pacific	1.01	0.99	1.04	0.87	0.86	0.94	2.66	2.70	2.58
Washington	0.92	0.85	0.89	0.85	0.78	0.84	2.57	2.69	2.18
Oregon	0.86	0.83	0.88	0.83	0.81	0.85	*2.34	*1.93	*1.66
California	1.04	1.02	1.08	0.89	0.88	0.96	2.68	2.71	2.63
Alaska	0.84	0.87	0.97	0.76	0.73	0.85	*1.94	*2.08	*2.94
Hawaii	1.05	1.03	1.02	0.84	0.99	0.88	*2.56	*2.94	*2.89

* Data for States with fewer than 5,000 live births for the 3-year period are considered unreliable. Data for States with fewer than 1,000 live births are considered highly unreliable and are not shown.

SOURCE: Centers for Disease Control and Prevention, National Center for Health Statistics. Data computed by the Division of Health and Utilization Analysis from data compiled by the Division of Vital Statistics.

Table 15. Legal abortion ratios, according to selected patient characteristics: United States, selected years 1973–95

[Data are based on reporting by State health departments and by hospitals and other medical facilities]

Characteristic	1973	1975	1980	1985	1987	1988	1989	1990	1991	1992	1993	1994	1995
	Abortions per 100 live births[1]												
Total	19.6	27.2	35.9	35.4	35.6	35.2	34.6	34.5	33.9	33.5	33.4	32.1	31.1
Age													
Under 15 years	123.7	119.3	139.7	137.6	127.5	94.9	88.6	84.4	76.7	79.0	74.4	70.4	66.7
15–19 years.	53.9	54.2	71.4	68.8	66.8	62.4	56.0	51.5	46.2	44.0	44.0	41.5	39.9
20–24 years.	29.4	28.9	39.5	38.6	38.6	37.4	36.6	37.7	37.8	37.6	38.4	36.4	34.9
25–29 years.	20.7	19.2	23.7	21.7	21.8	21.4	21.1	22.0	22.1	22.2	22.7	22.2	22.1
30–34 years.	28.0	25.0	23.7	19.9	19.6	18.8	18.7	19.1	18.7	18.3	18.0	17.2	16.5
35–39 years.	45.1	42.2	41.0	33.6	29.7	28.0	27.1	27.3	26.2	25.6	24.8	23.4	22.4
40 years and over	68.4	66.8	80.7	62.3	55.5	51.4	49.6	50.1	46.9	45.4	43.0	41.2	38.7
Race													
White[2]	32.6	27.7	33.2	27.7	26.7	25.9	25.2	25.8	24.6	23.6	23.1	21.7	20.4
Black[3]	42.0	47.6	54.3	47.2	50.0	48.9	49.6	52.1	50.2	51.8	55.2	53.8	53.4
Hispanic origin[4]													
Hispanic	- - -	- - -	- - -	- - -	- - -	- - -	- - -	- - -	30.0	30.7	28.9	27.8	26.5
Non-Hispanic	- - -	- - -	- - -	- - -	- - -	- - -	- - -	- - -	33.2	32.6	30.9	29.0	28.0
Marital status													
Married	7.6	9.6	10.5	8.0	9.6	8.8	8.1	8.9	8.9	8.4	8.4	7.9	7.8
Unmarried	139.8	161.0	147.6	117.4	101.9	102.7	92.1	87.9	81.5	79.0	78.9	68.9	64.5
Previous live births[5]													
0	43.7	38.4	45.7	45.1	41.0	37.7	36.8	35.8	34.8	32.7	32.4	30.9	28.6
1	23.5	22.0	20.2	21.6	22.2	21.8	21.2	23.0	23.2	22.9	23.1	22.3	22.1
2	36.8	36.8	29.5	29.9	31.5	30.4	28.9	31.7	31.9	31.9	32.2	30.9	30.9
3	46.9	47.7	29.8	18.2	30.9	29.1	26.5	30.2	31.0	30.8	31.5	30.8	31.0
4 or more[6]	44.7	43.5	24.3	21.5	24.7	21.9	22.3	27.1	22.6	25.5	23.4	23.3	23.9

- - - Data not available.

[1]For calculation of ratios according to each characteristic, abortions with the characteristic unknown have been distributed in proportion to abortions with the characteristic known.

[2]For 1989 and later years, white race includes women of Hispanic ethnicity.

[3]Reported as black and other races before 1989.

[4]Includes data for 20–22 States, the District of Columbia, and New York City in 1991–95. States with large Hispanic populations that are not included are California, Florida, and Illinois.

[5]For 1973–75 data indicate number of living children.

[6]For 1975 data refer to four previous live births, not four or more. For five or more previous live births, the ratio is 47.3.

NOTES: For each year since 1969 the Centers for Disease Control and Prevention has compiled total abortion data from 50 States, the District of Columbia (DC), and New York City (NYC). The number of States reporting each characteristic varies from year to year. For 1992–95 the number of States reporting each characteristic was as follows: age, 41–42 States, DC, and NYC; race, 34–35 States, DC, and NYC; marital status, 32–37 States, DC (in 1992), and NYC; previous live births, 36–38 States and NYC. Some data for 1993 and 1994 have been revised and differ from the previous edition of *Health, United States*.

SOURCES: Centers for Disease Control and Prevention: Abortion Surveillance, 1973, 1975, 1979–80. Public Health Service, DHHS, Atlanta, Ga., May 1975, April 1977, May 1983; CDC Surveillance Summaries. Abortion Surveillance, United States, 1982–83, Vol. 36, No. 1SS, Public Health Service, DHHS, Atlanta, Ga., Feb. 1987; 1984 and 1985, Vol. 38, No. SS–2, Sept. 1989; 1986 and 1987, Vol. 39, No. SS–2, June 1990; 1988, Vol. 40, No. SS–2, July 1991; 1989, Vol. 41, No. SS–5, Sept. 1992; 1990, Vol. 42, No. SS–6, Dec. 1993; 1991, Vol. 44, No. SS–2, May 1995; 1992, Vol. 45, No. SS–3, May 1996; 1993 and 1994, Vol. 46, No. SS–4, Aug. 1997; 1995, in press, 1998.

Table 16. Legal abortions, according to selected characteristics: United States, selected years 1973–95

[Data are based on reporting by State health departments and by hospitals and other facilities]

Characteristic	1973	1975	1980	1985	1987	1988	1989	1990	1991	1992	1993	1994	1995
	Number of legal abortions reported in thousands												
Centers for Disease Control and Prevention	616	855	1,298	1,329	1,354	1,371	1,397	1,430	1,389	1,359	1,330	1,267	1,211
Alan Guttmacher Institute[1]	745	1,034	1,554	1,589	1,559	1,591	1,567	1,609	1,557	1,529	- - -	1,400	- - -
	Percent distribution[2]												
Total	100.0	100.0	100.0	100.0	100.0	100.0	100.0	100.0	100.0	100.0	100.0	100.0	100.0
Period of gestation													
Under 9 weeks	36.1	44.6	51.7	50.3	50.4	48.7	49.8	51.6	52.3	52.1	52.3	53.7	54.0
Under 7 weeks	- - -	- - -	- - -	- - -	- - -	- - -	- - -	- - -	- - -	14.3	14.7	15.7	15.7
7 weeks	- - -	- - -	- - -	- - -	- - -	- - -	- - -	- - -	- - -	15.6	16.2	16.5	17.1
8 weeks	- - -	- - -	- - -	- - -	- - -	- - -	- - -	- - -	- - -	22.2	21.6	21.6	21.2
9–10 weeks	29.4	28.4	26.2	26.6	26.0	26.4	25.8	25.3	25.1	24.2	24.4	23.5	23.1
11–12 weeks	17.9	14.9	12.2	12.5	12.4	12.7	12.6	11.7	11.5	12.0	11.6	10.9	10.9
13–15 weeks	6.9	5.0	5.1	5.9	6.2	6.6	6.6	6.4	6.1	6.0	6.3	6.3	6.3
16–20 weeks	8.0	6.1	3.9	3.9	4.2	4.5	4.2	4.0	3.9	4.2	4.1	4.3	4.3
21 weeks and over	1.7	1.0	0.9	0.8	0.8	1.1	1.0	1.0	1.1	1.5	1.3	1.3	1.4
Type of procedure													
Curettage	88.4	90.9	95.5	97.5	97.2	98.6	98.8	98.8	98.9	98.9	99.0	99.1	98.9
Intrauterine instillation	10.4	6.2	3.1	1.7	1.3	1.1	0.9	0.8	0.7	0.7	0.6	0.5	0.5
Other[3]	1.2	2.8	1.4	0.8	1.5	0.3	0.3	0.4	0.4	0.4	0.4	0.4	0.6
Location of facility													
In State of residence	74.8	89.2	92.6	92.4	91.7	91.4	91.0	91.8	91.6	92.0	91.4	91.5	91.7
Out of State of residence	25.2	10.8	7.4	7.6	8.3	8.6	9.0	8.2	8.4	8.0	8.6	8.5	8.3
Previous induced abortions													
0	- - -	81.9	67.6	60.1	58.5	57.8	58.1	57.1	56.1	55.1	54.9	54.8	55.2
1	- - -	14.9	23.5	25.7	26.5	26.9	26.5	26.9	27.2	27.4	27.3	27.2	27.0
2	- - -	2.5	6.6	9.8	10.3	10.4	9.9	10.1	10.6	11.0	11.0	11.1	10.9
3 or more	- - -	0.7	2.3	4.4	4.7	4.9	5.5	5.9	6.1	6.5	6.7	7.0	6.9

- - - Data not available.

[1]No survey was conducted in 1983, 1986, 1989, 1990, 1993, or 1994; data for these years are estimated.
[2]Excludes cases for which selected characteristic is unknown.
[3]Includes hysterotomy and hysterectomy.

NOTES: For a discussion of the differences in reported legal abortions between the Centers for Disease Control and Prevention and the Alan Guttmacher Institute, see Appendix I. For each year since 1969 the Centers for Disease Control and Prevention has compiled total abortion data from 50 States, the District of Columbia (DC), and New York City (NYC). The number of States reporting each characteristic varies from year to year. For 1992–95 the number of States reporting each characteristic was as follows: gestational age, 37–39 States, DC (in 1992–94), and NYC; detailed gestational age under 9 weeks, 35–37 States and NYC; type of procedure, 38–39 States, DC, and NYC; location of facility, 40–42 States, DC, and NYC; previous induced abortions, 35–37 States, DC (in 1992), and NYC.

SOURCES: Centers for Disease Control and Prevention: Abortion Surveillance, 1973, 1975, 1979–80. Public Health Service, DHHS, Atlanta, Ga., May 1975, April 1977, May 1983; CDC Surveillance Summaries. Abortion Surveillance, United States, 1982–83, Vol. 36, No. 1SS, Public Health Service, DHHS, Atlanta, Ga., Feb. 1987; 1984 and 1985, Vol. 38, No. SS–2, Sept. 1989; 1986 and 1987, Vol. 39, No. SS–2, June 1990; 1988, Vol. 40, No. SS–2, July 1991; 1989, Vol. 41, No. SS–5, Sept. 1992; 1990, Vol. 42, No. SS–6, Dec. 1993; 1991, Vol. 44, No. SS–2, May 1995; 1992, Vol. 45, No. SS–3, May 1996; 1993 and 1994, Vol. 46, No. SS–4, Aug. 1997; 1995, in press, 1998; Henshaw, S. K. and Van Vort, J.: Abortion services in the United States, 1991 and 1992. Fam. Plann. Perspect. 26(3), May–June 1994; unpublished data.

Table 17. Legal abortions, abortion-related deaths, and abortion-related death rates, according to period of gestation: United States, 1974–76 through 1989–91

[Data are based primarily on reporting by State health departments and by facilities]

Period of gestation and year	Number of legal abortions reported	Abortion-related deaths	
		Number	Rate per 100,000 abortions
Total			
1974–76	2,606,596	66	2.5
1977–79[1]	3,489,127	48	1.4
1980–82[2]	3,902,346	28	0.7
1983–85[3]	3,931,078	34	0.9
1986–88[4]	4,053,068	34	0.8
1989–91[5]	4,215,172	28	0.7
Under 9 weeks			
1974–76	1,170,991	8	0.7
1977–79	1,808,026	10	0.6
1980–82	1,996,665	7	0.4
1983–85	1,972,385	3	0.2
1986–88	2,027,403	5	0.2
1989–91	2,159,611	3	0.1
9–10 weeks			
1974–76	739,599	10	1.4
1977–79	941,986	9	1.0
1980–82	1,036,739	5	0.5
1983–85	1,045,538	6	0.6
1986–88	1,056,627	2	0.2
1989–91	1,070,644	–	–
11–12 weeks			
1974–76	387,259	10	2.6
1977–79	446,562	7	1.6
1980–82	477,393	4	0.8
1983–85	496,525	3	0.6
1986–88	504,038	2	0.4
1989–91	502,967	–	–
13 weeks and over			
1974–76	308,748	38	12.3
1977–79	292,553	20	6.8
1980–82	391,548	11	2.8
1983–85	416,630	19	4.6
1986–88	465,000	16	3.4
1989–91	481,949	17	3.5

– Quantity zero.

[1]Includes two deaths with weeks of gestation unknown.
[2]Includes one death with weeks of gestation unknown.
[3]Includes three deaths with weeks of gestation unknown.
[4]Includes nine deaths with weeks of gestation unknown.
[5]Includes eight deaths with weeks of gestation unknown.

SOURCE: Centers for Disease Control and Prevention. Surveillance summaries, Abortion surveillance, United States, 1992. Vol 45, no SS–3. Atlanta, Georgia: Public Health Service. 1996; unpublished data.

Table 18. Methods of contraception for women 15–44 years of age, according to race and age: United States, 1982, 1988, and 1995

[Data are based on household interviews of samples of women in the childbearing ages]

Method of contraception and age	All races 1982	All races 1988	All races 1995	White 1982	White 1988	White 1995	Black 1982	Black 1988	Black 1995
	1982	*1988*	*1995*	*1982*	*1988*	*1995*	*1982*	*1988*	*1995*
				Number of women in thousands					
15–44 years	54,099	57,900	60,201	45,367	47,076	47,981	6,985	7,679	8,460
15–19 years	9,521	9,179	8,961	7,815	7,313	6,838	1,416	1,409	1,454
20–24 years	10,629	9,413	9,041	8,855	7,401	7,015	1,472	1,364	1,386
25–34 years	19,644	21,726	20,758	16,485	17,682	16,609	2,479	2,865	2,861
35–44 years	14,305	17,582	21,440	12,212	14,681	17,519	1,618	2,041	2,758
All methods			Percent of women using contraception						
15–44 years	55.7	60.3	64.2	56.7	61.8	65.5	52.0	56.7	61.5
15–19 years	24.2	32.1	29.8	23.4	32.2	30.0	30.0	35.1	34.5
20–24 years	55.8	59.0	63.5	56.6	60.2	63.3	52.5	61.1	66.9
25–34 years	66.7	66.3	71.1	67.7	67.7	72.6	64.0	63.8	66.4
35–44 years	61.6	68.3	72.3	63.1	70.2	73.4	52.3	58.9	68.0
Female sterilization			Percent of contracepting women						
15–44 years	23.2	27.5	27.7	22.1	26.1	25.7	30.0	38.1	39.9
15–19 years	–	*1.5	*0.3	–	*1.6	–	–	*1.6	–
20–24 years	4.5	4.6	4.0	*3.8	3.9	3.5	9.8	9.1	7.2
25–34 years	22.1	25.0	23.8	20.2	23.2	21.3	33.5	39.9	40.3
35–44 years	43.5	47.6	45.0	41.9	44.7	41.7	56.8	70.5	66.3
Male sterilization									
15–44 years	10.9	11.7	10.9	12.2	13.6	12.7	*1.4	*0.9	1.7
15–19 years	*0.4	*0.2	–	*0.5	*0.3	–	–	–	–
20–24 years	*3.6	*1.8	*1.1	*4.2	*2.3	*1.3	*0.5	–	*0.2
25–34 years	10.1	10.2	7.8	11.3	11.7	8.9	*1.4	*1.1	*1.5
35–44 years	19.9	20.8	19.4	21.6	23.7	22.1	*3.1	*1.5	3.1
Birth control pill									
15–44 years	28.0	30.7	26.9	26.7	29.8	28.0	38.0	38.0	23.8
15–19 years	63.9	58.8	43.8	62.1	55.9	47.5	70.8	74.2	33.2
20–24 years	55.1	68.2	52.1	53.5	67.9	55.4	65.0	70.3	41.5
25–34 years	25.7	32.6	33.3	24.8	32.4	35.0	33.7	35.7	26.6
35–44 years	3.7	4.3	8.7	3.7	4.5	8.9	*5.1	*4.2	9.6
Intrauterine device									
15–44 years	7.1	2.0	0.8	6.9	1.8	0.8	9.1	3.1	*0.8
15–19 years	*1.3	–	–	*0.5	–	–	*4.9	–	–
20–24 years	4.2	*0.3	*0.3	*3.5	*0.3	*0.4	*6.2	*0.9	*0.2
25–34 years	9.7	2.1	0.8	9.4	1.7	0.7	13.0	*4.1	*1.5
35–44 years	6.9	3.1	1.1	7.0	3.0	1.2	*6.5	*4.3	*0.6
Diaphragm									
15–44 years	8.1	5.7	1.9	8.8	6.2	2.1	3.5	1.9	*0.8
15–19 years	*6.0	*1.0	*0.1	*7.1	*1.3	*0.2	*1.8	–	–
20–24 years	10.2	3.7	*0.6	11.3	4.1	*0.6	*2.8	*1.6	*0.7
25–34 years	10.3	7.3	1.7	11.3	8.0	1.8	*3.0	*1.7	*1.0
35–44 years	4.0	6.0	2.8	3.8	6.2	3.2	*6.0	*3.3	*0.9
Condom									
15–44 years	12.0	14.6	20.4	12.7	14.9	19.7	6.2	10.3	20.5
15–19 years	20.8	32.8	36.7	22.6	34.2	36.8	*12.6	22.7	37.8
20–24 years	10.7	14.5	26.4	11.4	15.8	23.8	*6.4	9.6	33.8
25–34 years	11.4	13.7	21.1	12.0	14.0	20.6	5.3	9.4	17.7
35–44 years	11.3	11.2	14.7	12.0	11.3	14.6	*4.5	7.0	12.2

– Quantity zero.

* Relative standard error greater than 30 percent.

NOTES: Method of contraception used in the month of interview. If multiple methods were reported, only the most effective method is shown in the table.

SOURCE: Centers for Disease Control and Prevention, National Center for Health Statistics, Division of Vital Statistics. Data from the National Survey of Family Growth.

Table 19. Breastfeeding by mothers 15–44 years of age by year of baby's birth, according to selected characteristics of mother: United States, 1972–74 to 1993–94

[Data are based on household interviews of samples of women in the childbearing ages]

Selected characteristics of mother	1972–74	1975–77	1978–80	1981–83	1984–86	1987–89	1990–92	1993–94
	Percent of babies breastfed							
Total	30.1	36.7	47.5	58.1	54.5	52.3	54.2	58.1
Race								
White, non-Hispanic	32.5	38.9	53.2	64.3	59.7	58.3	59.1	61.2
Black, non-Hispanic	12.5	16.8	19.6	26.0	22.9	21.0	22.9	27.5
Hispanic	33.1	42.9	46.3	52.8	58.9	51.3	58.8	67.4
Education[1]								
No high school diploma or GED[2] . . .	14.0	19.4	27.6	31.4	36.8	30.0	38.6	43.0
High school diploma or GED[2]	25.0	33.6	40.2	54.3	46.7	46.6	46.0	51.2
Some college, no bachelor's degree.	35.2	43.5	63.2	66.7	66.1	57.8	60.7	65.9
Bachelor's degree or higher.	65.5	66.9	71.3	83.2	75.3	79.2	80.8	80.6
Geographic region								
Northeast.	29.9	34.7	49.3	68.2	55.3	49.9	54.0	56.7
Midwest.	22.3	30.9	34.4	46.0	50.9	50.4	51.6	49.7
South	30.6	33.1	49.5	57.9	45.3	42.5	43.6	49.7
West	47.1	54.5	66.6	69.9	70.9	69.1	70.5	79.3
Age at baby's birth								
Under 20 years	17.0	22.1	31.4	31.0	30.6	26.2	35.2	45.3
20–24 years.	28.7	33.5	44.7	50.8	50.2	46.7	44.7	50.9
25–29 years.	38.7	45.9	53.6	62.2	59.8	57.1	56.5	55.9
30–44 years.	43.1	47.5	55.2	73.1	65.9	65.3	67.5	71.1
	Percent of breastfed babies who were breastfed 3 months or more[3]							
Total	62.3	66.2	64.7	68.3	63.2	61.5	61.0	56.2
Race								
White, non-Hispanic	62.1	66.7	67.6	68.1	62.5	62.3	62.6	56.8
Black, non-Hispanic	47.8	60.7	58.5	61.1	56.8	46.9	56.7	45.4
Hispanic	64.7	62.7	46.3	65.6	66.4	64.3	58.2	55.5
Education[1]								
No high school diploma or GED[2] . . .	54.4	54.7	53.7	50.5	59.8	57.3	55.5	44.5
High school diploma or GED[2]	53.7	62.5	59.4	59.6	58.0	58.3	58.2	49.7
Some college, no bachelor's degree.	69.5	77.2	63.8	73.3	63.4	60.7	53.8	60.2
Bachelor's degree or higher.	69.2	65.3	79.9	80.9	72.2	68.1	73.8	68.1
Geographic region								
Northeast.	64.6	68.2	71.2	75.0	64.8	59.7	72.7	58.7
Midwest.	44.4	54.3	53.1	64.4	60.4	58.6	63.1	56.7
South	72.6	74.1	67.6	65.0	60.3	55.2	50.8	50.9
West	69.0	70.6	66.8	69.6	66.9	69.9	60.4	59.0
Age at baby's birth								
Under 20 years	50.0	61.0	48.2	49.1	62.5	56.3	31.9	22.6
20–24 years.	57.7	59.4	60.0	63.7	51.9	51.6	54.0	50.6
25–29 years.	68.3	71.5	65.1	70.8	65.6	58.3	59.7	63.7
30–44 years.	79.4	72.8	81.5	72.8	73.2	73.5	71.8	62.3

[1]For women 22–44 years of age. Education is as of year of interview. See NOTES below.
[2]General equivalency diploma.
[3]For mothers interviewed in the first 3 months of 1995, only babies age 3 months and over are included so they would be eligible for breastfeeding for 3 months or more.

NOTES: Data on breastfeeding during 1972–83 are based on responses to questions in the National Survey of Family Growth (NSFG) Cycle 4, conducted in 1988. Data for 1984–94 are based on the NSFG Cycle 5, conducted in 1995. Data are based on all births to mothers 15–44 years of age at interview, including those births that occurred when the mothers were younger than 15 years of age.

SOURCE: Centers for Disease Control and Prevention, National Center for Health Statistics, Division of Vital Statistics. Data from the National Survey of Family Growth, Cycle 4 1988, Cycle 5 1995.

Table 20. Infant, neonatal, and postneonatal mortality rates, according to detailed race of mother and Hispanic origin of mother: United States, selected birth cohorts 1983–95

[Data are based on National Linked Birth/Infant Death Data Sets]

Race of mother and Hispanic origin of mother	Birth cohort								
	1983	1985	1988	1990	1991	1995[1]	1983–85	1986–88	1989–91
	Infant deaths per 1,000 live births								
All mothers	10.9	10.4	9.6	8.9	8.6	7.6	10.6	9.8	9.0
White	9.3	8.9	8.0	7.3	7.1	6.3	9.0	8.2	7.4
Black	19.2	18.6	17.8	16.9	16.6	14.6	18.7	17.9	17.1
American Indian or Alaska Native	15.2	13.1	12.7	13.1	11.3	9.0	13.9	13.2	12.6
Asian or Pacific Islander	8.3	7.8	6.8	6.6	5.8	5.3	8.3	7.3	6.6
Chinese	9.5	5.8	5.5	4.3	4.6	3.8	7.4	5.8	5.1
Japanese	*	*6.0	*7.0	*5.5	*4.2	*5.3	6.0	6.9	5.3
Filipino	8.4	7.7	6.9	6.0	5.1	5.6	8.2	6.9	6.4
Hawaiian and part Hawaiian	*	*	*	*	*	*	11.3	11.1	9.0
Other Asian or Pacific Islander	8.1	8.5	7.0	7.4	6.3	5.5	8.6	7.6	7.0
Hispanic origin[2,3]	9.5	8.8	8.3	7.5	7.1	6.3	9.2	8.3	7.6
Mexican	9.1	8.5	7.9	7.2	6.9	6.0	8.8	7.9	7.2
Puerto Rican	12.9	11.1	11.6	9.9	9.7	8.9	12.3	11.1	10.4
Cuban	*7.5	8.5	7.2	7.2	5.2	5.3	8.0	7.3	6.2
Central and South American	8.5	8.0	7.2	6.8	5.9	5.5	8.2	7.6	6.6
Other and unknown Hispanic	10.6	9.5	9.1	8.0	8.2	7.4	9.9	9.0	8.2
White, non-Hispanic[3]	9.2	8.7	8.0	7.2	7.0	6.3	8.9	8.1	7.3
Black, non-Hispanic[3]	19.1	18.3	18.1	16.9	16.6	14.7	18.5	17.9	17.2
	Neonatal deaths per 1,000 live births								
All mothers	7.1	6.8	6.1	5.7	5.4	4.9	6.9	6.3	5.7
White	6.1	5.8	5.0	4.6	4.4	4.1	5.9	5.2	4.7
Black	12.5	12.3	11.5	11.1	10.7	9.6	12.2	11.7	11.1
American Indian or Alaska Native	7.5	6.1	5.4	6.1	5.5	4.0	6.7	5.9	5.9
Asian or Pacific Islander	5.2	4.8	4.3	3.9	3.6	3.4	5.2	4.5	3.9
Chinese	5.5	3.3	3.1	2.3	2.3	2.3	4.3	3.3	2.7
Japanese	*	*3.1	*4.5	*3.5	*3.2	*3.3	3.4	4.4	3.0
Filipino	5.6	5.1	4.4	3.5	3.4	3.4	5.3	4.5	4.0
Hawaiian and part Hawaiian	*	*	*	*	*	*	7.4	7.1	4.8
Other Asian or Pacific Islander	5.0	5.4	4.4	4.4	4.1	3.7	5.5	4.7	4.2
Hispanic origin[2,3]	6.2	5.7	5.2	4.8	4.5	4.1	6.0	5.3	4.8
Mexican	5.9	5.4	4.8	4.5	4.3	3.9	5.7	5.0	4.5
Puerto Rican	8.7	7.6	7.3	6.9	6.1	6.1	8.3	7.2	7.0
Cuban	*5.0	6.2	5.5	5.3	4.0	3.6	5.9	5.3	4.6
Central and South American	5.8	5.6	4.8	4.4	4.0	3.7	5.7	5.0	4.4
Other and unknown Hispanic	6.4	5.6	5.9	5.0	5.1	4.8	6.2	5.8	5.2
White, non-Hispanic[3]	6.0	5.7	5.0	4.5	4.3	4.0	5.8	5.1	4.6
Black, non-Hispanic[3]	12.1	11.9	11.5	11.0	10.7	9.6	11.8	11.4	11.1
	Postneonatal deaths per 1,000 live births								
All mothers	3.8	3.6	3.5	3.2	3.2	2.6	3.7	3.5	3.3
White	3.2	3.1	3.0	2.7	2.6	2.2	3.1	3.0	2.7
Black	6.7	6.3	6.3	5.9	5.9	5.0	6.4	6.2	6.0
American Indian or Alaska Native	7.7	7.0	7.4	7.0	5.8	5.1	7.2	7.3	6.7
Asian or Pacific Islander	3.1	2.9	2.6	2.7	2.2	1.9	3.1	2.8	2.6
Chinese	*	*2.5	2.4	2.0	2.3	1.5	3.1	2.5	2.4
Japanese	*	*	*	*	*	*	2.6	2.5	2.2
Filipino	*2.8	*2.7	2.5	2.5	1.8	2.2	2.9	2.4	2.3
Hawaiian and part Hawaiian	*	*	*	*	*	*	*	*4.0	*4.1
Other Asian or Pacific Islander	3.0	3.0	2.6	3.0	2.3	1.9	3.1	2.9	2.8
Hispanic origin[2,3]	3.3	3.2	3.1	2.7	2.6	2.1	3.2	3.0	2.7
Mexican	3.2	3.2	3.1	2.7	2.6	2.1	3.2	2.9	2.7
Puerto Rican	4.2	3.5	4.2	3.0	3.5	2.8	4.0	3.9	3.4
Cuban	*	*	*	*	*	*	2.2	2.0	1.6
Central and South American	2.6	2.4	2.4	2.4	1.9	1.9	2.5	2.6	2.2
Other and unknown Hispanic	4.1	3.9	3.2	3.0	3.1	2.6	3.7	3.2	3.0
White, non-Hispanic[3]	3.2	3.0	3.0	2.7	2.7	2.2	3.1	3.0	2.7
Black, non-Hispanic[3]	7.0	6.4	6.6	5.9	5.9	5.0	6.7	6.4	6.1

* Infant and neonatal mortality rates for groups with fewer than 10,000 births are considered unreliable. Postneonatal mortality rates for groups with fewer than 20,000 births are considered unreliable. Infant and neonatal mortality rates for groups with fewer than 7,500 births are considered highly unreliable and are not shown. Postneonatal mortality rates for groups with fewer than 15,000 births are considered highly unreliable and are not shown.

[1]Rates based on a period file using weighted data. Data for 1995 not strictly comparable with unweighted birth cohort data for earlier years (see Appendix I, National Vital Statistics System). The 1995 weighted mortality rates shown in this table are less than 1 percent to 5 percent higher than unweighted rates for 1995.

[2]Includes mothers of all races.

[3]Data shown only for States with an Hispanic-origin item on their birth certificates. The number of States reporting the item increased from 23 and the District of Columbia (DC) in 1983–87, to 30 and DC in 1988, 47 and DC in 1989, 48 and DC in 1990, 49 and DC in 1991, and 50 and DC in 1995 (see Appendix I).

NOTES: The race groups, white, black, American Indian or Alaska Native, and Asian or Pacific Islander, include persons of Hispanic and non-Hispanic origin. Conversely, persons of Hispanic origin may be of any race. National linked files do not exist for 1992–94 birth cohorts.

SOURCE: Centers for Disease Control and Prevention, National Center for Health Statistics. Data computed by the Division of Health and Utilization Analysis from data compiled by the Division of Vital Statistics for the National Linked Birth/Infant Death Data Sets.

Table 21. Infant mortality rates for mothers 20 years of age and over, according to educational attainment, detailed race of mother, and Hispanic origin of mother: United States, selected birth cohorts 1983–95

[Data are based on National Linked Birth/Infant Death Data Sets]

Education of mother, race of mother, and Hispanic origin of mother	Birth cohort								
	1983	1985	1988	1990	1991	1995[1]	1983–85	1986–88	1989–91
Less than 12 years of education	Infant deaths per 1,000 live births								
All mothers	15.0	14.3	13.6	10.8	10.5	8.9	14.6	13.8	11.1
White	12.5	12.2	11.2	9.0	8.8	7.6	12.4	11.4	9.2
Black	23.4	21.5	21.0	19.5	19.6	17.0	21.8	21.1	20.3
American Indian or Alaska Native	*	*	*	*14.3	*12.9	*	15.2	16.8	13.8
Asian or Pacific Islander[2]	*9.7	*8.0	*8.6	6.6	6.3	5.7	9.5	8.2	6.9
Hispanic origin[3,4]	10.9	10.4	10.2	7.3	6.9	6.0	10.6	9.9	7.5
Mexican	8.7	10.0	7.9	7.0	6.6	5.8	9.5	8.3	7.1
Puerto Rican	*15.3	*11.8	14.3	10.1	10.3	10.6	14.1	12.8	11.7
Cuban	*	*	*	*	*	*	*	*	*
Central and South American	*	*	*8.9	7.0	5.8	5.1	8.6	9.2	6.8
Other and unknown Hispanic	*	*	*	9.9	9.9	*7.3	10.1	10.6	10.0
White, non-Hispanic[4]	12.8	12.5	11.5	10.9	10.8	9.9	12.6	11.8	11.0
Black, non-Hispanic[4]	24.7	21.6	21.9	19.7	19.9	17.3	22.6	21.6	20.6
12 years of education									
All mothers	10.2	9.9	9.6	8.8	8.6	7.8	10.0	9.6	8.9
White	8.7	8.5	7.9	7.1	6.9	6.4	8.5	8.0	7.2
Black	17.8	17.6	17.0	16.0	16.2	14.7	17.7	17.1	16.4
American Indian or Alaska Native	*15.5	*10.9	11.2	13.4	11.0	7.9	13.4	11.6	12.3
Asian or Pacific Islander[2]	10.0	8.0	7.5	7.5	6.6	5.5	9.3	7.9	7.5
Hispanic origin[3,4]	8.4	9.1	8.7	7.0	6.5	5.9	9.1	8.3	6.8
Mexican	*6.9	*9.3	9.4	6.8	6.4	5.7	7.8	8.2	6.5
Puerto Rican	*9.5	*11.1	10.9	8.5	8.3	6.5	10.8	10.1	8.6
Cuban	*	*	*	*	*	*	*8.6	*6.6	7.6
Central and South American	*	*7.5	6.9	6.5	5.5	6.1	8.7	7.4	6.3
Other and unknown Hispanic	8.8	8.3	8.1	7.4	6.3	6.5	8.8	7.7	7.0
White, non-Hispanic[4]	8.7	8.2	7.8	7.1	7.0	6.5	8.3	7.9	7.3
Black, non-Hispanic[4]	17.8	18.3	17.3	16.1	16.3	14.8	17.9	17.4	16.5
13 years or more of education									
All mothers	8.1	7.7	7.0	6.4	6.1	5.4	7.8	7.2	6.4
White	7.2	6.6	5.9	5.4	5.2	4.7	6.9	6.2	5.5
Black	15.3	15.8	14.5	13.7	13.1	11.9	15.3	14.9	13.7
American Indian or Alaska Native	*	*	*	*	*	*5.9	10.4	8.4	8.1
Asian or Pacific Islander[2]	6.6	6.2	5.6	5.1	4.5	4.4	6.7	5.9	5.1
Hispanic origin[3,4]	9.0	6.4	7.0	5.7	5.5	5.0	7.4	7.0	5.8
Mexican	*	*	*	5.5	5.7	5.2	7.6	6.4	5.7
Puerto Rican	*	*	*7.1	7.3	6.6	6.3	8.1	6.9	7.8
Cuban	*	*	*	*	*	*	*5.5	5.9	4.2
Central and South American	*	*	*	5.6	4.8	3.7	7.2	7.6	5.4
Other and unknown Hispanic	*	*	*	5.4	5.8	5.2	7.9	7.5	5.6
White, non-Hispanic[4]	7.0	6.6	6.0	5.4	5.2	4.6	6.8	6.1	5.4
Black, non-Hispanic[4]	14.8	15.1	14.7	13.7	13.2	12.0	14.7	14.9	13.8

* Infant mortality rates for groups with fewer than 10,000 births are considered unreliable. Infant mortality rates for groups with fewer than 7,500 births are considered highly unreliable and are not shown.

[1] Rates based on a period file using weighted data. Data for 1995 not strictly comparable with unweighted birth cohort data for earlier years (see Appendix I, National Vital Statistics System). The 1995 weighted mortality rates shown in this table are less than 1 percent to 4 percent higher than unweighted rates for 1995.

[2] The States not reporting maternal education on the birth certificate accounted for 49–51 percent of the Asian or Pacific Islander births in the United States in 1983–87, 59 percent in 1988, and 12 percent in 1989–91.

[3] Includes mothers of all races.

[4] Data shown only for States with an Hispanic-origin item and education of mother on their birth certificates. The number of States reporting both items increased from 21 and the District of Columbia (DC) in 1983–87, to 26 and DC in 1988, 45 and DC in 1989, 47 and DC in 1990–91, and 50 and DC in 1995 (see Appendix I, National Vital Statistics System). The Hispanic reporting States that did not report maternal education on the birth certificate during 1983–88 together accounted for 28–85 percent of the births in each Hispanic subgroup (except Cuban, 11–16 percent and Puerto Rican, 6–7 percent in 1983–87); and in 1989–91 accounted for 27–39 percent of Central and South American and Puerto Rican births and 2–9 percent of births in other Hispanic subgroups.

NOTES: Data for all mothers and by race based on data for 47 States and the District of Columbia (DC) in 1983–87, 46 States and DC in 1988, 48 States and DC in 1989–91, and 50 States and DC in 1995. Excludes data for California and Texas (1983–88), Washington (1983–91), and New York (1988–91), which did not require the reporting of maternal education on the birth certificate (see Appendix I). The race groups, white, black, American Indian or Alaska Native, and Asian or Pacific Islander, include persons of Hispanic and non-Hispanic origin. Conversely, persons of Hispanic origin may be of any race. National linked files do not exist for 1992–94 birth cohorts.

SOURCE: Centers for Disease Control and Prevention, National Center for Health Statistics. Data computed by the Division of Health and Utilization Analysis from data compiled by the Division of Vital Statistics for the National Linked Birth/Infant Death Data Sets.

Table 22. Infant mortality rates according to birthweight: United States, selected birth cohorts 1983–95

[Data are based on National Linked Birth/Infant Death Data Sets]

| Birthweight | \multicolumn{10}{c}{Birth cohort} |
	1983	1984	1985	1986	1987	1988	1989	1990	1991	1995[1]
	\multicolumn{10}{c}{Infant deaths per 1,000 live births[2]}
All birthweights	10.9	10.4	10.4	10.1	9.8	9.6	9.5	8.9	8.6	7.6
Less than 2,500 grams.	95.9	94.1	93.9	89.9	86.5	84.2	83.1	78.1	74.3	65.3
Less than 1,500 grams	400.6	390.5	387.7	371.8	358.0	348.7	343.1	317.6	305.4	270.7
Less than 500 grams	890.3	883.4	895.9	889.9	890.4	878.4	905.6	898.2	889.9	904.9
500–999 grams	584.2	570.9	559.2	537.4	507.9	502.0	480.4	440.1	422.6	351.0
1,000–1,499 grams	162.3	151.4	145.4	132.8	122.2	121.3	118.5	97.9	91.3	69.6
1,500–1,999 grams	58.4	57.4	54.0	51.9	48.8	48.9	46.0	43.8	40.4	33.5
2,000–2,499 grams	22.5	21.4	20.9	20.7	19.5	18.7	17.9	17.8	17.0	13.7
2,500 grams or more	4.7	4.4	4.3	4.3	4.1	4.0	4.0	3.7	3.6	3.0
2,500–2,999 grams	8.8	8.0	7.9	7.9	7.5	7.6	7.4	6.7	6.7	5.5
3,000–3,499 grams	4.4	4.2	4.3	4.1	4.0	3.9	3.8	3.7	3.5	2.9
3,500–3,999 grams	3.2	3.0	3.0	2.9	2.8	2.8	2.8	2.6	2.5	2.0
4,000 grams or more	3.3	3.4	3.2	3.0	3.0	2.9	2.6	2.4	2.4	2.0
4,000–4,499 grams	2.9	3.0	2.9	2.5	2.6	2.4	2.3	2.2	2.2	1.8
4,500–4,999 grams	3.9	3.5	3.8	3.6	3.4	3.4	3.1	2.5	3.0	2.2
5,000 grams or more[3]	14.4	19.0	14.7	16.3	15.8	20.7	9.6	9.8	8.2	8.5

[1]Rates based on a period file using weighted data; not stated birthweight imputed when period of gestation is known and proportionately distributed when period of gestation is unknown. Data for 1995 not strictly comparable with unweighted and unimputed birth cohort data for earlier years (see Appendix I, National Vital Statistics System). The 1995 weighted mortality rates with imputed birthweight shown in this table are less than 1 percent to 3 percent higher than unweighted rates with unimputed birthweight for 1995.

[2]For calculation of birthweight-specific infant mortality rates, unknown birthweight has been distributed in proportion to known birthweight separately for live births (denominator) and infant deaths (numerator).

[3]In 1989 a birthweight-gestational age consistency check instituted for the natality file resulted in a decrease in the number of deaths to infants coded with birthweights of 5,000 grams or more and a discontinuity in the mortality trend for infants weighing 5,000 grams or more at birth. Starting with 1989 the rates are believed to be more accurate.

NOTE: National linked files do not exist for 1992–94 birth cohorts.

SOURCE: Centers for Disease Control and Prevention, National Center for Health Statistics. Data computed by the Division of Health and Utilization Analysis from data compiled by the Division of Vital Statistics for the National Linked Birth/Infant Death Data Sets.

Table 23. Infant mortality rates, fetal mortality rates, and perinatal mortality rates, according to race: United States, selected years 1950–96

[Data are based on the National Vital Statistics System]

Race and year	Infant[1]	Neonatal[1] Under 28 days	Neonatal[1] Under 7 days	Postneonatal[1]	Fetal mortality rate[2]	Late fetal mortality rate[3]	Perinatal mortality rate[4]
All races		Deaths per 1,000 live births					
1950[5]	29.2	20.5	17.8	8.7	18.4	14.9	32.5
1960[5]	26.0	18.7	16.7	7.3	15.8	12.1	28.6
1970	20.0	15.1	13.6	4.9	14.0	9.5	23.0
1980	12.6	8.5	7.1	4.1	9.1	6.2	13.2
1985	10.6	7.0	5.8	3.7	7.8	4.9	10.7
1988	10.0	6.3	5.2	3.6	7.5	4.5	9.7
1989	9.8	6.2	5.1	3.6	7.5	4.5	9.6
1990	9.2	5.8	4.8	3.4	7.5	4.3	9.1
1991	8.9	5.6	4.6	3.4	7.3	4.1	8.7
1992	8.5	5.4	4.4	3.1	7.4	4.1	8.5
1993	8.4	5.3	4.3	3.1	7.1	3.8	8.1
1994	8.0	5.1	4.2	2.9	7.0	3.7	7.9
1995	7.6	4.9	4.0	2.7	7.0	3.6	7.6
1996	7.3	4.8	3.8	2.5	6.9	3.6	7.4
Race of child:[6] White							
1950[5]	26.8	19.4	17.1	7.4	16.6	13.3	30.1
1960[5]	22.9	17.2	15.6	5.7	13.9	10.8	26.2
1970	17.8	13.8	12.5	4.0	12.3	8.6	21.0
1980	11.0	7.5	6.2	3.5	8.1	5.7	11.9
Race of mother:[7] White							
1980	10.9	7.4	6.1	3.5	8.1	5.7	11.8
1985	9.2	6.0	5.0	3.2	6.9	4.5	9.5
1988	8.4	5.3	4.3	3.1	6.4	4.0	8.3
1989	8.1	5.1	4.2	2.9	6.4	4.0	8.2
1990	7.6	4.8	3.9	2.8	6.4	3.8	7.7
1991	7.3	4.5	3.7	2.8	6.2	3.7	7.4
1992	6.9	4.3	3.5	2.6	6.2	3.7	7.2
1993	6.8	4.3	3.5	2.5	6.1	3.4	6.9
1994	6.6	4.2	3.4	2.4	6.0	3.3	6.7
1995	6.3	4.1	3.3	2.2	5.9	3.3	6.5
1996	6.1	4.0	3.2	2.1	5.9	3.3	6.4
Race of child:[6] Black							
1950[5]	43.9	27.8	23.0	16.1	32.1	- - -	- - -
1960[5]	44.3	27.8	23.7	16.5	- - -	- - -	- - -
1970	32.6	22.8	20.3	9.9	23.2	- - -	34.5
1980	21.4	14.1	11.9	7.3	14.4	8.9	20.7
Race of mother:[7] Black							
1980	22.2	14.6	12.3	7.6	14.7	9.1	21.3
1985	19.0	12.6	10.8	6.4	12.8	7.2	17.9
1988	18.5	12.1	10.3	6.5	13.0	6.9	17.1
1989	18.6	11.9	10.1	6.7	13.1	6.8	16.8
1990	18.0	11.6	9.7	6.4	13.3	6.7	16.4
1991	17.6	11.2	9.4	6.3	12.8	6.4	15.7
1992	16.8	10.8	9.0	6.0	13.3	6.4	15.4
1993	16.5	10.7	9.0	5.8	12.8	5.8	14.7
1994	15.8	10.2	8.6	5.6	12.5	5.8	14.3
1995	15.1	9.8	8.2	5.3	12.7	5.7	13.8
1996	14.7	9.6	7.8	5.1	12.5	5.5	13.3

- - - Data not available.

[1]Infant (under 1 year of age), neonatal (under 28 days), early neonatal (under 7 days), and postneonatal (28–365 days).
[2]Number of fetal deaths of 20 weeks or more gestation per 1,000 live births plus fetal deaths.
[3]Number of fetal deaths of 28 weeks or more gestation per 1,000 live births plus late fetal deaths.
[4]Number of late fetal deaths plus infant deaths within 7 days of birth per 1,000 live births plus late fetal deaths.
[5]Includes births and deaths of persons who were not residents of the 50 States and the District of Columbia.
[6]Infant deaths are tabulated by race of decedent; live births and fetal deaths are tabulated by race of child (see Appendix II, Race).
[7]Infant deaths are tabulated by race of decedent; fetal deaths and live births are tabulated by race of mother (see Appendix II, Race).

NOTES: Infant mortality rates in this table are based on infant deaths from the mortality file (numerator) and live births from the natality file (denominator). Inconsistencies in reporting race for the same infant between the birth and death certificate can result in underestimated infant mortality rates for races other than white or black. Infant mortality rates for minority population groups are available from the national linked files of live births and infant deaths and are presented in tables 20–22.

SOURCES: Centers for Disease Control and Prevention, National Center for Health Statistics: Vital statistics of the United States, vol. II, mortality, part A, for data years 1950–96. Public Health Service. Washington. U.S. Government Printing Office; Peters KD, Kochanek KD, Murphy SL. Report of final mortality statistics, 1996. Monthly vital statistics report; vol 45. Hyattsville, Maryland: 1998; and data computed by the Division of Health and Utilization Analysis from data compiled by the Division of Vital Statistics.

Table 24. Infant mortality rates, according to race, geographic division, and State: United States, average annual 1984–86, 1989–91, and 1994–96

[Data are based on the National Vital Statistics System]

Geographic division and State	All races 1984–86	1989–91	1994–96	White[1] 1984–86	1989–91	1994–96	Black[1] 1984–86	1989–91	1994–96
				Infant[2] deaths per 1,000 live births					
United States	10.6	9.3	7.6	9.1	7.6	6.3	19.0	18.0	15.2
New England	9.2	7.4	6.0	8.4	6.7	5.5	20.2	15.2	11.9
Maine	8.8	6.8	5.7	8.8	6.7	5.6	*	*	*
New Hampshire	9.5	7.1	5.6	9.5	7.1	5.5	*	*	*
Vermont	9.1	6.4	6.9	9.0	6.5	6.9	*	*	*
Massachusetts	8.8	7.1	5.4	8.1	6.5	5.0	19.9	13.5	9.6
Rhode Island	9.1	8.8	5.8	8.7	8.3	5.4	*16.0	*16.8	*10.5
Connecticut	9.8	8.0	7.2	8.4	6.6	6.1	21.1	17.5	15.3
Middle Atlantic	10.7	9.6	7.5	9.0	7.5	6.0	18.6	18.9	14.8
New York	10.8	9.9	7.5	9.3	7.8	6.0	17.1	18.2	13.6
New Jersey	10.4	9.0	7.1	8.5	6.7	5.5	19.5	18.7	14.9
Pennsylvania	10.5	9.6	8.0	8.9	7.6	6.3	21.9	20.9	17.8
East North Central	11.1	10.2	8.5	9.2	8.1	6.7	21.5	20.5	18.1
Ohio	10.5	9.7	8.4	9.2	8.1	6.9	18.3	18.7	17.1
Indiana	11.1	9.7	8.6	10.0	8.6	7.5	21.0	18.8	18.5
Illinois	12.0	11.1	9.1	9.2	8.2	6.8	22.7	21.7	18.6
Michigan	11.5	10.7	8.3	9.1	7.8	6.1	23.6	21.9	17.8
Wisconsin	9.4	8.5	7.5	8.6	7.7	6.3	18.7	16.6	19.2
West North Central	9.6	8.6	7.4	8.9	7.5	6.5	18.4	19.3	16.2
Minnesota	9.0	7.3	6.6	8.7	6.5	5.8	*18.9	22.7	16.8
Iowa	8.9	8.1	7.5	8.8	7.8	7.1	*16.5	*19.0	*22.3
Missouri	10.4	9.9	7.7	9.0	8.0	6.4	18.5	19.1	15.3
North Dakota	8.4	8.0	6.6	8.0	7.4	6.1	*	*	*
South Dakota	11.0	9.7	8.3	9.2	7.8	6.7	*	*	*
Nebraska	9.8	7.9	8.0	9.1	7.0	7.6	*19.6	*18.5	*13.5
Kansas	9.4	8.7	7.7	8.8	7.9	6.8	18.1	17.9	18.8
South Atlantic	12.0	10.6	8.7	9.3	7.8	6.4	19.2	17.8	14.9
Delaware	12.4	11.2	7.3	9.8	8.8	5.7	21.3	19.3	12.5
Maryland	11.8	9.7	8.8	9.3	7.1	5.9	18.4	15.9	14.8
District of Columbia	21.0	21.5	16.5	9.9	11.4	7.2	24.2	25.5	19.5
Virginia	11.6	10.0	7.9	9.3	7.4	6.1	19.5	18.8	14.7
West Virginia	10.7	9.2	7.4	10.2	9.0	7.0	*23.0	*14.4	*17.0
North Carolina	11.9	10.9	9.5	9.4	8.2	7.1	18.3	17.2	15.9
South Carolina	14.0	11.9	9.1	10.2	8.5	6.3	20.3	17.5	14.1
Georgia	12.7	12.0	9.6	9.5	8.5	6.6	18.9	18.4	15.4
Florida	11.0	9.5	7.7	8.8	7.4	6.1	18.6	16.6	13.4
East South Central	12.1	10.5	9.3	9.7	8.2	7.1	18.7	16.8	15.5
Kentucky	10.9	8.9	7.6	10.2	8.2	7.1	17.9	16.0	13.0
Tennessee	11.4	10.4	8.9	9.1	7.9	6.6	19.5	18.4	17.1
Alabama	12.9	11.4	10.2	9.9	8.5	7.4	18.8	16.9	15.7
Mississippi	13.5	11.7	10.8	9.4	8.2	7.4	18.3	15.5	14.7
West South Central	10.4	8.9	7.5	9.2	7.5	6.4	16.7	15.5	13.3
Arkansas	11.0	9.9	9.1	9.6	8.2	7.8	15.6	15.5	13.8
Louisiana	11.9	11.0	9.8	8.7	7.9	6.5	17.3	15.6	14.7
Oklahoma	10.7	9.1	8.4	10.2	8.6	8.0	18.1	15.2	14.6
Texas	9.9	8.3	6.7	9.0	7.2	6.0	16.4	15.4	12.0
Mountain	9.6	8.5	6.8	9.2	8.0	6.5	18.2	19.1	15.8
Montana	9.6	9.1	7.1	9.0	8.0	7.0	*	*	*
Idaho	10.5	9.0	6.8	10.4	8.8	6.7	*	*	*
Wyoming	11.4	8.6	6.9	11.3	8.6	6.5	*	*	*
Colorado	9.4	8.6	6.7	9.0	8.1	6.3	19.7	18.0	17.3
New Mexico	9.9	8.5	6.9	9.5	8.1	6.7	*18.1	*20.8	*10.7
Arizona	9.5	8.9	7.7	8.9	8.2	7.2	18.4	20.9	18.0
Utah	9.1	7.2	5.9	9.0	6.9	5.7	*	*	*
Nevada	9.4	8.6	6.1	9.0	7.8	5.7	*15.8	18.3	11.9
Pacific	9.5	8.0	6.4	8.8	7.4	5.9	18.5	17.7	14.7
Washington	10.2	8.2	6.0	9.9	7.7	5.7	20.1	18.8	15.5
Oregon	9.7	8.1	6.2	9.5	7.8	6.0	*20.3	*21.8	*18.1
California	9.3	8.0	6.4	8.6	7.4	5.9	18.4	17.6	14.5
Alaska	10.9	9.5	7.5	9.2	7.5	6.3	*20.1	*12.0	*14.6
Hawaii	9.4	7.4	6.1	6.0	4.9	4.1	*22.0	*19.8	*18.8

* Data for States with fewer than 5,000 live births for the 3-year period are considered unreliable. Data for States with fewer than 1,000 live births are considered highly unreliable and are not shown.

[1]Deaths are tabulated by race of decedent; live births are tabulated by race of mother.

[2]Under 1 year of age.

NOTES: Infant mortality rates in this table are based on infant deaths from the mortality file (numerator) and live births from the natality file (denominator). Inconsistencies in reporting race for the same infant between the birth and death certificate can result in underestimated infant mortality rates for races other than white or black. Infant mortality rates for minority population groups are available from the national linked files of live births and infant deaths, tables 20–22.

SOURCE: Centers for Disease Control and Prevention, National Center for Health Statistics. Data computed by the Division of Health and Utilization Analysis from data compiled by the Division of Vital Statistics.

Health, United States, 1998

Table 25. Neonatal mortality rates, according to race, geographic division, and State: United States, average annual 1984–86, 1989–91, and 1994–96

[Data are based on the National Vital Statistics System]

Geographic division and State	All races 1984–86	All races 1989–91	All races 1994–96	White[1] 1984–86	White[1] 1989–91	White[1] 1994–96	Black[1] 1984–86	Black[1] 1989–91	Black[1] 1994–96
	Neonatal[2] deaths per 1,000 live births								
United States	6.9	5.9	4.9	5.9	4.8	4.1	12.4	11.6	9.9
New England	6.4	5.1	4.2	5.9	4.7	3.9	14.6	10.7	8.5
Maine	5.7	4.7	3.9	5.8	4.6	3.9	*	*	*
New Hampshire	6.4	4.3	3.8	6.4	4.3	3.8	*	*	*
Vermont	6.1	4.1	4.5	6.1	4.2	4.6	*	*	*
Massachusetts	6.2	4.9	3.8	5.7	4.5	3.6	13.6	9.7	6.7
Rhode Island	6.5	6.4	4.4	6.2	6.1	4.2	*11.6	*11.5	*7.5
Connecticut	7.3	5.8	5.2	6.3	4.8	4.4	16.1	12.2	11.2
Middle Atlantic	7.3	6.5	5.2	6.3	5.2	4.3	12.0	12.4	9.6
New York	7.4	6.7	5.2	6.6	5.4	4.3	10.9	12.1	8.8
New Jersey	7.1	6.0	4.9	6.1	4.7	4.0	12.1	11.6	9.4
Pennsylvania	7.2	6.4	5.4	6.1	5.2	4.4	14.7	13.7	11.7
East North Central	7.4	6.5	5.6	6.1	5.2	4.5	14.3	13.0	11.6
Ohio	6.8	6.1	5.6	6.0	5.1	4.6	11.7	11.6	11.5
Indiana	7.4	6.1	5.6	6.6	5.4	4.9	14.3	12.4	11.8
Illinois	8.1	7.2	6.0	6.4	5.5	4.6	14.6	13.6	11.7
Michigan	7.9	7.0	5.5	6.1	5.0	4.0	17.0	14.7	11.8
Wisconsin	5.9	5.1	4.7	5.3	4.7	4.1	12.3	8.5	11.1
West North Central	6.0	5.0	4.7	5.6	4.5	4.2	11.5	10.9	10.0
Minnesota	5.5	4.3	4.1	5.4	4.0	3.7	*11.4	12.4	9.7
Iowa	5.8	4.9	4.9	5.7	4.6	4.6	*10.9	*13.2	*12.3
Missouri	6.6	6.0	4.8	5.7	5.0	3.9	11.4	10.8	9.6
North Dakota	4.7	4.9	4.3	4.6	4.8	4.1	*	*	*
South Dakota	6.0	5.1	4.5	5.4	4.4	3.8	*	*	*
Nebraska	6.3	4.5	5.2	5.9	4.0	5.1	*12.5	*11.0	*8.9
Kansas	5.9	5.0	5.0	5.5	4.6	4.5	11.4	9.6	11.6
South Atlantic	8.1	7.0	5.8	6.3	5.1	4.2	13.0	12.0	10.3
Delaware	9.0	7.8	4.8	7.3	6.3	3.6	14.8	12.7	8.6
Maryland	8.2	6.3	6.0	6.3	4.4	3.9	13.1	10.7	10.5
District of Columbia	16.0	15.4	11.8	7.3	7.4	4.9	18.6	18.3	14.0
Virginia	8.1	6.9	5.6	6.5	4.9	4.1	13.6	13.4	10.7
West Virginia	7.0	5.9	4.8	6.7	5.8	4.6	*16.4	*8.8	*11.5
North Carolina	7.8	7.3	6.6	6.3	5.2	4.9	12.0	12.2	11.3
South Carolina	9.5	7.7	6.2	7.0	5.4	4.1	13.6	11.4	10.1
Georgia	8.6	7.9	6.3	6.5	5.5	4.2	12.8	12.3	10.5
Florida	7.2	6.2	4.9	5.8	4.8	3.9	11.7	10.7	8.6
East South Central	7.9	6.6	5.8	6.4	5.0	4.3	12.1	10.8	10.0
Kentucky	7.1	5.1	4.7	6.6	4.7	4.4	11.9	9.4	8.3
Tennessee	7.5	6.5	5.3	5.8	4.9	3.9	13.4	12.0	10.6
Alabama	8.7	7.5	6.6	6.9	5.7	4.6	12.3	11.1	10.7
Mississippi	8.4	7.3	6.6	6.2	5.1	4.5	11.1	9.7	9.1
West South Central	6.6	5.3	4.5	5.8	4.5	3.8	10.4	9.3	8.0
Arkansas	6.5	5.4	5.3	5.8	4.5	4.6	9.0	8.5	7.6
Louisiana	7.8	6.9	6.4	5.9	5.1	4.2	11.1	9.5	9.5
Oklahoma	6.7	5.0	5.0	6.4	4.8	4.8	11.2	8.0	8.8
Texas	6.2	5.0	3.9	5.7	4.3	3.5	10.1	9.5	7.0
Mountain	5.6	4.8	4.2	5.5	4.6	4.0	10.8	11.5	9.1
Montana	5.0	4.5	4.1	4.8	4.1	3.9	*	*	*
Idaho	6.0	5.3	4.1	5.9	5.2	4.1	*	*	*
Wyoming	6.4	4.1	3.9	6.5	4.1	3.7	*	*	*
Colorado	5.5	5.0	4.2	5.2	4.6	3.9	11.7	11.9	11.2
New Mexico	5.9	5.2	4.3	5.9	5.1	4.4	*8.7	*12.2	*4.7
Arizona	5.7	5.3	4.9	5.5	5.0	4.8	11.4	12.7	10.5
Utah	5.4	3.8	3.5	5.3	3.6	3.5	*	*	*
Nevada	5.2	4.3	3.1	5.0	3.9	2.8	*8.8	9.5	6.1
Pacific	5.8	4.8	3.9	5.4	4.5	3.7	11.4	10.3	8.7
Washington	5.7	4.4	3.6	5.5	4.2	3.5	12.4	11.1	8.5
Oregon	4.9	4.4	3.5	4.8	4.3	3.4	*11.5	*11.5	*8.8
California	5.9	4.9	4.0	5.5	4.6	3.8	11.3	10.3	8.7
Alaska	5.7	4.3	3.8	5.0	3.8	3.2	*9.7	*5.7	*5.1
Hawaii	6.2	4.4	3.8	4.1	3.1	2.8	*12.3	*10.1	*12.9

* Data for States with fewer than 5,000 live births for the 3-year period are considered unreliable. Data for States with fewer than 1,000 live births are considered highly unreliable and are not shown.

[1] Deaths are tabulated by race of decedent; live births are tabulated by race of mother.

[2] Infants under 28 days of age.

NOTES: Infant mortality rates in this table are based on infant deaths from the mortality file (numerator) and live births from the natality file (denominator). Inconsistencies in reporting race for the same infant between the birth and death certificate can result in underestimated infant mortality rates for races other than white or black. Infant mortality rates for minority population groups are available from the national linked files of live births and infant deaths, tables 20–22.

SOURCE: Centers for Disease Control and Prevention, National Center for Health Statistics. Data computed by the Division of Health and Utilization Analysis from data compiled by the Division of Vital Statistics.

Table 26. Postneonatal mortality rates, according to race, geographic division, and State: United States, average annual 1984–86, 1989–91, and 1994–96

[Data are based on the National Vital Statistics System]

Geographic division and State	All races 1984–86	All races 1989–91	All races 1994–96	White[1] 1984–86	White[1] 1989–91	White[1] 1994–96	Black[1] 1984–86	Black[1] 1989–91	Black[1] 1994–96
	Postneonatal[2] deaths per 1,000 live births								
United States	3.7	3.4	2.7	3.2	2.8	2.2	6.6	6.5	5.3
New England	2.7	2.3	1.7	2.5	2.1	1.6	5.6	4.5	3.4
Maine	3.0	2.1	1.8	3.1	2.0	1.7	*	*	*
New Hampshire	3.1	2.8	1.8	3.1	2.8	1.7	*	*	*
Vermont	2.9	2.3	2.3	2.9	2.3	2.3	*	*	*
Massachusetts	2.7	2.2	1.6	2.4	2.1	1.4	6.3	3.8	3.0
Rhode Island	2.7	2.4	1.4	2.5	2.2	1.2	*4.4	*5.3	*3.1
Connecticut	2.4	2.2	2.0	2.1	1.8	1.7	5.0	5.3	4.1
Middle Atlantic	3.4	3.1	2.4	2.7	2.3	1.7	6.6	6.6	5.2
New York	3.4	3.2	2.3	2.7	2.4	1.7	6.1	6.1	4.8
New Jersey	3.3	3.0	2.2	2.4	2.0	1.5	7.4	7.1	5.5
Pennsylvania	3.3	3.2	2.5	2.8	2.5	1.9	7.1	7.2	6.1
East North Central	3.7	3.7	2.9	3.1	2.9	2.3	7.2	7.5	6.4
Ohio	3.7	3.6	2.8	3.2	3.0	2.3	6.6	7.0	5.7
Indiana	3.7	3.6	3.0	3.4	3.2	2.6	6.7	6.5	6.6
Illinois	3.9	3.9	3.1	2.8	2.7	2.2	8.1	8.1	6.9
Michigan	3.6	3.7	2.9	3.0	2.8	2.2	6.6	7.2	5.9
Wisconsin	3.6	3.5	2.8	3.3	2.9	2.3	6.4	8.1	8.1
West North Central	3.6	3.5	2.7	3.3	3.0	2.4	7.0	8.3	6.2
Minnesota	3.5	3.0	2.5	3.3	2.5	2.1	*7.5	*10.3	*7.1
Iowa	3.1	3.3	2.7	3.1	3.2	2.5	*5.6	*5.8	*10.0
Missouri	3.9	3.9	2.9	3.3	3.0	2.5	7.1	8.2	5.6
North Dakota	3.7	3.1	2.2	3.4	2.7	2.0	*	*	*
South Dakota	5.1	4.6	3.7	3.8	3.4	2.9	*	*	*
Nebraska	3.5	3.5	2.8	3.1	3.0	2.6	*7.1	*7.6	*4.6
Kansas	3.6	3.7	2.7	3.3	3.3	2.3	*6.7	*8.2	*7.2
South Atlantic	3.9	3.6	2.8	3.0	2.7	2.2	6.2	5.8	4.6
Delaware	3.4	3.5	2.5	2.5	2.5	2.1	*6.5	*6.6	*3.9
Maryland	3.6	3.4	2.8	3.0	2.7	2.0	5.3	5.2	4.3
District of Columbia	4.9	6.2	4.8	*2.6	*4.0	*2.3	5.6	7.2	5.5
Virginia	3.5	3.1	2.4	2.8	2.5	2.0	5.8	5.4	4.0
West Virginia	3.6	3.3	2.5	3.5	3.2	2.4	*6.6	*	*
North Carolina	4.0	3.6	2.9	3.1	3.0	2.2	6.4	5.0	4.6
South Carolina	4.5	4.2	2.9	3.2	3.0	2.2	6.7	6.2	4.0
Georgia	4.1	4.1	3.3	3.0	3.0	2.5	6.1	6.1	4.9
Florida	3.8	3.3	2.8	2.9	2.5	2.2	6.9	5.9	4.8
East South Central	4.2	3.9	3.5	3.3	3.1	2.8	6.6	6.0	5.6
Kentucky	3.8	3.8	2.9	3.6	3.5	2.8	6.0	6.6	4.7
Tennessee	3.9	3.8	3.6	3.3	3.0	2.7	6.1	6.5	6.5
Alabama	4.2	3.8	3.6	3.0	2.8	2.8	6.6	5.7	5.0
Mississippi	5.1	4.5	4.2	3.2	3.1	3.0	7.2	5.9	5.6
West South Central	3.8	3.6	3.0	3.3	3.0	2.6	6.3	6.2	5.2
Arkansas	4.4	4.4	3.8	3.8	3.7	3.2	6.6	7.0	6.1
Louisiana	4.1	4.2	3.4	2.8	2.9	2.3	6.2	6.1	5.2
Oklahoma	4.1	4.1	3.4	3.8	3.7	3.2	6.8	7.2	5.8
Texas	3.7	3.3	2.8	3.3	2.9	2.5	6.3	5.9	5.0
Mountain	4.0	3.7	2.7	3.8	3.4	2.4	7.4	7.6	6.7
Montana	4.6	4.7	3.1	4.2	3.9	3.1	*	*	*
Idaho	4.5	3.7	2.7	4.5	3.7	2.6	*	*	*
Wyoming	4.9	4.5	3.0	4.8	4.5	2.8	*	*	*
Colorado	3.9	3.7	2.5	3.7	3.6	2.4	*7.9	*6.1	*6.1
New Mexico	4.0	3.3	2.6	3.6	3.0	2.2	*	*	*
Arizona	3.9	3.6	2.8	3.4	3.1	2.4	*7.1	*8.1	*7.5
Utah	3.8	3.4	2.4	3.7	3.3	2.2	*	*	*
Nevada	4.1	4.2	3.0	4.0	3.9	2.9	*6.9	*8.8	*5.9
Pacific	3.7	3.3	2.4	3.4	2.9	2.2	7.2	7.4	6.0
Washington	4.6	3.8	2.4	4.4	3.6	2.2	*7.7	*7.6	*7.0
Oregon	4.8	3.7	2.8	4.7	3.5	2.6	*	*10.4	*9.2
California	3.4	3.1	2.4	3.1	2.8	2.2	7.0	7.3	5.8
Alaska	5.3	5.2	3.7	4.2	3.7	3.0	*	*	*
Hawaii	3.1	3.1	2.3	1.9	1.8	1.2	*	*	*

* Data for States with fewer than 10,000 live births for the 3-year period are considered unreliable. Data for States with fewer than 2,500 live births are considered highly unreliable and are not shown.

[1]Deaths are tabulated by race of decedent; live births are tabulated by race of mother.

[2]Infants 28–365 days of age.

NOTES: Infant mortality rates in this table are based on infant deaths from the mortality file (numerator) and live births from the natality file (denominator). Inconsistencies in reporting race for the same infant between the birth and death certificate can result in underestimated infant mortality rates for races other than white or black. Infant mortality rates for minority population groups are available from the national linked files of live births and infant deaths, tables 20–22.

SOURCE: Centers for Disease Control and Prevention, National Center for Health Statistics. Data computed by the Division of Health and Utilization Analysis from data compiled by the Division of Vital Statistics.

Table 27. Infant mortality rates, feto-infant mortality rates, and postneonatal mortality rates, and average annual percent change: Selected countries, 1989 and 1994

[Data are based on reporting by countries]

Country[4]	Infant mortality rate[1] 1989[5]	1994[6]	Average annual percent change	Feto-infant mortality rate[2] 1989[7]	1994[8]	Average annual percent change	Postneonatal mortality rate[3] 1989[9]	1994[10]	Average annual percent change
Japan	4.59	4.25	−1.5	8.65	7.52	−2.8	2.01	1.92	−0.9
Singapore	6.61	4.34	−8.1	10.97	7.71	−6.8	2.01	1.88	−1.3
Hong Kong	7.43	4.43	−9.8	11.99	9.14	−5.3	2.64	1.79	−7.5
Sweden	5.77	4.45	−5.1	9.42	7.54	−4.4	2.03	1.46	−6.4
Finland	6.03	4.72	−4.8	10.57	7.08	−7.7	1.91	1.24	−8.3
Switzerland	7.34	5.12	−7.0	11.43	8.57	−5.6	2.91	1.85	−8.7
Norway	7.72	5.23	−7.5	12.65	9.77	−5.0	3.96	1.65	−16.1
Denmark	7.95	5.45	−7.3	13.07	9.90	−5.4	3.31	1.45	−15.2
Germany	- - -	5.60	- - -	- - -	9.64	- - -	- - -	2.38	- - -
Netherlands	6.78	5.64	−3.6	12.60	11.04	−2.6	2.20	1.63	−5.8
Ireland	7.55	5.93	−4.7	13.92	11.87	−3.9	3.21	1.96	−9.4
Australia	8.46	6.05	−6.5	12.80	9.53	−5.7	3.45	1.95	−10.8
Northern Ireland	6.90	6.05	−2.6	12.00	11.28	−1.2	2.91	1.89	−8.3
England and Wales	8.45	6.20	−6.0	13.15	10.58	−4.3	3.69	2.06	−11.0
Scotland	8.73	6.20	−6.6	13.75	10.75	−4.8	4.00	2.21	−11.2
Austria	8.31	6.25	−5.5	12.18	9.58	−4.7	3.45	2.39	−7.1
Canada	7.13	6.30	−3.0	11.28	10.16	−2.6	2.47	2.15	−3.4
France	7.54	6.47	−3.8	13.75	11.48	−4.4	3.70	3.32	−2.7
Italy	8.77	6.63	−5.4	14.72	11.59	−5.8	1.94	2.06	1.5
Spain	7.78	6.69	−3.0	12.19	11.09	−2.3	2.67	2.44	−1.8
New Zealand	10.32	7.24	−8.5	14.92	10.26	−8.9	5.78	3.53	−11.6
Israel	10.06	7.80	−6.2	15.01	11.13	−7.2	3.47	3.09	−2.9
Greece	9.78	7.93	−4.1	17.88	13.70	−4.3	3.15	2.33	−5.9
Czech Republic	9.97	7.95	−4.4	14.10	11.10	−4.7	3.02	3.21	1.2
United States	9.81	8.02	−3.9	14.13	11.76	−3.6	3.59	2.90	−4.2
Portugal	12.18	8.06	−7.9	20.16	16.30	−5.2	4.12	3.25	−4.6
Belgium	8.53	8.20	−1.3	14.44	13.42	−1.5	3.87	4.01	1.2
Cuba	11.08	9.40	−4.0	22.94	21.10	−2.7	3.91	4.13	2.8
Slovakia	13.46	11.19	−3.6	18.02	15.32	−3.2	4.24	3.84	−2.0
Puerto Rico	14.27	11.47	−4.3	23.57	21.51	−1.8	3.09	2.83	−1.7
Hungary	15.74	11.55	−6.0	21.04	15.08	−6.4	4.05	3.60	−2.3
Chile	17.06	11.99	−6.8	23.51	18.34	−6.0	7.96	5.15	−8.3
Kuwait	17.33	12.68	−4.4	25.39	21.51	−2.1	5.22	3.34	−6.2
Costa Rica	13.90	13.71	−0.3	23.20	21.99	−2.6	5.32	5.20	−0.8
Poland	15.96	15.13	−1.1	21.49	20.77	−0.7	4.44	3.84	−2.9
Bulgaria	14.37	16.31	2.6	20.33	22.51	2.1	7.05	7.54	1.4
Russian Federation	18.06	18.58	0.6	27.14	26.46	−0.5	7.34	6.74	−1.7
Romania	26.90	23.89	−2.3	35.16	30.47	−2.8	19.95	14.84	−5.7

- - - Data not available.

[1]Number of deaths of infants under 1 year per 1,000 live births.
[2]Number of late fetal deaths plus infant deaths under 1 year per 1,000 live births plus late fetal deaths.
[3]Number of postneonatal deaths per 1,000 live births.
[4]Refers to countries, territories, cities, or geographic areas.
[5]Data for Spain are for 1988 and data for Kuwait are for 1987. As German unification did not take place until 1990, no data are available for prior years.
[6]Data for Canada, Cuba, France, Israel, New Zealand, and Spain are for 1993. Data for Belgium are for 1992.
[7]Data for Greece and Spain are for 1988, data for Belgium are for 1987, and data for Kuwait are for 1986.
[8]Data for Canada, Chile, France, Ireland, Israel, Italy, New Zealand, and Portugal are for 1993. Data for Belgium, Cuba, and Spain are for 1992. Data for Costa Rica are for 1991.
[9]Data for Costa Rica and Italy are for 1988 and data for Kuwait and Spain are for 1987.
[10]Data for Canada, France, Israel, and New Zealand are for 1993. Data for Belgium, Italy, and Spain are for 1992. Data for Costa Rica and Cuba are for 1991.

NOTES: Rankings are from lowest to highest infant mortality rates based on the latest data available for countries or geographic areas with at least 1 million population and with "complete" counts of live births and infant deaths as indicated in the United Nations Demographic Yearbook, 1995 edition. Some of the international variation in infant mortality rates (IMR) is due to differences among countries in distinguishing between fetal and infant deaths. The feto-infant mortality rate (FIMR) is an alternative measure of pregnancy outcome that reduces the effect of international differences in distinguishing between fetal and infant deaths. The United States ranks 25th on the IMR, 23rd on the FIMR, and 22nd on the postneonatal mortality rate.

SOURCES: World Health Organization: World Health Statistics Annuals. Vols. 1990–1995. Geneva; United Nations: Demographic Yearbook 1990 and 1995. New York; Centers for Disease Control and Prevention, National Center for Health Statistics. Vital statistics of the United States, 1989 and 1994, vol II, mortality, part A. Washington: Public Health Service. 1993 and unpublished.

Table 28 (page 1 of 2). Life expectancy at birth and at 65 years of age, according to sex: Selected countries, 1989 and 1994

[Data are based on reporting by countries]

Country[1]	At birth		At 65 years	
	1989[2]	1994[3]	1989[2]	1994[3]
Male	Life expectancy in years			
Japan	76.2	76.6	16.5	16.8
Sweden	74.2	76.1	15.0	16.0
Greece	74.3	75.2	15.6	16.2
Switzerland	74.1	75.1	15.5	16.1
Australia	73.3	75.1	14.7	15.8
Israel	73.9	75.1	15.2	15.8
Canada	73.7	74.8	15.3	15.8
Netherlands	73.7	74.6	14.3	14.8
Norway	73.3	74.2	14.7	14.8
Italy	73.3	74.0	14.7	15.5
England and Wales	72.9	73.8	14.0	14.4
France	73.1	73.8	15.8	16.2
Spain	73.6	73.7	15.6	15.8
Singapore	71.4	73.5	13.3	15.2
Austria	72.1	73.3	14.5	15.1
New Zealand	71.4	73.3	14.0	15.0
Germany[4]	- - -	73.0	- - -	14.7
Finland	70.9	72.8	13.9	14.7
Denmark	72.2	72.7	14.0	14.1
Ireland	71.7	72.6	13.0	13.6
Northern Ireland	71.4	72.5	12.9	13.6
United States	71.7	72.4	15.0	15.5
Portugal	71.1	71.5	14.5	12.7
Scotland	70.6	71.4	12.7	13.1
Chile	69.4	71.4	14.0	14.7
Puerto Rico	69.1	69.6	14.9	16.3
Czech Republic	68.1	69.5	11.7	12.9
Slovakia	- - -	68.3	- - -	12.9
Poland	66.7	67.4	12.5	12.7
Bulgaria	68.3	67.1	12.8	12.7
Romania	66.4	66.0	12.8	12.7
Hungary	65.5	64.9	12.1	12.0
Russian Federation[5]	64.8	57.7	- - -	10.6
Female				
Japan	82.5	83.3	20.7	21.3
France	81.5	82.1	20.5	21.0
Switzerland	81.3	81.9	20.0	20.5
Sweden	80.1	81.4	18.8	19.8
Spain	80.3	81.1	19.1	19.6
Canada	80.6	81.0	19.8	19.9
Australia	79.6	80.9	18.7	19.7
Italy	79.9	80.7	18.7	19.3
Netherlands	81.1	80.4	19.1	18.8
Norway	80.0	80.3	18.9	18.8
Greece	79.4	80.2	17.9	18.5
Finland	79.0	80.2	17.8	18.7
Austria	78.9	79.8	18.0	18.6
England and Wales	78.4	79.7	17.8	18.6
Northern Ireland	77.3	79.7	16.8	18.6
Germany[4]	- - -	79.6	- - -	18.4
United States	78.5	79.0	18.8	19.0
Singapore	76.7	79.0	16.4	18.3
Puerto Rico	77.2	78.9	17.5	19.4
New Zealand	77.3	78.9	17.7	18.6

See footnotes at end of table.

Table 28 (page 2 of 2). Life expectancy at birth and at 65 years of age, according to sex: Selected countries, 1989 and 1994

[Data are based on reporting by countries]

Country[1]	At birth		At 65 years	
	1989[2]	1994[3]	1989[2]	1994[3]
Female—Con.	Life expectancy in years			
Israel	77.6	78.9	16.9	17.7
Portugal	78.2	78.6	17.9	17.9
Ireland	77.2	78.2	16.5	17.3
Denmark	77.9	77.9	18.0	17.6
Scotland	76.2	77.7	16.3	17.3
Czech Republic	75.4	76.6	15.2	16.2
Slovakia	- - -	76.5	- - -	16.5
Chile	76.5	76.3	17.6	17.6
Poland	75.5	76.0	16.2	16.4
Bulgaria	74.8	74.7	15.1	15.4
Hungary	73.9	74.3	15.6	15.7
Romania	72.3	73.3	14.7	15.0
Russian Federation[5]	74.4	73.1	- - -	15.6

- - - Data not available.

[1]Refers to countries, territories, cities, or geographic areas.

[2]Data for Israel, Italy, Romania, Russian Federation, and Sweden are for 1988. Data for Denmark are for 1990.

[3]Data for Australia, Canada, Denmark, New Zealand, and Norway are for 1993. Data for Chile, Ireland, Italy, Puerto Rico, Romania, and Spain are for 1992.

[4]As German unification did not take place until 1990, no data are available for prior years.

[5]Life expectancy for 1988 from Goskomstat (Russian national figures).

NOTES: Rankings are from highest to lowest life expectancy based on the latest available data for countries or geographic areas with at least 1 million population. This table is based on official mortality data from the country concerned, as submitted to the United Nations Demographic Yearbook or the World Health Statistics Annual.

SOURCES: World Health Organization: World Health Statistics Annuals. Vols. 1990–1995. Geneva; United Nations: Demographic Yearbook 1990 and 1995. New York; Centers for Disease Control and Prevention, National Center for Health Statistics. Vital statistics of the United States, 1989 and 1994, vol II, mortality, part A. Washington: Public Health Service. 1993 and unpublished.

Table 29. Life expectancy at birth, at 65 years of age, and at 75 years of age, according to race and sex: United States, selected years 1900–96

[Data are based on the National Vital Statistics System]

Specified age and year	All races			White			Black		
	Both sexes	Male	Female	Both sexes	Male	Female	Both sexes	Male	Female
At birth	Remaining life expectancy in years								
1900[1,2]	47.3	46.3	48.3	47.6	46.6	48.7	[3]33.0	[3]32.5	[3]33.5
1950[2]	68.2	65.6	71.1	69.1	66.5	72.2	60.7	58.9	62.7
1960[2]	69.7	66.6	73.1	70.6	67.4	74.1	63.2	60.7	65.9
1970	70.8	67.1	74.7	71.7	68.0	75.6	64.1	60.0	68.3
1980	73.7	70.0	77.4	74.4	70.7	78.1	68.1	63.8	72.5
1985	74.7	71.1	78.2	75.3	71.8	78.7	69.3	65.0	73.4
1986	74.7	71.2	78.2	75.4	71.9	78.8	69.1	64.8	73.4
1987	74.9	71.4	78.3	75.6	72.1	78.9	69.1	64.7	73.4
1988	74.9	71.4	78.3	75.6	72.2	78.9	68.9	64.4	73.2
1989	75.1	71.7	78.5	75.9	72.5	79.2	68.8	64.3	73.3
1990	75.4	71.8	78.8	76.1	72.7	79.4	69.1	64.5	73.6
1991	75.5	72.0	78.9	76.3	72.9	79.6	69.3	64.6	73.8
1992	75.8	72.3	79.1	76.5	73.2	79.8	69.6	65.0	73.9
1993	75.5	72.2	78.8	76.3	73.1	79.5	69.2	64.6	73.7
1994	75.7	72.4	79.0	76.5	73.3	79.6	69.5	64.9	73.9
1995	75.8	72.5	78.9	76.5	73.4	79.6	69.6	65.2	73.9
1996	76.1	73.1	79.1	76.8	73.9	79.7	70.2	66.1	74.2
At 65 years									
1900–1902[1,2]	11.9	11.5	12.2	- - -	11.5	12.2	- - -	10.4	11.4
1950[2]	13.9	12.8	15.0	- - -	12.8	15.1	13.9	12.9	14.9
1960[2]	14.3	12.8	15.8	14.4	12.9	15.9	13.9	12.7	15.1
1970	15.2	13.1	17.0	15.2	13.1	17.1	14.2	12.5	15.7
1980	16.4	14.1	18.3	16.5	14.2	18.4	15.1	13.0	16.8
1985	16.7	14.5	18.5	16.8	14.5	18.7	15.2	13.0	16.9
1986	16.8	14.6	18.6	16.9	14.7	18.7	15.2	13.0	17.0
1987	16.9	14.7	18.7	17.0	14.8	18.8	15.2	13.0	17.0
1988	16.9	14.7	18.6	17.0	14.8	18.7	15.1	12.9	16.9
1989	17.1	15.0	18.8	17.2	15.1	18.9	15.2	13.0	16.9
1990	17.2	15.1	18.9	17.3	15.2	19.1	15.4	13.2	17.2
1991	17.4	15.3	19.1	17.5	15.4	19.2	15.5	13.4	17.2
1992	17.5	15.4	19.2	17.6	15.5	19.3	15.7	13.5	17.4
1993	17.3	15.3	18.9	17.4	15.4	19.0	15.5	13.4	17.1
1994	17.4	15.5	19.0	17.5	15.6	19.1	15.7	13.6	17.2
1995	17.4	15.6	18.9	17.6	15.7	19.1	15.6	13.6	17.1
1996	17.5	15.7	19.0	17.6	15.8	19.1	15.8	13.9	17.2
At 75 years									
1980	10.4	8.8	11.5	10.4	8.8	11.5	9.7	8.3	10.7
1985	10.6	9.0	11.7	10.6	9.0	11.7	10.1	8.7	11.1
1986	10.7	9.1	11.7	10.7	9.1	11.8	10.1	8.6	11.1
1987	10.7	9.1	11.8	10.7	9.1	11.8	10.1	8.6	11.1
1988	10.6	9.1	11.7	10.7	9.1	11.7	10.0	8.5	11.0
1989	10.9	9.3	11.9	10.9	9.3	11.9	10.1	8.6	11.0
1990	10.9	9.4	12.0	11.0	9.4	12.0	10.2	8.6	11.2
1991	11.1	9.5	12.1	11.1	9.5	12.1	10.2	8.7	11.2
1992	11.2	9.6	12.2	11.2	9.6	12.2	10.4	8.9	11.4
1993	10.9	9.5	11.9	11.0	9.5	12.0	10.2	8.7	11.1
1994	11.0	9.6	12.0	11.1	9.6	12.0	10.3	8.9	11.2
1995	11.0	9.7	11.9	11.1	9.7	12.0	10.2	8.8	11.1
1996	11.1	9.8	12.0	11.1	9.8	12.0	10.3	9.0	11.2

- - - Data not available.

[1]Death registration area only. The death registration area increased from 10 States and the District of Columbia in 1900 to the coterminous United States in 1933.
[2]Includes deaths of persons who were not residents of the 50 States and the District of Columbia.
[3]Figure is for the all other population.

SOURCES: U.S. Bureau of the Census: U.S. Life Tables 1890, 1901, 1910, and 1901–1910, by Glover JW. Washington. U.S. Government Printing Office, 1921; Centers for Disease Control and Prevention, National Center for Health Statistics: Vital Statistics Rates in the United States, 1940–1960, by Grove RD and Hetzel AM. DHEW Pub. No. (PHS) 1677. Public Health Service. Washington. U.S. Government Printing Office, 1968; Peters KD, Kochanek KD, Murphy SL. Report of final mortality statistics, 1996. Monthly vital statistics report; vol 45. Hyattsville, Maryland: 1998; unpublished data from the Division of Vital Statistics; data for 1960 and earlier years for the black population were computed by the Office of Research and Methodology from data compiled by the Division of Vital Statistics.

Table 30 (page 1 of 2). Age-adjusted death rates, according to detailed race, Hispanic origin, geographic division, and State: United States, average annual 1984–86, 1989–91, and 1994–96

[Data are based on the National Vital Statistics System]

Geographic division and State	All persons			White	Black	American Indian or Alaska Native	Asian or Pacific Islander	Hispanic	White, non-Hispanic
	1984–86	1989–91	1994–96	1994–96	1994–96	1994–96	1994–96	1994–96	1994–96
	Deaths per 100,000 resident population[1]								
United States	547.7	522.0	500.7	474.5	758.7	461.7	282.8	376.1	473.6
New England	514.4	473.0	453.3	445.9	657.2	*	239.3	324.3	440.6
Maine	530.2	490.3	474.3	475.4	*	*	*	*	461.2
New Hampshire	519.8	473.7	451.7	452.8	*	*	*	219.2	436.9
Vermont	528.5	480.5	458.3	459.0	*	*	*	*	459.5
Massachusetts..........	518.7	475.0	451.5	446.5	609.1	*	267.2	336.8	443.6
Rhode Island...........	517.3	478.8	448.0	440.6	686.9	*	275.9	245.2	435.6
Connecticut	497.3	461.4	451.9	432.2	716.7	*	166.9	343.9	427.4
Middle Atlantic............	566.2	537.2	506.3	477.4	737.3	*	247.1	414.3	466.3
New York...............	573.0	549.7	508.8	482.7	686.6	*	262.3	443.8	459.3
New Jersey	553.6	522.3	495.3	461.1	789.0	*	194.2	313.7	461.5
Pennsylvania	562.5	525.8	507.2	479.2	817.0	*	273.6	476.2	476.7
East North Central..........	553.0	525.3	507.3	475.9	792.6	*	230.8	316.8	474.8
Ohio	561.6	528.1	511.4	489.3	728.8	*	195.9	338.0	488.1
Indiana	551.2	524.1	514.1	495.1	778.6	*	228.3	296.6	496.3
Illinois	559.5	541.5	522.1	476.8	852.6	*	221.7	310.0	476.0
Michigan	569.6	534.3	512.1	471.1	788.9	*	268.2	355.7	466.9
Wisconsin	488.5	463.9	446.6	433.1	740.0	*	288.3	255.9	434.0
West North Central	497.1	471.9	464.3	448.4	762.5	*	290.5	343.7	445.8
Minnesota	462.6	431.2	419.8	411.7	679.6	787.7	318.8	412.4	409.5
Iowa	472.7	448.9	436.9	433.2	719.9	*	325.4	348.3	432.8
Missouri...............	549.7	527.8	527.9	501.7	790.9	*	267.4	355.1	501.6
North Dakota	449.6	435.9	425.4	411.0	*	959.0	*	*	400.5
South Dakota..........	497.2	459.4	452.3	418.4	*	1,149.8	*	*	418.3
Nebraska..............	484.1	464.1	446.6	436.2	739.0	893.7	246.5	301.5	432.2
Kansas	494.0	467.6	463.6	450.7	729.9	*	260.3	326.8	442.1
South Atlantic	565.0	540.0	523.2	472.6	775.0	*	226.7	342.6	477.2
Delaware...............	573.9	549.4	529.3	488.5	780.7	*	157.3	325.2	488.0
Maryland...............	577.6	544.9	528.4	461.9	761.1	*	256.7	113.4	468.9
District of Columbia	765.8	824.5	816.8	430.5	1,054.5	*	188.0	116.1	466.1
Virginia	564.2	528.6	506.2	465.5	731.2	*	227.7	197.5	468.3
West Virginia	593.6	576.5	549.7	545.2	763.6	*	*	*	546.4
North Carolina	576.9	556.7	540.5	484.8	778.8	605.3	256.4	182.4	485.5
South Carolina..........	618.6	596.4	581.1	511.8	792.1	*	255.5	187.0	512.9
Georgia................	614.9	592.6	566.4	506.9	775.5	*	255.5	212.5	506.8
Florida.................	521.2	497.9	489.3	458.2	760.2	*	183.2	375.8	466.0
East South Central	598.3	584.0	575.5	534.3	790.1	*	257.8	324.7	534.4
Kentucky...............	592.6	571.0	553.8	542.4	752.0	*	277.5	443.8	542.3
Tennessee..............	583.7	566.9	566.7	529.9	818.0	*	280.0	347.8	529.8
Alabama	604.5	593.7	582.4	530.3	777.0	*	190.3	318.6	530.8
Mississippi.............	625.3	621.3	614.9	539.1	794.4	*	280.1	187.2	539.6
West South Central	564.6	548.6	524.8	499.0	743.2	*	228.2	413.6	501.4
Arkansas...............	575.7	564.7	558.2	528.1	785.8	*	317.0	186.5	528.3
Louisiana...............	623.7	621.1	594.9	523.2	791.0	*	252.2	232.3	529.5
Oklahoma	550.4	534.1	541.1	538.7	711.1	*	300.7	- - -	- - -
Texas	549.4	530.1	499.8	481.7	711.4	*	216.8	419.9	489.0
Mountain	502.4	479.1	465.6	458.3	618.3	627.9	294.2	437.7	452.6
Montana	513.7	484.1	463.1	448.4	*	826.2	*	368.9	445.1
Idaho	488.7	456.8	437.5	436.7	*	545.2	336.6	307.8	437.7
Wyoming...............	507.5	484.7	469.2	464.4	*	789.7	*	455.5	462.3
Colorado...............	478.9	456.1	436.6	433.9	587.0	377.2	249.6	446.4	427.6
New Mexico.............	518.5	497.3	479.7	471.2	490.8	600.9	305.3	475.5	456.2
Arizona	511.9	488.4	481.7	469.9	648.4	677.9	269.0	441.4	463.7
Utah	465.8	426.8	412.9	410.4	599.7	559.2	368.7	409.1	407.0
Nevada	586.6	569.3	555.2	553.2	694.2	427.3	328.2	268.8	557.1

See footnotes at end of table.

Table 30 (page 2 of 2). Age-adjusted death rates, according to detailed race, Hispanic origin, geographic division, and State: United States, average annual 1984–86, 1989–91, and 1994–96

[Data are based on the National Vital Statistics System]

Geographic division and State	All persons			White	Black	American Indian or Alaska Native	Asian or Pacific Islander	Hispanic	White, non-Hispanic
	1984–86	1989–91	1994–96	1994–96	1994–96	1994–96	1994–96	1994–96	1994–96
	Deaths per 100,000 resident population[1]—Con.								
Pacific	516.6	491.9	458.8	460.3	708.0	*	310.1	342.7	470.8
Washington	496.9	463.7	444.0	441.8	648.1	550.7	305.2	285.6	441.9
Oregon	510.9	479.9	468.0	466.9	683.6	*	293.6	288.6	468.3
California................	523.4	500.7	463.0	464.8	718.0	*	289.3	345.2	481.2
Alaska..................	561.8	525.6	483.9	448.0	496.9	762.2	273.4	277.6	449.8
Hawaii..................	418.6	405.5	389.4	383.5	321.3	*	394.4	318.7	390.1

* Data for States with population under 10,000 in the middle year of a 3-year period or fewer than 50 deaths for the 3-year period are considered unreliable and are not shown. Data for American Indians or Alaska Natives in States with more than 10 percent misclassification of American Indian or Alaska Native deaths on death certificates or without information on misclassification are also not shown. (Support Services International, Inc. Methodology for adjusting IHS mortality data for miscoding race-ethnicity of American Indians and Alaska Natives on State death certificates. Report submitted to Indian Health Service. 1996.) Division death rates for American Indians or Alaska Natives are not shown when any State within the division does not meet reliability criteria.

- - - Data not available.

[1]Average annual death rate.

NOTES: The race groups, white, black, American Indian or Alaska Native, and Asian or Pacific Islander, include persons of Hispanic and non-Hispanic origin. Conversely, persons of Hispanic origin may be of any race. Consistency of race identification between the death certificate (source of data for numerator of death rates) and data from the Census Bureau (denominator) is high for individual white and black persons; however, persons identified as American Indian, Asian, or Hispanic origin in data from the Census Bureau are sometimes misreported as white or non-Hispanic on the death certificate, causing death rates to be underestimated by 22–30 percent for American Indians, about 12 percent for Asians, and about 7 percent for persons of Hispanic origin. (Sorlie PD, Rogot E, and Johnson NJ: Validity of demographic characteristics on the death certificate, *Epidemiology* 3(2):181–184, 1992.) Denominators for rates are population estimates for the middle year of each 3-year period, multiplied by 3.

SOURCE: Centers for Disease Control and Prevention, National Center for Health Statistics. Data computed by the Division of Health and Utilization Analysis from data compiled by the Division of Vital Statistics.

Table 31 (page 1 of 4). Age-adjusted death rates for selected causes of death, according to sex, detailed race, and Hispanic origin: United States, selected years 1950–96

[Data are based on the National Vital Statistics System]

Sex, race, Hispanic origin, and cause of death	1950[1]	1960[1]	1970	1980	1985	1990	1993	1994	1995	1996
All persons	\multicolumn{10}{c}{Deaths per 100,000 resident population}									
All causes	841.5	760.9	714.3	585.8	548.9	520.2	513.3	507.4	503.9	491.6
Natural causes	766.6	695.2	636.9	519.7	493.0	465.1	459.7	454.4	451.7	440.6
Diseases of heart	307.2	286.2	253.6	202.0	181.4	152.0	145.3	140.4	138.3	134.5
Ischemic heart disease	- - -	- - -	- - -	149.8	126.1	102.6	94.9	91.4	89.5	86.7
Cerebrovascular diseases	88.8	79.7	66.3	40.8	32.5	27.7	26.5	26.5	26.7	26.4
Malignant neoplasms	125.4	125.8	129.8	132.8	134.4	135.0	132.6	131.5	129.9	127.9
Respiratory system	12.8	19.2	28.4	36.4	39.1	41.4	40.8	40.1	39.7	39.3
Colorectal	- - -	17.7	16.8	15.5	14.9	13.6	12.9	12.8	12.7	12.2
Prostate[2]	13.4	13.1	13.3	14.4	14.7	16.7	16.4	16.0	15.4	14.9
Breast[3]	22.2	22.3	23.1	22.7	23.3	23.1	21.5	21.3	21.0	20.2
Chronic obstructive pulmonary diseases	4.4	8.2	13.2	15.9	18.8	19.7	21.4	21.0	20.8	21.0
Pneumonia and influenza	26.2	28.0	22.1	12.9	13.5	14.0	13.5	13.0	12.9	12.8
Chronic liver disease and cirrhosis	8.5	10.5	14.7	12.2	9.7	8.6	7.9	7.9	7.6	7.5
Diabetes mellitus	14.3	13.6	14.1	10.1	9.7	11.7	12.4	12.9	13.3	13.6
Human immunodeficiency virus infection	- - -	- - -	- - -	- - -	- - -	9.8	13.8	15.4	15.6	11.1
External causes	73.9	65.7	77.4	66.1	55.9	55.1	53.6	53.0	52.2	50.9
Unintentional injuries	57.5	49.9	53.7	42.3	34.8	32.5	30.3	30.3	30.5	30.4
Motor vehicle-related injuries	23.3	22.5	27.4	22.9	18.8	18.5	16.0	16.1	16.3	16.2
Suicide	11.0	10.6	11.8	11.4	11.5	11.5	11.3	11.2	11.2	10.8
Homicide and legal intervention	5.4	5.2	9.1	10.8	8.3	10.2	10.7	10.3	9.4	8.5
Male										
All causes	1,001.6	949.3	931.6	777.2	723.0	680.2	664.9	654.6	646.3	623.7
Natural causes	- - -	- - -	- - -	675.5	637.9	595.8	583.2	573.6	567.0	547.2
Diseases of heart	383.8	375.5	348.5	280.4	250.1	206.7	195.5	188.5	184.9	178.8
Ischemic heart disease	- - -	- - -	- - -	214.8	179.6	144.0	132.3	127.0	123.9	119.3
Cerebrovascular diseases	91.9	85.4	73.2	44.9	35.5	30.2	29.0	29.0	28.9	28.5
Malignant neoplasms	130.8	143.0	157.4	165.5	166.1	166.3	161.9	159.6	156.8	153.8
Respiratory system	21.3	34.8	50.6	59.7	60.7	61.0	58.1	56.5	55.3	54.2
Colorectal	- - -	18.6	18.7	18.3	17.9	16.8	15.7	15.6	15.3	14.8
Prostate	13.4	13.1	13.3	14.4	14.7	16.7	16.4	16.0	15.4	14.9
Chronic obstructive pulmonary diseases	6.0	13.7	23.4	26.1	28.1	27.2	27.8	26.9	26.3	25.9
Pneumonia and influenza	30.6	35.0	28.8	17.4	18.4	18.5	17.5	16.7	16.5	16.2
Chronic liver disease and cirrhosis	11.4	14.5	20.2	17.1	13.7	12.2	11.3	11.3	11.0	10.7
Diabetes mellitus	11.4	12.0	13.5	10.2	10.0	12.3	13.4	13.9	14.4	14.9
Human immunodeficiency virus infection	- - -	- - -	- - -	- - -	- - -	17.7	24.1	26.4	26.2	18.1
External causes	- - -	- - -	- - -	101.7	85.2	84.4	81.7	81.0	79.3	76.5
Unintentional injuries	83.7	73.9	80.7	64.0	51.8	47.7	44.2	44.0	44.1	43.3
Motor vehicle-related injuries	36.4	34.5	41.1	34.3	27.3	26.3	22.5	22.5	22.7	22.3
Suicide	17.3	16.6	17.3	18.0	18.8	19.0	18.7	18.7	18.6	18.0
Homicide and legal intervention	8.4	7.9	14.9	17.4	12.8	16.3	17.0	16.4	14.7	13.3
Female										
All causes	688.4	590.6	532.5	432.6	410.3	390.6	388.3	385.2	385.2	381.0
Natural causes	- - -	- - -	- - -	400.1	382.2	363.5	361.9	359.2	359.1	354.8
Diseases of heart	233.9	205.7	175.2	140.3	127.4	108.9	105.0	101.6	100.4	98.2
Ischemic heart disease	- - -	- - -	- - -	98.8	84.2	70.2	65.4	63.1	61.9	60.4
Cerebrovascular diseases	86.0	74.7	60.8	37.6	30.0	25.7	24.5	24.5	24.8	24.6
Malignant neoplasms	120.8	111.2	108.8	109.2	111.7	112.7	111.4	111.1	110.4	108.8
Respiratory system	4.6	5.2	10.1	18.3	22.5	26.2	27.2	27.3	27.5	27.5
Colorectal	- - -	16.9	15.4	13.4	12.6	11.3	10.8	10.6	10.6	10.2
Breast	22.2	22.3	23.1	22.7	23.3	23.1	21.5	21.3	21.0	20.2
Chronic obstructive pulmonary diseases	2.9	3.5	5.4	8.9	12.5	14.7	17.1	17.1	17.1	17.6
Pneumonia and influenza	22.0	21.8	16.7	9.8	10.1	11.0	10.7	10.4	10.4	10.4
Chronic liver disease and cirrhosis	5.8	6.9	9.8	7.9	6.1	5.3	4.9	4.8	4.6	4.5
Diabetes mellitus	17.1	15.0	14.4	10.0	9.4	11.1	11.7	12.1	12.4	12.5
Human immunodeficiency virus infection	- - -	- - -	- - -	- - -	- - -	2.1	3.8	4.8	5.2	4.2
External causes	- - -	- - -	- - -	32.5	28.1	27.0	26.4	26.1	26.1	26.2
Unintentional injuries	31.7	26.8	28.2	21.8	18.7	17.9	17.0	17.2	17.5	17.9
Motor vehicle-related injuries	10.7	11.0	14.4	11.8	10.5	10.7	9.6	9.9	10.0	10.2
Suicide	4.9	5.0	6.8	5.4	4.9	4.5	4.3	4.2	4.1	4.0
Homicide and legal intervention	2.5	2.6	3.7	4.5	3.9	4.2	4.5	4.0	4.0	3.6

See footnotes at end of table.

Table 31 (page 2 of 4). Age-adjusted death rates for selected causes of death, according to sex, detailed race, and Hispanic origin: United States, selected years 1950–96

[Data are based on the National Vital Statistics System]

Sex, race, Hispanic origin, and cause of death	1950[1]	1960[1]	1970	1980	1985	1990	1993	1994	1995	1996
White				Deaths per 100,000 resident population						
All causes	800.4	727.0	679.6	559.4	524.9	492.8	485.1	479.8	476.9	466.8
Natural causes	- - -	- - -	- - -	497.7	471.9	442.0	436.5	431.4	428.5	419.2
Diseases of heart	300.5	281.5	249.1	197.6	176.6	146.9	139.9	135.4	133.1	129.8
Ischemic heart disease	- - -	- - -	- - -	150.6	126.6	102.5	94.6	91.1	89.0	86.4
Cerebrovascular diseases	83.2	74.2	61.8	38.0	30.1	25.5	24.5	24.5	24.7	24.5
Malignant neoplasms	124.7	124.2	127.8	129.6	131.2	131.5	129.4	128.6	127.0	125.2
Respiratory system	13.0	19.1	28.0	35.6	38.4	40.6	40.2	39.7	39.3	38.9
Colorectal	- - -	17.9	16.9	15.4	14.7	13.3	12.6	12.5	12.3	11.8
Prostate[2]	13.1	12.4	12.3	13.2	13.4	15.3	14.9	14.6	14.0	13.5
Breast[3]	22.5	22.4	23.4	22.8	23.4	22.9	21.2	20.9	20.5	19.8
Chronic obstructive pulmonary diseases	4.3	8.2	13.4	16.3	19.2	20.1	21.9	21.6	21.3	21.5
Pneumonia and influenza	22.9	24.6	19.8	12.2	12.9	13.4	12.9	12.5	12.4	12.2
Chronic liver disease and cirrhosis	8.6	10.3	13.4	11.0	8.9	8.0	7.6	7.5	7.4	7.3
Diabetes mellitus	13.9	12.8	12.9	9.1	8.6	10.4	11.0	11.5	11.7	12.0
Human immunodeficiency virus infection	- - -	- - -	- - -	- - -	- - -	8.0	10.5	11.2	11.1	7.2
External causes	- - -	- - -	- - -	61.9	53.0	50.8	48.6	48.5	48.4	47.5
Unintentional injuries	55.7	47.6	51.0	41.5	34.2	31.8	29.6	29.5	29.9	29.9
Motor vehicle-related injuries	23.1	22.3	26.9	23.4	19.1	18.6	16.1	16.2	16.4	16.3
Suicide	11.6	11.1	12.4	12.1	12.3	12.2	12.0	11.9	11.9	11.6
Homicide and legal intervention	2.6	2.7	4.7	6.9	5.4	5.9	6.0	5.8	5.5	4.9
Black										
All causes	1,236.7	1,073.3	1,044.0	842.5	793.6	789.2	785.2	772.1	765.7	738.3
Natural causes	- - -	- - -	- - -	740.2	713.5	701.3	696.4	686.5	685.8	662.3
Diseases of heart	379.6	334.5	307.6	255.7	240.6	213.5	208.9	198.8	198.8	191.5
Ischemic heart disease	- - -	- - -	- - -	150.5	130.9	113.2	108.3	103.8	103.4	99.4
Cerebrovascular diseases	150.9	140.3	114.5	68.5	55.8	48.4	45.0	45.4	45.0	44.2
Malignant neoplasms	129.1	142.3	156.7	172.1	176.6	182.0	177.2	173.8	171.6	167.8
Respiratory system	10.4	20.3	33.5	46.5	50.3	54.0	51.8	50.6	49.9	48.9
Colorectal	- - -	15.2	16.6	16.9	17.9	17.9	17.4	17.2	17.3	16.8
Prostate[2]	16.9	22.2	25.4	29.1	31.2	35.3	35.8	35.3	34.0	33.8
Breast[3]	19.3	21.3	21.5	23.3	25.5	27.5	27.1	26.9	27.5	26.5
Chronic obstructive pulmonary diseases	- - -	- - -	- - -	12.5	15.3	16.9	17.8	17.7	17.6	17.8
Pneumonia and influenza	57.0	56.4	40.4	19.2	18.8	19.8	18.6	17.5	17.8	17.8
Chronic liver disease and cirrhosis	7.2	11.7	24.8	21.6	16.3	13.7	10.9	10.7	9.9	9.2
Diabetes mellitus	17.2	22.0	26.5	20.3	20.1	24.8	26.8	27.4	28.5	28.8
Human immunodeficiency virus infection	- - -	- - -	- - -	- - -	- - -	25.7	41.6	49.4	51.8	41.4
External causes	- - -	- - -	- - -	101.2	80.1	87.8	88.7	85.6	79.8	76.0
Unintentional injuries	70.9	66.4	74.4	51.2	42.3	39.7	38.4	38.1	37.4	36.7
Motor vehicle-related injuries	24.7	23.4	30.6	19.7	17.4	18.4	16.3	16.6	16.6	16.7
Suicide	4.2	4.7	6.1	6.4	6.4	7.0	7.2	7.1	6.9	6.6
Homicide and legal intervention	30.5	27.4	46.1	40.6	29.2	39.5	40.9	38.2	33.4	30.6
American Indian or Alaska Native										
All causes	- - -	- - -	- - -	564.1	468.2	445.1	468.9	460.7	468.5	456.7
Natural causes	- - -	- - -	- - -	436.5	375.1	360.3	386.3	374.9	385.4	374.5
Diseases of heart	- - -	- - -	- - -	131.2	119.6	107.1	108.9	104.9	104.5	100.8
Ischemic heart disease	- - -	- - -	- - -	87.4	77.3	66.6	68.5	65.8	65.4	63.8
Cerebrovascular diseases	- - -	- - -	- - -	26.6	22.5	19.3	20.7	20.2	21.6	21.1
Malignant neoplasms	- - -	- - -	- - -	70.6	72.0	75.0	79.2	78.1	80.8	84.9
Respiratory system	- - -	- - -	- - -	15.0	18.8	20.5	22.6	23.7	23.7	24.4
Colorectal	- - -	- - -	- - -	5.6	6.3	6.4	7.1	7.5	7.6	8.5
Prostate[2]	- - -	- - -	- - -	9.6	8.9	7.7	10.3	9.2	8.8	9.8
Breast[3]	- - -	- - -	- - -	8.1	8.0	10.0	9.4	10.4	10.4	12.7
Chronic obstructive pulmonary diseases	- - -	- - -	- - -	7.5	9.8	12.8	14.9	13.3	13.8	12.6
Pneumonia and influenza	- - -	- - -	- - -	19.4	14.9	15.2	14.7	14.8	14.2	14.0
Chronic liver disease and cirrhosis	- - -	- - -	- - -	38.6	23.6	19.8	21.0	21.4	24.3	20.7
Diabetes mellitus	- - -	- - -	- - -	20.0	18.7	20.8	24.7	25.9	27.3	27.8
Human immunodeficiency virus infection	- - -	- - -	- - -	- - -	- - -	1.8	4.6	5.4	7.0	4.2
External causes	- - -	- - -	- - -	127.6	93.1	84.8	82.6	85.8	83.0	82.1
Unintentional injuries	- - -	- - -	- - -	95.1	66.2	59.0	58.1	58.3	56.7	57.6
Motor vehicle-related injuries	- - -	- - -	- - -	54.4	36.3	33.2	32.3	31.4	33.1	34.0
Suicide	- - -	- - -	- - -	12.8	12.1	12.4	12.1	14.0	12.2	13.0
Homicide and legal intervention	- - -	- - -	- - -	16.0	12.2	11.1	11.0	11.9	11.9	10.1

See footnotes at end of table.

Table 31 (page 3 of 4). Age-adjusted death rates for selected causes of death, according to sex, detailed race, and Hispanic origin: United States, selected years 1950–96

[Data are based on the National Vital Statistics System]

Sex, race, Hispanic origin, and cause of death	1950[1]	1960[1]	1970	1980	1985	1990	1993	1994	1995	1996
Asian or Pacific Islander				Deaths per 100,000 resident population						
All causes	- - -	- - -	- - -	315.6	305.7	297.6	295.9	299.2	298.9	277.4
Natural causes	- - -	- - -	- - -	280.7	274.4	266.7	266.4	269.5	269.2	250.3
Diseases of heart	- - -	- - -	- - -	93.9	88.6	78.5	79.0	79.7	78.9	71.7
Ischemic heart disease	- - -	- - -	- - -	67.5	58.8	49.7	49.5	50.5	49.3	44.8
Cerebrovascular diseases	- - -	- - -	- - -	29.0	25.5	25.0	24.5	25.4	25.8	23.9
Malignant neoplasms	- - -	- - -	- - -	77.2	80.2	79.8	81.4	81.8	81.1	76.3
Respiratory system	- - -	- - -	- - -	18.1	17.2	18.3	19.1	18.5	18.5	17.4
Colorectal	- - -	- - -	- - -	9.3	9.6	8.3	8.5	8.4	8.2	7.7
Prostate[2]	- - -	- - -	- - -	4.0	5.9	6.9	7.1	6.4	7.4	5.8
Breast[3]	- - -	- - -	- - -	9.2	9.6	10.0	9.5	10.5	11.0	8.9
Chronic obstructive pulmonary diseases	- - -	- - -	- - -	5.9	8.4	8.7	8.7	8.5	9.0	8.6
Pneumonia and influenza	- - -	- - -	- - -	9.1	9.1	10.4	11.2	10.5	10.8	9.9
Chronic liver disease and cirrhosis	- - -	- - -	- - -	4.5	4.2	3.7	2.8	3.2	2.7	2.6
Diabetes mellitus	- - -	- - -	- - -	6.9	6.1	7.4	7.1	8.0	9.2	8.8
Human immunodeficiency virus infection	- - -	- - -	- - -	- - -	- - -	2.1	2.8	3.5	3.1	2.2
External causes	- - -	- - -	- - -	34.9	31.4	30.9	29.5	29.7	29.7	27.1
Unintentional injuries	- - -	- - -	- - -	21.7	20.1	19.3	16.0	17.2	17.1	16.1
Motor vehicle-related injuries	- - -	- - -	- - -	12.6	12.0	12.5	9.5	10.3	10.8	9.5
Suicide	- - -	- - -	- - -	6.7	6.4	6.0	6.4	6.6	6.6	6.0
Homicide and legal intervention	- - -	- - -	- - -	5.6	4.2	5.2	6.4	5.4	5.4	4.6
Hispanic										
All causes	- - -	- - -	- - -	- - -	397.4	400.2	385.3	383.8	386.8	365.9
Natural causes	- - -	- - -	- - -	- - -	342.7	342.4	329.3	330.3	334.0	316.9
Diseases of heart	- - -	- - -	- - -	- - -	116.0	102.8	94.7	91.9	92.1	88.6
Ischemic heart disease	- - -	- - -	- - -	- - -	77.8	68.0	62.1	59.9	60.1	58.2
Cerebrovascular diseases	- - -	- - -	- - -	- - -	23.8	21.0	19.4	19.5	20.3	19.5
Malignant neoplasms	- - -	- - -	- - -	- - -	75.8	82.4	78.7	79.5	79.7	77.8
Respiratory system	- - -	- - -	- - -	- - -	14.3	16.9	15.5	15.5	15.6	15.4
Colorectal	- - -	- - -	- - -	- - -	7.5	8.2	7.5	7.9	7.6	7.3
Prostate[2]	- - -	- - -	- - -	- - -	8.5	9.5	10.6	11.0	10.9	9.9
Breast[3]	- - -	- - -	- - -	- - -	11.8	14.1	12.4	12.6	12.7	12.8
Chronic obstructive pulmonary diseases	- - -	- - -	- - -	- - -	8.2	8.7	9.1	9.0	9.4	8.9
Pneumonia and influenza	- - -	- - -	- - -	- - -	12.0	11.5	10.7	9.8	9.9	9.7
Chronic liver disease and cirrhosis	- - -	- - -	- - -	- - -	16.3	14.2	13.4	13.7	12.9	12.6
Diabetes mellitus	- - -	- - -	- - -	- - -	12.8	15.7	16.8	18.0	19.3	18.8
Human immunodeficiency virus infection	- - -	- - -	- - -	- - -	- - -	15.5	20.1	23.6	23.9	16.3
External causes	- - -	- - -	- - -	- - -	54.7	57.8	56.0	53.6	52.9	49.0
Unintentional injuries	- - -	- - -	- - -	- - -	31.8	32.2	30.6	29.2	29.8	29.0
Motor vehicle-related injuries	- - -	- - -	- - -	- - -	16.9	19.3	16.8	16.6	16.6	16.1
Suicide	- - -	- - -	- - -	- - -	6.1	7.3	7.3	7.2	7.2	6.7
Homicide and legal intervention	- - -	- - -	- - -	- - -	15.7	17.7	17.0	16.1	15.0	12.4

See footnotes at end of table.

Table 31 (page 4 of 4). Age-adjusted death rates for selected causes of death, according to sex, detailed race, and Hispanic origin: United States, selected years 1950–96

[Data are based on the National Vital Statistics System]

Sex, race, Hispanic origin, and cause of death	1950[1]	1960[1]	1970	1980	1985	1990	1993	1994	1995	1996
White, non-Hispanic					Deaths per 100,000 resident population					
All causes	---	---	---	---	510.7	493.1	479.5	478.1	475.2	466.7
Natural causes	---	---	---	---	460.7	444.2	433.5	431.7	428.8	420.7
Diseases of heart	---	---	---	---	173.0	148.2	139.5	136.4	134.1	131.0
Ischemic heart disease	---	---	---	---	125.4	103.7	94.3	91.9	89.8	87.4
Cerebrovascular diseases	---	---	---	---	29.2	25.7	24.3	24.4	24.6	24.4
Malignant neoplasms	---	---	---	---	128.3	134.2	130.7	130.7	129.2	127.6
Respiratory system	---	---	---	---	38.0	41.9	41.2	40.9	40.5	40.2
Colorectal	---	---	---	---	14.4	13.6	12.7	12.7	12.5	12.1
Prostate[2]	---	---	---	---	13.0	15.6	14.9	14.7	14.1	13.6
Breast[3]	---	---	---	---	23.3	23.5	21.5	21.3	20.9	20.1
Chronic obstructive pulmonary diseases	---	---	---	---	19.7	20.7	22.3	22.1	21.8	22.1
Pneumonia and influenza	---	---	---	---	13.2	13.3	12.7	12.4	12.3	12.2
Chronic liver disease and cirrhosis	---	---	---	---	8.5	7.5	7.0	6.9	6.8	6.7
Diabetes mellitus	---	---	---	---	8.0	10.1	10.6	11.0	11.2	11.5
Human immunodeficiency virus infection	---	---	---	---	---	7.0	9.0	9.6	9.4	6.0
External causes	---	---	---	---	50.0	48.9	46.0	46.4	46.4	46.0
Unintentional injuries	---	---	---	---	31.9	31.3	28.5	28.9	29.3	29.3
Motor vehicle-related injuries	---	---	---	---	17.8	18.4	15.6	15.8	16.0	16.0
Suicide	---	---	---	---	12.7	12.7	12.2	12.2	12.2	12.0
Homicide and legal intervention	---	---	---	---	4.5	4.2	4.1	4.1	3.8	3.5

- - - Data not available.

[1]Includes deaths of persons who were not residents of the 50 States and the District of Columbia.
[2]Male only.
[3]Female only.

NOTES: For data years shown, code numbers for cause of death are based on the current revision of *International Classification of Diseases*. See Appendix II, tables IV, V. Categories for coding human immunodeficiency virus infection deaths were introduced in the United States in 1987. Consistency of race identification between the death certificate (source of data for numerator of death rates) and data from the Census Bureau (denominator) is high for individual white and black persons; however, persons identified as American Indian, Asian, or Hispanic origin in data from the Census Bureau are sometimes misreported as white or non-Hispanic on the death certificate, causing death rates to be underestimated by 22–30 percent for American Indians, about 12 percent for Asians, and about 7 percent for persons of Hispanic origin. (Sorlie PD, Rogot E, and Johnson NJ: Validity of demographic characteristics on the death certificate, *Epidemiology* 3(2):181–184, 1992.)

SOURCES: Centers for Disease Control and Prevention, National Center for Health Statistics: Grove, RD, Hetzel, AM. *Vital statistics rates in the United States, 1940–1960.* Washington: U.S. Government Printing Office. 1968; *Vital statistics of the United States, vol II, mortality, part A,* for data years 1960–96. Washington: Public Health Service; data computed by Division of Health and Utilization Analysis from data compiled by Division of Vital Statistics and table 1 and unpublished Hispanic population estimates prepared by the Housing and Household Economic Statistics Division, U.S. Bureau of the Census.

Table 32 (page 1 of 5). Years of potential life lost before age 75 for selected causes of death, according to sex, detailed race, and Hispanic origin: United States, selected years 1980–96

[Data are based on the National Vital Statistics System]

Sex, race, Hispanic origin, and cause of death	Crude					Age-adjusted				
	1980	1985	1990	1995	1996	1980	1985	1990	1995	1996
All persons	Years lost before age 75 per 100,000 population under 75 years of age									
All causes	10,267.6	9,255.3	8,997.0	8,595.8	8,210.0	9,813.5	8,793.2	8,518.3	8,128.2	7,748.0
Diseases of heart	2,065.3	1,842.3	1,517.6	1,430.2	1,396.8	1,877.5	1,664.1	1,363.0	1,259.2	1,222.6
Ischemic heart disease.	1,454.3	1,207.4	942.1	841.8	820.4	1,307.4	1,078.5	834.8	727.9	704.9
Cerebrovascular diseases	332.9	277.3	246.2	241.1	240.7	302.9	250.8	221.1	211.5	210.2
Malignant neoplasms.	1,932.4	1,911.8	1,863.4	1,779.4	1,755.1	1,815.2	1,776.2	1,713.9	1,587.7	1,554.2
Respiratory system	521.1	536.1	538.0	495.9	490.2	479.5	488.1	486.3	432.7	424.1
Colorectal	175.8	168.8	153.4	146.8	142.2	158.5	151.0	137.3	128.3	123.5
Prostate[1]	78.8	81.5	89.5	77.8	75.5	67.2	69.2	76.6	66.6	64.6
Breast[2]	408.5	417.1	416.5	389.0	375.5	393.0	392.7	381.9	340.0	324.3
Chronic obstructive pulmonary diseases.	164.5	182.6	182.5	188.0	187.9	141.4	156.2	156.9	161.4	161.1
Pneumonia and influenza.	156.4	139.3	139.9	126.5	125.6	149.1	130.4	128.5	115.3	114.5
Chronic liver disease and cirrhosis	254.1	199.4	178.4	166.4	164.1	259.1	196.0	168.8	149.7	145.7
Diabetes mellitus.	124.6	120.3	147.0	169.6	174.6	115.1	109.8	133.0	149.9	153.5
Human immunodeficiency virus infection	- - -	- - -	391.2	615.0	435.1	- - -	- - -	366.2	570.3	401.9
Unintentional injuries	1,688.7	1,344.6	1,221.2	1,098.1	1,079.1	1,688.3	1,365.8	1,263.0	1,155.5	1,136.5
Motor vehicle-related injuries.	1,017.6	803.1	752.4	634.1	626.9	1,010.8	817.0	788.8	687.9	680.8
Suicide.	401.6	407.5	404.8	395.0	380.8	402.8	404.5	405.9	405.6	387.8
Homicide and legal intervention	459.5	358.0	452.3	399.1	360.4	460.9	357.1	466.4	436.4	394.7
White male										
All causes	12,454.3	11,168.6	10,629.4	10,120.3	9,558.1	11,877.4	10,594.8	10,064.6	9,546.4	8,980.1
Diseases of heart	2,907.1	2,551.2	2,058.7	1,918.4	1,866.2	2,681.9	2,329.5	1,856.8	1,678.9	1,623.5
Ischemic heart disease.	2,241.0	1,839.3	1,416.9	1,254.8	1,214.9	2,060.2	1,673.2	1,269.3	1,085.7	1,044.7
Cerebrovascular diseases	309.0	258.0	222.9	224.3	223.6	280.2	231.6	198.6	195.7	194.4
Malignant neoplasms.	2,087.1	2,042.3	1,970.9	1,868.5	1,842.6	1,939.8	1,875.4	1,793.9	1,653.5	1,620.7
Respiratory system	744.8	725.9	700.1	621.6	611.2	680.6	655.6	627.7	537.8	525.5
Colorectal	194.2	191.0	174.7	166.6	160.9	176.2	170.9	155.7	144.8	138.8
Prostate	72.6	75.6	85.0	72.3	70.1	59.1	60.5	68.3	58.1	56.3
Chronic obstructive pulmonary diseases.	219.3	222.4	208.9	200.7	198.3	187.1	187.6	177.2	169.4	167.5
Pneumonia and influenza.	156.0	146.5	143.3	131.1	128.1	147.4	135.2	130.5	117.9	115.1
Chronic liver disease and cirrhosis	306.4	249.1	233.5	235.2	233.7	307.9	242.6	219.1	208.8	205.1
Diabetes mellitus.	114.7	114.7	141.0	165.6	174.8	107.4	105.4	127.5	145.7	153.0
Human immunodeficiency virus infection	- - -	- - -	589.3	775.8	492.5	- - -	- - -	544.3	707.8	448.0
Unintentional injuries	2,553.8	1,990.3	1,766.9	1,556.2	1,513.5	2,523.6	2,004.5	1,821.5	1,638.4	1,591.5
Motor vehicle-related injuries.	1,579.9	1,198.9	1,085.4	878.7	857.6	1,549.8	1,209.7	1,134.9	957.0	933.1
Suicide.	663.0	691.5	694.0	687.4	657.0	656.4	680.2	692.2	703.8	665.7
Homicide and legal intervention	455.2	341.8	384.7	344.0	303.6	452.6	338.0	391.6	372.5	327.7
Black male										
All causes	21,081.4	18,896.4	20,744.8	19,543.6	18,140.3	22,338.5	20,016.3	21,250.2	20,272.8	18,994.6
Diseases of heart	3,383.9	3,166.8	2,769.2	2,718.5	2,585.5	4,179.5	3,864.5	3,338.2	3,151.1	2,969.9
Ischemic heart disease.	1,805.9	1,538.7	1,249.8	1,180.7	1,125.5	2,283.2	1,929.9	1,561.4	1,411.1	1,326.2
Cerebrovascular diseases	714.1	597.6	546.4	522.4	509.5	870.2	727.3	655.6	601.0	583.0
Malignant neoplasms.	2,495.1	2,474.9	2,444.5	2,236.3	2,197.8	3,070.6	3,058.0	3,021.7	2,654.4	2,576.8
Respiratory system	911.8	916.1	899.8	766.2	759.6	1,160.8	1,167.2	1,150.8	941.0	918.1
Colorectal	176.1	183.8	188.6	187.7	192.1	215.9	226.0	234.0	223.7	225.6
Prostate	136.9	141.1	143.7	135.4	130.8	159.1	170.0	177.6	166.5	160.2
Chronic obstructive pulmonary diseases.	223.3	236.1	241.4	244.6	239.0	258.7	273.9	278.7	275.3	266.7
Pneumonia and influenza.	467.1	391.5	399.2	305.8	311.3	492.6	424.3	416.8	321.2	328.4
Chronic liver disease and cirrhosis	610.1	480.8	390.5	285.3	265.8	791.8	588.5	461.4	320.5	293.5
Diabetes mellitus.	199.8	204.8	263.0	319.5	310.7	245.5	249.4	317.8	373.8	357.4
Human immunodeficiency virus infection	- - -	- - -	1,622.4	2,939.3	2,293.6	- - -	- - -	1,625.8	2,928.0	2,270.3
Unintentional injuries	2,934.4	2,420.2	2,308.7	2,049.3	1,985.9	2,931.3	2,395.9	2,265.6	2,042.6	1,983.7
Motor vehicle-related injuries.	1,289.2	1,127.6	1,163.1	1,008.0	994.4	1,281.2	1,099.4	1,143.1	1,007.9	997.1
Suicide.	415.7	432.5	482.3	482.0	459.7	428.1	428.6	478.0	489.3	465.6
Homicide and legal intervention	2,872.4	2,128.4	3,197.7	2,635.6	2,417.8	2,939.9	2,079.8	3,096.6	2,663.5	2,448.4

See footnotes at end of table.

[Data are based on the National Vital Statistics System]

Sex, race, Hispanic origin, and cause of death	Crude					Age-adjusted				
	1980	1985	1990	1995	1996	1980	1985	1990	1995	1996
American Indian or Alaska Native male[3]	Years lost before age 75 per 100,000 population under 75 years of age									
All causes	16,368.1	12,443.4	11,879.5	11,670.7	11,023.5	16,915.2	12,848.9	12,125.2	12,349.1	11,607.8
Diseases of heart	1,667.6	1,391.3	1,287.0	1,285.5	1,285.0	2,299.7	1,887.9	1,660.5	1,592.9	1,564.5
Ischemic heart disease	1,024.5	846.3	712.6	792.0	771.1	1,511.6	1,207.8	985.1	1,016.3	965.7
Cerebrovascular diseases	190.2	165.1	160.3	225.5	200.3	256.4	220.3	194.1	270.1	234.2
Malignant neoplasms	661.4	799.1	725.2	839.5	821.9	912.9	1,056.6	948.4	1,053.0	1,030.9
Respiratory system	174.5	202.9	206.2	243.2	267.5	256.6	297.1	293.1	325.1	358.1
Colorectal	44.9	75.3	53.1	77.7	80.0	64.6	105.5	68.9	97.4	103.6
Prostate	34.2	35.2	22.5	30.5	42.1	53.1	53.3	33.5	43.0	58.3
Chronic obstructive pulmonary diseases	78.2	98.9	100.3	106.5	80.6	106.2	128.8	128.2	134.3	99.1
Pneumonia and influenza	343.1	222.4	230.2	225.8	261.7	370.1	233.4	227.5	240.0	274.9
Chronic liver disease and cirrhosis	943.9	526.0	445.9	669.3	504.7	1,259.9	658.7	530.2	735.9	555.6
Diabetes mellitus	183.1	155.5	191.6	257.9	291.7	255.3	220.0	256.1	324.7	360.0
Human immunodeficiency virus infection	- - -	- - -	130.2	436.2	271.0	- - -	- - -	130.3	429.3	264.8
Unintentional injuries	5,731.6	4,092.4	3,600.0	3,321.2	3,175.7	5,509.9	3,897.0	3,508.2	3,289.7	3,130.9
Motor vehicle-related injuries	3,329.6	2,374.8	2,095.9	1,934.5	1,955.5	3,146.2	2,240.8	2,047.2	1,936.6	1,925.0
Suicide	984.6	961.7	968.2	879.2	877.2	921.0	900.9	945.1	880.4	867.0
Homicide and legal intervention	1,029.4	821.3	778.2	829.3	682.3	1,003.6	805.3	754.5	823.3	677.3
Asian or Pacific Islander male[4]										
All causes	6,131.1	5,582.4	5,414.5	5,158.3	4,981.1	6,342.7	5,841.0	5,638.0	5,310.0	5,101.5
Diseases of heart	1,027.0	870.9	740.6	763.5	804.5	1,237.1	1,059.4	877.9	852.2	873.7
Ischemic heart disease	697.6	532.9	413.4	429.6	445.4	863.6	675.0	507.1	487.2	493.2
Cerebrovascular diseases	201.0	154.2	176.2	212.5	202.5	238.4	188.3	208.1	234.7	219.3
Malignant neoplasms	969.1	996.4	965.7	975.0	952.8	1,160.1	1,193.0	1,132.1	1,072.9	1,031.3
Respiratory system	239.3	211.9	192.8	199.9	199.7	304.7	275.8	245.4	231.4	227.6
Colorectal	84.1	89.0	85.6	98.4	80.4	104.8	112.8	103.7	109.2	89.1
Prostate	10.3	11.5	18.6	16.1	18.3	12.9	15.6	25.0	20.1	21.9
Chronic obstructive pulmonary diseases	67.1	66.8	61.6	65.7	79.4	76.8	83.5	77.7	75.1	88.3
Pneumonia and influenza	94.1	76.9	72.2	69.3	72.4	93.9	81.3	79.4	73.3	75.5
Chronic liver disease and cirrhosis	94.7	92.6	84.8	62.5	60.1	112.1	106.7	95.7	64.4	61.8
Diabetes mellitus	63.6	49.8	60.2	71.3	89.9	76.6	63.5	74.1	82.2	98.5
Human immunodeficiency virus infection	- - -	- - -	145.8	221.5	146.2	- - -	- - -	134.5	202.4	133.0
Unintentional injuries	1,196.8	1,058.1	986.7	789.5	776.6	1,143.8	1,020.4	957.1	797.1	788.6
Motor vehicle-related injuries	732.6	668.3	657.3	494.3	466.3	699.8	641.6	634.9	505.4	477.7
Suicide	320.0	326.0	336.5	355.5	326.4	308.9	311.9	320.5	361.0	324.6
Homicide and legal intervention	317.1	257.3	347.5	359.0	317.4	304.4	244.2	330.7	371.5	323.8
Hispanic male[5]										
All causes	- - -	9,338.3	10,217.2	9,583.2	8,477.9	- - -	9,872.6	10,469.6	9,989.4	8,861.4
Diseases of heart	- - -	975.8	897.3	846.4	825.4	- - -	1,478.3	1,301.8	1,155.8	1,124.6
Ischemic heart disease	- - -	564.7	483.5	445.2	432.8	- - -	917.1	759.4	650.8	631.2
Cerebrovascular diseases	- - -	189.8	168.7	183.5	183.6	- - -	275.8	228.9	232.4	233.5
Malignant neoplasms	- - -	753.2	810.1	838.1	791.9	- - -	1,055.9	1,131.3	1,104.4	1,042.3
Respiratory system	- - -	138.0	169.2	158.4	149.3	- - -	226.0	267.9	235.0	224.2
Colorectal	- - -	56.1	64.1	68.8	64.7	- - -	91.7	98.7	98.5	91.8
Prostate	- - -	24.4	22.0	29.3	27.2	- - -	43.8	37.8	46.9	44.4
Chronic obstructive pulmonary diseases	- - -	50.8	54.6	60.9	53.6	- - -	76.5	74.8	79.0	72.2
Pneumonia and influenza	- - -	151.5	139.4	118.8	111.6	- - -	173.3	152.5	129.1	119.0
Chronic liver disease and cirrhosis	- - -	418.8	340.2	309.6	301.7	- - -	572.1	454.0	395.8	377.9
Diabetes mellitus	- - -	77.4	107.2	144.2	142.5	- - -	125.1	160.0	206.8	204.0
Human immunodeficiency virus infection	- - -	- - -	964.3	1,332.9	871.8	- - -	- - -	972.6	1,330.6	869.6
Unintentional injuries	- - -	2,092.0	2,120.1	1,794.7	1,679.3	- - -	1,936.0	1,972.7	1,757.9	1,632.1
Motor vehicle-related injuries	- - -	1,182.8	1,305.0	1,024.3	951.4	- - -	1,076.4	1,202.0	1,002.9	922.9
Suicide	- - -	412.7	450.2	462.7	420.5	- - -	391.0	434.3	464.3	413.3
Homicide and legal intervention	- - -	1,261.3	1,466.4	1,209.1	993.2	- - -	1,152.2	1,330.1	1,182.4	949.7

See footnotes at end of table.

Table 32 (page 3 of 5). Years of potential life lost before age 75 for selected causes of death, according to sex, detailed race, and Hispanic origin: United States, selected years 1980–96

[Data are based on the National Vital Statistics System]

Sex, race, Hispanic origin, and cause of death	Crude					Age-adjusted				
	1980	1985	1990	1995	1996	1980	1985	1990	1995	1996
White, non-Hispanic male[5]	Years lost before age 75 per 100,000 population under 75 years of age									
All causes	- - -	10,733.3	10,530.0	9,992.3	9,528.0	- - -	10,091.2	9,803.6	9,226.3	8,744.4
Diseases of heart	- - -	2,528.2	2,175.5	2,034.3	1,988.3	- - -	2,246.8	1,877.0	1,697.9	1,643.2
Ischemic heart disease	- - -	1,827.2	1,515.2	1,346.6	1,309.8	- - -	1,614.6	1,294.4	1,107.3	1,065.8
Cerebrovascular diseases	- - -	244.9	228.8	226.0	224.6	- - -	213.1	195.0	188.5	185.9
Malignant neoplasms	- - -	2,046.9	2,102.1	1,988.6	1,974.6	- - -	1,833.5	1,835.5	1,679.9	1,651.4
Respiratory system	- - -	732.9	760.4	677.3	671.3	- - -	642.8	649.2	554.8	544.1
Colorectal	- - -	194.4	187.9	178.6	173.5	- - -	168.7	159.8	147.5	141.5
Prostate	- - -	74.7	92.8	77.8	75.8	- - -	57.7	70.4	58.6	56.8
Chronic obstructive pulmonary diseases	- - -	234.5	227.2	216.7	216.1	- - -	192.6	183.2	173.2	172.0
Pneumonia and influenza	- - -	147.7	141.3	130.1	127.6	- - -	134.6	125.3	113.6	110.9
Chronic liver disease and cirrhosis	- - -	234.4	219.1	219.5	218.4	- - -	221.8	198.2	187.3	183.8
Diabetes mellitus	- - -	107.7	144.7	166.4	176.7	- - -	96.0	125.9	140.0	147.5
Human immunodeficiency virus infection	- - -	- - -	531.4	684.0	425.7	- - -	- - -	485.9	618.2	384.0
Unintentional injuries	- - -	1,829.1	1,689.9	1,484.3	1,451.1	- - -	1,858.9	1,769.3	1,581.6	1,549.9
Motor vehicle-related injuries	- - -	1,097.8	1,041.9	837.9	821.8	- - -	1,122.2	1,111.0	928.0	914.2
Suicide	- - -	702.9	719.4	705.2	681.0	- - -	689.1	720.9	723.2	692.1
Homicide and legal intervention	- - -	254.3	239.2	207.0	189.1	- - -	253.0	242.3	219.0	200.3
White female										
All causes	6,655.6	6,116.8	5,740.0	5,533.7	5,443.6	6,185.7	5,606.7	5,225.3	5,005.0	4,899.9
Diseases of heart	1,142.1	1,044.2	864.1	811.8	798.8	915.3	832.2	689.3	648.9	637.1
Ischemic heart disease	758.1	653.5	521.1	464.1	459.5	584.8	501.0	399.6	356.1	352.2
Cerebrovascular diseases	275.0	226.7	200.1	193.4	193.7	231.4	188.8	165.4	156.8	157.3
Malignant neoplasms	1,774.6	1,793.5	1,760.8	1,701.4	1,684.0	1,595.5	1,584.0	1,528.7	1,425.7	1,403.1
Respiratory system	305.8	360.5	391.8	393.1	392.3	267.5	307.0	326.9	316.0	312.3
Colorectal	165.1	151.3	133.2	125.6	120.8	137.5	124.5	109.5	101.2	96.8
Breast	418.8	426.2	420.7	383.8	369.1	390.0	388.3	373.0	324.1	308.5
Chronic obstructive pulmonary diseases	117.4	152.8	164.6	183.6	183.7	94.8	120.9	128.9	143.4	142.0
Pneumonia and influenza	103.6	91.7	92.3	89.8	90.8	97.0	83.4	81.8	78.8	79.8
Chronic liver disease and cirrhosis	145.2	110.8	95.5	89.4	91.4	138.7	102.0	84.6	75.9	77.1
Diabetes mellitus	108.0	101.4	121.8	135.8	136.5	91.4	84.5	101.0	110.3	110.9
Human immunodeficiency virus infection	- - -	- - -	43.4	102.6	76.4	- - -	- - -	41.8	98.1	73.2
Unintentional injuries	793.0	656.1	610.1	577.6	584.4	816.8	690.3	654.1	629.2	634.9
Motor vehicle-related injuries	525.0	440.1	426.7	382.7	387.6	539.1	465.5	464.8	429.5	434.7
Suicide	193.0	181.0	166.1	153.4	153.8	196.1	181.2	165.3	154.0	153.6
Homicide and legal intervention	132.0	119.0	117.2	114.0	102.5	136.1	122.7	123.5	124.0	111.1
Black female										
All causes	11,795.1	10,576.5	10,966.0	10,373.3	10,054.1	11,863.1	10,630.9	10,662.7	10,179.7	10,012.6
Diseases of heart	2,020.0	1,867.5	1,665.2	1,594.1	1,618.1	2,189.5	1,993.1	1,756.0	1,627.8	1,636.2
Ischemic heart disease	987.7	852.4	711.9	661.6	670.3	1,078.5	917.5	762.1	680.9	682.3
Cerebrovascular diseases	600.9	506.3	458.3	415.6	425.1	656.7	544.5	481.2	417.3	422.9
Malignant neoplasms	1,855.8	1,833.0	1,893.9	1,856.4	1,822.9	2,085.5	2,019.3	2,041.9	1,911.8	1,845.0
Respiratory system	279.5	306.7	344.9	330.9	328.6	322.0	344.7	382.4	347.6	337.5
Colorectal	162.6	171.6	164.0	160.7	157.5	179.2	187.1	178.3	165.8	160.8
Breast	382.8	424.0	465.4	484.2	484.4	448.6	479.8	505.6	495.9	484.0
Chronic obstructive pulmonary diseases	109.0	132.4	149.0	169.6	185.7	116.3	139.7	157.4	172.8	187.4
Pneumonia and influenza	252.3	204.3	214.2	189.1	179.1	245.2	203.9	206.1	184.0	177.2
Chronic liver disease and cirrhosis	323.8	227.1	193.2	128.9	121.7	378.0	250.2	203.4	130.0	119.8
Diabetes mellitus	248.3	229.2	279.1	307.2	321.9	271.6	246.7	299.0	318.0	329.5
Human immunodeficiency virus infection	- - -	- - -	427.1	956.6	801.2	- - -	- - -	402.5	913.5	757.5
Unintentional injuries	898.9	769.7	767.7	740.1	753.1	876.0	754.6	748.3	730.1	751.9
Motor vehicle-related injuries	362.9	349.5	381.2	367.2	389.4	354.7	342.3	376.7	370.2	396.9
Suicide	88.3	76.4	90.0	77.6	74.1	91.2	76.8	89.0	77.5	74.7
Homicide and legal intervention	605.3	491.6	619.7	505.1	467.1	593.1	474.9	596.5	505.6	470.5

See footnotes at end of table.

[Data are based on the National Vital Statistics System]

Sex, race, Hispanic origin, and cause of death	Crude					Age-adjusted				
	1980	1985	1990	1995	1996	1980	1985	1990	1995	1996
American Indian or Alaska Native female[3]	Years lost before age 75 per 100,000 population under 75 years of age									
All causes	9,077.4	6,853.0	6,086.8	6,586.7	6,560.8	9,126.7	6,974.6	6,192.2	6,788.9	6,797.2
Diseases of heart	714.8	664.1	647.0	679.4	651.4	870.8	811.5	753.2	781.6	738.7
Ischemic heart disease.	323.4	320.0	299.7	342.6	315.7	442.1	422.4	381.1	408.3	376.3
Cerebrovascular diseases	158.3	163.8	167.1	178.3	175.5	204.2	196.0	191.7	199.2	194.6
Malignant neoplasms.	775.0	690.8	860.2	875.1	994.6	980.9	856.7	1,012.8	978.0	1,105.9
Respiratory system	67.2	97.1	138.6	146.8	152.3	94.9	125.3	177.3	170.1	178.1
Colorectal	45.8	40.4	56.2	83.4	73.3	63.9	50.8	68.3	92.3	85.7
Breast.	125.9	108.9	150.1	158.5	188.8	173.5	138.8	178.3	179.5	210.0
Chronic obstructive pulmonary diseases.	*	54.7	80.1	107.7	95.6	*	69.1	94.2	126.1	110.1
Pneumonia and influenza.	216.4	146.3	152.9	143.5	137.6	210.9	140.3	154.4	144.7	141.1
Chronic liver disease and cirrhosis	681.0	461.1	381.8	396.6	411.4	842.4	537.3	415.9	427.7	428.0
Diabetes mellitus.	190.5	199.5	186.6	270.1	276.6	260.4	256.1	233.0	318.5	317.8
Human immunodeficiency virus infection	- - -	- - -	*	96.5	*	- - -	- - -	*	96.8	*
Unintentional injuries	2,170.7	1,521.9	1,185.9	1,354.1	1,360.0	2,056.6	1,461.4	1,155.4	1,337.2	1,350.9
Motor vehicle-related injuries.	1,486.8	967.6	778.5	955.7	923.7	1,412.6	924.3	772.9	955.5	924.6
Suicide.	211.6	202.5	153.9	172.3	238.5	212.9	192.6	152.8	176.3	243.1
Homicide and legal intervention	342.9	192.8	226.8	242.9	218.9	345.9	194.4	219.8	238.7	211.8
Asian or Pacific Islander female[4]										
All causes	3,893.8	3,520.2	3,264.7	3,178.5	2,990.8	3,918.3	3,580.2	3,308.2	3,159.5	2,949.8
Diseases of heart	378.1	361.4	318.1	353.5	319.1	420.4	396.9	343.0	358.9	318.8
Ischemic heart disease.	167.1	174.1	148.3	151.7	137.8	200.5	199.5	164.1	157.6	139.0
Cerebrovascular diseases	192.2	164.8	175.3	153.3	161.6	215.6	184.1	190.0	157.3	158.6
Malignant neoplasms.	870.0	881.9	847.0	960.6	910.8	949.9	946.4	893.7	959.1	886.9
Respiratory system	98.1	92.9	110.7	126.7	106.7	113.1	106.1	121.6	129.8	106.4
Colorectal	79.7	79.6	69.7	71.3	78.6	89.9	86.6	75.7	70.0	77.5
Breast.	175.7	156.8	173.1	215.9	175.9	190.0	171.0	182.0	211.1	164.1
Chronic obstructive pulmonary diseases.	22.1	47.6	47.4	42.0	52.6	23.2	53.4	50.4	41.5	52.8
Pneumonia and influenza.	49.6	42.9	59.6	47.4	46.7	52.3	43.5	60.7	46.6	45.8
Chronic liver disease and cirrhosis	34.0	30.8	30.3	24.8	19.0	39.6	35.0	32.2	25.1	18.8
Diabetes mellitus.	53.1	30.9	44.5	61.8	61.6	62.6	35.0	50.2	64.7	61.4
Human immunodeficiency virus infection	- - -	- - -	*	25.6	20.4	- - -	- - -	*	23.3	18.2
Unintentional injuries	486.4	472.6	419.6	380.0	340.0	481.7	467.1	424.0	398.0	349.5
Motor vehicle-related injuries.	338.1	307.2	325.0	281.5	241.5	333.1	301.2	328.3	297.2	246.4
Suicide.	159.2	145.6	114.7	129.4	119.8	151.0	144.7	111.3	132.2	116.5
Homicide and legal intervention	131.0	123.2	117.9	113.3	93.8	124.8	121.0	113.0	113.0	97.4
Hispanic female[5]										
All causes	- - -	4,427.9	4,753.5	4,395.2	4,219.0	- - -	4,567.2	4,662.3	4,378.8	4,211.1
Diseases of heart	- - -	478.8	442.2	402.6	385.0	- - -	641.5	556.9	485.5	458.9
Ischemic heart disease.	- - -	246.6	219.8	193.8	189.3	- - -	356.7	297.0	249.6	241.9
Cerebrovascular diseases	- - -	143.8	151.9	140.8	130.0	- - -	184.0	182.8	165.6	155.1
Malignant neoplasms.	- - -	740.9	828.7	793.1	807.4	- - -	944.4	1,014.7	937.1	942.3
Respiratory system	- - -	49.3	66.3	64.5	68.3	- - -	68.7	88.9	82.1	85.3
Colorectal	- - -	48.4	54.4	54.8	52.1	- - -	65.8	70.9	67.2	64.8
Breast.	- - -	164.1	201.4	180.0	187.8	- - -	218.2	254.2	217.8	220.2
Chronic obstructive pulmonary diseases.	- - -	41.3	50.6	55.0	49.6	- - -	52.4	61.6	64.2	58.0
Pneumonia and influenza.	- - -	89.4	93.0	73.3	78.2	- - -	87.5	87.7	71.2	74.8
Chronic liver disease and cirrhosis	- - -	105.4	93.1	75.3	82.1	- - -	139.7	115.7	90.2	95.5
Diabetes mellitus.	- - -	83.4	103.4	132.4	131.1	- - -	115.9	137.0	168.8	164.2
Human immunodeficiency virus infection	- - -	- - -	152.9	312.6	225.8	- - -	- - -	146.0	309.8	224.2
Unintentional injuries	- - -	549.6	556.5	515.8	536.9	- - -	513.7	526.1	501.7	520.7
Motor vehicle-related injuries.	- - -	347.7	382.4	354.7	361.9	- - -	330.7	368.1	349.7	355.6
Suicide.	- - -	61.8	89.8	73.8	82.3	- - -	64.4	88.4	75.9	84.8
Homicide and legal intervention	- - -	203.1	227.5	202.4	165.4	- - -	188.4	214.0	197.1	158.8

See footnotes at end of table.

Table 32 (page 5 of 5). Years of potential life lost before age 75 for selected causes of death, according to sex, detailed race, and Hispanic origin: United States, selected years 1980–96

[Data are based on the National Vital Statistics System]

Sex, race, Hispanic origin, and cause of death	Crude					Age-adjusted				
	1980	1985	1990	1995	1996	1980	1985	1990	1995	1996
White, non-Hispanic female[5]	Years lost before age 75 per 100,000 population under 75 years of age									
All causes	- - -	6,037.6	5,788.3	5,591.3	5,519.7	- - -	5,495.7	5,189.9	4,968.7	4,874.5
Diseases of heart	- - -	1,046.7	902.4	853.4	842.8	- - -	816.2	691.9	654.2	643.8
Ischemic heart disease.	- - -	660.4	549.4	492.7	489.0	- - -	493.7	402.7	360.4	356.9
Cerebrovascular diseases	- - -	219.7	205.5	197.5	199.2	- - -	178.2	163.4	153.7	155.6
Malignant neoplasms.	- - -	1,807.8	1,861.9	1,804.2	1,787.1	- - -	1,560.5	1,563.0	1,453.5	1,429.5
Respiratory system	- - -	377.8	428.1	433.3	433.2	- - -	314.4	343.6	333.1	328.9
Colorectal	- - -	151.7	142.6	134.1	128.9	- - -	122.0	112.6	103.3	98.6
Breast.	- - -	436.1	444.4	407.0	390.3	- - -	387.9	381.3	330.9	313.4
Chronic obstructive pulmonary diseases.	- - -	164.5	176.9	198.4	199.8	- - -	126.9	132.5	147.7	147.0
Pneumonia and influenza.	- - -	96.2	90.2	90.4	91.0	- - -	86.9	78.1	77.7	78.0
Chronic liver disease and cirrhosis	- - -	115.8	95.6	90.1	91.9	- - -	104.0	82.0	74.0	74.9
Diabetes mellitus.	- - -	97.7	123.2	134.4	135.2	- - -	80.2	98.9	105.1	105.7
Human immunodeficiency virus infection.	- - -	- - -	29.1	72.2	53.4	- - -	- - -	28.2	69.4	51.2
Unintentional injuries	- - -	639.9	607.4	574.7	577.0	- - -	682.3	661.1	636.4	637.3
Motor vehicle-related injuries.	- - -	419.7	425.1	378.8	381.4	- - -	450.2	470.9	433.2	436.7
Suicide.	- - -	195.6	172.6	161.0	161.0	- - -	194.5	170.9	160.7	159.8
Homicide and legal intervention	- - -	115.0	102.3	96.1	90.9	- - -	119.3	108.3	105.9	99.5

- - - Data not available.

* Based on fewer than 20 deaths.

[1] Male only.

[2] Female only.

[3] Interpretation of trends should take into account that population estimates for American Indians increased by 45 percent between 1980 and 1990, partly due to better enumeration techniques in the 1990 decennial census and to the increased tendency for people to identify themselves as American Indian in 1990.

[4] Interpretation of trends should take into account that the Asian population in the United States more than doubled between 1980 and 1990, primarily due to immigration.

[5] Excludes data from States lacking an Hispanic-origin item on their death certificates. See Appendix I, National Vital Statistics System.

NOTES: For data years shown, the code numbers for cause of death are based on the *International Classification of Diseases, Ninth Revision*, described in Appendix II, table V. Categories for coding human immunodeficiency virus infection were introduced in the United States in 1987. Years of potential life lost (YPLL) before age 75 provides a measure of the impact of mortality on the population under 75 years of age. These data are presented as YPLL–75 because the average life expectancy in the United States is over 75 years. YPLL–65 was calculated in *Health, United States, 1995* and earlier editions. See Appendix II, YPLL, for method of calculation. The race groups, white, black, Asian or Pacific Islander, and American Indian or Alaska Native, include persons of Hispanic and non-Hispanic origin. Conversely, persons of Hispanic origin may be of any race. Consistency of race identification between the death certificate (source of data for numerator of death rates) and data from the Census Bureau (denominator) is high for individual white and black persons; however, persons identified as American Indian, Asian, or Hispanic origin in data from the Census Bureau are sometimes misreported as white or non-Hispanic on the death certificate, causing death rates to be underestimated by 22–30 percent for American Indians, about 12 percent for Asians, and about 7 percent for persons of Hispanic origin. (Sorlie PD, Rogot E, and Johnson NJ: Validity of demographic characteristics on the death certificate, *Epidemiology* 3(2):181–184, 1992.) YPLL rates for minority groups may also be underestimated.

SOURCES: Centers for Disease Control and Prevention, National Center for Health Statistics. *Vital statistics of the United States, vol II, mortality, part A*, for data years 1980–96. Washington: Public Health Service; data computed by the Division of Health and Utilization Analysis from data compiled by the Division of Vital Statistics and from unrounded national population estimates for race groups from table 1 and unpublished Hispanic population estimates prepared by the Housing and Household Economic Statistics Division, U.S. Bureau of the Census.

Table 33 (page 1 of 4). Leading causes of death and numbers of deaths, according to sex, detailed race, and Hispanic origin: United States, 1980 and 1996

[Data are based on the National Vital Statistics System]

Sex, race, Hispanic origin, and rank order	1980 Cause of death	1980 Deaths	1996 Cause of death	1996 Deaths
All persons				
. . .	All causes	1,989,841	All causes	2,314,690
1.	Diseases of heart	761,085	Diseases of heart	733,361
2.	Malignant neoplasms	416,509	Malignant neoplasms	539,533
3.	Cerebrovascular diseases	170,225	Cerebrovascular diseases	159,942
4.	Unintentional injuries	105,718	Chronic obstructive pulmonary diseases	106,027
5.	Chronic obstructive pulmonary diseases	56,050	Unintentional injuries	94,948
6.	Pneumonia and influenza	54,619	Pneumonia and influenza	83,727
7.	Diabetes mellitus	34,851	Diabetes mellitus	61,767
8.	Chronic liver disease and cirrhosis	30,583	Human immunodeficiency virus infection	31,130
9.	Atherosclerosis	29,449	Suicide	30,903
10.	Suicide	26,869	Chronic liver disease and cirrhosis	25,047
Male				
. . .	All causes	1,075,078	All causes	1,163,569
1.	Diseases of heart	405,661	Diseases of heart	360,075
2.	Malignant neoplasms	225,948	Malignant neoplasms	281,898
3.	Unintentional injuries	74,180	Cerebrovascular diseases	62,475
4.	Cerebrovascular diseases	69,973	Unintentional injuries	61,589
5.	Chronic obstructive pulmonary diseases	38,625	Chronic obstructive pulmonary diseases	54,485
6.	Pneumonia and influenza	27,574	Pneumonia and influenza	37,991
7.	Suicide	20,505	Diabetes mellitus	27,646
8.	Chronic liver disease and cirrhosis	19,768	Human immunodeficiency virus infection	25,277
9.	Homicide and legal intervention	19,088	Suicide	24,998
10.	Diabetes mellitus	14,325	Chronic liver disease and cirrhosis	16,311
Female				
. . .	All causes	914,763	All causes	1,151,121
1.	Diseases of heart	355,424	Diseases of heart	373,286
2.	Malignant neoplasms	190,561	Malignant neoplasms	257,635
3.	Cerebrovascular diseases	100,252	Cerebrovascular diseases	97,467
4.	Unintentional injuries	31,538	Chronic obstructive pulmonary diseases	51,542
5.	Pneumonia and influenza	27,045	Pneumonia and influenza	45,736
6.	Diabetes mellitus	20,526	Diabetes mellitus	34,121
7.	Atherosclerosis	17,848	Unintentional injuries	33,359
8.	Chronic obstructive pulmonary diseases	17,425	Alzheimer's disease	14,426
9.	Chronic liver disease and cirrhosis	10,815	Nephritis, nephrotic syndrome, and nephrosis	12,662
10.	Certain conditions originating in the perinatal period	9,815	Septicemia	12,177
White				
. . .	All causes	1,738,607	All causes	1,992,966
1.	Diseases of heart	683,347	Diseases of heart	645,514
2.	Malignant neoplasms	368,162	Malignant neoplasms	469,406
3.	Cerebrovascular diseases	148,734	Cerebrovascular diseases	138,296
4.	Unintentional injuries	90,122	Chronic obstructive pulmonary diseases	97,889
5.	Chronic obstructive pulmonary diseases	52,375	Unintentional injuries	79,405
6.	Pneumonia and influenza	48,369	Pneumonia and influenza	74,194
7.	Diabetes mellitus	28,868	Diabetes mellitus	49,511
8.	Atherosclerosis	27,069	Suicide	27,856
9.	Chronic liver disease and cirrhosis	25,240	Chronic liver disease and cirrhosis	21,422
10.	Suicide	24,829	Alzheimer's disease	20,198
Black				
. . .	All causes	233,135	All causes	282,089
1.	Diseases of heart	72,956	Diseases of heart	77,641
2.	Malignant neoplasms	45,037	Malignant neoplasms	60,766
3.	Cerebrovascular diseases	20,135	Cerebrovascular diseases	18,481
4.	Unintentional injuries	13,480	Human immunodeficiency virus infection	13,997
5.	Homicide and legal intervention	10,283	Unintentional injuries	12,655
6.	Certain conditions originating in the perinatal period	6,961	Diabetes mellitus	10,800
7.	Pneumonia and influenza	5,648	Homicide and legal intervention	9,983
8.	Diabetes mellitus	5,544	Pneumonia and influenza	7,963
9.	Chronic liver disease and cirrhosis	4,790	Chronic obstructive pulmonary diseases	6,924
10.	Nephritis, nephrotic syndrome, and nephrosis	3,416	Certain conditions originating in the perinatal period	4,711

See footnotes at end of table.

Table 33 (page 2 of 4). Leading causes of death and numbers of deaths, according to sex, detailed race, and Hispanic origin: United States, 1980 and 1996

[Data are based on the National Vital Statistics System]

Sex, race, Hispanic origin, and rank order	1980		1996	
	Cause of death	Deaths	Cause of death	Deaths
American Indian or Alaska Native				
...	All causes	6,923	All causes	10,127
1............	Diseases of heart	1,494	Diseases of heart	2,256
2............	Unintentional injuries	1,290	Malignant neoplasms	1,750
3............	Malignant neoplasms	770	Unintentional injuries	1,287
4............	Chronic liver disease and cirrhosis	410	Diabetes mellitus	553
5............	Cerebrovascular diseases	322	Cerebrovascular diseases	506
6............	Pneumonia and influenza	257	Chronic liver disease and cirrhosis	423
7............	Homicide and legal intervention	219	Pneumonia and influenza	354
8............	Diabetes mellitus	210	Suicide	291
9............	Certain conditions originating in the perinatal period	199	Chronic obstructive pulmonary diseases	289
10............	Suicide	181	Homicide and legal intervention	225
Asian or Pacific Islander				
...	All causes	11,071	All causes	29,508
1............	Diseases of heart	3,265	Diseases of heart	7,950
2............	Malignant neoplasms	2,522	Malignant neoplasms	7,611
3............	Cerebrovascular diseases	1,028	Cerebrovascular diseases	2,659
4............	Unintentional injuries	810	Unintentional injuries	1,601
5............	Pneumonia and influenza	342	Pneumonia and influenza	1,216
6............	Suicide	249	Chronic obstructive pulmonary diseases	925
7............	Certain conditions originating in the perinatal period	246	Diabetes mellitus	903
8............	Diabetes mellitus	227	Suicide	592
9............	Homicide and legal intervention	211	Homicide and legal intervention	446
10............	Chronic obstructive pulmonary diseases	207	Nephritis, nephrotic syndrome, and nephrosis	328
Hispanic[1]				
...		---	All causes	94,957
1............		---	Diseases of heart	22,986
2............		---	Malignant neoplasms	18,043
3............		---	Unintentional injuries	7,958
4............		---	Cerebrovascular diseases	5,125
5............		---	Human immunodeficiency virus infection	4,364
6............		---	Diabetes mellitus	4,361
7............		---	Homicide and legal intervention	3,504
8............		---	Pneumonia and influenza	2,891
9............		---	Chronic liver disease and cirrhosis	2,809
10............		---	Chronic obstructive pulmonary diseases	2,392
White male				
...	All causes	933,878	All causes	991,984
1............	Diseases of heart	364,679	Diseases of heart	316,889
2............	Malignant neoplasms	198,188	Malignant neoplasms	243,952
3............	Unintentional injuries	62,963	Cerebrovascular diseases	53,016
4............	Cerebrovascular diseases	60,095	Unintentional injuries	51,061
5............	Chronic obstructive pulmonary diseases	35,977	Chronic obstructive pulmonary diseases	49,822
6............	Pneumonia and influenza	23,810	Pneumonia and influenza	32,924
7............	Suicide	18,901	Diabetes mellitus	22,829
8............	Chronic liver disease and cirrhosis	16,407	Suicide	22,547
9............	Diabetes mellitus	12,125	Human immunodeficiency virus infection	14,662
10............	Atherosclerosis	10,543	Chronic liver disease and cirrhosis	13,992
Black male				
...	All causes	130,138	All causes	149,472
1............	Diseases of heart	37,877	Diseases of heart	37,335
2............	Malignant neoplasms	25,861	Malignant neoplasms	32,973
3............	Unintentional injuries	9,701	Human immunodeficiency virus infection	10,329
4............	Cerebrovascular diseases	9,194	Unintentional injuries	8,642
5............	Homicide and legal intervention	8,385	Homicide and legal intervention	8,183
6............	Certain conditions originating in the perinatal period	3,869	Cerebrovascular diseases	7,972
7............	Pneumonia and influenza	3,386	Pneumonia and influenza	4,170
8............	Chronic liver disease and cirrhosis	3,020	Diabetes mellitus	4,132
9............	Chronic obstructive pulmonary diseases	2,429	Chronic obstructive pulmonary diseases	3,928
10............	Diabetes mellitus	2,010	Certain conditions originating in the perinatal period	2,631

See footnotes at end of table.

Table 33 (page 3 of 4). Leading causes of death and numbers of deaths, according to sex, detailed race, and Hispanic origin: United States, 1980 and 1996

[Data are based on the National Vital Statistics System]

Sex, race, Hispanic origin, and rank order	1980		1996	
	Cause of death	Deaths	Cause of death	Deaths
American Indian or Alaska Native male				
. . .	All causes	4,193	All causes	5,563
1.	Unintentional injuries	946	Diseases of heart	1,257
2.	Diseases of heart	917	Unintentional injuries	877
3.	Malignant neoplasms	408	Malignant neoplasms	862
4.	Chronic liver disease and cirrhosis	239	Diabetes mellitus	242
5.	Homicide and legal intervention	164	Chronic liver disease and cirrhosis	230
6.	Cerebrovascular diseases	163	Suicide	226
7.	Pneumonia and influenza	148	Cerebrovascular diseases	212
8.	Suicide	147	Pneumonia and influenza	195
9.	Certain conditions originating in the perinatal period	107	Homicide and legal intervention	174
10.	Diabetes mellitus	86	Chronic obstructive pulmonary diseases	135
Asian or Pacific Islander male				
. . .	All causes	6,809	All causes	16,550
1.	Diseases of heart	2,174	Diseases of heart	4,594
2.	Malignant neoplasms	1,485	Malignant neoplasms	4,111
3.	Unintentional injuries	556	Cerebrovascular diseases	1,275
4.	Cerebrovascular diseases	521	Unintentional injuries	1,009
5.	Pneumonia and influenza	227	Pneumonia and influenza	702
6.	Suicide	159	Chronic obstructive pulmonary diseases	600
7.	Chronic obstructive pulmonary diseases	158	Diabetes mellitus	443
8.	Homicide and legal intervention	151	Suicide	405
9.	Certain conditions originating in the perinatal period	128	Homicide and legal intervention	342
10.	Diabetes mellitus	103	Human immunodeficiency virus infection	207
Hispanic male[1]				
. . .		- - -	All causes	55,217
1.		- - -	Diseases of heart	12,426
2.		- - -	Malignant neoplasms	9,523
3.		- - -	Unintentional injuries	6,039
4.		- - -	Human immunodeficiency virus infection	3,546
5.		- - -	Homicide and legal intervention	3,026
6.		- - -	Cerebrovascular diseases	2,433
7.		- - -	Chronic liver disease and cirrhosis	2,083
8.		- - -	Diabetes mellitus	1,988
9.		- - -	Suicide	1,528
10.		- - -	Pneumonia and influenza	1,468
White female				
. . .	All causes	804,729	All causes	1,000,982
1.	Diseases of heart	318,668	Diseases of heart	328,625
2.	Malignant neoplasms	169,974	Malignant neoplasms	225,454
3.	Cerebrovascular diseases	88,639	Cerebrovascular diseases	85,280
4.	Unintentional injuries	27,159	Chronic obstructive pulmonary diseases	48,067
5.	Pneumonia and influenza	24,559	Pneumonia and influenza	41,270
6.	Diabetes mellitus	16,743	Unintentional injuries	28,344
7.	Atherosclerosis	16,526	Diabetes mellitus	26,682
8.	Chronic obstructive pulmonary diseases	16,398	Alzheimer's disease	13,634
9.	Chronic liver disease and cirrhosis	8,833	Nephritis, nephrotic syndrome, and nephrosis	10,147
10.	Certain conditions originating in the perinatal period	6,512	Septicemia	9,883
Black female				
. . .	All causes	102,997	All causes	132,617
1.	Diseases of heart	35,079	Diseases of heart	40,306
2.	Malignant neoplasms	19,176	Malignant neoplasms	27,793
3.	Cerebrovascular diseases	10,941	Cerebrovascular diseases	10,509
4.	Unintentional injuries	3,779	Diabetes mellitus	6,668
5.	Diabetes mellitus	3,534	Unintentional injuries	4,013
6.	Certain conditions originating in the perinatal period	3,092	Pneumonia and influenza	3,793
7.	Pneumonia and influenza	2,262	Human immunodeficiency virus infection	3,668
8.	Homicide and legal intervention	1,898	Chronic obstructive pulmonary diseases	2,996
9.	Chronic liver disease and cirrhosis	1,770	Nephritis, nephrotic syndrome, and nephrosis	2,271
10.	Nephritis, nephrotic syndrome, and nephrosis	1,722	Septicemia	2,152

See footnotes at end of table.

Table 33 (page 4 of 4). Leading causes of death and numbers of deaths, according to sex, detailed race, and Hispanic origin: United States, 1980 and 1996

[Data are based on the National Vital Statistics System]

Sex, race, Hispanic origin, and rank order	1980		1996	
	Cause of death	Deaths	Cause of death	Deaths
American Indian or Alaska Native female				
. . .	All causes	2,730	All causes	4,564
1.	Diseases of heart	577	Diseases of heart	999
2.	Malignant neoplasms	362	Malignant neoplasms	888
3.	Unintentional injuries	344	Unintentional injuries	410
4.	Chronic liver disease and cirrhosis	171	Diabetes mellitus	311
5.	Cerebrovascular diseases	159	Cerebrovascular diseases	294
6.	Diabetes mellitus	124	Chronic liver disease and cirrhosis	193
7.	Pneumonia and influenza	109	Pneumonia and influenza	159
8.	Certain conditions originating in the perinatal period	92	Chronic obstructive pulmonary diseases	154
9.	Nephritis, nephrotic syndrome, and nephrosis	56	Nephritis, nephrotic syndrome, and nephrosis	68
10.	Homicide and legal intervention	55	Suicide	65
Asian or Pacific Islander female				
. . .	All causes	4,262	All causes	12,958
1.	Diseases of heart	1,091	Malignant neoplasms	3,500
2.	Malignant neoplasms	1,037	Diseases of heart	3,356
3.	Cerebrovascular diseases	507	Cerebrovascular diseases	1,384
4.	Unintentional injuries	254	Unintentional injuries	592
5.	Diabetes mellitus	124	Pneumonia and influenza	514
6.	Certain conditions originating in the perinatal period	118	Diabetes mellitus	460
7.	Pneumonia and influenza	115	Chronic obstructive pulmonary diseases	325
8.	Congenital anomalies	104	Suicide	187
9.	Suicide	90	Nephritis, nephrotic syndrome, and nephrosis	176
10.	Homicide and legal intervention	60	Congenital anomalies	138
Hispanic female[1]				
. . .	- - -	- - -	All causes	39,740
1.	- - -	- - -	Diseases of heart	10,560
2.	- - -	- - -	Malignant neoplasms	8,520
3.	- - -	- - -	Cerebrovascular diseases	2,692
4.	- - -	- - -	Diabetes mellitus	2,373
5.	- - -	- - -	Unintentional injuries	1,919
6.	- - -	- - -	Pneumonia and influenza	1,423
7.	- - -	- - -	Chronic obstructive pulmonary diseases	1,136
8.	- - -	- - -	Human immunodeficiency virus infection	818
9.	- - -	- - -	Chronic liver disease and cirrhosis	726
10.	- - -	- - -	Certain conditions originating in the perinatal period	722

. . . Category not applicable.

- - - Data not available.

[1]Excludes data from Oklahoma that did not include an Hispanic-origin item on the death certificate. See Appendix I, National Vital Statistics System.

NOTES: For data years shown, the code numbers for cause of death are based on the *International Classification of Diseases, 9th Revision*, described in Appendix II, table V. Categories for the coding and classification of human immunodeficiency virus infection were introduced in the United States beginning with mortality data for 1987.

SOURCES: Centers for Disease Control and Prevention, National Center for Health Statistics. *Vital statistics of the United States, vol II, mortality, part A,* 1980. Washington: Public Health Service. 1985; Peters KD, Kochanek KD, Murphy SL. Report of final mortality statistics, 1996. Monthly vital statistics report; vol 45. Hyattsville, Maryland: 1998; and data computed by the Division of Health and Utilization Analysis from data compiled by the Division of Vital Statistics.

Table 34 (page 1 of 2). Leading causes of death and numbers of deaths, according to age: United States, 1980 and 1996

[Data are based on the National Vital Statistics System]

Age and rank order	1980		1996	
	Cause of death	Deaths	Cause of death	Deaths
Under 1 year				
. . .	All causes	45,526	All causes	28,487
1.	Congenital anomalies	9,220	Congenital anomalies	6,381
2.	Sudden infant death syndrome	5,510	Disorders relating to short gestation and unspecified low birthweight	3,902
3.	Respiratory distress syndrome	4,989	Sudden infant death syndrome	3,050
4.	Disorders relating to short gestation and unspecified low birthweight	3,648	Respiratory distress syndrome	1,362
5.	Newborn affected by maternal complications of pregnancy	1,572	Newborn affected by maternal complications of pregnancy	1,249
6.	Intrauterine hypoxia and birth asphyxia	1,497	Newborn affected by complications of placenta, cord, and membranes	949
7.	Unintentional injuries	1,166	Unintentional injuries	804
8.	Birth trauma	1,058	Infections specific to the perinatal period	756
9.	Pneumonia and influenza	1,012	Pneumonia and influenza	496
10.	Newborn affected by complications of placenta, cord, and membranes	985	Intrauterine hypoxia and birth asphyxia	428
1–4 years				
. . .	All causes	8,187	All causes	5,948
1.	Unintentional injuries	3,313	Unintentional injuries	2,147
2.	Congenital anomalies	1,026	Congenital anomalies	638
3.	Malignant neoplasms	573	Malignant neoplasms	424
4.	Diseases of heart	338	Homicide and legal intervention	420
5.	Homicide and legal intervention	319	Diseases of heart	217
6.	Pneumonia and influenza	267	Pneumonia and influenza	168
7.	Meningitis	223	Human immunodeficiency virus infection	147
8.	Meningococcal infection	110	Septicemia	83
9.	Certain conditions originating in the perinatal period	84	Benign neoplasms	70
10.	Septicemia	71	Certain conditions originating in the perinatal period	60
5–14 years				
. . .	All causes	10,689	All causes	8,330
1.	Unintentional injuries	5,224	Unintentional injuries	3,433
2.	Malignant neoplasms	1,497	Malignant neoplasms	1,028
3.	Congenital anomalies	561	Homicide and legal intervention	514
4.	Homicide and legal intervention	415	Congenital anomalies	457
5.	Diseases of heart	330	Diseases of heart	334
6.	Pneumonia and influenza	194	Suicide	302
7.	Suicide	142	Human immunodeficiency virus infection	177
8.	Benign neoplasms	104	Chronic obstructive pulmonary diseases	165
9.	Cerebrovascular diseases	95	Pneumonia and influenza	136
10.	Chronic obstructive pulmonary diseases	85	Benign neoplasms	85
15–24 years				
. . .	All causes	49,027	All causes	32,443
1.	Unintentional injuries	26,206	Unintentional injuries	13,809
2.	Homicide and legal intervention	6,647	Homicide and legal intervention	6,548
3.	Suicide	5,239	Suicide	4,358
4.	Malignant neoplasms	2,683	Malignant neoplasms	1,632
5.	Diseases of heart	1,223	Diseases of heart	969
6.	Congenital anomalies	600	Human immunodeficiency virus infection	413
7.	Cerebrovascular diseases	418	Congenital anomalies	382
8.	Pneumonia and influenza	348	Chronic obstructive pulmonary diseases	237
9.	Chronic obstructive pulmonary diseases	141	Pneumonia and influenza	203
10.	Anemias	133	Cerebrovascular diseases	167

See footnotes at end of table.

[Data are based on the National Vital Statistics System]

Age and rank order	1980		1996	
	Cause of death	Deaths	Cause of death	Deaths
25–44 years				
. . .	All causes	108,658	All causes	147,180
1.	Unintentional injuries	26,722	Unintentional injuries	27,092
2.	Malignant neoplasms	17,551	Malignant neoplasms	21,894
3.	Diseases of heart	14,513	Human immunodeficiency virus infection	21,685
4.	Homicide and legal intervention	11,136	Diseases of heart	16,567
5.	Suicide	9,855	Suicide	12,602
6.	Chronic liver disease and cirrhosis	4,782	Homicide and legal intervention	9,322
7.	Cerebrovascular diseases	3,154	Chronic liver disease and cirrhosis	4,210
8.	Diabetes mellitus	1,472	Cerebrovascular diseases	3,442
9.	Pneumonia and influenza	1,467	Diabetes mellitus	2,526
10.	Congenital anomalies	817	Pneumonia and influenza	2,029
45–64 years				
. . .	All causes	425,338	All causes	378,054
1.	Diseases of heart	148,322	Malignant neoplasms	131,455
2.	Malignant neoplasms	135,675	Diseases of heart	102,369
3.	Cerebrovascular diseases	19,909	Unintentional injuries	16,717
4.	Unintentional injuries	18,140	Cerebrovascular diseases	15,468
5.	Chronic liver disease and cirrhosis	16,089	Chronic obstructive pulmonary diseases	12,847
6.	Chronic obstructive pulmonary diseases	11,514	Diabetes mellitus	12,687
7.	Diabetes mellitus	7,977	Chronic liver disease and cirrhosis	10,743
8.	Suicide	7,079	Human immunodeficiency virus infection	8,053
9.	Pneumonia and influenza	5,804	Suicide	7,762
10.	Homicide and legal intervention	4,057	Pneumonia and influenza	5,706
65 years and over				
. . .	All causes	1,341,848	All causes	1,713,725
1.	Diseases of heart	595,406	Diseases of heart	612,199
2.	Malignant neoplasms	258,389	Malignant neoplasms	382,988
3.	Cerebrovascular diseases	146,417	Cerebrovascular diseases	140,488
4.	Pneumonia and influenza	45,512	Chronic obstructive pulmonary diseases	91,470
5.	Chronic obstructive pulmonary diseases	43,587	Pneumonia and influenza	74,979
6.	Atherosclerosis	28,081	Diabetes mellitus	46,376
7.	Diabetes mellitus	25,216	Unintentional injuries	30,830
8.	Unintentional injuries	24,844	Alzheimer's disease	21,077
9.	Nephritis, nephrotic syndrome, and nephrosis	12,968	Nephritis, nephrotic syndrome, and nephrosis	20,869
10.	Chronic liver disease and cirrhosis	9,519	Septicemia	17,337

. . . Category not applicable.

NOTES: For data years shown, the code numbers for cause of death are based on the *International Classification of Diseases, 9th Revision*, described in Appendix II, table V. Categories for the coding and classification of human immunodeficiency virus infection were introduced in the United States beginning with mortality data for 1987.

SOURCES: Centers for Disease Control and Prevention, National Center for Health Statistics. *Vital statistics of the United States, vol II, mortality, part A*, 1980. Washington: Public Health Service. 1985; Peters KD, Kochanek KD, Murphy SL. Report of final mortality statistics, 1996. Monthly vital statistics report; vol 45. Hyattsville, Maryland: 1998; and data computed by the Division of Health and Utilization Analysis from data compiled by the Division of Vital Statistics.

Table 35 (page 1 of 2). Age-adjusted death rates, according to race, sex, region, and urbanization: United States, average annual 1984–86, 1989–91, and 1993–95

[Data are based on the National Vital Statistics System]

Sex, region, and urbanization[1]	All races			White			Black		
	1984–86	1989–91	1993–95	1984–86	1989–91	1993–95	1984–86	1989–91	1993–95
Both sexes	Deaths per 100,000 resident population[2]								
All regions:									
Large core metropolitan........	575.2	556.5	538.2	536.9	510.8	491.9	810.4	826.5	810.5
Large fringe metropolitan.......	511.5	474.1	459.7	504.0	464.6	449.3	710.5	691.7	682.2
Medium/small metropolitan......	538.2	509.2	500.7	517.7	486.0	477.4	785.2	777.8	760.0
Urban nonmetropolitan.........	549.8	529.4	519.1	531.1	509.0	499.4	791.6	793.7	761.9
Rural.....................	549.4	534.1	526.4	528.7	511.1	503.9	755.9	758.8	737.1
Northeast:									
Large core metropolitan........	592.7	577.4	556.3	552.5	528.1	508.2	799.0	811.6	782.5
Large fringe metropolitan.......	515.2	472.4	456.1	509.2	464.7	448.6	694.6	670.8	655.6
Medium/small metropolitan......	527.4	486.8	475.5	519.0	476.2	463.4	761.4	737.7	748.0
Urban nonmetropolitan.........	543.3	501.2	483.7	542.8	500.6	482.9	726.4	667.9	662.4
Rural.....................	527.7	497.5	474.5	528.7	497.8	474.5	*	*	*
South:									
Large core metropolitan........	587.5	577.7	561.7	522.8	500.5	481.3	834.7	857.8	857.3
Large fringe metropolitan.......	522.6	491.1	475.7	506.8	472.4	455.7	710.9	695.6	681.3
Medium/small metropolitan......	559.4	534.7	527.5	522.6	494.6	488.6	797.5	792.2	770.2
Urban nonmetropolitan.........	594.4	579.4	571.5	560.0	542.4	536.8	799.9	803.7	773.3
Rural.....................	595.7	583.8	576.3	566.8	553.5	547.6	757.8	759.1	739.9
Midwest:									
Large core metropolitan........	600.9	582.4	570.7	544.9	512.1	496.4	824.8	841.3	833.1
Large fringe metropolitan.......	519.4	478.5	468.1	510.8	467.8	456.4	751.9	727.8	732.7
Medium/small metropolitan......	522.1	490.4	482.5	510.0	475.3	466.2	752.8	748.2	746.0
Urban nonmetropolitan.........	503.8	484.4	473.8	501.5	481.1	470.5	718.3	721.0	669.4
Rural.....................	503.4	488.0	481.4	493.6	475.4	468.6	704.1	782.8	626.6
West:									
Large core metropolitan........	527.5	504.0	483.6	523.4	499.9	481.0	757.8	768.1	733.8
Large fringe metropolitan.......	475.9	445.2	430.6	479.9	448.0	432.0	661.2	661.8	661.5
Medium/small metropolitan......	508.5	487.1	476.7	510.1	488.8	478.6	714.5	710.9	665.4
Urban nonmetropolitan.........	515.3	493.8	481.8	508.7	486.4	475.0	654.1	660.3	557.3
Rural.....................	502.6	468.6	458.5	502.1	465.2	454.9	*	*	*
Male									
All regions:									
Large core metropolitan........	757.7	733.5	703.9	707.5	671.9	640.8	1,092.0	1,130.3	1,101.1
Large fringe metropolitan.......	664.1	607.8	580.3	655.4	595.6	566.6	918.7	899.6	880.1
Medium/small metropolitan......	709.8	663.5	644.1	685.5	633.7	613.9	1,029.6	1,035.8	999.9
Urban nonmetropolitan.........	729.7	695.0	670.2	707.8	669.7	645.0	1,042.4	1,054.4	1,011.7
Rural.....................	730.3	704.7	678.3	704.7	675.2	649.3	1,005.9	1,016.6	979.2
Northeast:									
Large core metropolitan........	784.9	767.6	731.1	730.3	699.5	665.0	1,095.2	1,127.6	1,075.2
Large fringe metropolitan.......	671.2	607.9	578.6	663.8	597.8	568.6	910.3	881.3	858.7
Medium/small metropolitan......	697.0	635.0	612.4	686.6	621.3	596.7	996.3	982.0	976.5
Urban nonmetropolitan.........	712.7	652.1	617.2	713.1	652.2	616.4	868.0	808.6	820.4
Rural.....................	696.7	651.2	600.6	699.0	651.3	600.5	*	*	*
South:									
Large core metropolitan........	778.7	772.0	742.0	693.6	668.2	632.9	1,124.5	1,179.1	1,176.6
Large fringe metropolitan.......	683.6	636.4	605.7	664.4	611.9	579.6	926.3	915.0	884.9
Medium/small metropolitan......	742.2	702.4	684.8	697.4	649.6	633.8	1,053.6	1,066.2	1,026.1
Urban nonmetropolitan.........	800.1	772.2	749.0	760.2	725.6	703.7	1,064.3	1,082.9	1,040.5
Rural.....................	799.1	778.8	751.3	764.2	740.2	713.4	1,011.1	1,021.8	987.8
Midwest:									
Large core metropolitan........	798.5	769.5	748.9	725.8	674.0	647.2	1,107.7	1,147.9	1,134.8
Large fringe metropolitan.......	674.9	611.2	588.7	664.9	598.2	574.3	957.4	929.9	929.3
Medium/small metropolitan......	689.7	638.2	618.4	675.5	619.2	598.0	974.4	979.6	962.5
Urban nonmetropolitan.........	667.9	635.4	610.5	665.7	632.1	607.0	880.0	874.5	828.0
Rural.....................	666.2	639.7	616.2	653.9	624.4	600.9	891.7	945.5	741.3
West:									
Large core metropolitan........	684.5	652.2	624.9	679.9	646.9	620.4	994.0	1,011.4	951.9
Large fringe metropolitan.......	607.8	561.4	535.3	613.8	565.4	535.9	810.0	812.3	809.4
Medium/small metropolitan......	657.4	620.9	599.8	661.6	624.4	601.2	881.1	874.2	800.7
Urban nonmetropolitan.........	661.0	624.5	602.4	653.2	615.4	594.0	782.9	763.5	629.0
Rural.....................	646.2	596.0	572.0	646.4	590.4	568.1	*	*	*

See footnotes at end of table.

Table 35 (page 2 of 2). Age-adjusted death rates, according to race, sex, region, and urbanization: United States, average annual 1984–86, 1989–91, and 1993–95

[Data are based on the National Vital Statistics System]

Sex, region, and urbanization[1]	All races			White			Black		
	1984–86	1989–91	1993–95	1984–86	1989–91	1993–95	1984–86	1989–91	1993–95
Female	Deaths per 100,000 resident population[2]								
All regions:									
Large core metropolitan.	432.6	413.5	401.6	403.7	379.9	367.6	599.4	598.2	589.1
Large fringe metropolitan.	391.1	367.3	361.2	384.9	360.2	353.5	544.3	526.3	522.7
Medium/small metropolitan.	402.6	385.4	383.0	385.3	367.6	365.2	597.9	580.6	573.4
Urban nonmetropolitan.	402.6	393.3	392.0	386.4	376.6	376.5	598.1	594.9	570.1
Rural	391.6	385.4	391.0	374.8	367.4	373.6	550.4	551.1	541.0
Northeast:									
Large core metropolitan.	446.7	428.3	416.9	417.1	392.6	381.3	589.3	585.4	571.3
Large fringe metropolitan.	395.3	367.0	358.5	390.5	361.4	353.0	527.6	507.3	496.9
Medium/small metropolitan.	398.9	372.8	366.1	392.3	365.1	357.3	575.4	545.3	559.6
Urban nonmetropolitan.	408.0	379.9	373.2	407.2	379.2	372.8	592.0	532.7	490.7
Rural	383.7	366.8	363.4	383.5	367.0	363.3	*	*	*
South:									
Large core metropolitan.	436.5	420.2	412.4	386.9	362.9	353.8	617.0	616.0	615.7
Large fringe metropolitan.	392.5	372.4	367.5	379.1	358.2	352.2	539.7	523.9	520.5
Medium/small metropolitan.	414.5	399.7	398.8	383.1	368.9	368.6	605.6	587.8	577.6
Urban nonmetropolitan.	428.4	423.7	425.5	397.2	392.8	397.8	600.1	596.6	574.0
Rural	421.7	417.3	424.1	397.2	392.6	401.9	550.8	549.2	541.4
Midwest:									
Large core metropolitan.	451.7	438.3	430.3	410.7	389.0	379.1	610.0	611.5	604.1
Large fringe metropolitan.	398.8	375.2	372.3	391.5	366.8	363.2	586.8	565.3	570.8
Medium/small metropolitan.	394.0	375.7	375.0	383.8	364.0	362.5	578.4	567.5	570.9
Urban nonmetropolitan.	371.5	361.9	360.1	369.1	358.9	357.1	575.5	585.1	528.4
Rural	360.7	355.1	360.1	353.4	345.2	349.9	*	*	*
West:									
Large core metropolitan.	398.8	377.2	360.5	395.2	373.3	357.5	564.9	565.2	546.4
Large fringe metropolitan.	368.9	348.9	341.8	371.5	351.0	343.5	525.6	519.5	518.5
Medium/small metropolitan.	380.7	370.5	367.1	381.3	371.3	369.0	551.3	552.7	529.7
Urban nonmetropolitan.	384.3	376.0	370.4	379.8	370.8	365.4	521.7	566.7	478.8
Rural	364.6	345.9	347.4	363.6	345.2	344.3	*	*	*

* Data for groups with population under 5,000 in the middle year of a 3-year period are considered unreliable and are not shown.

[1]Urbanization categories for county of residence of decedent are based on a modification of the 1993 classification of counties by the Department of Agriculture. See Appendix II, Urbanization.

[2]Average annual death rate.

NOTE: Denominators for rates are population estimates for the middle year of each 3-year period multiplied by 3.

SOURCE: Centers for Disease Control and Prevention, National Center for Health Statistics. Data computed by the Division of Health and Utilization Analysis using the Compressed Mortality File. See Appendix I, National Vital Statistics System.

Table 36. Death rates for persons 25–64 years of age, for all races and the white population, according to sex, age, and educational attainment: Selected States, 1994–96

[Data are based on the National Vital Statistics System]

Sex, age, and educational attainment[1]	All races			White		
	1994	1995	1996	1994	1995	1996
Both sexes	Deaths per 100,000 resident population					
25–64 years of age:[2]						
Less than 12 years	571.0	581.2	556.0	520.1	529.9	515.1
12 years	486.1	491.7	472.4	439.6	443.7	426.1
13 years or more	243.4	240.4	230.4	230.6	227.2	218.1
25–44 years of age:						
Less than 12 years	316.2	322.8	297.4	267.0	273.3	253.6
12 years	249.8	256.6	236.9	213.5	219.9	204.4
13 years or more	109.0	107.4	96.6	99.5	98.1	88.2
45–64 years of age:						
Less than 12 years	1,043.7	1,062.7	1,035.8	994.4	1,011.5	1,004.4
12 years	876.6	880.8	858.7	819.9	819.2	796.0
13 years or more	427.3	419.5	409.4	411.0	402.5	392.6
Male						
25–64 years of age:[2]						
Less than 12 years	762.6	770.5	733.0	694.5	696.2	670.5
12 years	679.2	684.9	642.6	614.2	619.6	582.1
13 years or more	309.9	303.0	287.2	294.6	287.7	273.2
25–44 years of age:						
Less than 12 years	432.4	434.4	386.3	364.9	367.8	329.7
12 years	354.8	360.8	323.6	306.3	311.9	283.1
13 years or more	152.9	149.6	129.4	140.7	137.7	119.1
45–64 years of age:						
Less than 12 years	1,365.9	1,384.5	1,364.0	1,303.6	1,301.9	1,297.1
12 years	1,197.5	1,202.2	1,154.4	1,115.2	1,117.0	1,071.4
13 years or more	527.8	513.7	498.3	509.9	495.9	480.9
Female						
25–64 years of age:[2]						
Less than 12 years	379.8	391.3	379.4	343.4	357.0	353.4
12 years	327.6	332.4	328.9	295.3	298.6	294.7
13 years or more	173.3	174.5	171.4	161.0	161.5	158.8
25–44 years of age:						
Less than 12 years	186.1	196.0	192.9	151.7	159.1	159.0
12 years	145.2	151.5	147.5	119.9	126.4	123.0
13 years or more	66.7	67.2	65.8	58.9	59.6	58.4
45–64 years of age:						
Less than 12 years	743.3	762.2	733.2	705.3	733.6	723.9
12 years	636.2	639.8	631.7	596.6	595.4	585.0
13 years or more	317.4	316.3	313.0	299.2	296.8	293.7

[1]Educational attainment for the numerator is based on the death certificate item "highest grade completed." Educational attainment for the denominator is based on answers to the Current Population Survey question "What is the highest level of school completed or highest degree received?" (Kominski R, Adams A. Educational Attainment in the United States: March 1993 and 1992, U.S. Bureau of the Census, Current Population Reports, P20–476, Washington DC. 1994.)
[2]Age adjusted.

NOTES: Based on data from 45 States and the District of Columbia (DC). See Appendix I. Death records with education not stated are not included in the calculation of rates. Therefore the levels of the rates are underestimated by approximately the percent not stated, which ranges from 3 to 5 percent for rates shown in this table. Misreporting of education on the death certificate tends to overstate the death rate for high school graduates (12 years of education) because there is a tendency for some people who did not graduate from high school to be reported as high school graduates on the death certificate; by extension, the death rate for the group with less than 12 years of education tends to be understated. Data for the elderly population and black population are not shown because percent with education not stated is somewhat higher for these groups and because of possible bias due to misreporting of education on the death certificate. (Sorlie PD, Johnson NJ: Validity of education information on the death certificate, *Epidemiology* 7(4):437–439, 1996.)

SOURCES: Centers for Disease Control and Prevention, National Center for Health Statistics. Rates computed by the Division of Health and Utilization Analysis from vital statistics data compiled by the Division of Vital Statistics; and from unpublished population estimates prepared by the Housing and Household Economic Statistics Division, U.S. Bureau of the Census.

Table 37 (page 1 of 4). Death rates for all causes, according to sex, detailed race, Hispanic origin, and age: United States, selected years 1950–96

[Data are based on the National Vital Statistics System]

Sex, race, Hispanic origin, and age	1950[1]	1960[1]	1970	1980	1985	1990	1994	1995	1996	1994–96[2]
All persons				Deaths per 100,000 resident population						
All ages, age adjusted	841.5	760.9	714.3	585.8	548.9	520.2	507.4	503.9	491.6	500.9
All ages, crude	963.8	954.7	945.3	878.3	876.9	863.8	875.4	880.0	872.5	876.0
Under 1 year	3,299.2	2,696.4	2,142.4	1,288.3	1,088.1	971.9	819.3	768.8	755.7	781.5
1–4 years	139.4	109.1	84.5	63.9	51.8	46.8	42.9	40.6	38.3	40.6
5–14 years	60.1	46.6	41.3	30.6	26.5	24.0	22.5	22.5	21.7	22.2
15–24 years	128.1	106.3	127.7	115.4	94.9	99.2	98.0	95.3	89.6	94.3
25–34 years	178.7	146.4	157.4	135.5	124.4	139.2	143.3	141.3	126.7	137.2
35–44 years	358.7	299.4	314.5	227.9	207.7	223.2	238.8	240.8	221.3	233.5
45–54 years	853.9	756.0	730.0	584.0	519.3	473.4	461.6	460.1	445.9	455.7
55–64 years	1,901.0	1,735.1	1,658.8	1,346.3	1,294.2	1,196.9	1,128.2	1,114.5	1,094.1	1,112.2
65–74 years	4,104.3	3,822.1	3,582.7	2,994.9	2,862.8	2,648.6	2,584.9	2,563.5	2,538.4	2,562.3
75–84 years	9,331.1	8,745.2	8,004.4	6,692.6	6,398.7	6,007.2	5,860.2	5,851.8	5,803.1	5,837.9
85 years and over	20,196.9	19,857.5	16,344.9	15,980.3	15,712.4	15,327.4	15,296.7	15,469.5	15,327.2	15,364.7
Male										
All ages, age adjusted	1,001.6	949.3	931.6	777.2	723.0	680.2	654.6	646.3	623.7	641.4
All ages, crude	1,106.1	1,104.5	1,090.3	976.9	948.6	918.4	915.0	914.1	896.4	908.4
Under 1 year	3,728.0	3,059.3	2,410.0	1,428.5	1,219.9	1,082.8	899.4	843.8	828.0	857.4
1–4 years	151.7	119.5	93.2	72.6	58.5	52.4	47.3	44.8	42.2	44.8
5–14 years	70.9	55.7	50.5	36.7	31.8	28.5	26.9	26.7	25.4	26.3
15–24 years	167.9	152.1	188.5	172.3	138.9	147.4	145.8	140.5	130.6	138.9
25–34 years	216.5	187.9	215.3	196.1	179.6	204.3	208.8	204.7	178.6	197.5
35–44 years	428.8	372.8	402.6	299.2	278.9	310.4	332.9	333.0	298.1	321.1
45–54 years	1,067.1	992.2	958.5	767.3	671.6	610.3	599.4	598.9	573.8	590.3
55–64 years	2,395.3	2,309.5	2,282.7	1,815.1	1,711.4	1,553.4	1,444.3	1,416.7	1,388.7	1,416.4
65–74 years	4,931.4	4,914.4	4,873.8	4,105.2	3,856.3	3,491.5	3,332.3	3,284.6	3,233.4	3,283.4
75–84 years	10,426.0	10,178.4	10,010.2	8,816.7	8,501.6	7,888.6	7,440.9	7,377.1	7,249.8	7,353.8
85 years and over	21,636.0	21,186.3	17,821.5	18,801.1	18,614.1	18,056.6	17,972.3	17,978.9	17,547.7	17,826.3
Female										
All ages, age adjusted	688.4	590.6	532.5	432.6	410.3	390.6	385.2	385.2	381.0	383.8
All ages, crude	823.5	809.2	807.8	785.3	809.1	812.0	837.6	847.3	849.7	844.9
Under 1 year	2,854.6	2,321.3	1,863.7	1,141.7	950.6	855.7	735.5	690.1	680.0	702.1
1–4 years	126.7	98.4	75.4	54.7	44.8	41.0	38.2	36.2	34.3	36.3
5–14 years	48.9	37.3	31.8	24.2	21.0	19.3	17.9	18.2	17.8	17.9
15–24 years	89.1	61.3	68.1	57.5	49.6	49.0	48.2	48.1	46.2	47.5
25–34 years	142.7	106.6	101.6	75.9	69.4	74.2	77.8	77.9	74.7	76.8
35–44 years	290.3	229.4	231.1	159.3	138.7	137.9	146.4	150.1	145.4	147.3
45–54 years	641.5	526.7	517.2	412.9	375.2	342.7	330.1	327.6	323.3	326.9
55–64 years	1,404.8	1,196.4	1,098.9	934.3	925.6	878.8	842.2	840.8	826.7	836.5
65–74 years	3,333.2	2,871.8	2,579.7	2,144.7	2,096.9	1,991.2	1,990.3	1,986.1	1,979.0	1,985.1
75–84 years	8,399.6	7,633.1	6,677.6	5,440.1	5,162.1	4,883.1	4,870.9	4,882.7	4,868.3	4,873.9
85 years and over	19,194.7	19,008.4	15,518.0	14,746.9	14,553.9	14,274.3	14,265.3	14,492.4	14,444.7	14,402.4
White male										
All ages, age adjusted	963.1	917.7	893.4	745.3	693.3	644.3	617.9	610.5	591.4	606.5
All ages, crude	1,089.5	1,098.5	1,086.7	983.3	963.6	930.9	931.6	932.1	918.1	927.2
Under 1 year	3,400.5	2,694.1	2,113.2	1,230.3	1,056.5	896.1	740.1	717.5	683.3	713.7
1–4 years	135.5	104.9	83.6	66.1	52.8	45.9	40.5	38.8	37.1	38.8
5–14 years	67.2	52.7	48.0	35.0	30.1	26.4	24.2	24.5	23.2	24.0
15–24 years	152.4	143.7	170.8	167.0	134.2	131.3	124.2	122.3	113.9	120.1
25–34 years	185.3	163.2	176.6	171.3	158.8	176.1	179.7	177.7	154.8	170.8
35–44 years	380.9	332.6	343.5	257.4	243.1	268.2	287.1	287.7	259.6	278.0
45–54 years	984.5	932.2	882.9	698.9	611.7	548.7	535.8	534.6	515.5	528.3
55–64 years	2,304.4	2,225.2	2,202.6	1,728.5	1,625.8	1,467.2	1,364.5	1,330.8	1,305.2	1,333.4
65–74 years	4,864.9	4,848.4	4,810.1	4,035.7	3,770.7	3,397.7	3,247.3	3,199.0	3,158.3	3,201.5
75–84 years	10,526.3	10,299.6	10,098.8	8,829.8	8,486.1	7,844.9	7,385.8	7,320.6	7,205.5	7,302.1
85 years and over	22,116.3	21,750.0	18,551.7	19,097.3	18,980.1	18,268.3	18,196.4	18,152.9	17,870.5	18,068.8

See footnotes at end of table.

Table 37 (page 2 of 4). Death rates for all causes, according to sex, detailed race, Hispanic origin, and age: United States, selected years 1950–96

[Data are based on the National Vital Statistics System]

Sex, race, Hispanic origin, and age	1950[1]	1960[1]	1970	1980	1985	1990	1994	1995	1996	1994–96[2]
Black male				Deaths per 100,000 resident population						
All ages, age adjusted	1,373.1	1,246.1	1,318.6	1,112.8	1,053.4	1,061.3	1,029.9	1,016.7	967.0	1,004.1
All ages, crude	1,260.3	1,181.7	1,186.6	1,034.1	989.3	1,008.0	987.8	980.7	939.9	969.2
Under 1 year	- - -	5,306.8	4,298.9	2,586.7	2,219.9	2,112.4	1,797.0	1,590.8	1,748.2	1,710.4
1–4 years	- - -	208.5	150.5	110.5	90.1	85.8	84.1	77.5	71.4	77.7
5–14 years	95.1	75.1	67.1	47.4	42.3	41.2	42.2	40.2	38.1	40.2
15–24 years	289.7	212.0	320.6	209.1	173.6	252.2	277.5	249.2	233.0	253.1
25–34 years	503.5	402.5	559.5	407.3	351.9	430.8	433.8	416.5	361.0	403.8
35–44 years	878.1	762.0	956.6	689.8	630.2	699.6	732.1	721.2	629.2	693.2
45–54 years	1,905.0	1,624.8	1,777.5	1,479.9	1,292.9	1,261.0	1,267.6	1,273.0	1,190.6	1,242.4
55–64 years	3,773.2	3,316.4	3,256.9	2,873.0	2,779.8	2,618.0	2,422.9	2,437.5	2,395.1	2,418.4
65–74 years	5,310.3	5,798.7	5,803.2	5,131.1	5,172.4	4,946.1	4,653.6	4,610.5	4,431.5	4,564.2
75–84 years	- - -	8,605.1	9,454.9	9,231.6	9,262.3	9,129.5	8,829.5	8,778.8	8,614.9	8,739.1
85 years and over	- - -	14,844.8	12,222.3	16,098.8	15,774.2	16,954.9	16,266.9	16,728.7	16,006.3	16,329.1
American Indian or Alaska Native male[3]										
All ages, age adjusted	- - -	- - -	- - -	732.5	602.6	573.1	585.9	580.4	555.9	573.7
All ages, crude	- - -	- - -	- - -	597.1	492.5	476.4	502.6	502.3	489.8	498.2
Under 1 year	- - -	- - -	- - -	1,598.1	1,080.0	1,056.6	951.6	689.3	874.4	837.7
1–4 years	- - -	- - -	- - -	82.7	105.3	77.4	81.0	81.2	72.9	78.5
5–14 years	- - -	- - -	- - -	43.7	39.2	33.4	30.9	30.3	37.8	33.0
15–24 years	- - -	- - -	- - -	311.1	214.4	219.8	189.1	203.2	174.7	188.5
25–34 years	- - -	- - -	- - -	360.6	275.0	256.1	293.0	284.2	260.0	278.9
35–44 years	- - -	- - -	- - -	556.8	363.5	365.4	385.0	420.5	370.0	391.6
45–54 years	- - -	- - -	- - -	871.3	687.9	619.9	661.8	668.1	580.2	635.5
55–64 years	- - -	- - -	- - -	1,547.5	1,319.1	1,211.3	1,320.9	1,369.5	1,348.0	1,346.3
65–74 years	- - -	- - -	- - -	2,968.4	2,692.3	2,461.7	2,815.2	2,605.2	2,640.7	2,685.4
75–84 years	- - -	- - -	- - -	5,607.0	5,572.7	5,389.2	4,734.4	4,780.0	4,633.8	4,713.7
85 years and over	- - -	- - -	- - -	12,635.2	8,900.0	11,243.9	8,325.9	7,404.3	7,686.7	7,789.3
Asian or Pacific Islander male[4]										
All ages, age adjusted	- - -	- - -	- - -	416.6	396.9	377.8	386.5	384.4	355.8	373.8
All ages, crude	- - -	- - -	- - -	375.3	344.6	334.3	354.0	354.9	350.7	353.2
Under 1 year	- - -	- - -	- - -	816.5	750.0	605.3	496.7	427.3	457.6	460.4
1–4 years	- - -	- - -	- - -	50.9	43.4	45.0	30.7	26.8	24.6	27.3
5–14 years	- - -	- - -	- - -	23.4	22.5	20.7	19.9	18.8	17.1	18.6
15–24 years	- - -	- - -	- - -	80.8	76.0	76.0	82.5	81.2	73.2	78.9
25–34 years	- - -	- - -	- - -	83.5	77.3	79.6	87.4	80.5	75.6	81.1
35–44 years	- - -	- - -	- - -	128.3	114.4	130.8	128.9	131.4	125.0	128.4
45–54 years	- - -	- - -	- - -	342.3	284.8	287.1	305.3	286.9	277.0	289.1
55–64 years	- - -	- - -	- - -	881.1	869.4	789.1	748.1	745.1	726.3	739.3
65–74 years	- - -	- - -	- - -	2,236.1	2,102.0	2,041.4	1,984.3	1,975.8	1,948.4	1,969.0
75–84 years	- - -	- - -	- - -	5,389.5	5,551.2	5,008.6	5,175.7	5,182.4	4,844.3	5,055.5
85 years and over	- - -	- - -	- - -	13,753.6	12,750.0	12,446.3	16,148.0	17,273.0	11,637.4	14,498.7
Hispanic male[5]										
All ages, age adjusted	- - -	- - -	- - -	- - -	524.8	531.2	516.4	515.0	474.8	501.1
All ages, crude	- - -	- - -	- - -	- - -	374.6	411.6	411.4	412.1	381.3	401.1
Under 1 year	- - -	- - -	- - -	- - -	1,041.8	921.8	731.6	687.2	686.2	701.4
1–4 years	- - -	- - -	- - -	- - -	53.8	53.8	43.6	39.7	37.3	40.1
5–14 years	- - -	- - -	- - -	- - -	23.0	26.0	24.7	25.3	23.5	24.5
15–24 years	- - -	- - -	- - -	- - -	147.5	159.3	166.9	168.7	140.3	157.9
25–34 years	- - -	- - -	- - -	- - -	202.0	234.0	222.3	215.7	175.0	203.8
35–44 years	- - -	- - -	- - -	- - -	290.3	341.8	353.3	343.3	279.7	323.5
45–54 years	- - -	- - -	- - -	- - -	495.4	533.9	531.6	533.3	493.7	518.5
55–64 years	- - -	- - -	- - -	- - -	1,129.2	1,123.7	1,045.3	1,058.7	1,032.0	1,045.1
65–74 years	- - -	- - -	- - -	- - -	2,488.9	2,368.2	2,362.0	2,322.2	2,245.4	2,307.9
75–84 years	- - -	- - -	- - -	- - -	5,724.6	5,369.1	5,080.1	5,199.0	4,966.4	5,078.0
85 years and over	- - -	- - -	- - -	- - -	11,856.1	12,272.1	12,183.5	12,242.7	10,617.7	11,609.5

See footnotes at end of table.

Table 37 (page 3 of 4). **Death rates for all causes, according to sex, detailed race, Hispanic origin, and age: United States, selected years 1950–96**

[Data are based on the National Vital Statistics System]

Sex, race, Hispanic origin, and age	1950[1]	1960[1]	1970	1980	1985	1990	1994	1995	1996	1994–96[2]
White, non-Hispanic male[5]					Deaths per 100,000 resident population					
All ages, age adjusted	- - -	- - -	- - -	- - -	669.7	643.1	613.4	605.7	589.5	602.8
All ages, crude	- - -	- - -	- - -	- - -	956.3	985.9	988.1	989.0	982.1	986.4
Under 1 year	- - -	- - -	- - -	- - -	1,002.5	865.4	718.8	695.7	654.6	689.9
1–4 years	- - -	- - -	- - -	- - -	48.8	43.8	38.8	37.5	36.2	37.5
5–14 years	- - -	- - -	- - -	- - -	28.9	25.7	23.7	23.6	22.5	23.3
15–24 years	- - -	- - -	- - -	- - -	125.0	123.4	112.9	110.6	105.6	109.7
25–34 years	- - -	- - -	- - -	- - -	151.2	165.3	168.5	166.4	147.2	160.9
35–44 years	- - -	- - -	- - -	- - -	231.8	257.1	274.3	275.9	252.3	267.4
45–54 years	- - -	- - -	- - -	- - -	587.6	544.5	528.2	526.1	509.0	520.9
55–64 years	- - -	- - -	- - -	- - -	1,550.8	1,479.7	1,373.0	1,337.0	1,308.7	1,339.4
65–74 years	- - -	- - -	- - -	- - -	3,648.0	3,434.5	3,271.9	3,221.9	3,181.1	3,225.0
75–84 years	- - -	- - -	- - -	- - -	8,364.2	7,920.4	7,425.8	7,368.2	7,274.5	7,354.7
85 years and over	- - -	- - -	- - -	- - -	18,637.2	18,505.4	18,192.3	18,157.7	18,110.1	18,152.5
White female										
All ages, age adjusted	645.0	555.0	501.7	411.1	391.0	369.9	364.9	364.9	361.9	363.9
All ages, crude	803.3	800.9	812.6	806.1	840.1	846.9	880.1	891.3	896.2	889.2
Under 1 year	2,566.8	2,007.7	1,614.6	962.5	799.3	690.0	604.8	571.6	558.0	578.2
1–4 years	112.2	85.2	66.1	49.3	40.0	36.1	32.3	31.2	28.5	30.7
5–14 years	45.1	34.7	29.9	22.9	19.5	17.9	16.2	16.6	16.4	16.4
15–24 years	71.5	54.9	61.6	55.5	48.1	45.9	44.2	44.3	42.7	43.7
25–34 years	112.8	85.0	84.1	65.4	59.4	61.5	63.7	64.3	62.7	63.6
35–44 years	235.8	191.1	193.3	138.2	121.9	117.4	121.5	125.8	121.6	123.0
45–54 years	546.4	458.8	462.9	372.7	341.7	309.3	297.1	294.4	290.5	293.9
55–64 years	1,293.8	1,078.9	876.2	869.1	822.7	792.4	788.4	779.5	786.8	
65–74 years	3,242.8	2,779.3	2,470.7	2,066.6	2,027.1	1,923.5	1,930.4	1,924.5	1,919.8	1,924.9
75–84 years	8,481.5	7,696.6	6,698.7	5,401.7	5,111.6	4,839.1	4,822.1	4,831.1	4,826.5	4,826.6
85 years and over	19,679.5	19,477.7	15,980.2	14,979.6	14,745.4	14,400.6	14,416.1	14,639.1	14,642.9	14,568.0
Black female										
All ages, age adjusted	1,106.7	916.9	814.4	631.1	594.8	581.6	572.0	571.0	561.0	567.9
All ages, crude	1,002.0	905.0	829.2	733.3	734.2	747.9	752.9	759.0	753.5	755.2
Under 1 year	- - -	4,162.2	3,368.8	2,123.7	1,821.4	1,735.5	1,452.9	1,342.0	1,444.0	1,411.6
1–4 years	- - -	173.3	129.4	84.4	71.1	67.6	70.1	62.9	63.7	65.6
5–14 years	72.8	53.8	43.8	30.5	28.6	27.5	27.1	26.5	25.9	26.5
15–24 years	213.1	107.5	111.9	70.5	59.6	68.7	72.1	70.3	66.8	69.7
25–34 years	393.3	273.2	231.0	150.0	137.6	159.5	168.4	166.6	153.8	163.0
35–44 years	758.1	568.5	533.0	323.9	276.5	298.6	327.3	327.7	316.4	323.7
45–54 years	1,576.4	1,177.0	1,043.9	768.2	667.6	639.4	628.5	619.0	610.1	618.9
55–64 years	3,089.4	2,510.9	1,986.2	1,561.0	1,532.5	1,452.6	1,341.8	1,350.3	1,311.7	1,334.4
65–74 years	4,000.2	4,064.2	3,057.4	2,967.8	2,865.7	2,815.5	2,823.7	2,787.0	2,808.7	
75–84 years	- - -	6,730.0	6,691.5	6,212.1	6,078.0	5,688.3	5,778.9	5,840.3	5,775.9	5,798.3
85 years and over	- - -	13,052.6	10,706.6	12,367.2	12,703.0	13,309.5	13,165.5	13,472.2	13,398.5	13,348.2
American Indian or Alaska Native female[3]										
All ages, age adjusted	- - -	- - -	- - -	414.1	353.3	335.1	350.8	368.0	367.7	362.3
All ages, crude	- - -	- - -	- - -	380.1	342.5	330.4	371.0	390.6	396.0	386.0
Under 1 year	- - -	- - -	- - -	1,352.6	910.5	688.7	809.3	756.5	718.2	762.0
1–4 years	- - -	- - -	- - -	87.5	54.8	37.8	67.7	60.0	67.1	64.9
5–14 years	- - -	- - -	- - -	33.5	23.0	25.5	25.2	22.5	23.7	23.8
15–24 years	- - -	- - -	- - -	90.3	72.8	69.0	63.5	64.8	62.5	63.6
25–34 years	- - -	- - -	- - -	178.5	121.5	102.3	124.8	115.5	108.9	116.4
35–44 years	- - -	- - -	- - -	286.0	185.6	156.4	167.8	194.2	196.3	186.3
45–54 years	- - -	- - -	- - -	491.4	415.5	380.9	352.1	386.9	435.4	392.6
55–64 years	- - -	- - -	- - -	837.1	851.9	805.9	889.4	917.6	862.2	889.5
65–74 years	- - -	- - -	- - -	1,765.5	1,630.3	1,679.4	1,749.0	1,894.3	1,878.8	1,841.3
75–84 years	- - -	- - -	- - -	3,612.9	3,200.0	3,073.2	3,368.9	3,591.1	3,657.1	3,542.1
85 years and over	- - -	- - -	- - -	8,567.4	7,740.0	8,201.1	6,731.8	6,521.3	6,193.5	6,464.8

See footnotes at end of table.

Table 37 (page 4 of 4). Death rates for all causes, according to sex, detailed race, Hispanic origin, and age: United States, selected years 1950–96

[Data are based on the National Vital Statistics System]

Sex, race, Hispanic origin, and age	1950[1]	1960[1]	1970	1980	1985	1990	1994	1995	1996	1994–96[2]
Asian or Pacific Islander female[4]					Deaths per 100,000 resident population					
All ages, age adjusted	- - -	- - -	- - -	224.6	228.5	228.9	229.3	231.4	214.4	224.3
All ages, crude	- - -	- - -	- - -	222.5	224.9	234.3	252.2	257.7	257.9	256.0
Under 1 year	- - -	- - -	- - -	755.8	622.0	518.2	410.2	359.9	347.4	372.4
1–4 years	- - -	- - -	- - -	35.4	36.8	32.0	19.6	23.8	25.6	23.1
5–14 years	- - -	- - -	- - -	21.5	19.1	13.0	12.4	14.7	11.4	12.9
15–24 years	- - -	- - -	- - -	32.3	30.7	28.8	31.4	33.5	30.6	31.9
25–34 years	- - -	- - -	- - -	45.4	36.5	37.5	39.3	38.1	35.4	37.5
35–44 years	- - -	- - -	- - -	89.7	77.8	69.9	73.1	68.6	68.7	70.1
45–54 years	- - -	- - -	- - -	214.1	184.9	182.7	182.0	191.2	173.8	182.1
55–64 years	- - -	- - -	- - -	440.8	468.0	483.4	457.0	475.6	417.7	449.3
65–74 years	- - -	- - -	- - -	1,027.7	1,130.8	1,089.2	1,075.9	1,061.5	1,090.8	1,076.4
75–84 years	- - -	- - -	- - -	2,833.6	2,873.9	3,127.9	3,323.2	3,278.9	3,118.8	3,233.0
85 years and over	- - -	- - -	- - -	7,923.3	9,808.3	10,254.0	10,705.8	11,256.4	8,599.1	9,981.9
Hispanic female[5]										
All ages, age adjusted	- - -	- - -	- - -	- - -	286.6	284.9	268.6	274.4	268.0	270.3
All ages, crude	- - -	- - -	- - -	- - -	251.9	285.4	281.1	290.8	289.8	287.4
Under 1 year	- - -	- - -	- - -	- - -	793.0	746.6	627.6	575.0	540.2	580.2
1–4 years	- - -	- - -	- - -	- - -	42.3	42.1	34.4	33.5	29.6	32.5
5–14 years	- - -	- - -	- - -	- - -	16.0	17.3	15.3	15.5	16.9	15.9
15–24 years	- - -	- - -	- - -	- - -	36.3	40.6	40.0	40.6	39.2	39.9
25–34 years	- - -	- - -	- - -	- - -	56.3	62.9	69.0	63.1	61.1	64.4
35–44 years	- - -	- - -	- - -	- - -	100.0	109.3	115.8	121.0	108.2	114.8
45–54 years	- - -	- - -	- - -	- - -	251.3	253.3	244.7	238.9	231.8	238.2
55–64 years	- - -	- - -	- - -	- - -	620.3	607.5	571.9	586.2	580.9	579.8
65–74 years	- - -	- - -	- - -	- - -	1,449.3	1,453.8	1,359.8	1,399.6	1,400.0	1,387.0
75–84 years	- - -	- - -	- - -	- - -	3,549.8	3,351.3	3,149.8	3,275.0	3,279.4	3,236.6
85 years and over	- - -	- - -	- - -	- - -	10,216.9	10,098.7	8,826.9	9,613.6	8,783.9	9,066.0
White, non-Hispanic female[5]										
All ages, age adjusted	- - -	- - -	- - -	- - -	385.3	372.2	366.1	366.4	364.1	365.5
All ages, crude	- - -	- - -	- - -	- - -	861.7	903.6	944.3	956.7	965.0	955.4
Under 1 year	- - -	- - -	- - -	- - -	762.8	655.3	578.3	550.2	541.1	556.7
1–4 years	- - -	- - -	- - -	- - -	36.6	34.0	31.3	30.0	27.8	29.7
5–14 years	- - -	- - -	- - -	- - -	19.0	17.6	16.3	16.4	15.9	16.2
15–24 years	- - -	- - -	- - -	- - -	47.9	46.0	44.0	44.0	42.4	43.5
25–34 years	- - -	- - -	- - -	- - -	59.0	60.6	61.7	62.8	61.7	62.1
35–44 years	- - -	- - -	- - -	- - -	122.8	116.8	120.0	124.0	121.1	121.7
45–54 years	- - -	- - -	- - -	- - -	335.7	312.1	297.7	296.1	292.0	295.2
55–64 years	- - -	- - -	- - -	- - -	853.3	834.5	801.9	797.2	787.6	795.5
65–74 years	- - -	- - -	- - -	- - -	1,997.8	1,940.2	1,945.0	1,940.3	1,937.1	1,940.8
75–84 years	- - -	- - -	- - -	- - -	5,058.5	4,887.3	4,862.2	4,860.2	4,868.1	4,863.5
85 years and over	- - -	- - -	- - -	- - -	14,561.4	14,533.1	14,437.4	14,724.6	14,826.1	14,665.2

- - - Data not available.

[1]Includes deaths of persons who were not residents of the 50 States and the District of Columbia.

[2]Average annual death rate.

[3]Interpretation of trends should take into account that population estimates for American Indians increased by 45 percent between 1980 and 1990, partly due to better enumeration techniques in the 1990 decennial census and to the increased tendency for people to identify themselves as American Indian in 1990.

[4]Interpretation of trends should take into account that the Asian population in the United States more than doubled between 1980 and 1990, primarily due to immigration.

[5]Excludes data from States lacking an Hispanic-origin item on their death certificates. See Appendix I, National Vital Statistics System.

NOTES: The race groups, white, black, Asian or Pacific Islander, and American Indian or Alaska Native, include persons of Hispanic and non-Hispanic origin. Conversely, persons of Hispanic origin may be of any race. Consistency of race identification between the death certificate (source of data for numerator of death rates) and data from the Census Bureau (denominator) is high for individual white and black persons; however, persons identified as American Indian, Asian, or Hispanic origin in data from the Census Bureau are sometimes misreported as white or non-Hispanic on the death certificate, causing death rates to be underestimated by 22–30 percent for American Indians, about 12 percent for Asians, and about 7 percent for persons of Hispanic origin. (Sorlie PD, Rogot E, and Johnson NJ: Validity of demographic characteristics on the death certificate, *Epidemiology* 3(2):181–184, 1992.)

SOURCES: Centers for Disease Control and Prevention, National Center for Health Statistics. Grove RD and Hetzel AM. *Vital statistics rates in the United States, 1940–60*. Washington: Public Health Service, 1968; *Vital statistics of the United States, vol II, mortality, part A*, for data years 1950–96. Washington: Public Health Service; data computed by the Division of Health and Utilization Analysis from data compiled by the Division of Vital Statistics and from national population estimates for race groups from table 1 and unpublished Hispanic population estimates prepared by the Housing and Household Economic Statistics Division, U.S. Bureau of the Census.

Table 38 (page 1 of 3). Death rates for diseases of heart, according to sex, detailed race, Hispanic origin, and age: United States, selected years 1950–96

[Data are based on the National Vital Statistics System]

Sex, race, Hispanic origin, and age	1950[1]	1960[1]	1970	1980	1985	1990	1993	1994	1995	1996	1994–96[2]
All persons					Deaths per 100,000 resident population						
All ages, age adjusted	307.2	286.2	253.6	202.0	181.4	152.0	145.3	140.4	138.3	134.5	137.7
All ages, crude	355.5	369.0	362.0	336.0	324.1	289.5	288.4	281.3	280.7	276.4	279.5
Under 1 year	3.5	6.6	13.1	22.8	25.0	20.1	16.9	17.7	17.1	16.6	17.1
1–4 years	1.3	1.3	1.7	2.6	2.2	1.9	1.9	1.8	1.6	1.4	1.6
5–14 years	2.1	1.3	0.8	0.9	1.0	0.9	0.8	0.9	0.8	0.9	0.8
15–24 years	6.8	4.0	3.0	2.9	2.8	2.5	2.7	2.8	2.9	2.7	2.8
25–34 years	19.4	15.6	11.4	8.3	8.3	7.6	8.5	8.5	8.5	8.3	8.4
35–44 years	86.4	74.6	66.7	44.6	38.1	31.4	32.2	31.8	32.0	30.5	31.4
45–54 years	308.6	271.8	238.4	180.2	153.8	120.5	114.0	112.6	111.0	108.2	110.5
55–64 years	808.1	737.9	652.3	494.1	443.0	367.3	344.3	329.9	322.9	315.2	322.6
65–74 years	1,839.8	1,740.5	1,558.2	1,218.6	1,089.8	894.3	848.2	817.4	799.9	776.2	797.9
75–84 years	4,310.1	4,089.4	3,683.8	2,993.1	2,693.1	2,295.7	2,182.9	2,093.0	2,064.7	2,010.2	2,055.3
85 years and over	9,150.6	9,317.8	7,891.3	7,777.1	7,384.1	6,739.9	6,668.9	6,494.9	6,484.1	6,314.5	6,429.1
Male											
All ages, age adjusted	383.8	375.5	348.5	280.4	250.1	206.7	195.5	188.5	184.9	178.8	184.0
All ages, crude	423.4	439.5	422.5	368.6	344.1	297.6	292.1	284.3	282.7	277.4	281.4
Under 1 year	4.0	7.8	15.1	25.5	27.8	21.9	18.3	18.6	17.5	17.4	17.8
1–4 years	1.4	1.4	1.9	2.8	2.2	1.9	2.0	1.8	1.7	1.4	1.6
5–14 years	2.0	1.4	0.9	1.0	0.9	0.9	0.8	0.9	0.8	0.9	0.9
15–24 years	6.8	4.2	3.7	3.7	3.5	3.1	3.4	3.4	3.6	3.3	3.4
25–34 years	22.9	20.1	15.2	11.4	11.6	10.3	11.3	11.0	11.4	11.0	11.1
35–44 years	118.4	112.7	103.2	68.7	58.6	48.1	47.4	46.6	47.2	44.2	46.0
45–54 years	440.5	420.4	376.4	282.6	237.8	183.0	172.8	170.6	168.6	161.8	166.9
55–64 years	1,104.5	1,066.9	987.2	746.8	659.1	537.3	499.2	478.1	465.4	453.8	465.7
65–74 years	2,292.3	2,291.3	2,170.3	1,728.0	1,535.8	1,250.0	1,175.3	1,133.1	1,102.3	1,065.0	1,100.1
75–84 years	4,825.0	4,742.4	4,534.8	3,834.3	3,496.9	2,968.2	2,788.7	2,655.1	2,615.0	2,529.4	2,598.6
85 years and over	9,659.8	9,788.9	8,426.2	8,752.7	8,251.8	7,418.4	7,331.9	7,123.0	7,039.6	6,834.0	6,994.5
Female											
All ages, age adjusted	233.9	205.7	175.2	140.3	127.4	108.9	105.0	101.6	100.4	98.2	100.0
All ages, crude	288.4	300.6	304.5	305.1	305.2	281.8	284.9	278.5	278.8	275.5	277.6
Under 1 year	2.9	5.4	10.9	20.0	22.0	18.3	15.5	16.7	16.7	15.7	16.4
1–4 years	1.2	1.1	1.6	2.5	2.2	1.9	1.7	1.8	1.5	1.4	1.6
5–14 years	2.2	1.2	0.8	0.9	1.0	0.8	0.9	0.8	0.7	0.8	0.8
15–24 years	6.7	3.7	2.3	2.1	2.1	1.8	2.0	2.1	2.2	2.0	2.1
25–34 years	16.2	11.3	7.7	5.3	5.0	5.0	5.6	6.0	5.6	5.6	5.7
35–44 years	55.1	38.2	32.2	21.4	18.3	15.1	17.2	17.2	17.1	16.8	17.0
45–54 years	177.2	127.5	109.9	84.5	74.4	61.0	57.9	57.1	56.0	56.9	56.7
55–64 years	510.0	429.4	351.6	272.1	252.1	215.7	204.5	195.8	193.9	189.3	193.0
65–74 years	1,419.3	1,261.3	1,082.7	828.6	746.1	616.8	589.3	566.3	557.8	543.8	556.0
75–84 years	3,872.0	3,582.7	3,120.8	2,497.0	2,220.4	1,893.8	1,808.2	1,741.3	1,715.2	1,674.7	1,710.0
85 years and over	8,796.1	9,016.8	7,591.8	7,350.5	7,037.6	6,478.1	6,414.6	6,252.7	6,267.8	6,108.0	6,208.1
White male											
All ages, age adjusted	381.1	375.4	347.6	277.5	246.2	202.0	190.3	183.8	179.7	174.5	179.2
All ages, crude	433.0	454.6	438.3	384.0	360.3	312.7	307.6	300.1	297.9	293.3	297.1
45–54 years	423.6	413.2	365.7	269.8	225.5	170.6	159.9	157.7	155.7	149.8	154.3
55–64 years	1,081.7	1,056.0	979.3	730.6	640.1	516.7	475.6	458.6	443.0	431.8	444.4
65–74 years	2,308.3	2,297.9	2,177.2	1,729.7	1,522.7	1,230.5	1,154.6	1,114.7	1,080.5	1,049.5	1,081.5
75–84 years	4,907.3	4,839.9	4,617.6	3,883.2	3,527.0	2,983.4	2,795.3	2,661.8	2,616.1	2,536.0	2,603.3
85 years and over	9,950.5	10,135.8	8,818.0	8,958.0	8,481.7	7,558.7	7,466.9	7,262.2	7,165.5	7,014.5	7,144.1
Black male											
All ages, age adjusted	415.5	381.2	375.9	327.3	310.8	275.9	267.9	254.0	255.9	242.6	250.7
All ages, crude	348.4	330.6	330.3	301.0	288.6	256.8	251.4	240.4	244.2	234.8	239.8
45–54 years	624.1	514.0	512.8	433.4	385.2	328.9	324.2	316.5	317.1	297.7	310.1
55–64 years	1,434.0	1,236.8	1,135.4	987.2	935.3	824.0	813.4	742.3	757.8	740.9	747.0
65–74 years	2,140.1	2,281.4	2,237.8	1,847.2	1,839.2	1,632.9	1,565.2	1,479.3	1,482.9	1,381.3	1,447.4
75–84 years	- - -	3,533.6	3,783.4	3,578.8	3,436.6	3,107.1	2,975.6	2,874.5	2,881.4	2,762.0	2,838.2
85 years and over	- - -	6,037.9	5,367.6	6,819.5	6,393.5	6,479.6	6,240.0	5,919.4	5,985.7	5,675.4	5,856.3

See footnotes at end of table.

Table 38 (page 2 of 3). Death rates for diseases of heart, according to sex, detailed race, Hispanic origin, and age: United States, selected years 1950–96

[Data are based on the National Vital Statistics System]

Sex, race, Hispanic origin, and age	1950[1]	1960[1]	1970	1980	1985	1990	1993	1994	1995	1996	1994–96[2]
American Indian or Alaska Native male[3]				Deaths per 100,000 resident population							
All ages, age adjusted	---	---	---	180.9	162.2	144.6	149.0	145.5	136.7	131.6	137.7
All ages, crude	---	---	---	130.6	117.9	108.0	119.0	116.7	110.4	110.7	112.5
45–54 years	---	---	---	238.1	209.1	173.8	175.8	181.2	151.4	157.5	163.0
55–64 years	---	---	---	496.3	438.3	411.0	433.0	414.2	403.2	404.9	407.4
65–74 years	---	---	---	1,009.4	984.6	839.1	892.0	937.5	918.5	778.0	876.6
75–84 years	---	---	---	2,062.2	2,118.2	1,788.8	1,733.2	1,628.4	1,534.9	1,546.5	1,568.6
85 years and over	---	---	---	4,413.7	2,766.7	3,860.3	3,525.5	3,072.1	2,308.7	2,660.1	2,671.0
Asian or Pacific Islander male[4]											
All ages, age adjusted	---	---	---	136.7	123.4	102.6	107.6	107.6	106.2	98.1	103.3
All ages, crude	---	---	---	119.8	103.5	88.7	96.3	96.9	96.9	97.3	97.0
45–54 years	---	---	---	112.0	81.1	70.4	68.9	80.4	73.4	75.4	76.3
55–64 years	---	---	---	306.7	291.2	226.1	210.4	229.1	214.3	220.7	221.2
65–74 years	---	---	---	852.4	753.5	623.5	600.5	623.5	605.8	581.2	602.9
75–84 years	---	---	---	2,010.9	2,025.6	1,642.2	1,842.2	1,576.3	1,680.5	1,534.8	1,594.6
85 years and over	---	---	---	5,923.0	4,937.5	4,617.8	5,934.4	6,158.3	6,372.3	4,338.0	5,423.9
Hispanic male[5]											
All ages, age adjusted	---	---	---	---	152.3	136.3	126.3	123.5	121.9	117.6	120.8
All ages, crude	---	---	---	---	92.1	91.0	88.2	87.4	87.5	85.8	86.9
45–54 years	---	---	---	---	128.0	116.4	97.9	102.1	103.0	98.7	101.1
55–64 years	---	---	---	---	398.8	363.0	322.6	308.3	306.0	310.0	308.1
65–74 years	---	---	---	---	972.6	829.9	793.2	769.4	750.0	725.7	747.7
75–84 years	---	---	---	---	2,160.8	1,971.3	1,812.4	1,770.0	1,734.5	1,688.6	1,728.9
85 years and over	---	---	---	---	4,791.2	4,711.9	4,756.7	4,726.9	4,699.7	4,078.6	4,472.7
White, non-Hispanic male[5]											
All ages, age adjusted	---	---	---	---	240.3	204.1	190.0	185.3	181.2	176.2	180.9
All ages, crude	---	---	---	---	362.8	336.5	328.5	324.2	322.0	318.9	321.7
45–54 years	---	---	---	---	219.9	172.8	161.4	160.1	157.5	152.1	156.5
55–64 years	---	---	---	---	610.6	521.3	475.9	464.2	448.0	435.1	449.0
65–74 years	---	---	---	---	1,471.3	1,243.4	1,153.4	1,123.6	1,088.3	1,056.4	1,089.5
75–84 years	---	---	---	---	3,514.1	3,007.7	2,782.5	2,674.1	2,635.6	2,559.8	2,622.1
85 years and over	---	---	---	---	8,539.3	7,663.4	7,353.7	7,260.9	7,166.3	7,109.2	7,177.1
White female											
All ages, age adjusted	223.6	197.1	167.8	134.6	121.7	103.1	99.2	96.1	94.9	92.9	94.6
All ages, crude	289.4	306.5	313.8	319.2	321.8	298.4	302.8	296.8	297.4	294.2	296.1
45–54 years	141.9	103.4	91.4	71.2	62.5	50.2	47.5	47.0	45.9	46.9	46.6
55–64 years	460.2	383.0	317.7	248.1	227.1	192.4	181.7	174.7	173.1	167.8	171.9
65–74 years	1,400.9	1,229.8	1,044.0	796.7	713.3	583.6	557.4	535.6	526.3	515.1	525.7
75–84 years	3,925.2	3,629.7	3,143.5	2,493.6	2,207.5	1,874.3	1,780.8	1,717.6	1,689.8	1,652.9	1,686.4
85 years and over	9,084.7	9,280.8	7,839.9	7,501.6	7,170.0	6,563.4	6,495.0	6,342.8	6,352.6	6,211.4	6,301.1
Black female											
All ages, age adjusted	349.5	292.6	251.7	201.1	188.3	168.1	165.3	158.0	156.3	153.4	155.9
All ages, crude	289.9	268.5	261.0	249.7	250.3	237.0	240.2	230.6	231.1	229.0	230.2
45–54 years	526.8	360.7	290.9	202.4	176.2	155.3	150.8	146.4	143.1	144.7	144.7
55–64 years	1,210.7	952.3	710.5	530.1	510.7	442.0	418.6	392.2	384.9	388.4	388.5
65–74 years	1,659.4	1,680.5	1,553.2	1,210.3	1,149.9	1,017.5	983.7	941.7	933.7	890.0	921.6
75–84 years	---	2,926.9	2,964.1	2,707.2	2,533.4	2,250.9	2,278.5	2,158.1	2,163.1	2,097.7	2,139.3
85 years and over	---	5,650.0	5,003.8	5,796.5	5,686.5	5,766.1	5,785.8	5,531.8	5,614.8	5,493.6	5,546.2

See footnotes at end of table.

Table 38 (page 3 of 3). Death rates for diseases of heart, according to sex, detailed race, Hispanic origin, and age: United States, selected years 1950–96

[Data are based on the National Vital Statistics System]

Sex, race, Hispanic origin, and age	1950[1]	1960[1]	1970	1980	1985	1990	1993	1994	1995	1996	1994–96[2]
American Indian or Alaska Native female[3]					Deaths per 100,000 resident population						
All ages, age adjusted	- - -	- - -	- - -	88.4	83.7	76.6	75.4	71.3	77.3	74.9	74.5
All ages, crude	- - -	- - -	- - -	80.3	84.3	77.5	84.8	82.1	87.0	86.7	85.3
45–54 years	- - -	- - -	- - -	65.2	59.2	62.0	60.2	48.7	69.2	61.1	59.8
55–64 years	- - -	- - -	- - -	193.5	230.8	197.0	186.1	196.8	210.2	192.5	199.8
65–74 years	- - -	- - -	- - -	577.2	472.7	492.8	500.9	429.9	503.3	512.8	482.2
75–84 years	- - -	- - -	- - -	1,364.3	1,258.8	1,050.3	1,084.9	1,055.6	1,045.6	1,030.0	1,043.4
85 years and over	- - -	- - -	- - -	2,893.3	3,180.0	2,868.7	2,879.8	2,490.9	2,209.8	2,108.8	2,257.8
Asian or Pacific Islander female[4]											
All ages, age adjusted	- - -	- - -	- - -	55.8	59.6	58.3	56.2	57.7	57.7	50.9	55.0
All ages, crude	- - -	- - -	- - -	57.0	60.3	62.0	63.7	66.7	68.2	66.8	67.2
45–54 years	- - -	- - -	- - -	28.6	23.8	17.5	18.8	22.1	21.6	17.2	20.2
55–64 years	- - -	- - -	- - -	92.9	103.0	99.0	97.2	93.3	93.0	82.3	89.3
65–74 years	- - -	- - -	- - -	313.3	341.0	323.9	270.8	295.7	294.9	282.0	290.6
75–84 years	- - -	- - -	- - -	1,053.2	1,056.5	1,130.9	1,080.4	1,110.7	1,063.0	1,009.8	1,057.8
85 years and over	- - -	- - -	- - -	3,211.0	4,208.3	4,161.2	4,505.2	4,376.5	4,717.9	3,394.7	4,064.3
Hispanic female[5]											
All ages, age adjusted	- - -	- - -	- - -	- - -	86.5	76.0	69.6	67.0	68.1	64.7	66.5
All ages, crude	- - -	- - -	- - -	- - -	75.0	79.4	77.4	75.6	78.9	77.0	77.2
45–54 years	- - -	- - -	- - -	- - -	46.6	43.5	34.8	31.8	32.0	31.3	31.7
55–64 years	- - -	- - -	- - -	- - -	184.8	153.2	132.7	134.3	137.3	125.1	132.1
65–74 years	- - -	- - -	- - -	- - -	534.0	460.4	422.5	399.3	402.4	387.6	396.3
75–84 years	- - -	- - -	- - -	- - -	1,456.5	1,259.7	1,210.1	1,163.5	1,150.1	1,152.8	1,155.3
85 years and over	- - -	- - -	- - -	- - -	4,523.4	4,440.3	3,986.3	3,783.1	4,243.9	3,673.8	3,892.0
White, non-Hispanic female[5]											
All ages, age adjusted	- - -	- - -	- - -	- - -	120.2	103.7	98.5	96.5	95.4	93.6	95.2
All ages, crude	- - -	- - -	- - -	- - -	334.2	320.0	322.4	320.6	321.4	318.9	320.3
45–54 years	- - -	- - -	- - -	- - -	61.3	50.2	47.3	47.5	46.6	47.5	47.2
55–64 years	- - -	- - -	- - -	- - -	219.6	193.6	181.2	175.5	173.6	169.0	172.7
65–74 years	- - -	- - -	- - -	- - -	700.4	584.7	552.7	537.2	529.1	518.0	528.1
75–84 years	- - -	- - -	- - -	- - -	2,201.4	1,890.2	1,771.4	1,728.0	1,697.8	1,663.5	1,696.1
85 years and over	- - -	- - -	- - -	- - -	7,164.7	6,615.2	6,425.5	6,354.2	6,384.5	6,285.4	6,340.9

- - - Data not available.

[1]Includes deaths of persons who were not residents of the 50 States and the District of Columbia.

[2]Average annual death rate.

[3]Interpretation of trends should take into account that population estimates for American Indians increased by 45 percent between 1980 and 1990, partly due to better enumeration techniques in the 1990 decennial census and to the increased tendency for people to identify themselves as American Indian in 1990.

[4]Interpretation of trends should take into account that the Asian population in the United States more than doubled between 1980 and 1990, primarily due to immigration.

[5]Excludes data from States lacking an Hispanic-origin item on their death certificates. See Appendix I, National Vital Statistics System.

NOTES: For data years shown, the code numbers for cause of death are based on the then current *International Classification of Diseases*, which are described in Appendix II, tables IV and V. Age groups were selected to minimize the presentation of unstable age-specific death rates based on small numbers of deaths and for consistency among comparison groups. The race groups, white, black, Asian or Pacific Islander, and American Indian or Alaska Native, include persons of Hispanic and non-Hispanic origin. Conversely, persons of Hispanic origin may be of any race. Consistency of race identification between the death certificate (source of data for numerator of death rates) and data from the Census Bureau (denominator) is high for individual white and black persons; however, persons identified as American Indian, Asian, or Hispanic origin in data from the Census Bureau are sometimes misreported as white or non-Hispanic on the death certificate, causing death rates to be underestimated by 22–30 percent for American Indians, about 12 percent for Asians, and about 7 percent for persons of Hispanic origin. (Sorlie PD, Rogot E, and Johnson NJ: Validity of demographic characteristics on the death certificate, *Epidemiology* 3(2):181–184, 1992.)

SOURCES: Centers for Disease Control and Prevention, National Center for Health Statistics. *Vital statistics of the United States, vol II, mortality, part A*, for data years 1950–96. Washington: Public Health Service; data computed by the Division of Health and Utilization Analysis from data compiled by the Division of Vital Statistics and from national population estimates for race groups from table 1 and unpublished Hispanic population estimates prepared by the Housing and Household Economic Statistics Division, U.S. Bureau of the Census.

Table 39 (page 1 of 3). Death rates for cerebrovascular diseases, according to sex, detailed race, Hispanic origin, and age: United States, selected years 1950–96

[Data are based on the National Vital Statistics System]

Sex, race, Hispanic origin, and age	1950[1]	1960[1]	1970	1980	1985	1990	1993	1994	1995	1996	1994–96[2]
All persons				Deaths per 100,000 resident population							
All ages, age adjusted	88.8	79.7	66.3	40.8	32.5	27.7	26.5	26.5	26.7	26.4	26.5
All ages, crude	104.0	108.0	101.9	75.1	64.3	57.9	58.2	58.9	60.1	60.3	59.8
Under 1 year	5.1	4.1	5.0	4.4	3.7	3.8	5.5	5.1	5.8	6.2	5.7
1–4 years	0.9	0.8	1.0	0.5	0.3	0.3	0.3	0.3	0.4	0.3	0.3
5–14 years	0.5	0.7	0.7	0.3	0.2	0.2	0.2	0.2	0.2	0.2	0.2
15–24 years	1.6	1.8	1.6	1.0	0.8	0.6	0.6	0.5	0.5	0.5	0.5
25–34 years	4.2	4.7	4.5	2.6	2.2	2.2	1.9	1.9	1.8	1.8	1.8
35–44 years	18.7	14.7	15.6	8.5	7.2	6.5	6.2	6.5	6.5	6.3	6.4
45–54 years	70.4	49.2	41.6	25.2	21.3	18.7	17.6	17.9	17.6	17.9	17.8
55–64 years	194.2	147.3	115.8	65.2	54.8	48.0	46.0	45.6	46.1	45.3	45.6
65–74 years	554.7	469.2	384.1	219.5	172.8	144.4	135.8	135.7	137.2	135.5	136.1
75–84 years	1,499.6	1,491.3	1,254.2	788.6	601.5	499.3	479.1	480.2	481.4	477.0	479.5
85 years and over	2,990.1	3,680.5	3,014.3	2,288.9	1,865.1	1,633.9	1,607.7	1,604.1	1,636.5	1,612.7	1,617.8
Male											
All ages, age adjusted	91.9	85.4	73.2	44.9	35.5	30.2	29.0	29.0	28.9	28.5	28.8
All ages, crude	102.5	104.5	94.5	63.6	52.5	46.8	46.9	47.4	48.0	48.1	47.8
Under 1 year	6.4	5.0	5.8	5.0	4.6	4.4	5.9	5.8	6.3	6.5	6.2
1–4 years	1.1	0.9	1.2	0.4	0.4	0.3	0.3	0.4	0.4	0.3	0.4
5–14 years	0.5	0.7	0.8	0.3	0.2	0.2	0.3	0.2	0.2	0.2	0.2
15–24 years	1.8	1.9	1.8	1.1	0.7	0.7	0.5	0.5	0.5	0.5	0.5
25–34 years	4.2	4.5	4.4	2.6	2.2	2.1	2.0	1.8	1.9	1.7	1.8
35–44 years	17.5	14.6	15.7	8.7	7.4	6.8	6.8	7.1	7.1	6.7	6.9
45–54 years	67.9	52.2	44.4	27.3	23.2	20.5	19.6	20.1	19.8	20.0	20.0
55–64 years	205.2	163.8	138.7	74.7	63.5	54.4	52.5	52.5	53.4	52.5	52.8
65–74 years	589.6	530.7	449.5	259.2	201.4	166.8	157.4	156.0	155.9	154.7	155.6
75–84 years	1,543.6	1,555.9	1,361.6	868.3	661.2	552.7	523.7	524.6	517.1	508.7	516.6
85 years and over	3,048.6	3,643.1	2,895.2	2,199.2	1,730.1	1,533.2	1,541.9	1,521.8	1,537.7	1,512.7	1,523.9
Female											
All ages, age adjusted	86.0	74.7	60.8	37.6	30.0	25.7	24.5	24.5	24.8	24.6	24.7
All ages, crude	105.6	111.4	109.0	86.1	75.5	68.6	69.0	69.8	71.7	71.9	71.2
Under 1 year	3.7	3.2	4.0	3.8	2.7	3.1	5.0	4.3	5.2	5.9	5.1
1–4 years	0.7	0.7	0.7	0.5	0.3	0.3	0.3	*	0.3	0.3	0.3
5–14 years	0.4	0.6	0.6	0.3	0.3	0.2	0.2	0.2	0.2	0.2	0.2
15–24 years	1.5	1.6	1.4	0.8	0.8	0.6	0.6	0.5	0.4	0.4	0.4
25–34 years	4.3	4.9	4.7	2.6	2.1	2.2	1.8	2.1	1.7	1.8	1.9
35–44 years	19.9	14.8	15.6	8.4	6.9	6.1	5.6	5.9	6.0	5.9	5.9
45–54 years	72.9	46.3	39.0	23.3	19.4	17.0	15.8	15.8	15.5	15.9	15.8
55–64 years	183.1	131.8	95.3	56.9	47.2	42.2	40.1	39.3	39.4	38.8	39.2
65–74 years	522.1	415.7	333.3	189.0	150.7	126.9	118.7	119.5	122.2	120.1	120.6
75–84 years	1,462.2	1,441.1	1,183.1	741.6	566.3	467.4	451.6	452.4	458.7	456.5	455.9
85 years and over	2,949.4	3,704.4	3,081.0	2,328.2	1,918.9	1,672.7	1,632.9	1,635.9	1,675.0	1,652.4	1,654.6
White male											
All ages, age adjusted	87.0	80.3	68.8	41.9	33.0	27.7	26.8	26.6	26.5	26.3	26.5
All ages, crude	100.5	102.7	93.5	63.3	52.7	47.0	47.7	48.1	48.6	49.1	48.6
45–54 years	53.7	40.9	35.6	21.7	18.1	15.4	14.9	15.2	14.8	15.2	15.1
55–64 years	182.2	139.0	119.9	64.2	54.6	45.8	44.1	44.1	44.7	43.4	44.1
65–74 years	569.7	501.0	420.0	240.4	186.4	153.2	145.8	143.6	143.5	142.0	143.0
75–84 years	1,556.3	1,564.8	1,361.6	854.8	650.0	540.7	511.2	511.0	503.1	500.1	504.6
85 years and over	3,127.1	3,734.8	3,018.1	2,236.9	1,765.6	1,549.8	1,562.0	1,539.8	1,550.0	1,537.7	1,542.5
Black male											
All ages, age adjusted	146.2	141.2	122.5	77.5	62.7	56.1	51.9	52.4	52.2	50.9	51.8
All ages, crude	122.0	122.9	108.8	73.1	59.2	53.1	49.8	50.5	51.0	50.1	50.5
45–54 years	211.9	166.1	136.1	82.1	71.1	68.4	63.2	64.7	64.1	62.1	63.6
55–64 years	522.8	439.9	343.4	189.8	160.7	141.8	134.9	134.2	134.1	137.5	135.3
65–74 years	783.6	899.2	780.1	472.8	379.7	327.2	291.5	293.2	291.5	292.2	292.3
75–84 years	- - -	1,475.2	1,445.7	1,067.6	814.4	723.7	696.0	702.0	700.2	653.0	684.6
85 years and over	- - -	2,700.0	1,963.1	1,873.2	1,429.0	1,430.5	1,361.7	1,319.8	1,393.9	1,329.5	1,347.7

See footnotes at end of table.

Table 39 (page 2 of 3). **Death rates for cerebrovascular diseases, according to sex, detailed race, Hispanic origin, and age: United States, selected years 1950–96**

[Data are based on the National Vital Statistics System]

Sex, race, Hispanic origin, and age	1950[1]	1960[1]	1970	1980	1985	1990	1993	1994	1995	1996	1994–96[2]
American Indian or Alaska Native male[3]				Deaths per 100,000 resident population							
All ages, age adjusted	- - -	- - -	- - -	30.7	24.9	20.5	21.1	22.0	23.5	21.4	22.3
All ages, crude	- - -	- - -	- - -	23.2	18.5	16.0	17.2	18.7	20.1	18.7	19.2
45–54 years	- - -	- - -	- - -	*	*	*	*	*	28.4	19.9	21.7
55–64 years	- - -	- - -	- - -	72.0	*	39.8	59.4	43.3	45.7	42.9	43.9
65–74 years	- - -	- - -	- - -	170.5	200.0	120.3	119.5	141.3	153.1	139.1	144.5
75–84 years	- - -	- - -	- - -	535.1	372.7	325.9	359.7	333.2	290.1	319.4	314.1
85 years and over	- - -	- - -	- - -	1,384.7	733.3	949.8	667.0	845.9	748.8	550.4	705.0
Asian or Pacific Islander male[4]											
All ages, age adjusted	- - -	- - -	- - -	32.3	28.0	26.9	27.8	30.1	31.2	26.9	29.2
All ages, crude	- - -	- - -	- - -	28.7	24.0	23.4	24.9	27.2	28.6	27.0	27.6
45–54 years	- - -	- - -	- - -	17.0	13.9	15.6	18.7	20.3	17.3	19.5	19.0
55–64 years	- - -	- - -	- - -	59.9	48.8	51.8	49.8	49.8	62.1	55.6	55.9
65–74 years	- - -	- - -	- - -	197.9	155.6	167.9	154.2	166.9	162.3	161.4	163.5
75–84 years	- - -	- - -	- - -	619.5	583.7	485.7	512.2	564.9	571.8	430.0	517.3
85 years and over	- - -	- - -	- - -	1,399.0	1,387.5	1,196.6	1,537.4	1,702.9	1,808.5	1,348.7	1,578.3
Hispanic male[5]											
All ages, age adjusted	- - -	- - -	- - -	- - -	27.7	22.7	22.7	23.3	23.1	22.3	22.8
All ages, crude	- - -	- - -	- - -	- - -	17.2	15.6	16.5	16.9	17.1	16.8	16.9
45–54 years	- - -	- - -	- - -	- - -	23.6	20.0	21.2	21.9	20.5	23.1	21.8
55–64 years	- - -	- - -	- - -	- - -	63.9	49.4	47.4	48.4	46.1	50.7	48.4
65–74 years	- - -	- - -	- - -	- - -	163.5	126.4	124.5	133.5	132.2	114.8	126.5
75–84 years	- - -	- - -	- - -	- - -	396.7	356.6	340.1	343.3	349.9	348.6	347.4
85 years and over	- - -	- - -	- - -	- - -	1,152.1	866.3	916.5	980.0	996.3	866.3	942.2
White, non-Hispanic male[5]											
All ages, age adjusted	- - -	- - -	- - -	- - -	31.6	27.9	26.4	26.4	26.3	26.1	26.3
All ages, crude	- - -	- - -	- - -	- - -	52.2	50.7	50.9	51.7	52.3	53.0	52.3
45–54 years	- - -	- - -	- - -	- - -	16.0	14.9	14.1	14.5	14.1	14.2	14.3
55–64 years	- - -	- - -	- - -	- - -	50.5	45.2	42.9	43.4	43.9	42.0	43.1
65–74 years	- - -	- - -	- - -	- - -	178.5	154.8	145.0	143.2	143.1	142.0	142.8
75–84 years	- - -	- - -	- - -	- - -	637.0	548.8	512.6	514.7	507.4	505.1	509.0
85 years and over	- - -	- - -	- - -	- - -	1,735.1	1,583.6	1,557.3	1,544.5	1,552.4	1,560.6	1,552.7
White female											
All ages, age adjusted	79.7	68.7	56.2	35.2	27.9	23.8	22.7	22.8	23.1	22.9	22.9
All ages, crude	103.3	110.1	109.8	88.8	78.4	71.8	72.8	73.9	76.0	76.3	75.4
45–54 years	55.0	33.8	30.5	18.7	15.5	13.5	12.6	12.3	12.7	12.8	12.6
55–64 years	156.9	103.0	78.1	48.7	40.0	35.8	34.1	33.7	33.6	33.3	33.5
65–74 years	498.1	383.3	303.2	172.8	137.9	116.3	108.5	109.7	112.6	110.2	110.8
75–84 years	1,471.3	1,444.7	1,176.8	730.3	552.9	457.6	442.1	442.8	449.5	446.7	446.3
85 years and over	3,017.9	3,795.7	3,167.6	2,367.8	1,944.9	1,691.4	1,652.0	1,656.7	1,690.0	1,679.3	1,675.5
Black female											
All ages, age adjusted	155.6	139.5	107.9	61.7	50.6	42.7	39.9	40.1	39.6	39.2	39.6
All ages, crude	128.3	127.7	112.2	77.9	68.6	60.7	58.8	59.3	60.4	59.7	59.8
45–54 years	248.9	166.2	119.4	61.9	50.8	44.1	40.5	43.1	36.4	38.6	39.3
55–64 years	567.7	452.0	272.4	138.7	113.6	97.0	89.2	84.8	85.5	82.9	84.4
65–74 years	754.4	830.5	673.5	362.2	285.6	236.8	220.8	217.9	221.2	216.4	218.5
75–84 years	- - -	1,413.1	1,338.3	918.6	753.8	596.0	582.3	582.2	583.2	586.5	584.0
85 years and over	- - -	2,578.9	2,210.5	1,896.3	1,657.1	1,496.5	1,449.8	1,447.9	1,568.8	1,443.6	1,486.6

See footnotes at end of table.

Table 39 (page 3 of 3). Death rates for cerebrovascular diseases, according to sex, detailed race, Hispanic origin, and age: United States, selected years 1950–96

[Data are based on the National Vital Statistics System]

Sex, race, Hispanic origin, and age	1950[1]	1960[1]	1970	1980	1985	1990	1993	1994	1995	1996	1994–96[2]
American Indian or Alaska Native female[3]					Deaths per 100,000 resident population						
All ages, age adjusted	- - -	- - -	- - -	23.3	20.6	18.5	20.3	18.8	19.9	20.6	19.8
All ages, crude	- - -	- - -	- - -	22.1	21.8	19.3	23.3	21.9	23.8	25.5	23.8
45–54 years	- - -	- - -	- - -	*	*	*	*	*	*	24.6	17.7
55–64 years	- - -	- - -	- - -	*	40.4	40.7	50.3	44.4	43.5	29.7	39.1
65–74 years	- - -	- - -	- - -	128.3	121.2	100.5	116.8	121.6	112.3	127.7	120.6
75–84 years	- - -	- - -	- - -	404.2	317.6	282.0	314.3	296.9	321.7	354.9	325.2
85 years and over	- - -	- - -	- - -	1,123.6	1,000.0	776.2	817.7	654.9	697.3	700.0	685.5
Asian or Pacific Islander female[4]											
All ages, age adjusted	- - -	- - -	- - -	25.9	23.6	23.4	21.8	21.8	21.6	21.5	21.6
All ages, crude	- - -	- - -	- - -	26.5	23.3	24.3	24.2	24.9	24.9	27.5	25.8
45–54 years	- - -	- - -	- - -	20.3	15.1	19.7	16.9	14.8	16.2	16.2	15.8
55–64 years	- - -	- - -	- - -	44.5	49.0	42.5	37.5	35.4	39.1	36.3	36.9
65–74 years	- - -	- - -	- - -	136.1	130.8	124.0	113.1	111.7	103.3	111.2	108.8
75–84 years	- - -	- - -	- - -	449.6	387.0	396.6	363.8	394.3	405.2	409.2	403.4
85 years and over	- - -	- - -	- - -	1,545.2	1,383.3	1,395.0	1,487.9	1,452.4	1,432.5	1,243.3	1,358.4
Hispanic female[5]											
All ages, age adjusted	- - -	- - -	- - -	- - -	20.6	19.5	16.8	16.5	18.1	17.1	17.3
All ages, crude	- - -	- - -	- - -	- - -	18.3	20.2	18.0	18.2	20.1	19.6	19.3
45–54 years	- - -	- - -	- - -	- - -	15.8	15.2	15.7	14.2	15.1	15.3	14.9
55–64 years	- - -	- - -	- - -	- - -	35.8	38.8	32.4	32.3	35.7	35.2	34.4
65–74 years	- - -	- - -	- - -	- - -	108.6	102.9	91.3	84.7	98.2	90.3	91.1
75–84 years	- - -	- - -	- - -	- - -	339.8	309.5	266.9	274.2	287.4	284.3	282.1
85 years and over	- - -	- - -	- - -	- - -	1,191.5	1,060.4	807.0	825.7	932.4	837.8	864.8
White, non-Hispanic female[5]											
All ages, age adjusted	- - -	- - -	- - -	- - -	27.2	23.9	22.6	22.8	23.1	23.0	23.0
All ages, crude	- - -	- - -	- - -	- - -	81.0	77.4	78.3	80.0	82.2	82.9	81.7
45–54 years	- - -	- - -	- - -	- - -	14.3	13.2	12.0	12.0	12.4	12.4	12.3
55–64 years	- - -	- - -	- - -	- - -	37.8	35.7	33.7	33.5	33.0	32.7	33.0
65–74 years	- - -	- - -	- - -	- - -	133.5	117.1	108.0	110.1	112.4	110.7	111.1
75–84 years	- - -	- - -	- - -	- - -	551.6	463.1	445.0	447.3	452.9	450.4	450.2
85 years and over	- - -	- - -	- - -	- - -	1,926.2	1,720.4	1,657.3	1,666.4	1,704.8	1,707.4	1,693.1

- - - Data not available.

* Based on fewer than 20 deaths.

[1]Includes deaths of persons who were not residents of the 50 States and the District of Columbia.

[2]Average annual death rate.

[3]Interpretation of trends should take into account that population estimates for American Indians increased by 45 percent between 1980 and 1990, partly due to better enumeration techniques in the 1990 decennial census and to the increased tendency for people to identify themselves as American Indian in 1990.

[4]Interpretation of trends should take into account that the Asian population in the United States more than doubled between 1980 and 1990, primarily due to immigration.

[5]Excludes data from States lacking an Hispanic-origin item on their death certificates. See Appendix I, National Vital Statistics System.

NOTES: For data years shown, the code numbers for cause of death are based on the then current *International Classification of Diseases*, which are described in Appendix II, tables IV and V. Age groups were selected to minimize the presentation of unstable age-specific death rates based on small numbers of deaths and for consistency among comparison groups. The race groups, white, black, Asian or Pacific Islander, and American Indian or Alaska Native, include persons of Hispanic and non-Hispanic origin. Conversely, persons of Hispanic origin may be of any race. Consistency of race identification between the death certificate (source of data for numerator of death rates) and data from the Census Bureau (denominator) is high for individual white and black persons; however, persons identified as American Indian, Asian, or Hispanic origin in data from the Census Bureau are sometimes misreported as white or non-Hispanic on the death certificate, causing death rates to be underestimated by 22–30 percent for American Indians, about 12 percent for Asians, and about 7 percent for persons of Hispanic origin. (Sorlie PD, Rogot E, and Johnson NJ: Validity of demographic characteristics on the death certificate, *Epidemiology* 3(2):181–184, 1992.)

SOURCES: Centers for Disease Control and Prevention, National Center for Health Statistics. Grove RD and Hetzel AM. *Vital statistics rates in the United States, 1940–60*. Washington: Public Health Service, 1968; *Vital statistics of the United States, vol II, mortality, part A*, for data years 1950–96. Washington: Public Health Service; data computed by the Division of Health and Utilization Analysis from data compiled by the Division of Vital Statistics and from national population estimates for race groups from table 1 and unpublished Hispanic population estimates prepared by the Housing and Household Economic Statistics Division, U.S. Bureau of the Census.

Table 40 (page 1 of 4). Death rates for malignant neoplasms, according to sex, detailed race, Hispanic origin, and age: United States, selected years 1950–96

[Data are based on the National Vital Statistics System]

Sex, race, Hispanic origin, and age	1950[1]	1960[1]	1970	1980	1985	1990	1993	1994	1995	1996	1994–96[2]
All persons				Deaths per 100,000 resident population							
All ages, age adjusted	125.4	125.8	129.8	132.8	134.4	135.0	132.6	131.5	129.9	127.9	129.7
All ages, crude	139.8	149.2	162.8	183.9	194.0	203.2	205.6	205.2	204.9	203.4	204.5
Under 1 year	8.7	7.2	4.7	3.2	3.1	2.3	2.2	1.5	1.8	2.3	1.9
1–4 years	11.7	10.9	7.5	4.5	3.8	3.5	3.3	3.3	3.1	2.7	3.0
5–14 years	6.7	6.8	6.0	4.3	3.5	3.1	2.9	2.8	2.7	2.7	2.7
15–24 years	8.6	8.3	8.3	6.3	5.4	4.9	4.8	4.8	4.6	4.5	4.6
25–34 years	20.0	19.5	16.5	13.7	13.2	12.6	12.1	12.2	11.9	12.0	12.1
35–44 years	62.7	59.7	59.5	48.6	45.9	43.3	41.1	40.4	40.3	39.3	40.0
45–54 years	175.1	177.0	182.5	180.0	170.1	158.9	147.9	145.9	142.2	137.9	141.9
55–64 years	390.7	396.8	423.0	436.1	454.6	449.6	433.4	424.6	416.0	406.5	415.6
65–74 years	698.8	713.9	751.2	817.9	845.5	872.3	876.1	875.4	868.2	861.6	868.4
75–84 years	1,153.3	1,127.4	1,169.2	1,232.3	1,271.8	1,348.5	1,366.9	1,367.4	1,364.8	1,351.5	1,361.1
85 years and over	1,451.0	1,450.0	1,320.7	1,594.6	1,615.4	1,752.9	1,807.7	1,789.0	1,823.8	1,798.3	1,803.8
Male											
All ages, age adjusted	130.8	143.0	157.4	165.5	166.1	166.3	161.9	159.6	156.8	153.8	156.7
All ages, crude	142.9	162.5	182.1	205.3	213.4	221.3	222.1	220.7	219.5	217.2	219.1
Under 1 year	9.7	7.7	4.4	3.7	3.0	2.4	2.8	1.4	1.8	2.2	1.8
1–4 years	12.5	12.4	8.3	5.2	4.3	3.7	3.7	3.5	3.6	3.1	3.4
5–14 years	7.4	7.6	6.7	4.9	3.9	3.5	3.3	3.1	3.0	3.0	3.0
15–24 years	9.7	10.2	10.4	7.8	6.4	5.7	5.5	5.8	5.5	5.1	5.5
25–34 years	17.7	18.8	16.3	13.4	13.2	12.6	11.9	12.1	11.7	11.5	11.8
35–44 years	45.6	48.9	53.0	44.0	42.4	38.5	38.0	36.7	36.5	35.6	36.3
45–54 years	156.2	170.8	183.5	188.7	175.2	162.5	150.7	148.8	143.7	140.7	144.3
55–64 years	413.1	459.9	511.8	520.8	536.9	532.9	507.4	495.3	480.5	469.1	481.6
65–74 years	791.5	890.5	1,006.8	1,093.2	1,105.2	1,122.2	1,113.3	1,102.5	1,089.9	1,080.9	1,091.1
75–84 years	1,332.6	1,389.4	1,588.3	1,790.5	1,839.7	1,914.4	1,885.4	1,862.6	1,842.3	1,802.7	1,835.2
85 years and over	1,668.3	1,741.2	1,720.8	2,369.5	2,451.8	2,739.9	2,830.7	2,805.8	2,837.3	2,733.1	2,790.9
Female											
All ages, age adjusted	120.8	111.2	108.8	109.2	111.7	112.7	111.4	111.1	110.4	108.8	110.1
All ages, crude	136.8	136.4	144.4	163.6	175.7	186.0	189.8	190.5	191.0	190.2	190.6
Under 1 year	7.6	6.8	5.0	2.7	3.2	2.2	1.7	1.6	1.8	2.4	1.9
1–4 years	10.8	9.3	6.7	3.7	3.4	3.2	2.9	3.0	2.6	2.3	2.6
5–14 years	6.0	6.0	5.2	3.6	3.1	2.8	2.6	2.4	2.4	2.4	2.4
15–24 years	7.6	6.5	6.2	4.8	4.3	4.1	4.1	3.9	3.6	3.8	3.8
25–34 years	22.2	20.1	16.7	14.0	13.2	12.6	12.3	12.3	12.2	12.6	12.3
35–44 years	79.3	70.0	65.6	53.1	49.2	48.1	44.1	44.1	44.0	42.9	43.7
45–54 years	194.0	183.0	181.5	171.8	165.3	155.5	145.2	143.1	140.7	135.2	139.6
55–64 years	368.2	337.7	343.2	361.7	381.8	375.2	366.7	360.7	357.5	349.6	355.9
65–74 years	612.3	560.2	557.9	607.1	645.3	677.4	688.4	694.7	690.7	685.2	690.2
75–84 years	1,000.7	924.1	891.9	903.1	937.8	1,010.3	1,046.1	1,057.5	1,061.5	1,060.0	1,059.7
85 years and over	1,299.7	1,263.9	1,096.7	1,255.7	1,281.4	1,372.1	1,415.3	1,397.1	1,429.1	1,426.8	1,417.9
White male											
All ages, age adjusted	130.9	141.6	154.3	160.5	160.4	160.3	156.4	154.4	151.8	149.2	151.7
All ages, crude	147.2	166.1	185.1	208.7	218.1	227.7	229.8	228.9	228.1	225.8	227.6
25–34 years	17.7	18.8	16.2	13.6	13.1	12.3	11.6	11.8	11.3	11.3	11.5
35–44 years	44.5	46.3	50.1	41.1	39.8	35.8	35.9	34.5	34.2	33.5	34.0
45–54 years	150.8	164.1	172.0	175.4	162.0	149.9	139.0	138.0	134.3	131.8	134.6
55–64 years	409.4	450.9	498.1	497.4	512.0	508.2	486.0	474.7	460.0	448.9	461.2
65–74 years	798.7	887.3	997.0	1,070.7	1,076.5	1,090.7	1,084.2	1,074.6	1,064.6	1,057.3	1,065.5
75–84 years	1,367.6	1,413.7	1,592.7	1,779.7	1,817.1	1,883.2	1,850.3	1,831.2	1,810.9	1,771.0	1,803.7
85 years and over	1,732.7	1,791.4	1,772.2	2,375.6	2,449.1	2,715.1	2,794.4	2,780.3	2,805.2	2,723.9	2,769.0
Black male											
All ages, age adjusted	126.1	158.5	198.0	229.9	239.9	248.1	238.9	232.6	226.8	221.9	227.0
All ages, crude	106.6	136.7	171.6	205.5	214.9	221.9	216.8	212.1	209.1	207.3	209.5
25–34 years	18.0	18.4	18.8	14.1	14.9	15.7	15.0	15.5	15.2	14.0	14.9
35–44 years	55.7	72.9	81.3	73.8	69.9	64.3	58.4	57.2	57.5	55.0	56.6
45–54 years	211.7	244.7	311.2	333.0	315.9	302.6	281.4	269.5	250.7	242.7	253.8
55–64 years	490.8	579.7	689.2	812.5	851.3	859.2	794.1	772.7	755.3	741.2	756.3
65–74 years	636.4	938.5	1,168.9	1,417.2	1,532.8	1,613.9	1,582.1	1,547.8	1,509.6	1,473.2	1,509.9
75–84 years	- - -	1,053.3	1,624.8	2,029.6	2,229.6	2,478.3	2,516.5	2,456.3	2,426.8	2,421.8	2,434.6
85 years and over	- - -	1,155.2	1,387.0	2,393.9	2,629.0	3,238.3	3,400.9	3,274.6	3,338.2	3,209.7	3,273.0

See footnotes at end of table.

Table 40 (page 2 of 4). Death rates for malignant neoplasms, according to sex, detailed race, Hispanic origin, and age: United States, selected years 1950–96

[Data are based on the National Vital Statistics System]

Sex, race, Hispanic origin, and age	1950[1]	1960[1]	1970	1980	1985	1990	1993	1994	1995	1996	1994–96[2]
American Indian or Alaska Native male[3]				Deaths per 100,000 resident population							
All ages, age adjusted	---	---	---	82.1	87.1	83.5	92.9	91.3	94.0	94.0	93.2
All ages, crude	---	---	---	58.1	62.8	61.4	71.5	70.7	74.2	75.9	73.6
25–34 years	---	---	---	*	*	*	*	*	*	*	6.8
35–44 years	---	---	---	*	28.8	22.8	21.4	18.9	16.0	18.4	17.8
45–54 years	---	---	---	86.9	89.4	86.9	83.8	79.8	88.0	76.0	81.2
55–64 years	---	---	---	213.4	276.6	246.2	314.1	287.8	300.3	325.5	304.8
65–74 years	---	---	---	613.0	584.6	530.6	608.6	728.3	670.4	680.1	692.5
75–84 years	---	---	---	936.4	963.6	1,038.4	1,138.0	892.8	1,111.9	1,036.6	1,015.9
85 years and over	---	---	---	1,471.2	1,133.3	1,654.4	1,119.6	1,135.4	1,081.5	1,284.2	1,172.8
Asian or Pacific Islander male[4]											
All ages, age adjusted	---	---	---	96.4	101.0	99.6	99.9	100.9	98.3	93.8	97.3
All ages, crude	---	---	---	81.9	82.6	82.7	86.5	88.1	87.1	87.1	87.4
25–34 years	---	---	---	6.3	10.0	9.2	8.9	9.9	8.8	7.8	8.8
35–44 years	---	---	---	29.4	25.7	27.7	27.5	27.8	27.4	27.4	27.6
45–54 years	---	---	---	108.2	98.0	92.6	91.3	95.4	86.6	85.7	89.0
55–64 years	---	---	---	298.5	315.0	274.6	266.6	270.3	255.4	247.5	257.3
65–74 years	---	---	---	581.2	631.3	687.2	650.7	659.5	640.6	663.6	654.6
75–84 years	---	---	---	1,147.6	1,251.2	1,229.9	1,285.9	1,288.8	1,278.9	1,199.8	1,252.7
85 years and over	---	---	---	1,798.7	1,800.0	1,837.0	2,513.6	2,385.5	2,712.8	1,668.4	2,165.9
Hispanic male[5]											
All ages, age adjusted	---	---	---	---	92.1	99.8	97.4	97.4	98.6	93.1	96.3
All ages, crude	---	---	---	---	56.1	65.5	66.7	67.4	68.9	65.8	67.3
25–34 years	---	---	---	---	9.7	8.0	8.1	9.3	9.2	8.0	8.8
35–44 years	---	---	---	---	23.0	22.5	27.8	22.5	25.4	22.0	23.3
45–54 years	---	---	---	---	83.4	96.6	80.4	85.5	85.8	81.6	84.2
55–64 years	---	---	---	---	259.0	294.0	282.8	269.9	276.8	262.2	269.5
65–74 years	---	---	---	---	599.1	655.5	648.2	663.9	667.1	647.9	659.4
75–84 years	---	---	---	---	1,216.6	1,233.4	1,236.1	1,241.4	1,272.1	1,178.3	1,228.7
85 years and over	---	---	---	---	1,700.7	2,019.4	1,960.5	1,962.5	1,858.7	1,637.8	1,806.5
White, non-Hispanic male[5]											
All ages, age adjusted	---	---	---	---	156.0	163.3	157.5	156.8	154.0	151.7	154.1
All ages, crude	---	---	---	---	217.4	246.2	246.6	248.1	247.1	246.2	247.1
25–34 years	---	---	---	---	13.5	12.8	11.9	12.1	11.4	11.8	11.7
35–44 years	---	---	---	---	39.1	36.8	35.7	35.4	34.7	34.4	34.9
45–54 years	---	---	---	---	159.9	153.9	141.6	141.0	137.0	134.9	137.5
55–64 years	---	---	---	---	496.4	520.6	492.1	486.4	469.9	458.6	471.6
65–74 years	---	---	---	---	1,044.2	1,109.0	1,093.6	1,091.2	1,081.1	1,073.6	1,082.0
75–84 years	---	---	---	---	1,766.1	1,906.6	1,847.8	1,846.0	1,825.6	1,791.6	1,820.5
85 years and over	---	---	---	---	2,327.6	2,744.4	2,767.1	2,776.3	2,814.6	2,764.3	2,785.0
White female											
All ages, age adjusted	119.4	109.5	107.6	107.7	110.5	111.2	110.1	109.9	108.9	107.6	108.8
All ages, crude	139.9	139.8	149.4	170.3	184.4	196.1	200.9	201.9	202.4	201.8	202.1
25–34 years	20.9	18.8	16.3	13.5	12.7	11.9	11.8	11.8	11.5	12.1	11.8
35–44 years	74.5	66.6	62.4	50.9	47.3	46.2	41.8	41.8	42.0	40.5	41.4
45–54 years	185.8	175.7	177.3	166.4	161.6	150.9	140.2	139.4	136.1	131.0	135.4
55–64 years	362.5	329.0	338.6	355.5	376.3	368.5	363.4	356.5	352.6	347.3	352.1
65–74 years	616.5	562.1	554.7	605.2	644.9	675.1	686.2	694.3	689.6	684.6	689.5
75–84 years	1,026.6	939.3	903.5	905.4	938.2	1,011.8	1,044.6	1,056.5	1,060.2	1,059.9	1,058.9
85 years and over	1,348.3	1,304.9	1,126.6	1,266.8	1,285.4	1,372.3	1,413.4	1,395.6	1,428.2	1,430.1	1,418.3

See footnotes at end of table.

Table 40 (page 3 of 4). Death rates for malignant neoplasms, according to sex, detailed race, Hispanic origin, and age: United States, selected years 1950–96

[Data are based on the National Vital Statistics System]

Sex, race, Hispanic origin, and age	1950[1]	1960[1]	1970	1980	1985	1990	1993	1994	1995	1996	1994–96[2]
Black female					Deaths per 100,000 resident population						
All ages, age adjusted	131.9	127.8	123.5	129.7	131.8	137.2	135.3	133.7	134.1	130.7	132.8
All ages, crude	111.8	113.8	117.3	136.5	145.2	156.1	158.4	157.6	159.1	157.9	158.2
25–34 years	34.3	31.0	20.9	18.3	17.2	18.7	17.2	16.3	16.8	16.4	16.5
35–44 years	119.8	102.4	94.6	73.5	69.0	67.4	63.9	64.6	62.2	62.8	63.2
45–54 years	277.0	254.8	228.6	230.2	212.4	209.9	205.6	192.0	192.7	182.8	189.1
55–64 years	484.6	442.7	404.8	450.4	474.9	482.4	441.6	445.8	443.6	422.2	437.1
65–74 years	477.3	541.6	615.8	662.4	704.2	773.2	796.9	794.5	799.6	790.6	794.9
75–84 years	- - -	696.3	763.3	923.9	986.3	1,059.9	1,140.2	1,139.3	1,154.1	1,150.9	1,148.1
85 years and over	- - -	728.9	791.5	1,159.9	1,284.2	1,431.3	1,486.5	1,469.2	1,490.3	1,507.2	1,489.3
American Indian or Alaska Native female[3]											
All ages, age adjusted	- - -	- - -	- - -	62.1	60.5	69.6	68.9	68.0	70.7	78.6	72.5
All ages, crude	- - -	- - -	- - -	50.4	52.5	62.1	65.5	65.8	69.9	77.1	71.0
25–34 years	- - -	- - -	- - -	*	*	*	*	*	11.1	*	9.6
35–44 years	- - -	- - -	- - -	36.9	23.4	31.0	23.4	24.1	33.5	38.5	32.1
45–54 years	- - -	- - -	- - -	96.9	90.1	104.5	92.7	86.4	85.2	111.2	94.6
55–64 years	- - -	- - -	- - -	198.4	192.3	213.3	222.7	224.9	223.2	249.2	232.6
65–74 years	- - -	- - -	- - -	350.8	378.8	438.9	435.7	440.7	427.7	487.3	452.1
75–84 years	- - -	- - -	- - -	446.4	505.9	554.3	628.5	618.5	723.9	721.4	689.0
85 years and over	- - -	- - -	- - -	786.5	700.0	843.7	829.6	708.6	736.6	638.0	692.0
Asian or Pacific Islander female[4]											
All ages, age adjusted	- - -	- - -	- - -	59.8	62.8	63.6	67.0	67.3	68.4	63.2	66.2
All ages, crude	- - -	- - -	- - -	54.1	57.5	60.5	67.7	69.7	71.5	69.7	70.3
25–34 years	- - -	- - -	- - -	9.5	9.9	7.3	7.5	10.1	10.6	9.6	10.1
35–44 years	- - -	- - -	- - -	38.7	33.1	29.8	32.9	30.1	28.6	29.9	29.5
45–54 years	- - -	- - -	- - -	99.8	91.3	93.9	83.5	90.2	98.0	88.7	92.3
55–64 years	- - -	- - -	- - -	174.7	195.5	196.2	215.4	198.4	211.4	179.6	196.1
65–74 years	- - -	- - -	- - -	301.9	330.8	346.2	365.2	352.2	351.2	347.8	350.3
75–84 years	- - -	- - -	- - -	522.1	589.1	641.4	689.0	769.7	722.6	703.6	729.9
85 years and over	- - -	- - -	- - -	800.0	908.3	971.7	1,218.3	1,214.4	1,307.7	917.8	1,117.2
Hispanic female[5]											
All ages, age adjusted	- - -	- - -	- - -	- - -	64.1	70.0	65.4	67.1	66.1	66.7	66.6
All ages, crude	- - -	- - -	- - -	- - -	49.8	60.7	58.7	60.7	60.5	62.1	61.1
25–34 years	- - -	- - -	- - -	- - -	9.7	9.7	9.5	10.3	9.2	10.3	9.9
35–44 years	- - -	- - -	- - -	- - -	30.9	34.8	29.6	33.4	31.2	30.0	31.5
45–54 years	- - -	- - -	- - -	- - -	90.1	100.5	86.4	95.2	89.7	85.3	89.9
55–64 years	- - -	- - -	- - -	- - -	199.4	205.4	195.5	200.0	197.6	202.4	200.0
65–74 years	- - -	- - -	- - -	- - -	356.3	404.8	390.8	384.5	382.3	405.3	391.0
75–84 years	- - -	- - -	- - -	- - -	599.7	663.0	636.6	628.4	659.6	637.8	642.0
85 years and over	- - -	- - -	- - -	- - -	906.1	1,022.7	913.4	912.9	938.2	913.9	921.5

See footnotes at end of table.

Table 40 (page 4 of 4). Death rates for malignant neoplasms, according to sex, detailed race, Hispanic origin, and age: United States, selected years 1950–96

[Data are based on the National Vital Statistics System]

Sex, race, Hispanic origin, and age	1950[1]	1960[1]	1970	1980	1985	1990	1993	1994	1995	1996	1994–96[2]
White, non-Hispanic female[5]					Deaths per 100,000 resident population						
All ages, age adjusted	- - -	- - -	- - -	- - -	108.9	113.6	111.3	111.7	111.1	109.8	110.9
All ages, crude	- - -	- - -	- - -	- - -	187.1	210.6	214.7	217.5	218.4	218.3	218.1
25–34 years	- - -	- - -	- - -	- - -	12.2	11.9	11.9	11.8	11.7	12.2	11.9
35–44 years	- - -	- - -	- - -	- - -	47.2	47.0	41.9	42.1	42.7	41.2	42.0
45–54 years	- - -	- - -	- - -	- - -	158.8	154.9	142.4	141.7	139.3	133.9	138.2
55–64 years	- - -	- - -	- - -	- - -	372.7	379.5	370.8	366.1	362.7	356.6	361.8
65–74 years	- - -	- - -	- - -	- - -	638.3	688.5	693.2	706.8	703.1	697.9	702.6
75–84 years	- - -	- - -	- - -	- - -	917.7	1,027.2	1,050.4	1,069.6	1,070.5	1,075.3	1,071.8
85 years and over	- - -	- - -	- - -	- - -	1,241.6	1,385.7	1,404.4	1,397.7	1,438.4	1,448.8	1,428.6

- - - Data not available.

* Based on fewer than 20 deaths.

[1]Includes deaths of persons who were not residents of the 50 States and the District of Columbia.

[2]Average annual death rate.

[3]Interpretation of trends should take into account that population estimates for American Indians increased by 45 percent between 1980 and 1990, partly due to better enumeration techniques in the 1990 decennial census and to the increased tendency for people to identify themselves as American Indian in 1990.

[4]Interpretation of trends should take into account that the Asian population in the United States more than doubled between 1980 and 1990, primarily due to immigration.

[5]Excludes data from States lacking an Hispanic-origin item on their death certificates. See Appendix I, National Vital Statistics System.

NOTES: For data years shown, the code numbers for cause of death are based on the then current International Classification of Diseases, which are described in Appendix II, tables IV and V. Age groups were selected to minimize the presentation of unstable age-specific death rates based on small numbers of deaths and for consistency among comparison groups. The race groups, white, black, Asian or Pacific Islander, and American Indian or Alaska Native, include persons of Hispanic and non-Hispanic origin. Conversely, persons of Hispanic origin may be of any race. Consistency of race identification between the death certificate (source of data for numerator of death rates) and data from the Census Bureau (denominator) is high for individual white and black persons; however, persons identified as American Indian, Asian, or Hispanic origin in data from the Census Bureau are sometimes misreported as white or non-Hispanic on the death certificate, causing death rates to be underestimated by 22–30 percent for American Indians, about 12 percent for Asians, and about 7 percent for persons of Hispanic origin. (Sorlie PD, Rogot E, and Johnson NJ: Validity of demographic characteristics on the death certificate, Epidemiology 3(2):181–184, 1992.)

SOURCES: Centers for Disease Control and Prevention, National Center for Health Statistics. Grove RD and Hetzel AM. Vital statistics rates in the United States, 1940–60. Washington: Public Health Service, 1968; Vital statistics of the United States, vol II, mortality, part A, for data years 1950–96. Washington: Public Health Service; data computed by the Division of Health and Utilization Analysis from data compiled by the Division of Vital Statistics and from national population estimates for race groups from table 1 and unpublished Hispanic population estimates prepared by the Housing and Household Economic Statistics Division, U.S. Bureau of the Census.

Table 41 (page 1 of 3). Death rates for malignant neoplasms of respiratory system, according to sex, detailed race, Hispanic origin, and age: United States, selected years 1950–96

[Data are based on the National Vital Statistics System]

Sex, race, Hispanic origin, and age	1950[1]	1960[1]	1970	1980	1985	1990	1993	1994	1995	1996	1994–96[2]
All persons					Deaths per 100,000 resident population						
All ages, age adjusted	12.8	19.2	28.4	36.4	39.1	41.4	40.8	40.1	39.7	39.3	39.7
All ages, crude	14.1	22.2	34.2	47.9	53.5	58.9	59.8	59.4	59.5	59.3	59.4
Under 25 years	0.1	0.1	0.1	0.1	0.1	0.1	0.1	0.1	0.1	0.0	0.1
25–34 years	0.9	1.1	1.0	0.8	0.8	0.8	0.7	0.7	0.7	0.8	0.7
35–44 years	5.1	7.3	11.6	9.6	8.2	7.2	6.6	6.5	6.4	6.5	6.5
45–54 years	22.9	32.0	46.2	56.5	53.1	48.8	42.9	40.9	39.8	38.5	39.7
55–64 years	55.2	81.5	116.2	144.3	159.8	166.5	158.9	153.5	148.2	144.3	148.7
65–74 years	69.3	117.2	174.6	243.1	270.3	298.1	306.1	305.9	306.1	305.2	305.7
75–84 years	69.3	102.9	175.1	251.4	292.4	344.1	363.3	367.4	372.7	375.1	371.8
85 years and over	64.0	79.1	113.5	184.5	205.0	252.9	280.8	278.7	294.0	290.9	288.0
Male											
All ages, age adjusted	21.3	34.8	50.6	59.7	60.7	61.0	58.1	56.5	55.3	54.2	55.3
All ages, crude	23.1	38.5	57.0	71.9	75.6	78.3	76.8	75.4	74.6	73.6	74.5
Under 25 years	0.2	0.1	0.1	0.1	0.1	0.1	0.1	0.1	0.1	0.0	0.1
25–34 years	1.3	1.7	1.5	1.0	0.9	1.0	0.9	0.8	0.8	0.9	0.8
35–44 years	8.1	11.4	17.0	12.6	10.6	9.1	8.3	8.0	7.6	7.8	7.8
45–54 years	39.3	54.7	72.1	79.8	71.0	63.0	54.6	51.9	49.9	48.5	50.1
55–64 years	94.2	150.2	202.3	223.8	233.6	232.6	216.0	206.8	196.1	190.7	197.8
65–74 years	116.3	221.7	340.7	422.0	432.5	447.3	441.2	434.5	432.4	424.6	430.5
75–84 years	105.1	188.5	354.2	511.5	558.9	594.4	584.8	576.7	573.4	566.9	572.2
85 years and over	95.4	132.2	215.3	386.3	457.3	538.0	559.7	556.1	567.6	543.2	555.4
Female											
All ages, age adjusted	4.6	5.2	10.1	18.3	22.5	26.2	27.2	27.3	27.5	27.5	27.4
All ages, crude	5.2	6.2	12.6	25.2	32.6	40.4	43.7	44.2	45.1	45.6	45.0
Under 25 years	0.1	0.1	0.1	0.1	0.1	0.0	0.1	*	0.0	*	0.0
25–34 years	0.6	0.6	0.6	0.6	0.7	0.6	0.6	0.6	0.7	0.7	0.6
35–44 years	2.3	3.4	6.5	6.8	5.8	5.4	5.0	4.9	5.1	5.3	5.1
45–54 years	6.7	10.1	22.2	34.8	36.2	35.3	31.6	30.4	30.1	29.0	29.8
55–64 years	15.4	17.0	38.9	74.5	94.5	107.6	107.3	105.3	104.8	102.2	104.1
65–74 years	26.7	26.2	45.6	106.1	145.3	181.7	199.2	203.6	205.0	209.0	205.9
75–84 years	38.8	36.5	56.5	98.0	135.7	194.5	226.3	236.4	245.1	251.1	244.3
85 years and over	42.0	45.2	56.5	96.3	104.2	142.8	173.9	171.8	187.5	190.6	183.5
White male											
All ages, age adjusted	21.6	34.6	49.9	58.0	58.7	59.0	56.3	54.8	53.7	52.6	53.7
All ages, crude	24.1	39.6	58.3	73.4	77.6	81.0	79.7	78.5	77.8	76.8	77.7
45–54 years	39.1	53.0	67.6	74.3	65.5	57.9	49.5	47.4	46.0	45.0	46.1
55–64 years	95.9	149.8	199.3	215.0	223.3	222.5	208.5	199.4	188.2	182.4	189.9
65–74 years	119.4	225.1	344.8	418.4	425.2	438.2	432.4	427.0	426.1	419.1	424.1
75–84 years	109.1	191.9	360.7	516.1	561.7	593.6	579.6	571.8	569.2	562.7	567.8
85 years and over	102.7	133.9	221.8	391.5	463.8	540.4	559.8	552.3	565.3	547.5	555.0
Black male											
All ages, age adjusted	16.9	36.6	60.8	82.0	87.7	91.0	86.0	82.8	80.5	78.5	80.6
All ages, crude	14.3	31.1	51.2	70.8	75.5	77.8	74.7	72.5	71.2	70.1	71.3
45–54 years	41.1	75.0	123.5	142.8	133.1	125.0	113.5	104.2	96.4	92.5	97.5
55–64 years	78.8	161.8	250.3	340.3	373.2	377.5	331.1	322.2	315.0	310.8	316.0
65–74 years	65.2	184.6	322.2	499.4	565.9	613.4	608.2	581.1	573.9	550.0	568.2
75–84 years	- - -	126.3	290.6	499.6	579.0	669.9	711.2	708.1	695.3	692.3	698.4
85 years and over	- - -	110.3	154.4	337.7	409.7	535.7	596.8	623.2	607.3	566.3	598.1
American Indian or Alaska Native male[3]											
All ages, age adjusted	- - -	- - -	- - -	23.2	28.4	29.7	31.0	31.1	32.7	34.5	32.8
All ages, crude	- - -	- - -	- - -	15.7	19.6	21.1	23.1	23.0	25.1	26.4	24.8
45–54 years	- - -	- - -	- - -	*	*	26.6	26.6	22.6	28.4	26.2	25.8
55–64 years	- - -	- - -	- - -	80.0	95.7	106.8	100.2	119.8	114.3	142.9	125.8
65–74 years	- - -	- - -	- - -	221.2	234.6	206.7	233.4	290.8	258.7	273.1	274.0
75–84 years	- - -	- - -	- - -	*	281.8	371.4	418.6	220.1	368.6	325.0	306.2
85 years and over	- - -	- - -	- - -	*	*	*	*	*	*	*	216.9

See footnotes at end of table.

Table 41 (page 2 of 3). Death rates for malignant neoplasms of respiratory system, according to sex, detailed race, Hispanic origin, and age: United States, selected years 1950–96

[Data are based on the National Vital Statistics System]

Sex, race, Hispanic origin, and age	1950[1]	1960[1]	1970	1980	1985	1990	1993	1994	1995	1996	1994–96[2]
Asian or Pacific Islander male[4]				Deaths per 100,000 resident population							
All ages, age adjusted	- - -	- - -	- - -	27.6	26.9	26.8	28.4	28.0	25.8	25.8	26.4
All ages, crude	- - -	- - -	- - -	22.9	21.3	21.7	23.8	23.9	22.4	23.4	23.2
45–54 years	- - -	- - -	- - -	34.0	23.8	19.3	23.6	23.6	20.2	17.3	20.2
55–64 years	- - -	- - -	- - -	98.0	101.2	79.7	91.4	76.4	69.6	71.8	72.5
65–74 years	- - -	- - -	- - -	179.9	188.9	222.6	210.5	218.8	197.0	213.4	209.7
75–84 years	- - -	- - -	- - -	308.1	297.7	319.7	361.8	369.3	341.7	350.8	353.6
85 years and over	- - -	- - -	- - -	*	375.0	438.2	461.2	535.8	607.6	352.2	476.1
Hispanic male[5]											
All ages, age adjusted	- - -	- - -	- - -	- - -	24.0	27.7	25.1	24.8	25.2	23.9	24.6
All ages, crude	- - -	- - -	- - -	- - -	13.9	17.4	16.5	16.5	16.9	16.1	16.5
45–54 years	- - -	- - -	- - -	- - -	18.3	23.4	17.0	21.1	19.8	20.7	20.5
55–64 years	- - -	- - -	- - -	- - -	73.8	88.0	82.7	73.0	75.2	72.3	73.5
65–74 years	- - -	- - -	- - -	- - -	181.3	210.7	186.7	187.6	196.9	189.6	191.4
75–84 years	- - -	- - -	- - -	- - -	306.6	328.8	329.9	323.6	324.5	297.0	314.3
85 years and over	- - -	- - -	- - -	- - -	418.8	458.1	400.9	410.8	385.4	302.6	361.7
White, non-Hispanic male[5]											
All ages, age adjusted	- - -	- - -	- - -	- - -	57.2	60.5	57.3	56.3	55.0	54.0	55.1
All ages, crude	- - -	- - -	- - -	- - -	77.5	88.1	86.3	85.7	85.0	84.5	85.1
45–54 years	- - -	- - -	- - -	- - -	65.4	60.4	51.4	49.1	47.7	46.6	47.8
55–64 years	- - -	- - -	- - -	- - -	218.3	229.8	213.8	206.9	194.7	188.8	196.7
65–74 years	- - -	- - -	- - -	- - -	413.7	447.5	439.7	437.0	435.1	429.0	433.7
75–84 years	- - -	- - -	- - -	- - -	538.4	602.5	579.6	577.5	575.2	571.0	574.5
85 years and over	- - -	- - -	- - -	- - -	433.2	544.3	552.5	547.8	565.3	556.1	556.5
White female											
All ages, age adjusted	4.6	5.1	10.1	18.2	22.7	26.5	27.6	27.7	27.9	28.0	27.9
All ages, crude	5.4	6.4	13.1	26.5	34.8	43.4	47.3	47.9	48.9	49.6	48.8
45–54 years	6.5	9.8	22.1	33.9	36.2	35.2	31.5	30.5	30.1	29.1	29.9
55–64 years	15.5	16.7	39.3	74.2	94.7	108.0	109.4	107.1	106.8	105.1	106.3
65–74 years	27.2	26.5	45.4	108.1	149.0	185.3	203.7	207.9	208.7	213.9	210.2
75–84 years	40.0	36.5	56.8	99.3	138.7	199.0	231.6	241.2	250.8	256.3	249.5
85 years and over	44.0	45.2	57.4	96.8	103.2	143.2	173.9	173.2	188.4	193.1	185.1
Black female											
All ages, age adjusted	4.1	5.5	10.9	19.5	22.8	27.5	27.3	27.7	27.8	27.6	27.7
All ages, crude	3.4	4.9	10.1	19.3	23.5	29.2	30.2	30.8	31.3	31.6	31.2
45–54 years	8.8	12.8	25.3	46.4	41.5	43.4	40.0	36.0	36.6	34.9	35.8
55–64 years	15.3	20.7	36.4	83.8	107.8	122.8	110.1	111.6	110.0	103.2	108.2
65–74 years	16.4	20.7	49.3	91.7	120.6	169.9	184.2	196.4	202.0	203.0	200.5
75–84 years	- - -	33.1	52.6	81.1	105.6	153.8	184.0	198.2	195.3	213.6	202.4
85 years and over	- - -	44.7	47.6	90.5	117.3	138.1	169.5	157.3	171.4	167.0	165.4
American Indian or Alaska Native female[3]											
All ages, age adjusted	- - -	- - -	- - -	8.1	11.1	13.5	16.1	17.7	16.4	16.0	16.7
All ages, crude	- - -	- - -	- - -	6.4	9.2	11.3	14.6	16.5	15.5	15.4	15.8
45–54 years	- - -	- - -	- - -	*	*	22.9	*	23.0	*	*	17.1
55–64 years	- - -	- - -	- - -	*	38.5	53.7	62.5	66.6	49.3	62.3	59.4
65–74 years	- - -	- - -	- - -	*	100.0	80.9	143.8	123.7	136.1	102.1	120.6
75–84 years	- - -	- - -	- - -	*	*	111.8	124.8	181.4	193.0	196.7	190.6
85 years and over	- - -	- - -	- - -	*	*	*	*	*	*	*	81.2

See footnotes at end of table.

Table 41 (page 3 of 3). Death rates for malignant neoplasms of respiratory system, according to sex, detailed race, Hispanic origin, and age: United States, selected years 1950–96

[Data are based on the National Vital Statistics System]

Sex, race, Hispanic origin, and age	1950[1]	1960[1]	1970	1980	1985	1990	1993	1994	1995	1996	1994–96[2]
Asian or Pacific Islander female[4]					Deaths per 100,000 resident population						
All ages, age adjusted	- - -	- - -	- - -	9.5	9.2	11.3	11.7	11.2	13.0	10.9	11.7
All ages, crude	- - -	- - -	- - -	8.4	8.2	10.6	11.7	11.4	13.6	12.2	12.4
45–54 years	- - -	- - -	- - -	13.5	12.8	11.6	11.5	11.2	12.1	11.2	11.5
55–64 years	- - -	- - -	- - -	25.4	26.0	39.5	39.8	36.3	39.1	30.1	35.0
65–74 years	- - -	- - -	- - -	62.4	63.2	71.6	79.3	72.7	87.8	76.9	79.2
75–84 years	- - -	- - -	- - -	117.7	100.0	139.4	127.7	147.7	165.0	150.4	154.3
85 years and over	- - -	- - -	- - -	*	*	172.9	228.1	174.9	291.1	185.5	213.8
Hispanic female[5]											
All ages, age adjusted	- - -	- - -	- - -	- - -	6.7	8.7	8.2	8.5	8.2	8.6	8.4
All ages, crude	- - -	- - -	- - -	- - -	5.2	7.5	7.3	7.7	7.5	8.1	7.8
45–54 years	- - -	- - -	- - -	- - -	6.8	9.0	7.6	9.2	7.3	6.3	7.5
55–64 years	- - -	- - -	- - -	- - -	18.7	26.0	25.3	26.9	25.1	27.2	26.4
65–74 years	- - -	- - -	- - -	- - -	51.4	68.1	62.1	62.5	57.8	67.6	62.7
75–84 years	- - -	- - -	- - -	- - -	79.1	95.8	93.3	88.9	106.7	102.0	99.4
85 years and over	- - -	- - -	- - -	- - -	121.4	125.1	120.9	138.8	120.5	125.8	128.0
White, non-Hispanic female[5]											
All ages, age adjusted	- - -	- - -	- - -	- - -	23.2	27.5	28.6	28.8	29.1	29.2	29.0
All ages, crude	- - -	- - -	- - -	- - -	36.5	47.2	51.4	52.5	53.7	54.6	53.6
45–54 years	- - -	- - -	- - -	- - -	37.5	37.2	33.1	32.1	32.0	30.9	31.6
55–64 years	- - -	- - -	- - -	- - -	95.5	113.7	114.4	112.5	112.7	110.6	111.9
65–74 years	- - -	- - -	- - -	- - -	152.7	190.5	208.9	214.6	215.9	221.5	217.3
75–84 years	- - -	- - -	- - -	- - -	141.8	203.5	234.5	246.8	255.2	262.1	254.8
85 years and over	- - -	- - -	- - -	- - -	104.5	143.9	172.7	172.1	189.6	195.8	186.0

- - - Data not available.

* Based on fewer than 20 deaths.

0.0 Quantity more than zero but less than 0.05.

[1]Includes deaths of persons who were not residents of the 50 States and the District of Columbia.

[2]Average annual death rate.

[3]Interpretation of trends should take into account that population estimates for American Indians increased by 45 percent between 1980 and 1990, partly due to better enumeration techniques in the 1990 decennial census and to the increased tendency for people to identify themselves as American Indian in 1990.

[4]Interpretation of trends should take into account that the Asian population in the United States more than doubled between 1980 and 1990, primarily due to immigration.

[5]Excludes data from States lacking an Hispanic-origin item on their death certificates. See Appendix I, National Vital Statistics System.

NOTES: For data years shown, the code numbers for cause of death are based on the then current *International Classification of Diseases*, which are described in Appendix II, tables IV and V. Age groups were selected to minimize the presentation of unstable age-specific death rates based on small numbers of deaths and for consistency among comparison groups. The race groups, white, black, Asian or Pacific Islander, and American Indian or Alaska Native, include persons of Hispanic and non-Hispanic origin. Conversely, persons of Hispanic origin may be of any race. Consistency of race identification between the death certificate (source of data for numerator of death rates) and data from the Census Bureau (denominator) is high for individual white and black persons; however, persons identified as American Indian, Asian, or Hispanic origin in data from the Census Bureau are sometimes misreported as white or non-Hispanic on the death certificate, causing death rates to be underestimated by 22–30 percent for American Indians, about 12 percent for Asians, and about 7 percent for persons of Hispanic origin. (Sorlie PD, Rogot E, and Johnson NJ: Validity of demographic characteristics on the death certificate, *Epidemiology* 3(2):181–184, 1992.)

SOURCES: Centers for Disease Control and Prevention, National Center for Health Statistics. Grove RD and Hetzel AM. *Vital statistics rates in the United States, 1940–60*. Washington: Public Health Service, 1968; *Vital statistics of the United States, vol II, mortality, part A*, for data years 1950–96. Washington: Public Health Service; data computed by the Division of Health and Utilization Analysis from data compiled by the Division of Vital Statistics and from national population estimates for race groups from table 1 and unpublished Hispanic population estimates prepared by the Housing and Household Economic Statistics Division, U.S. Bureau of the Census.

Table 42 (page 1 of 2). Death rates for malignant neoplasm of breast for females, according to detailed race, Hispanic origin, and age: United States, selected years 1950–96

[Data are based on the National Vital Statistics System]

Race, Hispanic origin, and age	1950[1]	1960[1]	1970	1980	1985	1990	1993	1994	1995	1996	1994–96[2]
All persons	Deaths per 100,000 resident population										
All ages, age adjusted	22.2	22.3	23.1	22.7	23.3	23.1	21.5	21.3	21.0	20.2	20.8
All ages, crude	24.7	26.1	28.4	30.6	32.8	34.0	33.0	32.7	32.6	31.8	32.4
Under 25 years	*	*	*	*	0.0	*	*	*	*	0.0	0.0
25–34 years	3.8	3.8	3.9	3.3	3.0	2.9	2.6	2.7	2.7	2.7	2.7
35–44 years	20.8	20.2	20.4	17.9	17.5	17.8	15.2	15.2	15.0	14.2	14.8
45–54 years	46.9	51.4	52.6	48.1	47.1	45.4	42.0	41.6	41.4	38.8	40.6
55–64 years	70.4	70.8	77.6	80.5	84.2	78.6	72.2	69.8	69.8	67.4	69.0
65–74 years	94.0	90.0	93.8	101.1	107.8	111.7	105.7	105.6	103.3	99.1	102.7
75–84 years	139.8	129.9	127.4	126.4	136.2	146.3	146.4	145.9	142.0	139.8	142.5
85 years and over	195.5	191.9	157.1	169.3	178.5	196.8	206.0	197.5	203.7	204.9	202.1
White											
All ages, age adjusted	22.5	22.4	23.4	22.8	23.4	22.9	21.2	20.9	20.5	19.8	20.4
All ages, crude	25.7	27.2	29.9	32.3	34.7	35.9	34.7	34.4	34.1	33.3	34.0
35–44 years	20.8	19.7	20.2	17.3	16.8	17.1	14.1	14.2	14.1	12.9	13.7
45–54 years	47.1	51.2	53.0	48.1	46.8	44.3	40.6	40.2	39.2	36.9	38.7
55–64 years	70.9	71.8	79.3	81.3	84.7	78.5	72.1	69.1	68.7	67.2	68.3
65–74 years	96.3	91.6	95.9	103.7	109.9	113.3	106.8	106.5	103.9	99.8	103.4
75–84 years	143.6	132.8	129.6	128.4	138.8	148.2	147.3	147.1	143.0	140.6	143.5
85 years and over	204.2	199.7	161.9	171.7	180.9	198.0	207.8	197.8	205.9	207.1	203.7
Black											
All ages, age adjusted	19.3	21.3	21.5	23.3	25.5	27.5	27.1	26.9	27.5	26.5	27.0
All ages, crude	16.4	18.7	19.7	22.9	25.9	29.0	29.5	29.6	30.2	29.9	29.9
35–44 years	21.0	24.8	24.4	24.1	26.1	25.8	24.7	24.6	23.1	24.6	24.1
45–54 years	46.5	54.4	52.0	52.7	55.5	60.5	60.4	58.3	62.6	59.1	60.0
55–64 years	64.3	63.2	64.7	79.9	90.4	93.1	86.0	87.5	88.8	82.9	86.4
65–74 years	67.0	72.3	77.3	84.3	100.7	112.2	114.4	116.0	117.3	109.9	114.4
75–84 years	- - -	87.5	101.8	114.1	117.6	140.5	154.9	150.7	151.6	152.9	151.7
85 years and over	- - -	92.1	112.1	149.9	159.4	201.5	207.9	209.9	198.6	206.9	205.1
American Indian or Alaska Native[3]											
All ages, age adjusted	- - -	- - -	- - -	8.1	8.0	10.0	9.4	10.4	10.4	12.7	11.2
All ages, crude	- - -	- - -	- - -	6.1	6.9	8.6	8.6	9.6	9.8	12.1	10.5
35–44 years	- - -	- - -	- - -	*	*	*	*	*	*	*	7.4
45–54 years	- - -	- - -	- - -	*	*	23.9	22.0	22.1	24.0	28.0	24.8
55–64 years	- - -	- - -	- - -	*	*	*	32.0	29.6	39.1	43.9	37.6
65–74 years	- - -	- - -	- - -	*	*	*	*	60.8	45.4	66.0	57.4
75–84 years	- - -	- - -	- - -	*	*	*	*	*	*	*	58.6
85 years and over	- - -	- - -	- - -	*	*	*	*	*	*	*	87.7
Asian or Pacific Islander[4]											
All ages, age adjusted	- - -	- - -	- - -	9.2	9.6	10.0	9.5	10.5	11.0	8.9	10.1
All ages, crude	- - -	- - -	- - -	8.2	8.6	9.3	9.4	10.7	11.1	9.6	10.4
35–44 years	- - -	- - -	- - -	10.4	7.2	8.4	9.8	8.5	8.3	8.8	8.5
45–54 years	- - -	- - -	- - -	23.4	21.9	26.4	20.9	26.4	30.2	22.0	26.1
55–64 years	- - -	- - -	- - -	35.7	39.5	33.8	33.0	33.5	39.4	23.0	31.7
65–74 years	- - -	- - -	- - -	*	32.5	38.5	36.6	35.5	37.4	40.2	37.8
75–84 years	- - -	- - -	- - -	*	50.0	48.0	56.6	63.3	44.9	51.0	52.8
85 years and over	- - -	- - -	- - -	*	*	*	*	111.7	*	*	72.7
Hispanic[5]											
All ages, age adjusted	- - -	- - -	- - -	- - -	11.8	14.1	12.4	12.6	12.7	12.8	12.7
All ages, crude	- - -	- - -	- - -	- - -	8.8	11.5	10.4	10.7	10.9	11.4	11.0
35–44 years	- - -	- - -	- - -	- - -	10.4	11.7	9.7	11.6	9.7	11.0	10.8
45–54 years	- - -	- - -	- - -	- - -	26.4	32.8	26.6	28.0	27.7	27.4	27.7
55–64 years	- - -	- - -	- - -	- - -	43.5	45.8	44.5	43.0	43.8	39.7	42.1
65–74 years	- - -	- - -	- - -	- - -	40.9	64.8	51.3	51.2	55.7	56.5	54.5
75–84 years	- - -	- - -	- - -	- - -	64.5	67.2	70.7	72.8	75.5	85.6	78.2
85 years and over	- - -	- - -	- - -	- - -	85.7	102.8	88.1	76.2	105.4	104.5	96.1

See footnotes at end of table.

Table 42 (page 2 of 2). Death rates for malignant neoplasm of breast for females, according to detailed race, Hispanic origin, and age: United States, selected years 1950–96

[Data are based on the National Vital Statistics System]

Race, Hispanic origin, and age	1950[1]	1960[1]	1970	1980	1985	1990	1993	1994	1995	1996	1994–96[2]
White, non-Hispanic[5]					Deaths per 100,000 resident population						
All ages, age adjusted	- - -	- - -	- - -	- - -	23.3	23.5	21.5	21.3	20.9	20.1	20.8
All ages, crude	- - -	- - -	- - -	- - -	35.6	38.5	37.1	37.0	36.8	35.9	36.6
35–44 years	- - -	- - -	- - -	- - -	16.9	17.5	14.2	14.3	14.4	12.9	13.8
45–54 years	- - -	- - -	- - -	- - -	46.8	45.2	41.1	40.8	39.9	37.5	39.4
55–64 years	- - -	- - -	- - -	- - -	85.1	80.6	72.9	70.5	70.2	69.0	69.9
65–74 years	- - -	- - -	- - -	- - -	108.6	115.7	108.3	109.0	106.2	102.0	105.7
75–84 years	- - -	- - -	- - -	- - -	139.4	151.4	148.7	149.2	145.2	142.6	145.6
85 years and over	- - -	- - -	- - -	- - -	175.6	201.5	207.7	200.0	208.3	211.7	206.7

* Based on fewer than 20 deaths.
0.0 Quantity more than zero but less than 0.05.
- - - Data not available.
[1]Includes deaths of persons who were not residents of the 50 States and the District of Columbia.
[2]Average annual death rate.
[3]Interpretation of trends should take into account that population estimates for American Indians increased by 45 percent between 1980 and 1990, partly due to better enumeration techniques in the 1990 decennial census and to the increased tendency for people to identify themselves as American Indian in 1990.
[4]Interpretation of trends should take into account that the Asian population in the United States more than doubled between 1980 and 1990, primarily due to immigration.
[5]Excludes data from States lacking an Hispanic-origin item on their death certificates. See Appendix I, National Vital Statistics System.

NOTES: For data years shown, the code numbers for cause of death are based on the then current *International Classification of Diseases*, which are described in Appendix II, tables IV and V. Age groups were selected to minimize the presentation of unstable age-specific death rates based on small numbers of deaths and for consistency among comparison groups. The race groups, white, black, Asian or Pacific Islander, and American Indian or Alaska Native, include persons of Hispanic and non-Hispanic origin. Conversely, persons of Hispanic origin may be of any race. Consistency of race identification between the death certificate (source of data for numerator of death rates) and data from the Census Bureau (denominator) is high for individual white and black persons; however, persons identified as American Indian, Asian, or Hispanic origin in data from the Census Bureau are sometimes misreported as white or non-Hispanic on the death certificate, causing death rates to be underestimated by 22–30 percent for American Indians, about 12 percent for Asians, and about 7 percent for persons of Hispanic origin. (Sorlie PD, Rogot E, and Johnson NJ: Validity of demographic characteristics on the death certificate, *Epidemiology* 3(2):181–184, 1992.)

SOURCES: Centers for Disease Control and Prevention, National Center for Health Statistics. *Vital statistics of the United States, vol II, mortality, part A*, for data years 1950–96. Washington: Public Health Service; data computed by the Division of Health and Utilization Analysis from data compiled by the Division of Vital Statistics and from national population estimates for race groups from table 1 and unpublished Hispanic population estimates prepared by the Housing and Household Economic Statistics Division, U.S. Bureau of the Census.

Table 43 (page 1 of 3). Death rates for chronic obstructive pulmonary diseases, according to sex, detailed race, Hispanic origin, and age: United States, selected years 1980–96

[Data are based on the National Vital Statistics System]

Sex, race, Hispanic origin, and age	1980	1985	1989	1990	1991	1992	1993	1994	1995	1996	1994–96[1]
All persons				Deaths per 100,000 resident population							
All ages, age adjusted	15.9	18.8	19.6	19.7	20.1	19.9	21.4	21.0	20.8	21.0	20.9
All ages, crude	24.7	31.4	34.2	34.9	35.9	36.0	39.2	39.0	39.2	40.0	39.4
Under 1 year	1.6	1.4	1.2	1.4	1.5	1.1	1.4	1.4	1.1	1.0	1.2
1–4 years	0.4	0.3	0.4	0.4	0.3	0.4	0.3	0.3	0.2	0.3	0.3
5–14 years	0.2	0.3	0.3	0.3	0.3	0.3	0.4	0.3	0.4	0.4	0.4
15–24 years	0.3	0.5	0.5	0.5	0.6	0.5	0.6	0.6	0.7	0.7	0.7
25–34 years	0.5	0.6	0.7	0.7	0.8	0.7	0.7	0.9	0.9	0.9	0.9
35–44 years	1.6	1.6	1.7	1.6	1.7	1.8	1.8	1.8	2.0	2.0	1.9
45–54 years	9.8	10.2	9.3	9.1	9.1	8.3	8.7	9.0	8.9	8.7	8.8
55–64 years	42.7	47.9	50.6	48.9	49.7	48.3	51.0	49.2	47.3	47.0	47.8
65–74 years	129.1	149.2	151.5	152.5	156.3	155.5	167.8	163.8	160.6	161.6	162.0
75–84 years	224.4	289.5	310.9	321.1	327.0	326.5	357.3	351.9	351.8	358.3	354.1
85 years and over	274.0	365.4	413.5	433.3	446.9	460.9	493.9	509.7	527.8	540.9	526.5
Male											
All ages, age adjusted	26.1	28.1	26.9	27.2	27.0	26.4	27.8	26.9	26.3	25.9	26.4
All ages, crude	35.1	40.3	40.1	40.8	41.1	40.5	43.2	42.3	42.0	42.0	42.1
Under 1 year	1.9	2.0	1.8	1.6	1.6	1.7	1.5	1.7	1.4	1.3	1.5
1–4 years	0.5	*	0.4	0.5	0.4	0.4	0.4	0.3	0.2	0.4	0.3
5–14 years	0.2	0.3	0.4	0.4	0.4	0.3	0.4	0.4	0.5	0.5	0.5
15–24 years	0.4	0.4	0.5	0.5	0.6	0.6	0.7	0.8	0.7	0.7	0.7
25–34 years	0.6	0.6	0.8	0.7	0.8	0.7	0.6	0.9	0.9	0.8	0.9
35–44 years	1.7	1.6	1.9	1.7	1.8	1.8	1.8	1.8	1.7	1.9	1.8
45–54 years	12.1	11.3	9.5	9.4	9.3	8.7	9.5	9.3	9.0	8.9	9.0
55–64 years	59.9	60.8	60.0	58.6	57.5	56.3	58.1	55.9	52.9	52.2	53.6
65–74 years	210.0	218.9	201.5	204.0	202.4	199.7	208.4	202.0	196.9	192.6	197.2
75–84 years	437.4	505.2	488.3	500.0	495.4	478.6	512.1	490.4	482.5	478.8	483.8
85 years and over	583.4	758.1	792.3	815.1	830.8	830.9	883.1	874.9	896.2	878.6	883.3
Female											
All ages, age adjusted	8.9	12.5	14.7	14.7	15.5	15.5	17.1	17.1	17.1	17.6	17.3
All ages, crude	15.0	23.0	28.6	29.2	31.1	31.8	35.4	35.9	36.4	38.0	36.8
Under 1 year	1.3	*	*	1.2	1.4	*	1.2	1.1	*	*	0.9
1–4 years	*	*	0.4	*	*	0.4	*	*	*	*	0.2
5–14 years	0.3	0.4	0.3	0.3	0.3	0.3	0.3	0.2	0.2	0.4	0.3
15–24 years	0.3	0.5	0.4	0.5	0.5	0.5	0.4	0.5	0.6	0.6	0.6
25–34 years	0.5	0.6	0.7	0.7	0.7	0.6	0.8	0.9	0.9	0.9	0.9
35–44 years	1.5	1.5	1.6	1.5	1.7	1.7	1.8	1.7	2.2	2.1	2.0
45–54 years	7.7	9.2	9.1	8.8	8.9	7.9	8.0	8.7	8.8	8.4	8.6
55–64 years	27.6	36.6	42.3	40.3	42.7	41.0	44.6	43.1	42.2	42.4	42.6
65–74 years	67.1	95.5	112.6	112.3	120.2	120.7	135.6	133.4	131.5	136.7	133.9
75–84 years	98.7	162.7	205.3	214.2	225.1	233.4	261.5	265.2	268.8	280.4	271.6
85 years and over	138.7	208.6	266.2	286.0	298.6	317.6	344.6	368.8	384.3	406.7	387.0
White male											
All ages, age adjusted	26.7	28.7	27.2	27.4	27.4	26.8	28.2	27.3	26.6	26.3	26.7
All ages, crude	37.9	43.7	43.4	44.3	44.9	44.4	47.3	46.4	46.1	46.1	46.2
35–44 years	1.2	1.3	1.3	1.3	1.4	1.5	1.3	1.4	1.4	1.5	1.4
45–54 years	11.4	10.5	8.7	8.6	8.4	8.3	9.0	8.7	8.3	8.5	8.5
55–64 years	60.0	60.6	60.2	58.7	57.8	56.6	58.5	56.7	53.2	52.3	54.1
65–74 years	218.4	225.2	204.5	208.1	206.7	204.6	213.3	206.9	201.6	198.4	202.3
75–84 years	459.8	525.5	502.2	513.5	511.8	494.1	525.2	504.2	496.3	491.1	497.1
85 years and over	611.2	798.1	824.9	847.0	867.4	862.5	917.6	907.7	924.0	917.5	916.5
Black male											
All ages, age adjusted	20.9	24.8	26.5	26.5	25.9	24.8	26.6	25.7	25.4	24.8	25.3
All ages, crude	19.3	23.4	25.2	25.2	24.5	23.8	25.7	24.9	24.9	24.7	24.8
35–44 years	5.8	5.3	6.5	5.3	5.5	4.7	5.4	4.9	4.3	5.2	4.8
45–54 years	19.7	19.5	18.1	18.8	19.8	15.1	16.9	16.6	17.3	15.4	16.4
55–64 years	66.6	69.6	66.6	67.4	66.7	64.8	65.9	61.0	62.0	63.2	62.1
65–74 years	142.0	178.2	192.8	184.5	183.2	175.1	184.9	181.7	175.1	161.6	172.7
75–84 years	229.8	321.8	373.5	390.9	357.8	354.5	407.1	374.1	366.5	380.7	373.8
85 years and over	271.6	374.2	481.8	498.0	482.6	559.8	560.6	561.7	613.6	579.5	585.1

See footnotes at end of table.

Table 43 (page 2 of 3). Death rates for chronic obstructive pulmonary diseases, according to sex, detailed race, Hispanic origin, and age: United States, selected years 1980–96

[Data are based on the National Vital Statistics System]

Sex, race, Hispanic origin, and age	1980	1985	1989	1990	1991	1992	1993	1994	1995	1996	1994–96[1]
American Indian or Alaska Native male[2]				Deaths per 100,000 resident population							
All ages, age adjusted	11.2	14.1	20.1	18.5	15.5	14.7	17.3	16.5	16.4	13.7	15.5
All ages, crude	8.4	10.5	14.4	13.8	11.8	11.3	13.4	13.4	13.4	11.9	12.9
35–44 years	*	*	*	*	*	*	*	*	*	*	*
45–54 years	*	*	*	*	*	*	*	*	*	*	*
55–64 years	*	46.8	47.2	*	38.6	39.8	42.4	33.3	39.2	*	33.1
65–74 years	*	*	161.3	135.7	132.4	102.9	138.9	130.4	129.3	115.9	125.1
75–84 years	*	272.7	330.8	363.8	221.4	276.8	313.9	301.8	253.8	229.7	260.4
85 years and over	*	*	*	*	*	*	*	*	*	421.9	400.0
Asian or Pacific Islander male[3]											
All ages, age adjusted	9.8	12.0	12.9	13.1	12.2	11.6	13.5	12.8	13.5	13.0	13.0
All ages, crude	8.7	10.1	11.2	11.3	10.8	10.3	11.9	11.5	12.3	12.7	12.2
35–44 years	*	*	*	*	*	*	*	*	*	*	1.1
45–54 years	*	*	*	*	*	*	*	*	*	*	3.4
55–64 years	*	24.4	21.2	22.1	15.5	19.6	19.8	15.7	16.4	19.2	17.2
65–74 years	70.6	72.7	82.7	91.4	86.9	94.6	94.1	85.5	91.7	89.9	89.1
75–84 years	155.7	246.5	250.9	258.6	250.8	206.1	278.2	264.2	263.6	294.8	275.3
85 years and over	472.4	462.5	600.0	615.2	561.5	483.8	645.7	660.6	847.8	421.7	609.9
Hispanic male[4]											
All ages, age adjusted	---	11.8	13.3	12.2	12.8	11.3	12.4	12.4	12.7	11.4	12.2
All ages, crude	---	7.2	9.1	8.4	9.0	8.1	9.0	9.0	9.4	8.7	9.0
35–44 years	---	*	1.5	*	*	2.1	1.3	1.3	1.1	1.1	1.2
45–54 years	---	5.9	6.9	4.1	4.7	4.5	3.1	4.6	3.9	4.0	4.2
55–64 years	---	21.5	21.6	17.2	21.9	16.5	21.1	18.2	18.8	18.8	18.6
65–74 years	---	67.5	86.6	81.0	82.9	76.7	77.1	80.3	78.8	68.4	75.7
75–84 years	---	261.8	259.7	252.4	255.1	223.9	244.4	253.5	273.8	240.3	255.4
85 years and over	---	462.5	574.2	613.9	566.7	483.5	666.5	616.2	634.5	579.5	608.1
White, non-Hispanic male[4]											
All ages, age adjusted	---	29.1	27.6	28.2	27.7	27.2	28.5	27.8	27.1	26.9	27.3
All ages, crude	---	45.3	47.4	48.5	48.4	48.2	51.5	50.7	50.4	50.9	50.7
35–44 years	---	1.3	1.3	1.4	1.4	1.4	1.3	1.4	1.4	1.5	1.4
45–54 years	---	10.7	8.7	9.0	8.5	8.3	9.2	8.9	8.5	8.7	8.7
55–64 years	---	61.6	62.2	61.3	59.2	58.5	60.1	58.8	55.2	54.1	56.0
65–74 years	---	229.9	208.6	213.4	209.5	208.4	217.6	211.5	206.5	204.0	207.3
75–84 years	---	528.7	508.6	523.7	514.1	498.2	529.8	510.3	501.9	499.5	503.8
85 years and over	---	782.4	828.4	860.6	876.1	873.1	909.1	908.6	924.5	928.0	920.6
White female											
All ages, age adjusted	9.2	12.9	15.2	15.2	16.1	16.1	17.8	17.8	17.8	18.3	18.0
All ages, crude	16.4	25.5	31.9	32.8	35.0	35.8	40.0	40.6	41.2	43.0	41.6
35–44 years	1.3	1.3	1.3	1.2	1.3	1.3	1.4	1.3	1.7	1.7	1.6
45–54 years	7.6	9.1	8.8	8.3	8.4	7.5	7.6	8.3	8.4	8.0	8.2
55–64 years	28.7	37.8	43.7	41.9	44.7	43.2	47.0	45.2	44.3	44.6	44.7
65–74 years	71.0	101.1	118.6	118.8	127.0	127.7	143.8	141.8	139.8	145.3	142.3
75–84 years	104.0	171.0	216.2	226.3	238.3	246.9	276.1	280.1	282.8	296.4	286.6
85 years and over	144.2	217.6	278.1	298.4	311.6	330.7	361.2	384.9	402.0	423.6	403.8
Black female											
All ages, age adjusted	6.3	8.8	11.1	10.7	11.3	11.2	12.2	12.4	12.5	13.1	12.7
All ages, crude	6.8	10.0	13.1	12.6	13.4	13.7	14.9	15.4	15.8	17.0	16.1
35–44 years	3.4	2.8	4.2	3.8	4.1	4.3	5.3	5.1	5.4	5.0	5.2
45–54 years	9.3	11.2	12.8	14.0	15.0	13.3	12.6	13.5	12.9	13.2	13.2
55–64 years	20.8	30.6	37.4	33.4	34.0	32.1	35.2	35.8	34.7	34.8	35.1
65–74 years	32.7	48.3	68.5	64.7	70.4	73.5	78.3	79.2	78.3	84.3	80.6
75–84 years	41.1	76.6	99.2	96.0	96.0	105.6	120.2	122.1	136.6	137.6	132.2
85 years and over	63.2	94.0	130.7	133.0	142.3	169.0	163.5	195.0	191.4	236.5	208.2

See footnotes at end of table.

Table 43 (page 3 of 3). Death rates for chronic obstructive pulmonary diseases, according to sex, detailed race, Hispanic origin, and age: United States, selected years 1980–96

[Data are based on the National Vital Statistics System]

Sex, race, Hispanic origin, and age	1980	1985	1989	1990	1991	1992	1993	1994	1995	1996	1994–96[1]
American Indian or Alaska Native female[2]				Deaths per 100,000 resident population							
All ages, age adjusted	4.5	6.5	9.0	8.9	9.4	9.3	13.3	11.1	12.0	11.8	11.7
All ages, crude	3.8	5.9	8.4	8.7	9.6	9.3	12.9	11.5	12.5	13.4	12.4
35–44 years	*	*	*	*	*	*	*	*	*	*	*
45–54 years	*	*	*	*	*	*	*	*	*	*	8.3
55–64 years	*	*	*	*	*	*	38.1	34.0	40.6	32.6	35.7
65–74 years	*	*	69.2	56.4	71.4	62.3	114.6	73.8	77.8	78.7	76.8
75–84 years	*	*	110.0	116.7	150.0	128.9	172.2	189.7	168.9	192.9	183.9
85 years and over	*	*	*	*	*	*	*	*	*	265.8	207.9
Asian or Pacific Islander female[3]											
All ages, age adjusted	2.5	5.4	4.7	5.2	5.5	4.5	5.0	5.3	5.8	5.3	5.4
All ages, crude	2.6	5.1	4.6	5.2	5.7	4.9	5.4	5.8	6.5	6.5	6.3
35–44 years	*	*	*	*	*	*	*	*	*	*	1.2
45–54 years	*	*	*	*	*	*	*	*	3.6	*	3.0
55–64 years	*	13.5	13.0	15.2	12.1	9.2	7.8	9.4	10.0	11.1	10.2
65–74 years	*	35.0	27.4	26.5	38.4	29.6	31.0	29.4	29.8	32.7	30.7
75–84 years	*	76.1	78.7	80.6	86.3	79.7	102.4	105.5	120.1	81.1	101.2
85 years and over	*	208.3	168.8	232.5	226.3	190.7	191.8	238.0	272.6	240.9	249.5
Hispanic female[4]											
All ages, age adjusted	- - -	5.7	6.9	6.4	6.4	5.9	6.9	6.7	7.1	7.2	7.0
All ages, crude	- - -	4.8	6.7	6.3	6.7	6.3	7.3	7.3	7.9	8.3	7.8
35–44 years	- - -	*	1.6	*	*	1.3	1.2	1.3	1.5	1.3	1.4
45–54 years	- - -	*	5.7	4.9	4.7	4.2	3.6	4.1	4.6	4.1	4.3
55–64 years	- - -	13.8	14.9	14.4	12.7	10.8	12.2	12.1	12.5	13.0	12.6
65–74 years	- - -	35.0	41.6	36.6	37.4	34.5	44.8	41.2	41.4	40.9	41.2
75–84 years	- - -	99.1	107.7	101.1	106.3	109.2	123.0	114.5	116.7	134.1	122.1
85 years and over	- - -	175.0	249.1	269.0	293.9	250.2	290.5	308.4	367.2	342.8	340.2
White, non-Hispanic female[4]											
All ages, age adjusted	- - -	13.6	15.5	15.7	16.4	16.4	18.2	18.3	18.3	18.9	18.5
All ages, crude	- - -	27.7	34.6	35.7	37.6	38.7	43.3	44.4	45.0	47.2	45.5
35–44 years	- - -	1.2	1.3	1.2	1.3	1.3	1.4	1.3	1.7	1.7	1.5
45–54 years	- - -	9.6	9.1	8.5	8.5	7.5	7.7	8.5	8.6	8.2	8.5
55–64 years	- - -	39.8	44.9	43.7	46.3	44.8	49.0	47.3	46.6	46.8	46.9
65–74 years	- - -	107.6	121.6	122.8	129.6	130.8	147.0	146.2	144.0	150.4	146.9
75–84 years	- - -	179.4	218.4	231.9	240.4	250.1	280.1	285.6	288.4	302.5	292.2
85 years and over	- - -	221.4	279.3	302.1	310.6	330.9	358.7	383.6	401.2	426.8	404.1

* Based on fewer than 20 deaths.

- - - Data not available.

[1]Average annual death rate.

[2]Interpretation of trends should take into account that population estimates for American Indians increased by 45 percent between 1980 and 1990, partly due to better enumeration techniques in the 1990 decennial census and to the increased tendency for people to identify themselves as American Indian in 1990.

[3]Interpretation of trends should take into account that the Asian population in the United States more than doubled between 1980 and 1990, primarily due to immigration.

[4]Excludes data from States lacking an Hispanic-origin item on their death certificates. See Appendix I, National Vital Statistics System.

NOTES: For data years shown, the code numbers for cause of death are based on the then current *International Classification of Diseases*, which are described in Appendix II, tables IV and V. Age groups were selected to minimize the presentation of unstable age-specific death rates based on small numbers of deaths and for consistency among comparison groups. The race groups, white, black, Asian or Pacific Islander, and American Indian or Alaska Native, include persons of Hispanic and non-Hispanic origin. Conversely, persons of Hispanic origin may be of any race. Consistency of race identification between the death certificate (source of data for numerator of death rates) and data from the Census Bureau (denominator) is high for individual white and black persons; however, persons identified as American Indian, Asian, or Hispanic origin in data from the Census Bureau are sometimes misreported as white or non-Hispanic on the death certificate, causing death rates to be underestimated by 22–30 percent for American Indians, about 12 percent for Asians, and about 7 percent for persons of Hispanic origin. (Sorlie PD, Rogot E, and Johnson NJ: Validity of demographic characteristics on the death certificate, *Epidemiology* 3(2):181–184, 1992.)

SOURCES: Centers for Disease Control and Prevention, National Center for Health Statistics. *Vital statistics of the United States, vol II, mortality, part A*, for data years 1980–96. Washington: Public Health Service; data computed by the Division of Health and Utilization Analysis from data compiled by the Division of Vital Statistics and from national population estimates for race groups from table 1 and unpublished Hispanic population estimates prepared by the Housing and Household Economic Statistics Division, U.S. Bureau of the Census.

Table 44 (page 1 of 2). Death rates for human immunodeficiency virus (HIV) infection, according to sex, detailed race, Hispanic origin, and age: United States, 1987–96

[Data are based on the National Vital Statistics System]

Sex, race, Hispanic origin, and age	1987	1988	1989	1990	1991	1992	1993	1994	1995	1996	1994–96[1]
All persons					Deaths per 100,000 resident population						
All ages, age adjusted	5.5	6.7	8.7	9.8	11.3	12.6	13.8	15.4	15.6	11.1	14.0
All ages, crude	5.6	6.8	8.9	10.1	11.7	13.2	14.5	16.2	16.4	11.7	14.8
Under 1 year	2.3	2.2	3.1	2.7	2.3	2.5	2.2	2.5	1.5	1.1	1.7
1–4 years	0.7	0.8	0.8	0.8	1.0	1.0	1.3	1.3	1.3	0.9	1.2
5–14 years	0.1	0.2	0.2	0.2	0.3	0.3	0.4	0.5	0.5	0.5	0.5
15–24 years	1.3	1.4	1.6	1.5	1.7	1.6	1.7	1.8	1.7	1.1	1.6
25–34 years	11.7	14.0	17.9	19.7	22.1	24.6	27.0	29.3	29.1	19.9	26.2
35–44 years	14.0	17.6	23.5	27.4	31.2	35.6	39.1	44.1	44.4	31.4	39.9
45–54 years	8.0	9.8	13.3	15.2	18.4	20.3	22.6	25.6	26.3	19.3	23.7
55–64 years	3.5	4.0	5.4	6.2	7.4	8.5	8.8	10.4	11.0	8.4	9.9
65–74 years	1.3	1.6	1.8	2.0	2.4	2.8	2.9	3.1	3.6	2.7	3.2
75–84 years	0.8	0.8	0.7	0.7	0.9	0.8	0.8	0.9	0.7	0.8	0.8
85 years and over	*	*	*	*	*	*	*	*	*	*	0.4
Male											
All ages, age adjusted	10.0	12.1	15.8	17.7	20.1	22.3	24.1	26.4	26.2	18.1	23.5
All ages, crude	10.2	12.4	16.4	18.5	21.2	23.6	25.5	28.0	28.0	19.5	25.1
Under 1 year	2.2	2.5	2.7	2.4	2.1	2.3	2.1	2.1	1.7	1.1	1.6
1–4 years	0.7	0.8	0.7	0.8	1.0	1.1	1.3	1.2	1.2	0.9	1.1
5–14 years	0.2	0.2	0.2	0.3	0.3	0.4	0.4	0.5	0.5	0.5	0.5
15–24 years	2.2	2.3	2.6	2.2	2.4	2.3	2.3	2.3	2.1	1.4	1.9
25–34 years	20.7	24.5	31.5	34.5	38.3	42.2	46.0	48.5	47.1	31.4	42.4
35–44 years	26.3	32.6	43.6	50.2	56.9	63.5	68.5	76.2	75.9	51.8	67.8
45–54 years	15.5	19.0	25.6	29.1	34.4	38.1	41.7	46.3	46.9	33.6	42.1
55–64 years	6.8	7.8	10.5	12.0	14.0	15.9	16.5	19.1	19.9	14.9	18.0
65–74 years	2.4	2.9	3.3	3.7	4.5	5.3	5.4	5.8	6.4	5.1	5.8
75–84 years	1.2	1.5	1.2	1.1	1.5	1.6	1.4	1.4	1.3	1.5	1.4
85 years and over	*	*	*	*	*	*	*	*	*	*	*
Female											
All ages, age adjusted	1.1	1.4	1.8	2.1	2.7	3.2	3.8	4.8	5.2	4.2	4.7
All ages, crude	1.1	1.4	1.8	2.2	2.7	3.2	3.9	4.9	5.3	4.3	4.8
Under 1 year	2.5	1.7	3.5	3.0	2.4	2.7	2.4	2.9	1.2	*	1.7
1–4 years	0.7	0.7	0.8	0.8	1.1	1.0	1.3	1.3	1.5	1.0	1.3
5–14 years	*	0.1	0.1	0.2	0.2	0.2	0.4	0.5	0.5	0.4	0.5
15–24 years	0.3	0.5	0.6	0.7	0.9	0.9	1.1	1.3	1.4	1.0	1.2
25–34 years	2.8	3.5	4.4	4.9	6.0	6.9	8.0	10.1	11.1	8.5	9.9
35–44 years	2.1	3.0	3.9	5.2	6.1	8.2	10.2	12.5	13.4	11.3	12.4
45–54 years	0.8	1.1	1.6	1.9	3.1	3.4	4.4	5.8	6.7	5.7	6.0
55–64 years	0.5	0.7	0.8	1.1	1.5	1.9	1.9	2.6	2.9	2.5	2.6
65–74 years	0.5	0.6	0.7	0.8	0.8	0.9	1.0	1.0	1.4	0.8	1.1
75–84 years	0.5	0.4	0.4	0.4	0.5	0.4	0.4	0.6	0.3	0.3	0.4
85 years and over	*	*	*	*	*	*	*	*	*	*	0.3
All ages, age adjusted											
White male	8.4	10.0	13.2	15.0	16.7	18.1	19.0	20.1	19.6	12.5	17.4
Black male	25.4	31.6	40.3	44.2	52.9	61.8	70.0	81.7	84.3	66.4	77.4
American Indian or Alaska Native male	*	2.8	2.9	3.3	6.5	4.9	8.3	9.3	11.3	6.9	9.2
Asian or Pacific Islander male	2.2	2.9	3.6	4.0	4.0	4.3	5.1	6.6	5.8	4.1	5.5
Hispanic male[2]	17.8	20.3	27.0	27.2	30.1	33.0	33.6	39.3	39.0	26.0	34.5
White, non-Hispanic male[2]	6.4	10.7	12.2	13.4	14.8	15.9	16.7	17.7	17.1	10.7	15.2
White female	0.6	0.7	0.9	1.1	1.3	1.6	1.9	2.3	2.5	1.8	2.2
Black female	4.7	6.2	8.1	9.9	12.0	14.3	17.3	21.8	24.0	20.2	22.0
American Indian or Alaska Native female	*	*	*	*	*	*	*	*	2.7	*	1.9
Asian or Pacific Islander female	*	*	*	*	*	0.5	0.7	0.7	0.6	0.5	0.6
Hispanic female[2]	2.1	3.1	4.0	3.7	4.8	5.6	6.5	7.7	8.5	6.2	7.5
White, non-Hispanic female[2]	0.2	0.5	0.6	0.7	0.9	1.0	1.2	1.6	1.8	1.3	1.6

See footnotes at end of table.

Table 44 (page 2 of 2). Death rates for human immunodeficiency virus (HIV) infection, according to sex, detailed race, Hispanic origin, and age: United States, 1987–96

[Data are based on the National Vital Statistics System]

Sex, race, Hispanic origin, and age	1987	1988	1989	1990	1991	1992	1993	1994	1995	1996	1994–96[1]
Age 25–44 years	Deaths per 100,000 resident population										
All races	12.7	15.6	20.5	23.2	26.5	29.9	32.9	36.7	36.9	25.9	33.2
White male	19.2	23.0	30.8	35.0	39.3	42.8	45.5	48.4	46.9	29.6	41.6
Black male	60.2	74.3	94.1	102.0	117.9	137.4	155.3	178.0	182.0	139.1	166.2
American Indian or Alaska Native male	*	*	7.4	7.7	13.9	13.4	20.9	23.6	31.3	18.4	24.3
Asian or Pacific Islander male	4.1	6.3	7.5	8.1	9.0	9.4	10.8	13.8	12.8	8.1	11.5
Hispanic male[2]	36.8	43.5	58.2	59.3	63.9	68.9	71.0	78.0	78.9	50.5	68.6
White, non-Hispanic male[2]	14.3	24.7	28.2	31.6	34.9	38.1	40.2	43.4	41.5	25.8	36.9
White female	1.2	1.6	1.9	2.3	3.0	3.6	4.4	5.5	6.0	4.4	5.3
Black female	11.6	15.5	20.1	23.6	27.2	34.4	40.4	49.8	54.5	46.6	50.3
American Indian or Alaska Native female	*	*	*	*	*	*	*	*	*	*	4.5
Asian or Pacific Islander female	*	*	*	*	*	*	1.2	1.5	1.2	*	1.3
Hispanic female[2]	4.9	7.2	9.3	8.9	10.1	12.5	14.2	17.3	18.0	12.8	16.0
White, non-Hispanic female[2]	0.3	1.2	1.3	1.5	1.9	2.3	2.9	3.9	4.2	3.1	3.7
Age 45–64 years											
All races	5.8	7.1	9.7	11.1	13.4	15.2	16.8	19.3	20.1	15.0	18.1
White male	9.9	11.9	16.4	18.6	21.2	23.4	24.7	26.4	26.3	17.4	23.3
Black male	27.3	34.5	46.1	53.0	71.4	86.4	101.2	127.1	136.6	114.1	125.8
American Indian or Alaska Native male	*	*	*	*	*	*	*	*	*	*	8.2
Asian or Pacific Islander male	*	4.3	6.1	6.5	5.3	7.1	9.2	10.6	9.5	8.2	9.4
Hispanic male[2]	25.8	29.0	37.0	37.9	45.0	52.5	52.2	69.2	67.1	48.8	61.2
White, non-Hispanic male[2]	8.0	13.0	15.3	16.9	18.8	20.3	21.5	22.6	22.6	14.3	19.8
White female	0.5	0.6	0.7	0.9	1.2	1.5	1.8	2.1	2.4	1.9	2.1
Black female	2.6	4.0	5.6	7.5	12.2	12.9	16.5	24.1	27.2	24.4	25.2
American Indian or Alaska Native female	*	*	*	*	*	*	*	*	*	*	*
Asian or Pacific Islander female	*	*	*	*	*	*	*	*	*	*	0.7
Hispanic female[2]	*	2.6	3.5	3.1	6.2	6.8	8.2	9.9	12.4	9.7	10.7
White, non-Hispanic female[2]	0.3	0.4	0.5	0.7	0.8	1.0	1.1	1.4	1.5	1.2	1.4

* Based on fewer than 20 deaths.

[1] Average annual death rate.

[2] Data shown only for States with an Hispanic-origin item on their death certificates. See Appendix I, National Vital Statistics System.

NOTES: Categories for the coding and classification of human immunodeficiency virus infection were introduced in the United States beginning with mortality data for 1987. Age groups were selected to minimize the presentation of unstable age-specific death rates based on small numbers of deaths and for consistency among comparison groups. The race groups, white, black, Asian or Pacific Islander, and American Indian or Alaska Native, include persons of Hispanic and non-Hispanic origin. Conversely, persons of Hispanic origin may be of any race. Consistency of race identification between the death certificate (source of data for numerator of death rates) and data from the Census Bureau (denominator) is high for individual white and black persons; however, persons identified as American Indian, Asian, or Hispanic origin in data from the Census Bureau are sometimes misreported as white or non-Hispanic on the death certificate, causing death rates to be underestimated by 22–30 percent for American Indians, about 12 percent for Asians, and about 7 percent for persons of Hispanic origin. (Sorlie PD, Rogot E, and Johnson NJ: Validity of demographic characteristics on the death certificate, *Epidemiology* 3(2):181–184, 1992.)

SOURCES: Centers for Disease Control and Prevention, National Center for Health Statistics. *Vital statistics of the United States, vol II, mortality, part A*, for data years 1987–96. Washington: Public Health Service; data computed by the Division of Health and Utilization Analysis from data compiled by the Division of Vital Statistics and from national population estimates for race groups from table 1 and unpublished Hispanic population estimates prepared by the Housing and Household Economic Statistics Division, U.S. Bureau of the Census.

Table 45. Maternal mortality for complications of pregnancy, childbirth, and the puerperium, according to race, Hispanic origin, and age: United States, selected years 1950–96

[Data are based on the National Vital Statistics System]

Race, Hispanic origin, and age	1950[1]	1960[1]	1970	1980	1985	1990	1993	1994	1995	1996
					Number of deaths					
All persons.	2,960	1,579	803	334	295	343	302	328	277	294
White.	1,873	936	445	193	156	177	152	193	129	159
Black.	1,041	624	342	127	124	153	135	118	133	121
American Indian or Alaska Native	- - -	- - -	- - -	3	7	4	3	–	1	6
Asian or Pacific Islander	- - -	- - -	- - -	11	8	9	12	17	14	8
Hispanic.	- - -	- - -	- - -	- - -	29	47	48	64	43	39
White, non-Hispanic	- - -	- - -	- - -	- - -	60	125	104	127	84	114
All persons					Deaths per 100,000 live births					
All ages, age adjusted	73.7	32.1	21.5	9.4	7.6	7.6	6.7	7.9	6.3	6.4
All ages, crude	83.3	37.1	21.5	9.2	7.8	8.2	7.5	8.3	7.1	7.6
Under 20 years.	70.7	22.7	18.9	7.6	6.9	7.5	4.5	6.9	3.9	*
20–24 years	47.6	20.7	13.0	5.8	5.4	6.1	5.9	7.6	5.7	5.0
25–29 years	63.5	29.8	17.0	7.7	6.4	6.0	5.9	7.1	6.0	6.6
30–34 years	107.7	50.3	31.6	13.6	8.9	9.5	7.7	6.5	7.3	7.6
35 years and over[2]	222.0	104.3	81.9	36.3	25.0	20.7	19.6	18.3	15.9	19.0
White										
All ages, age adjusted	53.1	22.4	14.4	6.7	4.9	5.1	4.2	5.8	3.6	4.1
All ages, crude	61.1	26.0	14.3	6.6	5.1	5.4	4.8	6.2	4.2	5.1
Under 20 years.	44.9	14.8	13.8	5.8	*	*	*	6.2	*	*
20–24 years	35.7	15.3	8.4	4.2	3.3	3.9	3.5	4.7	3.5	*
25–29 years	45.0	20.3	11.1	5.4	4.6	4.8	3.6	6.1	4.0	4.0
30–34 years	75.9	34.3	18.7	9.3	5.1	5.0	5.5	5.0	4.0	5.0
35 years and over[2]	174.1	73.9	59.3	25.5	17.5	12.6	11.7	12.0	9.1	14.9
Black										
All ages, age adjusted	- - -	92.0	65.5	24.9	22.1	21.7	20.0	18.1	20.9	19.9
All ages, crude	- - -	103.6	60.9	22.4	21.3	22.4	20.5	18.5	22.1	20.3
Under 20 years.	- - -	54.8	32.3	13.1	*	*	*	*	*	*
20–24 years	- - -	56.9	41.9	13.9	14.6	14.7	14.4	18.2	15.3	15.1
25–29 years	- - -	92.8	65.2	22.4	19.4	14.9	21.1	*	21.0	25.5
30–34 years	- - -	150.6	117.8	44.0	38.0	44.2	25.8	*	31.2	28.6
35 years and over[2]	- - -	299.5	207.5	100.6	77.2	79.7	69.9	64.5	61.4	49.9
Hispanic[3]										
All ages, age adjusted	- - -	- - -	- - -	- - -	7.1	7.4	6.6	9.1	5.4	4.8
All ages, crude	- - -	- - -	- - -	- - -	7.8	7.9	7.3	9.6	6.3	5.6
White, non-Hispanic										
All ages, age adjusted	- - -	- - -	- - -	- - -	4.0	4.4	3.8	4.9	3.3	3.9
All ages, crude	- - -	- - -	- - -	- - -	4.3	4.8	4.2	5.2	3.5	4.8

- - - Data not available.
– Quantity zero.
* Based on fewer than 20 deaths.
[1]Includes deaths of persons who were not residents of the 50 States and the District of Columbia.
[2]Rates computed by relating deaths of women 35 years and over to live births to women 35–49 years.
[3]Age-specific maternal mortality rates are not calculated because rates based on fewer than 20 deaths are unreliable.

NOTES: For data years shown, the code numbers for cause of death are based on the then current *International Classification of Diseases*, described in Appendix II, tables IV and V. For 1950 and 1960, rates are based on live births by race of child; for all other years, rates are based on live births by race of mother. See Appendix II, Race. Rates are not calculated for American Indian or Alaska Native and Asian or Pacific Islander mothers because rates based on fewer than 20 deaths are unreliable. Hispanic and White, non-Hispanic data exclude data from States lacking an Hispanic-origin item on their death and birth certificates. See Appendix I, National Vital Statistics System.

SOURCES: Centers for Disease Control and Prevention, National Center for Health Statistics. *Vital statistics of the United States, vol II, mortality, part A*, for data years 1950–96. Washington: Public Health Service. *Vital statistics of the United States, vol I, natality*, for data years 1950–96. Washington: Public Health Service; data computed by the Division of Health and Utilization Analysis from data compiled by the Division of Vital Statistics.

Table 46 (page 1 of 4). Death rates for motor vehicle-related injuries, according to sex, detailed race, Hispanic origin, and age: United States, selected years 1950–96

[Data are based on the National Vital Statistics System]

Sex, race, Hispanic origin, and age	1950[1]	1960[1]	1970	1980	1985	1990	1993	1994	1995	1996	1994–96[2]
All persons					Deaths per 100,000 resident population						
All ages, age adjusted	23.3	22.5	27.4	22.9	18.8	18.5	16.0	16.1	16.3	16.2	16.2
All ages, crude	23.1	21.3	26.9	23.5	19.3	18.8	16.3	16.3	16.5	16.5	16.4
Under 1 year	8.4	8.1	9.8	7.0	4.9	4.9	4.9	4.8	4.7	5.7	5.1
1–14 years	9.8	8.6	10.5	8.2	7.0	6.0	5.4	5.6	5.3	5.2	5.4
1–4 years	11.5	10.0	11.5	9.2	7.2	6.3	5.6	6.0	5.2	5.3	5.5
5–14 years	8.8	7.9	10.2	7.9	6.9	5.9	5.3	5.4	5.4	5.2	5.3
15–24 years	34.4	38.0	47.2	44.8	35.7	34.1	29.1	29.7	29.5	29.2	29.4
25–34 years	24.6	24.3	30.9	29.1	23.0	23.6	19.6	18.8	19.8	19.1	19.2
35–44 years	20.3	19.3	24.9	20.9	17.2	16.9	14.9	14.8	15.4	15.6	15.3
45–64 years	25.2	23.0	26.5	18.0	15.4	15.7	13.5	13.9	14.2	14.4	14.2
45–54 years	22.2	21.4	25.5	18.6	15.2	15.6	13.3	14.0	13.9	14.1	14.0
55–64 years	29.0	25.1	27.9	17.4	15.6	15.9	13.9	13.9	14.6	15.0	14.5
65 years and over	43.1	34.7	36.2	22.5	21.7	23.1	22.3	22.9	22.7	23.0	22.9
65–74 years	39.1	31.4	32.8	19.2	17.9	18.6	16.7	18.1	17.6	18.3	18.0
75–84 years	52.7	41.8	43.5	28.1	27.4	29.1	29.8	29.2	28.6	28.3	28.7
85 years and over	45.1	37.9	34.2	27.6	26.5	31.2	29.7	29.1	31.4	30.1	30.2
Male											
All ages, age adjusted	36.4	34.5	41.1	34.3	27.3	26.3	22.5	22.5	22.7	22.3	22.5
All ages, crude	35.4	31.8	39.7	35.3	28.0	26.7	22.7	22.5	22.7	22.4	22.6
Under 1 year	9.1	8.6	9.3	7.3	5.0	5.0	4.8	4.8	4.9	5.7	5.1
1–14 years	12.3	10.7	13.0	10.0	8.5	7.0	6.3	6.5	6.2	5.9	6.2
1–4 years	13.0	11.5	12.9	10.2	8.3	6.9	6.1	6.6	5.6	5.7	6.0
5–14 years	11.9	10.4	13.1	9.9	8.6	7.0	6.3	6.5	6.4	6.0	6.3
15–24 years	56.7	61.2	73.2	68.4	52.7	49.5	41.8	41.8	41.4	40.7	41.3
25–34 years	40.8	40.1	49.4	46.3	35.9	35.7	29.1	27.7	29.1	27.5	28.1
35–44 years	32.5	29.9	37.7	31.7	25.2	24.7	21.6	21.4	21.9	21.8	21.7
45–64 years	37.7	33.3	38.9	26.5	22.0	21.9	18.9	19.2	19.7	19.8	19.6
45–54 years	33.6	31.6	37.2	27.6	21.9	22.0	18.8	19.4	19.6	19.6	19.5
55–64 years	43.1	35.6	40.9	25.4	22.1	21.7	19.0	18.9	19.8	20.1	19.6
65 years and over	66.6	52.1	54.4	33.9	30.4	32.1	30.6	31.2	30.8	31.4	31.1
65–74 years	59.1	45.8	47.3	27.3	23.0	24.2	21.3	23.1	22.3	23.9	23.1
75–84 years	85.0	66.0	68.2	44.3	41.3	41.2	41.8	40.5	39.7	38.7	39.6
85 years and over	78.1	62.7	63.1	56.1	55.3	64.5	62.8	59.6	61.9	59.0	60.1
Female											
All ages, age adjusted	10.7	11.0	14.4	11.8	10.5	10.7	9.6	9.9	10.0	10.2	10.1
All ages, crude	10.9	11.0	14.7	12.3	11.0	11.3	10.1	10.4	10.6	10.7	10.6
Under 1 year	7.6	7.5	10.4	6.7	4.7	4.9	4.9	4.8	4.4	5.8	5.0
1–14 years	7.2	6.3	7.9	6.3	5.4	4.9	4.5	4.5	4.5	4.4	4.5
1–4 years	10.0	8.4	10.0	8.1	6.0	5.6	5.2	5.4	4.8	4.8	5.0
5–14 years	5.7	5.4	7.2	5.7	5.1	4.7	4.2	4.2	4.3	4.2	4.2
15–24 years	12.6	15.1	21.6	20.8	18.2	17.9	16.0	17.0	17.1	17.1	17.1
25–34 years	9.3	9.2	13.0	12.2	10.1	11.5	10.2	9.9	10.4	10.7	10.4
35–44 years	8.5	9.1	12.9	10.4	9.4	9.2	8.3	8.5	9.0	9.4	9.0
45–64 years	12.6	13.1	15.3	10.3	9.5	10.1	8.5	9.1	9.1	9.4	9.2
45–54 years	10.9	11.6	14.5	10.2	9.0	9.6	8.0	8.8	8.5	8.8	8.7
55–64 years	14.9	15.2	16.2	10.5	9.9	10.8	9.3	9.4	9.9	10.3	9.9
65 years and over	21.9	20.3	23.1	15.0	15.8	17.2	16.7	17.3	17.2	17.2	17.2
65–74 years	20.6	19.0	21.6	13.0	14.0	14.1	13.1	14.1	13.8	13.9	13.9
75–84 years	25.2	23.0	27.2	18.5	19.2	21.9	22.3	22.1	21.5	21.5	21.7
85 years and over	22.1	22.0	18.0	15.2	15.0	18.3	17.1	17.4	19.6	18.6	18.5
White male											
All ages, age adjusted	35.9	34.0	40.1	34.8	27.6	26.3	22.5	22.5	22.6	22.2	22.4
All ages, crude	35.1	31.5	39.1	35.9	28.3	26.7	22.7	22.5	22.6	22.4	22.5
Under 1 year	9.1	8.8	9.1	7.0	4.6	4.8	4.4	4.3	4.3	5.2	4.6
1–14 years	12.4	10.6	12.5	9.8	8.3	6.6	5.9	6.2	5.9	5.7	5.9
15–24 years	58.3	62.7	75.2	73.8	56.5	52.5	43.8	43.6	43.2	42.2	43.0
25–34 years	39.1	38.6	47.0	46.6	35.8	35.4	29.3	28.0	28.8	27.0	27.9
35–44 years	30.9	28.4	35.2	30.7	24.3	23.7	20.9	21.1	21.1	21.4	21.2
45–64 years	36.2	31.7	36.5	25.2	20.8	20.6	17.9	18.3	18.9	19.2	18.8
65 years and over	67.1	52.1	54.2	32.7	29.9	31.4	30.1	30.5	30.2	31.1	30.6

See footnotes at end of table.

Table 46 (page 2 of 4). **Death rates for motor vehicle-related injuries, according to sex, detailed race, Hispanic origin, and age: United States, selected years 1950–96**

[Data are based on the National Vital Statistics System]

Sex, race, Hispanic origin, and age	1950[1]	1960[1]	1970	1980	1985	1990	1993	1994	1995	1996	1994–96[2]
Black male					Deaths per 100,000 resident population						
All ages, age adjusted	39.8	38.2	50.1	32.9	28.0	28.9	25.3	24.7	25.3	24.9	25.0
All ages, crude	37.2	33.1	44.3	31.1	27.1	28.1	24.6	23.9	24.6	24.3	24.3
Under 1 year.	- - -	*	10.6	7.8	*	*	7.2	8.0	8.3	7.6	8.0
1–14 years	- - -	11.2	16.3	11.4	9.7	8.9	8.3	8.7	7.8	7.6	8.0
15–24 years	41.6	46.4	58.1	34.9	32.0	36.1	34.3	35.0	34.3	35.2	34.8
25–34 years	57.4	51.0	70.4	44.9	37.7	39.5	30.9	29.1	32.9	32.5	31.5
35–44 years	45.9	43.6	59.5	41.2	34.7	33.5	28.6	25.3	28.9	26.6	26.9
45–64 years	54.6	47.8	61.7	39.5	32.9	33.3	28.4	27.3	26.9	26.8	27.0
65 years and over	52.6	48.2	53.4	42.4	35.2	36.3	37.4	37.7	36.3	35.6	36.5
American Indian or Alaska Native male[3]											
All ages, age adjusted	- - -	- - -	- - -	77.4	52.3	49.0	42.4	43.8	45.4	45.4	44.9
All ages, crude	- - -	- - -	- - -	74.6	51.7	47.6	40.7	41.8	43.8	44.2	43.3
1–14 years	- - -	- - -	- - -	15.1	16.2	11.6	9.6	9.5	8.5	13.5	10.5
15–24 years	- - -	- - -	- - -	126.1	77.3	75.2	71.5	68.0	76.6	69.6	71.4
25–34 years	- - -	- - -	- - -	107.0	84.0	78.2	61.1	58.4	73.1	70.5	67.4
35–44 years	- - -	- - -	- - -	82.8	55.8	57.0	44.7	52.9	50.4	48.8	50.7
45–64 years	- - -	- - -	- - -	77.4	52.2	45.9	40.8	49.5	42.5	39.8	43.8
65 years and over	- - -	- - -	- - -	97.0	*	43.0	45.1	*	*	43.5	35.3
Asian or Pacific Islander male[4]											
All ages, age adjusted	- - -	- - -	- - -	17.1	16.2	15.8	11.5	13.1	13.6	11.9	12.8
All ages, crude	- - -	- - -	- - -	17.1	16.0	15.8	11.1	12.5	13.1	11.5	12.3
1–14 years	- - -	- - -	- - -	8.2	5.2	6.3	3.7	3.8	4.3	2.9	3.7
15–24 years	- - -	- - -	- - -	27.2	28.1	25.7	19.2	22.3	20.6	22.4	21.8
25–34 years	- - -	- - -	- - -	18.8	18.4	17.0	10.9	11.0	13.2	13.3	12.5
35–44 years	- - -	- - -	- - -	13.1	12.0	12.2	8.8	8.5	10.4	9.9	9.6
45–64 years	- - -	- - -	- - -	13.7	13.4	15.1	13.4	13.0	15.0	9.7	12.5
65 years and over	- - -	- - -	- - -	37.3	37.3	33.6	21.6	39.3	34.4	23.9	32.2
Hispanic male[5]											
All ages, age adjusted	- - -	- - -	- - -	- - -	25.3	29.1	25.2	24.7	24.5	23.2	24.1
All ages, crude	- - -	- - -	- - -	- - -	25.6	29.2	24.7	23.9	23.5	22.3	23.2
1–14 years	- - -	- - -	- - -	- - -	7.7	7.2	6.7	6.9	5.8	5.6	6.1
15–24 years	- - -	- - -	- - -	- - -	44.9	48.2	43.5	42.4	42.4	37.5	40.7
25–34 years	- - -	- - -	- - -	- - -	31.2	41.0	32.8	31.0	31.6	28.0	30.2
35–44 years	- - -	- - -	- - -	- - -	26.3	28.0	26.5	24.8	23.8	23.9	24.1
45–64 years	- - -	- - -	- - -	- - -	25.9	28.9	23.0	23.0	23.0	23.8	23.3
65 years and over	- - -	- - -	- - -	- - -	22.9	35.3	32.0	33.2	35.1	35.2	34.5
White, non-Hispanic male[5]											
All ages, age adjusted	- - -	- - -	- - -	- - -	25.3	25.7	21.6	21.7	21.9	21.7	21.7
All ages, crude	- - -	- - -	- - -	- - -	25.9	26.0	21.8	21.8	22.0	21.9	21.9
1–14 years	- - -	- - -	- - -	- - -	7.8	6.4	5.6	6.0	5.8	5.5	5.8
15–24 years	- - -	- - -	- - -	- - -	53.3	52.3	42.7	42.6	42.3	42.0	42.3
25–34 years	- - -	- - -	- - -	- - -	33.2	34.0	28.0	26.7	27.5	26.1	26.8
35–44 years	- - -	- - -	- - -	- - -	21.6	23.1	19.8	20.1	20.3	20.5	20.3
45–64 years	- - -	- - -	- - -	- - -	18.0	19.8	17.0	17.5	18.2	18.4	18.1
65 years and over	- - -	- - -	- - -	- - -	27.6	31.1	29.4	30.0	29.6	30.5	30.0
White female											
All ages, age adjusted	10.6	11.1	14.4	12.3	10.8	11.0	9.7	10.0	10.3	10.4	10.2
All ages, crude	10.9	11.2	14.8	12.8	11.4	11.6	10.3	10.6	10.8	11.0	10.8
Under 1 year.	7.8	7.5	10.2	7.1	3.9	4.7	4.5	3.9	4.5	5.7	4.7
1–14 years	7.2	6.2	7.5	6.2	5.4	4.8	4.2	4.3	4.3	4.3	4.3
15–24 years	12.6	15.6	22.7	23.0	20.0	19.5	17.1	18.3	18.4	18.1	18.2
25–34 years	9.0	9.0	12.7	12.2	10.1	11.6	10.2	9.8	10.4	10.8	10.3
35–44 years	8.1	8.9	12.3	10.6	9.4	9.2	8.2	8.4	9.0	9.3	8.9
45–64 years	12.7	13.1	15.1	10.4	9.5	9.9	8.5	8.8	8.9	9.3	9.0
65 years and over	22.2	20.8	23.7	15.3	16.2	17.4	17.0	17.6	17.7	17.4	17.6

See footnotes at end of table.

Table 46 (page 3 of 4). Death rates for motor vehicle-related injuries, according to sex, detailed race, Hispanic origin, and age: United States, selected years 1950–96

[Data are based on the National Vital Statistics System]

Sex, race, Hispanic origin, and age	1950[1]	1960[1]	1970	1980	1985	1990	1993	1994	1995	1996	1994–96[2]
Black female				Deaths per 100,000 resident population							
All ages, age adjusted	10.3	10.0	13.8	8.4	8.2	9.3	8.5	9.5	8.9	9.4	9.3
All ages, crude	10.2	9.7	13.4	8.3	8.3	9.4	8.7	9.5	9.0	9.5	9.3
Under 1 year.	- - -	8.1	11.9	*	8.1	7.0	*	9.5	*	7.8	7.3
1–14 years	- - -	6.9	10.2	6.3	5.1	5.3	6.1	5.8	5.1	4.8	5.2
15–24 years	11.5	9.9	13.4	8.0	9.1	9.9	10.6	11.7	10.7	13.3	11.9
25–34 years	10.7	9.8	13.3	10.6	9.3	11.1	9.5	10.4	10.5	10.9	10.6
35–44 years	11.1	11.0	16.1	8.3	9.1	9.4	9.1	8.9	9.8	9.6	9.4
45–64 years	11.8	12.7	16.7	9.2	9.0	10.7	7.7	10.1	9.4	8.9	9.5
65 years and over	14.3	13.2	15.7	9.5	11.2	13.5	11.6	13.6	11.5	13.1	12.7
American Indian or Alaska Native female[3]											
All ages, age adjusted	- - -	- - -	- - -	32.5	20.9	17.8	22.4	19.3	21.0	22.6	21.0
All ages, crude	- - -	- - -	- - -	32.0	20.6	17.3	21.8	18.8	20.4	21.8	20.3
1–14 years	- - -	- - -	- - -	15.0	9.2	8.1	7.9	9.1	9.1	9.7	9.3
15–24 years	- - -	- - -	- - -	42.3	29.5	31.4	35.0	30.7	32.7	27.1	30.1
25–34 years	- - -	- - -	- - -	52.5	30.2	18.8	33.5	28.3	36.7	31.9	32.3
35–44 years	- - -	- - -	- - -	38.1	27.0	18.2	23.4	16.8	19.4	23.0	19.8
45–64 years	- - -	- - -	- - -	32.6	19.5	17.6	20.0	17.0	17.1	27.1	20.5
65 years and over	- - -	- - -	- - -	*	*	*	*	*	*	*	16.7
Asian or Pacific Islander female[4]											
All ages, age adjusted	- - -	- - -	- - -	8.4	8.0	9.2	7.6	7.7	8.2	7.2	7.7
All ages, crude	- - -	- - -	- - -	8.2	7.9	9.0	7.6	7.6	8.0	7.4	7.7
1–14 years	- - -	- - -	- - -	7.4	5.0	3.6	3.4	2.7	3.0	2.3	2.7
15–24 years	- - -	- - -	- - -	7.4	7.4	11.4	8.8	9.3	12.4	8.3	10.0
25–34 years	- - -	- - -	- - -	7.3	8.4	7.3	6.3	6.1	5.1	5.6	5.6
35–44 years	- - -	- - -	- - -	8.6	7.0	7.5	5.0	6.8	6.2	7.5	6.8
45–64 years	- - -	- - -	- - -	8.5	8.6	11.8	9.2	10.4	10.8	8.9	10.0
65 years and over	- - -	- - -	- - -	18.6	20.5	24.3	24.7	19.2	19.7	21.3	20.1
Hispanic female[5]											
All ages, age adjusted	- - -	- - -	- - -	- - -	8.3	9.2	8.2	8.3	8.5	8.7	8.5
All ages, crude	- - -	- - -	- - -	- - -	7.9	8.9	8.0	8.1	8.3	8.5	8.3
1–14 years	- - -	- - -	- - -	- - -	4.8	4.8	4.1	4.0	4.4	4.7	4.4
15–24 years	- - -	- - -	- - -	- - -	10.1	11.6	10.5	11.8	12.8	11.8	12.1
25–34 years	- - -	- - -	- - -	- - -	7.5	9.4	8.7	9.0	7.7	9.0	8.6
35–44 years	- - -	- - -	- - -	- - -	8.8	8.0	8.5	7.3	8.1	7.7	7.7
45–64 years	- - -	- - -	- - -	- - -	9.4	11.4	8.5	9.1	9.2	9.7	9.3
65 years and over	- - -	- - -	- - -	- - -	14.8	14.9	14.3	13.5	13.9	13.9	13.8

See footnotes at end of table.

Table 46 (page 4 of 4). Death rates for motor vehicle-related injuries, according to sex, detailed race, Hispanic origin, and age: United States, selected years 1950–96

[Data are based on the National Vital Statistics System]

Sex, race, Hispanic origin, and age	1950[1]	1960[1]	1970	1980	1985	1990	1993	1994	1995	1996	1994–96[2]
White, non-Hispanic female[5]					Deaths per 100,000 resident population						
All ages, age adjusted	- - -	- - -	- - -	- - -	10.4	11.1	9.7	10.1	10.3	10.4	10.2
All ages, crude	- - -	- - -	- - -	- - -	10.9	11.7	10.3	10.7	10.9	11.0	10.9
1–14 years	- - -	- - -	- - -	- - -	4.9	4.7	4.1	4.3	4.2	4.2	4.2
15–24 years	- - -	- - -	- - -	- - -	20.2	20.4	17.6	19.0	19.0	18.8	18.9
25–34 years	- - -	- - -	- - -	- - -	9.8	11.7	10.2	9.7	10.6	10.8	10.3
35–44 years	- - -	- - -	- - -	- - -	8.6	9.3	8.0	8.3	8.9	9.3	8.8
45–64 years	- - -	- - -	- - -	- - -	8.6	9.7	8.3	8.7	8.7	9.0	8.8
65 years and over	- - -	- - -	- - -	- - -	15.3	17.5	16.7	17.6	17.7	17.4	17.6

- - - Data not available.

* Based on fewer than 20 deaths.

[1]Includes deaths of persons who were not residents of the 50 States and the District of Columbia.

[2]Average annual death rate.

[3]Interpretation of trends should take into account that population estimates for American Indians increased by 45 percent between 1980 and 1990, partly due to better enumeration techniques in the 1990 decennial census and to the increased tendency for people to identify themselves as American Indian in 1990.

[4]Interpretation of trends should take into account that the Asian population in the United States more than doubled between 1980 and 1990, primarily due to immigration.

[5]Excludes data from States lacking an Hispanic-origin item on their death certificates. See Appendix I, National Vital Statistics System.

NOTES: For data years shown, the code numbers for cause of death are based on the then current *International Classification of Diseases*, which are described in Appendix II, tables IV and V. Age groups were selected to minimize the presentation of unstable age-specific death rates based on small numbers of deaths and for consistency among comparison groups. The race groups, white, black, Asian or Pacific Islander, and American Indian or Alaska Native, include persons of Hispanic and non-Hispanic origin. Conversely, persons of Hispanic origin may be of any race. Consistency of race identification between the death certificate (source of data for numerator of death rates) and data from the Census Bureau (denominator) is high for individual white and black persons; however, persons identified as American Indian, Asian, or Hispanic origin in data from the Census Bureau are sometimes misreported as white or non-Hispanic on the death certificate, causing death rates to be underestimated by 22–30 percent for American Indians, about 12 percent for Asians, and about 7 percent for persons of Hispanic origin. (Sorlie PD, Rogot E, and Johnson NJ: Validity of demographic characteristics on the death certificate, *Epidemiology* 3(2):181–184, 1992.) Recent data for the age group 65 years and over in all population groups have been revised and differ from the previous edition of *Health, United States*.

SOURCES: Centers for Disease Control and Prevention, National Center for Health Statistics. Grove RD and Hetzel AM. *Vital statistics rates in the United States, 1940–60*. Washington: Public Health Service, 1968; *Vital statistics of the United States, vol II, mortality, part A*, for data years 1950–96. Washington: Public Health Service; data computed by the Division of Health and Utilization Analysis from data compiled by the Division of Vital Statistics and from national population estimates for race groups from table 1 and unpublished Hispanic population estimates prepared by the Housing and Household Economic Statistics Division, U.S. Bureau of the Census.

Table 47 (page 1 of 3). Death rates for homicide and legal intervention, according to sex, detailed race, Hispanic origin, and age: United States, selected years 1950–96

[Data are based on the National Vital Statistics System]

Sex, race, Hispanic origin, and age	1950[1]	1960[1]	1970	1980	1985	1990	1993	1994	1995	1996	1994–96[2]
All persons				Deaths per 100,000 resident population							
All ages, age adjusted	5.4	5.2	9.1	10.8	8.3	10.2	10.7	10.3	9.4	8.5	9.3
All ages, crude	5.3	4.7	8.3	10.7	8.4	10.0	10.1	9.6	8.7	7.9	8.7
Under 1 year	4.4	4.8	4.3	5.9	5.4	8.4	8.8	8.1	8.1	8.8	8.3
1–14 years	0.6	0.6	1.1	1.5	1.6	1.8	2.1	2.0	1.9	1.7	1.9
1–4 years	0.6	0.7	1.9	2.5	2.5	2.6	2.9	3.0	2.9	2.7	2.9
5–14 years	0.5	0.5	0.9	1.2	1.2	1.5	1.8	1.5	1.5	1.3	1.4
15–24 years	6.3	5.9	11.7	15.6	11.9	19.9	23.4	22.6	20.3	18.1	20.3
25–44 years	9.3	8.9	15.2	17.6	13.3	14.9	14.3	13.8	12.3	11.1	12.4
25–34 years	9.9	9.7	16.6	19.6	14.8	17.7	17.4	16.7	15.1	13.4	15.1
35–44 years	8.8	8.1	13.7	15.1	11.3	11.8	11.1	10.9	9.7	9.0	9.8
45–64 years	5.2	5.3	8.8	9.1	7.0	6.4	6.1	5.6	5.5	5.2	5.4
45–54 years	6.1	6.2	10.1	11.1	8.1	7.6	7.2	6.5	6.2	5.9	6.2
55–64 years	4.0	4.2	7.1	7.0	5.7	5.0	4.7	4.3	4.5	4.1	4.3
65 years and over	3.0	2.7	4.6	5.6	4.3	4.0	3.7	3.5	3.2	3.0	3.2
65–74 years	3.2	2.8	5.0	5.7	4.3	3.8	3.7	3.4	3.3	3.0	3.2
75–84 years	2.6	2.4	4.0	5.2	4.3	4.3	3.5	3.6	3.1	2.9	3.2
85 years and over	2.3	2.4	4.2	5.3	4.2	4.6	4.1	3.5	3.3	3.0	3.2
Male											
All ages, age adjusted	8.4	7.9	14.9	17.4	12.8	16.3	17.0	16.4	14.7	13.3	14.8
All ages, crude	8.1	7.1	13.4	17.3	13.0	16.2	16.1	15.5	13.8	12.5	13.9
Under 1 year	4.5	4.7	4.5	6.3	5.6	8.8	9.6	9.0	8.9	8.7	8.9
1–14 years	0.6	0.6	1.2	1.6	1.8	2.0	2.5	2.3	2.3	1.9	2.1
1–4 years	0.5	0.7	1.9	2.7	2.5	2.7	3.4	3.3	3.1	2.7	3.0
5–14 years	0.6	0.5	1.0	1.2	1.4	1.7	2.2	1.9	1.9	1.6	1.8
15–24 years	9.6	9.1	19.0	24.5	18.6	32.9	39.2	38.3	33.9	30.4	34.2
25–44 years	14.7	13.6	25.0	29.4	21.0	24.0	22.3	21.7	19.1	17.3	19.4
25–34 years	15.5	14.9	27.6	32.5	23.3	28.3	27.2	26.5	23.7	21.4	23.9
35–44 years	13.8	12.3	22.2	24.9	17.9	19.0	17.2	17.0	14.6	13.5	15.0
45–64 years	8.4	8.3	14.9	15.4	11.1	10.3	9.7	8.9	8.6	8.0	8.5
45–54 years	9.9	9.6	17.0	18.6	12.9	12.1	11.4	10.3	9.6	8.9	9.6
55–64 years	6.5	6.6	12.2	11.9	9.2	8.1	7.4	6.9	7.2	6.6	6.9
65 years and over	4.9	4.3	7.8	8.9	6.2	5.8	5.0	5.0	4.3	4.1	4.5
65–74 years	5.3	4.6	8.6	9.3	6.5	5.8	5.3	5.0	4.6	4.3	4.7
75–84 years	4.0	3.7	6.0	8.1	5.8	5.7	4.5	4.9	3.7	3.8	4.1
85 years and over	2.5	3.6	7.4	7.5	5.0	6.8	5.7	5.6	4.2	3.7	4.5
Female											
All ages, age adjusted	2.5	2.6	3.7	4.5	3.9	4.2	4.5	4.0	4.0	3.6	3.9
All ages, crude	2.4	2.4	3.4	4.5	4.0	4.2	4.3	3.9	3.8	3.5	3.7
Under 1 year	4.2	4.9	4.1	5.6	5.2	8.0	7.9	7.1	7.2	8.9	7.7
1–14 years	0.6	0.5	1.0	1.4	1.4	1.6	1.7	1.6	1.5	1.6	1.5
1–4 years	0.7	0.7	1.9	2.2	2.4	2.4	2.5	2.7	2.6	2.7	2.7
5–14 years	0.5	0.4	0.7	1.1	1.0	1.2	1.4	1.2	1.0	1.1	1.1
15–24 years	3.1	2.8	4.6	6.6	5.1	6.3	6.9	6.2	6.0	5.1	5.8
25–44 years	4.2	4.3	5.9	6.4	5.7	6.0	6.4	5.8	5.7	5.0	5.5
25–34 years	4.5	4.6	6.0	7.0	6.4	7.2	7.6	6.8	6.5	5.5	6.3
35–44 years	3.8	4.1	5.7	5.7	4.9	4.8	5.2	4.9	4.9	4.5	4.8
45–64 years	1.9	2.5	3.1	3.4	3.2	2.8	2.7	2.5	2.6	2.5	2.5
45–54 years	2.3	2.9	3.7	4.1	3.7	3.2	3.1	2.8	3.0	3.0	2.9
55–64 years	1.4	2.0	2.5	2.8	2.7	2.3	2.2	2.0	2.1	1.9	2.0
65 years and over	1.4	1.3	2.3	3.3	3.0	2.8	2.8	2.4	2.4	2.1	2.3
65–74 years	1.3	1.3	2.2	3.0	2.6	2.2	2.5	2.1	2.2	1.9	2.0
75–84 years	1.4	1.3	2.7	3.5	3.4	3.4	3.0	2.7	2.7	2.4	2.6
85 years and over	2.1	1.6	2.5	4.3	3.8	3.8	3.4	2.6	2.9	2.7	2.8
White male											
All ages, age adjusted	3.9	3.9	7.3	10.9	8.1	8.9	8.9	8.8	8.2	7.3	8.1
All ages, crude	3.9	3.6	6.8	10.9	8.2	9.0	8.6	8.5	7.8	7.0	7.8
Under 1 year	4.3	3.8	2.9	4.3	3.8	6.4	7.0	6.0	7.1	6.5	6.6
1–14 years	0.4	0.5	0.7	1.2	1.3	1.3	1.6	1.5	1.5	1.4	1.5
15–24 years	3.7	4.4	7.9	15.5	11.0	15.4	17.1	17.4	16.5	14.0	16.0
25–44 years	5.9	5.9	12.0	17.4	12.9	13.3	12.3	12.3	11.0	9.9	11.1
25–34 years	5.4	6.2	13.0	18.9	14.0	15.1	14.4	14.3	12.9	11.5	12.9
35–44 years	6.4	5.5	11.0	15.5	11.5	11.4	10.1	10.4	9.2	8.4	9.3
45–64 years	5.0	4.7	8.4	9.9	7.5	7.0	6.7	6.3	5.8	5.5	5.8
65 years and over	3.9	3.2	5.5	6.7	4.5	4.1	3.5	3.6	3.0	3.2	3.3

See footnotes at end of table.

[Data are based on the National Vital Statistics System]

Sex, race, Hispanic origin, and age	1950[1]	1960[1]	1970	1980	1985	1990	1993	1994	1995	1996	1994–96[2]
Black male				Deaths per 100,000 resident population							
All ages, age adjusted	51.1	44.9	82.1	71.9	50.2	68.7	70.7	66.2	57.6	52.6	58.8
All ages, crude	47.3	36.6	67.6	66.6	49.0	69.2	69.7	65.1	56.3	51.5	57.5
Under 1 year	- - -	10.3	14.3	18.6	16.7	21.4	23.9	23.9	19.4	23.1	22.1
1–14 years	- - -	1.5	4.4	4.1	4.2	5.8	7.5	6.4	6.1	4.8	5.8
15–24 years	58.9	46.4	102.5	84.3	65.9	138.3	167.0	157.6	132.0	123.1	137.4
25–44 years	97.8	84.9	143.3	130.1	87.5	106.2	96.0	90.9	77.9	71.0	79.8
25–34 years	110.5	92.0	158.5	145.1	95.6	125.4	116.5	112.1	98.3	89.5	100.0
35–44 years	83.7	77.5	126.2	110.3	74.9	82.3	72.6	67.6	56.2	52.0	58.5
45–64 years	47.6	45.4	83.0	70.8	46.3	41.7	38.3	33.4	34.6	30.5	32.8
65 years and over	16.7	17.9	33.7	31.1	26.2	25.9	24.2	22.1	19.9	15.6	19.2
American Indian or Alaska Native male[3]											
All ages, age adjusted	- - -	- - -	- - -	23.9	20.0	17.5	17.0	18.4	18.0	15.7	17.3
All ages, crude	- - -	- - -	- - -	23.4	19.0	17.3	16.9	18.3	17.8	15.3	17.1
15–24 years	- - -	- - -	- - -	36.0	27.1	27.7	24.4	32.5	32.2	26.6	30.4
25–44 years	- - -	- - -	- - -	39.7	30.2	26.0	28.0	27.9	28.4	23.6	26.6
45–64 years	- - -	- - -	- - -	22.1	21.2	15.5	15.3	*	13.2	12.7	12.5
Asian or Pacific Islander male[4]											
All ages, age adjusted	- - -	- - -	- - -	8.5	5.8	7.7	9.9	8.5	8.3	7.3	8.0
All ages, crude	- - -	- - -	- - -	8.3	6.0	7.9	9.9	8.5	8.0	7.2	7.9
15–24 years	- - -	- - -	- - -	9.3	8.6	14.9	23.3	19.6	19.4	15.6	18.2
25–44 years	- - -	- - -	- - -	11.3	8.9	9.7	11.3	9.9	8.1	8.4	8.8
45–64 years	- - -	- - -	- - -	10.4	5.4	7.0	7.6	6.3	8.4	7.6	7.4
Hispanic male[5]											
All ages, age adjusted	- - -	- - -	- - -	- - -	26.7	29.8	28.4	27.3	25.1	20.4	24.1
All ages, crude	- - -	- - -	- - -	- - -	27.6	31.5	28.9	27.8	25.2	20.9	24.5
Under 1 year	- - -	- - -	- - -	- - -	*	8.7	6.8	7.9	5.9	6.4	6.8
1–14 years	- - -	- - -	- - -	- - -	1.5	3.1	3.1	2.9	3.3	2.5	2.9
15–24 years	- - -	- - -	- - -	- - -	42.9	56.2	63.9	64.0	63.5	48.9	58.4
25–44 years	- - -	- - -	- - -	- - -	47.3	47.2	38.6	37.1	31.7	26.4	31.6
25–34 years	- - -	- - -	- - -	- - -	51.4	51.9	43.3	43.2	37.1	31.2	37.0
35–44 years	- - -	- - -	- - -	- - -	40.1	39.9	31.8	28.7	24.2	20.2	24.2
45–64 years	- - -	- - -	- - -	- - -	19.9	20.9	19.7	17.4	14.8	13.9	15.3
65 years and over	- - -	- - -	- - -	- - -	9.3	9.4	9.1	7.1	5.5	4.0	5.5
White, non-Hispanic male[5]											
All ages, age adjusted	- - -	- - -	- - -	- - -	6.2	5.8	5.6	5.7	5.1	4.7	5.2
All ages, crude	- - -	- - -	- - -	- - -	6.4	6.0	5.6	5.7	5.1	4.7	5.2
Under 1 year	- - -	- - -	- - -	- - -	4.6	5.4	6.7	5.4	6.7	6.4	6.2
1–14 years	- - -	- - -	- - -	- - -	1.2	0.9	1.2	1.1	1.1	1.1	1.1
15–24 years	- - -	- - -	- - -	- - -	7.7	7.7	8.0	8.3	7.3	6.4	7.3
25–44 years	- - -	- - -	- - -	- - -	9.5	9.0	8.2	8.5	7.6	6.9	7.6
25–34 years	- - -	- - -	- - -	- - -	9.6	9.6	9.1	9.0	8.2	7.3	8.2
35–44 years	- - -	- - -	- - -	- - -	9.3	8.3	7.2	7.9	7.1	6.6	7.2
45–64 years	- - -	- - -	- - -	- - -	6.4	5.8	5.5	5.2	4.8	4.6	4.9
65 years and over	- - -	- - -	- - -	- - -	4.4	3.7	3.1	3.4	2.7	3.1	3.0
White female											
All ages, age adjusted	1.4	1.5	2.2	3.2	2.9	2.8	3.0	2.7	2.8	2.5	2.7
All ages, crude	1.4	1.4	2.1	3.2	2.9	2.8	3.0	2.6	2.7	2.5	2.6
Under 1 year	3.9	3.5	2.9	4.3	4.3	5.1	5.9	5.1	5.0	6.8	5.7
1–14 years	0.4	0.4	0.7	1.1	1.1	1.0	1.1	1.1	1.1	1.1	1.1
15–24 years	1.3	1.5	2.7	4.7	3.6	4.0	4.2	3.9	4.0	3.3	3.7
25–44 years	2.0	2.1	3.3	4.2	4.1	3.8	4.2	3.7	3.8	3.3	3.6
45–64 years	1.5	1.7	2.1	2.6	2.6	2.3	2.2	1.9	2.2	2.1	2.1
65 years and over	1.2	1.2	1.9	2.9	2.6	2.2	2.3	1.9	2.0	1.8	1.9

See footnotes at end of table.

Table 47 (page 3 of 3). Death rates for homicide and legal intervention, according to sex, detailed race, Hispanic origin, and age: United States, selected years 1950–96

[Data are based on the National Vital Statistics System]

Sex, race, Hispanic origin, and age	1950[1]	1960[1]	1970	1980	1985	1990	1993	1994	1995	1996	1994–96[2]
Black female				Deaths per 100,000 resident population							
All ages, age adjusted	11.7	11.8	15.0	13.7	10.9	13.0	13.4	12.3	11.0	10.2	11.2
All ages, crude	11.5	10.4	13.3	13.5	11.1	13.5	13.6	12.4	11.1	10.2	11.2
Under 1 year.	- - -	13.8	10.7	12.8	10.7	22.8	18.1	17.4	19.2	21.1	19.2
1–14 years	- - -	1.2	3.1	3.3	3.3	4.7	4.9	4.1	3.6	3.9	3.9
15–24 years	16.5	11.9	17.7	18.4	14.2	18.9	22.0	18.7	16.8	14.7	16.7
25–44 years	22.5	22.8	25.4	22.3	17.8	20.9	20.6	19.5	17.4	15.8	17.5
45–64 years	6.8	10.3	13.4	10.8	7.9	6.5	6.3	6.6	5.9	6.0	6.2
65 years and over	3.6	3.0	7.4	8.0	7.8	9.5	8.5	7.4	6.9	5.2	6.5
American Indian or Alaska Native female[3]											
All ages, age adjusted	- - -	- - -	- - -	8.3	4.8	4.9	5.1	5.4	5.6	4.5	5.2
All ages, crude	- - -	- - -	- - -	7.7	4.5	4.9	5.2	5.6	5.6	4.4	5.2
15–24 years	- - -	- - -	- - -	*	*	*	*	*	*	*	5.3
25–44 years	- - -	- - -	- - -	13.7	*	6.9	9.6	8.9	9.1	*	7.5
45–64 years	- - -	- - -	- - -	*	*	*	*	*	*	*	4.0
Asian or Pacific Islander female[4]											
All ages, age adjusted	- - -	- - -	- - -	3.0	2.7	2.7	2.9	2.4	2.6	2.1	2.4
All ages, crude	- - -	- - -	- - -	3.1	2.8	2.8	3.0	2.4	2.7	2.1	2.4
15–24 years	- - -	- - -	- - -	*	*	*	3.5	3.7	3.7	3.7	3.7
25–44 years	- - -	- - -	- - -	4.6	2.9	3.8	3.9	2.6	3.8	2.1	2.8
45–64 years	- - -	- - -	- - -	*	*	*	3.4	2.4	2.3	*	2.0
Hispanic female[5]											
All ages, age adjusted	- - -	- - -	- - -	- - -	4.2	4.6	4.8	4.2	4.4	3.4	4.0
All ages, crude	- - -	- - -	- - -	- - -	4.3	4.7	4.9	4.2	4.3	3.5	4.0
Under 1 year.	- - -	- - -	- - -	- - -	*	*	8.9	7.1	*	7.7	6.8
1–14 years	- - -	- - -	- - -	- - -	1.5	1.9	1.8	1.9	1.8	1.5	1.7
15–24 years	- - -	- - -	- - -	- - -	5.7	8.1	7.8	6.5	6.9	5.1	6.1
25–44 years	- - -	- - -	- - -	- - -	6.8	6.1	6.8	5.8	5.8	4.8	5.5
45–64 years	- - -	- - -	- - -	- - -	3.2	3.3	3.3	3.0	3.4	2.7	3.1
65 years and over	- - -	- - -	- - -	- - -	*	*	2.6	*	2.3	*	1.8
White, non-Hispanic female[5]											
All ages, age adjusted	- - -	- - -	- - -	- - -	2.8	2.5	2.6	2.4	2.4	2.2	2.4
All ages, crude	- - -	- - -	- - -	- - -	2.9	2.6	2.6	2.4	2.4	2.3	2.3
Under 1 year.	- - -	- - -	- - -	- - -	4.1	4.4	4.9	4.5	4.4	6.0	5.0
1–14 years	- - -	- - -	- - -	- - -	1.0	0.8	0.9	1.0	0.9	1.0	0.9
15–24 years	- - -	- - -	- - -	- - -	3.5	3.3	3.5	3.4	3.4	2.7	3.2
25–44 years	- - -	- - -	- - -	- - -	3.9	3.5	3.7	3.4	3.3	3.1	3.2
45–64 years	- - -	- - -	- - -	- - -	2.6	2.2	2.1	1.8	1.9	2.0	1.9
65 years and over	- - -	- - -	- - -	- - -	3.0	2.2	2.2	1.9	2.0	1.9	1.9

- - - Data not available.

* Based on fewer than 20 deaths.

[1]Includes deaths of persons who were not residents of the 50 States and the District of Columbia.

[2]Average annual death rate.

[3]Interpretation of trends should take into account that population estimates for American Indians increased by 45 percent between 1980 and 1990, partly due to better enumeration techniques in the 1990 decennial census and to the increased tendency for people to identify themselves as American Indian in 1990.

[4]Interpretation of trends should take into account that the Asian population in the United States more than doubled between 1980 and 1990, primarily due to immigration.

[5]Excludes data from States lacking an Hispanic-origin item on their death certificates. See Appendix I, National Vital Statistics System.

NOTES: For data years shown, the code numbers for cause of death are based on the then current *International Classification of Diseases*, which are described in Appendix II, tables IV and V. Age groups were selected to minimize the presentation of unstable age-specific death rates based on small numbers of deaths and for consistency among comparison groups. The race groups, white, black, Asian or Pacific Islander, and American Indian or Alaska Native, include persons of Hispanic and non-Hispanic origin. Conversely, persons of Hispanic origin may be of any race. Consistency of race identification between the death certificate (source of data for numerator of death rates) and data from the Census Bureau (denominator) is high for individual white and black persons; however, persons identified as American Indian, Asian, or Hispanic origin in data from the Census Bureau are sometimes misreported as white or non-Hispanic on the death certificate, causing death rates to be underestimated by 22–30 percent for American Indians, about 12 percent for Asians, and about 7 percent for persons of Hispanic origin. (Sorlie PD, Rogot E, and Johnson NJ: Validity of demographic characteristics on the death certificate, *Epidemiology* 3(2):181–184, 1992.)

SOURCES: Centers for Disease Control and Prevention, National Center for Health Statistics. Grove RD and Hetzel AM. *Vital statistics rates in the United States, 1940–60.* Washington: Public Health Service, 1968; *Vital statistics of the United States, vol II, mortality, part A,* for data years 1950–96. Washington: Public Health Service; data computed by the Division of Health and Utilization Analysis from data compiled by the Division of Vital Statistics and from national population estimates for race groups from table 1 and unpublished Hispanic population estimates prepared by the Housing and Household Economic Statistics Division, U.S. Bureau of the Census.

Table 48 (page 1 of 3). Death rates for suicide, according to sex, detailed race, Hispanic origin, and age: United States, selected years 1950–96

[Data are based on the National Vital Statistics System]

Sex, race, Hispanic origin, and age	1950[1]	1960[1]	1970	1980	1985	1990	1993	1994	1995	1996	1994–96[2]
All persons			Deaths per 100,000 resident population								
All ages, age adjusted	11.0	10.6	11.8	11.4	11.5	11.5	11.3	11.2	11.2	10.8	11.0
All ages, crude	11.4	10.6	11.6	11.9	12.4	12.4	12.1	12.0	11.9	11.6	11.8
Under 1 year.	. . .	. . .	. . .	. . .	. . .	. . .	. . .	. . .	. . .	. . .	. . .
1–4 years	. . .	. . .	. . .	. . .	. . .	. . .	. . .	. . .	. . .	. . .	. . .
5–14 years	0.2	0.3	0.3	0.4	0.8	0.8	0.9	0.9	0.9	0.8	0.8
15–24 years	4.5	5.2	8.8	12.3	12.8	13.2	13.5	13.8	13.3	12.0	13.0
25–44 years	11.6	12.2	15.4	15.6	15.0	15.2	15.1	15.3	15.3	15.0	15.2
25–34 years.	9.1	10.0	14.1	16.0	15.3	15.2	15.1	15.4	15.4	14.5	15.1
35–44 years.	14.3	14.2	16.9	15.4	14.6	15.3	15.1	15.3	15.2	15.5	15.4
45–64 years	23.5	22.0	20.6	15.9	16.3	15.3	14.6	14.0	14.1	14.4	14.2
45–54 years.	20.9	20.7	20.0	15.9	15.7	14.8	14.5	14.4	14.6	14.9	14.6
55–64 years.	27.0	23.7	21.4	15.9	16.8	16.0	14.6	13.4	13.3	13.7	13.4
65 years and over	30.0	24.5	20.8	17.6	20.4	20.5	18.9	18.1	18.1	17.3	17.8
65–74 years.	29.3	23.0	20.8	16.9	18.7	17.9	16.3	15.3	15.8	15.0	15.4
75–84 years.	31.1	27.9	21.2	19.1	23.9	24.9	22.3	21.3	20.7	20.0	20.7
85 years and over	28.8	26.0	19.0	19.2	19.4	22.2	22.8	23.0	21.6	20.2	21.6
Male											
All ages, age adjusted	17.3	16.6	17.3	18.0	18.8	19.0	18.7	18.7	18.6	18.0	18.4
All ages, crude	17.8	16.5	16.8	18.6	20.0	20.4	19.9	19.8	19.8	19.3	19.6
Under 1 year.	. . .	. . .	. . .	. . .	. . .	. . .	. . .	. . .	. . .	. . .	. . .
1–4 years	. . .	. . .	. . .	. . .	. . .	. . .	. . .	. . .	. . .	. . .	. . .
5–14 years	0.3	0.4	0.5	0.6	1.2	1.1	1.2	1.2	1.3	1.1	1.2
15–24 years	6.5	8.2	13.5	20.2	21.0	22.0	22.4	23.4	22.5	20.0	22.0
25–44 years	17.2	17.9	20.9	24.0	23.7	24.4	24.4	24.8	24.9	24.3	24.7
25–34 years.	13.4	14.7	19.8	25.0	24.7	24.8	24.9	25.6	25.6	24.0	25.1
35–44 years.	21.3	21.0	22.1	22.5	22.3	23.9	24.0	24.1	24.1	24.6	24.3
45–64 years	37.1	34.4	30.0	23.7	25.3	24.3	23.0	22.1	22.5	23.0	22.6
45–54 years.	32.0	31.6	27.9	22.9	23.6	23.2	22.4	22.1	22.8	23.3	22.8
55–64 years.	43.6	38.1	32.7	24.5	27.1	25.7	23.9	22.0	22.0	22.7	22.2
65 years and over	52.8	44.0	38.4	35.0	40.9	41.6	38.2	36.6	36.3	35.2	36.0
65–74 years.	50.5	39.6	36.0	30.4	33.9	32.2	29.4	27.7	28.7	27.7	28.0
75–84 years.	58.3	52.5	42.8	42.3	53.1	56.1	48.9	47.0	44.8	43.4	45.0
85 years and over	58.3	57.4	42.4	50.6	56.2	65.9	68.3	66.6	63.1	59.9	63.1
Female											
All ages, age adjusted	4.9	5.0	6.8	5.4	4.9	4.5	4.3	4.2	4.1	4.0	4.1
All ages, crude	5.1	4.9	6.6	5.5	5.2	4.8	4.6	4.5	4.4	4.4	4.4
Under 1 year.	. . .	. . .	. . .	. . .	. . .	. . .	. . .	. . .	. . .	. . .	. . .
1–4 years	. . .	. . .	. . .	. . .	. . .	. . .	. . .	. . .	. . .	. . .	. . .
5–14 years	0.1	0.1	0.2	0.2	0.4	0.4	0.5	0.5	0.4	0.4	0.4
15–24 years	2.6	2.2	4.2	4.3	4.3	3.9	4.1	3.7	3.7	3.6	3.7
25–44 years	6.2	6.6	10.2	7.7	6.5	6.2	5.8	5.9	5.8	5.8	5.9
25–34 years.	4.9	5.5	8.6	7.1	5.9	5.6	5.2	5.1	5.2	5.0	5.1
35–44 years.	7.5	7.7	11.9	8.5	7.1	6.8	6.5	6.7	6.5	6.6	6.6
45–64 years	9.9	10.2	12.0	8.9	8.0	7.1	6.7	6.4	6.1	6.4	6.3
45–54 years.	9.9	10.2	12.6	9.4	8.3	6.9	7.1	7.0	6.7	7.0	6.9
55–64 years.	9.9	10.2	11.4	8.4	7.8	7.3	6.3	5.6	5.3	5.5	5.5
65 years and over	9.4	8.4	8.1	6.1	6.6	6.4	5.8	5.5	5.5	4.8	5.2
65–74 years.	10.1	8.4	9.0	6.5	6.9	6.7	5.9	5.4	5.4	4.8	5.2
75–84 years.	8.1	8.9	7.0	5.5	6.7	6.3	5.8	5.3	5.5	5.0	5.2
85 years and over	8.2	6.0	5.9	5.5	4.7	5.4	5.4	6.2	5.5	4.4	5.3
White male											
All ages, age adjusted	18.1	17.5	18.2	18.9	19.9	20.1	19.7	19.7	19.7	19.1	19.5
All ages, crude	19.0	17.6	18.0	19.9	21.6	22.0	21.4	21.3	21.4	20.9	21.2
15–24 years	6.6	8.6	13.9	21.4	22.3	23.2	23.1	24.1	23.5	20.9	22.8
25–44 years	17.9	18.5	21.5	24.6	24.8	25.4	25.7	26.1	26.3	25.7	26.0
45–64 years	39.3	36.5	31.9	25.0	27.0	26.0	24.6	23.8	24.2	24.9	24.3
65 years and over	55.8	46.7	41.1	37.2	43.7	44.2	40.9	38.9	38.7	37.8	38.4
65–74 years.	53.2	42.0	38.7	32.5	35.8	34.2	31.4	29.3	30.3	29.6	29.8
75–84 years.	61.9	55.7	45.5	45.5	57.0	60.2	52.1	50.0	47.5	46.1	47.8
85 years and over	61.9	61.3	45.8	52.8	60.9	70.3	73.6	71.4	68.2	65.4	68.2

See footnotes at end of table.

Table 48 (page 2 of 3). **Death rates for suicide, according to sex, detailed race, Hispanic origin, and age: United States, selected years 1950–96**

[Data are based on the National Vital Statistics System]

Sex, race, Hispanic origin, and age	1950[1]	1960[1]	1970	1980	1985	1990	1993	1994	1995	1996	1994–96[2]
Black male					Deaths per 100,000 resident population						
All ages, age adjusted	7.0	7.8	9.9	11.1	11.5	12.4	12.9	12.7	12.4	11.8	12.3
All ages, crude	6.3	6.4	8.0	10.3	11.0	12.0	12.5	12.4	11.9	11.4	11.9
15–24 years	4.9	4.1	10.5	12.3	13.3	15.1	20.1	20.6	18.0	16.7	18.4
25–44 years	9.8	12.6	16.1	19.2	17.8	19.6	19.0	18.9	18.6	17.8	18.4
45–64 years	12.7	13.0	12.4	11.8	12.9	13.1	12.3	10.3	11.8	11.8	11.3
65 years and over	9.0	9.9	8.7	11.4	15.8	14.9	13.2	15.4	14.3	12.6	14.1
65–74 years	10.0	11.3	8.7	11.1	16.7	14.7	11.7	15.0	13.5	12.7	13.8
75–84 years	- - -	6.6	8.9	10.5	15.6	14.4	16.3	14.9	16.6	12.5	14.7
85 years and over	- - -	6.9	*	*	*	*	*	*	*	*	14.6
American Indian or Alaska Native male[3]											
All ages, age adjusted	- - -	- - -	- - -	20.8	19.9	21.0	18.7	23.8	20.1	20.0	21.3
All ages, crude	- - -	- - -	- - -	20.9	20.3	20.9	18.4	23.3	19.6	19.9	20.9
15–24 years	- - -	- - -	- - -	45.3	42.0	49.1	31.6	45.8	34.2	32.1	37.3
25–44 years	- - -	- - -	- - -	31.2	30.2	27.8	30.9	38.4	31.8	34.8	35.0
45–64 years	- - -	- - -	- - -	*	*	*	12.8	14.8	15.0	11.5	13.7
65 years and over	- - -	- - -	- - -	*	*	*	*	*	*	*	11.8
Asian or Pacific Islander male[4]											
All ages, age adjusted	- - -	- - -	- - -	9.0	8.5	8.8	9.2	9.7	9.7	8.6	9.3
All ages, crude	- - -	- - -	- - -	8.8	8.4	8.7	9.1	9.6	9.4	8.6	9.2
15–24 years	- - -	- - -	- - -	10.8	14.2	13.5	12.7	15.1	16.0	11.9	14.3
25–44 years	- - -	- - -	- - -	11.0	9.3	10.6	11.3	12.7	11.5	11.5	11.9
45–64 years	- - -	- - -	- - -	13.0	10.4	9.7	10.3	9.1	9.1	8.6	8.9
65 years and over	- - -	- - -	- - -	18.6	16.7	16.8	19.1	18.3	20.3	16.0	18.1
Hispanic male[5]											
All ages, age adjusted	- - -	- - -	- - -	- - -	10.4	12.4	12.6	12.5	12.3	11.1	11.9
All ages, crude	- - -	- - -	- - -	- - -	9.8	11.4	11.9	11.8	11.5	10.6	11.2
15–24 years	- - -	- - -	- - -	- - -	13.8	14.7	18.2	18.7	18.3	15.5	17.4
25–44 years	- - -	- - -	- - -	- - -	14.8	16.2	16.6	16.8	15.5	14.6	15.6
45–64 years	- - -	- - -	- - -	- - -	12.3	16.1	13.8	13.6	14.2	13.3	13.7
65 years and over	- - -	- - -	- - -	- - -	14.7	23.4	22.3	17.8	19.9	17.7	18.5
White, non-Hispanic male[5]											
All ages, age adjusted	- - -	- - -	- - -	- - -	20.3	20.8	20.0	20.1	20.2	19.7	20.0
All ages, crude	- - -	- - -	- - -	- - -	22.3	23.1	22.2	22.2	22.3	22.0	22.2
15–24 years	- - -	- - -	- - -	- - -	22.6	24.4	23.5	24.4	23.8	21.4	23.2
25–44 years	- - -	- - -	- - -	- - -	25.1	26.4	26.3	26.9	27.3	27.1	27.1
45–64 years	- - -	- - -	- - -	- - -	27.3	26.8	25.0	24.4	24.8	25.6	24.9
65 years and over	- - -	- - -	- - -	- - -	46.4	45.4	41.1	39.7	39.2	38.6	39.2
White female											
All ages, age adjusted	5.3	5.3	7.2	5.7	5.3	4.8	4.6	4.5	4.4	4.4	4.4
All ages, crude	5.5	5.3	7.1	5.9	5.6	5.3	5.0	4.9	4.8	4.8	4.8
15–24 years	2.7	2.3	4.2	4.6	4.7	4.2	4.3	3.8	3.9	3.8	3.8
25–44 years	6.6	7.0	11.0	8.1	7.0	6.6	6.3	6.5	6.3	6.4	6.4
45–64 years	10.6	10.9	13.0	9.6	8.7	7.7	7.4	7.0	6.7	7.0	6.9
65 years and over	9.9	8.8	8.5	6.4	6.9	6.8	6.1	5.8	5.7	5.0	5.5

See footnotes at end of table.

Table 48 (page 3 of 3). **Death rates for suicide, according to sex, detailed race, Hispanic origin, and age: United States, selected years 1950–96**

[Data are based on the National Vital Statistics System]

Sex, race, Hispanic origin, and age	1950[1]	1960[1]	1970	1980	1985	1990	1993	1994	1995	1996	1994–96[2]
Black female					Deaths per 100,000 resident population						
All ages, age adjusted	1.7	1.9	2.9	2.4	2.1	2.4	2.1	2.1	2.0	2.0	2.0
All ages, crude	1.5	1.6	2.6	2.2	2.1	2.3	2.1	2.0	2.0	2.0	2.0
15–24 years	1.8	*	3.8	2.3	2.0	2.3	2.7	2.7	2.2	2.3	2.4
25–44 years	2.3	3.0	4.8	4.3	3.2	3.8	3.1	3.1	3.4	2.9	3.1
45–64 years	2.7	3.1	2.9	2.5	2.8	2.9	2.4	2.3	2.0	2.3	2.2
65 years and over	2.0	1.9	2.6	*	2.7	1.9	2.3	2.0	2.2	2.1	2.1
American Indian or Alaska Native female[3]											
All ages, age adjusted	- - -	- - -	- - -	5.0	4.4	3.8	5.5	4.3	4.4	5.9	4.9
All ages, crude	- - -	- - -	- - -	4.7	4.4	3.7	5.3	4.0	4.2	5.6	4.6
15–24 years	- - -	- - -	- - -	*	*	*	10.9	*	*	10.2	7.7
25–44 years	- - -	- - -	- - -	10.7	*	*	7.0	*	7.1	9.0	7.1
45–64 years	- - -	- - -	- - -	*	*	*	*	*	*	*	4.9
65 years and over	- - -	- - -	- - -	*	*	*	*	*	*	*	*
Asian or Pacific Islander female[4]											
All ages, age adjusted	- - -	- - -	- - -	4.7	4.4	3.4	3.8	3.8	3.7	3.6	3.7
All ages, crude	- - -	- - -	- - -	4.7	4.3	3.4	3.9	3.9	3.8	3.7	3.8
15–24 years	- - -	- - -	- - -	*	5.8	3.9	5.0	5.7	5.2	3.0	4.6
25–44 years	- - -	- - -	- - -	5.4	4.2	3.8	4.5	4.2	3.8	4.5	4.2
45–64 years	- - -	- - -	- - -	7.9	5.4	5.0	4.6	5.4	4.9	5.2	5.1
65 years and over	- - -	- - -	- - -	*	13.6	8.5	8.9	6.8	9.0	8.4	8.1
Hispanic female[5]											
All ages, age adjusted	- - -	- - -	- - -	- - -	1.8	2.3	2.1	1.9	2.0	2.2	2.1
All ages, crude	- - -	- - -	- - -	- - -	1.6	2.2	2.0	1.8	1.9	2.1	1.9
15–24 years	- - -	- - -	- - -	- - -	2.1	3.1	2.9	2.8	2.6	3.3	2.9
25–44 years	- - -	- - -	- - -	- - -	2.1	3.1	2.6	2.6	2.7	2.8	2.7
45–64 years	- - -	- - -	- - -	- - -	3.2	2.5	2.2	2.1	2.7	2.6	2.5
65 years and over	- - -	- - -	- - -	- - -	*	*	*	2.4	*	2.5	2.4
White, non-Hispanic female[5]											
All ages, age adjusted	- - -	- - -	- - -	- - -	5.7	5.0	4.8	4.7	4.6	4.5	4.6
All ages, crude	- - -	- - -	- - -	- - -	6.2	5.6	5.3	5.2	5.1	5.0	5.1
15–24 years	- - -	- - -	- - -	- - -	4.7	4.3	4.4	3.9	4.0	3.8	3.9
25–44 years	- - -	- - -	- - -	- - -	7.7	7.0	6.6	6.9	6.7	6.7	6.8
45–64 years	- - -	- - -	- - -	- - -	9.2	8.0	7.6	7.3	7.0	7.3	7.2
65 years and over	- - -	- - -	- - -	- - -	7.5	7.0	6.2	5.9	5.8	5.1	5.6

. . . Category not applicable.

- - - Data not available.

* Based on fewer than 20 deaths.

[1] Includes deaths of persons who were not residents of the 50 States and the District of Columbia.

[2] Average annual death rate.

[3] Interpretation of trends should take into account that population estimates for American Indians increased by 45 percent between 1980 and 1990, partly due to better enumeration techniques in the 1990 decennial census and to the increased tendency for people to identify themselves as American Indian in 1990.

[4] Interpretation of trends should take into account that the Asian population in the United States more than doubled between 1980 and 1990, primarily due to immigration.

[5] Excludes data from States lacking an Hispanic-origin item on their death certificates. See Appendix I, National Vital Statistics System.

NOTES: For data years shown, the code numbers for cause of death are based on the then current *International Classification of Diseases*, which are described in Appendix II, tables IV and V. Age groups chosen to show data for American Indians, Asians, Hispanics, and non-Hispanic whites were selected to minimize the presentation of unstable age-specific death rates based on small numbers of deaths and for consistency among comparison groups. The race groups, white, black, Asian or Pacific Islander, and American Indian or Alaska Native, include persons of Hispanic and non-Hispanic origin. Conversely, persons of Hispanic origin may be of any race. Consistency of race identification between the death certificate (source of data for numerator of death rates) and data from the Census Bureau (denominator) is high for individual white and black persons; however, persons identified as American Indian, Asian, or Hispanic origin in data from the Census Bureau are sometimes misreported as white or non-Hispanic on the death certificate, causing death rates to be underestimated by 22–30 percent for American Indians, about 12 percent for Asians, and about 7 percent for persons of Hispanic origin. (Sorlie PD, Rogot E, and Johnson NJ: Validity of demographic characteristics on the death certificate, *Epidemiology* 3(2):181–184, 1992.)

SOURCES: Centers for Disease Control and Prevention, National Center for Health Statistics. Grove RD and Hetzel AM. *Vital statistics rates in the United States, 1940–60.* Washington: Public Health Service, 1968; *Vital statistics of the United States, vol II, mortality, part A,* for data years 1950–96. Washington: Public Health Service; data computed by the Division of Health and Utilization Analysis from data compiled by the Division of Vital Statistics and from national population estimates for race groups from table 1 and unpublished Hispanic population estimates prepared by the Housing and Household Economic Statistics Division, U.S. Bureau of the Census.

Table 49 (page 1 of 3). Death rates for firearm-related injuries, according to sex, detailed race, Hispanic origin, and age: United States, selected years 1970–96

[Data are based on the National Vital Statistics System]

Sex, race, Hispanic origin, and age	1970	1980	1985	1988	1990	1992	1993	1994	1995	1996	1994–96[1]
All persons					Deaths per 100,000 resident population						
All ages, age adjusted	14.0	14.8	12.8	13.4	14.6	14.9	15.6	15.1	13.9	12.9	14.0
All ages, crude	13.0	14.9	13.3	13.9	14.9	14.8	15.4	14.8	13.7	12.8	13.8
Under 1 year	*	*	*	*	*	*	*	*	*	*	0.3
1–14 years	1.6	1.4	1.4	1.5	1.5	1.7	1.8	1.6	1.6	1.3	1.5
1–4 years	1.0	0.7	0.7	0.6	0.6	0.7	0.6	0.6	0.6	0.5	0.6
5–14 years	1.7	1.6	1.8	1.9	1.9	2.1	2.3	2.0	2.0	1.6	1.9
15–24 years	15.5	20.6	17.2	20.6	25.8	29.1	31.1	30.8	27.2	24.2	27.4
25–44 years	20.9	22.5	17.9	18.3	19.3	18.6	19.3	18.8	17.2	16.1	17.4
25–34 years	22.2	24.3	19.3	20.4	21.8	21.3	22.4	21.9	20.1	18.3	20.1
35–44 years	19.6	20.0	16.0	15.8	16.3	15.6	16.0	15.6	14.4	14.0	14.7
45–64 years	17.6	15.2	14.3	13.4	13.6	13.0	13.2	12.2	11.8	11.9	12.0
45–54 years	18.1	16.4	14.7	13.5	13.9	13.3	13.7	12.8	12.1	12.3	12.4
55–64 years	17.0	13.9	13.9	13.3	13.3	12.5	12.5	11.4	11.4	11.2	11.3
65 years and over	13.8	13.5	15.6	16.2	16.0	14.8	15.1	14.3	14.2	13.9	14.1
65–74 years	14.5	13.8	15.1	14.9	14.4	13.6	13.5	12.6	12.9	12.6	12.7
75–84 years	13.4	13.4	17.7	19.3	19.4	17.2	17.7	16.9	16.4	15.9	16.4
85 years and over	10.2	11.6	12.2	13.6	14.7	14.4	15.4	15.1	14.6	14.5	14.7
Male											
All ages, age adjusted	23.8	25.3	21.9	23.0	25.4	25.9	26.9	26.2	24.1	22.4	24.2
All ages, crude	22.2	25.7	22.8	24.1	26.2	26.0	26.8	26.0	23.9	22.5	24.1
Under 1 year	*	*	*	*	*	*	*	*	*	*	*
1–14 years	2.3	2.0	2.1	2.2	2.2	2.5	2.6	2.3	2.3	1.8	2.1
1–4 years	1.2	0.9	0.8	0.8	0.7	0.8	0.8	0.7	0.8	0.5	0.7
5–14 years	2.7	2.5	2.7	2.8	2.9	3.2	3.4	3.0	2.9	2.4	2.8
15–24 years	26.4	34.8	29.1	35.5	44.7	50.9	54.0	54.0	47.6	42.2	47.9
25–44 years	34.1	38.1	29.7	30.5	32.6	31.5	32.2	31.7	28.9	27.0	29.2
25–34 years	36.5	41.4	32.1	34.2	37.0	36.4	37.8	37.4	34.3	31.4	34.4
35–44 years	31.6	33.2	26.6	26.0	27.4	26.1	26.4	26.0	23.7	22.9	24.2
45–64 years	31.0	25.9	24.5	22.9	23.4	22.4	22.7	21.0	20.2	20.4	20.5
45–54 years	30.7	27.3	24.4	22.4	23.2	22.4	23.1	21.3	20.4	20.5	20.7
55–64 years	31.3	24.5	24.6	23.5	23.7	22.3	22.2	20.5	20.0	20.2	20.2
65 years and over	29.7	29.7	34.2	35.5	35.3	32.3	32.8	31.2	30.9	30.2	30.8
65–74 years	29.5	27.8	30.0	29.4	28.2	26.5	26.2	24.6	25.3	24.8	24.9
75–84 years	31.0	33.0	42.7	47.0	46.9	40.6	41.9	39.9	37.7	36.4	37.9
85 years and over	26.2	34.9	38.2	43.1	49.3	47.3	50.5	49.7	47.4	46.7	47.9
Female											
All ages, age adjusted	4.8	4.8	4.2	4.2	4.3	4.1	4.6	4.2	4.0	3.6	3.9
All ages, crude	4.4	4.7	4.2	4.2	4.3	4.1	4.5	4.1	3.9	3.6	3.9
Under 1 year	*	*	*	*	*	*	*	*	*	*	*
1–14 years	0.8	0.7	0.7	0.8	0.8	0.9	0.9	0.9	0.8	0.7	0.8
1–4 years	0.9	0.5	0.5	0.5	0.5	0.6	0.5	0.5	0.5	0.4	0.5
5–14 years	0.8	0.7	0.8	0.9	1.0	1.0	1.1	1.0	0.9	0.8	0.9
15–24 years	4.8	6.1	5.0	5.1	6.0	6.2	7.1	6.5	6.0	5.1	5.9
25–44 years	8.3	7.4	6.2	6.3	6.1	5.8	6.4	6.0	5.6	5.2	5.6
25–34 years	8.4	7.5	6.6	6.7	6.7	6.2	7.1	6.5	5.9	5.2	5.9
35–44 years	8.2	7.2	5.8	5.8	5.4	5.3	5.8	5.5	5.3	5.1	5.3
45–64 years	5.4	5.4	5.0	4.7	4.5	4.2	4.4	4.1	4.0	3.9	4.0
45–54 years	6.4	6.2	5.6	5.1	4.9	4.6	4.8	4.6	4.3	4.4	4.4
55–64 years	4.2	4.6	4.5	4.3	4.0	3.7	3.8	3.3	3.5	3.1	3.3
65 years and over	2.4	2.5	3.2	3.2	3.1	3.0	3.0	2.7	2.8	2.6	2.7
65–74 years	2.8	3.1	3.6	3.7	3.6	3.4	3.4	3.0	3.0	2.8	2.9
75–84 years	1.7	1.7	3.0	2.9	2.9	2.9	2.8	2.5	2.8	2.6	2.7
85 years and over	*	1.3	1.8	2.1	1.3	1.6	1.9	1.8	1.8	1.7	1.8
White male											
All ages, age adjusted	18.2	21.1	19.4	19.3	20.5	20.4	20.7	20.4	19.3	18.0	19.2
All ages, crude	17.6	21.8	20.7	20.7	21.8	21.3	21.5	21.1	20.1	19.0	20.1
1–14 years	1.8	1.9	2.1	1.9	1.9	1.9	2.0	1.8	1.9	1.5	1.7
15–24 years	16.9	28.4	24.1	25.3	29.5	32.4	33.0	34.2	31.4	26.9	30.8
25–44 years	24.2	29.5	25.0	24.4	25.7	24.8	25.1	24.9	23.6	22.0	23.5
25–34 years	24.3	31.1	26.3	26.0	27.8	27.0	27.9	27.6	26.1	23.6	25.8
35–44 years	24.1	27.1	23.3	22.5	23.3	22.6	22.2	22.3	21.2	20.6	21.3
45–64 years	27.4	23.3	23.6	22.5	22.8	21.8	22.0	20.6	19.7	20.2	20.2
65 years and over	29.9	30.1	35.4	37.0	36.8	33.8	34.4	32.5	32.3	31.8	32.2

See footnotes at end of table.

Table 49 (page 2 of 3). Death rates for firearm-related injuries, according to sex, detailed race, Hispanic origin, and age: United States, selected years 1970–96

[Data are based on the National Vital Statistics System]

Sex, race, Hispanic origin, and age	1970	1980	1985	1988	1990	1992	1993	1994	1995	1996	1994–96[1]
Black male					Deaths per 100,000 resident population						
All ages, age adjusted	73.4	61.8	42.2	51.0	61.5	64.5	68.8	65.1	55.6	52.0	57.5
All ages, crude	60.6	57.7	41.3	51.7	61.9	63.9	67.6	63.8	54.0	50.6	56.1
1–14 years	5.3	3.0	2.7	4.0	4.4	5.8	6.1	5.2	4.6	3.6	4.4
15–24 years	97.3	77.9	61.3	99.0	138.0	162.3	179.0	169.6	140.2	131.6	147.0
25–44 years	126.2	114.1	71.8	82.1	90.3	85.6	88.2	84.5	71.2	67.0	74.2
25–34 years	145.6	128.4	79.8	97.1	108.6	108.3	110.7	109.0	94.4	88.6	97.4
35–44 years	104.2	92.3	59.2	60.7	66.1	58.6	62.3	57.7	46.6	44.7	49.5
45–64 years	71.1	55.6	36.9	30.7	34.5	32.1	33.4	29.1	29.1	27.0	28.4
65 years and over	30.6	29.7	26.3	24.8	23.9	22.0	22.0	23.2	21.4	19.1	21.2
American Indian or Alaska Native male[2]											
All ages, age adjusted	- - -	26.5	24.9	24.0	20.8	20.0	21.8	24.6	23.4	19.4	22.4
All ages, crude	- - -	27.5	24.4	24.1	20.5	19.6	21.2	24.1	22.9	19.1	22.0
15–24 years	- - -	55.3	39.8	48.1	49.1	43.2	37.3	54.6	45.5	40.0	46.6
25–44 years	- - -	43.9	40.3	34.4	25.4	25.0	32.7	33.8	34.1	26.7	31.5
45–64 years	- - -	*	21.2	*	*	*	*	18.5	13.6	15.6	13.8	14.3
65 years and over	- - -	*	*	*	*	*	*	*	*	*	11.2
Asian or Pacific Islander male[3]											
All ages, age adjusted	- - -	8.1	7.1	8.4	9.2	10.4	11.9	10.9	10.8	8.7	10.1
All ages, crude	- - -	8.2	7.3	8.6	9.4	10.5	11.7	10.8	10.4	8.6	9.9
15–24 years	- - -	10.8	12.6	14.2	21.0	25.0	27.6	26.9	27.1	19.6	24.4
25–44 years	- - -	12.8	9.8	11.0	10.9	11.7	13.5	13.0	11.3	10.0	11.4
45–64 years	- - -	10.4	6.7	9.3	8.1	8.8	9.7	7.4	8.6	7.7	7.9
65 years and over	- - -	*	*	*	*	*	*	*	*	*	5.5
Hispanic male[4]											
All ages, age adjusted	- - -	- - -	25.3	23.8	28.9	31.0	30.5	29.9	28.0	22.5	26.7
All ages, crude	- - -	- - -	26.0	24.5	29.9	31.7	30.8	30.0	27.6	22.6	26.6
1–14 years	- - -	- - -	1.4	1.4	2.6	2.5	2.7	2.3	2.9	1.9	2.4
15–24 years	- - -	- - -	42.0	40.4	55.5	72.6	70.3	72.0	70.7	54.4	65.3
25–44 years	- - -	- - -	43.2	37.4	42.7	41.6	40.0	38.8	33.5	27.5	33.1
25–34 years	- - -	- - -	47.3	39.9	47.3	46.8	46.0	45.5	39.9	32.8	39.2
35–44 years	- - -	- - -	35.9	33.0	35.4	33.8	31.2	29.5	24.9	20.8	24.9
45–64 years	- - -	- - -	19.2	20.6	21.4	19.2	21.1	19.2	17.2	16.2	17.5
65 years and over	- - -	- - -	12.4	15.3	19.1	16.1	16.7	14.7	15.6	11.7	13.9
White, non-Hispanic male[4]											
All ages, age adjusted	- - -	- - -	18.4	17.9	18.7	18.0	18.3	18.1	17.2	16.4	17.2
All ages, crude	- - -	- - -	19.9	19.7	20.4	19.4	19.8	19.5	18.6	18.0	18.7
1–14 years	- - -	- - -	2.0	1.8	1.6	1.7	1.8	1.6	1.6	1.4	1.5
15–24 years	- - -	- - -	22.0	22.1	24.1	24.3	25.3	26.3	23.3	20.4	23.3
25–44 years	- - -	- - -	23.0	22.0	23.3	22.0	22.4	22.4	21.6	20.6	21.5
25–34 years	- - -	- - -	23.7	23.0	24.7	23.2	24.1	23.9	22.9	21.2	22.7
35–44 years	- - -	- - -	22.0	20.8	21.6	20.8	20.6	20.9	20.4	20.1	20.5
45–64 years	- - -	- - -	23.0	21.9	22.7	21.6	21.7	20.5	19.7	20.2	20.1
65 years and over	- - -	- - -	37.3	38.6	37.4	34.0	34.7	33.2	32.7	32.6	32.8
White female											
All ages, age adjusted	4.0	4.2	3.9	3.7	3.7	3.6	3.9	3.6	3.5	3.1	3.4
All ages, crude	3.7	4.1	4.0	3.8	3.8	3.6	3.9	3.6	3.5	3.2	3.5
15–24 years	3.4	5.1	4.4	4.1	4.8	4.7	5.2	4.9	4.6	3.8	4.4
25–44 years	6.9	6.2	5.6	5.3	5.3	4.9	5.5	5.2	5.0	4.6	4.9
45–64 years	5.0	5.1	5.0	4.7	4.5	4.3	4.5	4.1	4.0	3.9	4.0
65 years and over	2.2	2.5	3.2	3.3	3.1	3.1	3.0	2.7	2.9	2.6	2.7

See footnotes at end of table.

Table 49 (page 3 of 3). Death rates for firearm-related injuries, according to sex, detailed race, Hispanic origin, and age: United States, selected years 1970–96

[Data are based on the National Vital Statistics System]

Sex, race, Hispanic origin, and age	1970	1980	1985	1988	1990	1992	1993	1994	1995	1996	1994–96[1]
Black female					Deaths per 100,000 resident population						
All ages, age adjusted	11.4	9.1	6.6	7.6	7.8	8.1	8.8	8.0	6.8	6.5	7.1
All ages, crude	10.0	8.8	6.5	7.7	7.8	8.0	8.6	7.8	6.6	6.4	6.9
15–24 years	15.2	12.3	8.3	11.2	13.3	15.3	18.3	15.5	13.5	12.0	13.7
25–44 years	19.4	16.1	11.4	13.1	12.4	12.4	12.9	11.9	10.0	9.8	10.5
45–64 years	10.2	8.2	5.8	5.2	4.8	4.1	4.0	4.6	4.1	4.1	4.2
65 years and over	4.3	3.1	3.7	2.8	3.1	2.7	3.0	2.9	2.6	3.0	2.8
American Indian or Alaska Native female[2]											
All ages, age adjusted	- - -	6.1	4.3	3.6	3.6	2.3	4.5	4.5	4.5	3.8	4.3
All ages, crude	- - -	5.8	4.1	3.8	3.4	2.2	4.5	4.4	4.4	3.7	4.2
15–24 years	- - -	*	*	*	*	*	*	*	*	*	6.0
25–44 years	- - -	10.2	*	6.9	*	*	7.8	7.5	7.7	5.9	7.0
45–64 years	- - -	*	*	*	*	*	*	*	*	*	*
65 years and over	- - -	*	*	*	*	*	*	*	*	*	*
Asian or Pacific Islander female[3]											
All ages, age adjusted	- - -	2.0	1.7	1.8	2.0	2.1	2.6	2.1	2.2	1.7	2.0
All ages, crude	- - -	2.1	1.7	2.0	2.1	2.1	2.6	2.1	2.2	1.7	2.0
15–24 years	- - -	*	*	*	*	3.4	3.8	4.0	4.2	3.7	4.0
25–44 years	- - -	3.2	2.2	3.4	2.7	2.7	3.5	2.6	2.9	2.1	2.5
45–64 years	- - -	*	*	*	*	*	2.9	*	*	*	1.9
65 years and over	- - -	*	*	*	*	*	*	*	*	*	*
Hispanic female[4]											
All ages, age adjusted	- - -	- - -	3.2	3.1	3.6	3.7	4.0	3.5	3.5	2.8	3.2
All ages, crude	- - -	- - -	3.2	3.1	3.6	3.6	3.9	3.4	3.4	2.7	3.1
15–24 years	- - -	- - -	5.1	5.5	6.9	6.2	7.8	6.9	6.6	5.0	6.1
25–44 years	- - -	- - -	5.5	4.7	5.1	5.3	5.2	5.0	4.9	4.1	4.6
45–64 years	- - -	- - -	2.2	2.1	2.4	3.0	2.6	2.4	2.4	2.3	2.4
65 years and over	- - -	- - -	*	*	*	*	*	*	*	*	1.1
White, non-Hispanic female[4]											
All ages, age adjusted	- - -	- - -	3.9	3.7	3.6	3.4	3.7	3.5	3.4	3.1	3.3
All ages, crude	- - -	- - -	4.1	3.8	3.7	3.5	3.8	3.6	3.5	3.2	3.4
15–24 years	- - -	- - -	4.5	3.9	4.3	4.3	4.6	4.5	4.1	3.5	4.0
25–44 years	- - -	- - -	5.6	5.3	5.1	4.8	5.4	5.1	4.8	4.5	4.8
45–64 years	- - -	- - -	5.1	4.9	4.6	4.4	4.5	4.1	4.1	4.0	4.1
65 years and over	- - -	- - -	3.4	3.6	3.2	3.1	3.0	2.7	2.9	2.7	2.8

* Based on fewer than 20 deaths.

- - - Data not available.

[1]Average annual death rate.

[2]Interpretation of trends should take into account that population estimates for American Indians increased by 45 percent between 1980 and 1990, partly due to better enumeration techniques in the 1990 decennial census and to the increased tendency for people to identify themselves as American Indian in 1990.

[3]Interpretation of trends should take into account that the Asian population in the United States more than doubled between 1980 and 1990, primarily due to immigration.

[4]Excludes data from States lacking an Hispanic-origin item on their death certificates. See Appendix I, National Vital Statistics System.

NOTES: For data years shown, the code numbers for cause of death are based on the then current *International Classification of Diseases*, which are described in Appendix II, tables IV and V. Age groups chosen to show data for American Indians, Asians, Hispanics, and non-Hispanic whites were selected to minimize the presentation of unstable age-specific death rates based on small numbers of deaths and for consistency among comparison groups. The race groups, white, black, Asian or Pacific Islander, and American Indian or Alaska Native, include persons of Hispanic and non-Hispanic origin. Conversely, persons of Hispanic origin may be of any race. Consistency of race identification between the death certificate (source of data for numerator of death rates) and data from the Census Bureau (denominator) is high for individual white and black persons; however, persons identified as American Indian, Asian, or Hispanic origin in data from the Census Bureau are sometimes misreported as white or non-Hispanic on the death certificate, causing death rates to be underestimated by 22–30 percent for American Indians, about 12 percent for Asians, and about 7 percent for persons of Hispanic origin. (Sorlie PD, Rogot E, and Johnson NJ: Validity of demographic characteristics on the death certificate, *Epidemiology* 3(2):181–184, 1992.)

SOURCES: Centers for Disease Control and Prevention, National Center for Health Statistics. *Vital statistics of the United States, vol II, mortality, part A,* for data years 1970–96. Washington: Public Health Service; data computed by the Division of Health and Utilization Analysis from data compiled by the Division of Vital Statistics and from national population estimates for race groups from table 1 and unpublished Hispanic population estimates prepared by the Housing and Household Economic Statistics Division, U.S. Bureau of the Census.

Table 50. Deaths from selected occupational diseases for males, according to age: United States, selected years 1970–96

[Data are based on the National Vital Statistics System]

Age and cause of death	1970	1975	1980	1985	1987	1988	1989	1990	1991	1992	1993	1994	1995	1996
25 years and over						Number of deaths[1]								
Malignant neoplasm of peritoneum and pleura (mesothelioma)	602	591	552	571	575	556	565	629	607	618	551	511	546	574
Coalworkers' pneumoconiosis	1,155	973	977	947	823	757	725	727	692	631	564	491	531	533
Asbestosis	25	43	96	130	195	206	261	282	247	270	308	325	342	345
Silicosis	351	243	202	138	153	128	130	146	150	110	123	113	110	95
25–64 years														
Malignant neoplasm of peritoneum and pleura (mesothelioma)	308	280	241	210	196	187	179	199	190	193	164	161	163	146
Coalworkers' pneumoconiosis	294	188	136	89	71	56	50	49	48	32	34	21	40	20
Asbestosis	17	22	30	29	32	38	31	50	35	34	32	35	32	33
Silicosis	90	64	49	30	32	26	21	35	29	25	25	25	15	19
65 years and over														
Malignant neoplasm of peritoneum and pleura (mesothelioma)	294	311	311	361	379	369	386	430	417	425	387	350	383	428
Coalworkers' pneumoconiosis	861	785	841	858	752	701	675	678	644	599	530	470	491	513
Asbestosis	8	21	66	101	163	168	230	232	212	236	276	290	310	312
Silicosis	261	179	153	108	121	102	109	111	121	85	98	88	95	76

[1]This table classifies deaths according to underlying cause. Additional deaths for which occupational diseases are classified as nonunderlying causes can be identified from multiple cause of death data from the National Vital Statistics System. The numbers of such deaths are shown below for males 25 years of age and over.

Nonunderlying cause of death	1980	1985	1987	1988	1989	1990	1991	1992	1993	1994	1995	1996
Malignant neoplasm of peritoneum and pleura (mesothelioma)	135	102	111	104	83	105	96	87	84	103	83	74
Coalworkers' pneumoconiosis	1,587	1,652	1,419	1,445	1,402	1,248	1,227	1,130	1,052	974	876	874
Asbestosis	228	382	488	536	588	619	660	653	661	701	796	778
Silicosis	232	187	173	162	156	152	155	130	145	109	122	111

NOTES: Selection of occupational diseases based on definitions in D. Rutstein et al.: Sentinel health events (occupational): A basis for physician recognition and public health surveillance, *Am. J. Public Health* 73(9):1054–1062, Sept. 1983. For data years shown, the code numbers for cause of death are based on the then current *International Classification of Diseases*, which are described in Appendix II, tables IV and V.

SOURCE: Data computed by the Centers for Disease Control and Prevention, National Center for Health Statistics, Office of Analysis, Epidemiology, and Health Promotion from data compiled by the Division of Vital Statistics.

Table 51. Occupational injury deaths, according to industry: United States, selected years 1980–93

[Data are based on information from death certificates]

Industry	1980	1985	1986	1987	1988	1989	1990	1991	1992[1]	1993
	Deaths per 100,000 workers[2]									
Total civilian work force.	7.6	5.8	5.2	5.2	5.0	4.9	4.6	4.4	4.1	4.2
Agriculture, forestry, and fishing.	24.4	23.7	20.9	21.5	20.7	20.6	18.0	18.1	17.5	18.5
Mining.	43.8	30.0	25.0	23.2	23.4	26.7	30.0	23.9	22.3	25.4
Construction	21.3	16.6	15.0	15.9	14.9	14.3	14.0	12.5	12.3	11.8
Manufacturing	4.7	4.0	3.8	4.0	3.8	3.7	4.0	3.9	3.6	3.6
Transportation, communication, and public utilities.	21.2	15.7	13.5	12.9	13.2	12.9	10.4	10.3	9.5	10.1
Wholesale trade.	4.4	2.8	2.6	2.6	2.9	2.3	3.6	3.6	3.1	3.6
Retail trade	3.7	2.7	2.2	2.4	2.3	2.2	2.8	3.0	2.7	2.9
Finance, insurance, and real estate.	1.4	1.0	1.1	1.2	0.9	1.0	0.9	1.1	0.9	1.0
Services	2.4	1.8	1.6	1.6	1.7	1.6	1.5	1.7	1.4	1.4
Public administration	7.7	6.4	6.2	6.8	6.1	5.3	3.8	3.2	4.2	4.2
Not classified.	- - -	- - -	- - -	- - -	- - -	- - -	- - -	- - -	- - -	- - -
	Number of deaths									
Total civilian work force.	7,405	6,250	5,672	5,884	5,751	5,714	5,384	5,192	4,810	5,029
Agriculture, forestry, and fishing.	848	791	701	730	687	695	603	614	592	602
Mining.	412	282	220	190	176	192	219	175	148	170
Construction	1,294	1,160	1,091	1,188	1,130	1,096	1,077	887	863	850
Manufacturing	1,014	834	802	831	810	791	838	789	726	699
Transportation, communication, and public utilities.	1,355	1,184	1,032	1,013	1,068	1,046	847	844	783	857
Wholesale trade.	167	122	113	120	135	107	168	169	149	164
Retail trade	595	489	407	449	443	430	543	575	521	588
Finance, insurance, and real estate.	84	69	79	94	72	81	75	89	68	78
Services	663	603	554	563	642	606	592	654	552	597
Public administration	401	319	318	359	333	292	213	179	238	255
Not classified.	572	397	355	347	255	378	209	217	170	169

- - - Data not available.

[1]Fatality data for 1992 were not available from Connecticut and New York City.

[2]Denominators are from the U.S. Bureau of Labor Statistics' annual average employment data.

NOTES: Includes deaths to United States workers, 16 years of age and over, that resulted from an "external" cause and the item "injury at work" was checked on the death certificate. Industry is coded based on *Standard Industrial Classification Manual*, 1987 Edition (see Appendix II, table VI). Rates for 1980–89 have been recalculated and may differ from the previous edition of *Health, United States*.

SOURCE: Centers for Disease Control and Prevention, National Institute for Occupational Safety and Health, Division of Safety Research. National Traumatic Occupational Fatalities (NTOF) surveillance system. Morgantown, West Virginia.

Table 52. Vaccinations of children 19–35 months of age for selected diseases, according to race, Hispanic origin, poverty status, and residence in metropolitan statistical area (MSA): United States, 1994–96

[Data are based on telephone interviews of a sample of the civilian noninstitutionalized population supplemented by a survey of immunization providers for interview participants]

| Vaccination and year | Total | Race and Hispanic origin | | | | | Poverty status[1] | | Location of residence | | |
| | | Hispanic | White, non-Hispanic | Black, non-Hispanic | Asian or Pacific Islander | American Indian or Alaska Native | Below poverty | At or above poverty | Inside MSA | | Outside MSA |
									Central city	Remaining areas	
					Percent of children 19–35 months of age						
Combined series (4:3:1:3):[2]											
1994	69	62	72	67	60	82	61	72	68	70	70
1995	74	69	77	70	75	70	67	77	73	76	75
1996	77	71	79	74	78	80	69	80	74	78	77
DTP (4 doses or more):[3]											
1994	76	70	80	72	84	84	69	79	75	77	78
1995	79	75	81	74	82	73	71	81	77	80	79
1996	81	77	83	79	84	83	73	84	80	83	81
Polio (3 doses or more):											
1994	83	81	85	79	92	90	78	85	83	84	83
1995	88	87	89	84	89	87	84	89	87	88	89
1996	91	89	92	90	90	89	88	92	89	92	92
Measles-containing:[4]											
1994	89	88	90	86	95	90	87	90	90	90	87
1995	90	88	91	86	95	88	85	91	89	91	90
1996	91	88	92	89	94	87	87	92	90	92	91
Hib (3 doses or more):[5]											
1994	86	84	87	85	70	90	81	88	86	87	86
1995	92	90	93	89	91	92	88	93	91	92	92
1996	92	89	93	90	92	90	88	93	90	93	92
Hepatitis B (3 doses or more):											
1994	37	33	40	29	39	43	25	41	36	40	28
1995	68	69	68	65	80	55	64	69	68	71	60
1996	82	80	82	82	84	78	78	83	81	83	80

| Vaccination and year | Race and Hispanic origin and poverty status[1] | | | | | |
| | Hispanic | | White, non-Hispanic | | Black, non-Hispanic | |
	Below poverty	At or above poverty	Below poverty	At or above poverty	Below poverty	At or above poverty
	Percent of children 19–35 months of age					
Combined series (4:3:1:3):[2]						
1995	65	72	68	79	66	75
1996	68	74	68	81	70	78

[1]Poverty status is based on family income and family size using Bureau of the Census poverty thresholds. Children missing information about poverty status were omitted from analysis by poverty level. In 1996, 21 percent of all children, 29 percent of Hispanic, 17 percent of non-Hispanic white, and 25 percent of non-Hispanic black children were missing information about poverty status and were omitted. See Appendix II.

[2]The 4:3:1:3 combined series consists of 4 doses of diphtheria-tetanus-pertussis (DTP) vaccine, 3 doses of polio vaccine, 1 dose of a measles-containing vaccine, and 3 doses of Haemophilus influenzae type b (Hib) vaccine.

[3]Diphtheria-tetanus-pertussis vaccine.

[4]Respondents were asked about measles-containing or MMR (measles-mumps-rubella) vaccines.

[5]Haemophilus influenzae type b (Hib) vaccine.

NOTES: Some numbers in this table have been revised and differ from previous editions of *Health, United States*. Final estimates of data from the National Immunization Survey include an adjustment for children with missing immunization provider data.

SOURCES: Centers for Disease Control and Prevention, National Center for Health Statistics and National Immunization Program. Data from the National Immunization Survey.

Table 53 (page 1 of 2). Vaccination coverage among children 19–35 months of age according to geographic division, State, and selected urban areas: United States, 1994–96

[Data are based on telephone interviews of a sample of the civilian noninstitutionalized population supplemented by a survey of immunization providers for interview participants]

Geographic division and State	1994	1995	1996
	Percent of children 19–35 months of age with 4:3:1:3 series[1]		
United States	69	74	77
New England:			
Maine	75	87	85
New Hampshire	78	86	83
Vermont	82	84	85
Massachusetts	77	80	86
Rhode Island	78	82	85
Connecticut	81	83	87
Middle Atlantic:			
New York	72	77	79
New Jersey	67	72	77
Pennsylvania	71	76	79
East North Central:			
Ohio	70	73	77
Indiana	69	75	70
Illinois	60	79	75
Michigan	55	67	74
Wisconsin	70	74	76
West North Central:			
Minnesota	74	76	83
Iowa	75	82	80
Missouri	59	75	74
North Dakota	73	81	81
South Dakota	67	79	80
Nebraska	62	75	80
Kansas	76	70	73
South Atlantic:			
Delaware	77	72	80
Maryland	75	78	78
District of Columbia	67	67	78
Virginia	76	71	77
West Virginia	62	71	71
North Carolina	75	80	77
South Carolina	78	80	84
Georgia	75	77	80
Florida	72	75	77
East South Central:			
Kentucky	74	79	76
Tennessee	68	73	77
Alabama	70	75	75
Mississippi	79	81	79
West South Central:			
Arkansas	64	73	72
Louisiana	66	76	79
Oklahoma	70	73	73
Texas	65	73	72
Mountain:			
Montana	69	71	77
Idaho	58	64	66
Wyoming	71	71	77
Colorado	66	77	76
New Mexico	66	76	79
Arizona	70	70	70
Utah	62	66	63
Nevada	63	65	70
Pacific:			
Washington	68	77	78
Oregon	64	72	70
California	67	69	76
Alaska	65	72	69
Hawaii	78	78	77

See footnotes at end of table.

Table 53 (page 2 of 2). Vaccination coverage among children 19–35 months of age according to geographic division, State, and selected urban areas: United States, 1994–96

[Data are based on telephone interviews of a sample of the civilian noninstitutionalized population supplemented by a survey of immunization providers for interview participants]

Geographic division and urban areas	1994	1995	1996
	Percent of children 19–35 months of age with 4:3:1:3 series[1]		
New England:			
Boston, Massachusetts	87	87	84
Middle Atlantic:			
New York City, New York.	73	78	75
Newark, New Jersey.	46	67	62
Philadelphia, Pennsylvania	67	67	75
East North Central:			
Cuyahoga County (Cleveland), Ohio.	82	71	80
Franklin County (Columbus), Ohio	71	74	78
Marion County (Indianapolis), Indiana.	72	75	72
Chicago, Illinois	55	69	74
Detroit, Michigan	45	57	63
Milwaukee County (Milwaukee), Wisconsin	72	68	70
South Atlantic:			
Baltimore, Maryland	74	75	81
District of Columbia	67	67	78
Fulton/DeKalb Counties (Atlanta), Georgia	72	79	74
Dade County (Miami), Florida	73	77	76
Duval County (Jacksonville), Florida.	69	71	76
East South Central:			
Davidson County (Nashville), Tennessee	65	73	77
Shelby County (Memphis), Tennessee	67	68	70
Jefferson County (Birmingham), Alabama	72	85	77
West South Central:			
Orleans Parish (New Orleans), Louisiana	59	75	71
Bexar County (San Antonio), Texas	60	74	74
Dallas County (Dallas), Texas	62	70	71
El Paso County (El Paso), Texas	78	77	62
Houston, Texas	57	70	68
Mountain:			
Maricopa County (Phoenix), Arizona.	71	69	71
Pacific:			
King County (Seattle), Washington.	70	82	81
Los Angeles County (Los Angeles), California . .	65	70	79
San Diego County (San Diego), California	68	73	77
Santa Clara County (Santa Clara), California . .	78	74	79

[1]The 4:3:1:3 combined series consists of 4 doses of diphtheria-tetanus-pertussis (DTP) vaccine, 3 doses of polio vaccine, 1 dose of a measles-containing vaccine, and 3 doses of Haemophilus influenzae type b (Hib) vaccine.

NOTES: Urban areas were chosen because they were high risk for under-vaccination. Final estimates of data from the National Immunization Survey include an adjustment for children with missing immunization provider data.

SOURCES: Centers for Disease Control and Prevention, National Center for Health Statistics and National Immunization Program. Data from the National Immunization Survey.

Table 54. Selected notifiable disease rates, according to disease: United States, selected years 1950–96

[Data are based on reporting by State health departments]

Disease	1950	1960	1970	1980	1990	1993	1994	1995	1996
				Cases per 100,000 population					
Diphtheria	3.83	0.51	0.21	0.00	0.00	–	0.00	–	0.01
Hepatitis A	- - -	- - -	27.87	12.84	12.64	9.40	10.29	12.13	11.70
Hepatitis B	- - -	- - -	4.08	8.39	8.48	5.18	4.81	4.19	4.01
Mumps	- - -	- - -	55.55	3.86	2.17	0.66	0.60	0.35	0.29
Pertussis (whooping cough)	79.82	8.23	2.08	0.76	1.84	2.55	1.77	1.97	2.94
Poliomyelitis, total	22.02	1.77	0.02	0.00	0.00	0.00	0.00	0.00	0.01
Paralytic[1]	- - -	1.40	0.02	0.00	0.00	0.00	0.00	0.00	0.01
Rubella (German measles)	- - -	- - -	27.75	1.72	0.45	0.07	0.09	0.05	0.10
Rubeola (measles)	211.01	245.42	23.23	5.96	11.17	0.12	0.37	0.12	0.20
Salmonellosis, excluding typhoid fever	- - -	3.85	10.84	14.88	19.54	16.15	16.64	17.66	17.15
Shigellosis	15.45	6.94	6.79	8.41	10.89	12.48	11.44	12.32	9.80
Tuberculosis[2]	80.45	30.83	18.28	12.25	10.33	9.82	9.36	8.70	8.04
Sexually transmitted diseases:[3]									
Syphilis[4]	146.02	68.78	45.26	30.51	54.30	39.30	31.40	26.40	20.20
Primary and secondary	16.73	9.06	10.89	12.06	20.30	10.30	7.90	6.30	4.30
Early latent	39.71	10.11	8.08	9.00	22.30	16.30	12.30	10.10	7.70
Late and late latent	70.22	45.91	24.94	9.30	10.40	11.50	10.30	9.20	7.70
Congenital[5]	8.97	2.48	0.97	0.12	1.60	1.30	0.90	0.70	0.40
Chlamydia[6]	- - -	- - -	- - -	- - -	145.40	180.40	193.30	190.40	194.50
Gonorrhea[7]	192.50	145.40	297.22	445.10	278.00	172.00	165.10	149.40	124.00
Chancroid	3.34	0.94	0.70	0.30	1.70	0.50	0.30	0.20	0.10
				Number of cases					
Diphtheria	5,796	918	435	3	4	–	2	–	2
Hepatitis A	- - -	- - -	56,797	29,087	31,441	24,238	29,796	31,582	31,032
Hepatitis B	- - -	- - -	8,310	19,015	21,102	13,361	12,517	10,805	10,637
Mumps	- - -	- - -	104,953	8,576	5,292	1,692	1,537	906	751
Pertussis (whooping cough)	120,718	14,809	4,249	1,730	4,570	6,586	4,617	5,137	7,796
Poliomyelitis, total	33,300	3,190	33	9	6	4	8	6	5
Paralytic[1]	- - -	2,525	31	8	6	4	8	6	5
Rubella (German measles)	- - -	- - -	56,552	3,904	1,125	192	227	128	238
Rubeola (measles)	319,124	441,703	47,351	13,506	27,786	312	963	281	508
Salmonellosis, excluding typhoid fever	- - -	6,929	22,096	33,715	48,603	41,641	43,323	45,970	45,471
Shigellosis	23,367	12,487	13,845	19,041	27,077	32,198	29,769	32,080	25,978
Tuberculosis[2]	121,742	55,494	37,137	27,749	25,701	25,287	24,361	22,860	21,337
Sexually transmitted diseases:[3]									
Syphilis[4]	217,558	122,538	91,382	68,832	135,043	101,335	81,696	69,320	52,995
Primary and secondary	23,939	16,145	21,982	27,204	50,578	26,497	20,627	16,542	11,387
Early latent	59,256	18,017	16,311	20,297	55,397	41,902	32,012	26,655	20,187
Late and late latent	113,569	81,798	50,348	20,979	25,750	29,675	26,840	24,272	20,240
Congenital[5]	13,377	4,416	1,953	277	3,865	3,261	2,217	1,851	1,181
Chlamydia[6]	- - -	- - -	- - -	- - -	308,139	407,312	448,984	478,534	490,080
Gonorrhea[7]	286,746	258,933	600,072	1,004,029	691,368	443,278	418,068	392,622	325,883
Chancroid	4,977	1,680	1,416	788	4,212	1,237	773	607	386

- - - Data not available.

– Quantity zero.

[1] Data beginning in 1986 may be updated due to retrospective case evaluations or late reports.

[2] Data after 1974 are not comparable to prior years because of changes in reporting criteria effective in 1975.

[3] Newly reported civilian cases prior to 1991; includes military cases beginning in 1991 and adjustments to the number of cases through June 13, 1997. For 1950, data for Alaska and Hawaii not included.

[4] Includes stage of syphilis not stated.

[5] Data reported for 1989 and later years reflect change in case definition introduced in 1988. Through 1994, all cases of congenitally acquired syphilis; as of 1995, congenital syphilis less than 1 year of age.

[6] Chlamydia was non-notifiable in 1994 and earlier years (see Appendix I).

[7] Data for 1994 do not include cases from Georgia.

NOTES: Rates greater than 0 but less than 0.005 are shown as 0.00. The total resident population was used to calculate all rates except sexually transmitted diseases, for which the civilian resident population was used prior to 1991. Population data from those States where diseases were not notifiable or not available were excluded from rate calculation. See Appendix I for information on underreporting of notifiable diseases. Some numbers in this table have been revised and differ from previous editions of Health, United States.

SOURCES: Centers for Disease Control and Prevention. Summary of notifiable diseases, United States, 1996. Morbidity and mortality weekly report 1996; 45(53). Atlanta, Georgia: Public Health Service. 1997; National Center for HIV, STD, and TB Prevention, Division of STD Prevention. Sexually transmitted disease surveillance, 1996. Atlanta, Georgia: Public Health Service. Centers for Disease Control and Prevention, 1997.

Table 55. Acquired immunodeficiency syndrome (AIDS) cases, according to age at diagnosis, sex, detailed race, and Hispanic origin: United States, selected years 1985–97

[Data are based on reporting by State health departments]

Age at diagnosis, sex, race, and Hispanic origin	All years[1]	All years[1]	1985	1990	1992	1993	1994	1995	1996	January– June 1997	12 months ending June 30, 1997
	Percent distribution	Number, by year of report									Cases per 100,000 population[2]
All races	. . .	592,144	8,161	41,569	45,771	102,211	77,237	71,039	66,659	30,153	23.6
Male											
All males, 13 years and over . . .	100.0	496,642	7,509	36,314	39,069	85,393	62,935	57,231	52,781	23,336	47.0
White, non-Hispanic	51.6	256,246	4,756	20,894	20,832	43,346	29,556	26,260	23,270	9,164	26.1
Black, non-Hispanic	32.4	160,859	1,707	10,276	12,158	28,368	22,471	21,027	20,144	9,656	172.3
Hispanic	14.8	73,718	990	4,769	5,624	12,641	10,111	9,198	8,622	4,138	77.4
American Indian[3]	0.3	1,390	7	80	104	309	205	198	169	83	24.9
Asian or Pacific Islander[4]	0.8	3,831	49	265	295	660	527	486	478	198	12.8
13–19 years	0.4	1,769	28	108	91	362	226	229	202	108	1.5
20–29 years	16.8	83,548	1,505	6,951	6,495	14,653	9,689	8,434	7,085	3,011	34.7
30–39 years	45.9	227,984	3,585	16,727	17,879	38,941	28,996	25,904	23,954	10,468	101.0
40–49 years	26.3	130,444	1,636	8,865	10,303	22,909	17,259	16,335	15,540	6,931	74.5
50–59 years	7.9	39,074	596	2,652	3,067	6,428	5,066	4,749	4,463	2,094	35.3
60 years and over	2.8	13,823	159	1,011	1,234	2,100	1,699	1,580	1,537	724	7.9
Female											
All females, 13 years and over . .	100.0	87,976	524	4,532	5,953	15,947	13,330	13,061	13,222	6,551	11.8
White, non-Hispanic	24.2	21,311	141	1,225	1,468	4,048	3,090	3,067	2,875	1,327	3.3
Black, non-Hispanic	58.4	51,352	280	2,542	3,408	9,104	7,861	7,637	8,119	4,083	61.8
Hispanic	16.4	14,470	100	733	1,014	2,627	2,283	2,237	2,077	1,061	20.6
American Indian[3]	0.3	261	2	8	19	61	41	38	43	16	5.3
Asian or Pacific Islander[4]	0.5	476	1	19	39	97	49	72	80	34	2.2
13–19 years	1.2	1,055	4	65	56	198	174	155	176	89	1.3
20–29 years	22.5	19,820	178	1,118	1,386	3,726	2,945	2,684	2,684	1,266	14.4
30–39 years	46.0	40,442	233	2,078	2,731	7,528	6,007	5,987	5,927	2,934	26.8
40–49 years	21.2	18,690	45	780	1,234	3,215	3,088	3,082	3,274	1,665	16.6
50–59 years	5.8	5,130	26	272	337	850	771	816	836	418	6.4
60 years and over	3.2	2,839	38	219	209	430	345	337	325	179	1.3
Children											
All children, under 13 years	100.0	7,526	128	723	749	871	972	747	656	266	1.2
White, non-Hispanic	18.6	1,399	26	159	128	151	143	117	96	35	0.3
Black, non-Hispanic	60.8	4,579	84	387	485	535	633	483	427	178	5.2
Hispanic	19.5	1,465	18	168	129	175	181	136	127	51	1.4
American Indian[3]	0.3	26	–	5	3	3	2	2	3	1	0.8
Asian or Pacific Islander[4]	0.5	41	–	4	2	4	11	5	1	–	–
Under 1 year	40.2	3,029	63	315	329	351	350	271	219	85	4.8
1–12 years	59.8	4,497	65	408	420	520	622	476	437	181	0.9

. . . Category not applicable.

– Quantity zero.

[1]Includes cases prior to 1985.

[2]Computed using resident population estimates for 1996 based on extrapolation from 1990 census counts from the U.S. Bureau of the Census.

[3]Includes Aleut and Eskimo.

[4]Includes Chinese, Japanese, Filipino, Hawaiian and part Hawaiian, and other Asian or Pacific Islander.

NOTES: The AIDS case reporting definitions were expanded in 1985, 1987, and 1993. See Appendix II. Excludes data for U.S. dependencies and possessions and independent nations in free association with the United States. Data are updated periodically because of reporting delays. Data for all years have been updated through June 30, 1997. Data as of December 31, 1997, are available in the Centers for Disease Control and Prevention, HIV/AIDS Surveillance Report, Year-end edition, 1998.

SOURCE: Centers for Disease Control and Prevention, National Center for HIV, STD, and TB Prevention, Division of HIV/AIDS Prevention.

Table 56 (page 1 of 2). Acquired immunodeficiency syndrome (AIDS) cases, according to race, Hispanic origin, sex, and transmission category for persons 13 years of age and over at diagnosis: United States, selected years 1985–97

[Data are based on reporting by State health departments]

Race, Hispanic origin, sex, and transmission category	All years[1]	All years[1]	1985	1990	1992	1993	1994	1995	1996	January–June 1997
Race and Hispanic origin	Percent distribution	Number, by year of report								
All races	100.0	584,618	8,033	40,846	45,022	101,340	76,265	70,292	66,003	29,887
Men who have sex with men	50.5	295,355	5,357	23,826	24,467	49,600	35,291	30,939	27,316	10,625
Injecting drug use.	24.7	144,567	1,387	9,280	11,003	28,124	21,054	18,583	16,405	7,246
Men who have sex with men and injecting drug use	6.4	37,514	655	2,804	3,168	7,210	4,443	3,742	3,044	1,147
Hemophilia/coagulation disorder. . . .	0.8	4,508	71	348	334	1,080	505	443	321	107
Heterosexual contact[2].	8.6	50,356	151	2,261	3,523	9,054	8,240	8,112	8,609	3,843
Sex with injecting drug user	3.6	21,114	107	1,495	1,942	3,938	2,944	2,738	2,647	1,007
Transfusion[3]	1.3	7,860	166	788	602	1,097	688	622	548	211
Undetermined[4].	7.6	44,458	246	1,539	1,925	5,175	6,044	7,851	9,760	6,708
White, non-Hispanic	100.0	277,557	4,897	22,119	22,300	47,394	32,646	29,327	26,145	10,491
Men who have sex with men	69.9	193,985	3,983	16,589	16,051	32,055	21,755	18,922	16,349	6,019
Injecting drug use.	11.6	32,092	246	2,059	2,516	6,459	4,561	4,134	3,692	1,535
Men who have sex with men and injecting drug use	7.3	20,377	409	1,562	1,686	3,813	2,259	1,912	1,571	564
Hemophilia/coagulation disorder. . . .	1.3	3,531	59	280	256	878	371	320	211	78
Heterosexual contact[2].	4.4	12,206	33	650	899	2,300	1,937	1,899	1,856	785
Sex with injecting drug user	1.8	5,068	18	352	429	982	746	684	633	229
Transfusion[3]	1.7	4,774	125	512	368	596	320	295	221	91
Undetermined[4].	3.8	10,592	42	467	524	1,293	1,443	1,845	2,245	1,419
Black, non-Hispanic	100.0	212,211	1,987	12,818	15,566	37,472	30,332	28,664	28,263	13,739
Men who have sex with men	29.1	61,844	785	4,481	5,103	10,683	8,215	7,376	6,846	2,882
Injecting drug use.	38.2	81,025	740	5,172	6,125	15,727	11,984	10,499	9,312	4,126
Men who have sex with men and injecting drug use	5.8	12,239	161	900	1,050	2,419	1,571	1,329	1,085	444
Hemophilia/coagulation disorder. . . .	0.2	529	5	34	42	121	71	70	66	14
Heterosexual contact[2].	13.6	28,931	91	1,224	2,043	5,129	4,756	4,590	5,226	2,331
Sex with injecting drug user	5.6	11,979	65	857	1,166	2,188	1,661	1,500	1,522	592
Transfusion[3]	1.0	2,054	30	170	141	333	251	231	225	91
Undetermined[4].	12.1	25,589	175	837	1,062	3,060	3,484	4,569	5,503	3,851
Hispanic	100.0	88,188	1,090	5,502	6,638	15,268	12,394	11,435	10,699	5,199
Men who have sex with men	40.3	35,535	547	2,469	2,980	6,115	4,781	4,158	3,682	1,549
Injecting drug use.	34.8	30,673	394	2,014	2,312	5,782	4,406	3,823	3,296	1,511
Men who have sex with men and injecting drug use	5.1	4,523	83	320	399	896	553	454	348	122
Hemophilia/coagulation disorder. . . .	0.4	351	7	28	30	60	50	44	33	10
Heterosexual contact[2].	9.9	8,722	27	376	546	1,518	1,483	1,543	1,430	680
Sex with injecting drug user	4.4	3,905	24	281	336	726	514	535	467	177
Transfusion[3]	0.9	817	6	83	71	138	92	77	86	24
Undetermined[4].	8.6	7,567	26	212	300	759	1,029	1,336	1,824	1,303

See footnotes at end of table.

Table 56 (page 2 of 2). Acquired immunodeficiency syndrome (AIDS) cases, according to race, Hispanic origin, sex, and transmission category for persons 13 years of age and over at diagnosis: United States, selected years 1985–97

[Data are based on reporting by State health departments]

Race, Hispanic origin, sex, and transmission category	All years[1]	All years[1]	1985	1990	1992	1993	1994	1995	1996	January–June 1997
Sex	Percent distribution	Number, by year of report								
Male	100.0	496,642	7,509	36,314	39,069	85,393	62,935	57,231	52,781	23,336
Men who have sex with men	59.5	295,355	5,357	23,826	24,467	49,600	35,291	30,939	27,316	10,625
Injecting drug use.	21.2	105,175	1,101	6,956	8,038	20,100	15,162	13,319	11,718	5,158
Men who have sex with men and injecting drug use	7.6	37,514	655	2,804	3,168	7,210	4,443	3,742	3,044	1,147
Hemophilia/coagulation disorder. . . .	0.9	4,325	68	333	324	1,048	478	420	300	99
Heterosexual contact[2].	3.4	17,048	32	720	1,234	2,991	2,798	2,756	3,088	1,468
Sex with injecting drug user	1.3	6,455	25	459	624	1,172	920	871	811	348
Transfusion[3]	0.9	4,537	103	452	346	606	374	346	282	113
Undetermined[4].	6.6	32,688	193	1,223	1,492	3,838	4,389	5,709	7,033	4,726
Female	100.0	87,976	524	4,532	5,953	15,947	13,330	13,061	13,222	6,551
Injecting drug use.	44.8	39,392	286	2,324	2,965	8,024	5,892	5,264	4,687	2,088
Hemophilia/coagulation disorder. . . .	0.2	183	3	15	10	32	27	23	21	8
Heterosexual contact[2].	37.9	33,308	119	1,541	2,289	6,063	5,442	5,356	5,521	2,375
Sex with injecting drug user	16.7	14,659	82	1,036	1,318	2,766	2,024	1,867	1,836	659
Transfusion[3]	3.8	3,323	63	336	256	491	314	276	266	98
Undetermined[4].	13.4	11,770	53	316	433	1,337	1,655	2,142	2,727	1,982

[1]Includes cases before 1985.

[2]Includes persons who have had heterosexual contact with a person with human immunodeficiency virus (HIV) infection or at risk of HIV infection.

[3]Receipt of blood transfusion, blood components, or tissue.

[4]Includes persons for whom risk information is incomplete (because of death, refusal to be interviewed, or loss to followup), persons still under investigation, men reported only to have had heterosexual contact with prostitutes, and interviewed persons for whom no specific risk is identified.

NOTES: The AIDS case reporting definitions were expanded in 1985, 1987, and 1993. See Appendix II. Excludes data for U.S. dependencies and possessions and independent nations in free association with the United States. Data are updated periodically because of reporting delays. Data for all years have been updated through June 30, 1997. Data as of December 31, 1997, are available in the Centers for Disease Control and Prevention, HIV/AIDS Surveillance Report, Year-end edition, 1998.

SOURCE: Centers for Disease Control and Prevention, National Center for HIV, STD, and TB Prevention, Division of HIV/AIDS Prevention.

Table 57. Acquired immunodeficiency syndrome (AIDS) cases, according to geographic division and State: United States, selected years 1985–97

[Data are based on reporting by State health departments]

Geographic division and State of residence	All years[1]	1985	1990	1992	1993	1994	1995	1996	January–June 1997	12 months ending June 30, 1997
					Number, by year of report					Cases per 100,000 population[2]
United States[3]	592,144	8,161	41,569	45,771	102,211	77,237	71,039	66,659	30,153	23.6
New England	25,193	282	1,513	1,736	5,134	2,818	3,586	2,761	1,265	19.8
Maine.	783	11	65	43	149	116	129	50	28	4.4
New Hampshire.	729	3	65	46	122	94	110	93	17	5.8
Vermont	316	2	22	26	71	38	44	25	17	5.4
Massachusetts	12,523	170	845	865	2,697	1,376	1,438	1,307	467	18.5
Rhode Island.	1,668	11	89	106	341	275	221	177	79	16.4
Connecticut.	9,174	85	427	650	1,754	919	1,644	1,109	657	36.6
Middle Atlantic	166,808	3,153	11,948	11,589	25,519	22,081	19,138	18,305	9,568	48.2
New York	113,549	2,481	8,280	8,219	16,986	14,703	12,373	12,372	6,623	68.9
New Jersey.	34,871	474	2,448	2,020	5,364	4,866	4,396	3,591	1,972	47.3
Pennsylvania.	18,388	198	1,220	1,350	3,169	2,512	2,369	2,342	973	17.6
East North Central	44,893	354	3,041	4,041	7,965	6,227	5,371	5,171	2,040	10.2
Ohio.	9,109	53	693	787	1,530	1,175	1,098	1,152	396	8.3
Indiana	4,779	26	294	399	945	615	523	592	361	9.7
Illinois.	19,319	190	1,263	1,877	2,944	3,045	2,213	2,192	764	14.8
Michigan.	8,770	61	579	748	1,821	1,022	1,192	964	386	9.9
Wisconsin.	2,916	24	212	230	725	370	345	271	133	4.9
West North Central	14,579	127	1,055	1,303	3,130	1,609	1,702	1,622	541	7.3
Minnesota.	3,095	41	203	216	655	411	364	304	101	5.3
Iowa.	1,028	12	68	112	198	130	116	110	52	3.7
Missouri	7,487	50	579	708	1,718	706	784	852	237	12.9
North Dakota.	85	–	1	9	11	22	5	12	7	1.6
South Dakota	122	1	9	8	29	20	18	14	4	1.4
Nebraska	843	7	58	60	178	88	115	99	55	6.0
Kansas.	1,919	16	137	190	341	232	300	231	85	7.3
South Atlantic.	133,179	1,286	8,788	10,343	22,726	18,631	17,887	16,596	7,435	32.6
Delaware	1,922	12	93	138	370	267	317	285	144	36.4
Maryland	16,223	149	988	1,198	2,507	2,673	2,558	2,247	950	42.9
District of Columbia	9,946	177	733	710	1,588	1,397	1,026	1,258	537	220.2
Virginia.	9,699	107	745	780	1,619	1,153	1,602	1,193	604	18.8
West Virginia.	801	6	61	56	106	93	125	121	57	6.2
North Carolina.	7,742	67	570	584	1,371	1,186	1,001	897	428	11.7
South Carolina	6,661	37	372	393	1,475	1,151	977	865	389	22.0
Georgia	17,985	194	1,229	1,428	2,847	2,269	2,312	2,422	965	28.7
Florida	62,200	537	3,997	5,056	10,843	8,442	7,969	7,308	3,361	46.7
East South Central	15,902	73	1,060	1,320	2,691	2,079	2,264	2,280	1,022	13.4
Kentucky	2,401	18	192	215	321	317	296	401	177	10.4
Tennessee	5,947	19	340	408	1,198	752	891	822	418	15.0
Alabama.	4,504	28	239	441	731	582	637	607	237	12.2
Mississippi	3,050	8	289	256	441	428	440	450	190	16.5
West South Central.	57,001	612	4,427	4,292	9,965	7,599	6,100	6,812	3,176	22.8
Arkansas	2,270	10	209	276	398	286	276	267	120	9.7
Louisiana	9,660	104	700	822	1,415	1,223	1,079	1,464	545	28.3
Oklahoma.	2,886	20	205	268	722	268	295	272	155	8.7
Texas.	42,185	478	3,313	2,926	7,430	5,822	4,450	4,809	2,356	25.8
Mountain	18,287	158	1,128	1,330	3,870	2,277	2,258	2,012	880	11.9
Montana	249	–	17	19	32	29	25	34	22	4.8
Idaho	394	4	28	35	71	61	48	39	28	3.7
Wyoming	153	–	6	7	38	19	18	7	13	3.5
Colorado.	5,962	62	366	403	1,321	810	672	520	210	11.3
New Mexico	1,522	14	108	106	296	213	164	206	79	13.4
Arizona.	5,258	49	316	376	1,219	611	674	587	226	12.0
Utah.	1,449	17	98	135	264	153	163	193	68	7.9
Nevada.	3,300	12	189	249	629	381	494	426	234	29.1
Pacific.	115,933	2,115	8,587	9,797	21,137	13,850	12,662	11,047	4,204	22.4
Washington.	7,930	107	747	561	1,567	925	881	800	344	13.8
Oregon.	4,021	33	336	288	773	605	457	461	162	11.1
California	101,569	1,942	7,324	8,793	18,371	12,046	10,997	9,551	3,642	25.7
Alaska	385	4	24	18	69	58	69	36	22	7.2
Hawaii	2,028	29	156	137	357	216	258	199	34	12.2

– Quantity zero.

[1]Includes cases before 1985.

[2]Computed using resident population estimates for 1996 based on extrapolation from 1990 census counts from the U.S. Bureau of the Census.

[3]Includes unknown State of residence.

NOTES: The AIDS case reporting definitions were expanded in 1985, 1987, and 1993. See Appendix II. Excludes data for U.S. dependencies and possessions and independent nations in free association with the United States. Data are updated periodically because of reporting delays. Data for all years have been updated through June 30, 1997. Data as of December 31, 1997, are available in the Centers for Disease Control and Prevention, HIV/AIDS Surveillance Report, Year-end edition, 1998.

SOURCE: Centers for Disease Control and Prevention, National Center for HIV, STD, and TB Prevention, Division of HIV/AIDS Prevention.

Table 58. Age-adjusted cancer incidence rates for selected cancer sites, according to sex and race: Selected geographic areas, selected years 1973–95

[Data are based on the Surveillance, Epidemiology, and End Results Program's population-based registries in Atlanta, Detroit, Seattle-Puget Sound, San Francisco-Oakland, Connecticut, Iowa, New Mexico, Utah, and Hawaii]

Race, sex, and site	1973	1975	1980	1985	1990	1991	1992	1993	1994	1995
White male	Number of new cases per 100,000 population[1]									
All sites	364.3	379.7	407.5	431.2	481.9	518.9	535.3	502.1	475.0	452.3
Oral cavity and pharynx	17.6	18.3	17.0	16.8	16.4	16.1	15.7	16.0	14.7	14.2
Esophagus	4.8	4.8	4.9	5.3	6.1	5.7	6.2	5.9	6.0	5.6
Stomach	14.0	12.5	12.3	10.5	9.4	9.7	9.4	9.1	9.4	8.8
Colon and rectum	54.2	55.1	58.7	63.4	59.0	58.0	56.5	54.2	53.0	49.7
Colon	34.8	36.1	39.3	43.4	40.3	40.6	39.1	38.1	37.1	34.6
Rectum	19.5	19.0	19.4	20.1	18.7	17.4	17.4	16.1	15.9	15.1
Pancreas	12.8	12.5	11.1	10.7	10.1	10.0	10.4	9.6	9.8	9.3
Lung and bronchus	72.4	75.9	82.2	82.0	80.9	80.4	79.5	77.2	74.5	71.5
Prostate gland	62.6	68.9	78.8	87.1	133.0	169.1	188.3	163.4	140.0	129.8
Urinary bladder	27.3	28.8	31.5	31.2	32.4	32.4	32.0	32.0	31.7	30.6
Non-Hodgkin's lymphoma	10.3	11.4	12.6	15.9	19.6	20.5	19.6	20.0	20.6	20.7
Leukemia	14.3	14.2	14.6	14.8	14.4	14.2	14.5	13.6	13.3	13.4
Black male										
All sites	441.4	438.0	510.4	532.7	575.8	622.5	659.7	665.3	637.1	584.1
Oral cavity and pharynx	16.6	17.2	23.1	22.6	24.8	21.3	22.7	23.0	25.1	20.6
Esophagus	13.3	17.6	16.4	19.4	19.9	15.3	15.8	15.3	13.3	12.4
Stomach	25.9	19.9	21.4	18.8	18.2	20.2	16.2	18.7	19.4	14.3
Colon and rectum	42.8	47.6	63.5	60.8	59.7	62.6	62.4	62.1	59.8	54.0
Colon	31.7	34.7	45.8	47.0	46.2	46.6	47.1	47.2	44.5	41.1
Rectum	11.1	12.9	17.7	13.8	13.5	16.0	15.3	14.9	15.3	12.9
Pancreas	15.9	15.6	17.6	19.7	15.4	14.7	16.0	15.5	17.4	15.6
Lung and bronchus	104.8	101.0	131.0	131.3	118.6	126.0	128.7	115.7	113.3	114.7
Prostate gland	106.3	111.5	126.7	133.6	173.3	223.3	256.9	270.6	245.7	211.6
Urinary bladder	10.6	13.4	14.5	16.3	15.5	15.1	16.7	18.2	15.8	14.6
Non-Hodgkin's lymphoma	8.8	7.0	9.3	10.0	14.2	15.9	15.4	15.7	17.9	18.2
Leukemia	12.0	12.5	13.1	13.0	12.1	10.0	11.7	12.1	9.8	9.4
White female										
All sites	295.1	310.5	311.3	343.8	356.3	359.5	356.8	349.9	354.6	351.9
Colon and rectum	41.7	42.9	44.7	45.9	40.2	38.9	38.5	37.8	37.0	36.6
Colon	30.3	30.9	32.9	34.0	30.1	29.0	28.7	28.0	27.8	27.5
Rectum	11.5	12.0	11.8	12.0	10.1	9.9	9.8	9.8	9.3	9.0
Pancreas	7.5	7.1	7.3	8.1	7.7	7.6	8.0	7.3	7.6	7.3
Lung and bronchus	17.8	21.8	28.2	35.9	42.5	44.2	44.4	43.8	44.5	44.2
Melanoma of skin	5.9	6.9	9.4	10.5	11.4	12.2	11.9	11.7	12.1	12.9
Breast	84.4	90.0	87.8	107.2	114.4	116.4	114.4	112.2	114.8	115.0
Cervix uteri	12.8	11.1	9.1	7.6	8.3	7.7	7.9	7.7	7.2	6.5
Corpus uteri	29.5	33.7	25.3	23.1	23.1	22.5	22.8	22.2	22.8	22.7
Ovary	14.6	14.4	14.0	15.1	16.1	16.3	15.8	15.7	14.9	15.2
Non-Hodgkin's lymphoma	7.6	8.5	9.2	11.4	12.9	12.5	12.9	12.8	13.5	12.6
Black female										
All sites	283.7	296.5	304.8	323.7	342.7	344.5	345.3	338.5	345.5	330.0
Colon and rectum	41.8	43.5	49.6	45.9	49.5	46.3	46.1	44.8	46.9	43.9
Colon	30.0	32.7	41.2	36.0	38.6	37.8	36.2	36.6	37.1	35.3
Rectum	11.8	10.8	8.5	9.9	10.9	8.5	9.9	8.2	9.7	8.6
Pancreas	11.6	11.6	13.0	11.3	10.3	12.6	13.0	12.1	12.0	12.3
Lung and bronchus	20.9	20.6	33.8	40.2	46.9	49.8	49.1	46.0	49.3	42.9
Breast	69.0	78.5	74.3	92.5	97.7	98.1	102.6	101.0	101.9	101.3
Cervix uteri	29.9	28.0	19.0	15.9	13.9	13.4	11.3	11.3	11.6	11.4
Corpus uteri	15.0	17.1	14.1	15.4	14.6	14.7	14.6	14.8	15.8	15.7
Ovary	10.5	10.1	10.1	10.1	10.2	10.1	10.7	11.1	12.5	9.7
Non-Hodgkin's lymphoma	5.5	4.2	6.0	7.1	9.3	8.6	8.4	8.1	7.2	9.1

[1]Age adjusted by the direct method to the 1970 U.S. population.

NOTE: Numbers have been revised and differ from previous editions of *Health, United States*.

SOURCE: National Institutes of Health, National Cancer Institute, Cancer Statistics Branch, Bethesda, Maryland 20892.

Table 59. Five-year relative cancer survival rates for selected cancer sites, according to race and sex: Selected geographic areas, 1974–79, 1980–82, 1983–85, 1986–88, and 1989–94

[Data are based on the Surveillance, Epidemiology, and End Results Program's population-based registries in Atlanta, Detroit, Seattle-Puget Sound, San Francisco-Oakland, Connecticut, Iowa, New Mexico, Utah, and Hawaii]

Sex and site	White					Black				
	1974–79	1980–82	1983–85	1986–88	1989–94	1974–79	1980–82	1983–85	1986–88	1989–94
Male					Percent of patients					
All sites	43.3	46.6	49.1	52.8	60.0	31.9	34.2	34.7	37.7	45.1
Oral cavity and pharynx.	54.0	54.3	54.9	53.0	52.0	31.2	26.2	30.2	29.8	27.4
Esophagus.	5.0	6.7	7.9	11.7	12.5	2.3	4.6	5.2	7.1	8.2
Stomach	13.8	15.4	14.7	16.5	16.1	15.1	18.5	17.9	14.3	20.5
Colon	50.8	56.0	59.9	64.1	64.6	44.9	46.4	48.3	52.0	51.4
Rectum	48.9	51.5	56.0	60.3	61.0	36.6	36.1	42.8	47.1	53.3
Pancreas	2.7	2.6	2.5	3.0	3.7	2.4	3.7	4.8	6.6	3.3
Lung and bronchus.	11.6	12.2	12.2	12.4	13.0	9.9	11.0	10.4	11.9	9.7
Prostate gland	70.0	74.5	77.7	85.2	95.1	60.5	64.7	64.0	69.2	81.2
Urinary bladder.	75.7	79.9	80.7	84.4	86.3	58.6	62.4	64.3	67.5	66.5
Non-Hodgkin's lymphoma . . .	47.0	50.9	53.9	50.9	48.5	44.1	47.9	43.6	47.1	37.3
Leukemia.	35.4	39.3	41.6	45.3	45.3	31.1	30.2	32.3	35.3	27.5
Female										
All sites	57.2	57.0	59.1	61.9	63.1	46.7	45.9	45.5	47.8	48.8
Colon	52.4	55.4	58.5	61.7	63.1	48.6	51.3	50.0	53.4	53.1
Rectum	50.6	54.6	57.1	60.2	61.6	43.6	40.8	45.3	55.2	53.2
Pancreas	2.2	3.1	3.3	3.2	4.2	4.1	5.7	5.8	5.6	4.0
Lung and bronchus.	16.7	16.2	17.1	15.9	16.5	15.4	15.4	14.2	11.6	13.9
Melanoma of skin	85.7	88.2	89.4	91.4	91.2	68.9	- - -	71.6	- - -	77.3
Breast	75.2	77.1	79.7	84.6	86.7	63.1	65.9	63.7	69.6	70.6
Cervix uteri	69.4	67.8	70.5	71.9	71.5	63.0	61.1	60.0	55.0	59.0
Corpus uteri	87.5	82.8	84.9	85.1	86.5	59.2	54.1	54.2	56.7	54.4
Ovary	37.1	38.6	40.4	42.2	50.1	40.4	38.6	42.0	38.7	46.3
Non-Hodgkin's lymphoma . . .	49.1	52.8	55.7	56.5	57.3	56.9	53.3	46.8	54.3	46.9

- - - Data not available.

NOTES: Rates are based on followup of patients through 1995. The rate is the ratio of the observed survival rate for the patient group to the expected survival rate for persons in the general population similar to the patient group with respect to age, sex, race, and calendar year of observation. It estimates the chance of surviving the effects of cancer. Numbers have been revised and differ from previous editions of *Health, United States*.

SOURCE: National Institutes of Health, National Cancer Institute, Cancer Statistics Branch, Bethesda, Maryland 20892.

Table 60. Limitation of activity caused by chronic conditions, according to selected characteristics: United States, 1990 and 1995

[Data are based on household interviews of a sample of the civilian noninstitutionalized population]

Characteristic	Total with limitation of activity		Limited but not in major activity		Limited in amount or kind of major activity		Unable to carry on major activity	
	1990	1995	1990	1995	1990	1995	1990	1995
	Percent of population							
Total[1,2]	12.9	13.9	4.1	4.3	5.0	5.3	3.9	4.3
Age								
Under 15 years	4.7	5.6	1.2	1.5	3.1	3.5	0.4	0.6
Under 5 years	2.2	2.7	0.6	0.6	1.0	1.4	0.6	0.7
5–14 years	6.1	7.1	1.6	2.0	4.1	4.6	0.4	0.5
15–44 years	8.5	9.8	2.6	3.0	3.5	3.9	2.4	2.9
45–64 years	21.8	22.7	5.7	5.3	7.5	7.9	8.6	9.5
65 years and over	37.5	37.2	15.4	15.7	11.9	11.0	10.2	10.5
65–74 years	33.7	33.2	13.2	13.6	9.9	9.1	10.6	10.5
75 years and over	43.3	43.0	18.8	18.8	14.9	13.8	9.6	10.4
Sex and age								
Male[1]	12.9	14.2	3.8	4.2	4.7	5.2	4.4	4.8
Under 15 years	5.5	7.1	1.4	1.8	3.6	4.6	0.5	0.7
15–44 years	8.4	10.0	2.3	2.8	3.5	4.0	2.7	3.2
45–64 years	21.4	21.7	4.7	4.5	6.6	6.6	10.1	10.7
65–74 years	34.0	34.8	13.0	13.7	8.4	8.2	12.7	12.9
75 years and over	38.8	40.0	20.3	21.2	10.2	9.7	8.3	9.1
Female[1]	13.0	13.6	4.3	4.3	5.3	5.4	3.4	3.9
Under 15 years	3.9	4.1	1.0	1.2	2.5	2.4	0.4	0.5
15–44 years	8.7	9.7	2.9	3.1	3.6	3.9	2.2	2.7
45–64 years	22.2	23.6	6.6	6.0	8.4	9.1	7.2	8.4
65–74 years	33.5	31.9	13.4	13.6	11.1	9.8	8.9	8.6
75 years and over	46.0	44.8	17.9	17.3	17.7	16.4	10.4	11.2
Race and age								
White[1]	12.8	13.6	4.2	4.3	5.0	5.2	3.6	4.0
Under 15 years	4.7	5.5	1.3	1.5	3.0	3.4	0.4	0.5
15–44 years	8.5	9.7	2.7	3.1	3.6	3.9	2.2	2.7
45–64 years	21.2	22.0	5.8	5.3	7.6	7.9	7.9	8.8
65–74 years	33.2	32.4	13.4	13.6	9.8	8.9	10.0	9.9
75 years and over	42.9	42.7	19.2	19.2	14.7	13.5	9.0	10.0
Black[1]	15.5	17.4	3.8	4.1	5.3	6.3	6.5	7.1
Under 15 years	5.3	7.0	1.2	1.7	3.4	4.5	0.7	0.8
15–44 years	9.4	11.8	2.2	2.6	3.4	4.4	3.9	4.8
45–64 years	28.1	30.0	5.7	5.3	7.7	8.7	14.8	16.0
65–74 years	41.6	43.8	12.4	14.7	11.5	12.1	17.6	16.9
75 years and over	50.9	48.9	16.2	16.0	17.6	18.5	17.0	14.6
Family income[1,3]								
Less than $15,000	22.9	25.7	5.2	5.8	8.1	8.9	9.6	11.1
$15,000–$24,999	14.8	17.4	4.3	4.3	5.7	6.9	4.8	6.1
$25,000–$34,999	11.6	13.1	3.8	4.5	4.7	5.2	3.0	3.5
$35,000–$49,999	10.4	11.2	3.7	4.1	4.4	4.4	2.3	2.6
$50,000 or more	8.4	8.7	3.4	3.6	3.3	3.4	1.7	1.7
Geographic region[1]								
Northeast	11.9	12.9	3.9	3.8	4.5	5.1	3.6	3.9
Midwest	12.9	13.9	3.9	4.2	5.5	5.7	3.4	4.0
South	14.0	14.5	4.1	4.2	5.3	5.4	4.6	4.9
West	12.5	14.1	4.4	4.8	4.5	5.0	3.7	4.4
Location of residence[1]								
Within MSA[4]	12.4	13.6	4.0	4.2	4.7	5.3	3.7	4.2
Outside MSA[4]	14.9	14.8	4.3	4.2	6.1	5.6	4.5	5.0

[1]Age adjusted.
[2]Includes all other races not shown separately and unknown family income.
[3]Family income categories for 1995. In 1990 the two lowest income categories are less than $14,000 and $14,000–$24,999; the three higher income categories are as shown.
[4]Metropolitan statistical area.

SOURCE: Centers for Disease Control and Prevention, National Center for Health Statistics, Division of Health Interview Statistics. Data from the National Health Interview Survey.

Table 61. Respondent-assessed health status, according to selected characteristics: United States, 1987–95

[Data are based on household interviews of a sample of the civilian noninstitutionalized population]

Characteristic	Percent with fair or poor health								
	1987	1988	1989	1990	1991	1992	1993	1994	1995
Total[1,2]	9.5	9.4	9.1	8.9	9.3	9.7	9.7	9.6	9.4
Age									
Under 15 years	2.4	2.7	2.4	2.4	2.5	2.8	2.8	2.9	2.4
Under 5 years	2.6	3.4	2.6	2.9	2.6	2.9	3.3	2.9	2.8
5–14 years	2.3	2.4	2.3	2.2	2.4	2.8	2.6	2.9	2.3
15–44 years	5.4	5.5	5.6	5.4	5.8	6.4	6.6	6.4	6.3
45–64 years	17.4	17.1	16.1	16.0	16.7	17.2	17.1	16.6	16.7
65 years and over	30.8	29.4	28.5	27.7	29.0	28.7	28.0	28.0	28.3
65–74 years	28.2	26.6	26.3	25.1	26.0	25.7	25.0	25.6	25.6
75 years and over	34.9	33.8	32.0	31.7	33.6	33.2	32.4	31.3	32.2
Sex and age									
Male[1]	9.0	8.9	8.6	8.4	8.9	9.4	9.1	9.0	8.9
Under 15 years	2.5	2.7	2.6	2.6	2.5	2.9	2.9	3.1	2.7
15–44 years	4.5	4.6	4.6	4.5	5.0	5.7	5.6	5.4	5.2
45–64 years	16.6	16.5	15.4	15.5	16.1	16.5	16.0	15.3	15.7
65–74 years	28.9	27.0	27.2	25.0	26.7	26.8	25.4	26.6	26.3
75 years and over	36.0	33.0	33.0	31.7	33.7	33.5	31.9	31.9	32.9
Female[1]	9.9	9.9	9.5	9.3	9.7	10.1	10.4	10.1	9.9
Under 15 years	2.3	2.8	2.3	2.2	2.4	2.7	2.7	2.7	2.2
15–44 years	6.3	6.4	6.6	6.3	6.6	7.2	7.6	7.4	7.3
45–64 years	18.1	17.6	16.8	16.5	17.2	17.8	18.2	17.7	17.5
65–74 years	27.7	26.4	25.6	25.1	25.5	24.7	24.6	24.9	25.0
75 years and over	34.2	34.3	31.5	31.6	33.5	33.0	32.7	30.8	31.8
Race and age									
White[1]	8.5	8.5	8.2	8.1	8.6	8.9	8.8	8.6	8.7
Under 15 years	2.0	2.4	2.0	1.9	2.1	2.5	2.4	2.5	2.2
15–44 years	4.6	4.8	4.9	4.8	5.2	5.7	5.9	5.6	5.6
45–64 years	15.6	15.3	14.5	14.6	15.4	15.5	15.3	14.9	15.2
65–74 years	26.8	24.8	24.5	23.9	24.6	24.1	23.4	24.2	24.1
75 years and over	33.2	32.3	30.8	30.7	32.4	31.9	31.0	29.8	31.2
Black[1]	16.7	16.4	15.9	15.1	15.1	16.3	16.8	16.1	15.4
Under 15 years	4.1	4.6	4.4	4.8	4.5	4.4	4.9	4.9	3.8
15–44 years	10.5	9.9	10.2	9.9	9.7	10.7	11.1	10.6	10.9
45–64 years	32.9	30.9	29.6	28.3	27.2	30.9	32.0	30.2	28.1
65–74 years	42.9	46.8	44.7	38.4	41.2	42.1	41.1	40.3	40.5
75 years and over	52.4	50.8	45.2	42.9	48.2	48.4	48.2	46.8	44.3
Family income[1,3]									
Less than $15,000	20.5	19.8	19.4	18.6	19.9	20.7	21.4	20.4	20.6
$15,000–$24,999	14.1	12.0	10.1	10.8	10.8	11.6	12.1	12.3	13.1
$25,000–$34,999	11.0	9.0	6.9	7.5	7.1	8.1	8.2	7.9	8.1
$35,000–$49,999	7.1	6.5	5.1	5.3	5.5	6.0	5.7	6.2	5.9
$50,000 or more	4.7	4.0	3.7	4.0	3.9	3.8	3.9	3.9	3.7
Geographic region[1]									
Northeast	7.9	7.8	7.2	7.2	7.4	8.0	8.3	8.1	8.2
Midwest	8.8	8.6	8.3	7.9	8.1	8.6	8.7	8.6	8.6
South	11.7	11.5	11.2	11.2	11.7	11.8	11.6	11.2	11.0
West	8.2	8.4	8.5	8.1	8.8	9.5	9.3	9.4	9.0
Location of residence[1]									
Within MSA[4]	9.0	9.0	8.6	8.5	8.9	9.3	9.4	9.2	9.0
Outside MSA[4]	10.8	11.0	10.8	10.4	10.7	11.3	11.1	10.8	11.2

[1]Age adjusted.
[2]Includes all other races not shown separately and unknown family income.
[3]Family income categories for 1995. In 1989–94 the two lowest income categories are less than $14,000 and $14,000–$24,999; the three higher income categories are as shown. Income categories for 1988 are less than $13,000; $13,000–$18,999; $19,000–$24,999; $25,000–$44,999; and $45,000 or more. Income categories for 1987 are less than $10,000; $10,000–$14,999; $15,000–$19,999; $20,000–$34,999; and $35,000 or more.
[4]Metropolitan statistical area.

SOURCE: Centers for Disease Control and Prevention, National Center for Health Statistics, Division of Health Interview Statistics. Data from the National Health Interview Survey.

Table 62. Current cigarette smoking by persons 18 years of age and over, according to sex, race, and age: United States, selected years 1965–95

[Data are based on household interviews of a sample of the civilian noninstitutionalized population]

Sex, race, and age	1965	1974	1979	1983	1985	1990	1991	1992	1993	1994	1995
All persons	Percent of persons 18 years of age and over										
18 years and over, age adjusted	42.3	37.2	33.5	32.2	30.0	25.4	25.4	26.4	25.0	25.5	24.7
18 years and over, crude	42.4	37.1	33.5	32.1	30.1	25.5	25.6	26.5	25.0	25.5	24.7
All males											
18 years and over, age adjusted	51.6	42.9	37.2	34.7	32.1	28.0	27.5	28.2	27.5	27.8	26.7
18 years and over, crude	51.9	43.1	37.5	35.1	32.6	28.4	28.1	28.6	27.7	28.2	27.0
18–24 years	54.1	42.1	35.0	32.9	28.0	26.6	23.5	28.0	28.8	29.8	27.8
25–34 years	60.7	50.5	43.9	38.8	38.2	31.6	32.8	32.8	30.2	31.4	29.5
35–44 years	58.2	51.0	41.8	41.0	37.6	34.5	33.1	32.9	32.0	33.2	31.5
45–64 years	51.9	42.6	39.3	35.9	33.4	29.3	29.3	28.6	29.2	28.3	27.1
65 years and over	28.5	24.8	20.9	22.0	19.6	14.6	15.1	16.1	13.5	13.2	14.9
White:											
18 years and over, age adjusted.	50.8	41.7	36.5	34.1	31.3	27.6	27.0	28.0	27.0	27.5	26.4
18 years and over, crude.	51.1	41.9	36.8	34.5	31.7	28.0	27.4	28.2	27.0	27.7	26.6
18–24 years	53.0	40.8	34.3	32.5	28.4	27.4	25.1	30.0	30.4	31.8	28.4
25–34 years	60.1	49.5	43.6	38.6	37.3	31.6	32.1	33.5	29.9	32.5	29.9
35–44 years	57.3	50.1	41.3	40.8	36.6	33.5	32.1	30.9	31.2	32.0	31.2
45–64 years	51.3	41.2	38.3	35.0	32.1	28.7	28.0	28.1	27.8	26.9	26.3
65 years and over	27.7	24.3	20.5	20.6	18.9	13.7	14.2	14.9	12.5	11.9	14.1
Black:											
18 years and over, age adjusted.	59.2	54.0	44.1	41.3	39.9	32.2	34.7	32.0	33.2	33.5	28.5
18 years and over, crude.	60.4	54.3	44.1	40.6	39.9	32.5	35.0	32.2	32.7	33.7	28.5
18–24 years	62.8	54.9	40.2	34.2	27.2	21.3	15.0	16.2	19.9	18.7	14.6
25–34 years	68.4	58.5	47.5	39.9	45.6	33.8	39.4	29.5	30.7	29.8	25.1
35–44 years	67.3	61.5	48.6	45.5	45.0	42.0	44.4	47.5	36.9	44.5	36.3
45–64 years	57.9	57.8	50.0	44.8	46.1	36.7	42.0	35.4	42.4	41.2	33.9
65 years and over	36.4	29.7	26.2	38.9	27.7	21.5	24.3	28.3	27.9	25.6	28.5
All females											
18 years and over, age adjusted	34.0	32.5	30.3	29.9	28.2	23.1	23.6	24.8	22.7	23.3	22.8
18 years and over, crude	33.9	32.1	29.9	29.5	27.9	22.8	23.5	24.6	22.5	23.1	22.6
18–24 years	38.1	34.1	33.8	35.5	30.4	22.5	22.4	24.9	22.9	25.2	21.8
25–34 years	43.7	38.8	33.7	32.6	32.0	28.2	28.4	30.1	27.3	28.8	26.4
35–44 years	43.7	39.8	37.0	33.8	31.5	24.8	27.6	27.3	27.4	26.8	27.1
45–64 years	32.0	33.4	30.7	31.0	29.9	24.8	24.6	26.1	23.0	22.8	24.0
65 years and over	9.6	12.0	13.2	13.1	13.5	11.5	12.0	12.4	10.5	11.1	11.5
White:											
18 years and over, age adjusted.	34.3	32.3	30.6	30.1	28.3	23.9	24.2	25.7	23.7	24.3	23.6
18 years and over, crude.	34.0	31.7	30.1	29.4	27.7	23.4	23.7	25.1	23.1	23.7	23.1
18–24 years	38.4	34.0	34.5	36.5	31.8	25.4	25.1	28.5	26.8	28.5	24.9
25–34 years	43.4	38.6	34.1	32.2	32.0	28.5	28.4	31.5	28.4	30.2	27.3
35–44 years	43.9	39.3	37.2	34.8	31.0	25.0	27.0	27.6	27.3	27.1	27.0
45–64 years	32.7	33.0	30.6	30.6	29.7	25.4	25.3	25.8	23.4	23.2	24.3
65 years and over	9.8	12.3	13.8	13.2	13.3	11.5	12.1	12.6	10.5	11.1	11.7
Black:											
18 years and over, age adjusted.	32.1	35.9	30.8	31.8	30.7	20.4	23.1	23.9	19.8	21.1	22.8
18 years and over, crude.	33.7	36.4	31.1	32.2	31.0	21.2	24.4	24.2	20.8	21.7	23.5
18–24 years	37.1	35.6	31.8	32.0	23.7	10.0	11.8	10.3	8.2	11.8	8.8
25–34 years	47.8	42.2	35.2	38.0	36.2	29.1	32.4	26.9	24.7	24.8	26.7
35–44 years	42.8	46.4	37.7	32.7	40.2	25.5	35.3	32.4	31.5	28.2	31.9
45–64 years	25.7	38.9	34.2	36.3	33.4	22.6	23.4	30.9	21.3	23.5	27.5
65 years and over	7.1	8.9	8.5	13.1	14.5	11.1	9.6	11.1	10.2	13.6	13.3

NOTES: The definition of current smoker was revised in 1992 and 1993. See discussion of current smoker in Appendix II.

SOURCE: Centers for Disease Control and Prevention, National Center for Health Statistics, Division of Health Interview Statistics: Data from the National Health Interview Survey; data computed by the Division of Health and Utilization Analysis from data compiled by the Division of Health Interview Statistics.

Table 63. Age-adjusted prevalence of current cigarette smoking by persons 25 years of age and over, according to sex, race, and education: United States, selected years 1974–95

[Data are based on household interviews of a sample of the civilian noninstitutionalized population]

Sex, race, and education	1974	1979	1983	1985	1990	1991	1992	1993	1994	1995
	Percent of persons 25 years of age and over, age adjusted									
All persons[1]	37.1	33.3	31.7	30.2	25.6	26.0	26.5	24.8	25.1	24.6
Less than 12 years	43.8	41.1	40.8	41.0	36.7	37.4	36.7	35.8	37.5	35.7
12 years	36.4	33.7	33.6	32.1	29.3	29.7	30.7	28.3	29.2	29.0
13–15 years	35.8	33.2	30.3	29.7	23.5	24.7	24.6	24.5	24.9	22.9
16 or more years	27.5	22.8	20.7	18.6	14.1	13.9	15.3	13.6	11.9	13.6
All males[1]	43.0	37.6	35.1	32.9	28.3	28.4	28.2	27.2	27.4	26.4
Less than 12 years	52.4	48.1	47.2	46.0	41.8	42.4	41.2	41.0	43.9	39.7
12 years	42.6	39.1	37.4	35.6	33.2	32.9	33.3	30.5	31.7	32.6
13–15 years	41.6	36.5	33.0	33.0	25.9	27.2	26.1	27.4	27.3	24.0
16 or more years	28.6	23.1	21.8	19.7	14.6	14.8	15.8	14.6	13.2	13.9
White males[1]	41.9	36.9	34.5	31.9	27.7	27.3	27.6	26.3	26.6	26.0
Less than 12 years	51.6	48.0	47.9	45.2	41.7	41.8	41.4	39.7	42.6	38.8
12 years	42.2	38.6	37.1	34.8	33.0	32.4	32.9	29.7	31.7	32.7
13–15 years	41.4	36.4	32.6	32.3	25.4	26.0	25.9	26.9	26.9	23.6
16 or more years	28.1	22.8	21.1	19.2	14.5	14.7	15.0	14.1	12.7	13.4
Black males[1]	53.8	44.9	42.8	42.5	34.5	38.8	35.3	36.0	36.5	31.4
Less than 12 years	58.3	50.1	46.0	51.1	41.4	47.8	44.5	47.2	51.6	41.4
12 years	*51.2	48.4	47.2	41.9	37.4	39.6	38.7	36.4	37.1	36.4
13–15 years	*45.7	39.3	44.7	42.3	28.3	32.7	27.0	30.1	29.7	26.4
16 or more years	*41.8	*37.9	*31.3	*32.0	20.6	18.3	*26.9	*16.0	*25.9	*16.9
All females[1]	32.2	29.6	28.8	27.8	23.2	23.9	24.8	22.7	22.9	23.0
Less than 12 years	36.8	35.0	35.3	36.7	32.1	33.0	32.4	31.0	31.6	32.1
12 years	32.5	29.9	30.9	29.6	26.3	27.1	28.7	26.7	27.3	26.3
13–15 years	30.2	30.0	27.5	26.7	21.1	22.5	23.3	21.8	22.5	22.0
16 or more years	26.1	22.5	19.2	17.4	13.6	12.8	14.6	12.4	10.3	13.3
White females[1]	31.9	29.8	28.8	27.6	23.6	24.0	25.1	23.1	23.5	23.3
Less than 12 years	37.0	36.1	35.5	37.1	33.6	33.7	33.1	31.7	33.0	33.1
12 years	32.1	29.9	30.9	29.4	26.8	27.5	29.5	27.6	28.4	26.7
13–15 years	30.5	30.6	28.0	27.1	21.4	22.3	23.6	21.9	22.3	22.5
16 or more years	25.8	21.9	18.9	16.8	13.7	13.3	14.2	12.5	10.8	13.5
Black females[1]	35.9	30.6	31.8	32.1	22.6	25.5	26.8	22.2	23.0	25.7
Less than 12 years	36.4	31.9	36.9	39.2	26.8	33.3	33.2	29.8	30.1	31.6
12 years	41.9	33.0	35.2	32.3	24.0	26.0	25.9	23.9	22.5	27.9
13–15 years	33.2	*28.8	26.5	23.7	23.1	24.8	27.0	22.7	28.1	21.0
16 or more years	*35.2	*43.4	*38.7	27.5	16.9	14.4	*25.8	*13.3	*11.3	*18.0

* These age-adjusted percents should be considered unreliable because of small sample size. For age groups where percent smoking was 0 or 100, the age-adjustment procedure was modified to substitute the percent from the next lower education group.
[1]Includes unknown education.

NOTES: The definition of current smoker was revised in 1992 and 1993. See discussion of current smoker in Appendix II.

SOURCE: Data computed by the Centers for Disease Control and Prevention, National Center for Health Statistics, Division of Health and Utilization Analysis from data compiled by the Division of Health Interview Statistics.

Table 64 (page 1 of 2). Use of selected substances in the past month by persons 12 years of age and over, according to age, sex, race, and Hispanic origin: United States, selected years 1979–96

[Data are based on household interviews of a sample of the population 12 years of age and over]

Substance, age, sex, race, and Hispanic origin	1979	1982	1985	1988	1990	1991	1992	1993	1994	1995	1996
Cigarettes					Percent of population						
12–17 years	---	---	29	23	22	21	18	19	19	20	18
12–13 years	---	---	---	---	---	---	---	---	9	11	7
14–15 years	---	---	---	---	---	---	---	---	20	21	18
16–17 years	---	---	---	---	---	---	---	---	29	30	28
12–17 years:											
Male	---	---	31	24	24	23	18	18	20	21	18
Female	---	---	28	22	21	19	18	19	18	20	19
White, non-Hispanic	---	---	33	27	26	24	22	21	22	23	21
Black, non-Hispanic	---	---	17	10	*	8	6	8	12	12	12
Hispanic	---	---	21	15	21	17	14	16	14	16	15
18–25 years:											
Male	---	---	---	---	---	---	---	---	37	38	43
Female	---	---	---	---	---	---	---	---	32	32	33
White, non-Hispanic	---	---	---	---	---	---	---	---	39	39	43
Black, non-Hispanic	---	---	---	---	---	---	---	---	25	24	29
Hispanic	---	---	---	---	---	---	---	---	28	28	30
Alcohol											
12 years and over	63	57	60	55	53	52	49	51	54	52	51
12–17 years	50	35	41	33	33	27	21	24	22	21	19
12–13 years	---	---	---	---	---	---	---	---	9	8	5
14–15 years	---	---	---	---	---	---	---	---	22	21	19
16–17 years	---	---	---	---	---	---	---	---	36	34	31
18–25 years	75	67	70	65	63	63	59	59	63	61	60
26–34 years	72	72	71	65	64	63	62	64	65	63	62
35 years and over	60	53	58	63	50	50	47	50	54	53	52
12–17 years:											
Male	52	36	44	36	34	30	22	24	22	22	19
Female	47	34	38	31	31	24	19	23	21	20	18
White, non-Hispanic	53	39	46	36	37	27	22	26	24	23	20
Black, non-Hispanic	---	---	30	22	21	28	18	18	18	15	15
Hispanic	---	---	27	32	24	28	20	22	18	19	20
18–25 years:											
Male	---	---	---	---	---	---	---	---	71	68	67
Female	---	---	---	---	---	---	---	---	55	55	54
White, non-Hispanic	---	---	---	---	---	---	---	---	68	67	65
Black, non-Hispanic	---	---	---	---	---	---	---	---	52	48	50
Hispanic	---	---	---	---	---	---	---	---	54	49	50
Heavy alcohol[1]											
12 years and over	---	---	20	15	14	16	15	15	17	16	15
12–17 years	---	---	22	15	15	13	10	11	8	8	7
12–13 years	---	---	---	---	---	---	---	---	2	2	1
14–15 years	---	---	---	---	---	---	---	---	8	8	6
16–17 years	---	---	---	---	---	---	---	---	16	15	15
18–25 years	---	---	34	28	30	31	30	29	34	30	32
26–34 years	---	---	28	20	21	22	23	22	24	24	23
35 years and over	---	---	13	10	8	10	9	10	12	12	11
12–17 years:											
Male	---	---	29	19	19	17	13	15	10	9	9
Female	---	---	14	11	12	9	7	7	7	6	6
White, non-Hispanic	---	---	26	18	18	16	11	13	10	9	8
Black, non-Hispanic	---	---	6	3	*	6	6	3	4	3	4
Hispanic	---	---	15	13	11	11	9	12	5	7	8
18–25 years:											
Male	---	---	---	---	---	---	---	---	47	41	44
Female	---	---	---	---	---	---	---	---	21	19	21
White, non-Hispanic	---	---	---	---	---	---	---	---	40	34	37
Black, non-Hispanic	---	---	---	---	---	---	---	---	17	16	19
Hispanic	---	---	---	---	---	---	---	---	26	23	25

See footnotes at end of table.

Table 64 (page 2 of 2). Use of selected substances in the past month by persons 12 years of age and over, according to age, sex, race, and Hispanic origin: United States, selected years 1979–96

[Data are based on household interviews of a sample of the population 12 years of age and over]

Substance, age, sex, race, and Hispanic origin	1979	1982	1985	1988	1990	1991	1992	1993	1994	1995	1996
Marijuana					Percent of population						
12 years and over	13	12	10	6	5	5	5	5	5	5	5
12–17 years	14	10	10	5	4	4	3	4	6	8	7
12–13 years	---	---	---	---	---	---	---	---	2	2	1
14–15 years	---	---	---	---	---	---	---	---	5	10	7
16–17 years	---	---	---	---	---	---	---	---	12	13	13
18–25 years	36	27	22	15	13	13	11	11	12	12	13
26–34 years	20	19	19	12	10	8	9	8	7	7	6
35 years and over	3	4	3	2	2	3	2	2	2	2	2
12–17 years:											
Male	16	11	11	5	5	4	4	4	7	9	8
Female	12	9	9	6	4	3	3	4	5	7	7
White, non-Hispanic	16	11	12	6	5	4	4	4	6	8	7
Black, non-Hispanic	10	7	6	3	2	3	2	3	6	8	7
Hispanic	8	*	6	3	3	3	3	4	6	8	7
18–25 years:											
Male	---	---	---	---	---	---	---	---	16	15	17
Female	---	---	---	---	---	---	---	---	9	9	9
White, non-Hispanic	---	---	---	---	---	---	---	---	13	13	14
Black, non-Hispanic	---	---	---	---	---	---	---	---	12	12	14
Hispanic	---	---	---	---	---	---	---	---	8	7	8
Cocaine											
12 years and over	2.6	2.4	3.0	1.6	0.9	1.0	0.7	0.7	0.7	0.7	0.8
12–17 years	1.5	1.9	1.5	1.2	0.6	0.4	0.3	0.4	0.3	0.8	0.6
18–25 years	9.9	7.0	8.1	4.8	2.3	2.2	2.0	1.6	1.2	1.3	2.0
26–34 years	3.0	3.5	6.3	2.8	1.9	1.9	1.5	1.0	1.3	1.2	1.5
35 years and over	0.2	0.5	0.5	0.4	0.5	0.5	0.2	0.4	0.4	0.4	0.4
12–17 years:											
Male	2.2	2.4	1.9	0.9	0.8	0.5	0.3	0.5	0.3	0.8	0.4
Female	0.8	1.5	1.1	1.5	0.5	0.3	0.3	0.4	0.3	0.7	0.8
White, non-Hispanic	1.4	1.6	1.5	1.4	0.4	0.3	0.2	0.4	0.3	0.9	0.5
Black, non-Hispanic	*	*	1.3	0.5	0.8	0.5	0.3	0.3	0.1	0.1	0.1
Hispanic	2.1	*	2.6	1.4	2.0	1.4	1.3	1.1	0.8	0.8	1.1
18–25 years:											
Male	---	---	---	---	---	---	---	---	0.9	1.7	2.7
Female	---	---	---	---	---	---	---	---	0.6	0.9	1.4
White, non-Hispanic	---	---	---	---	---	---	---	---	1.2	1.5	2.3
Black, non-Hispanic	---	---	---	---	---	---	---	---	0.7	0.7	1.1
Hispanic	---	---	---	---	---	---	---	---	2.2	1.1	2.1

- - - Data not available.

* Estimates with relative standard error greater than 17.5 percent of the log transformation of the proportion are not shown.

[1]Five or more drinks on the same occasion at least once in the past month.

NOTES: In 1994 the survey underwent major changes. Estimates for 1993 and earlier years are adjusted to be comparable with data from the redesigned survey. See Appendix I, Substance Abuse and Mental Health Services Administration. Estimates of the use of substances from the National Household Survey on Drug Abuse and the Monitoring the Future Study differ because of different methodologies, sampling frames, and tabulation categories.

SOURCES: National Household Survey on Drug Abuse Series H–3: Preliminary Results from the 1996 National Household Survey on Drug Abuse; and H–4: National Household Survey on Drug Abuse: Population Estimates 1996.

Table 65 (page 1 of 2). Use of selected substances in the past month and heavy alcohol use in the past 2 weeks by high school seniors and eighth-graders, according to sex and race: United States, selected years 1980–97

[Data are based on a survey of high school seniors and eighth-graders in the coterminous United States]

Substance, sex, race, and grade in school	1980	1985	1987	1988	1989	1990	1991	1992	1993	1994	1995	1996	1997
Cigarettes						Percent using substance in the past month							
All seniors	30.5	30.1	29.4	28.7	28.6	29.4	28.3	27.8	29.9	31.2	33.5	34.0	36.5
Male	26.8	28.2	27.0	28.0	27.7	29.1	29.0	29.2	30.7	32.9	34.5	34.9	37.3
Female	33.4	31.4	31.4	28.9	29.0	29.2	27.5	26.1	28.7	29.2	32.0	32.4	35.2
White	31.0	31.7	32.2	32.3	32.1	32.5	31.8	31.8	34.6	35.9	37.3	38.9	42.5
Black	25.2	18.7	13.9	12.8	12.4	12.0	9.4	8.2	10.9	11.0	15.0	13.5	14.9
All eighth-graders	- - -	- - -	- - -	- - -	- - -	- - -	14.3	15.5	16.7	18.6	19.1	21.0	19.4
Male	- - -	- - -	- - -	- - -	- - -	- - -	15.5	14.9	17.2	19.3	18.8	20.6	19.1
Female	- - -	- - -	- - -	- - -	- - -	- - -	13.1	15.9	16.3	17.9	19.0	21.1	19.5
White	- - -	- - -	- - -	- - -	- - -	- - -	15.0	17.4	18.1	19.8	21.7	23.8	22.0
Black	- - -	- - -	- - -	- - -	- - -	- - -	5.3	5.3	7.7	9.6	8.2	11.3	10.4
Marijuana													
All seniors	33.7	25.7	21.0	18.0	16.7	14.0	13.8	11.9	15.5	19.0	21.2	21.9	23.7
Male	37.8	28.7	23.1	20.7	19.5	16.1	16.1	13.4	18.2	23.0	24.6	25.1	26.4
Female	29.1	22.4	18.6	15.2	13.8	11.5	11.2	10.2	12.5	15.1	17.2	18.3	20.3
White	34.2	26.4	22.3	19.9	18.6	15.6	15.0	13.1	16.7	20.1	21.5	22.5	24.6
Black	26.5	21.7	12.4	9.8	9.4	5.2	6.5	5.6	10.8	15.9	17.8	18.8	18.2
All eighth-graders	- - -	- - -	- - -	- - -	- - -	- - -	3.2	3.7	5.1	7.8	9.1	11.3	10.2
Male	- - -	- - -	- - -	- - -	- - -	- - -	3.8	3.8	6.1	9.5	9.8	12.1	11.4
Female	- - -	- - -	- - -	- - -	- - -	- - -	2.6	3.5	4.1	6.0	8.2	10.2	8.9
White	- - -	- - -	- - -	- - -	- - -	- - -	3.0	3.5	4.6	6.7	9.0	11.0	10.2
Black	- - -	- - -	- - -	- - -	- - -	- - -	2.1	1.9	3.7	6.2	7.0	9.3	8.7
Cocaine													
All seniors	5.2	6.7	4.3	3.4	2.8	1.9	1.4	1.3	1.3	1.5	1.8	2.0	2.3
Male	6.0	7.7	4.9	4.2	3.6	2.3	1.7	1.5	1.7	1.9	2.2	2.6	2.8
Female	4.3	5.6	3.7	2.6	2.0	1.3	0.9	0.9	0.9	1.1	1.3	1.4	1.6
White	5.4	7.0	4.4	3.7	2.9	1.8	1.3	1.2	1.2	1.5	1.7	2.1	2.4
Black	2.0	2.7	1.8	1.4	1.2	0.5	0.8	0.5	0.4	0.6	0.4	0.4	0.7
All eighth-graders	- - -	- - -	- - -	- - -	- - -	- - -	0.5	0.7	0.7	1.0	1.2	1.3	1.1
Male	- - -	- - -	- - -	- - -	- - -	- - -	0.7	0.6	0.9	1.2	1.1	1.2	1.2
Female	- - -	- - -	- - -	- - -	- - -	- - -	0.4	0.8	0.6	0.9	1.2	1.4	1.0
White	- - -	- - -	- - -	- - -	- - -	- - -	0.4	0.6	0.5	0.9	1.0	1.4	1.0
Black	- - -	- - -	- - -	- - -	- - -	- - -	0.4	0.4	0.3	0.3	0.4	0.4	0.3
Inhalants													
All seniors	1.4	2.2	2.8	2.6	2.3	2.7	2.4	2.3	2.5	2.7	3.2	2.5	2.5
Male	1.8	2.8	3.4	3.2	3.1	3.5	3.3	3.0	3.2	3.6	3.9	3.1	3.3
Female	1.0	1.7	2.2	2.0	1.5	2.0	1.6	1.6	1.7	1.9	2.5	2.0	1.8
White	1.4	2.4	3.0	2.9	2.4	3.0	2.4	2.4	2.7	2.9	3.7	2.9	3.1
Black	1.0	0.8	1.8	1.8	1.1	1.5	1.5	1.5	1.3	1.8	1.1	0.9	0.9
All eighth-graders	- - -	- - -	- - -	- - -	- - -	- - -	4.4	4.7	5.4	5.6	6.1	5.8	5.6
Male	- - -	- - -	- - -	- - -	- - -	- - -	4.1	4.4	4.9	5.4	5.6	4.8	5.1
Female	- - -	- - -	- - -	- - -	- - -	- - -	4.7	4.9	6.0	5.8	6.6	6.6	5.8
White	- - -	- - -	- - -	- - -	- - -	- - -	4.5	5.0	5.8	6.1	7.0	6.6	6.4
Black	- - -	- - -	- - -	- - -	- - -	- - -	2.3	2.4	2.9	2.6	2.3	1.7	2.2

See footnotes at end of table.

Table 65 (page 2 of 2). Use of selected substances in the past month and heavy alcohol use in the past 2 weeks by high school seniors and eighth-graders, according to sex and race: United States, selected years 1980–97

[Data are based on a survey of high school seniors and eighth-graders in the coterminous United States]

Substance, sex, race, and grade in school	1980	1985	1987	1988	1989	1990	1991	1992	1993	1994	1995	1996	1997
Alcohol[1]						Percent using substance in the past month							
All seniors	72.0	65.9	66.4	63.9	60.0	57.1	54.0	51.3	48.6	50.1	51.3	50.8	52.7
Male	77.4	69.8	69.9	68.0	65.1	61.3	58.4	55.8	54.2	55.5	55.7	54.8	56.2
Female	66.8	62.1	63.1	59.9	54.9	52.3	49.0	46.8	43.4	45.2	47.0	46.9	48.9
White	75.8	70.2	71.8	69.5	65.3	62.2	57.7	56.0	53.4	54.8	54.8	54.7	57.9
Black	47.7	43.6	38.5	40.9	38.1	32.9	34.4	29.5	35.1	33.1	37.4	35.7	33.1
All eighth-graders	- - -	- - -	- - -	- - -	- - -	- - -	25.1	26.1	24.3	25.5	24.6	26.2	24.5
Male	- - -	- - -	- - -	- - -	- - -	- - -	26.3	26.3	25.3	26.5	25.0	26.6	25.2
Female	- - -	- - -	- - -	- - -	- - -	- - -	23.8	25.9	28.7	24.7	24.0	25.8	23.9
White	- - -	- - -	- - -	- - -	- - -	- - -	26.0	27.3	25.1	25.4	25.4	27.7	25.7
Black	- - -	- - -	- - -	- - -	- - -	- - -	17.8	19.2	17.7	20.2	17.3	19.0	16.9
Heavy alcohol[2]						Percent in last 2 weeks							
All seniors	41.2	36.7	37.5	34.7	33.0	32.2	29.8	27.9	27.5	28.2	29.8	30.2	31.3
Male	52.1	45.3	46.1	43.0	41.2	39.1	37.8	35.6	34.6	37.0	36.9	37.0	37.9
Female	30.5	28.2	29.2	26.5	24.9	24.4	21.2	20.3	20.7	20.2	23.0	23.5	24.4
White	44.6	40.1	41.2	38.8	36.9	36.2	32.9	31.3	31.3	31.7	32.9	34.0	36.1
Black	17.0	16.7	15.5	14.9	16.6	11.6	11.8	10.8	14.6	14.2	15.5	15.1	12.0
All eighth-graders	- - -	- - -	- - -	- - -	- - -	- - -	12.9	13.4	13.5	14.5	14.5	15.6	14.5
Male	- - -	- - -	- - -	- - -	- - -	- - -	14.3	13.9	14.8	16.0	15.1	16.5	15.3
Female	- - -	- - -	- - -	- - -	- - -	- - -	11.4	12.8	12.3	13.0	13.9	14.5	13.5
White	- - -	- - -	- - -	- - -	- - -	- - -	12.6	12.9	12.4	13.4	14.5	15.7	14.6
Black	- - -	- - -	- - -	- - -	- - -	- - -	9.9	9.3	11.9	11.8	10.0	10.9	8.8

- - - Data not available.

[1]In 1993 the alcohol question was changed to indicate that a "drink" meant "more than a few sips." 1993 data based on a half sample.

[2]Five or more drinks in a row at least once in the prior 2-week period.

NOTES: Monitoring the Future Study excludes high school dropouts (see Appendix I) and absentees (about 16–17 percent of high school seniors, about 9–10 percent of eighth graders). High school dropouts and absentees have higher drug usage than those included in the survey. Estimates of the use of substances from the National Household Survey on Drug Abuse and the Monitoring the Future Study differ because of different methodologies, sampling frames, and tabulation categories. See Appendix I.

SOURCE: National Institute on Drug Abuse. Monitoring the Future Study. Annual surveys.

Table 66. Cocaine-related emergency room episodes, according to age, sex, race, and Hispanic origin: United States, selected years 1985–95

[Data are weighted national estimates based on a sample of emergency rooms]

Age, sex, race, and Hispanic origin	1985	1988	1989	1990	1991	1992	1993	1994	1995[1]
All races, both sexes[2]					Number of episodes				
All ages[3]	28,801	101,578	110,013	80,355	101,189	119,843	123,423	142,197	142,164
6–17 years	1,004	2,760	2,555	1,877	2,210	1,546	1,578	2,068	2,009
18–25 years	9,356	32,322	31,600	19,614	21,766	23,883	22,159	25,392	21,834
26–34 years	12,895	44,632	49,818	35,639	46,137	52,760	52,658	60,500	57,718
35 years and over	5,495	21,634	25,628	23,054	30,582	41,288	46,614	54,238	60,604
White, non-Hispanic male									
All ages[2]	7,540	23,372	24,789	15,512	19,385	21,360	21,193	27,179	26,783
6–17 years	354	531	885	527	486	264	371	409	509
18–25 years	2,785	8,096	7,455	3,810	5,284	5,297	5,155	5,877	5,672
26–34 years	3,236	10,306	11,397	6,724	8,777	9,175	8,828	11,908	10,958
35 years and over	1,149	4,396	4,967	4,432	4,747	6,585	6,818	8,985	9,644
Black, non-Hispanic male									
All ages[2]	8,159	31,891	33,070	27,745	36,597	46,064	46,218	51,483	51,513
6–17 years	94	386	365	241	244	246	213	273	301
18–25 years	1,714	8,107	7,430	5,104	5,743	6,308	5,661	6,698	5,006
26–34 years	3,888	14,212	14,862	12,160	16,232	19,952	18,542	20,978	19,667
35 years and over	2,444	9,146	10,342	10,202	14,110	19,416	21,709	23,533	26,539
Hispanic male									
All ages[2]	2,041	6,752	7,067	4,821	6,571	8,683	9,195	9,557	7,935
6–17 years	38	356	300	144	201	336	206	518	157
18–25 years	720	2,088	2,406	1,774	1,831	2,535	2,184	2,165	1,839
26–34 years	849	2,815	2,690	1,758	2,723	3,457	3,893	3,652	2,925
35 years and over	432	1,478	1,662	1,125	1,801	2,332	2,885	3,222	3,014
White, non-Hispanic female									
All ages[2]	4,111	10,843	13,226	8,331	9,541	10,132	11,263	13,229	14,116
6–17 years	338	682	505	486	529	204	323	357	449
18–25 years	1,690	4,601	4,802	2,663	2,765	2,817	2,832	3,400	3,035
26–34 years	1,757	4,166	5,846	3,636	4,427	4,571	5,472	5,905	6,352
35 years and over	323	1,377	2,009	1,539	1,808	2,531	2,562	3,566	4,280
Black, non-Hispanic female									
All ages[2]	3,959	16,518	17,657	14,833	19,149	22,687	22,186	25,034	25,201
6–17 years	91	304	249	177	210	100	134	102	151
18–25 years	1,249	5,302	4,954	3,820	3,892	4,247	3,674	3,908	3,458
26–34 years	1,927	7,751	8,705	7,418	9,481	11,078	10,381	11,551	11,317
35 years and over	686	3,138	3,659	3,369	5,512	7,198	7,953	9,472	10,275
Hispanic female									
All ages[2]	781	2,469	2,556	1,719	2,356	3,074	3,466	3,591	3,542
6–17 years	38	113	93	64	183	193	166	79	138
18–25 years	349	1,097	853	634	616	815	697	955	843
26–34 years	298	904	992	663	1,044	1,324	1,529	1,559	1,315
35 years and over	95	355	613	357	513	732	1,072	998	1,246

[1]Preliminary data.
[2]Includes other races and unknown race, Hispanic origin, and/or sex. Percent other and unknown ranges from 7–11 percent of episodes.
[3]Includes unknown age.

SOURCE: Substance Abuse and Mental Health Services Administration, Drug Abuse Warning Network.

Table 67. Alcohol consumption by persons 18 years of age and over, according to sex, race, Hispanic origin, and age: United States, 1985 and 1990

[Data are based on household interviews of a sample of the civilian noninstitutionalized population]

Alcohol consumption, race, Hispanic origin, and age	Both sexes 1985	Both sexes 1990	Male 1985	Male 1990	Female 1985	Female 1990
Drinking status	Percent distribution					
All	100.0	100.0	100.0	100.0	100.0	100.0
Abstainer	26.9	29.7	14.4	16.6	38.0	41.5
Former drinker	7.5	9.6	9.2	11.6	6.1	7.8
Current drinker	65.6	60.7	76.4	71.8	55.9	50.7
	Percent current drinkers among all persons					
All races:						
18–44 years	72.8	67.5	82.4	77.1	63.8	58.3
18–24 years	71.8	63.7	79.5	71.7	64.5	56.1
25–44 years	73.2	68.8	83.5	78.9	63.5	59.0
45 years and over	55.5	51.3	67.4	63.8	45.6	40.8
45–64 years	62.2	57.6	72.2	68.4	53.0	47.6
65 years and over	44.3	41.4	58.2	55.6	34.7	31.3
White, non-Hispanic:						
18–44 years	76.9	72.7	85.0	80.4	68.9	65.1
18–24 years	77.9	71.5	84.9	77.5	71.0	65.7
25–44 years	76.5	73.1	85.0	81.2	68.2	65.0
45 years and over	57.6	53.8	69.0	65.5	48.2	44.0
45–64 years	65.2	61.0	74.1	70.6	56.9	52.2
65 years and over	45.8	43.3	59.6	57.1	36.2	33.3
Black, non-Hispanic:						
18–44 years	59.0	51.5	72.2	68.1	48.2	37.9
45 years and over	41.5	36.0	57.1	51.3	29.9	24.5
Hispanic:						
18–44 years	58.7	55.7	73.2	71.3	45.6	42.0
45 years and over	48.5	43.4	64.3	63.3	35.4	27.8
Level of alcohol consumption in past 2 weeks for current drinkers	Percent distribution of current drinkers					
All drinking levels	100.0	100.0	100.0	100.0	100.0	100.0
None	21.6	24.1	18.0	20.3	26.1	29.1
Light	37.1	39.4	30.9	33.9	44.7	46.4
Moderate	29.5	27.4	34.0	32.3	24.0	21.1
Heavier	11.8	9.1	17.2	13.6	5.3	3.4
	Percent heavier drinkers among current drinkers					
All races:						
18–44 years	11.0	8.5	16.6	13.0	4.2	2.8
18–24 years	12.2	8.8	18.3	13.8	5.0	2.7
25–44 years	10.6	8.4	16.0	12.7	3.8	2.9
45 years and over	13.3	10.3	18.2	14.7	7.4	4.6
45–64 years	13.2	9.9	18.1	14.4	7.2	4.1
65 years and over	13.6	11.0	18.4	15.3	7.9	5.5
White, non-Hispanic:						
18–44 years	11.2	8.5	17.1	13.2	4.0	2.8
18–24 years	13.3	9.9	20.4	16.0	5.2	3.0
25–44 years	10.4	8.1	16.0	12.4	3.6	2.7
45 years and over	13.4	10.4	18.2	15.0	7.6	4.7
45–64 years	13.2	10.0	18.0	14.6	7.3	4.2
65 years and over	13.9	11.3	18.7	15.8	8.3	5.7
Black, non-Hispanic:						
18–44 years	9.6	10.3	13.4	14.7	5.1	3.9
45 years and over	10.3	7.7	16.2	10.1	*	*
Hispanic:						
18–44 years	10.6	7.9	15.2	11.3	*	*
45 years and over	15.7	12.1	*	17.2	*	*

* Estimates based on fewer than 30 subjects are not shown.

NOTES: Abstainers consumed fewer than 12 drinks in any single year. Former drinkers consumed 12 or more drinks in any single year, but no drinks in the past year. Current drinkers consumed 12 or more drinks in a single year and at least 1 drink in the past year. For current drinkers, drinking levels are classified according to the average daily consumption of absolute alcohol (ethanol), in ounces, in the previous 2-week period, assuming 0.5 ounce of ethanol per drink, as follows: none; light, .01–.21; moderate, .22–.99; and heavier, 1.00 or more. This corresponds to up to 3, 4–13, and 14 or more drinks per week for light, moderate, and heavier drinkers.

SOURCE: Data computed by the Alcohol Epidemiologic Data System of the National Institute on Alcohol Abuse and Alcoholism from data in the National Health Interview Survey compiled by the Division of Health Interview Statistics, National Center for Health Statistics, Centers for Disease Control and Prevention.

Table 68. Hypertension among persons 20 years of age and over, according to sex, age, race, and Hispanic origin: United States, 1960–62, 1971–74, 1976–80, and 1988–94

[Data are based on physical examinations of a sample of the civilian noninstitutionalized population]

Sex, age, race, and Hispanic origin[1]	1960–62	1971–74	1976–80[2]	1988–94
20–74 years, age adjusted		Percent of population		
Both sexes[3]	36.9	38.3	39.0	23.1
Male	40.0	42.4	44.0	25.3
Female[3]	33.7	34.3	34.0	20.8
White male	39.3	41.7	43.5	24.3
White female[3]	31.7	32.4	32.3	19.3
Black male	48.1	51.8	48.7	34.9
Black female[3]	50.8	50.3	47.5	33.8
White, non-Hispanic male	- - -	- - -	43.9	24.4
White, non-Hispanic female[3]	- - -	- - -	32.1	19.3
Black, non-Hispanic male	- - -	- - -	48.7	35.0
Black, non-Hispanic female[3]	- - -	- - -	47.6	34.2
Mexican male	- - -	- - -	25.0	25.2
Mexican female[3]	- - -	- - -	21.8	22.0
20–74 years, crude				
Both sexes[3]	39.0	39.7	39.7	23.1
Male	41.7	43.3	44.0	24.7
Female[3]	36.6	36.5	35.6	21.5
White male	41.0	42.8	43.8	24.3
White female[3]	34.9	34.9	34.2	20.4
Black male	50.5	52.1	47.4	31.5
Black female[3]	52.0	50.2	46.1	30.6
White, non-Hispanic male	- - -	- - -	44.3	25.0
White, non-Hispanic female[3]	- - -	- - -	34.4	20.9
Black, non-Hispanic male	- - -	- - -	47.5	31.6
Black, non-Hispanic female[3]	- - -	- - -	46.1	31.2
Mexican male	- - -	- - -	18.8	18.0
Mexican female[3]	- - -	- - -	16.7	15.8
Male				
20–34 years	22.8	24.8	28.9	8.6
35–44 years	37.7	39.1	40.5	20.9
45–54 years	47.6	55.0	53.6	34.1
55–64 years	60.3	62.5	61.8	42.9
65–74 years	68.8	67.2	67.1	57.3
75 years and over	- - -	- - -	- - -	64.2
Female[3]				
20–34 years	9.3	11.2	11.1	3.4
35–44 years	24.0	28.2	28.8	12.7
45–54 years	43.4	43.6	47.1	25.1
55–64 years	66.4	62.5	61.1	44.2
65–74 years	81.5	78.3	71.8	60.8
75 years and over	- - -	- - -	- - -	77.3

- - - Data not available.

[1]The race groups, white and black, include persons of Hispanic and non-Hispanic origin. Conversely, persons of Hispanic origin may be of any race.
[2]Data for Mexicans are for 1982–84. See Appendix I.
[3]Excludes pregnant women.

NOTES: A person with hypertension is defined by either having elevated blood pressure (systolic pressure of at least 140 mmHg or diastolic pressure of at least 90 mmHg) or taking antihypertensive medication. Percents are based on a single measurement of blood pressure to provide comparable data across the 4 time periods. In 1976–80, 31.3 percent of persons 20–74 years of age had hypertension, based on the average of 3 blood pressure measurements, in contrast to 39.7 percent when a single measurement is used.

SOURCE: Centers for Disease Control and Prevention, National Center for Health Statistics, Division of Health Examination Statistics. Unpublished data.

Table 69. Serum cholesterol levels among persons 20 years of age and over, according to sex, age, race, and Hispanic origin: United States, 1960–62, 1971–74, 1976–80, and 1988–94

[Data are based on physical examinations of a sample of the civilian noninstitutionalized population]

Sex, age, race, and Hispanic origin[1]	Percent of population with high serum cholesterol				Mean serum cholesterol level, mg/dL			
	1960–62	1971–74	1976–80[2]	1988–94	1960–62	1971–74	1976–80[2]	1988–94
20–74 years, age adjusted								
Both sexes	31.8	27.2	26.3	18.9	220	214	213	203
Male	28.7	25.8	24.6	17.5	217	213	211	202
Female	34.5	28.2	27.6	20.0	222	215	214	204
White male	29.4	25.9	24.6	17.8	218	213	211	202
White female	35.1	28.1	28.0	20.2	223	215	214	205
Black male	24.5	25.1	24.1	15.7	210	212	208	199
Black female	30.7	29.2	24.9	19.4	216	217	213	203
White, non-Hispanic male	- - -	- - -	24.7	17.3	- - -	- - -	211	202
White, non-Hispanic female	- - -	- - -	28.3	20.2	- - -	- - -	214	205
Black, non-Hispanic male	- - -	- - -	24.0	15.7	- - -	- - -	208	200
Black, non-Hispanic female	- - -	- - -	24.9	19.8	- - -	- - -	214	203
Mexican male	- - -	- - -	18.8	17.8	- - -	- - -	207	204
Mexican female	- - -	- - -	20.0	17.5	- - -	- - -	207	203
20–74 years, crude								
Both sexes	33.6	28.2	26.8	18.7	222	216	213	203
Male	30.7	26.8	24.9	17.6	220	214	211	202
Female	36.3	29.6	28.5	19.9	225	217	215	204
White male	31.4	26.9	25.0	18.1	221	215	211	203
White female	37.5	29.8	29.2	20.5	227	217	216	205
Black male	26.7	25.1	23.9	14.4	214	212	208	198
Black female	29.9	28.8	23.7	16.8	216	216	212	199
White, non-Hispanic male	- - -	- - -	25.1	17.9	- - -	- - -	211	203
White, non-Hispanic female	- - -	- - -	29.8	20.9	- - -	- - -	216	206
Black, non-Hispanic male	- - -	- - -	23.7	14.5	- - -	- - -	208	198
Black, non-Hispanic female	- - -	- - -	23.7	17.2	- - -	- - -	212	200
Mexican male	- - -	- - -	16.6	15.5	- - -	- - -	203	200
Mexican female	- - -	- - -	16.5	14.0	- - -	- - -	202	197
Male								
20–34 years	15.1	12.4	11.9	8.2	198	194	192	186
35–44 years	33.9	31.8	27.9	19.4	227	221	217	206
45–54 years	39.2	37.5	36.9	26.6	231	229	227	216
55–64 years	41.6	36.2	36.8	28.0	233	229	229	216
65–74 years	38.0	34.7	31.7	21.9	230	226	221	212
75 years and over	- - -	- - -	- - -	20.4	- - -	- - -	- - -	205
Female								
20–34 years	12.4	10.9	9.8	7.3	194	191	189	184
35–44 years	23.1	19.3	20.7	12.3	214	207	207	195
45–54 years	46.9	38.7	40.5	26.7	237	232	232	217
55–64 years	70.1	53.1	52.9	40.9	262	245	249	235
65–74 years	68.5	57.7	51.6	41.3	266	250	246	233
75 years and over	- - -	- - -	- - -	38.2	- - -	- - -	- - -	229

- - - Data not available.

[1]The race groups, white and black, include persons of Hispanic and non-Hispanic origin. Conversely, persons of Hispanic origin may be of any race.

[2]Data for Mexicans are for 1982–84. See Appendix I.

NOTES: High serum cholesterol is defined as greater than or equal to 240 mg/dL (6.20 mmol/L). Risk levels have been defined by the Second report of the National Cholesterol Education Program Expert Panel on Detection, Evaluation and Treatment of High Blood Cholesterol in Adults. National Heart, Lung, and Blood Institute, National Institutes of Health. September 1993. (Summarized in *JAMA* 269 (23): 3015–23. June 16, 1993.)

SOURCE: Centers for Disease Control and Prevention, National Center for Health Statistics, Division of Health Examination Statistics. Unpublished data.

Table 70. Overweight persons 20 years of age and over, according to sex, age, race, and Hispanic origin: United States, 1960–62, 1971–74, 1976–80, and 1988–94

[Data are based on physical examinations of a sample of the civilian noninstitutionalized population]

Sex, age, race, and Hispanic origin[1]	1960–62	1971–74	1976–80[2]	1988–94
20–74 years, age adjusted		Percent of	population	
Both sexes[3]	24.4	24.9	25.4	34.8
Male	22.9	23.6	24.0	33.7
Female[3]	25.6	25.9	26.5	35.9
White male	23.1	23.8	24.2	34.3
White female[3]	23.5	24.0	24.4	33.9
Black male	22.2	24.3	25.7	34.0
Black female[3]	41.7	42.9	44.3	53.0
White, non-Hispanic male	- - -	- - -	24.1	33.7
White, non-Hispanic female[3]	- - -	- - -	23.9	32.5
Black, non-Hispanic male	- - -	- - -	25.6	34.0
Black, non-Hispanic female[3]	- - -	- - -	44.1	53.3
Mexican male	- - -	- - -	31.0	40.1
Mexican female[3]	- - -	- - -	41.4	51.8
20–74 years, crude				
Both sexes[3]	25.5	25.5	25.7	35.1
Male	23.4	24.0	24.2	33.6
Female[3]	27.4	27.0	27.1	36.5
White male	23.7	24.2	24.4	34.5
White female[3]	25.4	25.2	25.1	34.8
Black male	22.5	24.5	25.7	33.5
Black female[3]	43.0	43.2	43.7	52.3
White, non-Hispanic male	- - -	- - -	24.4	34.1
White, non-Hispanic female[3]	- - -	- - -	24.8	33.5
Black, non-Hispanic male	- - -	- - -	25.6	33.6
Black, non-Hispanic female[3]	- - -	- - -	43.4	52.7
Mexican male	- - -	- - -	29.5	36.6
Mexican female[3]	- - -	- - -	39.1	50.4
Male				
20–34 years	19.6	19.2	17.3	25.4
35–44 years	22.8	29.4	28.9	34.9
45–54 years	28.1	27.6	31.0	37.7
55–64 years	26.9	24.8	28.1	43.7
65–74 years	21.8	23.0	25.2	42.9
75 years and over	- - -	- - -	- - -	27.7
Female[3]				
20–34 years	13.2	14.8	16.8	25.6
35–44 years	24.1	27.3	27.0	36.8
45–54 years	30.7	32.3	32.5	45.4
55–64 years	43.2	38.5	37.0	48.2
65–74 years	42.9	38.0	38.4	42.3
75 years and over	- - -	- - -	- - -	35.1

- - - Data not available.

[1]The race groups, white and black, include persons of Hispanic and non-Hispanic origin. Conversely, persons of Hispanic origin may be of any race.
[2]Data for Mexicans are for 1982–84. See Appendix I.
[3]Excludes pregnant women.

NOTES: Overweight is defined for men as body mass index greater than or equal to 27.8 kilograms/meter^2, and for women as body mass index greater than or equal to 27.3 kilograms/meter^2. These cut points were used because they represent the sex-specific 85th percentiles for persons 20–29 years of age in the 1976–80 National Health and Nutrition Examination Survey. Height was measured without shoes; two pounds are deducted from data for 1960–62 to allow for weight of clothing.

SOURCE: Centers for Disease Control and Prevention, National Center for Health Statistics, Division of Health Examination Statistics. Unpublished data.

Table 71. Overweight children and adolescents 6–17 years of age, according to sex, age, race, and Hispanic origin: United States, selected years 1963–65 through 1988–94

[Data are based on physical examinations of a sample of the civilian noninstitutionalized population]

Age, sex, race, and Hispanic origin[1]	1963–65 1966–70[2]	1971–74	1976–80[3]	1988–94[4]
6–11 years of age, age adjusted		Percent of population		
Both sexes	5.0	5.5	7.6	13.6
Boys	4.9	6.5	8.1	14.7
White	5.4	6.6	8.1	14.6
Black	1.7	5.6	8.6	15.1
White, non-Hispanic	- - -	- - -	7.4	13.1
Black, non-Hispanic	- - -	- - -	8.6	14.7
Mexican	- - -	- - -	14.5	18.8
Girls	5.2	4.4	7.1	12.6
White	5.1	4.4	6.5	11.7
Black	5.3	4.5	11.5	17.4
White, non-Hispanic	- - -	- - -	6.2	11.9
Black, non-Hispanic	- - -	- - -	11.6	17.7
Mexican	- - -	- - -	10.7	15.8
12–17 years of age, age adjusted				
Both sexes	5.0	6.2	5.6	11.4
Boys	5.0	5.3	5.3	12.4
White	5.2	5.5	5.3	13.1
Black	3.6	4.4	6.0	12.1
White, non-Hispanic	- - -	- - -	4.5	11.8
Black, non-Hispanic	- - -	- - -	6.1	12.5
Mexican	- - -	- - -	7.7	14.8
Girls[5]	5.0	7.2	6.0	10.5
White	4.8	6.6	5.4	10.0
Black	6.4	10.5	10.2	16.1
White, non-Hispanic	- - -	- - -	5.4	9.3
Black, non-Hispanic	- - -	- - -	10.5	16.0
Mexican	- - -	- - -	9.3	14.1
Boys				
6–8 years	5.1	6.3	8.1	15.4
9–11 years	4.8	6.7	8.1	14.0
12–14 years	5.2	5.4	5.4	11.5
15–17 years	4.8	5.2	5.1	13.1
Girls[5]				
6–8 years	5.1	4.1	7.1	14.6
9–11 years	5.2	4.7	7.1	10.8
12–14 years	5.0	8.6	7.8	13.9
15–17 years	4.9	6.0	4.5	7.5

- - - Data not available.

[1]The race groups, white and black, include persons of Hispanic and non-Hispanic origin. Conversely, persons of Hispanic origin may be of any race.

[2]Data for children 6–11 years of age are for 1963–65; data for adolescents 12–17 years of age are for 1966–70.

[3]Data for Mexicans are for 1982–84. See Appendix I.

[4]Excludes one non-Hispanic white adolescent boy age 12–14 years with an outlier sample weight.

[5]Excludes pregnant women starting with 1971–74. Pregnancy status not available for 1963–65/1966–70.

NOTES: Overweight is defined as body mass index (BMI) at or above the sex- and age-specific 95th percentile BMI cutoff points calculated at 6-month age intervals for children 6–11 years of age from the 1963–65 National Health Examination Survey (NHES) and for adolescents 12–17 years of age from the 1966–70 NHES. Age is at time of examination at mobile examination center. Some data for 1988–94 have been revised and differ from the previous edition of Health, United States.

SOURCE: Centers for Disease Control and Prevention, National Center for Health Statistics, Division of Health Examination Statistics. Unpublished data.

Table 72. Persons residing in counties that met national ambient air quality standards throughout the year, by race and Hispanic origin: United States, selected years 1988–96

[Data are based on air quality measurements in counties with monitoring devices]

Type of pollutant, race, and Hispanic origin	1988	1989	1990	1991	1992	1993	1994	1995	1996
All pollutants				Percent of population					
All persons	49.7	65.3	71.0	65.2	78.4	76.5	75.1	67.9	81.3
White	- - -	- - -	71.8	66.0	79.1	76.9	76.4	69.7	81.9
Black	- - -	- - -	71.5	63.4	76.5	75.2	70.4	59.4	80.8
American Indian or Alaska Native	- - -	- - -	76.8	75.2	83.0	82.4	80.0	77.9	83.2
Asian or Pacific Islander	- - -	- - -	49.6	46.7	64.4	62.8	55.6	48.2	64.4
Hispanic	- - -	- - -	49.3	45.2	56.8	57.7	54.8	44.5	56.3
Ozone									
All persons	53.6	72.6	76.3	71.9	81.9	79.5	79.9	71.6	83.3
White	- - -	- - -	76.9	72.7	82.7	79.9	80.0	73.0	83.9
Black	- - -	- - -	77.0	69.7	79.8	79.3	75.4	66.1	82.9
American Indian or Alaska Native	- - -	- - -	83.0	84.8	88.4	85.5	84.3	81.2	99.9
Asian or Pacific Islander	- - -	- - -	58.0	55.2	67.0	64.5	58.5	51.4	65.6
Hispanic	- - -	- - -	57.1	53.4	61.2	60.2	58.3	48.5	59.7
Carbon monoxide									
All persons	87.8	86.2	90.8	92.0	94.3	95.4	93.9	95.2	94.9
White	- - -	- - -	91.0	92.3	94.4	95.6	94.3	96.4	95.1
Black	- - -	- - -	93.4	93.5	95.5	96.0	92.6	96.1	96.0
American Indian or Alaska Native	- - -	- - -	88.7	89.9	92.9	95.1	93.2	94.2	93.8
Asian or Pacific Islander	- - -	- - -	73.7	78.0	84.7	85.8	84.6	85.9	85.5
Hispanic	- - -	- - -	72.5	75.6	79.8	82.2	81.4	82.6	80.9
Particulates (PM–10)[1]									
All persons	89.4	88.8	92.6	91.9	89.6	97.5	94.8	90.2	97.1
White	- - -	- - -	92.7	92.1	90.2	97.6	95.6	91.0	97.1
Black	- - -	- - -	94.2	93.6	87.9	96.8	94.0	87.1	96.8
American Indian or Alaska Native	- - -	- - -	92.4	90.6	89.9	97.4	96.2	90.4	96.8
Asian or Pacific Islander	- - -	- - -	82.7	80.8	79.3	98.5	93.2	80.7	96.9
Hispanic	- - -	- - -	76.1	76.3	71.3	97.4	91.0	75.2	92.7
Sulfur dioxide									
All persons	99.3	99.9	99.4	97.9	100.0	99.4	100.0	100.0	99.9
White	- - -	- - -	99.4	98.3	100.0	99.4	100.0	100.0	99.9
Black	- - -	- - -	99.5	95.6	100.0	99.5	100.0	100.0	100.0
American Indian or Alaska Native	- - -	- - -	99.8	99.4	100.0	100.0	100.0	100.0	100.0
Asian or Pacific Islander	- - -	- - -	99.8	97.4	100.0	99.8	100.0	100.0	100.0
Hispanic	- - -	- - -	99.9	96.9	100.0	100.0	100.0	100.0	100.0
Nitrogen dioxide									
All persons	96.6	96.5	96.4	96.4	100.0	100.0	100.0	100.0	100.0
White	- - -	- - -	96.8	96.8	100.0	100.0	100.0	100.0	100.0
Black	- - -	- - -	96.6	96.6	100.0	100.0	100.0	100.0	100.0
American Indian or Alaska Native	- - -	- - -	97.2	97.2	100.0	100.0	100.0	100.0	100.0
Asian or Pacific Islander	- - -	- - -	86.7	86.7	100.0	100.0	100.0	100.0	100.0
Hispanic	- - -	- - -	85.0	85.0	100.0	100.0	100.0	100.0	100.0
Lead									
All persons	99.3	99.4	94.1	94.1	98.1	97.8	98.3	98.1	98.3
White	- - -	- - -	94.9	94.8	98.5	98.2	98.7	98.3	98.6
Black	- - -	- - -	91.5	91.1	95.3	94.8	95.9	96.2	96.1
American Indian or Alaska Native	- - -	- - -	96.4	96.4	99.4	99.3	99.4	99.3	99.4
Asian or Pacific Islander	- - -	- - -	85.5	85.5	99.0	98.9	99.1	98.9	99.1
Hispanic	- - -	- - -	83.6	84.0	99.4	99.5	99.5	98.9	99.0

- - - Data not available.

[1]Particulate matter smaller than 10 microns.

NOTES: The race groups, white, black, American Indian or Alaska Native, and Asian or Pacific Islander, include persons of Hispanic and non-Hispanic origin. Conversely, persons of Hispanic origin may be of any race. Standard is met if the concentration of the pollutant does not exceed the criterion value more than once per calendar year. See Appendix II, National ambient air quality standards. 1988–89 data based on 1987 county population estimates; 1990–96 data based on 1990 county population estimates.

SOURCES: U.S. Environmental Protection Agency, Aerometric Information Retrieval System; data computed by the National Center for Health Statistics, Division of Health Promotion Statistics from data compiled by the U.S. Environmental Protection Agency, Office of Air Quality and Standards.

Table 73. Occupational injuries with lost workdays in the private sector, according to industry: United States, selected years 1980–96

[Data are based on employer records from a sample of business establishments]

Industry	1980	1985	1988	1989	1990	1991	1992	1993	1994	1995	1996
	Number of injuries with lost workdays in thousands										
Total private sector[1]	2,491.0	2,484.7	2,880.4	2,955.5	2,987.3	2,794.0	2,776.1	2,772.5	2,848.3	2,767.6	2,646.3
Agriculture, fishing, and forestry[1]	39.3	45.2	51.3	52.2	57.2	54.3	52.3	51.2	48.5	51.7	49.0
Mining	66.2	43.9	37.1	33.9	35.6	31.4	25.6	24.2	24.0	22.8	19.5
Construction	242.6	272.8	304.4	301.2	296.3	239.9	226.8	226.5	241.7	217.9	216.8
Manufacturing	1,009.5	825.1	1,007.3	1,007.4	975.0	886.0	833.7	819.5	859.4	838.1	782.9
Transportation, communication, and public utilities	263.0	243.5	261.3	273.9	293.3	283.5	266.1	284.1	301.5	289.2	293.0
Wholesale trade	191.1	188.4	214.7	230.3	211.5	204.1	205.3	205.3	214.0	214.7	203.9
Retail trade	330.2	399.9	461.6	480.6	483.9	457.0	476.7	480.4	477.7	459.6	433.9
Finance, insurance, and real estate	38.1	45.5	54.0	52.6	63.7	62.2	64.4	61.7	58.8	52.2	49.5
Services	311.1	420.6	488.6	523.4	570.8	575.6	625.1	619.6	622.8	621.4	597.8
	Injuries with lost workdays per 100 full-time equivalents[2]										
Total private sector[1]	3.9	3.6	3.8	3.9	3.9	3.7	3.6	3.5	3.5	3.4	3.1
Agriculture, fishing, and forestry[1]	5.6	5.6	5.5	5.6	5.7	5.2	5.2	4.8	4.6	4.2	3.8
Mining	6.4	4.7	5.1	4.8	4.9	4.4	4.0	3.8	3.8	3.8	3.2
Construction	6.5	6.8	6.8	6.7	6.6	6.0	5.7	5.4	5.4	4.8	4.4
Manufacturing	5.2	4.4	5.3	5.3	5.3	5.0	4.7	4.6	4.7	4.6	4.3
Transportation, communication, and public utilities	5.4	4.9	5.0	5.2	5.4	5.3	4.9	5.2	5.3	5.0	5.0
Wholesale trade	3.8	3.5	3.8	3.9	3.6	3.6	3.6	3.6	3.6	3.5	3.3
Retail trade	2.9	3.1	3.3	3.4	3.4	3.3	3.3	3.2	3.2	2.9	2.7
Finance, insurance, and real estate	0.8	0.9	0.9	0.9	1.1	1.0	1.1	1.0	0.9	0.9	0.8
Services	2.3	2.5	2.6	2.6	2.7	2.8	2.9	2.7	2.7	2.7	2.5

[1]Excludes farms with fewer than 11 employees.

[2]Incidence rate calculated as (N/EH) x 200,000, where N = total number of injuries with lost workdays in a calendar year, EH = total hours worked by all full-time and part-time employees in a calendar year, and 200,000 = base for 100 full-time equivalent employees working 40 hours per week, 50 weeks per year.

NOTES: Industry is coded based on various editions of the *Standard Industrial Classification Manual* as follows: data for 1980–87 are based on the 1972 edition, 1977 supplement; and data for 1988–96 are based on the 1987 edition (see Appendix II, Industry).

SOURCE: U.S. Department of Labor, Bureau of Labor Statistics. Occupational injuries and illnesses in the United States by industry, 1980–96 editions. 1982–98.

Table 74. Physician contacts, according to selected patient characteristics: United States, 1987–95

[Data are based on household interviews of a sample of the civilian noninstitutionalized population]

Characteristic	1987	1988	1989	1990	1991	1992	1993	1994	1995
	Physician contacts per person								
Total[1,2]	5.4	5.3	5.3	5.5	5.6	5.9	6.0	6.0	5.8
Age									
Under 15 years	4.5	4.6	4.6	4.5	4.7	4.6	4.9	4.6	4.5
Under 5 years	6.7	7.0	6.7	6.9	7.1	6.9	7.2	6.8	6.5
5–14 years	3.3	3.3	3.5	3.2	3.4	3.4	3.6	3.4	3.4
15–44 years	4.6	4.7	4.6	4.8	4.7	5.0	5.0	5.0	4.8
45–64 years	6.4	6.1	6.1	6.4	6.6	7.2	7.1	7.3	7.1
65 years and over	8.9	8.7	8.9	9.2	10.4	10.6	10.9	11.3	11.1
65–74 years	8.4	8.4	8.2	8.5	9.2	9.7	9.9	10.3	9.8
75 years and over	9.7	9.2	9.9	10.1	12.3	12.1	12.3	12.7	12.9
Sex and age									
Male[1]	4.6	4.6	4.8	4.7	4.9	5.1	5.2	5.2	4.9
Under 5 years	6.7	7.3	7.5	7.2	7.6	7.1	7.5	7.0	6.8
5–14 years	3.4	3.4	3.7	3.3	3.5	3.5	3.8	3.5	3.6
15–44 years	3.3	3.3	3.4	3.4	3.4	3.7	3.6	3.7	3.3
45–64 years	5.5	5.2	5.2	5.6	5.8	6.1	6.1	6.3	6.0
65–74 years	8.1	7.9	8.5	8.0	8.6	9.2	9.3	10.1	9.5
75 years and over	9.2	9.6	9.9	10.0	11.6	12.2	11.7	11.6	11.9
Female[1]	6.0	6.0	5.9	6.1	6.3	6.6	6.7	6.7	6.5
Under 5 years	6.7	6.8	5.9	6.5	6.6	6.7	6.9	6.5	6.3
5–14 years	3.1	3.3	3.3	3.2	3.2	3.3	3.4	3.3	3.1
15–44 years	5.8	6.0	5.9	6.0	5.9	6.2	6.4	6.2	6.2
45–64 years	7.2	6.9	7.0	7.1	7.4	8.2	8.1	8.3	8.1
65–74 years	8.6	8.8	7.9	9.0	9.7	10.1	10.4	10.5	10.1
75 years and over	10.0	9.0	9.9	10.2	12.7	12.1	12.8	13.4	13.5
Race and age									
White[1]	5.5	5.5	5.5	5.6	5.8	6.0	6.0	6.1	5.9
Under 5 years	7.1	7.6	7.1	7.1	7.4	7.3	7.5	7.1	6.7
5–14 years	3.5	3.6	3.8	3.5	3.7	3.7	3.9	3.7	3.6
15–44 years	4.7	4.8	4.8	4.9	4.9	5.0	5.1	5.1	4.9
45–64 years	6.4	6.1	6.2	6.4	6.6	7.2	7.0	7.4	7.0
65–74 years	8.4	8.3	8.0	8.5	9.4	9.6	9.7	10.5	9.9
75 years and over	9.7	9.3	9.7	10.1	12.1	12.0	12.2	12.4	13.1
Black[1]	5.1	4.8	4.9	5.1	5.2	5.9	6.0	5.7	5.5
Under 5 years	5.1	4.6	5.3	5.6	6.0	5.6	6.2	5.2	5.8
5–14 years	2.3	2.2	2.3	2.2	2.1	2.3	2.4	2.5	2.5
15–44 years	4.2	4.2	3.9	4.2	4.0	5.3	4.7	4.8	4.3
45–64 years	7.3	6.6	6.3	7.1	7.5	7.8	8.7	7.7	8.0
65–74 years	8.6	9.1	10.0	9.2	7.3	10.9	11.5	9.3	9.9
75 years and over	10.8	8.7	12.7	10.4	15.7	13.7	13.1	16.3	11.5
Family income[1,3]									
Less than $15,000	6.8	6.2	6.3	6.3	6.8	7.3	7.3	7.6	7.4
$15,000–$24,999	5.6	5.3	5.2	5.6	5.6	6.0	5.7	5.9	6.1
$25,000–$34,999	5.2	5.0	5.5	5.2	5.5	5.7	6.0	5.8	5.3
$35,000–$49,999	5.2	5.5	5.2	5.7	5.8	5.9	6.0	6.2	5.7
$50,000 or more	5.4	5.5	6.0	5.6	5.8	5.8	5.8	6.0	5.6
Geographic region[1]									
Northeast	5.2	5.0	5.3	5.2	5.4	5.9	5.9	5.9	5.6
Midwest	5.6	5.4	5.4	5.3	5.8	5.9	6.2	6.0	5.8
South	5.1	5.2	5.3	5.6	5.5	5.8	5.7	5.6	5.8
West	5.5	5.9	5.5	5.6	5.9	6.1	6.0	6.4	5.8
Location of residence[1]									
Within MSA[4]	5.5	5.5	5.4	5.6	5.8	6.0	6.1	6.0	5.9
Outside MSA[4]	4.8	4.9	5.2	4.9	5.1	5.6	5.6	5.7	5.3

[1]Age adjusted.

[2]Includes all other races not shown separately and unknown family income.

[3]Family income categories for 1995. In 1989–94 the two lowest income categories are less than $14,000 and $14,000–$24,999; the three higher income categories are as shown. Income categories for 1988 are less than $13,000; $13,000–$18,999; $19,000–$24,999; $25,000–$44,999; and $45,000 or more. Income categories for 1987 are less than $10,000; $10,000–$14,999; $15,000–$19,999; $20,000–$34,999; and $35,000 or more.

[4]Metropolitan statistical area.

SOURCE: Centers for Disease Control and Prevention, National Center for Health Statistics, Division of Health Interview Statistics. Data from the National Health Interview Survey.

Utilization of Health Resources

Table 75. Physician contacts, according to place of contact and selected patient characteristics: United States, 1990 and 1995

[Data are based on household interviews of a sample of the civilian noninstitutionalized population]

| | | Place of contact | | | | | | | | | |
| | | Doctor's office | | Hospital outpatient department[1] | | Telephone | | Home | | Other[2] | |
Characteristic	Total	1990	1995	1990	1995	1990	1995	1990	1995	1990	1995
					Percent distribution						
Total[3,4]	100.0	59.9	56.6	13.7	12.6	12.7	13.5	2.1	3.2	11.6	14.1
Age											
Under 15 years	100.0	60.7	59.3	13.6	12.4	14.9	14.6	0.9	*0.7	9.9	13.0
Under 5 years	100.0	59.1	58.9	14.0	12.5	15.9	15.0	*1.1	*1.2	9.8	12.4
5–14 years	100.0	62.6	59.6	13.1	12.2	13.7	14.2	*0.6	*0.3	10.0	13.6
15–44 years	100.0	59.4	55.7	14.3	13.1	12.0	14.0	0.6	1.8	13.7	15.5
45–64 years	100.0	60.4	55.4	14.1	13.0	12.2	12.7	2.0	4.4	11.4	14.5
65 years and over	100.0	58.7	54.4	11.1	10.4	9.9	10.3	11.8	14.1	8.4	10.8
65–74 years	100.0	60.2	57.7	13.7	12.5	9.7	10.8	7.0	6.5	9.4	12.5
75 years and over	100.0	56.8	50.7	7.8	8.2	10.2	9.7	18.1	22.4	7.0	9.0
Sex[3]											
Male	100.0	57.6	55.7	16.1	13.9	11.3	12.2	2.1	2.7	12.9	15.4
Female	100.0	61.6	57.0	12.2	11.8	13.4	14.2	2.0	3.5	10.9	13.5
Race[3]											
White	100.0	61.7	58.0	12.3	11.5	13.1	14.0	1.9	3.2	11.0	13.2
Black	100.0	48.2	48.3	24.3	19.5	9.1	10.1	2.8	3.3	15.6	18.8
Family income[3,5]											
Less than $15,000	100.0	48.9	46.4	19.9	15.7	11.5	11.0	3.2	5.0	16.4	21.9
$15,000–$24,999	100.0	56.9	54.3	16.0	15.0	11.8	11.4	1.7	3.6	13.5	15.7
$25,000–$34,999	100.0	60.9	56.7	13.8	13.0	13.2	13.9	1.6	2.5	10.4	14.1
$35,000–$49,999	100.0	62.0	58.7	11.5	10.6	14.6	16.2	1.1	3.0	10.9	11.5
$50,000 or more	100.0	66.1	62.1	8.9	10.0	14.1	16.1	1.5	2.0	9.5	9.7
Geographic region[3]											
Northeast	100.0	62.6	60.9	13.0	12.2	11.7	14.5	1.9	2.3	10.8	10.1
Midwest	100.0	55.8	52.9	14.7	13.8	15.4	15.8	1.9	1.8	12.3	15.7
South	100.0	61.1	57.3	13.6	12.4	11.3	12.7	2.6	4.5	11.3	13.1
West	100.0	60.4	55.8	13.6	12.0	12.8	11.3	1.4	3.4	12.0	17.4
Location of residence[3]											
Within MSA[6]	100.0	59.6	56.7	13.7	12.7	13.1	13.9	1.9	3.1	11.7	13.7
Outside MSA[6]	100.0	61.4	56.3	14.1	12.1	10.7	12.0	2.6	3.6	11.2	16.1

* Relative standard error greater than 30 percent.
[1] Includes hospital outpatient clinic, emergency room, and other hospital contacts.
[2] Includes clinics or other places outside a hospital.
[3] Age adjusted.
[4] Includes all other races not shown separately and unknown family income.
[5] Family income categories for 1995. In 1990 the two lowest income categories are less than $14,000 and $14,000–$24,999; the three higher income categories are as shown.
[6] Metropolitan statistical area.

SOURCE: Centers for Disease Control and Prevention, National Center for Health Statistics, Division of Health Interview Statistics. Data from the National Health Interview Survey.

Table 76. Physician contacts, according to respondent-assessed health status, age, sex, and poverty status: United States, 1987–89 and 1993–95

[Data are based on household interviews of a sample of the civilian noninstitutionalized population]

| | Respondent-assessed health status | | | | | |
| | All | | Good to excellent | | Fair or poor | |
Age, sex, and poverty status[1]	1987–89	1993–95	1987–89	1993–95	1987–89	1993–95
Total[2]	Physician contacts per person per year					
Male:						
Poor	5.2	6.1	3.4	3.9	11.1	13.7
Near poor	4.9	5.3	3.7	3.8	13.4	14.7
Nonpoor.......................	4.8	5.2	4.2	4.6	16.8	16.3
Female:						
Poor	7.0	8.2	4.7	5.4	13.6	16.2
Near poor	5.9	6.6	4.6	5.0	14.9	17.3
Nonpoor.......................	6.2	6.7	5.6	5.8	19.4	22.4
Under 15 years						
Poor..........................	4.0	4.5	3.6	4.0	10.8	14.2
Near poor	4.2	4.2	3.8	3.9	15.2	16.2
Nonpoor	5.3	5.1	5.0	4.9	22.6	20.7
15–44 years						
Male:						
Poor	3.6	4.3	2.8	3.0	9.8	12.2
Near poor	3.5	3.8	2.9	2.8	11.7	15.0
Nonpoor.......................	3.4	3.5	3.1	3.2	14.0	13.9
Female:						
Poor	6.4	6.8	5.1	5.1	14.0	15.0
Near poor	5.6	6.0	4.7	5.0	16.0	15.6
Nonpoor.......................	6.1	6.6	5.6	5.9	20.4	23.4
45–64 years						
Male:						
Poor	7.5	9.3	3.1	4.1	11.4	14.7
Near poor	6.5	7.4	3.5	3.6	12.8	15.1
Nonpoor.......................	5.1	5.8	4.1	4.8	13.8	15.3
Female:						
Poor	10.9	13.3	4.6	6.7	17.3	19.4
Near poor	7.6	8.5	4.7	5.1	14.5	16.4
Nonpoor.......................	6.8	7.7	5.7	6.2	16.1	21.0
65 years and over						
Male:						
Poor	9.7	11.0	5.5	6.6	13.2	15.2
Near poor	8.9	10.4	6.5	7.6	12.9	15.4
Nonpoor.......................	8.5	10.5	6.5	8.1	15.5	19.8
Female:						
Poor	10.6	14.2	6.5	8.8	16.0	21.5
Near poor	9.2	12.3	6.6	8.6	14.3	20.4
Nonpoor.......................	8.8	10.8	7.1	8.4	14.9	20.6

[1]Poverty status is based on family income and family size using Bureau of the Census poverty thresholds. Poor persons are defined as below the poverty threshold. Near poor persons have incomes of 100 percent to less than 200 percent of poverty threshold. Nonpoor persons have incomes of 200 percent or greater than the poverty threshold. See Appendix II.
[2]Age adjusted.

NOTES: Persons with unknown family income or unknown health status were eliminated from the analysis. Persons who reported their health to be good, very good, or excellent were categorized as good to excellent health. See Appendix II.

SOURCE: Centers for Disease Control and Prevention, National Center for Health Statistics. Data computed by the Division of Health and Utilization Analysis from data compiled by the Division of Health Interview Statistics.

Table 77. Interval since last physician contact, according to selected patient characteristics: United States, 1964, 1990, and 1995

[Data are based on household interviews of a sample of the civilian noninstitutionalized population]

Characteristic	Total	Less than 1 year			1 year–less than 2 years			2 years or more[1]		
		1964	1990	1995	1964	1990	1995	1964	1990	1995
		Percent distribution[2]								
Total[3,4]	100.0	66.9	78.2	79.5	14.0	10.1	9.5	19.1	11.7	11.0
Age										
Under 15 years	100.0	68.4	82.9	84.9	14.8	10.7	9.7	16.7	6.4	5.4
Under 5 years	100.0	80.7	93.6	94.9	11.1	5.0	4.1	8.2	1.4	0.9
5–14 years	100.0	61.7	77.2	79.7	16.9	13.7	12.5	21.4	9.1	7.8
15–44 years	100.0	66.3	73.3	73.1	15.0	11.6	11.5	18.7	15.0	15.4
45–64 years	100.0	64.5	77.3	79.9	13.0	8.6	7.8	22.5	14.1	12.4
65 years and over	100.0	69.7	87.1	90.0	9.3	4.7	4.0	21.0	8.2	6.0
65–74 years.	100.0	68.8	85.7	88.5	9.4	5.1	4.4	21.8	9.1	7.2
75 years and over	100.0	71.3	89.3	92.1	9.3	4.1	3.5	19.5	6.6	4.3
Sex and age										
Male[3]	100.0	63.5	73.3	74.6	15.0	11.3	10.7	21.5	15.4	14.7
Under 15 years	100.0	- - -	82.8	85.1	- - -	10.7	9.6	- - -	6.5	5.2
15–44 years.	100.0	- - -	64.2	63.5	- - -	13.8	13.9	- - -	22.0	22.5
45–64 years.	100.0	- - -	72.4	75.1	- - -	9.8	8.8	- - -	17.8	16.1
65–74 years.	100.0	- - -	84.2	87.4	- - -	5.8	4.7	- - -	10.0	7.9
75 years and over	100.0	- - -	86.9	91.4	- - -	4.7	3.3	- - -	8.4	5.3
Female[3]	100.0	69.9	82.9	84.2	13.1	9.0	8.3	17.0	8.1	7.5
Under 15 years	100.0	- - -	83.0	84.6	- - -	10.7	9.7	- - -	6.4	5.7
15–44 years.	100.0	- - -	82.1	82.3	- - -	9.5	9.2	- - -	8.3	8.5
45–64 years.	100.0	- - -	81.9	84.3	- - -	7.6	6.8	- - -	10.6	8.9
65–74 years.	100.0	- - -	86.9	89.3	- - -	4.6	4.2	- - -	8.4	6.6
75 years and over	100.0	- - -	90.7	92.6	- - -	3.7	3.7	- - -	5.6	3.7
Race and age										
White[3]	100.0	68.1	78.7	79.6	13.8	9.9	9.4	18.1	11.5	10.9
Under 15 years	100.0	- - -	83.6	85.0	- - -	10.3	9.5	- - -	6.1	5.4
15–44 years.	100.0	- - -	73.9	73.2	- - -	11.4	11.5	- - -	14.8	15.3
45–64 years.	100.0	- - -	77.3	79.6	- - -	8.7	7.8	- - -	14.1	12.5
65–74 years.	100.0	- - -	86.0	88.6	- - -	5.0	4.4	- - -	9.0	7.0
75 years and over	100.0	- - -	89.3	92.1	- - -	4.2	3.6	- - -	6.5	4.3
Black[3,5]	100.0	58.3	77.5	80.6	15.1	11.0	9.7	26.6	11.6	9.6
Under 15 years	100.0	- - -	79.9	84.5	- - -	12.6	10.6	- - -	7.5	4.9
15–44 years.	100.0	- - -	72.3	74.5	- - -	12.7	11.7	- - -	15.0	13.7
45–64 years.	100.0	- - -	80.2	83.0	- - -	8.0	7.3	- - -	11.8	9.7
65–74 years.	100.0	- - -	84.4	88.8	- - -	5.9	3.9	- - -	9.7	7.3
75 years and over	100.0	- - -	89.4	92.2	- - -	*3.4	*2.7	- - -	7.3	5.1
Family income[3,6]										
Less than $15,000.	100.0	58.6	77.3	78.2	13.2	9.8	9.5	28.2	12.9	12.3
$15,000–$24,999.	100.0	62.5	76.7	76.5	14.2	10.2	10.2	23.3	13.2	13.3
$25,000–$34,999.	100.0	66.8	78.7	77.9	14.5	10.0	10.4	18.7	11.4	11.8
$35,000–$49,999.	100.0	70.2	80.1	80.4	14.0	9.4	9.4	15.7	10.4	10.2
$50,000 or more	100.0	73.6	81.7	83.5	12.9	8.9	8.1	13.5	9.4	8.4
Geographic region[3]										
Northeast	100.0	68.0	81.6	83.4	14.1	9.1	7.9	17.9	9.3	8.7
Midwest	100.0	66.6	79.5	80.3	14.2	9.6	9.5	19.2	10.9	10.3
South.	100.0	65.2	76.0	77.8	13.9	11.3	10.5	20.9	12.7	11.7
West	100.0	69.0	77.5	78.0	13.7	9.4	9.3	17.3	13.1	12.7
Location of residence[3]										
Within MSA[7]	100.0	68.2	79.0	80.2	14.0	9.7	9.2	17.8	11.3	10.6
Outside MSA[7]	100.0	64.0	75.7	76.8	14.1	11.4	10.5	21.9	12.9	12.7

- - - Data not available.

* Relative standard error greater than 30 percent.

[1]Includes persons who never visited a physician.

[2]Denominator excludes persons with unknown interval.

[3]Age adjusted.

[4]Includes all other races not shown separately and unknown family income.

[5]1964 data include all other races.

[6]Family income categories for 1995. In 1990 the two lowest income categories are less than $14,000 and $14,000–$24,999; the three higher income categories are as shown. Income categories in 1964 are less than $2,000; $2,000–$3,999; $4,000–$6,999; $7,000–$9,999; and $10,000 or more.

[7]Metropolitan statistical area.

SOURCE: Centers for Disease Control and Prevention, National Center for Health Statistics, Division of Health Interview Statistics. Data from the National Health Interview Survey.

Table 78. No physician contact within the past 12 months among children under 6 years of age according to selected characteristics: United States, average annual 1993–94 and 1994–95

[Data are based on household interviews of a sample of the civilian noninstitutionalized population]

Characteristic	1993–94	1994–95
	Percent of children without a physician contact within the past 12 months	
All children[1]	8.3	8.8
Race and Hispanic origin		
White, non-Hispanic	7.3	8.1
Black, non-Hispanic	10.3	9.8
Hispanic	9.9	9.9
Poverty status[2]		
Poor	10.6	11.2
Near poor	9.9	10.1
Nonpoor	5.0	5.5
Race and Hispanic origin and poverty status[2]		
White, non-Hispanic:		
Poor	8.8	11.0
Near poor	10.0	9.9
Nonpoor	4.8	5.3
Black, non-Hispanic:		
Poor	12.2	10.9
Near poor	8.7	9.3
Nonpoor	*	7.1
Hispanic:		
Poor	10.7	10.8
Near poor	10.3	10.7
Nonpoor	*	5.0
Health insurance status[3]		
Insured	6.8	7.1
Private	6.5	6.6
Medicaid	7.2	7.9
Uninsured	15.6	17.1
Poverty status and health insurance status[2,3]		
Poor:		
Insured	7.9	8.4
Uninsured	21.5	23.3
Near poor:		
Insured	8.5	8.7
Uninsured	13.8	14.9
Nonpoor:		
Insured	4.8	5.1
Uninsured	8.9	11.8
Geographic region		
Northeast	4.4	5.4
Midwest	8.0	8.7
South	11.0	10.8
West	7.8	8.8
Location of residence		
Within MSA[4]	7.6	8.2
Outside MSA[4]	10.8	11.3

* Relative standard error greater than 30 percent.

[1]Includes all other races not shown separately and unknown poverty status and unknown health insurance status.

[2]Poverty status is based on family income and family size using Bureau of the Census poverty thresholds. Poor persons are defined as below the poverty threshold. Near poor persons have incomes of 100 percent to less than 200 percent of poverty threshold. Nonpoor persons have incomes of 200 percent or greater than the poverty threshold. See Appendix II, Poverty level.

[3]Health insurance categories are mutually exclusive. Persons who reported more than one type of health insurance coverage were classified to a single type of coverage according to the following hierarchy: Medicaid, private, other. Other health insurance includes Medicare, or Military coverage. See Appendix II, Health insurance coverage.

[4]MSA is metropolitan statistical area.

NOTES: See Appendix II for definition of Physician contact. In 1993–94 and 1994–95 about 10 percent of children have unknown health insurance status and about 13 percent of children have unknown poverty status.

SOURCE: Centers for Disease Control and Prevention, National Center for Health Statistics, data computed by the Division of Health and Utilization Analysis from the 1993, 1994, and 1995 National Health Interview Survey health insurance supplements.

Table 79. No usual source of health care among children under 18 years of age according to selected characteristics: United States, average annual 1993–94 and 1994–95

[Data are based on household interviews of a sample of the civilian noninstitutionalized population]

Characteristic	Under 6 years of age		6–17 years of age	
	1993–94	1994–95	1993–94	1994–95
	Percent of children without a usual source of health care			
All children[1]	4.3	4.0	8.1	7.5
Race and Hispanic origin				
White, non-Hispanic	3.4	3.2	6.1	5.7
Black, non-Hispanic	4.6	3.7	8.8	7.2
Hispanic	7.9	7.6	17.0	15.6
Poverty status[2]				
Poor	7.1	6.4	13.9	12.1
Near poor	5.7	5.9	10.1	10.1
Nonpoor	1.6	1.7	4.0	4.0
Race and Hispanic origin and poverty status[2]				
White, non-Hispanic:				
Poor	5.9	5.6	9.8	9.3
Near poor	6.0	5.4	9.2	8.9
Nonpoor	1.5	1.6	3.7	3.7
Black, non-Hispanic:				
Poor	6.9	5.3	11.4	8.7
Near poor	3.7	3.3	8.1	8.4
Nonpoor	*	1.4	4.3	4.5
Hispanic:				
Poor	9.6	8.4	22.8	19.4
Near poor	7.5	10.2	16.3	16.5
Nonpoor	*	2.9	5.9	6.6
Health insurance status[3]				
Insured	2.5	2.3	5.1	4.5
Private	1.7	1.7	4.2	3.8
Medicaid	4.0	3.6	8.1	6.9
Uninsured	16.3	15.6	24.0	23.4
Poverty status and health insurance status[2,3]				
Poor:				
Insured	3.9	3.6	8.3	6.8
Uninsured	22.4	20.7	28.5	27.1
Near poor:				
Insured	3.5	3.3	6.6	6.1
Uninsured	15.0	16.2	21.3	21.7
Nonpoor:				
Insured	1.3	1.3	3.3	3.2
Uninsured	6.5	7.8	13.9	15.6
Geographic region				
Northeast	2.7	2.3	3.9	3.7
Midwest	3.4	3.2	5.1	4.7
South	5.6	4.4	11.3	9.8
West	4.7	5.7	9.9	10.2
Location of residence				
Within MSA[4]	4.1	4.0	8.2	7.5
Outside MSA[4]	5.1	4.4	7.7	7.4

* Relative standard error greater than 30 percent.
[1]Includes all other races not shown separately and unknown poverty status and unknown health insurance status.
[2]Poverty status is based on family income and family size using Bureau of the Census poverty thresholds. Poor persons are defined as below the poverty threshold. Near poor persons have incomes of 100 percent to less than 200 percent of poverty threshold. Nonpoor persons have incomes of 200 percent or greater than the poverty threshold. See Appendix II, Poverty level.
[3]Health insurance categories are mutually exclusive. Persons who reported more than one type of health insurance coverage were classified to a single type of coverage according to the following hierarchy: Medicaid, private, other. Other health insurance includes Medicare, or Military coverage. See Appendix II, Health insurance coverage.
[4]MSA is metropolitan statistical area.

NOTES: See Appendix II for definition of usual source of care. In 1993–94 and 1994–95 about 10 percent of children have unknown health insurance status and about 13 percent of children have unknown poverty status.

SOURCE: Centers for Disease Control and Prevention, National Center for Health Statistics, data computed by the Division of Health and Utilization Analysis from the 1993, 1994, and 1995 National Health Interview Survey access to care and health insurance supplements.

Table 80 (page 1 of 2). Use of mammography for women 40 years of age and over according to selected characteristics: United States, selected years 1987–94

[Data are based on household interviews of a sample of the civilian noninstitutionalized population]

Characteristic	1987	1990	1991	1993	1994
Age					

Characteristic	1987	1990	1991	1993	1994
Age	Percent of women having a mammogram within the past 2 years[1]				
40 years and over...............	28.7	51.4	54.6	59.7	60.9
40–49 years	31.9	55.1	55.6	59.9	61.3
50 years and over	27.4	49.7	54.1	59.7	60.6
50–64 years.................	31.7	56.0	60.3	65.1	66.5
65 years and over.............	22.8	43.4	48.1	54.2	55.0
Age, race, and Hispanic origin					
40 years and over:					
White, non-Hispanic..............	30.3	52.7	56.0	60.6	61.3
Black, non-Hispanic	23.8	46.0	47.7	59.2	64.4
Hispanic	18.3	45.2	49.2	50.9	51.9
40–49 years:					
White, non-Hispanic	34.3	57.0	58.1	61.6	62.0
Black, non-Hispanic	27.9	48.4	48.0	55.6	67.2
Hispanic....................	15.3	45.1	44.0	52.6	47.5
50 years and over:					
White, non-Hispanic	28.8	50.7	55.1	60.2	61.0
Black, non-Hispanic	21.5	44.6	47.6	61.4	62.4
Hispanic....................	20.0	45.2	53.7	49.7	54.7
50–64 years:					
White, non-Hispanic..........	33.6	58.1	61.5	66.2	67.5
Black, non-Hispanic..........	26.4	48.4	52.4	65.5	63.6
Hispanic..................	23.0	47.5	61.7	59.2	60.1
65 years and over:					
White, non-Hispanic..........	24.0	43.8	49.1	54.7	54.9
Black, non-Hispanic..........	14.1	39.7	41.6	56.3	61.0
Hispanic..................	*13.7	41.1	40.9	35.7	48.0
Age and poverty status[2]					
40 years and over:					
Below poverty	15.0	28.7	36.5	40.8	44.4
At or above poverty	31.0	54.8	58.4	62.7	64.8
40–49 years:					
Below poverty................	19.0	33.2	33.7	35.8	44.0
At or above poverty...........	33.4	57.3	58.8	62.6	64.7
50 years and over:					
Below poverty................	13.8	27.0	37.6	42.9	44.5
At or above poverty...........	29.9	53.5	58.2	62.8	64.9
50–64 years:					
Below poverty...............	14.5	25.6	39.6	45.3	47.0
At or above poverty..........	34.1	59.5	64.3	67.8	70.3
65 years and over:					
Below poverty..............	13.4	28.0	36.0	41.2	43.2
At or above poverty..........	25.0	46.6	51.5	57.3	58.7

See footnotes at end of table.

Table 80 (page 2 of 2). Use of mammography for women 40 years of age and over according to selected characteristics: United States, selected years 1987–94

[Data are based on household interviews of a sample of the civilian noninstitutionalized population]

Characteristic	1987	1990	1991	1993	1994
Age and education	Percent of women having a mammogram within the past 2 years[1]				
40 years of age and over:					
Less than 12 years	17.8	36.4	40.0	46.4	48.2
12 years	31.3	52.7	55.8	59.0	61.0
13 years or more	37.7	62.8	65.2	69.5	69.7
40–49 years of age:					
Less than 12 years	15.1	38.5	40.8	43.6	50.4
12 years	32.6	53.1	52.0	56.6	55.8
13 years or more	39.2	62.3	63.7	66.1	68.7
50 years of age and over:					
Less than 12 years	18.4	36.0	39.9	46.9	47.7
12 years	30.6	52.6	57.7	60.1	63.6
13 years or more	36.8	63.2	66.3	72.5	70.5
50–64 years of age:					
Less than 12 years	21.2	41.0	43.6	51.4	51.6
12 years	33.8	56.5	60.8	62.4	67.8
13 years or more	40.5	68.0	72.7	78.5	74.7
65 years of age and over:					
Less than 12 years	16.5	33.0	37.7	44.2	45.6
12 years	25.9	47.5	54.0	57.4	59.1
13 years or more	32.3	56.7	57.9	64.8	64.3

* Relative standard error greater than 30 percent.

[1]Questions concerning use of mammography differed slightly on the National Health Interview Survey across the years for which data are shown. In 1987 and 1990 women were asked to report when they had their last mammogram. In 1991 women were asked whether they had a mammogram in the past 2 years. In 1993 and 1994 women were asked whether they had a mammogram within the past year, between 1 and 2 years ago, or over 2 years ago.

[2]Poverty status is based on family income and family size using Bureau of the Census poverty thresholds (see Appendix II).

NOTE: Some numbers in this table have been revised and differ from previous editions of *Health, United States*.

SOURCE: Centers for Disease Control and Prevention, National Center for Health Statistics, Division of Health Interview Statistics. Data from the National Health Interview Survey.

Table 81 (page 1 of 2). Ambulatory care visits to physician offices and hospital outpatient and emergency departments by selected patient characteristics: United States, 1993–96

[Data are based on reporting by a sample of office-based physician visits and hospital outpatient department and emergency department visits]

Age, sex, and race	All places[1]				Physician offices			
	1993	1994	1995	1996	1993	1994	1995	1996
	Number of visits in thousands							
Total..........................	869,992	841,205	860,858	892,025	717,191	681,457	697,082	734,493
Age								
Under 15 years....................	164,911	161,687	169,297	176,919	129,279	124,421	131,548	140,851
15–44 years......................	325,475	316,143	310,530	312,794	256,260	244,864	237,868	243,535
45–64 years......................	184,961	176,354	188,319	198,885	160,146	149,038	159,531	170,229
45–54 years.....................	99,119	93,963	104,891	112,393	85,532	78,280	88,266	95,689
55–64 years.....................	85,842	82,391	83,429	86,492	74,615	70,758	71,264	74,540
65 years and over..................	194,644	187,021	192,712	203,427	171,506	163,135	168,135	179,878
65–74 years.....................	105,132	99,213	102,605	105,624	93,873	87,461	90,544	93,879
75 years and over.................	89,512	87,808	90,106	97,803	77,633	75,674	77,591	85,999
	Number of visits per 100 persons							
Total, age adjusted.................	334	317	322	330	274	256	260	271
Total, crude.....................	342	324	329	337	282	262	266	278
Age								
Under 15 years....................	288	273	285	298	226	210	221	237
15–44 years	281	266	260	261	221	206	200	203
45–64 years......................	371	350	364	374	322	296	309	320
45–54 years.....................	345	316	339	349	298	263	286	297
55–64 years.....................	408	398	401	411	354	342	343	354
65 years and over	622	603	612	639	548	526	534	565
65–74 years.....................	565	544	560	579	504	479	494	515
75 years and over.................	707	687	683	719	613	592	588	632
Sex and age								
Male, age adjusted..................	289	275	280	289	234	219	223	235
Male, crude......................	286	272	277	285	232	216	220	232
Under 15 years..................	299	286	288	303	234	221	220	240
15–44 years....................	199	191	191	183	150	140	140	135
45–54 years....................	287	253	275	284	245	206	229	240
55–64 years....................	348	338	351	374	300	290	300	325
65–74 years....................	519	511	508	558	462	449	445	497
75 years and over................	716	688	711	767	621	602	616	683
Female, age adjusted...............	377	357	362	371	312	291	296	306
Female, crude....................	395	374	378	387	329	306	310	321
Under 15 years..................	277	260	281	292	217	199	222	233
15–44 years....................	361	339	329	338	290	270	258	270
45–54 years....................	399	377	400	411	348	318	339	352
55–64 years....................	462	453	446	445	404	389	382	382
65–74 years....................	602	570	603	597	538	504	534	530
75 years and over................	702	687	666	689	609	586	571	600
Race and age								
White, age adjusted.................	343	325	329	329	288	269	272	277
White, crude	354	335	338	339	299	278	281	286
Under 15 years..................	307	292	305	309	250	233	247	255
15–44 years....................	287	273	265	256	232	218	209	205
45–54 years....................	344	317	334	339	302	270	286	294
55–64 years....................	409	397	397	404	362	347	345	356
65–74 years....................	578	544	557	574	522	485	496	515
75 years and over................	719	681	689	716	629	590	598	634
Black, age adjusted	291	290	294	368	190	187	190	255
Black, crude	282	277	281	354	182	175	178	242
Under 15 years..................	208	201	198	276	113	110	103	172
15–44 years....................	257	244	249	307	154	143	150	197
45–54 years....................	340	351	387	461	247	245	281	346
55–64 years....................	429	409	414	481	325	295	294	350
65–74 years....................	421	510	553	613	322	390	429	492
75 years and over................	622	667	534	804	480	509	395	651

See notes at end of table.

Table 81 (page 2 of 2). Ambulatory care visits to physician offices and hospital outpatient and emergency departments by selected patient characteristics: United States, 1993–96

[Data are based on reporting by a sample of office-based physician visits and hospital outpatient department and emergency department visits]

Age, sex, and race	Hospital outpatient departments				Hospital emergency departments			
	1993	1994	1995	1996	1993	1994	1995	1996
	Number of visits in thousands							
Total...........................	62,534	66,345	67,232	67,186	90,266	93,402	96,545	90,347
Age								
Under 15 years...................	12,927	13,516	15,039	15,196	22,705	23,751	22,709	20,872
15–44 years.....................	26,810	27,648	26,895	26,857	42,404	43,630	45,767	42,402
45–64 years.....................	12,365	14,306	14,811	14,911	12,450	13,011	13,978	13,745
45–54 years....................	6,554	7,903	8,029	8,496	7,033	7,780	8,595	8,207
55–64 years....................	5,811	6,403	6,782	6,415	5,417	5,230	5,383	5,538
65 years and over.................	10,432	10,875	10,487	10,222	12,707	13,010	14,090	13,328
65–74 years....................	5,865	5,955	6,004	5,799	5,394	5,797	6,057	5,945
75 years and over.................	4,567	4,920	4,482	4,422	7,312	7,214	8,033	7,382
	Number of visits per 100 persons							
Total, age adjusted.................	24	25	26	25	35	36	36	34
Total, crude......................	25	26	26	25	35	36	37	34
Age								
Under 15 years...................	23	23	25	26	40	40	38	35
15–44 years.....................	23	23	23	22	37	37	38	35
45–64 years.....................	25	28	29	28	25	26	27	26
45–54 years....................	23	27	26	26	24	26	28	25
55–64 years....................	28	31	33	31	26	25	26	26
65 years and over	33	35	33	32	41	42	45	42
65–74 years....................	32	33	33	32	29	32	33	33
75 years and over.................	36	39	34	32	58	56	61	54
Sex and age								
Male, age adjusted.................	19	21	21	21	35	35	36	33
Male, crude......................	19	20	21	20	35	35	36	33
Under 15 years..................	22	23	27	26	42	42	41	36
15–44 years....................	14	15	14	14	35	35	37	33
45–54 years....................	19	21	20	20	23	26	26	24
55–64 years....................	23	24	26	24	25	24	25	26
65–74 years....................	29	30	29	29	28	32	34	32
75 years and over.................	35	35	34	30	60	50	61	54
Female, age adjusted.............	29	30	30	30	35	36	36	35
Female, crude....................	30	30	31	31	36	37	37	35
Under 15 years..................	23	23	24	25	37	38	36	34
15–44 years....................	32	31	31	31	39	38	40	38
45–54 years....................	26	32	32	32	26	26	29	27
55–64 years....................	31	37	38	37	27	27	26	27
65–74 years....................	34	35	36	34	30	31	32	33
75 years and over.................	37	40	34	34	56	60	61	55
Race and age								
White, age adjusted.................	21	23	23	21	33	34	34	31
White, crude......................	22	23	23	21	33	34	34	31
Under 15 years..................	20	21	23	21	37	38	35	33
15–44 years....................	21	21	21	19	34	34	36	32
45–54 years....................	20	23	23	22	23	24	25	23
55–64 years....................	24	27	28	25	24	24	24	24
65–74 years....................	28	29	29	28	28	30	32	31
75 years and over.................	33	35	31	29	57	55	60	53
Black, age adjusted	45	48	47	56	56	55	57	57
Black, crude	44	46	45	54	57	56	58	58
Under 15 years..................	37	36	40	52	58	56	56	52
15–44 years....................	41	41	38	48	62	60	62	63
45–54 years....................	49	60	55	62	45	46	51	54
55–64 years....................	60	70	73	79	44	44	47	51
65–74 years....................	60	71	77	74	39	49	47	47
75 years and over.................	73	82	66	73	69	75	73	80

[1] All places includes visits to physician offices and hospital outpatient and emergency departments.

NOTES: Rates are based on the civilian noninstitutionalized population. Rates will be overestimated to the extent that visits by institutionalized persons are counted in the numerator (for example, hospital emergency department visits by nursing home residents) and institutionalized persons are omitted from the denominator.

SOURCES: Centers for Disease Control and Prevention, National Center for Health Statistics, Division of Health Care Statistics. Data from the National Ambulatory Medical Care Survey and the National Hospital Ambulatory Medical Care Survey.

Table 82. Ambulatory care visits to physician offices, percent distribution according to selected patient characteristics and physician specialty: United States, 1975, 1985, and 1996

[Data are based on reporting by a sample of office-based physicians]

Age, sex, and race	All specialties	General and family practice			Internal medicine			Pediatrics			Obstetrics and gynecology		
		1975	1985	1996	1975	1985	1996	1975	1985	1996	1975	1985	1996
					Percent distribution								
Total	100.0	41.3	30.5	25.3	10.9	11.6	14.0	8.2	11.4	13.2	8.5	8.9	9.0
Age													
Under 15 years.	100.0	34.1	25.0	21.7	2.1	2.2	2.2	43.7	55.2	61.4	*	*	*
15–44 years.	100.0	40.9	33.0	27.1	8.1	8.3	12.5	1.4	2.6	3.6	17.5	19.1	21.5
45–64 years.	100.0	44.4	32.0	25.6	16.2	15.7	18.3	*	*	*	3.9	4.7	6.0
45–54 years.	100.0	44.5	32.9	26.3	15.0	14.3	18.4	*	*	*	5.3	6.5	7.3
55–64 years.	100.0	44.2	31.3	24.6	17.5	16.9	18.3	*	*	*	2.3	3.2	4.3
65 years and over.	100.0	45.5	29.1	25.5	19.3	22.1	21.3	*	*	*	1.2	1.4	1.8
65–74 years.	100.0	46.0	28.8	26.5	18.6	22.1	20.1	*	*	*	1.4	2.0	2.1
75 years and over	100.0	44.6	29.4	24.5	20.5	22.1	22.5	*	*	*	*	*	1.6
Sex and age													
Male:													
Under 15 years	100.0	34.8	24.7	21.5	2.0	1.9	2.4	43.2	53.9	60.9	. . .	. . .	. . .
15–44 years	100.0	45.9	36.4	31.4	10.0	9.9	15.7	1.9	2.5	6.1	. . .	. . .	. . .
45–64 years	100.0	43.4	31.0	25.2	17.3	16.0	20.2	*	*	*	. . .	. . .	. . .
65 years and over	100.0	45.7	28.1	25.3	17.5	20.8	20.7	*	*	*	. . .	. . .	. . .
Female:													
Under 15 years	100.0	33.3	25.3	22.1	2.2	2.5	1.9	44.3	56.5	61.9	*	*	*
15–44 years	100.0	38.3	31.3	25.0	7.1	7.5	10.9	1.1	2.6	2.3	26.4	28.4	32.1
45–64 years	100.0	45.0	32.7	25.9	15.5	15.5	17.0	*	*	*	6.4	7.7	10.1
65 years and over	100.0	45.4	29.7	25.7	20.4	23.0	21.7	*	*	*	1.9	2.3	3.2
Race													
White.	100.0	40.8	30.0	25.2	11.1	11.8	13.1	8.2	11.4	13.3	8.2	8.7	8.6
Black.	100.0	46.9	35.4	24.6	9.9	10.4	20.3	8.0	11.3	13.2	11.9	9.9	11.5

Age, sex, and race	General surgery			Ophthalmology			Orthopedic surgery			All others		
	1975	1985	1996	1975	1985	1996	1975	1985	1996	1975	1985	1996
						Percent distribution						
Total	7.3	4.7	2.5	4.4	6.3	5.5	3.4	5.0	4.9	16.0	21.7	25.5
Age												
Under 15 years.	2.6	1.4	*	3.4	2.6	1.8	3.4	2.9	2.2	9.6	10.4	9.8
15–44 years.	7.5	4.4	2.4	3.4	3.9	3.2	3.9	6.1	5.8	17.4	22.5	23.9
45–64 years.	9.7	6.6	3.5	4.9	7.1	5.5	3.7	6.1	6.6	17.3	27.4	34.0
45–54 years.	10.0	6.6	3.5	4.3	6.0	4.4	4.1	6.6	6.7	16.7	26.7	32.7
55–64 years.	9.3	6.6	3.5	5.4	7.9	6.9	3.3	5.7	6.4	17.9	28.0	35.6
65 years and over.	7.9	6.2	3.2	6.9	13.5	11.7	1.9	3.4	4.1	17.3	24.2	32.1
65–74 years.	7.9	6.4	3.7	6.4	11.2	9.9	2.1	3.6	4.4	17.4	25.9	33.0
75 years and over	7.8	6.0	2.6	7.8	16.6	13.8	1.4	3.1	3.7	17.0	21.9	31.1
Sex and age												
Male:												
Under 15 years	2.9	1.7	*	2.7	2.5	1.7	3.7	3.3	2.4	10.1	11.9	10.4
15–44 years	8.8	5.0	2.6	4.1	5.2	5.0	7.1	11.0	9.2	21.9	29.8	29.9
45–64 years	9.1	6.2	3.1	5.1	7.2	5.6	4.3	7.0	6.8	20.7	32.2	38.3
65 years and over	7.7	6.7	2.9	6.4	11.8	9.5	1.6	2.6	3.6	20.9	29.8	37.9
Female:												
Under 15 years	2.3	*	*	4.3	2.6	1.9	3.0	2.4	2.0	9.1	8.9	9.3
15–44 years	6.9	4.1	2.3	3.0	3.3	2.3	2.2	3.8	4.1	15.1	19.0	20.9
45–64 years	10.1	6.9	3.8	4.8	7.0	5.3	3.2	5.5	6.4	15.0	24.2	31.0
65 years and over	8.0	5.9	3.3	7.2	14.5	13.4	2.1	3.8	4.4	15.0	20.7	27.8
Race												
White.	7.5	4.6	2.5	4.3	6.4	6.0	3.5	5.0	5.1	16.5	22.3	26.2
Black.	6.1	6.2	2.5	3.2	4.7	2.8	2.8	4.8	3.9	11.0	17.2	21.3

* Relative standard error greater than 50 percent.
. . . Category not applicable.

NOTES: In 1975 and 1985 the survey excluded Alaska and Hawaii. Beginning in 1989 the survey included all 50 States. Specialty information based on the physician's self-designated primary area of practice. General and family practice includes general practice, family practice, and beginning in 1992 general and family practice includes subspecialties also. Internal medicine includes general internal medicine and excludes all subspecialties. Pediatrics and obstetrics and gynecology include physicians practicing in the general field and subspecialties.

SOURCE: Centers for Disease Control and Prevention, National Center for Health Statistics, Division of Health Care Statistics. Data from the National Ambulatory Medical Care Survey.

Health, United States, 1998

Table 83. Persons with a dental visit within the past year among persons 25 years of age and over, according to selected patient characteristics: United States, selected years 1983–93

[Data are based on household interviews of a sample of the civilian noninstitutionalized population]

Characteristic	1983[1]	1989[1]	1990	1991	1993
	Percent of persons with a visit within the past year				
Total[2,3]	53.9	58.9	62.3	58.2	60.8
Age					
25–34 years	59.0	60.9	65.1	59.1	60.3
35–44 years	60.3	65.9	69.1	64.8	66.9
45–64 years	54.1	59.9	62.8	59.2	62.0
65 years and over	39.3	45.8	49.6	47.2	51.7
65–74 years	43.8	50.0	53.5	51.1	56.3
75 years and over	31.8	39.0	43.4	41.3	44.9
Sex[3]					
Male	51.7	56.2	58.8	55.5	58.2
Female	55.9	61.4	65.6	60.8	63.4
Poverty status[3,4]					
Below poverty	30.4	33.3	38.2	33.0	35.9
At or above poverty	55.8	62.1	65.4	61.9	64.3
Race and Hispanic origin[3]					
White, non-Hispanic	56.6	61.8	64.9	61.5	64.0
Black, non-Hispanic	39.1	43.3	49.1	44.3	47.3
Hispanic	42.1	48.9	53.8	43.1	46.2
Education[3]					
Less than 12 years	35.1	36.9	41.2	35.2	38.0
12 years	54.8	58.2	61.3	56.7	58.7
13 years or more	70.9	73.9	75.7	72.2	73.8
Education, race, and Hispanic origin[3]					
Less than 12 years:					
White, non-Hispanic	36.1	39.1	41.8	38.1	41.2
Black, non-Hispanic	31.7	32.0	37.9	33.0	33.1
Hispanic	33.8	36.5	42.7	28.9	33.0
12 years:					
White, non-Hispanic	56.6	59.8	62.8	58.8	60.4
Black, non-Hispanic	40.5	44.8	51.1	43.1	48.2
Hispanic	48.7	56.5	59.9	49.5	54.6
13 years or more:					
White, non-Hispanic	72.6	75.8	77.3	74.2	75.8
Black, non-Hispanic	54.4	57.2	64.4	61.7	61.3
Hispanic	58.4	66.2	67.9	61.2	61.8

[1]Data for 1983 and 1989 are not strictly comparable with data for later years. Data for 1983 and 1989 are based on responses to the question "About how long has it been since you last went to a dentist?" Starting in 1990 data are based on the question "During the past 12 months, how many visits did you make to a dentist?"
[2]Includes all other races not shown separately and unknown poverty status and education level.
[3]Age adjusted.
[4]Poverty status is based on family income and family size using Bureau of the Census poverty thresholds. See Appendix II.

NOTES: Denominators exclude persons with unknown dental data. Estimates for 1983 and 1989 are based on data for all members of the sample household. Beginning in 1990 estimates are based on one adult member per sample household. Estimates for 1993 are based on responses during the last half of the year only.

SOURCE: Centers for Disease Control and Prevention, National Center for Health Statistics, Division of Health Interview Statistics. Data from the National Health Interview Survey.

Table 84. Substance abuse clients in specialty treatment units according to substance abused, geographic division, and State: United States, 1992 and 1995

[Data are based on a 1-day census of treatment providers]

Geographic division and State	All clients		Clients with both alcoholism and drug abuse		Alcoholism only clients		Drug abuse only clients	
	1992	1995	1992	1995	1992	1995	1992	1995
	Clients[1] per 100,000 population							
United States	436.0	457.4	167.1	212.4	160.1	139.0	108.8	106.0
New England	447.1	505.5	252.0	324.0	103.9	86.4	91.2	95.2
Maine	464.6	533.8	200.2	277.5	188.4	190.3	75.9	65.9
New Hampshire	188.0	355.3	99.7	256.4	63.1	75.9	25.1	23.0
Vermont	238.1	553.9	83.6	232.5	138.5	166.3	16.0	155.1
Massachusetts	474.2	525.0	341.8	451.4	64.6	47.6	67.8	26.0
Rhode Island	772.9	717.7	267.8	214.3	276.9	170.7	228.2	332.7
Connecticut	413.5	437.7	181.7	177.2	99.1	82.7	132.7	177.8
Middle Atlantic	590.3	596.0	240.2	265.2	124.3	141.8	225.8	189.0
New York	761.6	862.9	301.9	353.3	129.7	200.8	330.0	308.8
New Jersey	494.4	354.6	209.3	162.3	107.6	90.6	177.5	101.8
Pennsylvania	396.2	357.8	167.9	201.6	127.1	87.9	101.2	68.4
East North Central	411.6	461.2	170.8	211.8	156.5	147.0	84.3	102.4
Ohio	388.2	445.1	201.0	223.7	126.2	126.9	61.1	94.5
Indiana	345.1	297.1	129.3	150.5	167.4	93.0	48.4	53.7
Illinois	348.2	486.4	142.8	234.4	115.3	143.3	90.1	108.6
Michigan	574.2	600.7	203.6	221.5	226.1	211.1	144.5	168.1
Wisconsin	380.6	367.0	154.5	185.7	176.0	142.2	50.1	39.1
West North Central	278.2	278.9	129.1	143.9	109.1	94.3	39.9	40.6
Minnesota	175.6	179.1	102.8	92.4	52.4	59.2	20.4	27.4
Iowa	195.4	254.1	100.8	121.2	79.8	89.5	14.8	43.4
Missouri	259.6	262.7	130.5	143.0	79.6	69.2	49.5	50.6
North Dakota	285.0	249.9	116.9	118.3	151.4	114.2	16.6	17.5
South Dakota	279.1	341.1	86.9	134.0	157.0	185.3	35.2	21.8
Nebraska	443.1	413.2	185.5	219.5	221.2	144.8	36.4	48.9
Kansas	485.5	429.6	184.0	228.2	209.2	156.7	92.4	44.8
South Atlantic	349.1	418.5	135.0	192.2	130.4	132.3	83.7	94.0
Delaware	576.5	615.8	216.3	280.3	257.2	187.8	103.0	147.7
Maryland	630.6	668.2	226.1	269.8	213.2	172.6	191.3	225.8
District of Columbia	1,097.0	961.0	349.6	330.1	260.7	202.0	486.7	428.9
Virginia	313.8	329.6	125.7	187.9	121.3	87.4	66.8	54.4
West Virginia	250.2	283.2	42.9	98.6	178.0	154.2	29.3	30.4
North Carolina	318.9	287.9	128.6	152.8	139.3	89.7	51.0	45.4
South Carolina	399.1	422.0	121.1	149.0	222.1	201.6	55.9	71.4
Georgia	207.8	179.1	91.6	77.9	64.9	49.1	51.4	52.1
Florida	305.2	542.9	133.8	257.5	90.1	175.7	81.2	109.6
East South Central	227.5	301.3	85.6	127.4	91.7	115.3	50.2	58.6
Kentucky	363.2	584.1	123.4	203.7	185.6	298.9	54.2	81.6
Tennessee	183.6	147.5	64.7	82.6	67.1	36.0	51.8	29.0
Alabama	188.1	278.3	82.7	130.6	54.1	69.8	51.3	77.8
Mississippi	177.7	229.5	75.9	99.4	62.5	77.1	39.2	53.1
West South Central	265.7	257.8	144.9	147.4	53.8	49.8	66.9	60.6
Arkansas	153.3	167.8	49.5	65.6	46.1	44.0	57.7	58.2
Louisiana	351.2	315.2	190.7	179.5	77.1	68.5	83.4	67.3
Oklahoma	218.6	267.0	120.8	138.0	57.7	77.3	40.0	51.6
Texas	269.3	255.1	151.6	152.7	48.6	41.3	69.1	61.0
Mountain	475.3	494.6	163.9	207.1	210.2	191.7	101.3	95.7
Montana	286.7	224.9	137.5	103.0	121.0	96.5	28.2	25.4
Idaho	263.6	298.1	118.9	155.4	118.8	93.4	25.9	49.3
Wyoming	480.6	440.4	203.8	256.0	228.6	149.0	48.1	35.4
Colorado	768.0	615.1	266.2	288.2	380.5	240.5	121.2	86.4
New Mexico	659.4	680.2	164.5	179.9	336.3	344.7	158.7	155.6
Arizona	327.5	269.5	86.3	89.0	122.3	101.6	119.0	78.9
Utah	460.6	939.5	217.1	396.0	163.9	376.7	79.7	166.9
Nevada	223.6	388.5	89.1	211.2	51.7	69.1	82.8	108.2
Pacific	661.9	618.1	166.2	261.2	354.0	224.1	141.7	132.8
Washington	808.0	816.7	410.8	487.0	273.7	232.8	123.6	96.8
Oregon	689.4	840.5	274.5	560.3	298.5	139.7	116.5	140.4
California	655.3	566.7	115.5	193.5	387.5	232.9	152.2	140.4
Alaska	572.8	910.1	271.2	324.4	223.1	478.2	78.5	107.5
Hawaii	161.2	300.1	83.6	147.6	35.7	58.8	42.0	93.8

[1]Clients who are 12 years of age or over.

NOTES: Rates are based on the resident population 12 years of age or over as of July 1. Client data are as of September 30, 1992, and October 2, 1995.

SOURCES: Substance Abuse and Mental Health Services Administration. Office of Applied Studies, Advance Report No. 9, Overview of the National Drug and Alcoholism Treatment Unit Survey (NDATUS): 1992 and 1980–1992, January 1995; and Drug and Alcohol Services Information System (DASIS) Series S–2, Uniform Facility Data Set (UFDS): Data for 1995 and 1980–95, September 1997.

Table 85. Additions to mental health organizations according to type of service and organization: United States, selected years 1983–94

[Data are based on inventories of mental health organizations]

Service and organization	Additions in thousands				Additions per 100,000 civilian population			
	1983	1990	1992	1994	1983	1990	1992	1994
Inpatient and residential treatment								
All organizations	1,633	2,036	2,092	2,197	701.4	833.5	830.0	840.3
State and county mental hospitals	339	276	275	236	146.0	113.2	109.3	91.2
Private psychiatric hospitals	165	407	470	480	70.9	166.5	186.4	185.5
Non-Federal general hospital psychiatric services	786	960	951	1,067	336.8	393.2	377.4	411.9
Department of Veterans Affairs psychiatric services[1]	149	198	181	172	64.3	81.2	71.6	61.5
Residential treatment centers for emotionally disturbed children	17	42	36	39	7.1	17.0	14.4	15.0
All other[2]	177	153	179	203	76.3	62.4	70.9	75.2
Outpatient treatment								
All organizations	2,665	3,005	2,883	3,242	1,147.5	1,230.9	1,180.6	1,252.8
State and county mental hospitals	84	43	46	38	36.3	17.5	18.6	14.8
Private psychiatric hospitals	78	121	141	145	33.4	49.7	57.7	56.1
Non-Federal general hospital psychiatric services	469	605	429	443	202.1	247.8	175.8	171.0
Department of Veterans Affairs psychiatric services[1]	103	164	145	120	44.5	67.2	59.2	46.5
Residential treatment centers for emotionally disturbed children	33	86	113	156	14.1	35.3	46.2	60.3
Freestanding psychiatric outpatient clinics	538	462	464	567	231.7	189.3	190.3	218.9
All other[2]	1,360	1,524	1,545	1,773	585.4	624.1	632.8	685.2
Partial care treatment								
All organizations	177	293	281	273	76.3	120.2	115.8	105.3
State and county mental hospitals	4	5	4	3	1.6	2.2	1.7	1.3
Private psychiatric hospitals	6	42	65	68	2.4	17.2	26.8	26.4
Non-Federal general hospital psychiatric services	46	54	50	55	19.8	21.9	20.7	21.1
Department of Veterans Affairs psychiatric services[1]	10	19	14	12	4.4	8.0	5.9	4.6
Residential treatment centers for emotionally disturbed children	3	13	8	12	1.5	5.5	3.5	4.3
Freestanding psychiatric outpatient clinics[3]	5	...	...	...	2.3	...	...	...
All other[2,3,4]	103	160	140	123	44.3	65.4	57.2	47.6

... Category not applicable.

[1]Includes Department of Veterans Affairs neuropsychiatric hospitals, general hospital psychiatric services, and psychiatric outpatient clinics.
[2]Includes other multiservice mental health organizations with inpatient and residential treatment services that are not elsewhere classified.
[3]Beginning in 1986 outpatient psychiatric clinics providing partial care are counted as multiservice mental health organizations in the "all other" category.
[4]Includes freestanding psychiatric partial care organizations.

NOTES: See Appendix II for definition of Addition. Outpatient and partial care treatment exclude office-based mental health care (psychiatrists, psychologists, licensed clinical social workers, and psychiatric nurses).

SOURCES: Survey and Analysis Branch, Division of State and Community Systems Development, Center for Mental Health Services. Manderscheid RW, Sonnenschein MA. *Mental health, United States, 1996*. DHHS. 1996. Unpublished data.

Table 86. Home health care and hospice patients, according to selected characteristics: United States, 1992–96

[Data are based on a survey of current home health care and hospice patients]

Type of patient and characteristic	1992	1994	1996
Home health care patients	**Number of current patients**		
Total.	1,232,200	1,879,510	2,427,483
Age at admission[1]	**Percent distribution**		
Under 65 years.	24.1	27.2	27.5
65 years and over.	75.9	72.8	72.5
65–74 years.	24.5	22.0	21.8
75–84 years.	34.0	31.1	33.9
85 years and over	17.5	19.7	16.7
Sex			
Male.	33.2	32.5	32.9
Female.	66.8	67.5	67.1
Primary admission diagnosis[2]			
Malignant neoplasms.	5.7	5.7	4.8
Diabetes.	7.7	8.1	8.5
Diseases of the nervous system and sense organs.	6.3	8.0	5.8
Diseases of the circulatory system	25.9	27.2	25.6
Diseases of heart.	12.6	14.3	10.9
Cerebrovascular diseases.	5.8	6.1	7.8
Diseases of the respiratory system	6.6	6.1	7.7
Decubitus ulcers.	1.9	1.1	1.0
Diseases of the musculoskeletal system and connective tissue . . .	9.4	8.3	8.8
Osteoarthritis.	2.5	2.8	3.2
Fractures, all sites	3.8	3.7	3.3
Fracture of neck of femur (hip).	1.4	1.7	1.3
Other	32.7	31.8	34.6
Hospice patients	**Number of current patients**		
Total.	52,100	60,783	59,363
Age at admission[1]	**Percent distribution**		
Under 65 years.	20.4	31.2	22.1
65 years and over.	79.6	68.8	77.9
65–74 years.	27.4	23.1	24.6
75–84 years.	39.1	29.0	31.9
85 years and over	13.0	16.7	21.4
Sex			
Male.	46.1	44.7	44.9
Female.	53.9	55.3	55.1
Primary admission diagnosis[2]			
Malignant neoplasms.	65.7	57.2	58.3
Malignant neoplasms of large intestine and rectum	9.0	8.0	4.0
Malignant neoplasms of trachea, bronchus, and lung.	21.1	12.5	15.8
Malignant neoplasm of breast	3.9	4.8	6.2
Malignant neoplasm of prostate.	6.0	5.9	6.6
Diseases of heart	10.2	9.3	8.3
Diseases of the respiratory system	4.3	6.6	7.3
Other	19.8	27.0	26.1

[1]Denominator excludes persons with unknown age.
[2]Denominator excludes persons with unknown diagnosis.

NOTES: Current home health and hospice patients are those who were under the care of their agency on any given day during the survey period. Diagnostic categories are based on the *International Classification of Diseases, 9th Revision, Clinical Modification*. For a listing of the code numbers, see Appendix II, table VII.

SOURCE: Centers for Disease Control and Prevention, National Center for Health Statistics, Division of Health Care Statistics. Data from the National Home and Hospice Care Survey.

Table 87. Discharges, days of care, and average length of stay in short-stay hospitals, according to selected characteristics: United States, 1964, 1990, and 1995

[Data are based on household interviews of a sample of the civilian noninstitutionalized population]

Characteristic	Discharges			Days of care			Average length of stay		
	1964	1990	1995	1964	1990	1995	1964	1990	1995
	Number per 1,000 population						Number of days		
Total[1,2]	109.1	91.0	86.2	970.9	607.1	486.3	8.9	6.7	5.6
Age									
Under 15 years	67.6	46.7	40.5	405.7	271.3	207.1	6.0	5.8	5.1
Under 5 years	94.3	79.9	72.2	731.1	496.4	374.4	7.8	6.2	5.2
5–14 years	53.1	29.0	24.2	229.1	150.8	120.5	4.3	5.2	5.0
15–44 years	100.6	62.6	57.6	760.7	340.5	251.2	7.6	5.4	4.4
45–64 years	146.2	135.7	122.4	1,559.3	911.5	687.1	10.7	6.7	5.6
65 years and over	190.0	248.8	266.9	2,292.7	2,092.4	1,892.4	12.1	8.4	7.1
65–74 years.	181.2	215.4	235.1	2,150.4	1,719.3	1,533.4	11.9	8.0	6.5
75 years and over	206.7	300.6	311.8	2,560.4	2,669.9	2,401.9	12.4	8.9	7.7
Sex[1]									
Male.	103.8	91.0	88.5	1,010.2	622.7	529.5	9.7	6.8	6.0
Female.	113.7	91.7	84.8	933.4	592.9	450.2	8.2	6.5	5.3
Race[1]									
White	112.4	89.5	84.2	961.4	580.9	458.5	8.6	6.5	5.4
Black[3]	84.0	112.0	108.0	1,062.9	875.9	730.9	12.7	7.8	6.8
Family income[1,4]									
Less than $15,000	102.4	142.2	140.7	1,051.2	1,141.2	878.0	10.3	8.0	6.2
$15,000–$24,999.	116.4	98.4	104.1	1,213.9	594.5	628.2	10.4	6.0	6.0
$25,000–$34,999.	110.7	85.1	78.7	939.8	560.6	448.1	8.5	6.6	5.7
$35,000–$49,999.	109.2	73.2	68.9	882.6	380.3	315.2	8.1	5.2	4.6
$50,000 or more	110.7	72.5	61.6	918.9	446.2	301.3	8.3	6.2	4.9
Geographic region[1]									
Northeast	98.5	84.9	77.4	993.8	623.4	532.1	10.1	7.3	6.9
Midwest	109.2	91.5	85.4	944.9	570.8	424.7	8.7	6.2	5.0
South	117.8	106.4	97.6	968.0	713.6	543.9	8.2	6.7	5.6
West	110.5	70.5	76.2	985.9	444.6	412.2	8.9	6.3	5.4
Location of residence[1]									
Within MSA[5]	107.5	85.9	83.6	1,015.4	599.6	485.0	9.4	7.0	5.8
Outside MSA[5]	113.3	109.5	96.3	871.9	636.0	489.7	7.7	5.8	5.1

[1]Age adjusted.

[2]Includes all other races not shown separately and unknown family income.

[3]1964 data include all other races.

[4]Family income categories for 1995. In 1990 the two lowest income categories are less than $14,000 and $14,000–$24,999; the three higher income categories are as shown. Income categories in 1964 are less than $2,000; $2,000–$3,999; $4,000–$6,999; $7,000–$9,999; and $10,000 or more.

[5]Metropolitan statistical area.

NOTES: Estimates of hospital utilization from the National Health Interview Survey (NHIS) and the National Hospital Discharge Survey (NHDS) may differ because NHIS data are based on household interviews of the civilian noninstitutionalized population and exclude deliveries, whereas NHDS data are based on hospital discharge records of all persons. NHDS includes records for persons discharged alive or deceased and institutionalized persons, and excludes newborn infants. Differences in hospital utilization estimated by the two surveys are particularly evident for the elderly and for women. See Appendix I.

SOURCE: Centers for Disease Control and Prevention, National Center for Health Statistics, Division of Health Interview Statistics. Data from the National Health Interview Survey.

Table 88. Discharges, days of care, and average length of stay in non-Federal short-stay hospitals, according to selected characteristics: United States, selected years 1980–95

[Data are based on a sample of hospital records]

Characteristic	1980[1]	1985[1]	1988	1989	1990	1992	1993[2]	1994	1995
	Discharges per 1,000 population								
Total[3]	158.5	137.7	117.6	115.4	113.0	110.5	107.6	106.5	104.7
Sex[3]									
Male	140.3	124.4	106.9	105.1	100.9	98.6	95.2	94.2	92.3
Female	177.0	151.8	129.3	126.6	126.0	123.2	120.5	119.1	117.4
Age									
Under 15 years	71.6	57.7	49.8	48.8	44.6	45.2	37.7	39.2	41.7
15–44 years	150.1	125.0	103.9	102.7	101.6	96.0	95.4	93.2	89.8
45–64 years	194.8	170.8	142.1	136.8	135.0	131.0	126.8	124.1	118.2
65 years and over	383.7	369.8	336.8	333.4	330.9	336.5	341.6	341.6	344.6
65–74 years	315.8	297.2	266.8	261.9	259.1	264.5	262.2	261.6	257.6
75 years and over	489.3	475.6	435.5	433.1	429.9	432.7	446.3	445.3	455.2
Geographic region[3]									
Northeast	147.6	129.1	126.1	124.6	121.0	123.9	118.3	121.3	120.0
Midwest	175.4	143.4	120.3	117.2	115.1	105.3	102.2	102.6	99.5
South	165.1	143.5	118.9	119.0	119.2	116.3	116.9	111.8	110.9
West	136.9	130.3	103.0	97.7	92.1	93.7	87.6	87.6	86.0
	Days of care per 1,000 population								
Total[3]	1,129.0	872.1	750.8	727.5	705.0	659.3	626.9	594.0	544.3
Sex[3]									
Male	1,076.0	848.2	748.2	729.8	690.4	656.3	616.3	580.8	533.1
Female	1,187.1	902.0	760.6	734.0	725.3	667.5	640.5	609.5	556.7
Age									
Under 15 years	315.7	263.0	248.4	237.4	215.4	219.6	195.5	189.2	185.6
15–44 years	786.8	603.3	492.6	480.3	465.3	416.1	399.3	390.4	346.0
45–64 years	1,596.9	1,201.6	966.5	915.9	911.5	827.1	785.0	727.5	655.6
65 years and over	4,098.4	3,228.0	2,994.1	2,959.2	2,867.7	2,771.7	2,676.2	2,516.3	2,352.4
65–74 years	3,147.0	2,437.3	2,248.8	2,153.2	2,067.7	2,040.8	1,927.1	1,798.8	1,669.0
75 years and over	5,578.7	4,381.4	4,045.2	4,082.6	3,970.7	3,747.8	3,664.6	3,445.7	3,220.1
Geographic region[3]									
Northeast	1,204.7	953.5	922.4	909.1	878.0	838.6	787.2	774.9	722.1
Midwest	1,296.2	952.0	747.0	726.0	713.4	626.2	600.5	553.9	502.9
South	1,105.5	848.9	725.6	727.8	704.1	676.2	655.1	618.0	564.9
West	836.2	713.2	602.7	532.5	509.9	483.1	445.2	420.3	385.2
	Average length of stay in days								
Total[3]	7.1	6.3	6.4	6.3	6.2	6.0	5.8	5.6	5.2
Sex[3]									
Male	7.7	6.8	7.0	6.8	6.8	6.7	6.5	6.2	5.8
Female	6.7	5.9	5.9	5.9	5.8	5.4	5.3	5.1	4.7
Age									
Under 15 years	4.4	4.6	5.0	4.9	4.8	4.9	5.2	4.8	4.5
15–44 years	5.2	4.8	4.7	4.7	4.6	4.3	4.2	4.2	3.9
45–64 years	8.2	7.0	6.8	6.7	6.8	6.3	6.2	5.9	5.5
65 years and over	10.7	8.7	8.9	8.9	8.7	8.2	7.8	7.4	6.8
65–74 years	10.0	8.2	8.4	8.2	8.0	7.7	7.3	6.9	6.5
75 years and over	11.4	9.2	9.3	9.4	9.2	8.7	8.2	7.7	7.1
Geographic region[3]									
Northeast	8.2	7.4	7.3	7.3	7.3	6.8	6.7	6.4	6.0
Midwest	7.4	6.6	6.2	6.2	6.2	5.9	5.9	5.4	5.1
South	6.7	5.9	6.1	6.1	5.9	5.8	5.6	5.5	5.1
West	6.1	5.5	5.9	5.5	5.5	5.2	5.1	4.8	4.5

[1]Comparisons of data from 1980–85 with data from later years should be made with caution as estimates of change may reflect improvements in the design (see Appendix I) rather than true changes in hospital use.
[2]In 1993 children's hospitals had a high rate of nonresponse that may have resulted in underestimates of hospital utilization by children.
[3]Age adjusted.

NOTES: Rates are based on the civilian population as of July 1. Some numbers in this table have been revised and differ from previous editions of *Health, United States*. Estimates of hospital utilization from the National Health Interview Survey (NHIS) and the National Hospital Discharge Survey (NHDS) may differ because NHIS data are based on household interviews of the civilian noninstitutionalized population and exclude deliveries, whereas NHDS data are based on hospital discharge records of all persons. NHDS includes records for persons discharged alive or deceased and institutionalized persons, and excludes newborn infants. Differences in hospital utilization estimated by the two surveys are particularly evident for the elderly and for women. See Appendix I.

SOURCE: Centers for Disease Control and Prevention, National Center for Health Statistics, Division of Health Care Statistics. Data from the National Hospital Discharge Survey.

Table 89. Discharges, days of care, and average length of stay in non-Federal short-stay hospitals for discharges with the diagnosis of human immunodeficiency virus (HIV) and for all discharges: United States, 1986–95

[Data are based on a sample of hospital records]

Type of discharge, sex, and age	1986[1]	1987[1]	1988	1989	1990	1992	1993	1994	1995
	Discharges in thousands								
Discharges with diagnosis of HIV	44	67	95	140	146	194	225	234	249
Male, 20–49 years	35	51	73	102	102	141	158	155	162
Female, 20–49 years	*	*	13	19	27	31	44	49	55
All discharges	34,256	33,387	31,146	30,947	30,788	30,951	30,825	30,843	30,722
Male, 20–49 years	4,300	4,075	3,670	3,676	3,649	3,529	3,619	3,531	3,360
Female, 20–49 years	9,027	8,980	8,169	8,196	8,228	7,942	7,901	7,705	7,593
	Discharges per 1,000 population								
Discharges with diagnosis of HIV	0.18	0.28	0.39	0.57	0.59	0.76	0.88	0.90	0.95
Male, 20–49 years	0.67	0.96	1.36	1.87	1.84	2.47	2.76	2.68	2.79
Female, 20–49 years	*	*	0.23	0.34	0.47	0.54	0.74	0.83	0.93
All discharges	143.7	138.8	128.3	126.3	124.3	122.1	120.2	119.1	117.5
Male, 20–49 years	82.2	76.8	68.2	67.3	65.8	62.0	63.1	61.2	57.9
Female, 20–49 years	166.7	163.6	147.1	145.8	144.5	136.1	134.6	130.5	127.9
	Days of care in thousands								
Discharges with diagnosis of HIV	714	936	1,277	1,731	2,188	2,136	2,561	2,317	2,326
Male, 20–49 years	573	724	914	1,235	1,645	1,422	1,696	1,444	1,408
Female, 20–49 years	*	*	233	201	341	455	619	511	559
All discharges	218,496	214,942	203,678	200,827	197,422	190,386	184,601	177,179	164,627
Male, 20–49 years	26,488	26,295	22,697	22,967	22,539	21,614	21,348	20,448	17,984
Female, 20–49 years	40,620	39,356	34,800	35,007	34,473	30,886	29,555	28,740	26,596
	Days of care per 1,000 population								
Discharges with diagnosis of HIV	2.99	3.89	5.26	7.06	8.83	8.43	9.99	8.95	8.90
Male, 20–49 years	10.95	13.64	16.97	22.62	29.68	24.97	29.57	25.04	24.26
Female, 20–49 years	*	*	4.19	3.58	5.99	7.80	10.54	8.66	9.41
All discharges	916.5	893.6	838.8	819.3	796.9	751.0	719.9	684.3	629.8
Male, 20–49 years	506.4	495.2	421.5	420.7	406.6	379.5	372.2	354.6	309.8
Female, 20–49 years	750.2	717.1	626.5	622.8	605.4	529.3	503.4	486.7	447.9
	Average length of stay in days								
Discharges with diagnosis of HIV	16.4	14.1	13.4	12.4	14.9	11.0	11.4	9.9	9.3
Male, 20–49 years	16.4	14.1	12.5	12.1	16.2	10.1	10.7	9.3	8.7
Female, 20–49 years	*	*	18.0	10.6	12.6	14.6	14.2	10.5	10.2
All discharges	6.4	6.4	6.5	6.5	6.4	6.2	6.0	5.7	5.4
Male, 20–49 years	6.2	6.5	6.2	6.2	6.2	6.1	5.9	5.8	5.4
Female, 20–49 years	4.5	4.4	4.3	4.3	4.2	3.9	3.7	3.7	3.5

* Statistics based on fewer than 5,000 estimated discharges are not shown.

[1]Comparisons of data from 1986 and 1987 with data from later years should be made with caution as estimates of change may reflect improvements in the design (see Appendix I) rather than true changes in hospital use.

NOTES: Excludes newborn infants. Rates are based on the civilian population as of July 1. Some figures in this table have been revised and differ from previous editions of *Health, United States*. Discharges with diagnosis of HIV have at least one HIV diagnosis listed on the face sheet of the medical record and are not limited to the first-listed diagnosis. See Appendix II, Human immunodeficiency virus (HIV) infection.

SOURCE: Centers for Disease Control and Prevention, National Center for Health Statistics, Division of Health Care Statistics. Data from the National Hospital Discharge Survey.

Table 90 (page 1 of 3). Rates of discharges and days of care in non-Federal short-stay hospitals, according to sex, age, and selected first-listed diagnosis: United States, 1985, 1990, 1994, and 1995

[Data are based on a sample of hospital records]

Sex, age, and first-listed diagnosis	Discharges 1985[1]	1990	1994	1995	Days of care 1985[1]	1990	1994	1995
Both sexes				Number per 1,000 population				
Total[2,3]	137.7	113.0	106.5	104.7	872.1	705.0	594.0	544.3
Male								
All ages[2,3]	124.4	100.9	94.2	92.3	848.2	690.4	580.8	533.1
Under 15 years[3]	64.4	49.2	43.3	46.6	289.9	234.1	211.5	212.8
Bronchitis	1.7	0.8	0.6	0.7	5.4	2.4	1.6	2.1
Pneumonia	5.7	6.3	6.7	7.8	23.6	26.3	25.7	28.1
Asthma	3.5	3.9	3.6	4.5	12.0	11.0	9.1	12.1
Injuries and poisoning.	9.3	5.9	5.1	4.9	36.8	26.0	20.2	21.5
Fracture, all sites.	3.2	2.0	1.7	1.6	16.7	7.9	6.4	7.6
15–44 years[3]	75.3	57.8	53.8	50.2	458.2	353.6	313.3	269.5
Psychoses.	3.0	3.5	5.6	4.9	43.7	50.3	63.9	49.5
Diseases of heart	3.0	2.9	2.9	2.7	16.6	15.4	12.2	11.3
Intervertebral disc disorders.	2.9	2.4	1.8	1.6	18.7	10.0	7.3	4.0
Injuries and poisoning.	17.9	13.4	10.0	9.9	98.7	66.7	46.6	47.3
Fracture, all sites.	5.2	4.1	3.3	3.3	34.6	22.9	18.1	17.9
45–64 years[3]	177.6	140.2	127.1	121.2	1,229.0	943.6	740.9	682.2
Malignant neoplasms	13.1	10.6	8.1	7.6	120.6	99.1	66.1	53.4
Malignant neoplasms of trachea, bronchus, lung . .	3.6	2.7	1.6	1.5	31.9	19.1	12.2	10.2
Diabetes	3.4	2.9	2.7	3.4	26.5	21.2	17.5	22.3
Diseases of heart.	36.9	31.7	29.4	29.7	239.2	185.0	148.0	143.7
Ischemic heart disease	27.1	22.6	20.8	21.3	171.1	128.2	101.3	99.0
Acute myocardial infarction	9.2	7.4	7.3	7.5	82.4	55.8	42.8	42.5
Congestive heart failure	2.5	3.0	3.2	2.9	18.9	19.7	19.0	16.3
Cerebrovascular diseases	5.0	4.1	4.1	3.8	51.0	40.7	25.3	25.7
Pneumonia	3.4	3.5	4.4	3.0	27.4	27.4	31.9	20.6
Injuries and poisoning.	15.0	11.6	10.9	10.2	99.1	82.6	63.8	56.2
Fracture, all sites.	4.0	3.3	3.1	2.9	29.9	24.2	20.8	18.4
65–74 years[3]	325.5	285.9	280.9	274.5	2,622.0	2,237.2	1,878.8	1,759.0
Malignant neoplasms	38.8	27.7	28.3	24.3	352.8	275.8	231.7	190.7
Malignant neoplasms of large intestine and rectum.	3.9	3.0	3.2	2.6	54.9	34.0	33.4	27.8
Malignant neoplasms of trachea, bronchus, lung . .	10.8	6.3	5.5	5.2	89.5	55.4	47.8	39.8
Malignant neoplasms of prostate	6.6	5.0	6.2	5.0	48.2	32.9	34.6	26.5
Diabetes	4.3	4.3	4.6	5.3	42.6	39.6	33.9	46.8
Diseases of heart.	69.9	69.0	73.8	74.1	520.2	484.1	443.0	416.7
Ischemic heart disease	43.2	41.7	43.1	43.7	317.2	283.4	252.6	244.6
Acute myocardial infarction	17.6	13.9	14.9	15.4	160.4	121.7	112.8	101.7
Congestive heart failure	9.8	11.3	13.6	14.8	76.4	89.6	92.0	87.0
Cerebrovascular diseases	18.5	13.7	15.7	17.0	182.0	114.0	108.2	111.9
Pneumonia	10.9	11.3	12.1	12.6	104.9	107.1	88.5	86.8
Hyperplasia of prostate.	13.5	14.3	8.1	7.5	84.8	64.6	30.7	22.4
Osteoarthritis	3.4	5.0	5.5	5.9	36.9	44.6	36.5	33.4
Injuries and poisoning.	16.0	17.5	17.9	16.0	131.7	138.1	124.2	106.4
Fracture, all sites.	4.5	4.5	4.8	4.4	42.8	45.6	37.1	32.1
Fracture of neck of femur (hip)	1.4	1.5	1.8	1.8	21.6	18.0	16.7	14.6
75 years and over[3]	529.1	476.3	468.2	472.8	4,682.0	4,211.9	3,562.1	3,248.8
Malignant neoplasms	55.7	40.8	29.4	30.1	545.9	406.4	253.0	250.2
Malignant neoplasms of large intestine and rectum.	6.9	5.4	4.2	4.9	84.7	80.3	43.9	52.9
Malignant neoplasms of trachea, bronchus, lung . .	10.4	5.3	4.2	3.5	99.0	53.1	38.6	31.2
Malignant neoplasms of prostate	15.3	9.7	4.9	4.3	116.5	65.3	27.3	17.5
Diabetes	6.4	4.6	7.1	6.9	66.6	50.9	51.0	41.9
Diseases of heart.	108.6	105.7	113.2	113.4	841.2	851.7	736.4	674.6
Ischemic heart disease	51.3	48.9	49.0	51.6	413.2	396.2	313.8	320.6
Acute myocardial infarction	23.8	23.0	20.7	22.2	230.5	226.5	157.3	168.6
Congestive heart failure	27.8	30.9	35.3	31.2	220.5	241.2	231.5	192.6
Cerebrovascular diseases	37.9	30.0	31.5	31.9	380.7	296.9	219.3	214.4
Pneumonia	30.1	38.4	38.0	40.2	305.7	391.8	309.2	323.8
Hyperplasia of prostate.	19.7	17.8	10.1	9.4	141.0	108.7	44.1	32.7
Osteoarthritis	4.4	5.7	6.7	6.5	49.4	60.4	46.0	54.1
Injuries and poisoning.	31.8	31.1	30.4	32.5	358.8	339.7	247.8	222.6
Fracture, all sites.	14.3	13.7	13.1	16.1	223.9	144.4	123.5	114.5
Fracture of neck of femur (hip)	8.4	8.5	8.9	9.0	161.3	97.4	94.2	68.6

See footnotes at end of table.

[Data are based on a sample of hospital records]

	Discharges				Days of care			
Sex, age, and first-listed diagnosis	1985[1]	1990	1994	1995	1985[1]	1990	1994	1995
Female	Number per 1,000 population							
All ages[2,3]	151.8	126.0	119.1	117.4	902.0	725.3	609.5	556.7
Under 15 years[3]	50.6	39.7	34.9	36.5	234.8	195.8	165.7	157.1
Bronchitis	1.2	0.7	0.4	0.4	3.6	3.0	1.2	1.2
Pneumonia	4.7	4.8	4.5	5.4	20.9	20.5	18.3	20.0
Asthma	2.1	2.3	2.2	2.8	7.5	7.2	5.8	7.8
Injuries and poisoning	6.1	3.9	3.4	3.4	23.0	15.1	12.4	12.1
Fracture, all sites	1.9	1.3	1.2	0.9	8.9	6.0	4.6	4.0
15–44 years[3]	173.5	144.7	132.1	129.0	744.8	575.4	466.7	421.8
Delivery	67.9	68.5	65.7	63.3	222.6	191.0	157.3	135.0
Psychoses	3.2	3.8	5.4	5.3	50.7	56.3	56.9	51.5
Diseases of heart	1.5	1.3	1.4	1.9	8.8	6.8	6.5	9.1
Intervertebral disc disorders	1.8	1.4	1.3	1.1	13.5	6.8	4.8	2.9
Injuries and poisoning	9.2	6.9	6.0	5.8	48.0	36.5	26.4	24.8
Fracture, all sites	1.9	1.6	1.4	1.4	13.8	10.8	8.6	5.9
45–64 years[3]	164.6	130.2	121.3	115.4	1,176.5	881.9	715.0	630.9
Malignant neoplasms	15.4	12.6	9.4	9.6	128.8	106.8	63.1	60.5
Malignant neoplasms of trachea, bronchus, lung	2.4	1.7	1.3	1.5	22.3	14.7	8.2	8.0
Malignant neoplasms of breast	3.9	2.8	2.2	2.1	25.2	12.0	10.0	7.5
Diabetes	3.8	2.9	3.3	3.2	31.6	25.7	20.2	19.3
Diseases of heart	18.0	16.5	17.4	14.9	121.4	100.5	96.8	70.5
Ischemic heart disease	10.6	9.9	10.1	8.3	71.1	57.1	48.8	37.8
Acute myocardial infarction	3.0	2.8	3.0	2.5	33.5	21.5	18.8	15.0
Congestive heart failure	1.8	2.1	2.8	2.5	12.7	15.8	22.3	14.4
Cerebrovascular diseases	3.7	3.0	3.0	3.2	44.9	31.9	23.5	21.3
Pneumonia	3.3	3.3	3.6	3.3	29.2	26.4	26.4	21.8
Injuries and poisoning	12.2	9.4	9.0	8.4	82.4	62.9	54.1	45.1
Fracture, all sites	4.1	3.1	2.8	2.7	30.0	24.8	16.6	14.0
65–74 years[3]	275.5	238.2	246.2	244.0	2,294.9	1,935.3	1,735.1	1,597.0
Malignant neoplasms	29.1	20.6	19.2	20.1	274.8	187.5	153.7	146.9
Malignant neoplasms of large intestine and rectum	3.2	2.4	2.1	2.2	41.8	34.5	24.8	19.7
Malignant neoplasms of trachea, bronchus, lung	3.6	2.6	3.3	2.8	34.9	26.6	27.2	25.0
Malignant neoplasms of breast	5.1	3.9	3.3	3.2	44.6	17.4	10.0	9.9
Diabetes	6.8	5.8	5.5	4.7	65.5	46.3	54.1	35.8
Diseases of heart	49.4	44.6	50.8	47.8	375.1	313.1	311.0	273.6
Ischemic heart disease	27.5	24.1	25.2	24.0	205.1	151.9	152.1	133.8
Acute myocardial infarction	8.6	7.4	8.1	7.9	88.7	57.3	62.9	57.9
Congestive heart failure	8.2	9.1	10.6	10.2	67.9	80.8	78.3	66.8
Cerebrovascular diseases	15.0	11.2	12.1	10.4	155.1	94.8	87.3	71.1
Pneumonia	7.0	8.6	9.8	10.5	65.2	80.8	76.3	79.2
Osteoarthritis	4.3	6.8	8.3	8.5	45.2	68.1	56.7	48.4
Injuries and poisoning	19.7	17.6	18.0	17.9	178.8	164.2	130.3	112.5
Fracture, all sites	9.3	8.3	8.4	7.0	97.7	96.2	66.4	43.4
Fracture of neck of femur (hip)	3.5	3.5	3.3	2.8	48.0	58.8	28.1	21.2

See footnotes at end of table.

Table 90 (page 3 of 3). Rates of discharges and days of care in non-Federal short-stay hospitals, according to sex, age, and selected first-listed diagnosis: United States, 1985, 1990, 1994, and 1995

[Data are based on a sample of hospital records]

	Discharges				Days of care			
Sex, age, and first-listed diagnosis	1985[1]	1990	1994	1995	1985[1]	1990	1994	1995
Female—Con.	Number per 1,000 population							
75 years and over[3]	446.8	404.6	432.4	445.1	4,219.1	3,838.9	3,380.7	3,203.8
Malignant neoplasms	26.1	21.8	20.8	20.3	282.9	254.1	194.3	173.3
Malignant neoplasms of large intestine and rectum	5.3	4.6	4.0	3.6	69.3	68.9	51.0	48.0
Malignant neoplasms of trachea, bronchus, lung . .	1.8	2.1	2.6	1.8	24.9	20.3	27.5	16.0
Malignant neoplasms of breast	4.1	3.8	2.9	3.0	37.0	21.7	11.6	8.9
Diabetes	6.6	4.6	6.0	6.2	69.7	54.6	46.9	43.5
Diseases of heart	91.6	83.5	94.9	95.1	773.1	664.4	661.6	594.6
Ischemic heart disease	40.9	33.3	36.4	36.8	341.4	250.0	240.2	218.4
Acute myocardial infarction	17.0	12.9	14.9	15.0	170.3	124.3	130.3	114.7
Congestive heart failure	24.5	27.6	31.3	31.9	208.3	233.7	243.2	221.5
Cerebrovascular diseases	33.7	29.2	27.9	30.0	368.1	298.3	218.5	205.2
Pneumonia	18.4	23.6	25.6	27.7	184.8	256.9	225.7	224.8
Osteoarthritis	4.8	5.2	7.9	8.7	64.4	53.4	56.7	57.9
Injuries and poisoning	47.8	45.8	45.6	47.7	541.4	483.2	359.5	368.7
Fracture, all sites	31.9	31.1	30.7	31.2	402.9	348.4	263.7	248.7
Fracture of neck of femur (hip)	18.9	18.6	18.8	19.3	270.8	233.4	180.2	169.5

[1]Comparisons of data from 1985 with data from later years should be made with caution as estimates of change may reflect improvements in the design (see Appendix I) rather than true changes in hospital use.
[2]Age adjusted.
[3]Includes discharges with first-listed diagnoses not shown in table.

NOTES: Excludes newborn infants. Rates are based on the civilian population as of July 1. Diagnostic categories are based on the *International Classification of Diseases, 9th Revision, Clinical Modification*. For a listing of the code numbers, see Appendix II, table VII.

SOURCE: Centers for Disease Control and Prevention, National Center for Health Statistics, Division of Health Care Statistics. Data from the National Hospital Discharge Survey.

Table 91 (page 1 of 3). Discharges and average length of stay in non-Federal short-stay hospitals, according to sex, age, and selected first-listed diagnosis: United States, 1985, 1990, 1994, and 1995

[Data are based on a sample of hospital records]

Sex, age, and first-listed diagnosis	Discharges				Average length of stay			
	1985[1]	1990	1994	1995	1985[1]	1990	1994	1995
Both sexes	Number in thousands				Number of days			
Total[2,3]	35,056	30,788	30,843	30,722	6.3	6.2	5.6	5.2
Male								
All ages[2,3]	14,160	12,280	12,293	12,198	6.8	6.8	6.2	5.8
Under 15 years[3]	1,698	1,362	1,272	1,377	4.5	4.8	4.9	4.6
Bronchitis	45	22	16	21	3.2	3.1	2.8	3.0
Pneumonia	150	174	195	231	4.2	4.2	3.9	3.6
Asthma	93	107	107	134	3.4	2.8	2.5	2.7
Injuries and poisoning	245	164	150	144	4.0	4.4	3.9	4.4
Fracture, all sites	85	54	50	47	5.2	4.0	3.7	4.8
15–44 years[3]	4,153	3,330	3,146	2,949	6.1	6.1	5.8	5.4
Psychoses	167	200	325	287	14.4	14.5	11.5	10.1
Diseases of heart	165	166	170	159	5.5	5.3	4.2	4.2
Intervertebral disc disorders	161	138	103	95	6.4	4.2	4.1	2.5
Injuries and poisoning	988	772	584	581	5.5	5.0	4.7	4.8
Fracture, all sites	290	238	191	195	6.6	5.5	5.6	5.4
45–64 years[3]	3,776	3,115	3,120	3,053	6.9	6.7	5.8	5.6
Malignant neoplasms	279	235	199	191	9.2	9.4	8.2	7.0
Malignant neoplasms of trachea, bronchus, lung	76	60	39	37	8.9	7.1	7.6	6.9
Diabetes	71	65	65	86	7.9	7.3	6.6	6.5
Diseases of heart	784	704	721	749	6.5	5.8	5.0	4.8
Ischemic heart disease	577	502	509	537	6.3	5.7	4.9	4.6
Acute myocardial infarction	197	165	180	188	8.9	7.5	5.8	5.7
Congestive heart failure	53	66	78	73	7.6	6.7	6.0	5.6
Cerebrovascular diseases	107	91	100	96	10.2	10.0	6.2	6.8
Pneumonia	73	77	109	75	8.0	7.9	7.2	6.9
Injuries and poisoning	320	257	268	257	6.6	7.2	5.8	5.5
Fracture, all sites	85	74	77	74	7.5	7.2	6.7	6.3
65–74 years[3]	2,389	2,268	2,328	2,290	8.1	7.8	6.7	6.4
Malignant neoplasms	284	220	235	203	9.1	9.9	8.2	7.8
Malignant neoplasms of large intestine and rectum	29	24	26	22	14.0	11.4	10.6	10.7
Malignant neoplasms of trachea, bronchus, lung	79	50	45	44	8.3	8.7	8.7	7.6
Malignant neoplasms of prostate	49	40	52	41	7.3	6.5	5.6	5.3
Diabetes	31	34	38	44	9.9	9.1	7.3	8.8
Diseases of heart	513	547	612	618	7.4	7.0	6.0	5.6
Ischemic heart disease	317	331	357	365	7.3	6.8	5.9	5.6
Acute myocardial infarction	129	110	124	129	9.1	8.8	7.6	6.6
Congestive heart failure	72	90	113	123	7.8	7.9	6.8	5.9
Cerebrovascular diseases	136	108	130	141	9.8	8.3	6.9	6.6
Pneumonia	80	90	100	105	9.6	9.5	7.3	6.9
Hyperplasia of prostate	99	113	67	62	6.3	4.5	3.8	3.0
Osteoarthritis	25	39	45	49	10.9	9.0	6.7	5.7
Injuries and poisoning	118	139	148	133	8.2	7.9	6.9	6.7
Fracture, all sites	33	36	40	36	9.5	10.2	7.7	7.4
Fracture of neck of femur (hip)	10	12	15	15	15.2	11.8	9.5	8.1
75 years and over[3]	2,144	2,203	2,428	2,528	8.8	8.8	7.6	6.9
Malignant neoplasms	226	189	153	161	9.8	10.0	8.6	8.3
Malignant neoplasms of large intestine and rectum	28	25	22	26	12.3	15.0	10.4	10.8
Malignant neoplasms of trachea, bronchus, lung	42	25	22	19	9.5	10.0	9.3	8.9
Malignant neoplasms of prostate	62	45	26	23	7.6	6.8	5.6	4.1
Diabetes	26	21	37	37	10.5	11.0	7.2	6.1
Diseases of heart	440	489	587	606	7.7	8.1	6.5	5.9
Ischemic heart disease	208	226	254	276	8.1	8.1	6.4	6.2
Acute myocardial infarction	97	106	107	119	9.7	9.9	7.6	7.6
Congestive heart failure	113	143	183	167	7.9	7.8	6.6	6.2
Cerebrovascular diseases	154	139	163	171	10.0	9.9	7.0	6.7
Pneumonia	122	178	197	215	10.2	10.2	8.1	8.0
Hyperplasia of prostate	80	82	53	50	7.2	6.1	4.4	3.5
Osteoarthritis	18	27	35	35	11.3	10.5	6.9	8.3
Injuries and poisoning	129	144	158	174	11.3	10.9	8.1	6.8
Fracture, all sites	58	63	68	86	15.6	10.6	9.4	7.1
Fracture of neck of femur (hip)	34	39	46	48	19.2	11.5	10.5	7.7

See footnotes at end of table.

Table 91 (page 2 of 3). Discharges and average length of stay in non-Federal short-stay hospitals, according to sex, age, and selected first-listed diagnosis: United States, 1985, 1990, 1994, and 1995

[Data are based on a sample of hospital records]

Sex, age, and first-listed diagnosis	Discharges				Average length of stay			
	1985[1]	1990	1994	1995	1985[1]	1990	1994	1995
Female	Number in thousands				Number of days			
All ages[2,3]	20,896	18,508	18,550	18,525	5.9	5.8	5.1	4.7
Under 15 years[3]	1,274	1,049	978	1,028	4.6	4.9	4.7	4.3
Bronchitis	30	19	10	13	3.0	4.0	3.4	2.7
Pneumonia	119	125	127	152	4.4	4.3	4.0	3.7
Asthma	52	62	63	78	3.6	3.1	2.6	2.8
Injuries and poisoning	153	102	95	97	3.8	3.9	3.6	3.5
Fracture, all sites	47	33	33	27	4.8	4.8	3.8	4.2
15–44 years[3]	9,813	8,469	7,810	7,644	4.3	4.0	3.5	3.3
Delivery	3,838	4,008	3,885	3,752	3.3	2.8	2.4	2.1
Psychoses	180	222	318	316	15.9	14.9	10.6	9.7
Diseases of heart	85	73	83	110	5.8	5.4	4.6	4.9
Intervertebral disc disorders	104	85	79	63	7.4	4.7	3.6	2.7
Injuries and poisoning	521	402	356	344	5.2	5.3	4.4	4.3
Fracture, all sites	108	93	83	84	7.2	6.8	6.1	4.2
45–64 years[3]	3,834	3,129	3,191	3,115	7.1	6.8	5.9	5.5
Malignant neoplasms	359	303	246	258	8.4	8.5	6.7	6.3
Malignant neoplasms of trachea, bronchus, lung	56	41	33	39	9.3	8.6	6.4	5.5
Malignant neoplasms of breast	91	67	58	56	6.5	4.3	4.6	3.6
Diabetes	88	70	87	86	8.3	8.9	6.1	6.0
Diseases of heart	420	397	458	403	6.7	6.1	5.6	4.7
Ischemic heart disease	248	237	267	225	6.7	5.8	4.8	4.5
Acute myocardial infarction	71	68	79	68	11.0	7.6	6.3	6.0
Congestive heart failure	43	51	74	68	6.9	7.4	8.0	5.7
Cerebrovascular diseases	85	72	79	86	12.2	10.7	7.8	6.7
Pneumonia	76	80	96	88	8.9	7.9	7.3	6.7
Injuries and poisoning	283	225	236	225	6.8	6.7	6.0	5.4
Fracture, all sites	96	75	73	72	7.3	7.9	6.0	5.2
65–74 years[3]	2,623	2,421	2,566	2,542	8.3	8.1	7.0	6.5
Malignant neoplasms	277	210	201	209	9.4	9.1	8.0	7.3
Malignant neoplasms of large intestine and rectum	31	24	22	23	13.0	14.5	11.7	8.8
Malignant neoplasms of trachea, bronchus, lung	35	26	34	29	9.6	10.2	8.2	8.9
Malignant neoplasms of breast	49	40	34	33	8.7	4.5	3.1	3.1
Diabetes	64	59	58	49	9.7	8.0	9.8	7.7
Diseases of heart	470	453	529	497	7.6	7.0	6.1	5.7
Ischemic heart disease	262	245	263	250	7.5	6.3	6.0	5.6
Acute myocardial infarction	82	75	84	82	10.3	7.8	7.8	7.4
Congestive heart failure	78	92	110	106	8.3	8.9	7.4	6.5
Cerebrovascular diseases	143	114	126	109	10.3	8.5	7.2	6.8
Pneumonia	66	87	102	109	9.4	9.4	7.8	7.6
Osteoarthritis	40	69	86	89	10.6	10.0	6.8	5.7
Injuries and poisoning	188	179	187	187	9.1	9.3	7.2	6.3
Fracture, all sites	88	85	88	72	10.6	11.5	7.9	6.2
Fracture of neck of femur (hip)	33	36	35	29	13.9	16.7	8.4	7.5

See footnotes at end of table.

Table 91 (page 3 of 3). Discharges and average length of stay in non-Federal short-stay hospitals, according to sex, age, and selected first-listed diagnosis: United States, 1985, 1990, 1994, and 1995

[Data are based on a sample of hospital records]

Sex, age, and first-listed diagnosis	Discharges				Average length of stay			
	1985[1]	1990	1994	1995	1985[1]	1990	1994	1995
Female—Con.	Number in thousands				Number of days			
75 years and over[3]	3,352	3,440	4,005	4,196	9.4	9.5	7.8	7.2
Malignant neoplasms	196	185	192	191	10.8	11.7	9.4	8.5
Malignant neoplasms of large intestine and rectum	40	39	37	34	13.1	15.1	12.7	13.3
Malignant neoplasms of trachea, bronchus, lung . .	13	18	24	17	13.9	9.9	10.4	8.7
Malignant neoplasms of breast	31	33	27	29	9.1	5.7	4.0	2.9
Diabetes	49	39	55	58	10.6	11.9	7.9	7.1
Diseases of heart	688	711	879	896	8.4	8.0	7.0	6.3
Ischemic heart disease	307	283	337	347	8.3	7.5	6.6	5.9
Acute myocardial infarction	127	110	138	142	10.0	9.6	8.7	7.6
Congestive heart failure	184	235	290	301	8.5	8.5	7.8	6.9
Cerebrovascular diseases	253	249	258	283	10.9	10.2	7.8	6.8
Pneumonia	138	201	237	261	10.1	10.9	8.8	8.1
Osteoarthritis	36	45	73	82	13.5	10.2	7.1	6.6
Injuries and poisoning	358	389	422	449	11.3	10.6	7.9	7.7
Fracture, all sites	240	265	284	294	12.6	11.2	8.6	8.0
Fracture of neck of femur (hip)	142	158	175	182	14.3	12.5	9.6	8.8

[1]Comparisons of data from 1985 with data from later years should be made with caution as estimates of change may reflect improvements in the design (see Appendix I) rather than true changes in hospital use.
[2]Average length of stay is age-adjusted.
[3]Includes discharges with first-listed diagnoses not shown in table.

NOTES: Excludes newborn infants. Diagnostic categories are based on the *International Classification of Diseases, 9th Revision, Clinical Modification*. For a listing of the code numbers, see Appendix II, table VII.

SOURCE: Centers for Disease Control and Prevention, National Center for Health Statistics, Division of Health Care Statistics. Data from the National Hospital Discharge Survey.

Table 92 (page 1 of 3). Operations for inpatients discharged from non-Federal short-stay hospitals, according to sex, age, and surgical category: United States, 1985, 1990, 1994, and 1995

[Data are based on a sample of hospital records]

Sex, age, and surgical category	Operations in thousands				Operations per 1,000 population			
	1985[1]	1990	1994	1995	1985[1]	1990	1994	1995
Both sexes								
Total[2,3]	24,109	23,051	22,629	22,530	102.1	93.0	87.4	86.2
Male								
All ages[2,3]	8,737	8,538	8,369	8,388	76.5	71.1	66.5	66.0
Under 15 years[3]	827	598	507	518	31.4	21.6	17.3	17.5
Myringotomy.	53	30	16	15	2.0	1.1	0.5	0.5
Tonsillectomy, with or without adenoidectomy	97	33	14	15	3.7	1.2	0.5	0.5
Appendectomy[4]	41	40	38	31	1.6	1.4	1.3	1.0
Reduction of fracture (excluding skull and facial)	52	37	37	29	2.0	1.3	1.2	1.0
15–44 years[3]	2,705	2,257	1,980	1,899	49.1	39.1	33.9	32.4
Coronary angioplasty	10	17	26	23	0.2	0.3	0.4	0.4
Cardiac catheterization	58	68	62	62	1.0	1.2	1.1	1.1
Appendectomy[4]	88	80	90	80	1.6	1.4	1.5	1.4
Cholecystectomy	33	34	27	27	0.6	0.6	0.5	0.5
Reduction of fracture (excluding skull and facial)	160	137	119	121	2.9	2.4	2.0	2.1
Excision or destruction of intervertebral disc and spinal fusion.	119	147	131	130	2.2	2.5	2.2	2.2
Excision of semilunar cartilage of knee	48	25	21	19	0.9	0.4	0.4	0.3
45–64 years[3]	2,482	2,499	2,516	2,541	116.7	112.5	102.5	100.9
Coronary angioplasty	34	111	138	141	1.6	5.0	5.6	5.6
Direct heart revascularization (coronary bypass)[5].	102	132	165	192	4.8	6.0	6.7	7.6
Cardiac catheterization	241	306	286	294	11.4	13.8	11.7	11.7
Cholecystectomy	53	50	51	46	2.5	2.2	2.1	1.8
Prostatectomy	81	80	61	55	3.8	3.6	2.5	2.2
Reduction of fracture (excluding skull and facial)	47	41	51	53	2.2	1.9	2.1	2.1
Excision or destruction of intervertebral disc and spinal fusion.	60	80	94	87	2.8	3.6	3.8	3.4
65–74 years[3]	1,546	1,849	1,889	1,900	210.7	233.1	227.8	227.8
Coronary angioplasty	11	58	82	78	1.5	7.3	9.9	9.3
Direct heart revascularization (coronary bypass)[5].	45	100	127	151	6.1	12.6	15.3	18.1
Cardiac catheterization	102	170	184	196	13.9	21.4	22.2	23.4
Pacemaker insertion or replacement.	37	38	46	39	5.0	4.8	5.6	4.7
Carotid endarterectomy.	26	14	27	35	3.5	1.8	3.2	4.2
Cholecystectomy	34	33	37	37	4.6	4.2	4.4	4.4
Prostatectomy	150	159	117	102	20.4	20.0	14.1	12.3
Reduction of fracture (excluding skull and facial)	16	20	22	20	2.1	2.6	2.6	2.4
Arthroplasty and replacement of hip	20	24	20	29	2.7	3.0	2.4	3.4
75 years and over[3]	1,177	1,335	1,477	1,531	290.4	288.5	284.9	286.3
Coronary angioplasty	*	15	33	44	*	3.2	6.4	8.1
Direct heart revascularization (coronary bypass)[5].	12	37	55	67	3.0	8.1	10.7	12.5
Cardiac catheterization	24	66	93	102	5.9	14.3	18.0	19.1
Pacemaker insertion or replacement.	45	62	79	82	11.1	13.4	15.3	15.3
Carotid endarterectomy.	15	11	18	24	3.6	2.3	3.6	4.6
Cholecystectomy	27	30	32	30	6.6	6.5	6.2	5.5
Prostatectomy	134	125	83	81	33.2	27.0	16.1	15.2
Reduction of fracture (excluding skull and facial)	26	29	33	33	6.3	6.3	6.3	6.1
Arthroplasty and replacement of hip	20	27	26	33	4.9	5.8	5.1	6.2

See footnotes at end of table.

Table 92 (page 2 of 3). **Operations for inpatients discharged from non-Federal short-stay hospitals, according to sex, age, and surgical category: United States, 1985, 1990, 1994, and 1995**

[Data are based on a sample of hospital records]

Sex, age, and surgical category	Operations in thousands				Operations per 1,000 population			
	1985[1]	1990	1994	1995	1985[1]	1990	1994	1995
Female								
All ages[2,3]	15,372	14,513	14,260	14,142	126.0	113.7	107.1	105.3
Under 15 years[3]	548	413	366	362	21.8	15.6	13.1	12.9
Myringotomy	36	22	13	10	1.4	0.8	0.5	0.3
Tonsillectomy, with or without adenoidectomy	100	41	15	12	4.0	1.6	0.5	0.4
Appendectomy[4]	28	26	25	22	1.1	1.0	0.9	0.8
Reduction of fracture (excluding skull and facial)	32	18	18	17	1.3	0.7	0.7	0.6
15–44 years[3]	8,777	8,129	7,430	7,235	155.2	138.9	125.7	122.0
Cardiac catheterization	22	32	27	26	0.4	0.5	0.4	0.4
Appendectomy[4]	86	77	74	59	1.5	1.3	1.2	1.0
Cholecystectomy	134	172	124	134	2.4	2.9	2.1	2.3
Bilateral destruction or occlusion of fallopian tubes	461	418	360	326	8.1	7.1	6.1	5.5
Hysterectomy	421	349	298	325	7.4	6.0	5.0	5.5
Procedures to assist delivery	2,221	2,480	2,400	2,282	39.3	42.4	40.6	38.5
Cesarean section[6]	875	940	856	784	15.5	16.1	14.5	13.2
Repair of current obstetrical laceration	546	793	907	961	9.7	13.5	15.3	16.2
Reduction of fracture (excluding skull and facial)	71	60	59	63	1.3	1.0	1.0	1.1
Excision or destruction of intervertebral disc and spinal fusion	65	86	100	69	1.1	1.5	1.7	1.2
Excision of semilunar cartilage of knee	12	10	*9	8	0.2	0.2	*0.1	0.1
Mastectomy	17	13	14	13	0.3	0.2	0.2	0.2
45–64 years[3]	2,879	2,586	2,635	2,566	123.6	107.6	100.2	95.1
Coronary angioplasty	12	37	55	53	0.5	1.6	2.1	2.0
Direct heart revascularization (coronary bypass)[5]	24	37	52	45	1.0	1.5	2.0	1.7
Cardiac catheterization	108	151	158	144	4.7	6.3	6.0	5.3
Cholecystectomy	104	118	97	95	4.4	4.9	3.7	3.5
Hysterectomy	190	184	188	191	8.2	7.7	7.1	7.1
Reduction of fracture (excluding skull and facial)	66	53	56	60	2.8	2.2	2.1	2.2
Excision or destruction of intervertebral disc and spinal fusion	48	67	84	69	2.1	2.8	3.2	2.6
Mastectomy	49	52	42	41	2.1	2.1	1.6	1.5
65–74 years[3]	1,631	1,679	1,814	1,832	171.3	165.2	174.0	175.9
Coronary angioplasty	*9	31	51	48	*0.9	3.1	4.8	4.6
Direct heart revascularization (coronary bypass)[5]	23	40	52	63	2.4	3.9	5.0	6.1
Cardiac catheterization	76	126	130	127	8.0	12.4	12.5	12.2
Pacemaker insertion or replacement	27	32	44	40	2.8	3.1	4.2	3.8
Carotid endarterectomy	20	13	17	23	2.1	1.2	1.7	2.3
Cholecystectomy	49	48	53	47	5.2	4.7	5.1	4.5
Hysterectomy	43	38	48	45	4.5	3.7	4.6	4.3
Reduction of fracture (excluding skull and facial)	49	46	47	43	5.1	4.5	4.5	4.2
Arthroplasty and replacement of hip	36	42	47	43	3.7	4.1	4.5	4.2
Mastectomy	28	31	29	23	3.0	3.0	2.7	2.3

See footnotes at end of table.

Table 92 (page 3 of 3). Operations for inpatients discharged from non-Federal short-stay hospitals, according to sex, age, and surgical category: United States, 1985, 1990, 1994, and 1995

[Data are based on a sample of hospital records]

Sex, age, and surgical category	Operations in thousands				Operations per 1,000 population			
	1985[1]	1990	1994	1995	1985[1]	1990	1994	1995
Female—Con.								
75 years and over[3]	1,537	1,706	2,015	2,147	204.9	200.6	217.6	227.7
Coronary angioplasty	*	12	36	40	*	1.4	3.9	4.2
Direct heart revascularization (coronary bypass)[5]	*8	27	31	38	*1.1	3.1	3.3	4.1
Cardiac catheterization	26	59	95	105	3.4	6.9	10.3	11.1
Pacemaker insertion or replacement	59	67	105	94	7.9	7.9	11.4	10.0
Carotid endarterectomy	13	11	18	19	1.7	1.3	2.0	2.0
Cholecystectomy	40	36	39	52	5.3	4.2	4.2	5.5
Reduction of fracture (excluding skull and facial)	112	122	127	138	15.0	14.4	13.7	14.6
Arthroplasty and replacement of hip	73	86	93	94	9.7	10.1	10.1	9.9
Mastectomy	20	25	22	24	2.6	2.9	2.4	2.5

* Statistics based on fewer than 5,000 estimated discharges are not shown; those based on 5,000–9,000 estimated discharges are to be used with caution.

[1]Comparisons of data from 1985 with data from later years should be made with caution as estimates of change may reflect improvements in the design (see Appendix I) rather than true changes in hospital use.

[2]Rates are age adjusted.

[3]Includes operations not listed in table.

[4]Excludes appendectomies performed incidental to other abdominal surgery.

[5]Data are for all-listed direct heart revascularization (coronary bypass). Often, more than one coronary bypass procedure is performed during a single operation and for the purpose of this table would be counted more than once. The following table gives information based on the number of discharges with one or more coronary bypass procedures.

Sex and age	1985	1990	1994	1995
	Discharges per 1,000 population			
Males:				
45–64 years	4.1	3.8	4.1	4.5
65–74 years	5.5	8.3	9.3	11.2
75 years and over	2.6	6.4	7.6	8.9
Females:				
45–64 years	0.9	1.0	1.3	1.0
65–74 years	2.1	2.7	3.3	3.8
75 years and over	*	2.3	2.3	3.0

[6]Cesarean sections accounted for 16.5 percent of all deliveries in 1980, 22.7 percent in 1985, 23.5 percent in 1990, 22.0 percent in 1994, and 20.8 percent in 1995.

NOTES: Data in this table are for all inpatient operations (up to a maximum of four) listed on the face sheet of the medical record. Data in this table do not include operations for outpatients. Data from the 1994 National Survey of Ambulatory Surgery (NSAS), a national survey of hospital and freestanding ambulatory surgery centers, show that about one-half of all surgical operations occur on an outpatient basis. Surgical categories presented in this table that frequently occurred in the NSAS data as outpatient operations include reduction of fracture, tonsillectomy, myringotomy, cholecystectomy, excision of semilunar cartilage of the knee, cardiac catheterization, and bilateral destruction or occlusion of fallopian tubes. For further information see: Kozak LJ, Owings MF. Ambulatory and inpatient procedures in the United States, 1995. Series 13 no 135. Hyattsville, Maryland: National Center for Health Statistics, 1998. Excludes newborn infants. Rates are based on the civilian population as of July 1. Surgical categories are based on the *International Classification of Diseases, 9th Revision, Clinical Modification*. For a listing of the code numbers, see Appendix II, table VIII.

SOURCE: Centers for Disease Control and Prevention, National Center for Health Statistics, Division of Health Care Statistics. Data from the National Hospital Discharge Survey.

Table 93 (page 1 of 2). Diagnostic and other nonsurgical procedures for inpatients discharged from non-Federal short-stay hospitals, according to sex, age, and procedure category: United States, 1985, 1990, 1994, and 1995

[Data are based on a sample of hospital records]

Sex, age, and procedure category	Procedures in thousands				Procedures per 1,000 population			
	1985[1]	1990	1994	1995	1985[1]	1990	1994	1995
Both sexes								
Total[2,3]	12,650	17,455	18,081	17,278	53.6	70.5	69.8	66.1
Male								
All ages[2,3]	5,957	7,378	7,501	7,261	52.2	61.4	59.6	57.1
Under 15 years[3]	301	546	567	645	11.4	19.7	19.3	21.8
Spinal tap	62	94	72	86	2.4	3.4	2.5	2.9
Computerized axial tomography (CAT scan)	35	41	31	30	1.3	1.5	1.1	1.0
Diagnostic ultrasound	23	47	23	25	0.9	1.7	0.8	0.9
15–44 years[3]	1,306	1,584	1,649	1,538	23.7	27.5	28.2	26.2
Spinal tap	40	52	40	46	0.7	0.9	0.7	0.8
Endoscopy of large or small intestine without biopsy	114	77	62	55	2.1	1.3	1.1	0.9
Computerized axial tomography (CAT scan)	174	215	141	124	3.2	3.7	2.4	2.1
Angiocardiography using contrast material	55	102	96	98	1.0	1.8	1.6	1.7
Diagnostic ultrasound	96	118	104	76	1.7	2.0	1.8	1.3
Magnetic resonance imaging (MRI)	- - -	29	25	27	- - -	0.5	0.4	0.5
Radioisotope scan	67	47	27	23	1.2	0.8	0.5	0.4
45–64 years[3]	1,879	2,106	2,121	2,011	88.4	94.8	86.4	79.8
Endoscopy of large or small intestine without biopsy	153	116	114	95	7.2	5.2	4.6	3.8
Cystoscopy	114	80	37	29	5.4	3.6	1.5	1.1
Computerized axial tomography (CAT scan)	182	170	127	117	8.6	7.6	5.2	4.6
Arteriography using contrast material	94	65	56	57	4.4	2.9	2.3	2.3
Angiocardiography using contrast material	251	428	392	397	11.8	19.2	16.0	15.8
Diagnostic ultrasound	146	184	156	135	6.9	8.3	6.4	5.4
Magnetic resonance imaging (MRI)	- - -	24	38	32	- - -	1.1	1.5	1.3
Radioisotope scan	121	81	52	39	5.7	3.6	2.1	1.6
65–74 years[3]	1,360	1,646	1,625	1,578	185.3	207.5	196.0	189.2
Endoscopy of large or small intestine without biopsy	120	85	94	77	16.3	10.8	11.4	9.3
Cystoscopy	148	115	46	42	20.2	14.5	5.6	5.0
Computerized axial tomography (CAT scan)	145	144	90	91	19.7	18.1	10.9	11.0
Arteriography using contrast material	79	66	61	63	10.8	8.3	7.3	7.5
Angiocardiography using contrast material	101	225	255	253	13.8	28.4	30.8	30.3
Diagnostic ultrasound	114	151	123	129	15.5	19.1	14.8	15.4
Magnetic resonance imaging (MRI)	- - -	16	24	18	- - -	2.0	2.9	2.2
Radioisotope scan	97	68	39	38	13.3	8.6	4.7	4.6
75 years and over[3]	1,111	1,497	1,539	1,490	274.2	323.5	296.8	278.6
Endoscopy of large or small intestine without biopsy	108	122	113	122	26.6	26.3	21.8	22.8
Cystoscopy	140	117	56	50	34.6	25.2	10.7	9.3
Computerized axial tomography (CAT scan)	135	165	111	110	33.3	35.7	21.3	20.6
Arteriography using contrast material	56	43	38	48	13.7	9.2	7.4	8.9
Angiocardiography using contrast material	22	72	125	128	5.4	15.6	24.1	23.9
Diagnostic ultrasound	99	168	132	134	24.4	36.3	25.5	25.1
Magnetic resonance imaging (MRI)	- - -	19	15	17	- - -	4.2	3.0	3.2
Radioisotope scan	80	61	32	35	19.6	13.2	6.1	6.6

See footnotes at end of table.

Table 93 (page 2 of 2). Diagnostic and other nonsurgical procedures for inpatients discharged from non-Federal short-stay hospitals, according to sex, age, and procedure category: United States, 1985, 1990, 1994, and 1993

[Data are based on a sample of hospital records]

Sex, age, and procedure category	Procedures in thousands				Procedures per 1,000 population			
	1985[1]	1990	1994	1995	1985[1]	1990	1994	1995
Female								
All ages[2,3]	6,694	10,077	10,580	10,016	54.9	79.0	79.5	74.6
Under 15 years[3]	262	403	444	498	10.4	15.3	15.9	17.7
Spinal tap	50	71	64	71	2.0	2.7	2.3	2.5
Computerized axial tomography (CAT scan)	33	27	20	22	1.3	1.0	0.7	0.8
Diagnostic ultrasound	25	43	26	26	1.0	1.6	0.9	0.9
15–44 years[3]	2,169	4,217	4,316	3,980	38.3	72.1	73.0	67.1
Spinal tap	40	48	45	39	0.7	0.8	0.8	0.7
Endoscopy of large or small intestine without biopsy	125	87	60	51	2.2	1.5	1.0	0.9
Computerized axial tomography (CAT scan)	137	144	90	96	2.4	2.5	1.5	1.6
Angiocardiography using contrast material	21	45	38	39	0.4	0.8	0.6	0.7
Diagnostic ultrasound	283	309	219	182	5.0	5.3	3.7	3.1
Magnetic resonance imaging (MRI)	- - -	30	25	31	- - -	0.5	0.4	0.5
Radioisotope scan	83	58	31	22	1.5	1.0	0.5	0.4
45–64 years[3]	1,598	1,861	1,902	1,798	68.6	77.4	72.3	66.6
Endoscopy of large or small intestine without biopsy	167	130	101	94	7.2	5.4	3.9	3.5
Cystoscopy	48	37	26	17	2.1	1.5	1.0	0.6
Computerized axial tomography (CAT scan)	167	163	120	106	7.2	6.8	4.6	3.9
Arteriography using contrast material	64	59	41	53	2.7	2.5	1.6	2.0
Angiocardiography using contrast material	105	214	223	218	4.5	8.9	8.5	8.1
Diagnostic ultrasound	154	174	150	134	6.6	7.2	5.7	5.0
Magnetic resonance imaging (MRI)	- - -	28	34	29	- - -	1.1	1.3	1.1
Radioisotope scan	128	79	54	44	5.5	3.3	2.0	1.6
65–74 years[3]	1,252	1,603	1,568	1,525	131.5	157.7	150.4	146.3
Endoscopy of large or small intestine without biopsy	131	123	92	98	13.8	12.1	8.8	9.4
Cystoscopy	32	24	18	11	3.4	2.3	1.8	1.0
Computerized axial tomography (CAT scan)	156	165	103	94	16.4	16.3	9.9	9.0
Arteriography using contrast material	67	52	53	59	7.1	5.1	5.1	5.7
Angiocardiography using contrast material	73	171	186	180	7.6	16.8	17.8	17.3
Diagnostic ultrasound	121	167	147	124	12.7	16.5	14.1	11.9
Magnetic resonance imaging (MRI)	- - -	23	24	30	- - -	2.2	2.3	2.9
Radioisotope scan	116	85	47	37	12.2	8.4	4.5	3.6
75 years and over[3]	1,413	1,993	2,351	2,216	188.3	234.4	253.8	235.1
Endoscopy of large or small intestine without biopsy	183	201	207	182	24.4	23.7	22.4	19.4
Cystoscopy	45	32	23	23	6.0	3.8	2.4	2.4
Computerized axial tomography (CAT scan)	215	270	194	177	28.6	31.8	21.0	18.8
Arteriography using contrast material	48	39	51	34	6.4	4.6	5.5	3.6
Angiocardiography using contrast material	17	74	133	145	2.3	8.7	14.4	15.4
Diagnostic ultrasound	173	248	228	216	23.0	29.1	24.6	22.9
Magnetic resonance imaging (MRI)	- - -	20	27	30	- - -	2.3	2.9	3.2
Radioisotope scan	128	104	65	59	17.0	12.3	7.0	6.2

- - - Data not available.

[1]Comparisons of data from 1985 with data from later years should be made with caution as estimates of change may reflect improvements in the design (see Appendix I) rather than true changes in hospital use.

[2]Rates are age adjusted.

[3]Includes procedures not listed in table.

NOTES: Data in this table are for all inpatient procedures (up to a maximum of four) listed on the face sheet of the medical record. Data in this table do not include diagnostic and nonsurgical procedures for outpatient surgery centers, hospital outpatient or emergency departments or physician offices. For further information on procedures performed in outpatient surgery centers see: Kozak LJ, Owings MF. Ambulatory and inpatient procedures in the United States, 1995. Series 13 no 135. Hyattsville, Maryland: National Center for Health Statistics, 1998. For further information on procedures performed in hospital outpatient departments see: McCaig LF. National Hospital Ambulatory Medical Care Survey: 1995 Outpatient Department Summary. Advance data from vital and health statistics; no 284. Hyattsville, Maryland: National Center for Health Statistics, 1997. For further information on procedures performed in hospital emergency departments see: Stussman BJ. National Hospital Ambulatory Medical Care Survey: 1995 Emergency Department Summary. Advance data from vital and health statistics; no 285. Hyattsville, Maryland: National Center for Health Statistics, 1997. For further information on procedures performed in physician offices see: Woodwell DA. National Ambulatory Medical Care Survey: 1995 Summary. Advance data from vital and health statistics; no 286. Hyattsville, Maryland: National Center for Health Statistics, 1997. Excludes newborn infants. Rates are based on the civilian population as of July 1. Procedure categories are based on the *International Classification of Diseases, 9th Revision, Clinical Modification*. For a listing of the code numbers, see Appendix II, table IX.

SOURCE: Centers for Disease Control and Prevention, National Center for Health Statistics, Division of Health Care Statistics. Data from the National Hospital Discharge Survey.

Table 94. Hospital admissions, average length of stay, and outpatient visits, according to type of ownership and size of hospital, and percent outpatient surgery: United States, selected years 1975–96

[Data are based on reporting by a census of hospitals]

Type of ownership and size of hospital	1975	1980	1985	1990	1993	1994	1995	1996
Admissions				Number in thousands				
All hospitals	36,157	38,892	36,304	33,774	33,201	33,125	33,282	33,307
Federal	1,913	2,044	2,103	1,759	1,626	1,588	1,559	1,422
Non-Federal[1]	34,243	36,848	34,201	32,015	31,575	31,538	31,723	31,885
Community[2]	33,435	36,143	33,449	31,181	30,748	30,718	30,945	31,099
Nonprofit.	23,722	25,566	24,179	22,878	22,749	22,704	22,557	22,542
Proprietary	2,646	3,165	3,242	3,066	2,946	3,035	3,428	3,684
State-local government. . .	7,067	7,413	6,028	5,236	5,054	4,979	4,961	4,873
6–24 beds.	174	159	102	95	88	98	124	117
25–49 beds	1,431	1,254	1,009	870	854	881	944	925
50–99 beds	3,675	3,700	2,953	2,474	2,227	2,212	2,299	2,280
100–199 beds	7,017	7,162	6,487	5,833	5,927	5,983	6,288	6,456
200–299 beds	6,174	6,596	6,371	6,333	6,270	6,501	6,495	6,426
300–399 beds	4,739	5,358	5,401	5,091	5,086	4,843	4,693	4,856
400–499 beds	3,689	4,401	3,723	3,644	3,391	3,505	3,413	3,481
500 beds or more	6,537	7,513	7,401	6,840	6,905	6,695	6,690	6,558
Average length of stay				Number of days				
All hospitals	11.4	9.9	9.1	9.1	8.6	8.2	7.8	7.5
Federal	20.3	16.8	14.8	14.9	15.0	14.4	13.1	13.4
Non-Federal[1]	10.9	9.6	8.8	8.8	8.3	7.9	7.5	7.2
Community[2]	7.7	7.6	7.1	7.2	7.0	6.7	6.5	6.2
Nonprofit.	7.8	7.7	7.2	7.3	6.9	6.6	6.4	6.1
Proprietary	6.6	6.5	6.1	6.4	6.2	6.1	5.8	5.6
State-local government. . .	7.6	7.3	7.2	7.7	7.8	7.6	7.4	7.2
6–24 beds.	5.6	5.3	5.0	5.4	5.4	5.2	5.5	4.9
25–49 beds	6.0	5.8	5.3	6.1	5.9	5.7	5.7	5.3
50–99 beds	6.8	6.7	6.5	7.2	7.4	7.3	7.0	6.9
100–199 beds	7.1	7.0	6.7	7.1	6.9	6.7	6.4	6.2
200–299 beds	7.5	7.4	6.8	6.9	6.7	6.4	6.2	5.9
300–399 beds	7.8	7.6	7.0	7.0	6.6	6.4	6.1	5.9
400–499 beds	8.1	7.9	7.3	7.3	6.9	6.7	6.3	6.1
500 beds or more	9.1	8.7	8.1	8.1	7.8	7.4	7.1	6.7
Outpatient visits[3]				Number in thousands				
All hospitals	254,844	262,951	282,140	368,184	435,619	453,584	483,195	505,455
Federal	51,957	50,566	52,342	58,527	59,918	61,103	59,934	56,593
Non-Federal[1]	202,887	212,385	229,798	309,657	375,701	392,481	423,261	448,861
Community[2]	190,672	202,310	218,716	301,329	366,885	382,924	414,345	439,863
Nonprofit.	131,435	142,156	158,953	221,073	270,138	282,653	303,851	320,746
Proprietary	7,713	9,696	12,378	20,110	24,936	26,443	31,940	37,347
State-local government. . .	51,525	50,459	47,386	60,146	71,811	73,828	78,554	81,770
6–24 beds.	915	1,155	829	1,471	1,919	2,354	3,644	3,622
25–49 beds	5,855	6,227	6,623	10,812	14,654	16,749	19,465	20,960
50–99 beds	16,303	17,976	18,716	27,582	32,878	34,907	38,597	41,003
100–199 beds	35,156	36,453	41,049	58,940	75,766	79,420	91,312	99,999
200–299 beds	32,772	36,073	40,515	60,561	75,220	79,364	84,080	86,958
300–399 beds	29,169	30,495	33,773	43,699	53,941	54,324	54,277	60,190
400–499 beds	22,127	25,501	23,950	33,394	38,275	40,152	44,284	47,241
500 beds or more	48,375	48,430	53,262	64,870	74,232	75,654	78,685	79,891
Outpatient surgery				Percent of total surgeries[4]				
Community hospitals[2]	- - -	16.3	34.6	50.5	55.4	57.2	58.1	59.5

- - - Data not available.

[1]The category of non-Federal hospitals is comprised of psychiatric, tuberculosis and other respiratory diseases hospitals, and long-term and short-term hospitals.

[2]Community hospitals are short-term hospitals excluding hospital units in institutions such as prison and college infirmaries, facilities for the mentally retarded, and alcoholism and chemical dependency hospitals.

[3]Outpatient visits include visits to the emergency department, outpatient department, referred visits (pharmacy, EKG, radiology), and outpatient surgery.

[4]The American Hospital Association defines surgery as a surgical episode in the operating or procedure room. During a single episode, multiple surgical procedures may be performed. Outpatient surgery is performed on patients who do not remain in the hospital overnight. Outpatient surgery is performed in inpatient operating rooms or in procedure rooms located in an outpatient facility.

SOURCES: American Hospital Association: Hospital Statistics, 1976, 1981, 1986, 1991–98 Editions. Chicago, 1976, 1981, 1986, 1991–98. (Copyrights 1976, 1981, 1986, 1991–98: Used with the permission of the American Hospital Association and Healthcare InfoSource.)

Table 95. Nursing home and personal care home residents 65 years of age and over according to age, sex, and race: United States, 1963, 1973–74, 1985, and 1995

[Data are based on a sample of nursing home residents]

Age, sex, and race	Residents				Residents per 1,000 population			
	1963[1]	1973–74[2]	1985[2]	1995[2]	1963[1]	1973–74[2]	1985[2]	1995[2]
Age								
65 years and over	445,600	961,500	1,318,300	1,422,600	25.4	44.7	46.2	42.4
65–74 years	89,600	163,100	212,100	190,200	7.9	12.3	12.5	10.1
75–84 years	207,200	384,900	509,000	511,900	39.6	57.7	57.7	45.9
85 years and over	148,700	413,600	597,300	720,400	148.4	257.3	220.3	198.6
Male								
65 years and over	141,000	265,700	334,400	356,800	18.1	30.0	29.0	26.1
65–74 years	35,100	65,100	80,600	79,300	6.8	11.3	10.8	9.5
75–84 years	65,200	102,300	141,300	144,300	29.1	39.9	43.0	33.3
85 years and over	40,700	98,300	112,600	133,100	105.6	182.7	145.7	130.8
Female								
65 years and over	304,500	695,800	983,900	1,065,800	31.1	54.9	57.9	53.7
65–74 years	54,500	98,000	131,500	110,900	8.8	13.1	13.8	10.6
75–84 years	142,000	282,600	367,700	367,600	47.5	68.9	66.4	53.9
85 years and over	108,000	315,300	484,700	587,300	175.1	294.9	250.1	224.9
White[3]								
65 years and over	431,700	920,600	1,227,400	1,271,200	26.6	46.9	47.7	42.3
65–74 years	84,400	150,100	187,800	154,400	8.1	12.5	12.3	9.3
75–84 years	202,000	369,700	473,600	453,800	41.7	60.3	59.1	44.9
85 years and over	145,400	400,800	566,000	663,000	157.7	270.8	228.7	200.7
Black[4]								
65 years and over	13,800	37,700	82,000	122,900	10.3	22.0	35.0	45.2
65–74 years	5,200	12,200	22,500	29,700	5.9	11.1	15.4	18.4
75–84 years	5,300	13,400	30,600	47,300	13.8	26.7	45.3	57.2
85 years and over	3,300	12,100	29,000	45,800	41.8	105.7	141.5	167.1

[1]Includes residents in personal care or domiciliary care homes.
[2]Excludes residents in personal care or domiciliary care homes.
[3]For 1973–74 Hispanics were included in the white category.
[4]For 1963 black includes all other races.

NOTES: Age refers to age at time of interview. Rates are based on the resident population as of July 1.

SOURCES: Centers for Disease Control and Prevention: Wunderlich GS. Characteristics of residents in institutions for the aged and chronically ill, United States, April–June 1963. National Center for Health Statistics. Vital Health Stat 12(2). 1965; and Hing E, Sekscenski E, Strahan G. The National Nursing Home Survey: 1985 summary for the United States. National Center for Health Statistics. Vital Health Stat 13(97). 1989; and unpublished data from the 1995 National Nursing Home Survey.

Table 96. Nursing home residents 65 years of age and over, according to selected functional status and age, sex, and race: United States, 1985 and 1995

[Data are based on a sample of nursing home residents]

| Age, sex, and race | Residents | | Functional status[1] | | | | | | | |
| | | | Dependent mobility | | Incontinent | | Dependent eating | | Dependent mobility, eating, and incontinent | |
	1985	1995	1985	1995	1985	1995	1985	1995	1985	1995
All persons	Number		Percent							
65 years and over, age-adjusted[2]	...	...	75.7	79.0	55.0	63.8	40.9	44.9	32.5	36.5
65 years and over, crude	1,318,300	1,422,600	74.8	79.0	54.5	63.8	40.5	44.9	32.1	36.5
65–74 years	212,100	190,200	61.2	73.0	42.9	61.9	33.5	43.8	25.7	35.8
75–84 years	509,000	511,900	70.5	76.5	55.1	62.5	39.4	45.2	30.6	35.3
85 years and over	597,300	720,400	83.3	82.4	58.1	65.3	43.9	45.0	35.6	37.5
Male										
65 years and over, age-adjusted[2]	...	...	71.2	76.6	54.2	63.8	36.0	42.1	28.0	34.3
65 years and over, crude	334,400	356,800	67.8	75.8	51.9	63.9	34.9	42.7	26.9	34.8
65–74 years	80,600	79,300	55.8	70.6	38.8	63.4	32.8	44.2	24.1	36.9
75–84 years	141,300	144,300	65.7	76.6	54.4	64.6	32.6	44.1	25.5	35.5
85 years and over	112,600	133,100	79.2	78.2	58.1	63.4	39.2	40.2	30.9	32.7
Female										
65 years and over, age-adjusted[2]	...	...	77.3	79.7	55.4	63.6	42.4	45.6	33.9	36.9
65 years and over, crude	983,900	1,065,800	77.1	80.1	55.4	63.8	42.4	45.6	33.8	37.0
65–74 years	131,500	110,900	64.5	74.8	45.4	60.9	34.0	43.6	26.7	35.0
75–84 years	367,700	367,600	72.3	76.5	55.3	61.7	42.0	45.7	32.6	35.2
85 years and over	484,700	587,300	84.3	83.3	58.1	65.7	45.0	46.0	36.7	38.6
White										
65 years and over, age-adjusted[2]	...	...	75.2	78.5	54.6	63.2	40.4	44.2	32.1	35.7
65 years and over, crude	1,227,400	1,271,200	74.3	78.7	54.2	63.3	40.1	44.2	31.7	35.7
65–74 years	187,800	154,400	60.2	71.4	42.2	60.2	32.6	41.9	24.9	33.8
75–84 years	473,600	453,800	69.6	76.4	54.2	61.8	38.9	44.9	30.1	34.7
85 years and over	566,000	663,000	83.1	81.9	58.2	65.0	43.5	44.3	35.5	36.9
Black										
65 years and over, age-adjusted[2]	...	...	83.4	83.2	61.0	69.3	49.2	52.2	38.2	44.0
65 years and over, crude	82,000	122,900	81.1	82.1	59.9	69.1	47.9	51.7	37.7	43.7
65–74 years	22,500	29,700	70.9	79.6	48.6	68.3	43.1	51.2	33.8	43.1
75–84 years	30,600	47,300	82.5	77.8	70.1	68.9	47.9	49.5	40.6	42.3
85 years and over	29,000	45,800	87.4	88.0	57.9	69.8	51.7	54.3	37.6	45.5

... Category not applicable.

[1]Nursing home residents who are dependent in mobility and eating require the assistance of a person or special equipment. Nursing home residents who are incontinent have difficulty in controlling bowels and/or bladder or have an ostomy or indwelling catheter.

[2]Age-adjusted by the direct method to the 1995 National Nursing Home Survey population using the following 3 age groups: 65–74 years, 75–84 years, and 85 years and over.

NOTES: Some numbers in this table have been revised and differ from previous editions of *Health, United States*. Age refers to age at time of interview. Excludes residents in personal care or domiciliary care homes.

SOURCES: Centers for Disease Control and Prevention: Hing E, Sekscenski E, Strahan G. The National Nursing Home Survey: 1985 summary for the United States. National Center for Health Statistics. Vital Health Stat 13(97). 1989; and unpublished data from the 1995 National Nursing Home Survey.

Table 97. Additions to selected inpatient psychiatric organizations according to sex, age, and race: United States, 1975, 1980, and 1986

[Data are based on a sample survey of patients]

Sex, age, and race	State and county mental hospitals			Private psychiatric hospitals			Non-Federal general hospitals[1]		
	1975	1980	1986	1975	1980	1986	1975	1980	1986
Both sexes	Additions in thousands								
Total	385	369	343	130	141	222	516	564	851
Under 18 years...........	25	17	17	15	17	43	43	44	50
18–24 years.............	72	77	61	19	23	25	93	98	126
25–44 years.............	166	177	200	47	56	99	220	249	425
45–64 years.............	102	78	50	35	32	34	121	123	156
65 years and over.........	21	20	15	13	14	21	38	50	94
White..................	296	265	230	119	123	183	451	469	659
All other...............	89	104	113	10	18	39	65	95	192
Male									
Total	249	239	217	56	67	115	212	255	398
Under 18 years...........	16	11	10	8	9	23	20	20	22
18–24 years.............	52	56	41	10	13	16	45	52	59
25–44 years.............	107	119	134	20	27	56	85	115	222
45–64 years.............	61	43	25	14	13	14	48	46	66
65 years and over.........	13	11	7	5	5	6	14	21	29
White..................	191	171	145	51	58	89	184	213	292
All other...............	58	68	72	5	9	26	27	42	106
Female									
Total	136	130	126	74	74	107	304	309	453
Under 18 years...........	9	5	7	8	7	20	23	23	28
18–24 years.............	20	22	20	9	10	8	48	45	67
25–44 years.............	59	58	66	28	29	44	135	135	203
45–64 years.............	41	35	24	21	18	20	74	77	90
65 years and over.........	8	9	8	8	9	15	24	29	65
White..................	105	94	85	69	65	94	267	256	367
All other...............	31	36	41	5	9	13	37	53	86
Both sexes	Additions per 100,000 civilian population								
Total	182.2	163.6	143.4	61.4	62.6	92.5	243.8	250.0	355.4
Under 18 years...........	38.1	26.1	26.9	23.3	26.3	67.5	64.4	68.5	78.7
18–24 years.............	271.8	264.6	225.6	73.7	79.6	91.6	352.8	334.2	467.0
25–44 years.............	314.1	282.9	267.0	89.3	89.1	132.7	416.8	399.0	566.8
45–64 years.............	233.5	175.7	110.9	80.1	71.0	75.2	278.5	276.4	346.2
65 years and over.........	91.8	78.0	52.5	57.7	54.1	71.4	170.3	195.4	323.6
White..................	161.1	136.8	113.2	64.9	63.4	90.1	245.4	241.8	324.7
All other...............	321.9	328.0	311.4	37.9	57.5	106.1	233.3	300.0	526.2
Male									
Total	243.7	219.8	187.8	54.5	61.9	99.3	207.1	233.8	343.6
Under 18 years...........	48.3	35.4	32.2	22.5	28.9	69.8	59.1	62.6	67.5
18–24 years.............	409.0	387.9	307.5	78.0	92.2	124.2	350.8	365.3	446.2
25–44 years.............	418.4	388.1	363.0	76.6	86.8	151.2	332.8	374.7	602.9
45–64 years.............	291.5	202.3	118.6	66.8	63.2	65.5	228.6	219.1	306.1
65 years and over.........	136.4	105.3	59.4	50.3	47.3	52.1	152.0	203.4	245.6
White..................	214.2	182.2	147.2	57.0	61.7	90.3	206.9	226.3	296.4
All other...............	444.5	457.8	419.7	38.1	62.7	151.2	209.1	281.1	614.2
Female									
Total	124.7	111.1	101.8	67.8	63.3	86.2	278.1	265.1	366.4
Under 18 years...........	27.5	16.4	21.4	24.1	23.6	65.0	70.0	74.6	90.3
18–24 years.............	143.1	145.8	146.6	69.6	67.4	60.2	354.6	304.4	487.1
25–44 years.............	215.9	182.3	174.1	101.2	91.2	114.9	495.8	422.2	531.9
45–64 years.............	180.5	151.7	103.8	92.3	78.1	84.0	324.3	328.2	382.8
65 years and over.........	60.8	59.6	47.8	62.8	58.8	84.6	182.9	190.0	376.7
White..................	111.2	94.1	81.1	72.5	65.0	90.0	281.7	256.4	351.5
All other...............	212.0	212.6	214.2	37.7	52.8	65.5	254.9	316.7	447.0

[1]Non-Federal general hospitals include public and nonpublic facilities.

SOURCES: National Institute of Mental Health. Taube CA, Barrett SA. *Mental Health, United States, 1985.* DHHS. 1985; Manderscheid RW, Sonnenschein MA. *Mental Health, United States, 1992.* DHHS. 1992. Unpublished data.

Table 98. Additions to selected inpatient psychiatric organizations, according to selected primary diagnoses and age: United States, 1975, 1980, and 1986

[Data are based on a sample survey of patients]

Primary diagnosis and age	State and county mental hospitals			Private psychiatric hospitals			Non-Federal general hospitals[1]		
	1975	1980	1986	1975	1980	1986	1975	1980	1986
All diagnoses[2]	Additions per 100,000 civilian population								
All ages	182.2	163.6	143.4	61.4	62.6	92.5	243.8	250.0	355.4
Under 25 years	104.8	101.2	86.3	37.7	43.1	74.7	146.7	152.2	194.7
25–44 years	314.1	282.9	267.0	89.3	89.1	132.7	416.8	399.0	566.8
45–64 years	233.5	175.7	110.9	80.1	71.0	75.2	278.5	276.4	346.2
65 years and over	91.8	78.0	52.5	57.7	54.1	71.4	170.3	195.4	323.6
Alcohol related									
All ages	50.4	35.5	23.8	5.1	5.8	6.6	17.0	18.8	42.4
Under 25 years	10.7	12.4	16.8	0.4	1.4	2.2	2.4	4.4	13.7
25–44 years	86.2	64.0	45.4	7.6	9.3	10.0	31.0	34.3	94.8
45–64 years	110.0	57.7	15.3	12.5	10.9	11.0	34.5	30.6	32.9
65 years and over	14.8	11.5	*3.2	4.3	4.4	4.5	10.2	12.8	11.3
Drug related									
All ages	6.8	7.8	9.1	1.5	1.8	6.1	8.4	7.4	20.8
Under 25 years	7.2	9.4	6.3	1.5	1.8	7.5	7.7	7.8	18.8
25–44 years	12.6	12.9	14.8	2.3	3.0	9.3	13.8	9.3	42.0
45–64 years	*0.6	1.4	10.5	0.1	1.0	*1.8	6.5	7.1	*2.2
65 years and over	*3.5	*0.7	*0.8	0.4	0.6	- - -	*2.6	*2.0	*1.2
Organic disorders[3]									
All ages	9.6	6.8	4.5	2.5	2.2	2.0	9.0	7.4	10.7
Under 25 years	2.2	1.2	*0.2	0.7	0.5	*0.5	1.1	*0.8	1.7
25–44 years	6.4	4.7	3.0	1.1	0.9	*0.3	5.4	5.6	6.9
45–64 years	12.2	8.1	7.3	1.7	2.7	*1.5	9.3	6.9	6.8
65 years and over	43.3	30.0	17.2	14.5	10.8	11.7	49.3	36.4	54.5
Affective disorders									
All ages	21.3	22.0	23.6	26.0	26.8	45.4	91.9	79.2	135.9
Under 25 years	7.5	9.1	9.9	9.5	13.5	31.6	35.3	32.2	55.9
25–44 years	40.6	36.9	45.2	39.4	38.9	67.1	160.9	123.7	190.4
45–64 years	29.4	32.4	25.5	43.3	36.3	38.5	135.6	113.8	165.7
65 years and over	16.8	14.3	7.9	29.6	29.2	42.9	78.5	81.0	197.4
Schizophrenia									
All ages	61.2	62.1	53.2	13.4	13.3	11.0	58.9	59.9	66.2
Under 25 years	35.9	36.6	19.6	11.1	10.6	5.7	42.0	38.3	30.8
25–44 years	125.8	125.0	115.3	23.8	22.5	22.6	118.0	114.5	124.2
45–64 years	63.5	54.8	38.8	11.3	11.6	8.5	50.3	53.6	73.7
65 years and over	9.3	13.9	19.9	2.7	3.6	*1.8	5.6	16.3	15.3

* Based on 5 or fewer sample additions.
- - - Data not available.
[1]Non-Federal general hospitals include public and nonpublic facilities.
[2]Includes all other diagnoses not listed separately.
[3]Excludes alcohol and drug-related diagnoses.

NOTES: Primary diagnosis categories are based on the then current *International Classification of Diseases* and *Diagnostic and Statistical Manual of Mental Disorders*. For a listing of the code numbers, see Appendix II, table X.

SOURCES: National Institute of Mental Health. Taube CA, Barrett SA. *Mental Health, United States, 1985*. DHHS. 1985; Manderscheid RW, Sonnenschein MA. *Mental Health, United States, 1992*. DHHS. 1992. Unpublished data.

Table 99. Persons employed in health service sites: United States, selected years 1970–96

[Data are based on household interviews of a sample of the civilian noninstitutionalized population]

Site	1970	1975	1980	1985	1989	1990	1991	1992	1993	1994[1]	1995[1]	1996[1]
	Number of persons in thousands											
All employed civilians........	76,805	85,846	99,303	107,150	117,342	117,914	116,877	117,598	119,306	123,060	124,900	126,708
All health service sites........	4,246	5,945	7,339	7,910	9,110	9,447	9,817	10,271	10,553	10,587	10,928	11,199
Offices and clinics of physicians	477	618	777	894	1,039	1,098	1,128	1,434	1,450	1,404	1,512	1,501
Offices and clinics of dentists	222	331	415	480	560	580	574	583	567	596	644	614
Offices and clinics of chiropractors[2]..........	19	30	40	59	97	90	105	122	116	105	99	99
Hospitals.................	2,690	3,441	4,036	4,269	4,568	4,690	4,839	4,915	5,032	5,009	4,961	5,041
Nursing and personal care facilities...............	509	891	1,199	1,309	1,521	1,543	1,626	1,750	1,752	1,692	1,718	1,765
Other health service sites	330	634	872	899	1,325	1,446	1,545	1,467	1,635	1,781	1,995	2,178
	Percent of employed civilians											
All health service sites........	5.5	6.9	7.4	7.4	7.8	8.0	8.4	8.7	8.8	8.6	8.7	8.8
	Percent distribution											
All health service sites........	100.0	100.0	100.0	100.0	100.0	100.0	100.0	100.0	100.0	100.0	100.0	100.0
Offices and clinics of physicians	11.2	10.4	10.6	11.3	11.4	11.6	11.5	14.0	13.7	13.3	13.8	13.4
Offices and clinics of dentists	5.2	5.6	5.7	6.1	6.1	6.1	5.8	5.7	5.4	5.6	5.9	5.5
Offices and clinics of chiropractors[2]..........	0.4	0.5	0.5	0.7	1.1	1.0	1.1	1.2	1.1	1.0	0.9	0.9
Hospitals.................	63.4	57.9	55.0	54.0	50.1	49.6	49.3	47.9	47.7	47.3	45.4	45.0
Nursing and personal care facilities...............	12.0	15.0	16.3	16.5	16.7	16.3	16.6	17.0	16.6	16.0	15.7	15.8
Other health service sites	7.8	10.7	11.9	11.4	14.5	15.3	15.7	14.3	15.5	16.8	18.3	19.4

[1]Data for 1994 and later years are not strictly comparable with data from previous years due to a redesign of the Current Population Survey. See Appendix I, Department of Commerce.

[2]Data for 1980 are from the American Chiropractic Association; data for all other years are from the U.S. Bureau of Labor Statistics.

NOTES: Employment is full- or part-time work. Totals exclude persons in health-related occupations who are working in nonhealth industries, as classified by the U.S. Bureau of the Census, such as pharmacists employed in drugstores, school nurses, and nurses working in private households. Totals include Federal, State, and county health workers. In 1970–82, employed persons were classified according to the industry groups used in the 1970 Census of Population. In 1983–91, persons were classified according to the system used in the 1980 Census of Population. Beginning in 1992 persons were classified according to the system used in the 1990 Census of Population.

SOURCES: U.S. Bureau of the Census: 1970 Census of Population, occupation by industry. Subject Reports. Final Report PC(2)–7C. Washington. U.S. Government Printing Office, Oct. 1972; U.S. Bureau of Labor Statistics: Labor Force Statistics Derived from the Current Population Survey: A Databook, Vol. I. Washington. U.S. Government Printing Office, Sept. 1982; Employment and Earnings, January 1986–97. Vol. 32, No. 1, Vol. 33, No. 1, Vol. 35, No. 1, Vol. 36, No. 1, Vol. 37, No. 1, Vol. 38, No. 1, Vol. 39, No. 1, Vol. 40, No. 1, Vol. 41, No. 1, Vol. 42, No. 1, Vol. 43, No. 1, and Vol. 44, No. 1. Washington. U.S. Government Printing Office, Jan. 1986–97; American Chiropractic Association: Unpublished data.

Health Care Resources

Table 100 (page 1 of 2). Active non-Federal physicians and doctors of medicine in patient care, according to geographic division and State: United States, 1975, 1985, 1990, and 1996

[Data based on reporting by physicians]

Geographic division and State	Total physicians[1]				Doctors of medicine in patient care[2]			
	1975	1985	1990	1996[3]	1975	1985	1990	1996
	Number per 10,000 civilian population							
United States	15.3	20.7	22.2	24.7	13.5	18.0	19.5	21.7
New England	19.1	26.7	29.0	33.3	16.9	22.9	25.5	29.4
Maine.	12.8	18.7	20.1	23.4	10.7	15.6	16.6	19.1
New Hampshire.	14.3	18.1	20.1	22.5	13.1	16.7	18.6	20.6
Vermont	18.2	23.8	25.4	27.6	15.5	20.3	22.4	24.8
Massachusetts	20.8	30.2	32.8	38.2	18.3	25.4	28.6	33.8
Rhode Island.	17.8	23.3	26.0	31.5	16.1	20.2	22.6	27.6
Connecticut.	19.8	27.6	30.1	33.2	17.7	24.3	26.8	29.8
Middle Atlantic.	19.5	26.1	28.4	33.0	17.0	22.2	24.5	28.4
New York	22.7	29.0	31.1	36.0	20.2	25.2	27.6	32.1
New Jersey.	16.2	23.4	25.9	29.9	14.0	19.8	22.2	25.2
Pennsylvania.	16.6	23.6	26.0	30.5	13.9	19.2	21.3	24.8
East North Central.	13.9	19.3	20.6	23.9	12.0	16.4	17.6	20.3
Ohio.	14.1	19.9	21.4	24.4	12.2	16.8	18.0	20.4
Indiana	10.6	14.7	16.0	19.0	9.6	13.2	14.6	17.1
Illinois.	14.5	20.5	21.6	25.5	13.1	18.2	19.3	22.6
Michigan.	15.4	20.8	22.1	25.6	12.0	16.0	16.9	19.6
Wisconsin.	12.5	17.7	19.1	22.0	11.4	15.9	17.4	20.0
West North Central	13.3	18.3	19.8	22.3	11.4	15.6	17.1	19.2
Minnesota.	14.9	20.5	22.0	23.6	13.7	18.5	20.1	21.6
Iowa.	11.4	15.6	17.2	19.5	9.4	12.4	13.8	15.3
Missouri	15.0	20.5	22.0	24.6	11.6	16.3	17.7	20.2
North Dakota.	9.7	15.8	17.0	20.7	9.2	14.9	16.0	19.1
South Dakota	8.2	13.4	14.2	18.1	7.7	12.3	13.2	16.8
Nebraska	12.1	15.7	17.0	20.0	10.9	14.4	15.9	18.5
Kansas.	12.8	17.3	18.6	21.4	11.2	15.1	16.3	18.4
South Atlantic	14.0	19.7	21.7	24.1	12.6	17.6	19.3	21.6
Delaware	14.3	19.7	21.3	24.3	12.7	17.1	18.3	20.6
Maryland.	18.6	30.4	32.5	34.4	16.5	24.9	27.8	29.9
District of Columbia	39.6	55.3	60.0	66.6	34.6	45.6	50.1	55.9
Virginia.	12.9	19.5	21.2	23.0	11.9	17.8	19.5	21.2
West Virginia.	11.0	16.3	17.7	22.0	10.0	14.6	15.4	18.6
North Carolina.	11.7	16.9	18.9	22.0	10.6	15.0	17.2	20.2
South Carolina.	10.0	14.7	16.0	19.8	9.3	13.6	15.0	18.4
Georgia	11.5	16.2	17.6	20.2	10.6	14.7	16.2	18.4
Florida	15.2	20.2	21.6	23.8	13.4	17.8	19.2	21.1
East South Central	10.5	15.0	16.8	19.9	9.7	14.0	15.7	18.4
Kentucky.	10.9	15.1	16.8	19.5	10.1	13.9	15.7	18.2
Tennessee	12.4	17.7	19.5	23.3	11.3	16.2	18.1	21.5
Alabama	9.2	14.2	15.7	19.2	8.6	13.1	14.6	17.7
Mississippi	8.4	11.8	13.3	15.0	8.0	11.1	12.6	13.8
West South Central	11.9	16.4	17.8	20.0	10.5	14.5	15.8	17.7
Arkansas	9.1	13.8	15.1	18.3	8.5	12.8	14.1	16.9
Louisiana	11.4	17.3	18.6	22.7	10.5	16.1	17.4	21.3
Oklahoma.	11.6	16.1	17.1	19.3	9.4	12.9	13.6	15.1
Texas	12.5	16.8	18.1	19.7	11.0	14.7	16.0	17.4
Mountain	14.3	17.8	19.3	20.4	12.6	15.7	17.0	17.9
Montana.	10.6	14.0	16.0	18.8	10.1	13.2	15.2	17.5
Idaho	9.5	12.1	12.7	14.8	8.9	11.4	12.0	13.9
Wyoming.	9.5	12.9	13.9	16.5	8.9	12.0	13.1	14.9
Colorado.	17.3	20.7	22.1	23.5	15.0	17.7	19.2	20.4
New Mexico	12.2	17.0	18.9	20.9	10.1	14.7	16.7	18.5
Arizona.	16.7	20.2	21.5	21.4	14.1	17.1	18.4	18.2
Utah.	14.1	17.2	18.5	19.3	13.0	15.5	16.9	17.5
Nevada.	11.9	16.0	16.6	17.3	10.9	14.5	14.9	15.3

See footnotes at end of table.

Table 100 (page 2 of 2). Active non-Federal physicians and doctors of medicine in patient care, according to geographic division and State: United States, 1975, 1985, 1990, and 1996

[Data based on reporting by physicians]

Geographic division and State	Total physicians[1]				Doctors of medicine in patient care[2]			
	1975	1985	1990	1996[3]	1975	1985	1990	1996
	Number per 10,000 civilian population							
Pacific	17.9	22.5	23.4	23.5	16.3	20.5	21.3	21.4
Washington	15.3	20.2	21.5	22.9	13.6	17.9	19.3	20.5
Oregon	15.6	19.7	21.1	22.2	13.8	17.6	19.1	20.0
California	18.8	23.7	24.1	23.8	17.3	21.5	21.9	21.7
Alaska	8.4	13.0	14.8	16.4	7.8	12.1	13.7	14.6
Hawaii	16.2	21.5	23.8	25.6	14.7	19.8	21.9	23.4

[1]Includes active non-Federal doctors of medicine and active doctors of osteopathy.
[2]Excludes doctors of osteopathy; States with large numbers are Florida, Michigan, Missouri, New Jersey, Ohio, Pennsylvania, and Texas. Excludes doctors of medicine in medical teaching, administration, research, and other nonpatient care activities.
[3]Data for doctors of osteopathy are as of October 1996.

NOTES: Data for doctors of medicine are as of December 31, except for 1990 data, which are as of January 1. See Appendix II for physician definitions.

SOURCES: Compiled by Health Resources and Services Administration, Bureau of Health Professions based on data from the American Medical Association Physician Distribution and Licensure in the U.S., 1975, Physician Characteristics and Distribution in the U.S., 1986, 1992, and 1997/98 Editions; American Osteopathic Association: 1975–76 Yearbook and Directory of Osteopathic Physicians, 1985–86 Yearbook and Directory of Osteopathic Physicians; Rockville, Md., 1991. American Association of Colleges of Osteopathic Medicine: Annual Statistical Report, 1990 and 1996.

Table 101. Physicians, according to activity and place of medical education: United States and outlying U.S. areas, selected years 1975–96

[Data are based on reporting by physicians]

Activity and place of medical education	1975	1980	1985	1990	1994	1995	1996
	Number of physicians						
Doctors of medicine	393,742	467,679	552,716	615,421	684,414	720,325	737,764
Professionally active[1]	340,280	414,916	497,140	547,310	605,468	625,443	643,955
Place of medical education:							
U.S. medical graduates	- - -	333,325	392,007	432,884	467,092	481,137	495,463
International medical graduates[2]	- - -	81,591	105,133	114,426	138,376	144,306	148,492
Activity:[3]							
Non-Federal	312,089	397,129	475,573	526,835	583,014	604,364	623,526
Patient care	287,837	361,915	431,527	479,547	538,437	564,074	580,706
Office-based practice	213,334	271,268	329,041	359,932	407,044	427,275	445,765
General and family practice	46,347	47,772	53,862	57,571	58,210	59,932	61,760
Cardiovascular diseases	5,046	6,725	9,054	10,670	12,917	13,739	14,304
Dermatology	3,442	4,372	5,325	5,996	6,709	6,959	7,234
Gastroenterology	1,696	2,735	4,135	5,200	6,707	7,300	7,580
Internal medicine	28,188	40,514	52,712	57,799	67,897	72,612	77,929
Pediatrics	12,687	17,436	22,392	26,494	31,474	33,890	35,453
Pulmonary diseases	1,166	2,040	3,035	3,659	4,631	4,964	4,892
General surgery	19,710	22,409	24,708	24,498	24,209	24,086	25,425
Obstetrics and gynecology	15,613	19,503	23,525	25,475	28,211	29,111	29,872
Ophthalmology	8,795	10,598	12,212	13,055	14,297	14,596	14,931
Orthopedic surgery	8,148	10,719	13,033	14,187	16,580	17,136	17,637
Otolaryngology	4,297	5,262	5,751	6,360	6,856	7,139	7,152
Plastic surgery	1,706	2,437	3,299	3,835	4,313	4,612	5,012
Urological surgery	5,025	6,222	7,081	7,392	7,779	7,991	8,229
Anesthesiology	8,970	11,336	15,285	17,789	21,962	23,770	24,929
Diagnostic radiology	1,978	4,190	7,735	9,806	12,079	12,751	13,313
Emergency medicine	- - -	- - -	- - -	8,402	10,604	11,700	12,348
Neurology	1,862	3,245	4,691	5,587	7,131	7,623	7,898
Pathology, anatomical/clinical	4,195	5,952	6,877	7,269	8,715	9,031	9,661
Psychiatry	12,173	15,946	18,521	20,048	22,551	23,334	24,400
Radiology	6,970	7,791	7,355	6,056	5,885	5,994	6,276
Other specialty	15,320	24,064	28,453	22,784	27,327	29,005	29,530
Hospital-based practice	74,503	90,647	102,486	127,864	136,111	136,799	134,941
Residents and interns[4]	53,527	59,615	72,159	81,664	86,832	93,650	90,592
Full-time hospital staff	20,976	31,032	30,327	37,951	44,561	43,149	44,349
Other professional activity[5]	24,252	35,214	44,046	39,039	39,859	40,290	42,820
Federal[6]	28,191	17,787	21,567	20,475	22,454	21,079	20,429
Patient care	24,100	14,597	17,293	15,632	19,101	18,057	18,218
Office-based practice	2,095	732	1,156	1,063	. . .	. . .	. . .
Hospital-based practice	22,005	13,865	16,137	14,569	19,101	18,057	18,218
Residents and interns	4,275	2,427	3,252	1,725	3,443	2,702	5,749
Full-time hospital staff	17,730	11,438	12,885	12,844	15,658	15,355	12,469
Other professional activity[5]	4,091	3,190	4,274	4,843	3,353	3,022	2,211
Inactive	21,449	25,744	38,646	52,653	63,285	72,326	72,510
Not classified	26,145	20,629	13,950	12,678	14,283	20,579	19,998
Unknown address	5,868	6,390	2,980	2,780	1,378	1,977	1,311

- - - Data not available.

. . . Category not applicable.

[1]Excludes inactive, not classified, and address unknown.

[2]International medical graduates received their medical education in schools outside the United States and Canada.

[3]Specialty information based on the physician's self-designated primary area of practice. Categories include generalists and specialists.

[4]Beginning in 1990 clinical fellows are included in this category. In prior years clinical fellows were included in other professional activity.

[5]Includes medical teaching, administration, research, and other. Prior to 1990 this category included clinical fellows, also.

[6]Beginning in 1993 data collection for Federal physicians was revised.

NOTES: Data for doctors of medicine are as of December 31, except for 1990–94 data, which are as of January 1. See Appendix II for discussion of physician specialties. Outlying areas include Puerto Rico, Virgin Islands, and the Pacific islands of Canton, Caroline, Guam, Mariana, Marshall, American Samoa, and Wake.

SOURCES: Goodman LJ, Mason HR. Physician distribution and medical licensure in the U.S., 1975. Chicago. American Medical Association. 1976; Bidese CM, Danais DG. Physician characteristics and distribution in the U.S., 1981. Chicago. American Medical Association. 1982; Roback GA, Mead D, Randolph LL. Physician characteristics and distribution in the U.S., 1986. Chicago. American Medical Association. 1986; Roback GA, Randolph LL, Seidman B. Physician characteristics and distribution in the U.S., 1992; 1994; 1995–96; 1996–97; 1997–98. Chicago. American Medical Association. 1992; 1994; 1995–96; 1996–97; 1997–98. (Copyrights 1976, 1982, 1986, 1992, 1994, 1996, and 1997: Used with the permission of the American Medical Association).

Table 102. Primary care doctors of medicine, according to specialty: United States and outlying U.S. areas, selected years 1949–96

[Data are based on reporting by physicians]

Specialty	1949[1]	1960[1]	1970	1980	1985	1990	1994	1995	1996
					Number				
Total[2]	201,277	260,484	334,028	467,679	552,716	615,421	684,414	720,325	737,764
Active doctors of medicine[3] . . .	191,577	247,257	310,845	414,916	497,140	547,310	605,468	625,443	643,955
Primary care generalists . . .	113,222	125,359	115,822	146,093	170,741	183,294	200,020	207,810	216,446
General/family practice . . .	95,980	88,023	57,948	60,049	67,051	70,480	73,163	75,976	78,910
Internal medicine	12,453	26,209	39,924	58,462	70,691	76,295	84,951	88,240	92,321
Pediatrics	4,789	11,127	17,950	27,582	32,999	36,519	41,906	43,594	45,215
Primary care specialists	- - -	- - -	2,817	14,949	22,011	27,434	33,927	35,290	39,315
Internal medicine	- - -	- - -	1,948	13,069	18,171	22,054	26,476	26,928	29,804
Pediatrics	- - -	- - -	869	1,880	3,840	5,380	7,451	8,362	9,511
				Percent active doctors of medicine					
Primary care generalists . . .	59.1	50.7	37.3	35.2	34.3	33.5	33.0	33.2	33.6
General/family practice . . .	50.1	35.6	18.6	14.5	13.5	12.9	12.1	12.1	12.3
Internal medicine	6.5	10.6	12.8	14.1	14.2	13.9	14.0	14.1	14.3
Pediatrics	2.5	4.5	5.8	6.6	6.6	6.7	6.9	7.0	7.0
Primary care specialists	- - -	- - -	0.9	3.6	4.4	5.0	5.6	5.6	6.1
Internal medicine	- - -	- - -	0.6	3.1	3.7	4.0	4.4	4.3	4.6
Pediatrics	- - -	- - -	0.3	0.5	0.8	1.0	1.2	1.3	1.5

- - - Data not available.

[1]Estimated by the Bureau of Health Professions, Health Resources Administration. Active doctors of medicine (M.D.'s) include those with address unknown and primary specialty not classified.

[2]Includes M.D.'s engaged in Federal and non-Federal patient care (office-based or hospital-based) and other professional activities.

[3]Beginning in 1970, M.D.'s who are inactive, have unknown address, or primary specialty not classified are excluded.

NOTES: See Appendix II for definitions of physician specialties. Data are as of December 31 except for 1990–94 data, which are as of January 1 and 1949 data which are as of midyear. Outlying areas include Puerto Rico, Virgin Islands, and the Pacific islands of Canton, Caroline, Guam, Mariana, Marshall, American Samoa, and Wake.

SOURCES: Health Manpower Source Book: Medical Specialists, USDHEW, 1962; Roback GA, Randolph LL, Seidman B. Physician characteristics and distribution in the U.S., 1997–98. Chicago. American Medical Association. 1997–98. (Copyright 1997: Used with the permission of the American Medical Association).

Table 103. Active health personnel according to occupation and geographic region: United States, 1980, 1990, and 1995

[Data are compiled by the Bureau of Health Professions]

Year and occupation	Number of active health personnel	United States	Geographic region			
			Northeast	Midwest	South	West
1980		Number per 100,000 population[1]				
Physicians	427,122	189.8	- - -	- - -	- - -	- - -
Federal	17,642	7.8	- - -	- - -	- - -	- - -
Doctors of medicine[2]	16,585	7.4	- - -	- - -	- - -	- - -
Doctors of osteopathy	1,057	0.5	- - -	- - -	- - -	- - -
Non-Federal.	409,480	182.0	224.5	165.2	157.0	200.0
Doctors of medicine[2]	393,407	174.9	216.1	153.3	152.8	195.8
Doctors of osteopathy	16,073	7.1	8.4	11.9	4.2	4.2
Dentists[3]	121,240	53.5	66.2	52.7	42.6	59.2
Optometrists	22,330	9.8	9.9	10.9	7.7	11.6
Pharmacists	142,780	62.5	66.5	67.8	62.1	51.8
Podiatrists[4]	7,000	3.0	- - -	- - -	- - -	- - -
Registered nurses	1,272,900	560.0	736.0	583.6	443.4	533.7
Associate and diploma	908,300	399.9	536.0	429.2	316.5	351.1
Baccalaureate	297,300	130.9	161.0	127.8	103.8	148.1
Masters and doctorate	67,300	29.6	39.0	26.7	23.0	34.6
1990						
Physicians	567,611	230.2	- - -	- - -	- - -	- - -
Federal[2]	20,784	8.4	- - -	- - -	- - -	- - -
Doctors of medicine[2]	19,166	7.7	- - -	- - -	- - -	- - -
Doctors of osteopathy	1,618	0.7	- - -	- - -	- - -	- - -
Non-Federal.	546,826	221.8	285.5	203.9	195.5	223.3
Doctors of medicine[2]	520,450	211.1	271.6	186.8	188.6	216.9
Doctors of osteopathy	26,376	10.7	13.9	17.1	6.9	6.3
Dentists[3]	146,600	58.8	- - -	- - -	- - -	- - -
Optometrists	26,000	10.4	- - -	- - -	- - -	- - -
Pharmacists	161,900	64.4	- - -	- - -	- - -	- - -
Podiatrists[4]	10,600	4.2	- - -	- - -	- - -	- - -
Registered nurses	1,789,600	713.7	- - -	- - -	- - -	- - -
Associate and diploma	1,107,300	441.6	- - -	- - -	- - -	- - -
Baccalaureate	549,000	218.9	- - -	- - -	- - -	- - -
Masters and doctorate	133,300	53.2	- - -	- - -	- - -	- - -
1995						
Physicians	672,859	255.9	- - -	- - -	- - -	- - -
Federal	21,153	8.0	- - -	- - -	- - -	- - -
Doctors of medicine[2]	19,830	7.5	- - -	- - -	- - -	- - -
Doctors of osteopathy	1,323	0.5	- - -	- - -	- - -	- - -
Non-Federal.	651,706	247.9	336.6	235.1	218.3	229.5
Doctors of medicine[2]	617,362	234.8	318.3	214.7	209.8	221.8
Doctors of osteopathy	34,344	13.1	18.3	20.4	8.5	7.7
Dentists[3]	- - -	- - -	- - -	- - -	- - -	- - -
Optometrists	28,900	10.9	- - -	- - -	- - -	- - -
Pharmacists	182,300	68.9	- - -	- - -	- - -	- - -
Podiatrists[4]	10,300	3.9	- - -	- - -	- - -	- - -
Registered nurses	2,115,800	797.6	975.5	876.0	743.3	643.7
Associate and diploma	1,235,000	465.5	559.6	522.2	452.2	343.8
Baccalaureate	673,200	253.8	308.3	274.4	221.3	235.3
Masters and doctorate	207,500	78.2	107.6	79.4	69.8	64.6

- - - Data not available.

[1]Ratios for physicians and dentists are based on civilian population; ratios for all other health occupations are based on resident population.

[2]Excludes physicians not classified according to activity status and inactive from the number of active health personnel.

[3]Excludes dentists in military service, U.S. Public Health Service, and Department of Veterans Affairs.

[4]Patient care.

NOTES: Some numbers for 1990 have been revised and differ from previous editions of Health, United States. Starting in 1989 data for doctors of medicine are as of January 1; in earlier years these data are as of December 31. See Appendix II for physician definitions.

SOURCES: Division of Health Professions Analysis, Bureau of Health Professions: Supply and Characteristics of Selected Health Personnel. DHHS Pub. No. (HRA) 81–20. Health Resources Administration. Hyattsville, Md., June 1981; unpublished data; American Medical Association. Physician characteristics and distribution in the U.S., 1981, 1992, and 1996/97 editions. Chicago, 1982, 1992, and 1997; American Osteopathic Association. 1980–81 Yearbook and Directory of Osteopathic Physicians. Chicago, 1980. American Association of Colleges of Osteopathic Medicine. Annual statistical report, 1990 and 1996 editions. Rockville, Md., 1990 and 1996; unpublished data.

Table 104. Full-time equivalent employment in selected occupations for community hospitals: United States, selected years 1983–93

[Data are based on reporting by a census of registered hospitals]

Occupation	1983	1990	1991	1992	1993	Average annual percent change	
						1983–90	1990–93
All hospital personnel[1]	3,130,131	3,439,820	3,554,962	3,635,530	3,688,323	1.4	2.4
Administrators and assistant administrators[2]	28,805	37,015	39,505	52,575	57,811	3.6	16.0
Physicians	25,520	36,451	37,091	38,079	44,119	5.2	6.6
Physician assistants	2,222	3,543	3,940	4,320	4,676	6.9	9.7
Registered nurses	698,151	809,920	840,493	853,789	874,115	2.1	2.6
Licensed practical nurses	229,735	167,945	165,871	157,208	148,885	−4.4	−3.9
Ancillary nursing personnel	294,180	268,113	278,125	274,015	274,195	−1.3	0.8
Medical record administrators and technicians	39,115	50,723	51,380	53,033	53,531	3.8	1.8
Licensed pharmacists and pharmacy technicians	52,077	64,004	65,735	67,585	68,695	3.0	2.4
Medical technologists and other laboratory personnel	149,949	157,880	161,087	163,323	165,176	0.7	1.5
Dietitians and dietetic technicians	36,623	35,553	35,294	33,232	34,843	−0.4	−0.7
Radiologic service personnel	92,509	111,298	114,455	117,401	120,223	2.7	2.6
Occupational therapists, occupational therapy assistants, and recreational therapists	9,078	15,144	16,290	17,294	17,904	7.6	5.7
Physical therapists and physical therapy assistants and aides	28,759	35,455	38,004	38,956	40,678	3.0	4.7
Speech pathologists and audiologists	2,684	4,909	5,550	5,910	6,177	9.0	8.0
Respiratory therapists and respiratory therapy technicians	51,490	60,403	62,969	64,337	65,151	2.3	2.6
Medical social workers	14,489	21,389	23,077	23,515	25,488	5.7	6.0
Total trainee personnel[3]	66,515	69,111	71,570	73,324	77,561	0.5	3.9

[1]Includes occupational categories not shown.
[2]Beginning in 1992 the occupational definition of assistant administrator was expanded to include additional administrative job titles in more areas of the facility.
[3]This category is primarily composed of medical residents and interns.

SOURCE: Compiled by the Office of Data Analysis and Management, Bureau of Health Professions, Health Resources and Services Administration, from the American Hospital Association's 1983, 1990, 1991, 1992, and 1993 Annual Survey of Hospitals.

Table 105 (page 1 of 2). Full-time equivalent patient care staff in mental health organizations, according to type of organization and staff discipline: United States, selected years 1984–94

[Data are based on inventories of mental health organizations]

Organization and discipline	1984	1990	1992	1994	1984	1990	1992	1994
All organizations	Number				Percent distribution			
All patient care staff	313,243	416,282	434,620	457,503	100.0	100.0	100.0	100.0
Professional patient care staff	202,474	273,758	306,688	326,952	64.6	65.8	70.6	71.5
Psychiatrists	18,482	18,846	22,821	24,069	5.9	4.5	5.3	5.3
Psychologists	21,052	22,888	25,021	21,798	6.7	5.5	5.8	4.8
Social workers	36,397	53,487	57,201	55,493	11.6	12.8	13.2	12.1
Registered nurses	54,406	77,686	78,625	105,410	17.4	18.7	18.1	23.0
Other professional staff[1]	72,137	100,851	123,020	120,182	23.0	24.2	28.3	26.3
Other mental health workers	110,769	142,524	127,932	130,551	35.4	34.2	29.4	28.5
State and county mental hospitals								
All patient care staff	117,630	114,198	110,874	102,153	100.0	100.0	100.0	100.0
Professional patient care staff	51,290	50,035	56,953	41,359	43.6	43.8	51.4	40.5
Psychiatrists	4,108	3,849	4,457	3,177	3.5	3.4	4.0	3.1
Psychologists	3,239	3,324	3,620	2,697	2.8	2.9	3.3	2.6
Social workers	6,175	7,013	7,378	5,450	5.2	6.1	6.7	5.3
Registered nurses	16,051	20,848	21,119	17,685	13.6	18.3	19.0	17.3
Other professional staff[1]	21,717	15,001	20,379	12,350	18.5	13.1	18.4	12.1
Other mental health workers	66,340	64,163	53,921	60,794	56.4	56.2	48.6	59.5
Private psychiatric hospitals								
All patient care staff	26,359	57,200	56,877	58,262	100.0	100.0	100.0	100.0
Professional patient care staff	19,524	45,669	44,206	45,669	74.1	79.8	77.7	78.4
Psychiatrists	1,447	1,582	2,081	2,183	5.5	2.8	3.7	3.7
Psychologists	1,461	1,977	1,656	2,003	5.5	3.5	2.9	3.4
Social workers	2,179	4,044	4,587	5,473	8.3	7.1	8.1	9.4
Registered nurses	6,818	14,819	15,086	15,939	25.9	25.9	26.5	27.4
Other professional staff[1]	7,619	23,247	20,796	20,071	28.9	40.6	36.6	34.4
Other mental health workers	6,835	11,531	12,671	12,593	25.9	20.2	22.3	21.6
Non-Federal general hospitals' psychiatric services								
All patient care staff	59,848	72,214	72,880	87,304	100.0	100.0	100.0	100.0
Professional patient care staff	46,335	57,019	58,544	76,558	77.4	79.0	80.3	87.7
Psychiatrists	6,679	6,500	6,160	4,336	11.2	9.0	8.5	5.0
Psychologists	3,283	3,951	4,182	2,441	5.5	5.5	5.7	2.8
Social workers	4,898	7,241	7,985	5,355	8.2	10.0	11.0	6.1
Registered nurses	20,454	28,473	28,355	54,647	34.2	39.4	38.9	62.6
Other professional staff[1]	11,021	10,854	11,862	9,779	18.4	15.0	16.3	11.2
Other mental health workers	13,513	15,195	14,336	10,746	22.6	21.0	19.7	12.3
Department of Veterans Affairs psychiatric services								
All patient care staff	22,948	22,080	20,834	21,671	100.0	100.0	100.0	100.0
Professional patient care staff	16,265	14,619	16,274	18,393	70.9	66.2	78.1	84.9
Psychiatrists	2,463	2,103	3,403	6,272	10.7	9.5	16.3	28.9
Psychologists	1,247	1,476	2,479	587	5.4	6.7	11.9	2.7
Social workers	1,545	1,855	2,244	1,773	6.7	8.4	10.8	8.2
Registered nurses	5,699	5,888	5,485	8,475	24.8	26.7	26.3	39.1
Other professional staff[1]	5,311	3,297	2,663	1,286	23.1	14.9	12.8	5.9
Other mental health workers	6,683	7,461	4,560	3,278	29.1	33.8	21.9	15.1
Residential treatment centers for emotionally disturbed children								
All patient care staff	15,297	40,969	42,801	44,146	100.0	100.0	100.0	100.0
Professional patient care staff	10,551	26,032	30,207	31,079	69.0	63.5	70.6	70.4
Psychiatrists	240	498	748	840	1.6	1.2	1.7	1.9
Psychologists	820	1,492	1,641	1,707	5.4	3.6	3.8	3.9
Social workers	2,283	5,636	6,506	6,635	14.9	13.8	15.2	15.0
Registered nurses	485	1,238	1,367	1,468	3.2	3.0	3.2	3.3
Other professional staff[1]	6,723	17,168	19,945	20,429	43.9	41.9	46.6	46.3
Other mental health workers	4,746	14,937	12,594	13,067	31.0	36.5	29.4	29.6

See footnotes at end of table.

Table 105 (page 2 of 2). Full-time equivalent patient care staff in mental health organizations, according to type of organization and staff discipline: United States, selected years 1984–94

[Data are based on inventories of mental health organizations]

Organization and discipline	1984	1990	1992	1994	1984	1990	1992	1994
All other organizations[2]	Number				Percent distribution			
All patient care staff....................	71,161	109,621	130,354	143,967	100.0	100.0	100.0	100.0
Professional patient care staff	58,509	80,384	100,504	113,894	82.2	73.3	77.1	79.1
Psychiatrists.......................	3,545	4,314	5,972	7,261	5.0	3.9	4.6	5.0
Psychologists......................	11,002	10,668	11,443	12,363	15.5	9.7	8.8	8.6
Social workers	19,317	27,698	28,501	30,807	27.1	25.3	21.9	21.4
Registered nurses...................	4,899	6,420	7,213	7,196	6.9	5.9	5.5	5.0
Other professional staff[1]...............	19,746	31,284	47,375	56,267	27.7	28.5	36.3	39.1
Other mental health workers	12,652	29,237	29,850	30,073	17.8	26.7	22.9	20.9

[1]Includes occupational therapists, recreation therapists, vocational rehabilitation counselors, and teachers.
[2]Includes freestanding outpatient clinics, freestanding day–night organizations, multiservice organizations, and other residential organizations.

NOTES: Full-time equivalent figures presented in this table combine staffing data for inpatient, residential, outpatient, and partial care treatment programs. Some mental health organizations provide a mixture of inpatient and outpatient care (for example Private psychiatric hospitals and Department of Veterans Affairs), while others provide predominantly inpatient (State and county mental hospitals) or outpatient (All other organizations) care. Caution should be exercised in comparing levels of FTE staff between different types of mental health organizations due to the different types of care provided. Figures for nonpatient care staff (administrative, clerical, and maintenance staff) are not shown.

SOURCES: Survey and Analysis Branch, Division of State and Community Systems Development, Center for Mental Health Services. Manderscheid RW, Sonnenschein MA. *Mental health, United States, 1996*. DHHS. 1996; Unpublished data.

Table 106. First-year enrollment and graduates of health professions schools and number of schools, according to profession: United States, selected years 1950–96 and projections for year 2000

[Data are based on reporting by health professions schools]

Year	Medicine	Osteopathy	Registered nursing Total	Baccalaureate	Associate degree	Diploma	Licensed practical nursing	Dentistry	Optometry	Pharmacy	Chiropractic[1]
First-year enrollment											
1980	16,930	1,426	105,952	35,414	53,633	16,905	56,316	6,066	1,185	7,905	- - -
1985	16,997	1,750	118,224	39,573	63,776	14,875	47,034	4,983	1,177	6,749	1,383
1986[2]	16,963	1,737	100,791	34,310	56,635	9,846	44,477	4,777	1,154	6,584	1,712
1987[3]	16,819	1,724	90,693	28,026	54,330	8,337	42,452	4,494	1,210	7,081	1,598
1988[3]	16,713	1,692	94,269	28,505	57,375	8,389	43,774	4,316	1,234	7,309	1,507
1989[3]	16,868	1,780	103,025	29,042	63,973	10,010	47,602	4,148	1,271	8,067	1,531
1990	16,756	1,844	108,580	29,858	68,634	10,088	52,969	3,938	1,258	8,009	1,485
1991	16,876	1,950	113,526	33,437	69,869	10,220	56,176	3,961	1,207	- - -	1,467
1992	17,071	1,974	122,656	37,886	74,079	10,691	58,245	4,006	1,321	8,264	1,411
1993	17,079	2,035	126,837	41,290	75,382	10,165	60,749	4,029	1,359	8,664	1,743
1994	17,121	2,162	129,897	42,953	77,343	9,601	60,632	4,060	- - -	8,970	- - -
1995	17,085	2,217	127,184	43,451	76,016	7,717	57,906	4,078	1,354	9,091	- - -
1996	17,058	2,274	119,205	40,048	72,930	6,227	- - -	4,190	1,396	8,662	- - -
Graduates											
1950[4]	5,553	373	25,790	- - -	- - -	- - -	2,828	2,565	961	- - -	- - -
1960	7,081	427	30,113	4,136	789	25,188	16,491	3,253	364	3,497	660
1970	8,367	432	43,103	9,069	11,483	22,551	36,456	3,749	445	4,758	642
1980	15,135	1,059	75,523	24,994	36,034	14,495	41,892	5,256	1,073	7,432	2,049
1985	16,319	1,474	82,075	24,975	45,208	11,892	36,955	5,353	1,114	5,724	- - -
1986	16,125	1,560	77,027	25,170	41,333	10,524	29,599	4,957	1,085	5,800	1,924
1987	15,836	1,587	70,561	23,761	38,528	8,272	27,285	4,717	1,081	5,854	1,429
1988	15,887	1,572	64,839	21,504	37,397	5,938	26,912	4,581	1,106	6,171	1,650
1989[5]	15,620	1,609	61,660	18,997	37,837	4,826	30,368	4,312	1,143	6,557	1,753
1990	15,336	1,529	66,088	18,571	42,318	5,199	35,417	4,233	1,115	6,956	1,661
1991	15,481	1,534	72,230	19,264	46,794	6,172	38,100	3,995	1,136	7,122	1,631
1992	15,386	1,532	80,839	21,415	52,896	6,528	41,951	3,918	1,150	7,113	1,664
1993	15,512	1,606	88,149	24,442	56,770	6,937	44,822	3,744	1,161	7,380	1,591
1994	15,579	1,775	94,870	28,912	58,839	7,119	45,083	3,840	1,125	7,504	- - -
1995	15,911	1,843	97,052	31,254	58,749	7,049	44,234	3,840	1,219	7,837	- - -
1996	16,029	1,877	94,757	32,413	56,641	5,703	- - -	3,768	1,174	7,943	- - -
2000[6]	16,112	1,934	79,660	26,490	47,790	5,380	- - -	3,242	1,200	7,120	2,950
Schools[7]											
1950[4]	79	6	1,170	- - -	- - -	- - -	85	42	10	- - -	20
1960	86	6	1,137	172	57	908	661	47	10	76	12
1970	103	7	1,340	267	437	636	1,233	53	11	74	11
1980	126	14	1,385	377	697	311	1,299	60	15	72	14
1985	127	15	1,473	441	776	256	1,165	60	16	72	17
1986	127	15	1,469	455	776	238	1,087	59	16	73	17
1987	127	15	1,465	467	789	209	1,068	58	16	74	17
1988	127	15	1,442	479	792	171	1,095	58	16	74	17
1989	127	15	1,457	488	812	157	1,171	58	16	74	17
1990	126	15	1,470	489	829	152	1,154	56	16	74	17
1991	126	15	1,484	501	838	145	1,125	55	16	74	17
1992	126	15	1,484	501	848	135	1,154	55	16	74	17
1993	126	16	1,493	507	857	129	1,159	54	16	74	17
1994	125	16	1,501	509	868	124	1,185	54	16	74	17
1995	125	16	1,516	521	876	119	1,210	53	16	74	- - -
1996	125	17	1,508	523	876	109	- - -	53	16	78	- - -

- - - Data not available.

[1]Chiropractic first-year enrollment data are partial data from eight reporting schools.
[2]First-year enrollment data for optometry exclude Ohio State University.
[3]First-year enrollment data for pharmacy include the University of Puerto Rico.
[4]Data for total registered nursing graduates are for 1951.
[5]Data for chiropractic medicine are estimated.
[6]Projected.
[7]Some nursing schools offer more than one type of program. Numbers shown for nursing are number of nursing programs.

NOTE: Data on the number of schools are reported as of the beginning of the academic year while data on first-year enrollment and number of graduates are reported as of the end of the academic year.

SOURCES: Association of American Medical Colleges: AAMC Data Book, Statistical Information Related to Medical Education. Washington, DC. 1997; Bureau of Health Professions: Health Personnel in the United States, Eighth Report to Congress, 1991. Health Resources and Services Administration. DHHS Pub. No. HRS-P-OD–92–1, Rockville, Maryland. 1992 and unpublished data; National League for Nursing: Nursing data review, 1989 and 1996 and unpublished data; American Nurses Association: Facts About Nursing, 1951 and 1961; American Dental Association 1995/96 Survey of predoctoral dental educational institutions, Chicago. 1996; American Medical Association: Medical education in the United States. JAMA 276(9). September 4, 1996; American Association of Colleges of Osteopathic Medicine. Annual statistical report 1996. Rockville, Maryland. 1996; American Chiropractic Association: Unpublished data.

Table 107 (page 1 of 2). Total enrollment of minorities in schools for selected health occupations, according to detailed race and Hispanic origin: United States, academic years 1970–71, 1980–81, 1990–91, and 1995–96

[Data are based on reporting by health professions associations]

Occupation, detailed race, and Hispanic origin	1970–71[1]	1980–81	1990–91	1995–96[2]	1970–71[1]	1980–81	1990–91	1995–96[2]
Allopathic medicine	Number of students				Percent of students			
All races[3]	40,238	65,189	65,163	66,970	100.0	100.0	100.0	100.0
White, non-Hispanic	37,944	55,434	47,893	44,594	94.3	85.0	73.5	66.6
Black, non-Hispanic	1,509	3,708	4,241	5,337	3.8	5.7	6.5	8.0
Hispanic	196	2,761	3,538	4,349	0.5	4.2	5.4	6.5
Mexican	- - -	951	1,109	1,769	- - -	1.5	1.7	2.6
Mainland Puerto Rican	- - -	329	457	455	- - -	0.5	0.7	0.7
Other Hispanic[4]	- - -	1,481	1,972	2,125	- - -	2.3	3.0	3.2
American Indian	18	221	277	501	0.0	0.3	0.4	0.7
Asian	571	1,924	8,436	11,352	1.4	3.0	12.9	17.0
Osteopathic medicine								
All races	2,304	4,940	6,792	8,475	100.0	100.0	100.0	100.0
White, non-Hispanic[3]	2,241	4,688	5,680	6,808	97.3	94.9	83.6	80.3
Black, non-Hispanic	27	94	217	318	1.2	1.9	3.2	3.8
Hispanic	19	52	277	331	0.8	1.1	4.1	3.9
American Indian	6	19	36	85	0.3	0.4	0.5	1.0
Asian	11	87	582	933	0.5	1.8	8.6	11.0
Podiatry								
All races	1,268	2,577	2,226	2,312	100.0	100.0	100.0	100.0
White, non-Hispanic[3]	1,228	2,353	1,671	1,786	96.8	91.3	75.1	77.2
Black, non-Hispanic	27	110	237	112	2.1	4.3	10.6	4.8
Hispanic	5	39	148	99	0.4	1.5	6.6	4.3
American Indian	1	6	7	12	0.1	0.2	0.3	0.5
Asian	7	69	163	303	0.6	2.7	7.3	13.1
Dentistry[5]								
All races	19,187	22,842	15,770	16,374	100.0	100.0	100.0	100.0
White, non-Hispanic[3]	17,531	20,208	11,185	11,129	91.4	88.5	70.9	68.0
Black, non-Hispanic	872	1,022	940	951	4.5	4.5	6.0	5.8
Hispanic	185	519	1,073	788	1.0	2.3	6.8	4.8
American Indian	28	53	53	73	0.1	0.2	0.3	0.4
Asian	490	1,040	2,519	3,433	2.6	4.6	16.0	21.0
Optometry[5]								
All races	3,094	4,540	4,650	5,178	100.0	100.0	100.0	100.0
White, non-Hispanic[3]	2,913	4,148	3,706	3,903	94.1	91.4	79.7	75.4
Black, non-Hispanic	32	57	134	120	1.0	1.3	2.9	2.3
Hispanic	30	80	186	196	1.0	1.8	4.0	3.8
American Indian	2	12	21	22	0.1	0.3	0.5	0.4
Asian	117	243	603	937	3.8	5.4	13.0	18.1
Pharmacy[5,6]								
All races	17,909	21,628	22,764	33,205	100.0	100.0	100.0	100.0
White, non-Hispanic[3]	16,222	19,153	18,325	23,871	90.6	88.6	80.5	71.9
Black, non-Hispanic	659	945	1,301	2,548	3.7	4.4	5.7	7.7
Hispanic	254	459	945	940	1.4	2.1	4.2	2.8
American Indian	29	36	63	151	0.2	0.2	0.3	0.5
Asian	672	1,035	2,130	5,695	3.8	4.8	9.4	17.2

See footnotes at end of table.

Table 107 (page 2 of 2). Total enrollment of minorities in schools for selected health occupations, according to detailed race and Hispanic origin: United States, academic years 1970–71, 1980–81, 1990–91, and 1995–96

[Data are based on reporting by health professions associations]

Occupation, detailed race, and Hispanic origin	1970–71[1]	1980–81	1990–91	1995–96[2]	1970–71[1]	1980–81	1990–91	1995–96[2]
Registered nurses[5,7]		Number of students				Percent of students		
All races	211,239	230,966	221,170	261,219	100.0	100.0	100.0	100.0
White, non-Hispanic[3]	- - -	- - -	183,102	215,215	- - -	- - -	82.8	82.4
Black, non-Hispanic	- - -	- - -	23,094	24,621	- - -	- - -	10.4	9.4
Hispanic	- - -	- - -	6,580	9,039	- - -	- - -	3.0	3.5
American Indian	- - -	- - -	1,803	1,900	- - -	- - -	0.8	0.7
Asian	- - -	- - -	6,591	10,444	- - -	- - -	3.0	4.0

- - - Data not available.

[1]Data for osteopathic medicine, podiatry, and optometry are for 1971–72. Data for pharmacy and registered nurses are for 1972–73.

[2]Data for podiatry exclude New York College of Podiatric Medicine.

[3]Includes race and ethnicity unspecified.

[4]Includes Puerto Rican Commonwealth students.

[5]Excludes Puerto Rican schools.

[6]Prior to 1992–93 pharmacy total enrollment data are for students in the final 3 years of pharmacy education. Beginning in 1992–93 pharmacy data are for all students.

[7]In 1990 the National League for Nursing developed a new system for analyzing minority data. In evaluating the former system, much underreporting was noted. Therefore, race-specific data before 1990 would not be comparable and are not shown. Additional changes in the minority data question were introduced for academic years 1992–93 and 1993–94 resulting in a discontinuity in the trend.

NOTE: Total enrollment data are collected at the beginning of the academic year.

SOURCES: Association of American Medical Colleges: AAMC Data Book: Statistical Information Related to Medical Education. Washington, DC. 1997; American Association of Colleges of Osteopathic Medicine: 1996 Annual statistical report. Rockville, Maryland. 1996; Bureau of Health Professions: Minorities and women in the health fields, 1990 Edition; American Dental Association 1995/96 Survey of predoctoral dental educational institutions, Chicago. 1996; Association of Schools and Colleges of Optometry: Unpublished data; American Association of Colleges of Pharmacy: Profile of pharmacy students 1995, and unpublished data; American Association of Colleges of Podiatric Medicine: Unpublished data; National League for Nursing: Nursing datasource, vol 1, New York. 1996; Nursing data book. New York. 1982.

Table 108. First-year and total enrollment of women in schools for selected health occupations, according to detailed race and Hispanic origin: United States, academic years 1971–72, 1980–81, 1990–91, and 1995–96

[Data are based on reporting by health professions associations]

Enrollment, occupation, detailed race, and Hispanic origin	Both sexes				Women			
	1971–72[1]	1980–81	1990–91	1995–96[2]	1971–72[1]	1980–81	1990–91	1995–96[2]
First-year enrollment	Number of students				Percent of students			
Allopathic medicine[3]	12,361	17,186	16,876	17,058	13.7	28.9	38.8	43.1
White, non-Hispanic	- - -	14,262	11,830	10,907	- - -	27.4	37.7	41.1
Black, non-Hispanic	881	1,128	1,263	1,528	22.7	45.5	55.3	60.9
Hispanic	- - -	818	933	1,209	- - -	31.5	42.0	42.6
Mexican	118	258	285	535	8.5	30.6	39.3	42.6
Mainland Puerto Rican	40	95	120	127	15.0	43.2	43.3	39.4
Other Hispanic[4]	- - -	465	528	547	- - -	29.7	43.3	43.3
American Indian	23	67	76	150	34.8	35.8	40.8	44.7
Asian	217	572	2,527	3,046	19.4	31.5	40.3	42.0
Dentistry[5]	4,705	5,964	3,961	4,190	3.1	19.8	37.9	35.2
Osteopathic medicine	670	1,496	1,950	2,274	4.3	22.0	34.2	37.4
Podiatry[6]	399	695	622	630	- - -	- - -	- - -	- - -
Optometry[5]	906	1,174	1,207	1,396	5.3	25.3	50.6	52.4
Pharmacy[5,7]	6,532	7,442	8,009	8,662	25.8	48.4	- - -	63.3
Registered nurses[5]	93,344	110,201	113,526	127,184	94.5	92.7	89.3	86.7
Total enrollment								
Allopathic medicine[3]	43,650	65,189	65,163	66,970	10.9	26.5	37.3	41.9
White, non-Hispanic	- - -	55,434	47,893	44,594	- - -	25.0	35.4	39.8
Black, non-Hispanic	2,055	3,708	4,241	5,337	20.4	44.3	55.8	60.0
Hispanic	- - -	2,761	3,538	4,349	- - -	30.1	39.0	43.2
Mexican	252	951	1,109	1,769	9.5	26.4	38.5	42.1
Mainland Puerto Rican	76	329	457	455	17.1	35.9	43.1	44.4
Other Hispanic[4]	- - -	1,481	1,972	2,125	- - -	31.1	38.4	43.8
American Indian	42	221	277	501	23.8	28.5	42.6	44.5
Asian	647	1,924	8,436	11,352	17.9	30.4	37.7	41.2
Dentistry[5]	16,553	22,842	15,770	16,374	- - -	17.0	34.2	36.5
Osteopathic medicine	2,304	4,940	6,792	8,475	3.4	19.7	32.7	36.3
Podiatry[6]	1,268	2,577	2,226	2,312	1.2	11.9	- - -	- - -
Optometry[5]	3,094	4,540	4,650	5,178	- - -	- - -	47.3	53.0
Registered nurses[5]	211,239	230,966	221,170	261,219	95.5	94.3	- - -	86.9

- - - Data not available.

[1]Total enrollments for registered nurse students are for 1972–73.
[2]First-year enrollments for registered nurse students are for 1994–95.
[3]Includes race and ethnicity unspecified.
[4]Includes Puerto Rican Commonwealth students.
[5]Excludes Puerto Rican schools.
[6]Podiatry data for 1995–96 exclude New York College of Podiatric Medicine.
[7]Pharmacy first-year enrollment data are for students in the first year of the final 3 years of pharmacy education.

NOTES: Data not available on total enrollment of women in schools of pharmacy. Total enrollment data are collected at the beginning of the academic year while first-year enrollment data are collected during the academic year.

SOURCES: Association of American Medical Colleges: AAMC Data Book: Statistical Information Related to Medical Education. Washington, DC., 1997 and unpublished data; American Association of Colleges of Osteopathic Medicine: 1996 Annual Statistical Report. Rockville, Maryland. 1996; Bureau of Health Professions: Minorities and women in the health fields, 1990 edition; American Dental Association 1995/96 Survey of predoctoral dental educational institutions, Chicago. 1996; Association of Schools and Colleges of Optometry: Unpublished data; American Association of Colleges of Pharmacy: Unpublished data; American Association of Colleges of Podiatric Medicine: Unpublished data; National League for Nursing: Nursing datasource. New York. 1996; Nursing data book. New York. 1982; State-Approved Schools of Nursing-RN. New York. 1973.

Table 109. Hospitals, beds, and occupancy rates, according to type of ownership and size of hospital: United States, selected years 1975–96

[Data are based on reporting by a census of hospitals]

Type of ownership and size of hospital	1975	1980	1985	1990	1993	1994	1995	1996
Hospitals				Number				
All hospitals	7,156	6,965	6,872	6,649	6,467	6,374	6,291	6,201
Federal	382	359	343	337	316	307	299	290
Non-Federal[1]	6,774	6,606	6,529	6,312	6,151	6,067	5,992	5,911
Community[2]	5,875	5,830	5,732	5,384	5,261	5,229	5,194	5,134
Nonprofit	3,339	3,322	3,349	3,191	3,154	3,139	3,092	3,045
Proprietary	775	730	805	749	717	719	752	759
State-local government	1,761	1,778	1,578	1,444	1,390	1,371	1,350	1,330
6–24 beds	299	259	208	226	227	235	278	262
25–49 beds	1,155	1,029	982	935	894	900	922	906
50–99 beds	1,481	1,462	1,399	1,263	1,181	1,157	1,139	1,128
100–199 beds	1,363	1,370	1,407	1,306	1,337	1,331	1,324	1,338
200–299 beds	678	715	739	739	730	746	718	692
300–399 beds	378	412	439	408	402	377	354	361
400–499 beds	230	266	239	222	205	210	195	196
500 beds or more	291	317	319	285	285	273	264	251
Beds								
All hospitals	1,465,828	1,364,516	1,317,630	1,213,327	1,163,460	1,128,066	1,080,601	1,061,688
Federal	131,946	117,328	112,023	98,255	87,847	83,823	77,079	73,171
Non-Federal[1]	1,333,882	1,247,188	1,205,607	1,115,072	1,075,613	1,044,243	1,003,522	988,517
Community[2]	941,844	988,387	1,000,678	927,360	918,786	902,061	872,736	862,352
Nonprofit	658,195	692,459	707,451	656,755	651,272	636,949	609,729	598,162
Proprietary	73,495	87,033	103,921	101,377	98,964	100,667	105,737	109,197
State-local government	210,154	208,895	189,306	169,228	168,550	164,445	157,270	154,993
6–24 beds	5,615	4,932	4,031	4,427	4,323	4,388	5,085	4,770
25–49 beds	41,783	37,478	36,833	35,420	33,711	33,635	34,352	33,814
50–99 beds	106,776	105,278	101,680	90,394	84,950	83,018	82,024	81,185
100–199 beds	192,438	192,892	199,690	183,867	189,234	187,369	187,381	189,630
200–299 beds	164,405	172,390	180,165	179,670	178,864	182,111	175,240	168,977
300–399 beds	127,728	139,434	151,919	138,938	138,473	129,300	121,136	123,822
400–499 beds	101,278	117,724	106,653	98,833	91,389	93,415	86,459	86,913
500 beds or more	201,821	218,259	219,707	195,811	197,842	188,825	181,059	173,241
Occupancy rate				Percent of beds occupied				
All hospitals	76.7	77.7	69.0	69.5	67.3	66.0	65.7	64.5
Federal	80.7	80.1	76.3	72.9	76.0	74.9	72.6	71.4
Non-Federal[1]	76.3	77.4	68.4	69.2	66.6	65.3	65.1	64.0
Community[2]	75.0	75.6	64.8	66.8	64.4	62.9	62.8	61.5
Nonprofit	77.5	78.2	67.2	69.3	66.4	64.8	64.5	63.3
Proprietary	65.9	65.2	52.1	52.8	51.1	50.1	51.8	51.6
State-local government	70.4	71.1	62.9	65.3	64.5	63.5	63.7	61.7
6–24 beds	48.0	46.8	34.7	32.3	30.8	31.7	36.9	33.2
25–49 beds	56.7	52.8	40.0	41.3	41.4	40.9	42.6	40.0
50–99 beds	64.7	64.2	51.8	53.8	53.2	53.1	54.1	53.1
100–199 beds	71.2	71.4	59.7	61.5	59.3	58.2	58.8	57.8
200–299 beds	77.1	77.4	65.7	67.1	64.3	62.9	63.1	62.0
300–399 beds	79.7	79.7	68.4	70.0	66.9	65.5	64.8	63.6
400–499 beds	81.1	81.2	70.1	73.5	69.9	68.9	68.1	67.4
500 beds or more	80.9	82.1	74.6	77.3	74.6	71.8	71.4	69.7

[1]The category of non-Federal hospitals is comprised of psychiatric, tuberculosis and other respiratory disease hospitals, and long-term and short-term hospitals.
[2]Community hospitals are short-term hospitals excluding hospital units in institutions such as prison and college infirmaries, facilities for the mentally retarded, and alcoholism and chemical dependency hospitals.

SOURCES: American Hospital Association: Hospital Statistics, 1976, 1981, 1986, 1991–98 Editions. Chicago, 1976, 1981, 1986, 1991–98. (Copyrights 1976, 1981, 1986, 1991–98: Used with the permission of the American Hospital Association and Healthcare InfoSource.)

Table 110. Inpatient and residential mental health organizations and beds, according to type of organization: United States, selected years 1984–94

[Data are based on inventories of mental health organizations]

Type of organization	1984	1986	1988	1990	1992	1994
	Number of mental health organizations					
All organizations.	2,849	3,039	3,231	3,430	3,415	3,319
State and county mental hospitals	277	285	285	273	273	256
Private psychiatric hospitals.	220	314	444	462	475	430
Non-Federal general hospital psychiatric services . . .	1,259	1,287	1,425	1,571	1,517	1,531
Department of Veterans Affairs psychiatric services[1]	124	124	125	130	133	135
Residential treatment centers for emotionally disturbed children	322	437	440	501	497	459
All other[2]	647	592	512	493	520	508
	Number of beds					
All organizations.	262,673	267,613	271,923	272,253	270,867	252,333
State and county mental hospitals	130,411	119,033	107,109	98,789	93,058	79,294
Private psychiatric hospitals.	21,474	30,201	42,255	44,871	43,684	41,195
Non-Federal general hospital psychiatric services . . .	46,045	45,808	48,421	53,479	52,059	52,984
Department of Veterans Affairs psychiatric services[1]	23,546	26,874	25,742	21,712	22,466	21,146
Residential treatment centers for emotionally disturbed children	16,745	24,547	25,173	29,756	30,089	32,110
All other[2]	24,452	21,150	23,223	23,646	29,511	25,604
	Beds per 100,000 civilian population					
All organizations.	112.9	111.7	111.4	111.6	107.4	97.5
State and county mental hospitals	56.1	49.7	44.0	40.5	36.9	30.6
Private psychiatric hospitals.	9.2	12.6	17.3	18.4	17.3	15.9
Non-Federal general hospital psychiatric services . . .	19.8	19.1	19.8	21.9	20.7	20.5
Department of Veterans Affairs psychiatric services[1]	10.1	11.2	10.5	8.9	8.9	8.2
Residential treatment centers for emotionally disturbed children	7.2	10.3	10.3	12.2	11.9	12.4
All other[2]	10.5	8.8	9.5	9.7	11.7	9.9

[1]Includes Department of Veterans Affairs neuropsychiatric hospitals and general hospital psychiatric services.

[2]Includes other multiservice mental health organizations with inpatient and residential treatment services that are not elsewhere classified. See Appendix I.

SOURCES: Survey and Analysis Branch, Division of State and Community Systems Development, Center for Mental Health Services. Manderscheid RW, Sonnenschein MA. *Mental health, United States, 1996*. DHHS. 1996.

Table 111. Community hospital beds and average annual percent change, according to geographic division and State: United States, selected years 1940–96

[Data are based on reporting by facilities]

Geographic division and State	Beds per 1,000 civilian population							Average annual percent change				
	1940[1,2]	1950[1,2]	1960[2,3]	1970[2]	1980[2]	1990[4]	1996[4]	1940–60[1,2,3]	1960–70[2,3]	1970–80[2]	1980–90[5]	1990–96[4]
United States	3.2	3.3	3.6	4.3	4.5	3.7	3.3	0.6	1.8	0.5	−1.7	−1.9
New England	4.4	4.2	3.9	4.1	4.1	3.4	2.7	−0.6	0.5	0.0	−1.9	−3.8
Maine	3.0	3.2	3.4	4.7	4.7	3.7	3.1	0.6	3.3	0.0	−2.1	−2.9
New Hampshire	4.2	4.2	4.4	4.0	3.9	3.1	2.8	0.2	−0.9	−0.3	−2.3	−1.7
Vermont	3.3	4.0	4.5	4.5	4.4	3.0	2.8	1.6	0.0	−0.2	−3.4	−1.1
Massachusetts............	5.1	4.8	4.2	4.4	4.4	3.6	3.0	−1.0	0.5	0.0	−2.0	−3.0
Rhode Island	3.9	3.8	3.7	4.0	3.8	3.2	2.7	−0.3	0.8	−0.5	−1.7	−2.8
Connecticut	3.7	3.6	3.4	3.4	3.5	2.9	2.2	−0.4	0.0	0.3	−1.9	−4.5
Middle Atlantic.............	3.9	3.8	4.0	4.4	4.6	4.1	3.9	0.1	1.0	0.4	−0.9	−0.8
New York.................	4.3	4.1	4.3	4.6	4.5	4.1	4.0	0.0	0.7	−0.2	−0.7	−0.4
New Jersey	3.5	3.2	3.1	3.6	4.2	3.7	3.5	−0.6	1.5	1.6	−1.3	−0.9
Pennsylvania.............	3.5	3.8	4.1	4.7	4.8	4.4	3.9	0.8	1.4	0.2	−0.9	−2.0
East North Central...........	3.2	3.2	3.6	4.4	4.7	3.9	3.3	0.6	2.0	0.7	−1.8	−2.7
Ohio	2.7	2.9	3.4	4.2	4.7	4.0	3.3	1.2	2.1	1.1	−1.6	−3.2
Indiana	2.3	2.6	3.1	4.0	4.5	3.9	3.3	1.5	2.6	1.2	−1.4	−2.7
Illinois	3.4	3.6	4.0	4.7	5.1	4.0	3.4	0.8	1.6	0.8	−2.4	−2.7
Michigan	4.0	3.3	3.3	4.3	4.4	3.7	3.0	−1.0	2.7	0.2	−1.7	−3.4
Wisconsin	3.4	3.7	4.3	5.2	4.9	3.8	3.2	1.2	1.9	−0.6	−2.5	−2.8
West North Central	3.1	3.7	4.3	5.7	5.8	4.9	4.3	1.6	2.9	0.2	−1.7	−2.2
Minnesota	3.9	4.4	4.8	6.1	5.7	4.4	3.8	1.0	2.4	−0.7	−2.6	−2.4
Iowa....................	2.7	3.2	3.9	5.6	5.7	5.1	4.3	1.9	3.7	0.2	−1.1	−2.8
Missouri.................	2.9	3.3	3.9	5.1	5.7	4.8	4.0	1.5	2.7	1.1	−1.7	−3.0
North Dakota.............	3.5	4.3	5.2	6.8	7.4	7.0	6.6	2.0	2.7	0.8	−0.6	−1.0
South Dakota.............	2.8	4.4	4.5	5.6	5.5	6.1	6.1	2.4	2.2	−0.2	1.0	0.0
Nebraska................	3.4	4.2	4.4	6.2	6.0	5.5	5.0	1.3	3.5	−0.3	−1.0	−1.6
Kansas	2.8	3.4	4.2	5.4	5.8	4.8	4.3	2.0	2.5	0.7	−1.9	−1.8
South Atlantic	2.5	2.8	3.3	4.0	4.5	3.7	3.3	1.4	1.9	1.2	−1.9	−1.9
Delaware.................	4.4	3.9	3.7	3.7	3.6	3.0	2.2	−0.9	0.0	−0.3	−1.8	−5.0
Maryland................	3.9	3.6	3.3	3.1	3.6	2.8	2.5	−0.8	−0.6	1.5	−2.1	−1.9
District of Columbia	5.5	5.5	5.9	7.4	7.3	7.6	6.9	0.4	2.3	−0.1	0.3	−1.6
Virginia	2.2	2.5	3.0	3.7	4.1	3.3	2.8	1.6	2.1	1.0	−2.1	−2.7
West Virginia	2.7	3.1	4.1	5.4	5.5	4.7	4.4	2.1	2.8	0.2	−1.6	−1.1
North Carolina	2.2	2.6	3.4	3.8	4.2	3.3	3.1	2.2	1.1	1.0	−2.1	−1.0
South Carolina...........	1.8	2.4	2.9	3.7	3.9	3.3	3.0	2.4	2.5	0.5	−1.7	−1.6
Georgia.................	1.7	2.0	2.8	3.8	4.6	4.0	3.6	2.5	3.1	1.9	−1.4	−1.7
Florida..................	2.8	2.9	3.1	4.4	5.1	3.9	3.5	0.5	3.6	1.5	−2.4	−1.8
East South Central	1.7	2.1	3.0	4.4	5.1	4.7	4.2	2.9	3.9	1.5	−0.6	−1.9
Kentucky................	1.8	2.2	3.0	4.0	4.5	4.3	3.9	2.6	2.9	1.2	−0.2	−1.7
Tennessee...............	1.9	2.3	3.4	4.7	5.5	4.8	3.9	3.0	3.3	1.6	−1.1	−3.4
Alabama.................	1.5	2.0	2.8	4.3	5.1	4.6	4.4	3.2	4.4	1.7	−1.0	−0.8
Mississippi...............	1.4	1.7	2.9	4.4	5.3	5.0	4.9	3.7	4.3	1.9	0.0	−0.3
West South Central	2.1	2.7	3.3	4.3	4.7	3.8	3.3	2.3	2.7	0.9	−1.8	−2.2
Arkansas.................	1.4	1.6	2.9	4.2	5.0	4.6	4.1	3.7	3.8	1.8	−0.6	−1.9
Louisiana................	3.1	3.8	3.9	4.2	4.8	4.6	4.4	1.2	0.7	1.3	−0.4	−0.6
Oklahoma................	1.9	2.5	3.2	4.5	4.6	4.0	3.3	2.6	3.5	0.2	−1.4	−3.1
Texas	2.0	2.7	3.3	4.3	4.7	3.5	3.0	2.5	2.7	0.9	−2.9	−2.7
Mountain	3.6	3.8	3.5	4.3	3.8	3.1	2.5	−0.1	2.1	−1.2	−2.0	−3.3
Montana	4.9	5.3	5.1	5.8	5.9	5.8	4.8	0.2	1.3	0.2	−0.2	−3.1
Idaho	2.6	3.4	3.2	4.0	3.7	3.2	2.9	1.0	2.3	−0.8	−1.4	−1.6
Wyoming	3.5	3.9	4.6	5.5	3.6	4.8	4.2	1.4	1.8	−4.1	3.1	−2.3
Colorado.................	3.9	4.2	3.8	4.6	4.2	3.2	2.4	−0.1	1.9	−0.9	−2.7	−4.6
New Mexico..............	2.7	2.2	2.9	3.5	3.1	2.8	2.2	0.4	1.9	−1.2	−0.7	−4.1
Arizona..................	3.4	4.0	3.0	4.1	3.6	2.7	2.3	−0.6	3.2	−1.3	−2.8	−2.4
Utah....................	3.2	2.9	2.8	3.6	3.1	2.6	2.2	−0.7	2.5	−1.5	−1.7	−3.0
Nevada..................	5.0	4.4	3.9	4.2	4.2	2.8	2.2	−1.2	0.7	0.0	−3.6	−3.7
Pacific	4.1	3.2	3.1	3.7	3.5	2.7	2.3	−1.4	1.8	−0.6	−2.6	−2.4
Washington	3.4	3.6	3.3	3.5	3.1	2.5	2.0	−0.1	0.6	−1.2	−2.1	−3.5
Oregon	3.5	3.1	3.5	4.0	3.5	2.8	2.2	0.0	1.3	−1.3	−1.9	−3.7
California................	4.4	3.3	3.0	3.8	3.6	2.7	2.4	−1.9	2.4	−0.5	−2.8	−2.0
Alaska..................	...	...	2.4	2.3	2.7	2.3	1.9	...	−0.4	1.6	−1.6	−2.8
Hawaii..................	...	...	3.7	3.4	3.1	2.7	2.7	...	−0.8	−0.9	−1.0	−0.1

... Category not applicable.
[1] 1940 and 1950 data are estimated based on published figures.
[2] Data exclude facilities for the mentally retarded. See Appendix II, Hospital.
[3] 1960 data include hospital units of institutions.
[4] Starting with 1990, data exclude hospital units of institutions, facilities for the mentally retarded, and alcoholism and chemical dependency hospitals. See Appendix II.
[5] 1990 data used in this calculation (not shown in table) exclude only facilities for the mentally retarded, consistent with exclusions from 1980 data.

SOURCES: American Medical Association: Hospital service in United States. JAMA 116(11):1055–1144, 1941, and 146(2):109–184, 1951. (Copyright 1941, 1951: Used with permission of American Medical Association.); American Hospital Association: Hospitals. JAHA 35(15):383–430, Aug. 1, 1961. (Copyright 1961: Used with permission of American Hospital Association.); data computed by Centers for Disease Control and Prevention, National Center for Health Statistics, Division of Health and Utilization Analysis from data compiled by Division of Health Care Statistics, National Master Facility Inventory, and American Hospital Association annual surveys.

Table 112. Occupancy rates in community hospitals and average annual percent change, according to geographic division and State: United States, selected years 1940–96

[Data are based on reporting by facilities]

Geographic division and State	Percent of beds occupied						Average annual percent change				
	1940[1,2]	1960[2,3]	1970[2]	1980[2]	1990[4]	1996[4]	1940–60[1,2,3]	1960–70[2,3]	1970–80[2]	1980–90[5]	1990–96[4]
United States	69.9	74.7	77.3	75.2	66.8	61.6	0.3	0.3	–0.3	–1.2	–1.3
New England	72.5	75.2	79.7	80.1	74.0	67.6	0.2	0.6	0.1	–0.7	–1.5
Maine	72.4	73.2	73.0	74.5	71.5	64.5	0.1	–0.0	0.2	–0.4	–1.7
New Hampshire	65.3	66.5	73.4	73.2	66.8	59.8	0.1	1.0	–0.0	–0.9	–1.8
Vermont	68.8	68.5	76.3	73.7	67.3	74.0	–0.0	1.1	–0.3	–1.0	1.6
Massachusetts	71.8	75.8	80.3	81.7	74.2	67.4	0.3	0.6	0.2	–0.9	–1.6
Rhode Island	77.7	75.7	82.9	85.9	79.4	67.2	–0.1	0.9	0.4	–0.8	–2.7
Connecticut	75.9	78.2	82.6	80.4	77.0	71.6	0.1	0.5	–0.3	–0.4	–1.2
Middle Atlantic	75.5	78.1	82.4	83.2	80.5	72.4	0.2	0.5	0.1	–0.4	–1.8
New York	78.9	79.4	82.9	85.9	86.0	76.6	0.0	0.4	0.4	–0.0	–1.9
New Jersey	72.4	78.4	82.5	82.8	80.2	70.3	0.4	0.5	0.0	–0.3	–2.2
Pennsylvania	71.3	76.0	81.5	79.5	72.9	67.3	0.3	0.7	–0.2	–0.9	–1.3
East North Central	71.0	78.4	79.5	76.9	64.6	59.1	0.5	0.1	–0.3	–1.7	–1.5
Ohio	72.1	81.3	81.8	79.2	64.7	57.4	0.6	0.1	–0.3	–2.0	–2.0
Indiana	68.5	79.6	80.3	77.6	60.6	56.7	0.8	0.1	–0.3	–2.4	–1.1
Illinois	73.1	76.0	79.3	74.9	65.7	58.7	0.2	0.4	–0.6	–1.2	–1.9
Michigan	71.5	80.5	80.6	78.2	65.5	63.8	0.6	0.0	–0.3	–1.8	–0.4
Wisconsin	65.2	73.9	73.2	73.6	64.6	58.1	0.6	–0.1	0.1	–1.3	–1.8
West North Central	65.7	71.8	73.6	71.2	61.8	58.5	0.4	0.2	–0.3	–1.4	–0.9
Minnesota	71.0	72.3	73.9	73.7	66.8	65.4	0.1	0.2	–0.0	–1.0	–0.4
Iowa	63.6	72.6	71.9	68.7	61.7	57.0	0.7	–0.1	–0.5	–1.1	–1.3
Missouri	68.6	75.8	79.3	75.1	61.8	56.3	0.5	0.5	–0.5	–1.9	–1.5
North Dakota	61.9	71.3	67.1	68.6	64.2	62.4	0.7	–0.6	0.2	–0.6	–0.5
South Dakota	59.1	66.0	66.3	60.6	62.1	64.7	0.6	0.0	–0.9	0.2	0.7
Nebraska	59.0	65.6	69.9	67.4	57.6	55.4	0.5	0.6	–0.4	–1.4	–0.6
Kansas	60.4	69.1	71.4	68.8	55.6	51.6	0.7	0.3	–0.4	–2.1	–1.2
South Atlantic	66.7	74.8	77.9	75.5	67.4	62.0	0.6	0.4	–0.3	–1.2	–1.4
Delaware	59.2	70.2	78.8	81.8	76.5	79.0	0.9	1.2	0.4	–0.7	0.5
Maryland	74.6	73.9	79.3	84.0	78.6	68.0	–0.0	0.7	0.6	–0.7	–2.4
District of Columbia	76.2	80.8	77.7	83.0	75.3	75.9	0.3	–0.4	0.7	–0.9	0.1
Virginia	70.0	78.0	81.1	77.8	67.4	62.5	0.5	0.4	–0.4	–1.5	–1.3
West Virginia	62.1	74.5	79.3	75.6	62.7	59.1	0.9	0.6	–0.5	–1.9	–1.0
North Carolina	64.6	73.9	78.5	77.8	73.2	67.4	0.7	0.6	–0.1	–0.6	–1.4
South Carolina	69.1	76.9	76.4	77.0	70.9	63.2	0.5	–0.1	0.1	–0.9	–1.9
Georgia	62.7	71.7	76.5	70.4	65.8	60.0	0.7	0.7	–0.8	–0.8	–1.5
Florida	57.5	73.9	76.2	71.7	61.8	57.6	1.3	0.3	–0.6	–1.5	–1.2
East South Central	62.6	71.8	78.2	74.6	62.6	59.2	0.7	0.9	–0.5	–1.8	–0.9
Kentucky	61.6	73.4	79.6	77.4	62.4	57.5	0.9	0.8	–0.3	–2.2	–1.4
Tennessee	65.5	75.9	78.2	75.9	64.4	60.3	0.7	0.3	–0.3	–1.7	–1.1
Alabama	59.0	70.8	80.0	73.3	62.5	57.8	0.9	1.2	–0.9	–1.6	–1.3
Mississippi	63.8	62.8	73.6	70.5	59.4	61.6	–0.1	1.6	–0.4	–1.7	0.6
West South Central	62.5	68.7	73.2	69.7	57.8	54.3	0.5	0.6	–0.5	–1.9	–1.0
Arkansas	55.6	70.0	74.4	69.6	62.0	56.7	1.2	0.6	–0.7	–1.2	–1.5
Louisiana	75.0	67.9	73.6	69.7	57.4	53.1	–0.5	0.8	–0.5	–1.9	–1.3
Oklahoma	54.5	71.0	72.5	68.1	57.7	52.8	1.3	0.2	–0.6	–1.6	–1.5
Texas	59.6	68.2	73.0	70.1	57.2	54.6	0.7	0.7	–0.4	–2.0	–0.8
Mountain	60.9	69.9	71.2	69.6	60.5	58.2	0.7	0.2	–0.2	–1.4	–0.6
Montana	62.8	60.3	65.9	66.1	61.2	66.9	–0.2	0.9	0.0	–0.7	1.5
Idaho	65.4	55.9	66.1	65.2	55.7	55.8	–0.8	1.7	–0.1	–1.5	0.0
Wyoming	47.5	61.1	63.1	57.2	53.8	52.3	1.3	0.3	–1.0	–0.6	–0.5
Colorado	62.1	80.6	74.0	71.6	64.0	57.0	1.3	–0.9	–0.3	–1.2	–1.9
New Mexico	47.8	65.1	69.8	66.2	57.5	57.8	1.6	0.7	–0.5	–1.4	0.1
Arizona	61.2	74.2	73.3	74.2	61.8	59.7	1.0	–0.1	0.1	–1.7	–0.6
Utah	65.8	70.0	73.7	70.0	58.7	50.4	0.3	0.5	–0.5	–1.7	–2.5
Nevada	67.9	70.7	72.7	68.8	60.2	62.4	0.2	0.3	–0.5	–1.4	0.6
Pacific	69.7	71.4	71.0	69.0	63.8	58.5	0.1	–0.1	–0.3	–0.8	–1.4
Washington	67.5	63.4	69.7	71.7	62.7	54.8	–0.3	1.0	0.3	–1.4	–2.2
Oregon	71.2	65.8	69.3	69.3	56.7	51.8	–0.4	0.5	0.0	–2.0	–1.5
California	69.9	74.3	71.3	68.5	64.1	58.9	0.3	–0.4	–0.4	–0.7	–1.4
Alaska	. . .	53.8	59.1	58.3	49.5	56.7	. . .	0.9	–0.1	–1.5	2.3
Hawaii	. . .	61.5	75.7	74.7	85.1	76.9	. . .	2.1	–0.1	1.2	–1.7

0.0 Quantity more than zero but less than 0.05.   . . . Category not applicable.

[1] 1940 data are estimated based on published figures.
[2] Data exclude facilities for the mentally retarded. See Appendix II, Hospital.
[3] 1960 data include hospital units of institutions.
[4] Starting with 1990, data exclude hospital units of institutions, facilities for the mentally retarded, and alcoholism and chemical dependency hospitals. See Appendix II.
[5] 1990 data used in this calculation (not shown in table) exclude only facilities for the mentally retarded, consistent with exclusions from 1980 data.

NOTE: Occupancy rates exclude data for newborns from the numerator.

SOURCES: American Medical Association: Hospital service in United States. JAMA 116(11):1055–1144, 1941. (Copyright 1941: Used with permission of American Medical Association.); American Hospital Association: Hospitals. JAHA 35(15):383–430, Aug. 1, 1961. (Copyright 1961: Used with permission of American Hospital Association.); data computed by Centers for Disease Control and Prevention, National Center for Health Statistics, Division of Health and Utilization Analysis from data compiled by Division of Health Care Statistics, National Master Facility Inventory, and American Hospital Association annual surveys.

Table 113. Nursing homes with 3 or more beds, beds, and bed rates, according to geographic division and State: United States, 1976, 1986, and 1991

[Data are based on reporting by facilities]

Geographic division and State	Nursing homes			Beds			Bed rate[1]		
	1976	1986	1991	1976	1986	1991	1976	1986	1991
United States	16,091	16,388	14,744	1,298,968	1,504,683	1,559,394	685.3	542.1	494.5
New England	1,435	1,305	1,157	93,418	106,231	108,194	731.7	584.8	550.4
Maine	189	160	130	7,653	9,047	9,192	656.6	524.3	497.6
New Hampshire	99	92	79	6,110	6,901	7,493	761.6	550.5	545.7
Vermont	83	61	50	3,635	3,058	3,478	708.9	430.6	451.9
Massachusetts	694	641	554	46,436	50,675	50,133	732.4	580.2	540.3
Rhode Island	103	108	104	7,067	9,821	9,915	713.0	674.0	616.9
Connecticut	267	243	240	22,517	26,729	27,983	761.8	624.0	585.2
Middle Atlantic	1,607	1,643	1,497	178,323	211,274	220,241	527.4	447.7	423.9
New York	647	579	536	88,680	91,868	94,884	534.6	403.6	384.0
New Jersey	346	333	307	30,894	35,174	39,970	507.6	395.7	413.4
Pennsylvania	614	731	654	58,749	84,232	85,387	527.4	541.9	485.9
East North Central	3,184	3,254	3,029	288,352	324,442	331,278	806.5	654.6	602.1
Ohio	886	944	869	61,953	82,340	82,516	660.0	640.4	581.9
Indiana	466	454	528	36,029	47,081	55,701	752.3	721.4	759.1
Illinois	830	744	758	84,530	94,474	95,465	849.3	697.0	638.0
Michigan	543	690	469	56,858	50,552	48,886	824.5	511.3	446.7
Wisconsin	459	422	405	48,982	49,995	48,710	1,036.6	741.8	641.1
West North Central	2,185	2,139	2,108	163,231	182,256	187,639	803.2	663.5	610.4
Minnesota	456	400	399	41,313	43,574	42,001	932.9	685.0	600.3
Iowa	450	422	423	30,245	33,941	34,521	773.1	666.5	617.6
Missouri	439	575	525	32,677	48,262	51,652	605.0	665.3	619.7
North Dakota	80	67	70	6,015	5,904	6,056	845.9	625.2	519.3
South Dakota	133	115	122	8,154	7,800	8,448	909.5	643.1	626.6
Nebraska	264	209	209	22,484	17,288	17,846	1,097.6	634.4	599.3
Kansas	363	351	360	22,343	25,487	27,115	764.0	657.2	626.8
South Atlantic	1,749	2,150	1,883	140,161	187,935	210,534	531.3	428.4	393.0
Delaware	29	40	45	2,228	3,319	4,101	514.8	481.7	556.7
Maryland	183	207	212	18,804	24,330	27,163	695.0	573.6	567.6
District of Columbia	53	25	18	2,632	2,885	3,010	444.9	365.4	383.2
Virginia	244	235	217	23,251	24,440	26,324	680.3	463.1	426.0
West Virginia	102	95	107	5,152	7,753	9,792	298.0	334.1	376.9
North Carolina	414	357	283	19,891	26,159	28,259	541.5	432.2	387.3
South Carolina	108	182	132	8,224	13,471	13,122	501.8	496.0	410.3
Georgia	314	372	324	28,908	32,028	35,011	867.7	613.0	587.7
Florida	302	637	545	31,071	53,550	63,752	350.7	323.4	289.4
East South Central	867	970	890	65,037	86,124	93,932	562.1	517.1	490.5
Kentucky	258	331	271	18,215	22,886	25,685	590.9	538.1	536.7
Tennessee	267	279	275	19,125	28,077	32,493	547.6	534.8	534.6
Alabama	211	217	197	19,188	21,685	21,323	646.1	505.3	426.6
Mississippi	131	143	147	8,509	13,476	14,431	420.1	471.0	439.1
West South Central	1,758	1,889	1,935	157,492	187,267	199,056	913.9	726.0	665.5
Arkansas	212	231	221	19,357	21,448	21,706	862.7	688.3	601.9
Louisiana	203	276	298	19,030	32,615	36,644	716.2	833.0	829.4
Oklahoma	345	366	386	25,890	29,570	32,421	874.2	731.5	691.8
Texas	998	1,016	1,030	93,215	103,634	108,285	994.8	704.0	629.6
Mountain	630	642	611	47,662	53,564	59,113	680.5	472.1	423.4
Montana	89	63	70	4,944	4,898	5,713	611.4	501.1	517.3
Idaho	63	66	57	4,567	4,694	4,887	640.8	463.1	408.3
Wyoming	24	26	25	1,721	2,165	2,243	584.4	517.4	485.6
Colorado	225	197	176	22,005	17,323	17,609	1,079.9	574.4	516.3
New Mexico	46	63	62	3,011	4,902	5,933	435.5	415.4	399.2
Arizona	70	107	112	5,884	11,250	13,265	406.2	374.7	329.3
Utah	94	91	82	4,233	5,655	6,292	574.7	482.2	434.0
Nevada	19	29	27	1,297	2,677	3,171	473.2	474.2	384.9
Pacific	2,676	2,396	1,634	165,292	165,590	149,407	668.8	441.6	361.1
Washington	323	294	269	28,436	27,986	26,506	807.3	545.3	457.8
Oregon	233	199	183	15,317	16,068	14,382	641.6	457.1	358.2
California	2,031	1,831	1,133	118,145	118,848	105,781	646.1	425.6	348.3
Alaska	10	10	11	770	1,082	780	1,285.5	950.0	591.8
Hawaii	79	62	38	2,624	1,606	1,958	571.6	197.6	184.2

[1]Number of beds per 1,000 resident population 85 years of age and over.

NOTES: Estimates of nursing homes, nursing home beds, and utilization rates from the National Health Provider Inventory (NHPI) and the Online Survey and Certification and Reporting (OSCAR) database may differ because NHPI is a national survey of licensed nursing homes, including facilities managed by the Department of Veterans Affairs (DVA) and excluding hospital-based nursing homes, whereas the OSCAR database is a national census of currently-certified Medicare and/or Medicaid nursing homes and excludes licensed facilities that do not accept federal funding and facilities managed by DVA. See Appendix I.

SOURCES: Centers for Disease Control and Prevention, National Center for Health Statistics (NCHS): Strahan GW. Trends in nursing and related care homes and hospitals, United States, selected years 1969–80. Vital Health Stat 14(30). 1984; and Sirrocco A. Nursing home characteristics: 1986 Inventory of Long-Term Care Places. Vital Health Stat 14(33). 1989; unpublished data from the 1991 National Health Provider Inventory (National Master Facility Inventory); U.S. Bureau of the Census: Current Population Reports. Series P–25, No. 1106, March 1994. Washington; rates for 1976 and 1986 are based on data from Compressed Mortality File, a county-level national mortality and population database.

Table 114. Nursing homes, beds, occupancy, and residents, according to geographic division and State: United States, 1992 and 1996

[Data are based on a census of certified nursing facilities]

Geographic division and State	Nursing homes 1992	Nursing homes 1996	Beds 1992	Beds 1996	Occupancy rate[1] 1992	Occupancy rate[1] 1996	Resident rate[2] 1992[3]	Resident rate[2] 1996
United States[4]	15,846	17,208	1,692,123	1,839,686	86.0	82.7	442.9	407.0
New England	1,152	1,191	112,917	121,464	93.4	91.3	513.3	484.9
Maine	147	136	10,314	9,492	94.5	88.3	502.7	400.8
New Hampshire	76	81	7,349	8,075	93.2	91.5	469.1	455.1
Vermont	48	45	3,636	3,742	96.1	95.9	436.7	404.7
Massachusetts	535	567	52,103	57,426	93.1	89.8	500.1	485.7
Rhode Island	98	99	10,030	10,107	93.9	93.1	560.5	493.3
Connecticut	248	263	29,485	32,622	93.1	93.4	552.4	532.1
Middle Atlantic	1,617	1,774	240,485	261,041	93.0	92.5	412.2	395.4
New York	621	658	105,653	116,025	95.4	94.6	391.9	386.7
New Jersey	309	332	45,497	48,782	91.0	92.1	407.4	378.6
Pennsylvania	687	784	89,335	96,234	91.2	90.2	443.4	416.9
East North Central	3,176	3,327	356,414	390,048	83.0	77.3	517.4	479.2
Ohio	963	1,020	95,693	120,803	83.4	69.0	542.5	516.9
Indiana	565	576	60,952	61,594	74.2	73.2	597.6	549.0
Illinois	796	861	100,151	108,233	81.1	78.7	520.1	494.5
Michigan	439	447	50,371	51,448	88.8	86.7	392.7	353.0
Wisconsin	413	423	49,247	47,970	90.7	90.1	568.2	496.7
West North Central	2,268	2,398	205,186	214,523	82.7	79.7	535.2	501.3
Minnesota	458	457	46,938	46,118	93.4	92.4	610.3	547.5
Iowa	466	472	45,464	46,600	68.6	66.4	544.0	506.1
Missouri	493	598	49,156	57,643	76.5	73.3	433.9	452.8
North Dakota	84	88	7,068	7,121	94.9	95.5	554.7	504.1
South Dakota	114	115	8,335	8,268	94.3	94.0	571.8	525.6
Nebraska	234	236	18,292	18,358	88.9	87.3	532.8	490.2
Kansas	419	432	29,933	30,415	87.7	81.0	585.0	513.8
South Atlantic[4]	2,075	2,352	227,616	254,977	89.8	88.3	365.8	339.7
Delaware	40	42	4,729	4,857	72.6	80.0	449.9	443.6
Maryland	212	256	26,989	31,968	88.7	85.6	471.5	464.6
District of Columbia	- - -	- - -	- - -	- - -	- - -	- - -	- - -	- - -
Virginia	261	279	29,965	31,248	92.2	91.1	425.5	376.0
West Virginia	125	139	10,614	11,506	92.0	93.2	363.6	363.9
North Carolina	347	400	33,556	39,482	89.6	93.8	390.4	401.5
South Carolina	156	171	15,590	17,235	87.9	87.9	400.3	364.9
Georgia	344	359	36,960	39,497	93.7	91.6	548.1	480.1
Florida	590	706	69,213	79,184	88.4	83.7	261.4	236.2
East South Central	947	1,089	95,748	106,146	93.9	89.9	449.3	422.9
Kentucky	264	314	22,286	25,455	93.2	87.2	421.0	411.8
Tennessee	302	348	35,417	39,185	92.6	89.9	515.1	483.8
Alabama	215	223	22,348	24,389	94.6	90.9	403.1	367.8
Mississippi	166	204	15,697	17,117	96.5	92.7	438.7	409.8
West South Central	2,143	2,370	215,772	235,716	77.9	72.3	531.0	474.1
Arkansas	246	282	27,101	33,583	77.0	65.9	553.1	527.4
Louisiana	328	346	36,524	39,121	86.6	81.3	680.5	608.7
Oklahoma	407	430	34,042	36,055	80.0	74.9	554.1	501.3
Texas	1,162	1,312	118,105	126,957	74.8	70.6	482.4	423.3
Mountain	744	836	68,031	73,295	84.9	82.9	387.3	333.0
Montana	101	103	7,241	7,443	89.1	86.0	560.7	471.6
Idaho	68	83	5,266	6,215	85.2	78.7	355.8	319.2
Wyoming	37	38	2,986	3,125	85.1	83.9	513.8	439.1
Colorado	203	223	19,536	20,019	84.8	86.9	460.5	416.6
New Mexico	76	86	6,701	7,293	89.7	84.3	381.6	325.3
Arizona	134	162	15,588	17,468	82.3	77.4	292.9	243.2
Utah	88	96	6,962	7,556	81.2	80.1	367.7	324.6
Nevada	37	45	3,751	4,176	86.2	88.5	350.9	293.7
Pacific[4]	1,724	1,871	169,954	182,476	82.5	78.9	331.0	290.0
Washington	285	285	28,707	27,570	88.2	84.5	415.9	325.4
Oregon	163	164	14,100	14,101	87.3	81.2	290.4	231.4
California	1,276	1,422	127,147	140,805	80.7	77.6	320.3	291.0
Alaska	- - -	- - -	- - -	- - -	- - -	- - -	- - -	- - -
Hawaii	- - -	- - -	- - -	- - -	- - -	- - -	- - -	- - -

- - - Data not available.

[1]Percent of beds occupied.

[2]Number of nursing home residents (all ages) per 1,000 resident population 85 years of age and over.

[3]These numbers have been revised and differ from the previous edition of *Health, United States*.

[4]Occupancy and resident rates omit data for the District of Columbia, Alaska, and Hawaii from the numerator and denominator.

NOTES: Estimates of nursing homes, nursing home beds, and utilization rates from the National Health Provider Inventory (NHPI) and the Online Survey Certification and Reporting (OSCAR) database may differ because NHPI is a national survey of licensed nursing homes, including facilities managed by the Department of Veterans Affairs (DVA) and excluding hospital-based nursing homes, whereas the OSCAR database is a national census of currently-certified Medicare and/or Medicaid nursing homes and excludes licensed facilities that do not accept Federal funding and facilities managed by DVA. See Appendix I.

SOURCE: Health Care Financing Administration. Division of payment systems. Data from the Online Survey Certification and Reporting database.

Health, United States, 1998

Table 115. Gross domestic product, national health expenditures, and Federal and State and local government expenditures and average annual percent change: United States, selected years 1960–96

[Data are compiled by the Health Care Financing Administration]

Year	Gross domestic product in billions	National health expenditures Amount in billions	National health expenditures Percent of gross domestic product	National health expenditures Amount per capita	Federal government expenditures Total in billions	Federal government expenditures Health in billions	Federal government expenditures Health as a percent of total	State and local government expenditures Total in billions	State and local government expenditures Health in billions	State and local government expenditures Health as a percent of total
1960	$ 526.6	$ 26.9	5.1	$ 141	$ 89.6	$ 2.9	3.3	$ 38.4	$ 3.7	9.7
1965	719.1	41.1	5.7	202	122.4	4.8	3.9	57.2	5.5	9.5
1970	1,035.6	73.2	7.1	341	209.1	17.8	8.5	108.2	9.9	9.1
1971	1,125.4	81.0	7.2	373	228.6	20.4	8.9	123.7	10.8	8.7
1972	1,237.3	90.9	7.4	415	253.1	23.0	9.1	137.5	12.2	8.8
1973	1,382.7	100.8	7.3	456	275.1	25.2	9.2	152.0	14.1	9.3
1974	1,496.8	114.3	7.6	513	312.0	30.6	9.8	170.2	16.0	9.4
1975	1,630.6	130.7	8.0	582	371.3	36.4	9.8	198.0	18.6	9.4
1976	1,818.9	149.9	8.2	662	400.3	43.0	10.7	217.9	19.5	8.9
1977	2,026.8	170.4	8.4	746	435.9	47.7	10.9	237.1	22.5	9.5
1978	2,291.4	190.6	8.3	827	478.1	54.3	11.4	256.7	25.2	9.8
1979	2,557.5	215.2	8.4	924	529.5	61.4	11.6	278.3	28.8	10.3
1980	2,784.3	247.3	8.9	1,052	622.5	72.0	11.6	307.0	32.8	10.7
1981	3,115.9	286.9	9.2	1,208	707.1	83.7	11.8	335.4	37.5	11.2
1982	3,242.1	323.0	10.0	1,346	781.0	93.0	11.9	357.7	41.5	11.6
1983	3,514.5	355.3	10.1	1,466	846.3	103.1	12.2	378.8	44.4	11.7
1984	3,902.4	390.1	10.0	1,594	902.9	113.2	12.5	405.1	46.9	11.6
1985	4,180.7	428.7	10.3	1,735	974.2	123.2	12.6	437.8	51.0	11.7
1986	4,422.2	461.2	10.4	1,848	1,028	132.6	12.9	475.7	57.2	12.0
1987	4,692.3	500.5	10.7	1,986	1,066	143.1	13.4	511.1	64.1	12.5
1988	5,049.6	560.4	11.1	2,201	1,119	156.4	14.0	545.5	69.8	12.8
1989	5,438.7	623.5	11.5	2,423	1,193	174.8	14.7	585.9	77.4	13.2
1990	5,743.8	699.5	12.2	2,691	1,285	195.8	15.2	648.8	88.5	13.6
1991	5,916.7	766.8	13.0	2,920	1,345	225.8	16.8	708.4	95.9	13.5
1992	6,244.4	836.6	13.4	3,154	1,479	257.0	17.4	758.0	101.6	13.4
1993	6,558.1	895.1	13.6	3,341	1,526	279.6	18.3	807.0	109.3	13.5
1994	6,947.0	945.7	13.6	3,497	1,561	304.1	19.5	852.3	119.8	14.1
1995	7,265.4	991.4	13.6	3,633	1,638	328.7	20.1	895.9	126.5	14.1
1996	7,636.4	1,035.1	13.6	3,759	1,698	350.9	20.7	938.0	132.2	14.1
Average annual percent change										
1960–96	7.7	10.7	. . .	9.5	8.5	14.2	. . .	9.3	10.4	. . .
1960–65	6.4	8.9	. . .	7.4	6.4	10.6	. . .	8.3	7.9	. . .
1965–70	7.6	12.2	. . .	11.1	11.3	29.9	. . .	13.6	12.6	. . .
1970–75	9.5	12.3	. . .	11.3	12.2	15.4	. . .	12.8	13.5	. . .
1975–80	11.3	13.6	. . .	12.6	10.9	14.6	. . .	9.2	12.0	. . .
1980–85	8.5	11.6	. . .	10.5	9.4	11.3	. . .	7.4	9.2	. . .
1985–90	6.6	10.2	. . .	9.2	5.7	9.7	. . .	8.2	11.7	. . .
1990–95	4.8	7.2	. . .	6.2	5.0	10.9	. . .	6.7	7.4	. . .
1990–91	3.0	9.6	. . .	8.5	4.7	15.3	. . .	9.2	8.4	. . .
1991–92	5.5	9.1	. . .	8.0	10.0	13.8	. . .	7.0	5.9	. . .
1992–93	5.0	7.0	. . .	5.9	3.1	8.8	. . .	6.5	7.6	. . .
1993–94	5.9	5.7	. . .	4.7	2.3	8.8	. . .	5.6	9.6	. . .
1994–95	4.6	4.8	. . .	3.9	4.9	8.1	. . .	5.1	5.6	. . .
1995–96	5.1	4.4	. . .	3.5	3.7	6.8	. . .	4.7	4.5	. . .

. . . Category not applicable.

NOTES: These data include revisions in health expenditures and differ from previous editions of *Health, United States*. They reflect Social Security Administration population revisions as of July 1997.

SOURCE: National Health Statistics Group, Office of the Actuary. National health expenditures, 1996. Health Care Financing Review vol 19 no 1. HCFA pub no 03400. Health Care Financing Administration. Washington: U.S. Government Printing Office, Fall 1997.

Health Care Expenditures

Table 116. Total health expenditures as a percent of gross domestic product and per capita health expenditures in dollars: Selected countries and years 1960–95

[Data compiled by the Organization for Economic Cooperation and Development]

Country	1960	1965	1970	1975	1980	1985	1990	1992	1993	1994	1995[1]
Health expenditures as a percent of gross domestic product											
Australia	4.9	5.1	5.7	7.5	7.3	7.7	8.2	8.6	8.5	8.4	8.6
Austria	4.4	4.7	5.4	7.3	7.9	6.7	7.1	7.5	7.9	7.8	7.9
Belgium	3.4	3.9	4.1	5.9	6.6	7.4	7.6	8.1	8.2	8.1	8.0
Canada	5.5	6.0	7.1	7.2	7.3	8.4	9.2	10.2	10.2	9.9	9.7
Czechoslovakia	---	---	---	---	---	---	5.5	5.8	8.0	8.3	7.9
Denmark	3.6	4.8	6.1	6.5	6.8	6.3	6.5	6.6	6.8	6.6	6.4
Finland	3.9	4.9	5.7	6.4	6.5	7.3	8.0	9.3	8.4	7.9	7.7
France	4.2	5.2	5.8	7.0	7.6	8.5	8.9	9.4	9.8	9.7	9.9
Germany	4.3	4.6	5.7	8.0	8.1	8.5	8.2	10.2	10.1	10.3	10.4
Greece	2.4	2.6	3.3	3.4	3.6	4.0	4.2	4.5	5.0	5.5	5.8
Hungary	---	---	---	---	---	---	6.6	7.2	6.8	7.3	7.1
Iceland	3.3	3.9	5.0	5.8	6.2	7.3	8.0	8.2	8.3	8.1	8.2
Ireland	3.8	4.2	5.3	7.7	8.8	7.8	6.6	7.1	7.1	7.6	6.4
Italy	3.6	4.3	5.2	6.2	7.0	7.1	8.1	8.5	8.6	8.4	7.7
Japan	---	---	4.4	5.5	6.4	6.7	6.0	6.3	6.6	6.9	7.2
Korea	---	---	2.1	2.5	2.9	3.9	3.9	3.9	4.3	4.6	5.3
Luxembourg	---	---	3.7	5.1	6.2	6.1	6.6	6.6	6.7	6.5	7.0
Mexico	---	---	---	---	---	---	---	4.4	4.5	4.7	4.9
Netherlands	3.8	4.3	5.9	7.5	7.9	7.9	8.3	8.8	8.9	8.8	8.8
New Zealand	4.3	---	5.2	6.7	6.0	5.3	7.0	7.6	7.3	7.1	7.1
Norway	3.0	3.6	4.6	6.1	7.0	6.6	7.8	8.2	8.1	8.0	8.0
Poland	---	---	---	---	---	---	4.4	5.3	4.9	4.4	---
Portugal	---	---	2.8	5.6	5.8	6.3	6.5	7.4	7.7	7.8	8.2
Spain	1.5	2.6	3.7	4.9	5.7	5.7	6.9	7.2	7.3	7.3	7.6
Sweden	4.7	5.5	7.1	7.9	9.4	9.0	8.8	7.8	7.9	7.6	7.2
Switzerland	3.3	3.8	5.2	7.0	7.3	8.1	8.4	9.4	9.5	9.5	9.8
Turkey	---	---	2.4	2.7	3.3	2.2	2.5	2.7	2.5	5.2	---
United Kingdom	3.9	4.1	4.5	5.5	5.6	5.9	6.0	6.9	6.9	6.9	6.9
United States	5.1	5.7	7.1	8.0	8.9	10.3	12.2	13.4	13.6	13.6	13.6
Per capita health expenditures[2]											
Australia	$ 98	$125	$212	$443	$ 669	$ 989	$1,316	$1,468	$1,531	$1,609	$1,741
Austria	67	92	166	377	697	815	1,180	1,402	1,511	1,573	1,634
Belgium	53	82	131	311	588	890	1,247	1,526	1,600	1,653	1,665
Canada	105	151	255	433	729	1,206	1,691	1,939	1,979	2,005	2,069
Czechoslovakia	---	---	---	---	---	---	538	482	675	735	749
Denmark	67	120	215	348	595	816	1,069	1,210	1,300	1,344	1,368
Finland	55	92	165	312	521	852	1,292	1,392	1,310	1,289	1,373
France	73	121	208	398	716	1,088	1,539	1,794	1,838	1,868	1,972
Germany	91	127	230	498	860	1,274	1,642	1,900	1,885	2,020	2,134
Greece	16	27	60	106	190	288	389	480	549	634	703
Hungary	---	---	---	---	---	---	---	424	406	459	562
Iceland	50	85	139	295	637	929	1,375	1,510	1,555	1,571	1,774
Ireland	37	52	98	240	468	586	748	975	1,025	1,201	1,106
Italy	50	81	157	295	591	834	1,322	1,553	1,522	1,559	1,507
Japan	27	64	132	269	535	823	1,082	1,285	1,363	1,454	1,581
Korea	---	---	14	32	71	171	310	376	444	525	666
Luxembourg	---	---	150	315	617	895	1,499	1,764	1,900	1,962	2,206
Mexico	---	---	---	---	---	---	---	337	348	379	386
Netherlands	68	99	205	408	693	932	1,325	1,545	1,593	1,643	1,728
New Zealand	92	---	177	358	463	592	937	1,090	1,121	1,151	1,203
Norway	47	74	135	308	639	910	1,365	1,693	1,724	1,754	1,821
Poland	---	---	---	---	---	---	---	234	229	219	---
Portugal	---	---	45	154	264	387	616	812	874	939	1,035
Spain	14	37	83	190	332	455	813	959	971	992	1,075
Sweden	90	146	274	476	867	1,174	1,492	1,327	1,325	1,339	1,360
Switzerland	93	137	270	523	850	1,297	1,782	2,146	2,214	2,280	2,412
Turkey	---	---	23	41	77	73	119	141	140	272	---
United Kingdom	77	98	149	278	453	670	957	1,170	1,165	1,213	1,246
United States	141	202	341	582	1,052	1,735	2,691	3,154	3,341	3,497	3,633

- - - Data not available.
[1]Preliminary figures.
[2]Per capita health expenditures for each country have been adjusted to U.S. dollars using gross domestic product purchasing power parities for each year.

NOTE: Some numbers in this table have been revised and differ from previous editions of *Health, United States*.

SOURCES: Schieber GJ, Poullier JP, and Greenwald LG. U.S. health expenditure performance: An international comparison and data update. Health Care Financing Review vol 13 no 4. Washington: Health Care Financing Administration. September 1992; Office of National Health Statistics, Office of the Actuary. National health expenditures, 1995. Health Care Financing Review vol 18 no 1. Washington: Health Care Financing Administration. Fall 1996; Organization for Economic Cooperation and Development Health Data File: Unpublished data.

Table 117. Consumer Price Index and average annual percent change for all items and selected items: United States, selected years 1960–97

[Data are based on reporting by samples of providers and other retail outlets]

Year	All items	Medical care	Food	Apparel and upkeep	Housing	Energy	Personal care
			Consumer Price Index				
1960	29.6	22.3	30.0	45.7	- - -	22.4	34.6
1965	31.5	25.2	32.2	47.8	- - -	22.9	36.6
1970	38.8	34.0	39.2	59.2	36.4	25.5	43.5
1975	53.8	47.5	59.8	72.5	50.7	42.1	57.9
1976	56.9	52.0	61.6	75.2	53.8	45.1	61.7
1977	60.6	57.0	65.5	78.6	57.4	49.4	65.7
1978	65.2	61.8	72.0	81.4	62.4	52.5	69.9
1979	72.6	67.5	79.9	84.9	70.1	65.7	75.2
1980	82.4	74.9	86.8	90.9	81.1	86.0	81.9
1981	90.9	82.9	93.6	95.3	90.4	97.7	89.1
1982	96.5	92.5	97.4	97.8	96.9	99.2	95.4
1983	99.6	100.6	99.4	100.2	99.5	99.9	100.3
1984	103.9	106.8	103.2	102.1	103.6	100.9	104.3
1985	107.6	113.5	105.6	105.0	107.7	101.6	108.3
1986	109.6	122.0	109.0	105.9	110.9	88.2	111.9
1987	113.6	130.1	113.5	110.6	114.2	88.6	115.1
1988	118.3	138.6	118.2	115.4	118.5	89.3	119.4
1989	124.0	149.3	125.1	118.6	123.0	94.3	125.0
1990	130.7	162.8	132.4	124.1	128.5	102.1	130.4
1991	136.2	177.0	136.3	128.7	133.6	102.5	134.9
1992	140.3	190.1	137.9	131.9	137.5	103.0	138.3
1993	144.5	201.4	140.9	133.7	141.2	104.2	141.5
1994	148.2	211.0	144.3	133.4	144.8	104.6	144.6
1995	152.4	220.5	148.4	132.0	148.5	105.2	147.1
1996	156.9	228.2	153.3	131.7	152.8	110.1	150.1
1997	160.5	234.6	157.3	132.9	156.8	111.5	152.7
			Average annual percent change				
1960–97	4.7	6.6	4.6	2.9	[1]5.6	4.4	4.1
1960–65	1.3	2.5	1.4	0.9	- - -	0.4	1.1
1965–70	4.3	6.2	4.0	4.4	- - -	2.2	3.5
1970–75	6.8	6.9	8.8	4.1	6.9	10.5	5.9
1975–80	8.9	9.5	7.7	4.6	9.9	15.4	7.2
1980–85	5.5	8.7	4.0	2.9	5.8	3.4	5.7
1980–81	10.3	10.7	7.8	4.8	11.5	13.6	8.8
1981–82	6.2	11.6	4.1	2.6	7.2	1.5	7.1
1982–83	3.2	8.8	2.1	2.5	2.7	0.7	5.1
1983–84	4.3	6.2	3.8	1.9	4.1	1.0	4.0
1984–85	3.6	6.3	2.3	2.8	4.0	0.7	3.8
1985–90	4.0	7.5	4.6	3.4	3.6	0.1	3.8
1985–86	1.9	7.5	3.2	0.9	3.0	−13.2	3.3
1986–87	3.6	6.6	4.1	4.4	3.0	0.5	2.9
1987–88	4.1	6.5	4.1	4.3	3.8	0.8	3.7
1988–89	4.8	7.7	5.8	2.8	3.8	5.6	4.7
1989–90	5.4	9.0	5.8	4.6	4.5	8.3	4.3
1990–95	3.1	6.3	2.3	1.2	2.9	0.6	2.4
1990–91	4.2	8.7	2.9	3.7	4.0	0.4	3.5
1991–92	3.0	7.4	1.2	2.5	2.9	0.5	2.5
1992–93	3.0	5.9	2.2	1.4	2.7	1.2	2.3
1993–94	2.6	4.8	2.4	−0.2	2.5	0.4	2.2
1994–95	2.8	4.5	2.8	−1.0	2.6	0.6	1.7
1995–96	3.0	3.5	3.3	−0.2	2.9	4.7	2.0
1996–97	2.3	2.8	2.6	0.9	2.6	1.3	1.7

- - - Data not available.
[1]Data are for 1970–96.

NOTE: 1982–84=100.

SOURCE: U.S. Department of Labor, Bureau of Labor Statistics. Consumer Price Index. Various releases.

Table 118. Consumer Price Index and average annual percent change for all items and medical care components: United States, selected years 1960–97

[Data are based on reporting by samples of providers and other retail outlets]

Item and medical care component	1960	1965	1970	1975	1980	1985	1990	1994	1995	1996	1997
					Consumer Price Index						
CPI, all items	29.6	31.5	38.8	53.8	82.4	107.6	130.7	148.2	152.4	156.9	160.5
Less medical care.	30.2	32.0	39.2	54.3	82.8	107.2	128.8	144.7	148.6	152.8	156.3
CPI, all services	24.1	26.6	35.0	48.0	77.9	109.9	139.2	163.1	168.7	174.1	179.4
All medical care	22.3	25.2	34.0	47.5	74.9	113.5	162.8	211.0	220.5	228.2	234.6
Medical care services	19.5	22.7	32.3	46.6	74.8	113.2	162.7	213.4	224.2	232.4	239.1
Professional medical services	- - -	- - -	37.0	50.8	77.9	113.5	156.1	192.5	201.0	208.3	215.4
Physicians' services	21.9	25.1	34.5	48.1	76.5	113.3	160.8	199.8	208.8	216.4	222.9
Dental services	27.0	30.3	39.2	53.2	78.9	114.2	155.8	197.1	206.8	216.5	226.6
Eye care[1]	- - -	- - -	- - -	- - -	- - -	- - -	117.3	133.0	137.0	139.3	141.5
Services by other medical professionals[1]	- - -	- - -	- - -	- - -	- - -	- - -	120.2	141.3	143.9	146.6	151.8
Hospital and related services	- - -	- - -	- - -	- - -	69.2	116.1	178.0	245.6	257.8	269.5	278.4
Hospital services[2]	- - -	- - -	- - -	- - -	- - -	- - -	- - -	- - -	- - -	- - -	101.7
Inpatient services[2]	- - -	- - -	- - -	- - -	- - -	- - -	- - -	- - -	- - -	- - -	101.3
Outpatient services[1] . .	- - -	- - -	- - -	- - -	- - -	- - -	138.7	195.0	204.6	215.1	224.9
Hospital rooms.	9.3	12.3	23.6	38.3	68.0	115.4	175.4	239.2	251.2	261.0	- - -
Other inpatient services[1] .	- - -	- - -	- - -	- - -	- - -	- - -	142.7	197.1	206.8	216.9	- - -
Nursing home services[2] .	- - -	- - -	- - -	- - -	- - -	- - -	- - -	- - -	- - -	- - -	102.3
Medical care commodities . . .	46.9	45.0	46.5	53.3	75.4	115.2	163.4	200.7	204.5	210.4	215.3
Prescription drugs	54.0	47.8	47.4	51.2	72.5	120.1	181.7	230.6	235.0	242.9	249.3
Nonprescription drugs and medical supplies[1] . . .	- - -	- - -	- - -	- - -	- - -	- - -	120.6	138.1	140.5	143.1	145.4
Internal and respiratory over-the-counter drugs.	- - -	39.0	42.3	51.8	74.9	112.2	145.9	165.9	167.0	170.2	173.1
Nonprescription medical equipment and supplies.	- - -	- - -	- - -	- - -	79.2	109.6	138.0	160.0	166.3	169.1	171.5

Item and medical care component	1960–65	1965–70	1970–75	1975–80	1980–85	1985–90	1990–94	1994–95	1995–96	1996–97
				Average annual percent change						
CPI, all items	1.3	4.3	6.8	8.9	5.5	4.0	3.2	2.8	3.0	2.3
Less medical care	1.2	4.1	6.7	8.8	5.3	3.7	3.0	2.7	2.8	2.3
CPI, all services	2.0	5.6	6.5	10.2	7.1	4.8	4.0	3.4	3.2	3.0
All medical care.	2.5	6.2	6.9	9.5	8.7	7.5	6.7	4.5	3.5	2.8
Medical care services.	3.1	7.3	7.6	9.9	8.6	7.5	7.0	5.1	3.7	2.9
Professional medical services.	- - -	- - -	6.5	8.9	7.8	6.6	5.4	4.4	3.6	3.4
Physicians' services	2.8	6.6	6.9	9.7	8.2	7.3	5.6	4.5	3.6	3.0
Dental services	2.3	5.3	6.3	8.2	7.7	6.4	6.1	4.9	4.7	4.7
Eye care[1]	- - -	- - -	- - -	- - -	- - -	- - -	3.2	3.0	1.7	1.6
Services by other medical professionals[1]	- - -	- - -	- - -	- - -	- - -	- - -	4.1	1.8	1.9	3.5
Hospital and related services.	- - -	- - -	- - -	- - -	10.9	8.9	8.4	5.0	4.5	3.3
Hospital services[2]	- - -	- - -	- - -	- - -	- - -	- - -	- - -	- - -	- - -	- - -
Inpatient services[2]	- - -	- - -	- - -	- - -	- - -	- - -	- - -	- - -	- - -	- - -
Outpatient services[1]	- - -	- - -	- - -	- - -	- - -	- - -	8.9	4.9	5.1	4.6
Hospital rooms	5.8	13.9	10.2	12.2	11.2	8.7	8.1	5.0	3.9	- - -
Other inpatient services[1] . . .	- - -	- - -	- - -	- - -	- - -	- - -	8.4	4.9	4.9	- - -
Nursing home services[2]	- - -	- - -	- - -	- - -	- - -	- - -	- - -	- - -	- - -	- - -
Medical care commodities	-0.8	0.7	2.8	7.2	8.8	7.2	5.3	1.9	2.9	2.3
Prescription drugs	-2.4	-0.2	1.6	7.2	10.6	8.6	6.1	1.9	3.4	2.6
Nonprescription drugs and medical supplies[1]	- - -	- - -	- - -	- - -	- - -	- - -	3.4	1.7	1.9	1.6
Internal and respiratory over-the-counter drugs	- - -	1.6	4.1	7.7	8.4	5.4	3.3	0.7	1.9	1.7
Nonprescription medical equipment and supplies	- - -	- - -	- - -	- - -	6.7	4.7	3.8	3.9	1.7	1.4

- - - Data not available. [1] Dec. 1986=100. [2] Dec. 1996=100. NOTE: 1982–84=100, except where noted.

SOURCE: U.S. Department of Labor, Bureau of Labor Statistics. Consumer Price Index. Various releases.

Table 119. National health expenditures and average annual percent change, according to source of funds: United States, selected years 1929–96

[Data are compiled by the Health Care Financing Administration]

Year	All health expenditures in billions	Private funds Amount in billions	Private funds Amount per capita	Private funds Percent of total	Public funds Amount in billions	Public funds Amount per capita	Public funds Percent of total
1929	$ 3.6	$ 3.2	$ 25	86.4	$ 0.5	$ 4	13.6
1935	2.9	2.4	18	80.8	0.6	4	19.2
1940	4.0	3.2	24	79.7	0.8	6	20.3
1950	12.7	9.2	60	72.8	3.4	22	27.2
1955	17.7	13.2	78	74.3	4.6	27	25.7
1960	26.9	20.2	106	75.2	6.6	35	24.8
1965	41.1	30.9	151	75.0	10.3	50	25.0
1970	73.2	45.5	212	62.2	27.7	129	37.8
1975	130.7	75.7	337	57.9	55.0	245	42.1
1980	247.3	142.5	606	57.6	104.8	446	42.4
1981	286.9	165.7	698	57.8	121.2	510	42.2
1982	323.0	188.4	785	58.3	134.6	561	41.7
1983	355.3	207.7	857	58.5	147.5	609	41.5
1984	390.1	229.9	940	58.9	160.1	654	41.1
1985	428.7	254.5	1,030	59.4	174.2	705	40.6
1986	461.2	271.4	1,087	58.8	189.8	761	41.2
1987	500.5	293.3	1,164	58.6	207.2	822	41.4
1988	560.4	334.3	1,313	59.6	226.1	888	40.4
1989	623.5	371.4	1,444	59.6	252.1	980	40.4
1990	699.5	415.1	1,597	59.3	284.4	1,094	40.7
1991	766.8	445.2	1,695	58.1	321.7	1,225	41.9
1992	836.6	478.1	1,802	57.1	358.5	1,352	42.9
1993	895.1	506.2	1,889	56.5	389.0	1,452	43.5
1994	945.7	521.8	1,930	55.2	423.9	1,568	44.8
1995	991.4	536.2	1,965	54.1	455.2	1,668	45.9
1996	1,035.1	552.0	2,005	53.3	483.1	1,754	46.7
			Average annual percent change				
1929–65	7.0	6.5	5.1	. . .	8.8	7.3	. . .
1965–96	11.0	9.7	8.7	. . .	13.2	12.1	. . .
1929–35	–3.5	–4.7	–5.3	. . .	3.1	0.0	. . .
1935–40	6.6	5.9	5.9	. . .	5.9	8.4	. . .
1940–50	12.2	11.1	9.6	. . .	15.6	13.9	. . .
1950–55	6.9	7.5	5.4	. . .	6.2	4.2	. . .
1955–60	8.7	8.9	6.4	. . .	7.6	5.3	. . .
1960–65	8.9	8.8	7.3	. . .	9.1	7.6	. . .
1965–70	12.2	12.2	12.2	. . .	12.2	12.2	. . .
1970–75	12.3	12.3	12.3	. . .	12.3	12.3	. . .
1975–80	13.6	13.6	13.6	. . .	13.6	13.6	. . .
1980–85	11.6	12.3	11.2	. . .	10.7	9.6	. . .
1980–81	16.0	16.3	15.1	. . .	15.7	14.5	. . .
1981–82	12.6	13.7	12.5	. . .	11.0	9.9	. . .
1982–83	10.0	10.3	9.2	. . .	9.6	8.5	. . .
1983–84	9.8	10.7	9.6	. . .	8.5	7.5	. . .
1984–85	9.9	10.7	9.6	. . .	8.8	7.7	. . .
1985–90	10.3	10.3	9.2	. . .	10.3	9.2	. . .
1985–86	7.6	6.6	5.6	. . .	9.0	7.9	. . .
1986–87	8.5	8.1	7.0	. . .	9.2	8.1	. . .
1987–88	12.0	14.0	12.8	. . .	9.1	8.0	. . .
1988–89	11.3	11.1	10.0	. . .	11.5	10.3	. . .
1989–90	12.2	11.8	10.6	. . .	12.8	11.6	. . .
1990–95	7.2	5.3	4.2	. . .	9.9	8.8	. . .
1990–91	9.6	7.2	6.2	. . .	13.1	12.0	. . .
1991–92	9.1	7.4	6.3	. . .	11.5	10.3	. . .
1992–93	7.0	5.9	4.8	. . .	8.5	7.4	. . .
1993–94	5.6	3.1	2.1	. . .	9.0	8.0	. . .
1994–95	4.8	2.8	1.8	. . .	7.4	6.4	. . .
1995–96	4.4	3.0	2.0	. . .	6.1	5.2	. . .

. . . Category not applicable.

NOTES: These data include revisions in health expenditures and differ from previous editions of *Health, United States*. They reflect Social Security Administration population revisions as of July 1997.

SOURCE: National Health Statistics Group, Office of the Actuary. National health expenditures, 1996. Health Care Financing Review vol 19 no 1. HCFA pub no 03400. Health Care Financing Administration. Washington: U.S. Government Printing Office, Fall 1997.

Table 120 (page 1 of 2). National health expenditures, percent distribution, and average annual percent change, according to type of expenditure: United States, selected years 1960–96

[Data are compiled by the Health Care Financing Administration]

Type of expenditure	1960	1965	1970	1975	1980	1985	1990	1993	1994	1995	1996
	Amount in billions										
All expenditures	$ 26.9	$ 41.1	$ 73.2	$130.7	$247.3	$428.7	$699.5	$895.1	$945.7	$991.4	$1,035.1
Health services and supplies	25.2	37.7	67.9	122.3	235.6	412.3	675.0	866.1	915.2	960.7	1,003.6
Personal health care	23.6	35.2	63.8	114.5	217.0	376.4	614.7	787.0	828.5	869.0	907.2
Hospital care	9.3	14.0	28.0	52.6	102.7	168.3	256.4	323.0	335.7	346.7	358.5
Physician services	5.3	8.2	13.6	23.9	45.2	83.6	146.3	183.6	190.4	196.4	202.1
Dentist services	2.0	2.8	4.7	8.0	13.3	21.7	31.6	39.1	41.7	44.7	47.6
Nursing home care	0.8	1.5	4.2	8.7	17.6	30.7	50.9	66.3	70.9	75.2	78.5
Other professional services	0.6	0.9	1.4	2.7	6.4	16.6	34.7	46.3	50.3	54.3	58.0
Home health care	0.1	0.1	0.2	0.6	2.4	5.6	13.1	22.9	25.6	28.4	30.2
Drugs and other medical nondurables	4.2	5.9	8.8	13.0	21.6	37.1	59.9	75.6	79.5	84.9	91.4
Vision products and other medical durables	0.6	1.0	1.6	2.5	3.8	6.7	10.5	12.3	12.5	13.1	13.3
Other personal health care	0.7	0.8	1.3	2.5	4.0	6.1	11.2	18.0	21.9	25.3	27.6
Program administration and net cost of health insurance	1.2	1.9	2.7	4.9	11.9	24.3	40.7	53.8	58.2	60.1	60.9
Government public health activities[1]	0.4	0.6	1.3	2.9	6.7	11.6	19.6	25.3	28.5	31.5	35.5
Research and construction	1.7	3.4	5.3	8.4	11.6	16.4	24.5	29.0	30.5	30.7	31.5
Noncommercial research	0.7	1.5	2.0	3.3	5.5	7.8	12.2	14.5	15.9	16.7	17.0
Construction	1.0	1.9	3.4	5.1	6.2	8.5	12.3	14.5	14.6	14.0	14.5
	Percent distribution										
All expenditures	100.0	100.0	100.0	100.0	100.0	100.0	100.0	100.0	100.0	100.0	100.0
Health services and supplies	93.7	91.6	92.7	93.6	95.3	96.2	96.5	96.8	96.8	96.9	97.0
Personal health care	88.0	85.5	87.1	87.6	87.8	87.8	87.9	87.9	87.6	87.7	87.6
Hospital care	34.5	34.1	38.2	40.2	41.5	39.3	36.7	36.1	35.5	35.0	34.6
Physician services	19.7	19.9	18.5	18.3	18.3	19.5	20.9	20.5	20.1	19.8	19.5
Dentist services	7.3	6.8	6.4	6.1	5.4	5.0	4.5	4.4	4.4	4.5	4.6
Nursing home care	3.2	3.6	5.8	6.6	7.1	7.2	7.3	7.4	7.5	7.6	7.6
Other professional services	2.3	2.1	1.9	2.1	2.6	3.9	5.0	5.2	5.3	5.5	5.6
Home health care	0.2	0.2	0.3	0.5	1.0	1.3	1.9	2.6	2.7	2.9	2.9
Drugs and other medical nondurables	15.8	14.3	12.0	10.0	8.7	8.6	8.6	8.4	8.4	8.6	8.8
Vision products and other medical durables	2.4	2.4	2.2	2.0	1.5	1.6	1.5	1.4	1.3	1.3	1.3
Other personal health care	2.6	2.0	1.8	1.9	1.6	1.4	1.6	2.0	2.3	2.5	2.7
Program administration and net cost of health insurance	4.3	4.7	3.7	3.8	4.8	5.7	5.8	6.0	6.2	6.1	5.9
Government public health activities[1]	1.4	1.5	1.8	2.2	2.7	2.7	2.8	2.8	3.0	3.2	3.4
Research and construction	6.3	8.4	7.3	6.4	4.7	3.8	3.5	3.2	3.2	3.1	3.0
Noncommercial research	2.6	3.7	2.7	2.5	2.2	1.8	1.7	1.6	1.7	1.7	1.6
Construction	3.7	4.7	4.6	3.9	2.5	2.0	1.8	1.6	1.5	1.4	1.4

See footnotes at end of table.

Table 120 (page 2 of 2). National health expenditures, percent distribution, and average annual percent change, according to type of expenditure: United States, selected years 1960–96

[Data are compiled by the Health Care Financing Administration]

Type of expenditure	1960–65	1965–70	1970–75	1975–80	1980–85	1985–90	1990–93	1993–94	1994–95	1995–96
	Average annual percent change									
All expenditures	8.9	12.2	12.3	13.6	11.6	10.3	8.6	5.6	4.8	4.4
Health services and supplies	8.4	12.5	12.5	14.0	11.8	10.4	8.7	5.7	5.0	4.5
Personal health care	8.3	12.7	12.4	13.6	11.6	10.3	8.6	5.3	4.9	4.4
Hospital care	8.6	14.8	13.4	14.3	10.4	8.8	8.0	3.9	3.3	3.4
Physician services	9.2	10.6	12.0	13.6	13.1	11.8	7.8	3.7	3.1	2.9
Dentist services	7.3	10.8	11.2	10.9	10.2	7.8	7.4	6.6	7.3	6.4
Nursing home care	11.6	23.4	15.5	15.3	11.7	10.7	9.2	6.8	6.2	4.3
Other professional services	7.4	10.2	14.2	18.4	21.2	15.8	10.1	8.8	7.9	6.8
Home health care	9.6	19.7	23.2	30.7	18.9	18.4	20.3	12.2	10.9	6.2
Drugs and other medical nondurables	6.8	8.4	8.1	10.7	11.4	10.1	8.0	5.2	6.8	7.7
Vision products and other medical durables	9.1	10.2	9.5	8.1	12.4	9.2	5.6	1.5	4.9	1.4
Other personal health care	3.5	9.5	13.8	10.2	8.8	12.9	17.0	21.8	15.4	9.4
Program administration and net cost of health insurance	10.6	7.1	12.5	19.3	15.4	10.9	9.8	8.2	3.3	1.2
Government public health activities[1]	10.8	17.0	16.8	18.1	11.5	11.0	8.9	12.5	10.7	12.5
Research and construction	15.1	9.2	9.4	6.8	7.1	8.4	5.8	5.1	0.8	2.6
Noncommercial research	17.1	5.1	11.2	10.4	7.5	9.3	5.9	9.6	5.0	1.9
Construction	13.7	12.1	8.3	4.1	6.7	7.6	5.7	0.5	–3.8	3.4

[1]Includes personal care services delivered by government public health agencies.

NOTE: These data include revisions in health expenditures and differ from previous editions of *Health, United States*.

SOURCE: National Health Statistics Group, Office of the Actuary. National health expenditures, 1996. Health Care Financing Review vol 19 no 1. HCFA pub no 03400. Health Care Financing Administration. Washington: U.S. Government Printing Office, Fall 1997.

Table 121 (page 1 of 2). Expenditures for health services and supplies and percent distribution, by type of payer: United States, selected calendar years 1965–95

[Data are compiled by the Health Care Financing Administration]

Type of payer	1965	1970	1975	1980	1985	1990	1991	1992	1993	1994	1995
					Amount in billions						
Total[1]	$ 37.7	$ 67.9	$122.3	$235.6	$411.8	$672.9	$736.8	$806.7	$863.1	$906.7	$957.8
Private	29.8	48.9	83.7	158.4	282.2	450.8	483.4	522.4	547.0	569.5	597.4
Private business	5.9	13.6	27.5	61.7	108.6	185.8	200.1	217.9	229.5	239.0	249.4
Employer contribution to private health insurance premiums	4.9	9.7	19.7	45.3	79.1	138.4	148.2	162.4	172.3	177.1	183.8
Private employer contribution to Medicare hospital insurance trust fund[2]	0.0	2.1	5.0	10.5	20.3	29.5	32.7	34.3	36.0	40.2	43.1
Workers compensation and temporary disability insurance	0.8	1.4	2.4	5.1	7.7	15.7	16.7	18.5	18.4	18.6	19.3
Industrial inplant health services	0.2	0.3	0.5	0.9	1.4	2.2	2.4	2.6	2.8	3.1	3.3
Household	23.2	33.8	53.8	89.5	160.5	245.3	261.8	282.2	293.7	306.7	323.3
Employee contribution to private health insurance premiums and individual policy premiums	4.7	5.6	8.2	14.6	30.7	51.3	56.8	62.6	66.4	66.0	68.5
Employee and self-employment contributions and voluntary premiums paid to Medicare hospital insurance trust fund[2]	0.0	2.4	5.7	12.0	24.1	35.5	39.7	41.7	43.8	50.3	55.9
Premiums paid by individuals to Medicare supplementary medical insurance trust fund	0.0	1.0	1.7	2.7	5.2	10.1	10.3	12.1	11.9	14.4	16.3
Out-of-pocket health spending	18.5	24.9	38.1	60.3	100.6	148.4	155.0	165.8	171.6	176.0	182.6
Nonpatient revenues	0.6	1.5	2.4	7.2	13.1	19.8	21.6	22.4	23.8	23.7	24.7
Public	7.9	19.0	38.6	77.3	129.6	222.1	253.3	284.2	316.1	337.3	360.4
Federal Government	3.4	10.4	21.2	42.4	68.4	115.1	135.7	159.1	179.5	189.1	203.4
Employer contributions to private health insurance premiums	0.2	0.3	1.2	2.2	4.3	9.2	9.8	10.7	11.5	11.9	11.3
Medicaid[3]	0.0	2.9	7.6	14.7	23.1	43.4	57.8	69.2	78.2	83.2	88.7
Other[4]	3.2	7.2	12.4	25.5	41.0	62.5	68.1	79.2	89.8	94.0	103.4
State and local government	4.5	8.6	17.4	34.8	61.2	107.0	117.6	125.2	136.6	148.1	157.0
Employer contributions to private health insurance premiums	0.3	0.7	2.2	7.6	18.2	33.5	37.5	41.2	45.2	47.7	47.1
Medicaid[3]	0.0	2.5	6.1	11.7	18.6	33.2	37.9	39.2	43.9	49.8	55.6
Other[5]	4.2	5.4	9.1	15.5	24.4	40.2	42.2	44.8	47.5	50.6	54.3
					Percent distribution						
Total	100.0	100.0	100.0	100.0	100.0	100.0	100.0	100.0	100.0	100.0	100.0
Private	79.0	72.0	68.4	67.2	68.5	67.0	65.6	64.8	63.4	62.8	62.4
Private business	15.6	20.0	22.5	26.2	26.4	27.6	27.2	27.0	26.6	26.4	26.0
Employer contribution to private health insurance premiums	13.0	14.3	16.1	19.2	19.2	20.6	20.1	20.1	20.0	19.5	19.2
Private employer contribution to Medicare hospital insurance trust fund[2]	0.0	3.1	4.1	4.5	4.9	4.4	4.4	4.3	4.2	4.4	4.5
Workers compensation and temporary disability insurance	2.1	2.1	2.0	2.2	1.9	2.3	2.3	2.3	2.1	2.1	2.0
Industrial inplant health services	0.5	0.4	0.4	0.4	0.3	0.3	0.3	0.3	0.3	0.3	0.3
Household	61.5	49.8	44.0	38.0	39.0	36.5	35.5	35.0	34.0	33.8	33.7
Employee contribution to private health insurance premiums and individual policy premiums	12.5	8.2	6.7	6.2	7.5	7.6	7.7	7.8	7.7	7.3	7.1
Employee and self-employment contributions and voluntary premiums paid to Medicare hospital insurance trust fund[2]	0.0	3.5	4.7	5.1	5.9	5.3	5.4	5.2	5.1	5.6	5.8
Premiums paid by individuals to Medicare supplementary medical insurance trust fund	0.0	1.5	1.4	1.1	1.3	1.5	1.4	1.5	1.4	1.6	1.7
Out-of-pocket health spending	49.1	36.7	31.2	25.6	24.4	22.1	21.0	20.5	19.9	19.4	19.1
Nonpatient revenues	1.6	2.2	2.0	3.1	3.2	2.9	2.9	2.8	2.8	2.6	2.6

See footnotes at end of table.

Table 121 (page 2 of 2). Expenditures for health services and supplies and percent distribution, by type of payer: United States, selected calendar years 1965–95

[Data are compiled by the Health Care Financing Administration]

Type of payer	1965	1970	1975	1980	1985	1990	1991	1992	1993	1994	1995
						Percent distribution					
Public	21.0	28.0	31.6	32.8	31.5	33.0	34.4	35.2	36.6	37.2	37.6
Federal Government	9.0	15.3	17.3	18.0	16.6	17.1	18.4	19.7	20.8	20.9	21.2
Employer contributions to private health insurance premiums	0.5	0.4	1.0	0.9	1.0	1.4	1.3	1.3	1.3	1.3	1.2
Medicaid[3]	0.0	4.3	6.2	6.2	5.6	6.4	7.8	8.6	9.1	9.2	9.3
Other[4]	8.5	10.6	10.1	10.8	10.0	9.3	9.3	9.8	10.4	11.0	10.8
State and local government	11.9	12.7	14.2	14.8	14.9	15.9	16.0	15.5	15.8	16.3	16.4
Employer contributions to private health insurance premiums	0.8	1.0	1.8	3.2	4.4	5.0	5.1	5.1	5.2	5.3	4.9
Medicaid[3]	0.0	3.7	5.0	5.0	4.5	4.9	5.1	4.9	5.1	5.5	5.8
Other[5]	11.1	8.0	7.4	6.6	5.9	6.0	5.7	5.6	5.5	5.6	5.7

[1]Excludes research and construction.
[2]Includes one-half of self-employment contribution to Medicare hospital insurance trust fund.
[3]Includes Medicaid buy-in premiums for Medicare.
[4]Includes expenditures for Medicare with adjustments for contributions by employers and individuals and premiums paid to the Medicare insurance trust fund and maternal and child health, vocational rehabilitation, Substance Abuse and Mental Health Services Administration, Indian Health Service, Federal workers' compensation, and other miscellaneous general hospital and medical programs, public health activities, Department of Defense, and Department of Veterans Affairs.
[5]Includes other public and general assistance, maternal and child health, vocational rehabilitation, public health activities, hospital subsidies, and employer contributions to Medicare hospital insurance trust fund.

NOTES: This table disaggregates health expenditures according to four classes of payers: businesses, households (individuals), Federal Government, and State and local governments. Where businesses or households pay dedicated funds into government health programs (for example, Medicare) or employers and employees share in the cost of health premiums, these costs are assigned to businesses or households accordingly. This results in a lower share of expenditures being assigned to the Federal Government than for tabulations of expenditures by source of funds. Estimates of national health expenditure by source of funds aim to track government-sponsored health programs over time and do not delineate the role of business employers in paying for health care. Figures may not sum to totals due to rounding. These data include revisions and differ from previous editions of *Health, United States*.

SOURCE: Office of National Health Statistics, Office of the Actuary. Business, households, and government: Health spending 1995. Health Care Financing Review vol 18, no 3. Washington: Health Care Financing Administration. Spring 1997.

Table 122. Employers' costs per employee hour worked for total compensation, wages and salaries, and health insurance, according to selected characteristics: United States, selected years 1991–97

[Data are based on surveys of employers]

Characteristic	Total compensation				Wages and salaries			
	1991	1994	1996	1997	1991	1994	1996	1997
	Amount per employee-hour worked							
State and local government............	$22.31	$25.27	$25.73	$26.58	$15.52	$17.57	$17.95	$18.61
Total private industry	15.40	17.08	17.49	17.97	11.14	12.14	12.58	13.04
Industry:								
Goods producing................	18.48	20.85	21.27	21.86	12.70	13.87	14.38	14.92
Service producing	14.31	15.82	16.28	16.73	10.58	11.56	12.01	12.44
Manufacturing..................	18.22	20.72	20.99	21.84	12.40	13.69	14.13	14.79
Nonmanufacturing..............	14.67	16.19	16.69	17.10	10.81	11.76	12.23	12.64
Occupation:								
White collar....................	18.15	20.26	21.10	21.60	13.40	14.72	15.44	15.94
Blue collar.....................	15.15	16.92	17.04	17.19	10.37	11.31	11.61	11.80
Service........................	7.82	8.38	8.61	9.04	5.96	6.33	6.53	6.94
Region:								
Northeast	17.56	20.03	20.57	20.27	12.65	14.13	14.58	14.52
Midwest	15.05	16.26	16.30	17.33	10.70	11.34	11.59	12.33
South..........................	13.68	15.05	15.62	15.79	10.03	10.85	11.36	11.61
West..........................	15.97	18.08	18.78	19.68	11.62	13.01	13.72	14.57
Union status:								
Union..........................	19.76	23.26	23.31	23.48	13.02	14.76	14.93	15.13
Nonunion	14.54	16.04	16.61	17.21	10.78	11.70	12.23	12.75
Establishment employment size:								
1–99 employees	13.38	14.58	14.85	15.37	10.00	10.72	11.09	11.54
100 or more	17.34	19.45	20.09	20.61	12.23	13.48	14.05	14.55
100–499	14.31	15.88	16.61	16.97	10.32	11.37	11.90	12.29
500 or more..................	20.60	23.35	24.03	24.75	14.28	15.79	16.49	17.12

Characteristic	Health insurance				Health insurance as a percent of total compensation			
	1991	1994	1996	1997	1991	1994	1996	1997
	Amount per employee-hour worked							
State and local government............	$1.54	$2.06	$1.98	$1.99	6.9	8.2	7.7	7.5
Total private industry	0.92	1.14	1.04	0.99	6.0	6.7	5.9	5.5
Industry:								
Goods producing................	1.28	1.70	1.52	1.49	6.9	8.1	7.2	6.8
Service producing	0.79	0.95	0.88	0.83	5.5	6.0	5.4	4.9
Manufacturing..................	1.37	1.79	1.56	1.55	7.5	8.6	7.5	7.1
Nonmanufacturing..............	0.80	0.98	0.92	0.86	5.5	6.0	5.5	5.0
Occupation:								
White collar....................	1.02	1.25	1.16	1.07	5.6	6.2	5.5	5.0
Blue collar.....................	1.06	1.35	1.23	1.19	7.0	8.0	7.2	6.9
Service........................	0.36	0.45	0.41	0.40	4.6	5.4	4.8	4.5
Region:								
Northeast	1.08	1.37	1.28	1.17	6.2	6.9	6.2	5.8
Midwest	0.95	1.19	1.03	1.02	6.3	7.3	6.3	5.9
South..........................	0.76	0.95	0.92	0.86	5.5	6.3	5.9	5.4
West	0.92	1.10	0.97	0.95	5.8	6.1	5.2	4.8
Union status:								
Union..........................	1.63	2.28	2.05	2.01	8.2	9.8	8.8	8.5
Nonunion	0.78	0.94	0.88	0.85	5.4	5.9	5.3	4.9
Establishment employment size:								
1–99 employees	0.68	0.84	0.74	0.72	5.1	5.7	5.0	4.7
100 or more	1.14	1.42	1.33	1.26	6.6	7.3	6.6	6.1
100–499	0.90	1.03	1.05	0.98	6.3	6.5	6.3	5.8
500 or more..................	1.40	1.84	1.65	1.57	6.8	7.9	6.9	6.3

NOTE: Costs are calculated from March survey data each year.

SOURCES: U.S. Department of Labor, Bureau of Labor Statistics: Employment Cost Indexes and Levels, 1975–92. Bulletin 2413, Nov. 1992; U.S. Department of Labor: *News* pub nos 91–292, 94–290, 96–424, and 97–371. June 19, 1991, June 16, 1994, Oct. 10, 1996, and Oct. 21, 1997. Washington.

Table 123. Personal health care expenditures average annual percent increase and percent distribution of factors affecting growth: United States, 1960–96

[Data are compiled by the Health Care Financing Administration]

Period	Average annual percent increase	Factors affecting growth				
		All factors	Inflation[1]		Population	Intensity[2]
			Economy-wide	Medical		
		Percent distribution				
1960–96	10.7	100	43	15	10	32
1960–61	6.1	100	20	6	27	47
1961–62	7.6	100	17	11	21	51
1962–63	9.3	100	13	7	16	64
1963–64	9.9	100	15	15	14	56
1964–65	8.6	100	23	9	15	53
1965–66	10.4	100	29	21	11	39
1966–67	13.7	100	25	13	8	54
1967–68	12.9	100	35	11	8	46
1968–69	12.8	100	38	10	8	44
1969–70	13.5	100	40	8	8	43
1970–71	9.8	100	54	11	11	24
1971–72	11.4	100	39	–3	9	55
1972–73	11.6	100	50	–15	8	57
1973–74	14.7	100	62	1	6	30
1974–75	14.7	100	66	9	6	19
1975–76	14.0	100	44	21	6	29
1976–77	13.2	100	50	11	7	32
1977–78	11.6	100	64	5	9	22
1978–79	13.7	100	64	4	7	25
1979–80	15.8	100	60	13	7	20
1980–81	16.1	100	60	17	7	16
1981–82	12.4	100	52	35	9	4
1982–83	10.0	100	44	32	11	13
1983–84	9.6	100	39	40	11	10
1984–85	10.2	100	36	36	10	18
1985–86	9.0	100	29	26	11	34
1986–87	9.6	100	33	19	11	37
1987–88	11.0	100	34	24	10	32
1988–89	10.2	100	42	27	11	20
1989–90	11.7	100	38	21	9	31
1990–91	10.6	100	39	16	10	35
1991–92	9.0	100	32	28	12	28
1992–93	6.3	100	42	34	16	7
1993–94	5.3	100	43	30	18	9
1994–95	4.9	100	53	23	19	5
1995–96	4.4	100	55	13	21	11

[1]Total inflation is economy-wide and medical inflation is the medical inflation above economy-wide inflation.
[2]The residual percent of growth which cannot be attributed to price increases or population growth and represents changes in use or kinds of services and supplies.

NOTE: These data include revisions in health expenditures and in population back to 1960 and differ from previous editions of *Health, United States*.

SOURCE: National Health Statistics Group, Office of the Actuary. National health expenditures, 1996. Health Care Financing Review vol 19 no 1. HCFA pub no 03400. Washington: Health Care Financing Administration. Fall 1997.

Table 124. Personal health care expenditures and percent distribution, according to source of funds: United States, selected years 1929–96

[Data are compiled by the Health Care Financing Administration]

Year	Total in billions[1]	Per capita	All sources	Out-of-pocket payments	Private health insurance	Other private funds	Government Total	Federal	State and local
				Percent distribution					
1929	$ 3.2	$ 26	100.0	[2]88.4	([2])	2.6	9.0	2.7	6.3
1935	2.7	21	100.0	[2]82.4	([2])	2.8	14.7	3.4	11.3
1940	3.5	26	100.0	[2]81.3	([2])	2.6	16.1	4.1	12.0
1950	10.9	70	100.0	65.5	9.1	2.9	22.4	10.4	12.0
1955	15.7	93	100.0	58.1	16.1	2.8	23.0	10.5	12.5
1960	23.6	124	100.0	55.3	21.2	1.8	21.7	9.0	12.6
1965	35.2	172	100.0	52.7	24.7	2.0	20.6	8.4	12.2
1970	63.8	297	100.0	39.0	23.2	2.6	35.3	23.0	12.2
1971	70.1	323	100.0	37.7	23.5	2.6	36.2	24.1	12.1
1972	78.0	356	100.0	37.1	23.4	2.7	36.8	24.4	12.4
1973	87.1	394	100.0	36.7	23.7	2.5	37.1	24.3	12.8
1974	99.9	448	100.0	34.9	24.2	2.5	38.5	26.0	12.5
1975	114.5	510	100.0	33.3	24.8	2.4	39.6	27.0	12.5
1976	130.5	576	100.0	32.1	25.7	2.9	39.3	28.1	11.2
1977	147.7	647	100.0	31.4	26.4	2.8	39.3	27.9	11.4
1978	164.8	715	100.0	30.2	27.1	3.0	39.7	28.4	11.3
1979	187.5	805	100.0	29.0	28.1	3.1	39.8	28.7	11.2
1980	217.0	923	100.0	27.8	28.6	3.6	40.1	29.2	10.9
1981	252.0	1,061	100.0	27.2	28.9	3.7	40.2	29.6	10.6
1982	283.3	1,181	100.0	26.6	29.6	3.8	40.0	29.6	10.4
1983	311.5	1,285	100.0	26.4	29.8	3.7	40.1	29.9	10.2
1984	341.5	1,395	100.0	26.6	29.9	3.6	39.9	30.0	9.9
1985	376.4	1,523	100.0	26.7	30.3	3.7	39.2	29.5	9.7
1986	410.5	1,645	100.0	26.3	30.4	3.8	39.4	29.2	10.2
1987	449.7	1,784	100.0	25.8	31.2	3.8	39.2	28.8	10.4
1988	499.3	1,961	100.0	25.5	32.2	3.9	38.3	28.2	10.1
1989	550.1	2,138	100.0	24.2	33.3	3.7	38.8	28.7	10.1
1990	614.7	2,364	100.0	23.5	33.6	3.5	39.4	28.9	10.5
1991	679.6	2,588	100.0	22.3	33.5	3.4	40.8	30.4	10.4
1992	740.7	2,792	100.0	21.5	33.4	3.3	41.7	31.8	9.9
1993	787.0	2,937	100.0	20.8	33.2	3.4	42.6	32.6	10.0
1994	828.5	3,064	100.0	19.9	32.8	3.5	43.8	33.6	10.1
1995	869.0	3,185	100.0	19.2	32.5	3.6	44.7	34.7	10.0
1996	907.2	3,295	100.0	18.9	32.2	3.5	45.4	35.6	9.9

[1]Includes all expenditures for health services and supplies other than expenses for program administration and net cost of private health insurance and government public health activities.

[2]Out-of-pocket payments and private health insurance are combined for these years.

NOTES: These data include revisions in health expenditures and differ from previous editions of *Health, United States*. They reflect Social Security Administration population revisions as of July 1997.

SOURCE: National Health Statistics Group, Office of the Actuary. National health expenditures, 1996. Health Care Financing Review vol 19 no 1. HCFA pub no 03400. Health Care Financing Administration. Washington: U.S. Government Printing Office, Fall 1997.

Table 125. Expenditures on hospital care, nursing home care, physician services, and all other personal health care expenditures and percent distribution, according to source of funds: United States, selected years 1960–96

[Data are compiled by the Health Care Financing Administration]

Service and year	Total in billions	Out-of-pocket payments	Private health insurance	Other private funds	Government Total[1]	Government Medicaid	Government Medicare
Hospital care[2]			Percent distribution				
1960	$ 9.3	20.7	35.6	1.2	42.5	. . .	. . .
1965	14.0	19.6	40.9	1.9	37.6	. . .	. . .
1970	28.0	9.0	32.4	3.2	55.4	9.5	19.2
1975	52.6	8.3	32.9	2.7	56.0	10.0	22.0
1980	102.7	5.2	35.5	4.9	54.4	10.3	25.7
1985	168.3	5.2	35.0	4.9	54.8	9.3	29.1
1990	256.4	4.0	36.9	4.2	54.9	11.5	27.0
1991	282.3	4.0	35.3	4.1	56.6	13.4	27.3
1992	305.3	3.8	34.0	3.9	58.3	13.9	29.1
1993	323.0	3.7	33.8	4.0	58.5	14.6	28.9
1994	335.7	3.2	32.7	4.2	59.9	14.7	30.4
1995	346.7	2.8	32.2	4.3	60.7	14.7	31.9
1996	358.5	2.6	31.6	4.3	61.5	14.7	33.0
Nursing home care[3]							
1960	0.8	77.9	0.0	6.3	15.7	. . .	. . .
1965	1.5	60.1	0.1	5.7	34.1	. . .	. . .
1970	4.2	53.5	0.4	4.9	41.2	22.3	3.4
1975	8.7	42.6	0.8	4.8	51.9	47.1	2.5
1980	17.6	41.8	1.2	3.0	54.0	50.0	1.7
1985	30.7	44.3	2.7	1.8	51.2	47.2	1.5
1990	50.9	43.1	4.0	1.8	51.0	45.4	3.4
1991	57.2	40.2	4.1	1.8	53.8	48.1	3.6
1992	62.3	38.0	4.3	1.9	55.9	48.5	5.3
1993	66.3	35.3	4.5	1.8	58.4	48.9	7.2
1994	70.9	33.9	4.7	1.9	59.5	48.3	8.8
1995	75.2	33.4	4.9	1.9	59.9	47.2	10.4
1996	78.5	31.4	5.2	1.9	61.5	47.8	11.4
Physician services							
1960	5.3	62.7	30.2	0.1	7.1	. . .	. . .
1965	8.2	60.6	32.5	0.1	6.8	. . .	. . .
1970	13.6	42.2	35.2	0.1	22.5	4.8	12.2
1975	23.9	36.7	35.3	0.2	27.7	7.5	14.1
1980	45.2	32.4	37.9	0.8	28.9	5.5	17.6
1985	83.6	29.2	40.1	1.6	29.1	4.2	19.5
1990	146.3	22.1	45.6	1.8	30.5	4.8	20.0
1991	162.2	20.6	47.5	1.8	30.1	5.6	18.8
1992	175.9	19.3	49.2	1.8	29.7	6.3	17.8
1993	183.6	17.7	50.2	1.8	30.2	6.9	18.1
1994	190.4	16.0	51.1	1.9	31.0	7.1	19.0
1995	196.4	14.8	50.9	2.1	32.2	7.4	20.2
1996	202.1	14.6	50.4	2.1	32.9	7.5	21.1
All other personal health care[4]							
1960	8.2	87.4	1.5	3.0	8.1	. . .	. . .
1965	11.5	86.7	2.4	2.9	8.0	. . .	. . .
1970	18.0	79.9	5.0	2.8	12.3	4.5	0.7
1975	29.4	72.4	8.7	2.9	16.1	6.0	1.8
1980	51.5	63.9	15.9	3.6	16.5	5.5	3.2
1985	93.9	57.3	22.2	4.1	16.4	5.7	4.6
1990	161.0	49.6	26.9	4.3	19.2	7.3	5.5
1991	178.0	47.2	27.2	4.4	21.3	8.6	6.5
1992	197.1	45.8	27.6	4.2	22.4	9.0	7.4
1993	214.1	44.7	26.8	4.3	24.2	10.4	8.2
1994	231.5	43.0	26.5	4.3	26.2	11.3	9.1
1995	250.7	41.1	26.9	4.2	27.8	12.2	10.0
1996	268.1	40.2	27.3	4.0	28.5	12.8	10.4

. . . Category not applicable.

[1]Includes other government expenditures for these health care services, for example, care funded by the Department of Veterans Affairs and State and locally financed subsidies to hospitals.

[2]Includes expenditures for hospital-based nursing home care and home health agency care.

[3]Includes expenditures for care in freestanding nursing homes. Expenditures for care in facility-based nursing homes are included with hospital care.

[4]Includes expenditures for dental services, other professional services, home health care, drugs and other medical nondurables, vision products and other medical durables, and other personal health care.

NOTE: These data include revisions in health expenditures and differ from previous editions of *Health, United States*.

SOURCE: National Health Statistics Group, Office of the Actuary. National health expenditures, 1996. Health Care Financing Review vol 19 no 1. HCFA pub no 03400. Health Care Financing Administration. Washington: U.S. Government Printing Office, Fall 1997.

Table 126. Hospital expenses, according to type of ownership and size of hospital: United States, selected years 1975–96

[Data are based on reporting by a census of hospitals]

Type of ownership and size of hospital	1975	1980	1985	1990	1993	1994	1995	1996	1985–93	1993–96
Total expenses				Amount in billions					Average annual percent change	
All hospitals.	$ 48.7	$ 91.9	$153.3	$234.9	$301.5	$310.8	$320.3	$330.5	8.8	3.1
Federal	4.5	7.9	12.3	15.2	19.6	20.0	20.2	22.3	6.0	4.4
Non-Federal[1]	44.2	84.0	141.0	219.6	281.9	290.8	300.0	308.3	9.0	3.0
Community[2]	39.0	76.9	130.5	203.7	266.1	275.8	285.6	293.8	9.3	3.4
Nonprofit.	27.9	55.8	96.1	150.7	197.2	204.2	209.6	216.0	9.4	3.1
Proprietary.	2.6	5.8	11.5	18.8	23.1	23.4	26.7	28.4	9.1	7.1
State-local government	8.5	15.2	22.9	34.2	45.8	48.1	49.3	49.4	9.1	2.6
6–24 beds	0.1	0.2	0.3	0.5	0.7	0.8	1.1	1.1	11.2	16.3
25–49 beds	1.0	1.7	2.6	4.0	5.6	6.2	7.2	7.5	10.1	10.2
50–99 beds	2.9	5.4	8.6	12.6	15.8	16.6	17.8	18.4	7.9	5.2
100–199 beds	6.7	12.5	21.4	33.3	44.5	46.2	50.7	53.7	9.6	6.5
200–299 beds	6.8	13.4	23.3	38.7	50.6	54.3	55.8	56.5	10.2	3.7
300–399 beds	5.8	11.5	21.8	33.1	43.7	43.6	43.3	46.0	9.1	1.7
400–499 beds	4.8	10.5	15.7	25.3	30.4	33.5	33.7	35.5	8.6	5.3
500 beds or more.	11.0	21.6	36.8	56.2	74.9	74.6	76.1	75.0	9.3	0.0
Employee expenses as percent of total expenses[3]				Percent						
Federal	64.5	68.4	68.1	67.1	65.6	67.4	65.8	63.0	. . .	. . .
Non-Federal[1]	54.8	58.1	56.6	54.8	53.7	54.8	54.5	53.9	. . .	. . .
Community[2]	53.0	56.3	55.2	53.6	52.7	53.9	53.6	53.0	. . .	. . .
Nonprofit.	53.5	57.2	55.9	54.3	53.4	54.5	53.9	53.4	. . .	. . .
Proprietary.	43.5	45.7	45.2	43.7	45.7	47.3	47.9	48.2	. . .	. . .
State-local government	54.3	57.3	57.1	55.8	53.6	54.7	55.2	54.2	. . .	. . .
6–24 beds	51.3	54.9	55.0	54.4	53.9	53.6	54.2	54.1	. . .	. . .
25–49 beds	50.2	54.0	54.1	53.0	52.8	53.7	53.9	53.8	. . .	. . .
50–99 beds	50.6	53.7	52.9	51.8	52.4	53.8	53.7	53.0	. . .	. . .
100–199 beds	51.0	54.2	52.6	51.7	52.2	52.9	52.9	52.9	. . .	. . .
200–299 beds	52.8	55.6	54.6	53.0	52.6	53.8	53.3	52.8	. . .	. . .
300–399 beds	53.8	56.9	55.7	54.1	53.1	53.8	53.4	52.5	. . .	. . .
400–499 beds	54.2	57.8	56.2	55.1	53.2	54.7	54.1	53.9	. . .	. . .
500 beds or more.	54.3	57.9	56.9	54.5	52.9	54.5	54.1	53.1	. . .	. . .
Expenses per inpatient day				Amount						
Community[2]	$ 151	$ 245	$ 460	$ 687	$ 881	$ 931	$ 968	$1,006	8.5	4.5
Nonprofit.	150	246	463	692	898	950	994	1,042	8.6	5.1
Proprietary.	146	257	500	752	914	924	947	945	7.8	1.1
State-local government	157	239	433	634	800	859	878	903	8.0	4.1
6–24 beds	121	203	380	526	664	707	678	757	7.2	4.5
25–49 beds	111	197	379	489	635	675	696	749	6.7	5.7
50–99 beds	115	191	363	493	598	622	647	664	6.4	3.6
100–199 beds	134	215	402	585	729	760	796	827	7.7	4.3
200–299 beds	146	239	449	665	854	903	943	993	8.4	5.2
300–399 beds	156	248	484	731	956	1,031	1,070	1,109	8.9	5.1
400–499 beds	159	215	489	756	977	1,065	1,135	1,175	9.0	6.3
500 beds or more.	184	239	527	825	1,087	1,154	1,212	1,267	9.5	5.2
Expenses per inpatient stay										
Community[2]	$1,165	$1,851	$3,245	$4,947	$6,132	$6,230	$6,216	$6,225	8.3	0.5
Nonprofit.	1,178	1,902	3,307	5,001	6,178	6,257	6,279	6,344	8.1	0.9
Proprietary.	968	1,676	3,033	4,727	5,643	5,529	5,425	5,207	8.1	−2.6
State-local government	1,197	1,750	3,106	4,838	6,206	6,513	6,445	6,419	9.0	1.1
6–24 beds	684	1,072	1,876	2,701	3,471	3,419	3,578	3,630	8.0	1.5
25–49 beds	673	1,138	2,007	2,967	3,687	3,736	3,797	3,879	7.9	1.7
50–99 beds	785	1,271	2,342	3,461	4,312	4,438	4,427	4,474	7.9	1.2
100–199 beds	955	1,512	2,683	4,109	4,999	5,050	5,103	5,121	8.1	0.8
200–299 beds	1,096	1,767	3,044	4,618	5,713	5,797	5,851	5,917	8.2	1.2
300–399 beds	1,225	1,881	3,394	5,096	6,351	6,546	6,512	6,550	8.1	1.0
400–499 beds	1,290	2,090	3,571	5,500	6,706	7,118	7,164	7,253	8.2	2.6
500 beds or more.	1,677	2,517	4,254	6,667	8,460	8,511	8,531	8,450	9.0	0.0

. . . Category not applicable.

[1]The category of non-Federal hospitals is comprised of psychiatric, tuberculosis and other respiratory diseases hospitals, long-term, and short-term hospitals.
[2]Community hospitals are short-term hospitals excluding hospital units in institutions such as prison and college infirmaries, facilities for the mentally retarded, and alcoholism and chemical dependency hospitals.
[3]Includes employee payroll and benefit expenses. Does not include contracted labor services.

SOURCES: American Hospital Association: Hospital Statistics, 1976, 1981, 1986, 1991–98 Editions. Chicago, 1976, 1981, 1986, 1991–97. (Copyrights 1976, 1981, 1986, 1991–97: Used with the permission of the American Hospital Association.) and unpublished data.

Table 127. Nursing home average monthly charges per resident and percent of residents, according to selected facility and resident characteristics: United States, 1964, 1973–74, 1977, 1985, and 1995

[Data are based on reporting by a sample of nursing homes]

Facility and resident characteristic	Average monthly charge[1]					Percent of residents				
	1964	1973–74[2]	1977	1985	1995	1964	1973–74[2]	1977	1985	1995
Facility characteristic										
All facilities....................	$186	$479	$689	$1,456	$3,135	100.0	100.0	100.0	100.0	100.0
Ownership:										
Proprietary	205	489	670	1,379	3,047	60.2	69.8	68.2	68.7	63.6
Nonprofit and government	145	456	732	1,624	3,288	39.8	30.2	31.8	31.3	36.4
Certification:[3]										
Skilled nursing facility..........	. . .	566	880	1,905	- - -	. . .	39.8	20.7	18.5	- - -
Skilled nursing and intermediate facility....................	. . .	514	762	1,571	- - -	. . .	24.5	40.5	45.2	- - -
Intermediate facility	. . .	376	556	1,179	- - -	. . .	22.4	28.3	24.9	- - -
Not certified	. . .	329	390	875	- - -	. . .	13.3	10.6	11.4	- - -
Both Medicare and Medicaid......	- - -	- - -	- - -	- - -	3,317	- - -	- - -	- - -	- - -	78.4
Medicare only	- - -	- - -	- - -	- - -	4,211	- - -	- - -	- - -	- - -	3.0
Medicaid only	- - -	- - -	- - -	- - -	2,169	- - -	- - -	- - -	- - -	15.8
Neither.....................	- - -	- - -	- - -	- - -	2,323	- - -	- - -	- - -	- - -	2.8
Bed size:										
Less than 50 beds.............	- - -	397	546	1,036	4,978	- - -	15.2	12.9	8.9	4.5
50–99 beds..................	- - -	448	643	1,335	2,691	- - -	34.1	30.5	27.6	24.9
100–199 beds................	- - -	502	706	1,478	3,028	- - -	35.6	38.8	43.2	51.1
200 beds or more	- - -	576	837	1,759	3,560	- - -	15.1	17.9	20.2	19.5
Geographic region:										
Northeast	213	651	918	1,781	3,904	28.6	22.0	22.4	23.6	22.8
Midwest	171	433	640	1,399	2,740	36.6	34.6	34.5	32.5	32.3
South......................	161	410	585	1,256	2,752	18.1	26.0	27.2	29.4	32.0
West	204	454	653	1,458	3,710	16.7	17.4	15.9	14.5	12.9
Resident characteristic										
All residents..................	186	479	689	1,456	3,135	100.0	100.0	100.0	100.0	100.0
Age:										
Under 65 years	155	434	585	1,379	3,662	12.0	10.6	13.6	11.6	8.0
65–74 years	184	473	669	1,372	3,409	18.9	15.0	16.2	14.2	12.0
75–84 years	191	488	710	1,468	3,138	41.7	35.5	35.7	34.1	32.5
85 years and over	194	485	719	1,497	2,974	27.5	38.8	34.5	40.0	47.5
Sex:										
Male.......................	171	466	652	1,438	3,345	35.0	29.1	28.8	28.4	26.6
Female.....................	194	484	705	1,463	3,059	65.0	70.9	71.2	71.6	73.4

. . . Category not applicable.

- - - Data not available.

[1]Includes life-care residents and no-charge residents.

[2]Data exclude residents of personal care homes.

[3]Medicare extended care facilities and Medicaid skilled nursing homes from the 1973–74 survey were considered to be equivalent to Medicare or Medicaid skilled nursing facilities in 1977 and 1985 for the purposes of this comparison. In the 1995 survey the certification categories were based on Medicare and Medicaid certification.

SOURCES: Centers for Disease Control and Prevention: Van Nostrand JF, Sutton JF. Charges for care and sources of payment for residents in nursing homes, United States, June–August 1969. National Center for Health Statistics. Vital Health Stat 12(21). 1973; Hing E. Charges for care and sources of payment for residents in nursing homes, United States, National Nursing Home Survey, August 1973–April 1974. National Center for Health Statistics. Vital Health Stat 13(32). 1977; Van Nostrand JF, Zappolo A, Hing E, et al. The National Nursing Home Survey, 1977 summary for the United States. National Center for Health Statistics. Vital Health Stat 13(43). 1979; and Hing E, Sekscenski E, Strahan G. The National Nursing Home Survey: 1985 summary for the United States. National Center for Health Statistics. Vital Health Stat 13(97). 1989; and unpublished data.

Table 128. Nursing home average monthly charges per resident and percent of residents, according to primary source of payments and selected facility characteristics: United States, 1977, 1985, and 1995

[Data are based on reporting by a sample of nursing homes]

Facility characteristic	All sources 1995	Own income or family support[1] 1977	Own income or family support[1] 1985	Own income or family support[1] 1995	Medicare 1977	Medicare 1985	Medicare 1995	Medicaid 1977	Medicaid 1985	Medicaid 1995
					Average monthly charge[2]					
All facilities	$3,135	$ 690	$1,450	$3,081	$ 1,167	$ 2,141	$ 5,546	$ 720	$1,504	$2,769
Ownership										
Proprietary	3,047	686	1,444	3,190	1,048	2,058	5,668	677	1,363	2,560
Nonprofit and government	3,288	698	1,462	2,967	1,325	*2,456	5,304	825	1,851	3,201
Certification[3]										
Skilled nursing facility	- - -	866	1,797	- - -	1,136	2,315	- - -	955	2,000	- - -
Skilled nursing and intermediate facility	- - -	800	1,643	- - -	1,195	2,156	- - -	739	1,509	- - -
Intermediate facility	- - -	567	1,222	- - -	. . .	. . .	- - -	563	1,150	- - -
Not certified	- - -	447	999	- - -	. . .	. . .	- - -	. . .	. . .	- - -
Both Medicare and Medicaid	3,317	- - -	- - -	3,364	- - -	- - -	5,472	- - -	- - -	2,910
Medicare only	4,211	- - -	- - -	3,344	- - -	- - -	4*10,074	- - -	- - -	- - -
Medicaid only	2,169	- - -	- - -	2,352	- - -	- - -	. . .	- - -	- - -	2,069
Neither	2,323	- - -	- - -	2,390	- - -	- - -	. . .	- - -	- - -	- - -
Bed size										
Less than 50 beds	4,978	516	886	3,377	*869	*1,348	4*17,224	663	1,335	2,990
50–99 beds	2,691	686	1,388	2,849	*1,141	1,760	4,929	634	1,323	2,335
100–199 beds	3,028	721	1,567	3,138	1,242	2,192	4,918	691	1,413	2,659
200 beds or more	3,560	823	1,701	3,316	*1,179	2,767	4,523	925	1,919	3,520
Geographic region										
Northeast	3,904	909	1,645	4,117	1,369	2,109	4,883	975	2,035	3,671
Midwest	2,740	652	1,398	2,650	*1,160	2,745	5,439	639	1,382	2,478
South	2,752	585	1,359	2,945	*1,096	2,033	4,889	619	1,200	2,333
West	3,710	663	1,498	3,666	*868	1,838	8,825	663	1,501	2,848
					Percent of residents					
All facilities	100.0	38.4	41.6	27.8	2.0	1.4	9.9	47.8	50.4	60.2
Ownership										
Proprietary	100.0	37.5	40.1	24.1	1.7	1.6	10.4	49.6	52.1	63.8
Nonprofit and government	100.0	40.4	44.9	34.3	2.7	*0.9	9.2	43.8	46.6	54.0
Certification[3]										
Skilled nursing facility	- - -	41.5	39.1	- - -	4.6	2.6	- - -	41.4	53.7	- - -
Skilled nursing and intermediate facility	- - -	31.6	36.8	- - -	2.6	1.9	- - -	58.3	57.8	- - -
Intermediate facility	- - -	36.3	41.4	- - -	. . .	. . .	- - -	55.3	55.9	- - -
Not certified	- - -	64.2	65.5	- - -	. . .	. . .	- - -	. . .	. . .	- - -
Both Medicare and Medicaid	100.0	- - -	- - -	23.1	- - -	- - -	11.6	- - -	- - -	63.9
Medicare only	100.0	- - -	- - -	71.2	- - -	- - -	16.2	- - -	- - -	- - -
Medicaid only	100.0	- - -	- - -	32.1	- - -	- - -	- - -	- - -	- - -	63.0
Neither	100.0	- - -	- - -	91.0	- - -	- - -	- - -	- - -	- - -	- - -
Bed size										
Less than 50 beds	100.0	49.6	53.1	35.3	*1.8	*1.2	13.1	32.7	33.8	49.9
50–99 beds	100.0	39.5	49.5	34.5	*1.2	*1.3	6.2	46.5	42.9	57.6
100–199 beds	100.0	38.4	39.6	26.2	2.6	1.5	10.6	50.4	55.2	61.5
200 beds or more	100.0	28.6	30.1	22.0	2.3	*1.5	12.1	55.5	57.7	62.4
Geographic region										
Northeast	100.0	34.6	34.8	18.2	3.3	1.7	14.0	53.3	52.9	64.9
Midwest	100.0	44.5	49.1	36.3	1.5	*0.8	6.7	42.1	45.9	55.8
South	100.0	32.2	39.4	26.1	*1.4	*1.2	10.1	52.5	53.8	62.2
West	100.0	41.3	40.4	27.9	2.5	*2.7	10.5	44.7	49.2	57.9

* Relative standard error greater than 30 percent.
- - - Data not available.
. . . Category not applicable.
[1]Includes private health insurance.
[2]Includes life-care residents and no-charge residents.
[3]In the 1995 survey the certification categories were based on Medicare and Medicaid certification.
[4]Likely to include a high proportion of patients in subacute units of hospitals.

SOURCES: Centers for Disease Control and Prevention: Van Nostrand JF, Zappolo A, Hing E, et al. The National Nursing Home Survey, 1977 summary for the United States. National Center for Health Statistics. Vital Health Stat 13(43). 1979; and Hing E, Sekscenski E, Strahan G. The National Nursing Home Survey: 1985 summary for the United States. National Center for Health Statistics. Vital Health Stat 13(97). 1985; and unpublished data.

Table 129. Mental health expenditures, percent distribution, and per capita expenditures, according to type of mental health organization: United States, selected years 1975–94

[Data are based on inventories of mental health organizations]

Type of organization	1975	1979	1983	1986	1988	1990	1992	1994
	Amount in millions							
All organizations	$6,564	$8,764	$14,432	$18,458	$23,028	$28,410	$29,765	$33,136
State and county mental hospitals	3,185	3,757	5,491	6,326	6,978	7,774	7,970	7,825
Private psychiatric hospitals	467	743	1,712	2,629	4,588	6,101	5,302	6,468
Non-Federal general hospitals with separate psychiatric services.	621	723	2,176	2,878	3,610	4,662	5,193	5,344
Department of Veterans Affairs medical centers[1]	699	848	1,316	1,338	1,290	1,480	1,530	1,386
Residential treatment centers for emotionally disturbed children	279	436	573	978	1,305	1,969	2,167	2,360
Freestanding psychiatric outpatient clinics	422	589	430	518	657	671	821	878
All other organizations[2]	116	187	2,734	3,792	4,600	5,753	6,782	8,875
	Percent distribution							
All organizations	100.0	100.0	100.0	100.0	100.0	100.0	100.0	100.0
State and county mental hospitals	48.5	42.9	38.0	34.4	30.3	27.4	26.8	23.6
Private psychiatric hospitals	7.1	8.5	11.9	14.2	19.9	21.5	17.8	19.5
Non-Federal general hospitals with separate psychiatric services.	9.5	8.2	15.1	15.6	15.7	16.4	17.4	16.1
Department of Veterans Affairs medical centers[1]	10.6	9.7	9.1	7.2	5.6	5.2	5.1	4.2
Residential treatment centers for emotionally disturbed children	4.3	5.0	4.0	5.3	5.7	6.9	7.3	7.1
Freestanding psychiatric outpatient clinics	6.4	6.7	3.0	2.8	2.8	2.4	2.8	2.7
All other organizations[2]	1.8	2.1	18.9	20.5	20.0	20.2	22.8	26.8
	Amount per capita[3]							
All organizations	$ 31	$ 40	$ 62	$ 77	$ 95	$ 117	$ 117	$ 128
State and county mental hospitals	15	17	24	26	29	32	31	30
Private psychiatric hospitals	2	3	7	11	19	25	21	25
Non-Federal general hospitals with separate psychiatric services.	3	3	9	12	15	19	20	21
Department of Veterans Affairs medical centers[1]	3	4	6	6	5	6	6	5
Residential treatment centers for emotionally disturbed children	1	2	3	4	5	8	9	9
Freestanding psychiatric outpatient clinics	2	3	2	2	3	3	3	3
All other organizations[2]	1	1	12	16	19	24	27	35

[1]Includes Department of Veterans Affairs neuropsychiatric hospitals, general hospital psychiatric services, and psychiatric outpatient clinics.
[2]Includes freestanding outpatient clinics, freestanding day–night organizations, multiservice organizations, and other residential organizations. Multiservice mental health organizations were redefined in 1983; see Appendix I, Substance Abuse and Mental Health Services Administration.
[3]Civilian population.

NOTES: Comparisons of data from 1979 and 1983 with data from other years should be made with caution because changes in reporting procedures may affect the comparability of data. Mental health expenditures include salaries, other operating expenditures, and capital expenditures.

SOURCES: Survey and Analysis Branch, Division of State and Community Systems Development, Center for Mental Health Services. Manderscheid RW, Sonnenschein MA. Mental health, United States, 1996. U.S. Government Printing Office, 1996; unpublished data from the 1994 inventory of mental health organizations and general hospital mental health services.

Table 130. National funding for health research and development and average annual percent change, according to source of funds: United States, selected years 1960–95

[Data are compiled by the National Institutes of Health from multiple sources]

Year and period	All funding	Source of funds			
		Federal	State and local	Industry[1]	Private nonprofit organizations
	Amount in millions				
1960	$ 886	$ 448	$ 46	$ 253	$ 139
1965	1,890	1,174	90	450	176
1970	2,847	1,667	170	795	215
1975	4,701	2,832	286	1,319	264
1976	5,107	3,059	312	1,469	267
1977	5,568	3,396	338	1,614	220
1978	6,273	3,811	416	1,800	246
1979	7,162	4,321	465	2,093	284
1980	7,967	4,723	480	2,459	305
1981	8,738	4,848	564	2,998	328
1982	9,598	4,970	642	3,596	390
1983	10,786	5,399	718	4,213	456
1984	12,160	6,087	796	4,771	506
1985	13,567	6,791	878	5,360	538
1986	14,898	6,895	1,029	6,192	782
1987	16,933	7,847	1,182	7,105	800
1988	19,003	8,431	1,295	8,438	839
1989	20,918	9,163	1,466	9,407	882
1990	23,095	9,791	1,625	10,719	960
1991	25,886	10,602	1,833	12,261	1,090
1992	29,240	11,726	1,933	14,397	1,183
1993	31,088	12,108	2,054	15,711	1,215
1994	33,399	12,821	2,196	17,106	1,276
1995[2]	35,816	13,423	2,423	18,645	1,325
	Average annual percent change				
1960–95	11.1	10.2	12.0	13.1	6.7
1960–65	16.4	21.2	14.4	12.2	4.8
1965–70	8.5	7.3	13.6	12.1	4.1
1970–75	10.6	11.2	11.0	10.7	4.2
1975–80	11.1	10.8	10.9	13.3	2.9
1975–76	8.6	8.0	9.1	11.4	1.1
1976–77	9.0	11.0	8.3	9.9	−17.6
1977–78	12.7	12.2	23.1	11.5	11.8
1978–79	14.2	13.4	11.8	16.3	15.4
1979–80	11.2	9.3	3.2	17.5	7.4
1980–85	11.2	7.5	12.8	16.9	12.0
1980–81	9.7	2.6	17.5	21.9	7.5
1981–82	9.8	2.5	13.8	19.9	18.9
1982–83	12.4	8.6	11.8	17.2	16.9
1983–84	12.7	12.7	10.9	13.2	11.0
1984–85	11.6	11.6	10.3	12.3	6.3
1985–90	11.2	7.6	13.1	14.9	12.3
1985–86	9.8	1.5	17.2	15.5	45.4
1986–87	13.7	13.8	14.9	14.7	2.3
1987–88	12.2	7.4	9.6	18.8	4.9
1988–89	10.1	8.7	13.2	11.5	5.1
1989–90	10.4	6.9	10.8	13.9	8.8
1990–95	9.2	6.5	8.3	11.7	6.7
1990–91	12.1	8.3	12.8	14.4	13.5
1991–92	13.0	10.6	5.5	17.4	8.5
1992–93	6.3	3.3	6.3	9.1	2.7
1993–94	7.4	5.9	6.9	8.9	5.0
1994–95	7.2	4.7	10.3	9.0	3.8

[1]Includes expenditures for drug research. These expenditures are included in the "drugs and sundries" component of the Health Care Financing Administration's National Health Expenditure Series, not under "research."
[2]Preliminary figures.

SOURCE: National Institutes of Health, Office of Reports and Analysis.

Table 131. Federal funding for health research and development and percent distribution, according to agency: United States, selected fiscal years 1970–95

[Data are compiled by the National Institutes of Health from Federal Government sources]

Agency	1970	1975	1980	1985	1989	1990	1991	1992	1993[1]	1994	1995[2]
					Amount in millions						
Total	$1,667	$2,832	$4,723	$6,791	$9,163	$9,791	$10,602	$11,726	$12,108	$12,821	$13,423
					Percent distribution						
All Federal agencies	100.0	100.0	100.0	100.0	100.0	100.0	100.0	100.0	100.0	100.0	100.0
Department of Health and Human Services	70.6	77.6	78.2	79.7	84.9	85.2	85.7	85.8	85.0	85.6	85.1
National Institutes of Health	52.4	66.4	67.4	71.1	74.0	72.9	72.6	71.7	80.7	80.6	79.6
Centers for Disease Control and Prevention	- - -	1.5	1.8	0.7	1.3	1.0	1.1	1.3	1.3	1.6	2.4
Other Public Health Service	16.2	8.3	7.9	7.3	9.1	10.8	11.4	12.2	2.4	2.7	2.5
Other Department of Health and Human Services	2.0	1.3	1.1	0.6	0.6	0.5	0.7	0.7	0.6	0.6	0.6
Other agencies	29.4	22.4	21.8	20.3	15.1	14.8	14.3	14.2	15.0	14.4	14.9
Department of Agriculture	3.0	2.2	3.1	2.1	1.3	1.1	1.0	1.0	0.9	0.9	0.9
Department of Defense	7.5	4.1	4.5	6.5	4.2	4.4	3.8	4.1	5.6	5.3	5.3
Department of Education[3]	. . .	. . .	0.7	0.6	0.6	0.6	0.4	0.4	0.2	0.2	0.1
Department of Energy[4]	6.3	5.8	4.5	2.6	2.4	2.8	3.3	3.0	2.6	2.5	2.5
Department of the Interior	0.7	0.3	0.5	0.4	0.4	0.4	0.4	0.5	0.5	0.5	0.5
Department of Veterans Affairs	3.5	3.3	2.8	3.3	2.6	2.4	2.0	2.3	2.0	1.9	1.8
Environmental Protection Agency	. . .	1.3	1.7	0.8	0.6	0.3	0.5	0.3	0.4	0.3	0.2
International Development Cooperation Agency[5]	0.6	0.2	0.3	0.6	0.3	0.2	0.2	0.2	0.4	0.2	0.1
National Aeronautics and Space Administration	5.2	2.6	1.5	1.7	1.5	1.5	1.5	1.4	1.7	1.5	2.6
National Science Foundation	1.7	1.6	1.6	1.3	1.0	0.8	0.8	0.6	0.6	0.6	0.6
All other departments and agencies	0.9	1.0	0.4	0.4	0.3	0.2	0.3	0.3	0.4	0.4	0.3

- - - Data not available.

. . . Category not applicable.

[1]In fiscal year 1993 the Alcohol, Drug Abuse, and Mental Health Administration was reorganized and renamed the Substance Abuse and Mental Health Services Administration and its three research institutes were transferred into the National Institutes of Health.

[2]Preliminary figures.

[3]Office of Handicapped Research, formerly included in Other Department of Health and Human Services.

[4]Includes Atomic Energy Commission and Energy Research and Development Administration.

[5]Includes Department of State and Agency for International Development.

NOTES: Data for 1970 and 1975 fiscal years ending June 30; all other data for fiscal year ending September 30. These data include revisions and may differ from previous editions of *Health, United States*.

SOURCE: National Institutes of Health, Office of Reports and Analysis.

Table 132. Federal spending for human immunodeficiency virus (HIV)-related activities, according to agency and type of activity: United States, selected fiscal years 1985–97

[Data are compiled from Federal Government appropriations]

Agency and type of activity	1985	1989	1990	1991	1992	1993	1994	1995	1996	1997[1]
Agency					Amount in millions					
All Federal spending	$205	$2,297	$3,064	$3,806	$4,498	$5,328	$6,329	$6,821	$7,522	$8,451
Department of Health and Human Services, total	197	2,019	2,620	3,302	3,824	4,426	5,399	4,941	5,598	6,370
Department of Health and Human Services discretionary spending, total[2]	109	1,304	1,591	1,891	1,963	2,081	2,569	2,700	2,898	3,270
National Institutes of Health	66	717	907	1,014	1,047	1,073	1,296	1,334	1,411	1,501
Substance Abuse and Mental Health Services Administration	–	58	50	30	26	26	27	24	54	66
Centers for Disease Control and Prevention	33	378	443	497	480	498	543	590	584	617
Food and Drug Administration	9	74	57	63	72	73	72	73	73	73
Health Resources and Services Administration	–	60	113	266	317	390	608	661	762	1,001
Agency for Health Care Policy and Research	–	7	8	10	10	10	11	9	6	4
Office of the Assistant Secretary for Health	–	6	8	6	5	5	5	4	4	4
Indian Health Service	–	1	3	2	3	3	4	4	3	4
Other Department of Health and Human Services agencies	–	3	3	3	3	3	2	2	2	–
Health Care Financing Administration	75	545	780	1,050	1,360	1,675	1,990	2,240	2,700	3,100
Social Security Administration[3]	13	170	249	360	501	670	840	...	...	...
Social Security Administration[3]	...	...	...	...	...	...	...	940	976	1,070
Department of Veterans Affairs	8	136	220	258	279	325	312	317	331	350
Department of Defense	–	86	125	127	129	159	129	112	98	98
Agency for International Development	–	40	71	78	94	117	115	120	115	117
Department of Housing and Urban Development	–	–	–	–	107	196	258	171	171	196
Office of Personnel Management	–	12	21	34	58	98	108	212	226	241
Other departments	–	4	7	7	7	7	8	8	7	9
Activity										
Research	84	937	1,142	1,275	1,311	1,361	1,561	1,589	1,653	1,738
Department of Health and Human Services discretionary spending[2]	83	900	1,093	1,221	1,259	1,284	1,508	1,544	1,619	1,707
Department of Veterans Affairs	1	10	15	10	6	7	6	5	6	6
Department of Defense	–	27	34	44	46	70	47	40	28	25
Education and prevention	26	396	486	528	518	576	619	658	635	678
Department of Health and Human Services discretionary spending[2]	25	298	351	391	378	395	445	492	476	516
Department of Veterans Affairs	1	27	31	34	22	31	31	31	31	31
Department of Defense	–	26	28	19	18	27	22	12	11	11
Agency for International Development	–	40	71	78	94	117	115	120	115	117
Other	–	5	5	6	6	6	6	3	2	3
Medical care	81	794	1,187	1,642	2,061	2,523	3,051	3,462	4,087	4,769
Health Care Financing Administration:										
Medicaid (Federal share)	70	490	670	870	1,080	1,290	1,490	1,640	1,600	1,800
Medicare	5	55	110	180	280	385	500	600	1,100	1,300
Department of Health and Human Services discretionary spending[2]	–	103	144	274	323	397	613	664	803	1,047
Department of Veterans Affairs	6	99	174	214	251	287	275	281	294	313
Department of Defense	–	33	63	64	65	62	60	60	59	62
Office of Personnel Management	–	12	21	34	58	98	108	212	226	241
Other	–	2	5	4	4	4	5	5	5	6
Cash assistance	13	170	249	360	608	866	1,098	1,111	1,147	1,266
Social Security Administration:										
Disability Insurance	10	145	210	295	390	505	600	640	696	760
Supplemental Security Income	3	25	39	65	111	165	240	300	280	310
Department of Housing and Urban Development	–	–	–	–	107	196	258	171	171	196

– Quantity zero.

... Category not applicable.

[1]Preliminary figures.

[2]Department of Health and Human Services discretionary spending is spending that is not entitlement spending. Medicare and Medicaid are examples of entitlement spending.

[3]Prior to 1995 the Social Security Administration was part of the Department of Health and Human Services.

NOTES: These data include revisions and differ from the previous edition of Health, United States. Federal expenditures on HIV-related activities are estimated at about 35 to 40 percent of total HIV-related expenditures that include, for example, expenditures covered by private health insurance, out-of-pocket costs to patients, and the States' share of Medicaid, public hospital, and other local expenditures.

SOURCE: Budget Office, Public Health Service. Unpublished data.

[Data are based on household interviews of a sample of the civilian noninstitutionalized population]

Characteristic	Private insurance						Private insurance obtained through workplace[1]					
	1984	1989	1993[2]	1994	1995	1996[3]	1984	1989	1993[2]	1994	1995	1996[3]
	Number in millions											
Total[4]	157.5	162.7	159.9	160.7	165.0	165.9	141.8	146.3	146.4	146.7	151.4	151.4
	Percent of population											
Total, age adjusted[4]	76.6	75.7	71.3	69.9	71.2	71.1	68.9	68.1	65.3	63.8	65.4	64.8
Total, crude[4]	76.8	75.9	71.5	70.3	71.6	71.4	69.1	68.3	65.5	64.2	65.7	65.1
Age												
Under 18 years	72.6	71.8	66.5	63.8	65.7	66.4	66.5	65.8	61.8	59.0	60.9	61.1
Under 6 years	68.1	67.9	60.7	58.3	60.1	61.1	62.1	62.3	56.4	53.9	55.6	56.5
6–17 years	74.9	74.0	69.6	66.8	68.7	69.1	68.7	67.7	64.8	61.8	63.7	63.4
18–44 years	76.5	75.5	70.4	69.8	71.2	70.6	69.6	68.4	64.7	63.9	65.6	64.7
18–24 years	67.4	64.5	58.7	58.3	61.2	60.4	58.7	55.3	51.1	50.7	53.9	52.3
25–34 years	77.4	75.9	69.1	69.4	70.3	69.5	71.2	69.5	63.9	64.1	65.3	64.4
35–44 years	83.9	82.7	78.7	77.1	78.0	77.5	77.4	76.2	73.5	71.6	72.9	72.0
45–64 years	83.3	82.5	80.6	80.3	80.4	79.5	71.8	71.6	72.0	71.8	72.4	71.4
45–54 years	83.3	83.4	81.1	81.3	81.1	80.4	74.6	74.4	74.4	74.6	74.9	74.0
55–64 years	83.3	81.6	80.0	78.8	79.3	78.1	69.0	68.3	68.6	67.9	68.6	67.5
Sex[5]												
Male	77.1	76.0	71.5	70.4	71.6	71.4	69.7	68.6	65.6	64.3	65.9	65.2
Female	76.0	75.4	71.0	69.5	70.8	70.8	68.1	67.6	65.0	63.4	64.8	64.4
Race[5]												
White	79.7	79.0	75.1	73.5	74.4	74.2	71.9	71.1	68.8	67.0	68.4	67.6
Black	58.3	57.8	51.0	51.5	54.2	54.9	52.4	52.9	48.0	48.8	50.4	51.8
Asian or Pacific Islander	69.8	71.1	67.3	67.3	68.0	67.8	63.6	60.2	59.2	57.4	59.8	59.3
Hispanic origin and race[5]												
All Hispanic	56.3	52.6	48.3	48.6	47.3	47.5	52.3	48.0	44.0	44.5	44.0	43.8
Mexican	54.3	48.0	44.4	45.7	43.9	43.8	51.1	45.2	42.1	43.7	41.9	40.9
Puerto Rican	48.8	45.9	44.9	48.3	47.9	50.7	46.4	42.6	42.0	45.2	44.7	48.1
Cuban	71.7	69.0	68.3	63.9	62.4	65.4	57.7	55.8	52.8	46.5	53.1	54.4
Other Hispanic	61.6	61.9	56.2	52.3	52.2	52.6	57.4	55.4	50.3	46.2	47.1	47.6
White, non-Hispanic	82.3	82.4	78.7	77.3	78.6	78.5	74.0	74.1	72.0	70.4	72.1	71.5
Black, non-Hispanic	58.5	57.9	51.4	51.9	54.6	55.4	52.6	53.0	48.3	49.2	50.9	52.2
Age and percent of poverty level												
All ages:[5]												
Below 100 percent	32.4	26.7	22.8	21.3	21.9	20.0	23.7	19.4	17.3	16.1	17.0	15.5
100–149 percent	62.4	54.9	49.2	46.8	47.8	47.1	51.9	45.8	41.7	40.9	41.9	40.8
150–199 percent	77.7	71.3	69.6	65.7	66.5	67.9	69.5	62.9	62.7	59.0	60.4	60.9
200 percent or more	91.7	91.2	89.8	88.9	89.3	89.5	85.2	84.2	84.1	83.0	83.7	83.2
Under 18 years:												
Below 100 percent	28.7	22.3	17.3	14.9	16.8	16.1	23.2	17.5	14.9	12.4	13.4	13.4
100–149 percent	66.2	59.6	52.6	47.8	48.5	49.5	58.3	52.5	46.3	43.2	43.6	43.7
150–199 percent	80.9	75.9	74.2	69.3	68.5	73.0	75.8	70.1	69.3	64.0	63.0	67.4
200 percent or more	92.3	92.7	91.2	89.7	90.4	90.7	86.9	86.7	86.1	84.5	85.5	84.6
Geographic region[5]												
Northeast	80.1	81.8	75.9	74.8	75.1	74.9	73.8	74.9	70.7	69.5	69.5	68.7
Midwest	80.4	81.4	77.7	77.2	77.2	78.4	71.9	73.3	71.4	71.0	71.1	72.3
South	74.0	71.1	66.1	65.0	66.7	65.9	65.9	63.3	60.0	59.1	61.7	60.4
West	71.8	71.3	68.0	65.2	67.9	67.1	64.5	63.9	62.0	58.1	60.7	59.6
Location of residence[5]												
Within MSA[6]	77.2	76.3	71.5	70.4	72.1	72.5	70.6	69.5	65.9	64.8	66.6	66.5
Outside MSA[6]	75.1	73.6	70.5	68.1	67.7	65.8	65.1	63.4	63.1	60.4	60.5	58.6

See footnotes at end of table.

[Data are based on household interviews of a sample of the civilian noninstitutionalized population]

Characteristic	Medicaid or other public assistance[7]						Not covered[8]					
	1984	1989	1993[2]	1994	1995	1996[3]	1984	1989	1993[2]	1994	1995	1996[3]
	Number in millions											
Total[4]	14.0	15.4	22.7	24.1	25.3	25.0	29.8	33.4	38.4	40.4	37.4	38.9
	Percent of population											
Total, age adjusted[4]	7.3	7.8	11.1	11.5	12.0	11.7	14.2	15.2	16.5	17.1	15.6	16.1
Total, crude[4]	6.8	7.2	10.1	10.6	11.0	10.8	14.5	15.6	17.2	17.7	16.2	16.7
Age												
Under 18 years	11.9	12.6	19.3	20.0	20.6	20.1	13.9	14.7	14.1	15.3	13.6	13.4
Under 6 years	15.5	15.7	26.5	27.2	28.3	27.4	14.9	15.1	12.7	13.7	11.9	11.9
6–17 years	10.1	10.9	15.4	16.2	16.6	16.4	13.4	14.5	14.9	16.2	14.5	14.1
18–44 years	5.1	5.2	7.0	7.3	7.4	7.3	17.1	18.4	21.6	21.9	20.5	21.2
18–24 years	6.4	6.8	9.5	9.6	9.7	9.2	25.0	27.1	31.1	31.1	28.2	29.6
25–34 years	5.3	5.2	7.6	7.7	7.7	7.5	16.2	18.3	22.5	22.1	21.3	22.5
35–44 years	3.5	4.0	4.9	5.4	5.6	6.0	11.2	12.3	15.1	16.0	15.2	15.2
45–64 years	3.4	4.3	4.2	4.5	5.3	5.2	9.6	10.5	12.0	12.0	11.0	12.1
45–54 years	3.2	3.8	3.8	3.8	4.9	4.8	10.5	11.0	12.7	12.6	11.7	12.5
55–64 years	3.6	4.9	4.8	5.5	6.0	5.7	8.7	10.0	11.1	11.2	10.0	11.6
Sex[5]												
Male	6.1	6.5	9.4	9.8	10.3	10.1	14.8	16.1	17.6	18.1	16.7	17.2
Female	8.5	9.1	12.7	13.2	13.6	13.3	13.6	14.3	15.4	16.1	14.6	15.1
Race[5]												
White	5.0	5.6	8.1	8.7	9.4	9.3	13.3	14.1	15.6	16.4	15.0	15.4
Black	20.5	19.3	26.4	27.0	27.0	24.5	19.5	21.0	21.1	19.5	17.9	19.0
Asian or Pacific Islander	10.1	11.8	13.8	10.2	11.4	12.4	17.8	18.2	17.5	19.9	17.8	18.6
Hispanic origin and race[5]												
All Hispanic	13.1	13.5	18.7	19.6	21.2	20.1	29.0	32.4	32.6	31.4	30.8	31.6
Mexican	11.8	12.3	17.0	18.3	20.1	19.0	33.1	38.6	38.3	35.7	35.4	36.7
Puerto Rican	31.1	28.0	35.4	36.2	32.7	33.8	17.9	23.3	17.2	15.4	17.8	14.4
Cuban	5.0	8.0	16.4	9.8	15.3	13.9	21.6	21.8	15.7	26.1	21.6	17.6
Other Hispanic	8.0	11.2	14.0	16.2	18.4	16.3	27.1	24.8	30.1	30.2	29.0	29.8
White, non-Hispanic	4.0	4.6	6.6	7.1	7.5	7.5	11.6	11.7	13.4	14.2	12.7	12.9
Black, non-Hispanic	20.8	19.4	26.2	27.0	26.7	24.2	19.2	20.8	21.0	19.1	17.8	18.9
Age and percent of poverty level												
All ages:[5]												
Below 100 percent	32.1	37.0	44.3	45.0	46.9	46.8	34.0	35.2	33.2	32.7	30.9	32.7
100–149 percent	7.7	11.2	16.8	16.0	18.4	17.2	26.4	30.6	31.2	34.0	31.2	32.8
150–199 percent	3.3	5.1	5.4	5.9	7.7	7.7	16.7	21.0	22.6	24.9	22.8	22.5
200 percent or more	0.6	1.1	1.3	1.4	1.6	1.6	5.6	6.5	7.6	8.4	7.8	7.4
Under 18 years:												
Below 100 percent	43.1	47.8	62.2	63.6	65.6	65.9	28.9	31.6	24.3	23.3	20.6	21.3
100–149 percent	9.0	12.3	23.6	22.9	26.3	24.8	22.8	26.1	24.1	27.7	25.5	25.2
150–199 percent	4.4	6.1	8.2	8.6	11.7	10.8	12.7	15.8	16.1	19.0	17.7	16.1
200 percent or more	0.8	1.6	2.2	2.2	2.7	2.6	4.2	4.4	5.2	6.8	6.0	5.3
Geographic region[5]												
Northeast	9.4	7.4	11.4	12.0	12.5	12.3	9.8	10.5	13.0	13.3	12.7	13.2
Midwest	7.9	8.2	11.2	10.4	11.0	9.4	10.9	10.2	10.9	11.9	11.8	11.9
South	5.5	7.0	10.0	11.3	11.6	12.0	17.4	19.4	21.6	20.9	19.1	19.7
West	7.5	9.1	12.2	12.6	13.2	13.4	17.6	18.1	18.0	20.2	17.3	18.1
Location of residence[5]												
Within MSA[6]	7.8	7.7	11.4	11.7	11.8	11.1	13.2	14.7	16.0	16.6	14.9	15.3
Outside MSA[6]	6.4	8.3	10.1	11.1	12.8	13.9	16.3	16.7	18.2	18.8	18.4	19.2

[1]Private insurance originally obtained through a present or former employer or union.
[2]July 1 to Dec. 31, 1993. The questionnaire changed in 1993 compared with previous years.
[3]Preliminary data based on a five-eights sample.
[4]Includes all other races not shown separately and unknown family income.
[5]Age adjusted.   [6]Metropolitan statistical area.
[7]In 1996 the age-adjusted percent of the population under 65 years of age covered by Medicaid was 11.3 percent, and 0.4 percent were covered by public assistance.
[8]Includes persons not covered by private insurance, Medicaid or other public assistance, Medicare, or military plans. Estimates of persons lacking health care coverage based on the National Health Interview Survey (NHIS) are slightly higher than those based on the March Current Population Survey (CPS) (table 149). The NHIS questions ask about health insurance coverage over the previous month whereas the CPS asks about coverage over the previous calendar year. These differences result in higher estimates of Medicaid and other health insurance coverage and correspondingly lower estimates of persons without health care coverage in the CPS compared with the NHIS.

NOTE: Percents do not add to 100 because the percent with other types of health insurance (for example, Medicare, military) is not shown, and because persons with both private insurance and Medicaid appear in both columns.

SOURCES: Centers for Disease Control and Prevention, National Center for Health Statistics. Data computed by the Division of Health and Utilization Analysis from data compiled by the Division of Health Interview Statistics; and U.S. Bureau of the Census: Money Income of Households, Families, and Persons in the United States. Series P–60. Annual reports for 1989–96. Washington. U.S. Government Printing Office.

Table 134 (page 1 of 2). Health care coverage for persons 65 years of age and over, according to type of coverage and selected characteristics: United States, selected years 1984–96

[Data are based on household interviews of a sample of the civilian noninstitutionalized population]

Characteristic	Private insurance[1]						Private insurance obtained through workplace[1,2]					
	1984	1989	1993[3]	1994	1995	1996[4]	1984	1989	1993[3]	1994	1995	1996[4]
	Number in millions											
Total[5]	19.4	22.4	24.2	24.0	23.5	22.9	10.2	11.2	12.7	12.5	12.5	12.1
	Percent of population											
Total, age adjusted[5]	73.5	76.6	77.3	77.5	74.9	72.0	39.1	38.8	40.9	41.0	40.1	38.6
Total, crude[5]	73.3	76.5	77.1	77.3	74.8	72.0	38.8	38.4	40.3	40.4	39.6	38.1
Age												
65–74 years	76.5	78.2	78.9	78.4	75.3	72.4	45.1	43.7	45.9	45.6	43.3	41.5
75 years and over	68.1	73.9	74.4	75.8	74.2	71.3	28.6	30.2	32.1	33.0	34.3	33.3
75–84 years.	70.8	75.9	76.4	77.9	76.0	73.3	30.8	32.0	34.3	35.0	36.1	35.5
85 years and over	56.8	65.5	66.3	67.9	67.8	63.9	18.9	22.8	23.7	25.1	27.5	25.3
Sex[6]												
Male.	74.3	77.5	78.9	78.9	76.5	73.6	44.2	43.4	45.9	45.1	44.3	42.7
Female.	72.9	76.2	76.1	76.5	73.9	71.0	35.7	35.6	37.4	38.1	37.0	35.5
Race[6]												
White.	76.8	80.3	80.9	81.2	78.6	75.3	40.9	40.3	42.7	42.7	41.6	39.8
Black	42.3	43.0	45.0	44.7	41.9	44.0	24.0	24.9	25.7	26.5	26.4	30.1
Asian or Pacific Islander.	- - -	- - -	- - -	49.3	46.1	32.2	- - -	- - -	- - -	27.3	27.2	*13.1
Hispanic origin and race[6]												
All Hispanic.	40.5	44.6	39.8	51.2	40.9	38.6	25.4	24.3	18.8	22.1	20.1	19.4
Mexican.	41.4	36.6	34.9	44.6	33.0	35.6	25.5	22.4	23.5	23.1	17.4	18.7
Puerto Rican	- - -	- - -	- - -	48.4	42.2	39.0	- - -	- - -	- - -	15.1	17.1	28.5
Cuban.	- - -	- - -	- - -	58.1	44.7	49.9	- - -	- - -	- - -	*17.3	17.8	15.6
Other Hispanic.	- - -	- - -	- - -	58.2	50.0	35.2	- - -	- - -	- - -	27.8	27.4	19.5
White, non-Hispanic.	77.9	81.5	82.8	82.6	80.7	77.2	41.4	40.9	43.8	43.8	42.9	40.8
Black, non-Hispanic.	42.0	43.1	45.2	45.2	41.7	44.8	23.8	24.9	25.9	26.8	26.1	30.7
Percent of poverty level[6]												
Below 100 percent.	43.0	45.3	36.2	40.1	36.8	32.7	13.4	11.5	8.5	10.6	11.3	10.2
100–149 percent	67.3	66.7	63.9	68.0	67.4	58.8	27.8	22.4	23.2	25.2	25.3	22.3
150–199 percent	78.6	81.1	80.3	81.3	77.4	75.0	41.4	39.8	39.5	37.3	39.9	37.3
200 percent or more	85.7	86.2	88.9	88.9	86.6	84.0	52.8	51.5	53.8	54.0	51.7	49.9
Geographic region[6]												
Northeast	76.8	76.7	81.7	78.3	76.0	72.9	43.9	44.2	49.1	45.2	45.3	42.5
Midwest	79.6	82.3	83.1	84.6	82.5	80.8	40.6	41.4	44.3	43.6	46.0	42.3
South.	68.0	73.5	71.3	71.2	71.6	67.2	35.3	33.5	34.5	36.8	35.1	34.7
West	70.8	75.1	75.3	78.2	69.3	69.0	38.2	38.5	39.0	40.1	34.9	36.2
Location of residence[6]												
Within MSA[7].	74.5	77.2	77.6	78.0	75.1	72.2	42.3	41.6	42.7	42.6	42.0	40.5
Outside MSA[7].	71.8	75.1	76.4	76.0	74.4	71.3	33.7	31.3	35.8	36.5	33.5	32.2

See footnotes at end of table.

Table 134 (page 2 of 2). **Health care coverage for persons 65 years of age and over, according to type of coverage and selected characteristics: United States, selected years 1984–96**

[Data are based on household interviews of a sample of the civilian noninstitutionalized population]

Characteristic	Medicaid or other public assistance[1,8]						Medicare only[9]					
	1984	1989	1993[3]	1994	1995	1996[4]	1984	1989	1993[3]	1994	1995	1996[4]
	Number in millions											
Total[5].................	1.8	2.0	2.4	2.5	2.9	2.7	4.7	4.5	4.4	4.1	4.6	5.7
	Percent of population											
Total, age adjusted[5].........	6.9	7.0	7.4	7.8	9.0	8.3	17.7	15.3	14.0	13.1	14.7	18.1
Total, crude[5]...............	7.0	7.0	7.6	7.9	9.2	8.5	17.9	15.4	14.2	13.2	14.8	18.1
Age												
65–74 years...............	6.0	6.3	6.5	6.8	8.3	7.5	15.2	13.8	12.8	12.3	14.4	18.0
75 years and over...........	8.5	8.2	9.2	9.6	10.4	9.9	22.3	17.8	16.3	14.5	15.2	18.2
75–84 years..............	7.7	7.9	8.6	8.4	9.5	9.0	20.6	16.2	14.7	13.3	14.1	16.8
85 years and over	11.7	9.7	11.4	14.2	13.7	13.0	29.8	24.9	22.6	19.1	19.3	23.4
Sex[6]												
Male.....................	4.5	5.0	4.6	4.7	5.6	5.5	17.4	14.6	13.6	12.9	14.4	17.1
Female...................	8.6	8.4	9.5	10.0	11.5	10.4	18.1	15.6	14.4	13.3	14.9	18.7
Race[6]												
White....................	5.0	5.4	5.6	6.0	6.9	6.6	16.5	13.4	12.4	11.6	13.4	16.9
Black....................	24.9	20.4	20.5	21.7	26.8	21.8	30.7	34.5	29.9	28.7	28.6	30.1
Asian or Pacific Islander.......	- - -	- - -	- - -	27.8	32.9	38.8	- - -	- - -	- - -	17.5	14.2	21.0
Hispanic origin and race[6]												
All Hispanic...............	24.9	25.6	31.1	26.5	31.1	28.9	28.5	21.6	26.5	18.7	24.5	29.0
Mexican................	19.1	27.4	22.8	30.0	31.9	32.5	36.4	23.1	38.2	23.1	31.3	26.2
Puerto Rican..............	- - -	- - -	- - -	30.0	27.5	31.3	- - -	- - -	- - -	19.8	26.8	29.7
Cuban.................	- - -	- - -	- - -	30.5	42.3	19.9	- - -	- - -	- - -	9.4	15.8	34.7
Other Hispanic............	- - -	- - -	- - -	16.2	25.6	26.2	- - -	- - -	- - -	17.8	18.0	31.4
White, non-Hispanic..........	4.4	4.7	4.6	5.1	5.6	5.4	16.1	13.1	11.7	11.3	12.8	16.3
Black, non-Hispanic..........	25.2	20.4	20.5	21.2	27.0	21.7	30.8	34.5	29.7	28.8	28.7	29.3
Percent of poverty level[6]												
Below 100 percent...........	28.0	29.0	36.4	37.4	40.6	39.9	27.5	26.0	25.0	23.0	22.1	25.6
100–149 percent...........	6.9	9.2	11.0	10.8	13.3	12.5	22.5	21.1	22.4	19.0	18.3	26.6
150–199 percent...........	3.3	4.7	4.0	3.8	5.2	4.6	16.2	13.5	14.8	12.8	16.2	19.6
200 percent or more	1.8	2.3	2.1	1.8	1.8	1.9	11.0	10.4	8.3	7.8	9.9	12.4
Geographic region[6]												
Northeast.................	5.3	5.4	6.0	7.3	8.9	7.3	17.1	16.8	11.7	14.0	15.4	20.3
Midwest.................	4.2	3.6	4.3	3.7	5.6	5.1	15.2	13.4	11.8	10.7	10.9	12.8
South...................	9.5	9.1	9.5	10.3	10.8	9.9	19.8	16.3	17.1	16.0	15.8	19.7
West	7.9	9.3	9.6	9.4	10.8	10.8	18.4	13.8	14.2	10.3	17.3	18.6
Location of residence[6]												
Within MSA[7].............	6.2	6.4	7.4	7.3	8.4	7.7	17.6	15.3	14.0	12.9	14.9	18.7
Outside MSA[7].............	8.1	8.4	7.7	9.2	11.1	10.4	17.9	15.2	14.2	13.9	14.1	15.9

- - - Data not available.

* Relative standard error greater than 30 percent.

[1]Most persons are covered by Medicare also.

[2]Private insurance originally obtained through a present or former employer or union.

[3]July 1 to Dec. 31, 1993. The questionnaire changed in 1993 compared with previous years.

[4]Preliminary data based on a five-eights sample.

[5]Includes all other races not shown separately and unknown family income.

[6]Age adjusted.

[7]Metropolitan statistical area.

[8]In 1996 the age adjusted percent of the population 65 years of age and over covered by Medicaid was 7.9 percent, and 0.4 percent were covered by public assistance.

[9]Persons covered by Medicare but not covered by private health insurance, Medicaid, public assistance, or military plans.

NOTES: Percents do not add to 100 because persons with both private health insurance and Medicaid appear in more than one column. Persons with no health insurance (0.7 percent in 1996) are excluded from this table. Data for Asians or Pacific Islanders, Puerto Ricans, Cubans, and other Hispanics were not considered reliable for the years 1984, 1989, and 1993 and are not shown.

SOURCE: Centers for Disease Control and Prevention, National Center for Health Statistics. Data computed by the Division of Health and Utilization Analysis from data compiled by the Division of Health Interview Statistics; and U.S. Bureau of the Census: Money Income of Households, Families, and Persons in the United States. Series P–60. Annual reports for 1989–96. Washington. U.S. Government Printing Office.

Table 135. Health maintenance organizations (HMO's) and enrollment, according to model type, geographic region, and Federal program: United States, selected years 1976–97

[Data are based on a census of health maintenance organizations]

Plans and enrollment	1976	1980	1985[1]	1990	1991	1992	1993	1994[2]	1995[2]	1996[2]	1997[2]
Plans						Number					
All plans	174	235	478	572	553	555	551	543	562	630	651
Model type:[3]											
Individual practice association[4]	41	97	244	360	346	340	332	321	332	367	284
Group[5]	122	138	234	212	168	166	150	118	108	122	98
Mixed	- - -	- - -	- - -	- - -	39	49	69	104	122	141	258
Geographic region:											
Northeast	29	55	81	115	116	111	102	101	100	111	110
Midwest	52	72	157	160	157	165	169	159	157	182	184
South	23	45	141	176	163	161	167	173	196	218	236
West	70	63	99	121	117	118	113	110	109	119	121
Enrollment					Number of persons in millions						
Total	6.0	9.1	21.0	33.0	34.0	36.1	38.4	45.1	50.9	59.1	66.8
Model type:[3]											
Individual practice association[4]	0.4	1.7	6.4	13.7	13.6	14.7	15.3	17.8	20.1	26.0	26.7
Group[5]	5.6	7.4	14.6	19.3	17.1	16.5	15.4	13.9	13.3	14.1	11.0
Mixed	- - -	- - -	- - -	- - -	3.3	4.9	7.7	13.4	17.6	19.0	29.0
Federal program:[6]											
Medicaid[7]	- - -	0.3	0.6	1.2	1.4	1.7	1.7	2.6	3.5	4.7	5.5
Medicare	- - -	0.4	1.1	1.8	2.0	2.2	2.2	2.5	2.9	3.7	4.8
					Percent of HMO enrollees						
Model type:[3]											
Individual practice association[4]	6.6	18.7	30.4	41.6	40.1	40.7	39.8	39.4	39.4	44.1	39.9
Group[5]	93.4	81.3	69.6	58.4	50.2	45.9	40.1	30.7	26.0	23.7	16.5
Mixed	- - -	- - -	- - -	- - -	9.8	13.5	20.1	29.9	34.5	32.2	43.4
Federal program:[6]											
Medicaid[7]	- - -	2.9	2.7	3.5	4.3	4.8	4.4	5.8	6.9	8.0	8.2
Medicare	- - -	4.3	5.1	5.4	6.0	6.0	5.7	5.5	5.7	6.3	7.2
					Percent of population enrolled in HMO's						
Total	2.8	4.0	8.9	13.4	13.6	14.3	15.1	17.3	19.4	22.3	25.2
Geographic region:											
Northeast	2.0	3.1	7.9	14.6	15.4	16.1	18.0	20.8	24.4	25.9	32.4
Midwest	1.5	2.8	9.7	12.6	12.7	12.8	13.2	15.2	16.4	18.8	19.5
South	0.4	0.8	3.8	7.1	7.1	7.8	8.4	10.2	12.4	15.2	17.9
West	9.7	12.2	17.3	23.2	23.8	24.7	25.1	27.4	28.6	33.2	36.4

- - - Data not available.

[1]Increases partly due to changes in reporting methods. See Appendix I, InterStudy.

[2]Open-ended enrollment in HMO plans, amounting to 7.8 million on Jan. 1, 1997, is included from 1994 onwards. See Appendix II, Health maintenance organization.

[3]In 1976, 11 HMO's with 35,000 enrollment did not report model type. In 1997, 11 HMO's with 153,000 enrollment did not report model type.

[4]An HMO operating under an individual practice association model contracts with an association of physicians from various settings (a mixture of solo and group practices) to provide health services.

[5]Group includes staff, group, and network model types.

[6]Federal program enrollment in HMO's refers to enrollment by Medicaid or Medicare beneficiaries, where the Medicaid or Medicare program contracts directly with the HMO to pay the appropriate annual premium.

[7]Data for 1990 and later include enrollment in managed care health insuring organizations.

NOTES: Data as of June 30 in 1976–80, December 31 in 1985, and January 1 in 1990–97. Medicaid enrollment in 1990 is as of June 30. HMO's in Guam are included starting in 1994. Some numbers in this table have been revised and differ from previous editions of Health, United States.

SOURCES: Office of Health Maintenance Organizations: Summary of the National HMO census of prepaid plans—June 1976 and National HMO Census 1980. Public Health Service. Washington. U.S. Government Printing Office. DHHS Pub. No. (PHS) 80–50159; InterStudy: National HMO Census: Annual Report on the Growth of HMO's in the U.S., 1984–1985 Editions; The InterStudy Edge, 1990, vol. 2; Competitive Edge, vols. 1–7, 1991–1997; 1986 December Update of Medicare Enrollment in HMO's. 1988 January Update of Medicare Enrollment in HMO's. Excelsior, Minnesota (Copyrights 1983–95: Used with the permission of InterStudy); U.S. Bureau of the Census. Current Population Reports. Series P–25, Nos. 998 and 1058. Washington: U.S. Government Printing Office, Dec. 1986 and Mar. 1990. U.S. Dept. of Commerce. Press release CB 91–100. Mar. 11, 1991; Health Care Financing Administration: Unpublished data; Centers for Disease Control and Prevention, National Center for Health Statistics: Data computed by the Division of Health and Utilization Analysis.

Table 136. Medical care benefits for employees of private establishments by size of establishment and occupation: United States, selected years 1990–95

[Data are based on a survey of employers]

Size of establishment and type of benefit	All 1990	All 1992	All 1994	Professional, technical, and related 1990	Professional, technical, and related 1992	Professional, technical, and related 1994	Clerical and sales 1990	Clerical and sales 1992	Clerical and sales 1994	Blue-collar and service 1990	Blue-collar and service 1992	Blue-collar and service 1994
Small private establishments[1]				*Percent of all employees*								
Participation in medical care benefit:												
Full-time employees	69	71	66	82	83	80	75	78	70	60	61	57
Part-time employees	6	5	7	6	7	11	7	7	9	6	4	5
Type of medical care benefit among participating full-time employees				*Percent of participating full-time employees*								
Fee arrangement	100	100	100	100	100	100	100	100	100	100	100	100
Traditional fee-for-service	74	68	55	69	63	53	77	71	55	73	68	57
Preferred provider organization (PPO)	13	14	24	16	14	27	13	13	24	11	16	23
Health maintenance organization (HMO)	14	18	19	15	24	20	10	16	19	15	16	20
Other	0	0	1	0	0	0	0	0	2	0	0	0
Individual coverage:												
Employee contributions not required	58	53	47	56	52	49	53	51	44	62	55	48
Employee contributions required	42	47	53	44	48	51	47	49	56	38	45	52
Family coverage:												
Employee contributions not required	32	27	19	28	21	17	29	26	15	37	32	23
Employee contributions required	68	73	81	72	79	83	71	74	85	63	68	77
Individual coverage:				*Average monthly contribution*								
Average monthly employee contribution:												
Total	$ 25	$ 37	$ 41	$ 24	$ 35	$ 47	$ 24	$ 36	$ 41	$ 27	$ 38	$ 38
Non-HMO	25	36	39	24	35	46	24	36	38	28	36	36
HMO	25	39	49	24	35	48	27	37	50	25	42	47
Family coverage:												
Average monthly employee contribution:												
Total	109	151	160	112	147	181	106	151	160	111	152	149
Non-HMO	104	147	151	110	143	173	102	150	155	101	147	137
HMO	135	168	190	118	175	204	134	153	178	145	176	191

Size of establishment and type of benefit	All 1991	All 1993	All 1995	Professional, technical, and related 1991	Professional, technical, and related 1993	Professional, technical, and related 1995	Clerical and sales 1991	Clerical and sales 1993	Clerical and sales 1995	Blue-collar and service 1991	Blue-collar and service 1993	Blue-collar and service 1995
Medium and large private establishments[2]				*Percent of all employees*								
Participation in medical care benefit:												
Full-time employees	83	82	77	85	84	80	81	79	76	84	82	75
Part-time employees	28	24	19	42	33	31	26	22	20	26	24	15
Type of medical care benefit among participating full-time employees				*Percent of participating full-time employees*								
Fee arrangement	100	100	100	100	100	100	100	100	100	100	100	100
Traditional fee-for-service	67	50	37	62	41	29	59	42	30	73	59	45
Preferred provider organization (PPO)	16	26	34	19	29	36	21	30	36	12	22	33
Health maintenance organization (HMO)	17	23	27	18	28	33	19	27	32	14	18	21
Other	0	1	1	1	2	1	0	1	2	0	1	1
Individual coverage:												
Employee contributions not required	49	38	33	45	32	21	43	33	24	55	44	44
Employee contributions required	51	62	67	55	68	79	57	67	76	45	56	56
Family coverage:												
Employee contributions not required	31	22	22	25	15	11	27	18	15	37	29	33
Employee contributions required	69	78	78	75	85	89	73	82	85	63	71	67
Individual coverage:				*Average monthly contribution*								
Average monthly employee contribution:												
Total	$ 27	$ 32	$ 34	$ 26	$ 32	$ 35	$ 28	$ 34	$ 36	$ 26	$ 30	$ 32
Non-HMO	26	31	33	26	32	33	27	34	34	25	30	32
HMO	29	32	36	29	32	38	32	34	39	28	30	32
Family coverage:												
Average monthly employee contribution:												
Total	97	107	118	96	114	120	108	115	127	91	99	112
Non-HMO	92	102	112	93	113	116	104	112	120	84	92	106
HMO	118	122	133	110	117	128	121	125	141	122	124	130

[1]Less than 100 employees in all private nonfarm industries.
[2]100 or more employees in all private nonfarm industries.

NOTE: In 1992–93, 88 percent of full-time employees in private establishments were offered health care plans by their employers (96 percent in medium and large private establishments and 80 percent in small private establishments).

SOURCES: U.S. Department of Labor, Bureau of Labor Statistics, Employee benefits in small private establishments, 1990 Bulletin 2388, September 1991, 1992 Bulletin 2441, May 1994, and 1994 Bulletin 2475, April 1996. Employee benefits in medium and large private establishments, 1991 Bulletin 2422, May 1993, 1993 Bulletin 2456, Nov. 1994, and news release USDL 97–246. July 25, 1997. Blostin AP and Pfuntner JN. Employee medical care contributions on the rise. Compensation and Working Conditions, Spring 1998.

Table 137. Medicare enrollees and expenditures and percent distribution, according to type of service: United States and other areas, selected years 1967–96

[Data are compiled by the Health Care Financing Administration]

Type of service	1967	1970	1975	1980	1985	1990	1994	1995	1996[1]
Enrollees					Number in millions				
Total[2]	19.5	20.5	25.0	28.5	31.1	34.2	36.9	37.5	38.1
Hospital insurance	19.5	20.4	24.6	28.1	30.6	33.7	36.5	37.1	37.7
Supplementary medical insurance	17.9	19.6	23.9	27.4	30.0	32.6	35.2	35.7	36.1
Expenditures					Amount in millions				
Total	$4,737	$7,493	$16,316	$36,822	$72,294	$110,984	$164,862	$184,204	$200,338
Total hospital insurance[3]	3,430	5,281	11,581	25,577	48,414	66,997	104,545	117,604	129,929
Inpatient hospital	3,034	4,827	10,877	24,116	44,940	59,451	81,697	89,127	97,802
Skilled nursing facility	282	246	278	395	548	2,575	7,407	9,595	11,129
Home health agency	29	51	160	540	1,913	3,666	12,503	15,571	17,527
Hospice	...	...	...	...	43	358	1,486	1,883	1,999
Administrative expenses[4]	77	157	266	526	970	947	1,452	1,428	1,472
Total supplementary medical insurance	1,307	2,212	4,735	11,245	23,880	43,987	60,317	66,600	70,409
Physician	1,128	1,790	3,416	8,187	17,312	29,609	36,900	40,439	41,116
Outpatient hospital	33	114	643	1,897	4,319	8,482	14,034	15,392	16,529
Home health agency	10	34	95	234	38	74	154	197	215
Group practice prepayment	19	26	80	203	720	2,827	5,480	6,882	8,890
Independent laboratory	7	11	39	114	558	1,476	2,050	2,063	1,849
Administrative expenses[4]	110	237	462	610	933	1,519	1,699	1,627	1,810
					Percent distribution of expenditures				
Total hospital insurance[3]	100.0	100.0	100.0	100.0	100.0	100.0	100.0	100.0	100.0
Inpatient hospital	88.5	91.4	93.9	94.3	92.8	88.7	78.1	75.8	75.3
Skilled nursing facility	8.2	4.7	2.4	1.5	1.1	3.8	7.1	8.2	8.6
Home health agency	0.8	1.0	1.4	2.1	4.0	5.5	12.0	13.2	13.5
Hospice	...	...	...	...	0.1	0.5	1.4	1.6	1.5
Administrative expenses[4]	2.2	3.0	2.3	2.1	2.0	1.4	1.4	1.2	1.1
Total supplementary medical insurance	100.0	100.0	100.0	100.0	100.0	100.0	100.0	100.0	100.0
Physician	86.3	80.9	72.1	72.8	72.5	67.3	61.2	60.7	58.4
Outpatient hospital	2.5	5.2	13.6	16.9	18.1	19.3	23.3	23.1	23.5
Home health agency	0.8	1.5	2.0	2.1	0.2	0.2	0.3	0.3	0.3
Group practice prepayment	1.5	1.2	1.7	1.8	3.0	6.4	9.1	10.3	12.6
Independent laboratory	0.5	0.5	0.8	1.0	2.3	3.4	3.4	3.1	2.6
Administrative expenses[4]	8.4	10.7	9.8	5.4	3.9	3.5	2.8	2.4	2.6

... Category not applicable.
[1]Preliminary figures.
[2]Number enrolled in the hospital insurance and/or supplementary medical insurance programs on July 1.
[3]In 1967 includes coverage for outpatient hospital diagnostic services.
[4]Includes research, costs of experiments and demonstration projects, and peer review activity.

NOTES: Table includes data for Medicare enrollees residing in Puerto Rico, Virgin Islands, Guam, other outlying areas, foreign countries, and unknown residence. Some numbers in this table have been revised and differ from previous editions of Health, United States.

SOURCE: Health Care Financing Administration. Office of Medicare Cost Estimates, Office of the Actuary and Bureau of Data Management and Strategy. Washington.

Table 138. Medicare enrollment, persons served, and payments for Medicare enrollees 65 years of age and over, according to selected characteristics: United States and other areas, selected years 1977–95

[Data are compiled by the Health Care Financing Administration]

Characteristic	Enrollment in millions[1]				Persons served per 1,000 enrollees[2]				Payments per person served[3]				Payments per enrollee[3]			
	1977	1987	1994	1995	1977	1987	1994	1995	1977	1987	1994	1995	1977	1987	1994	1995
Total	23.8	29.4	32.8	33.1	570	754	830	826	$1,332	$3,025	$4,740	$5,074	$ 759	$2,281	$3,934	$4,193
Age																
65–66 years	3.3	4.0	3.9	3.8	533	700	819	809	1,075	2,214	3,014	3,146	573	1,550	2,467	2,546
67–68 years	3.2	3.7	3.8	3.8	511	667	749	746	1,173	2,536	3,735	3,936	599	1,691	2,799	2,937
69–70 years	2.9	3.4	3.8	3.7	531	705	773	773	1,211	2,700	3,929	4,205	643	1,902	3,039	3,249
71–72 years	2.6	3.1	3.5	3.6	555	740	801	790	1,228	2,904	4,281	4,538	681	2,150	3,430	3,586
73–74 years	2.3	2.9	3.3	3.3	576	762	810	817	1,319	3,048	4,629	4,911	759	2,322	3,747	4,010
75–79 years	4.5	5.7	6.4	6.6	597	787	857	845	1,430	3,312	5,174	5,464	853	2,608	4,435	4,616
80–84 years	3.0	3.7	4.4	4.5	623	828	890	890	1,549	3,496	5,823	6,299	965	2,894	5,184	5,603
85 years and over	2.1	3.0	3.7	3.8	652	841	910	911	1,636	3,708	6,416	6,980	1,068	3,119	5,841	6,356
Sex and age																
Male	9.6	11.8	13.3	13.4	546	712	790	784	1,505	3,432	5,125	5,450	821	2,443	4,047	4,275
65–66 years	- - -	1.8	1.8	1.8	- - -	640	764	755	- - -	2,560	3,404	3,516	- - -	1,639	2,600	2,655
67–68 years	- - -	1.6	1.7	1.7	- - -	623	711	707	- - -	2,955	4,121	4,401	- - -	1,841	2,929	3,110
69–70 years	- - -	1.5	1.7	1.7	- - -	667	737	737	- - -	3,116	4,383	4,740	- - -	2,078	3,230	3,491
71–72 years	- - -	1.3	1.5	1.5	- - -	711	767	757	- - -	3,399	4,800	5,032	- - -	2,416	3,682	3,810
73–74 years	- - -	1.2	1.4	1.4	- - -	735	779	782	- - -	3,587	5,125	5,420	- - -	2,635	3,992	4,241
75–79 years	- - -	2.2	2.6	2.6	- - -	764	831	816	- - -	3,775	5,738	6,026	- - -	2,883	4,767	4,915
80–84 years	- - -	1.3	1.5	1.6	- - -	806	872	869	- - -	3,997	6,451	6,895	- - -	3,222	5,524	5,994
85 years and over	- - -	0.8	1.0	1.1	- - -	808	875	874	- - -	4,227	7,106	7,636	- - -	3,417	6,217	6,671
Female	14.2	17.6	19.5	19.7	586	782	857	855	1,223	2,778	4,499	4,840	717	2,173	3,857	4,136
65–66 years	- - -	2.2	2.1	2.0	- - -	750	866	856	- - -	1,970	2,719	2,865	- - -	1,477	2,353	2,453
67–68 years	- - -	2.0	2.1	2.1	- - -	702	781	779	- - -	2,236	3,444	3,584	- - -	1,569	2,690	2,793
69–70 years	- - -	1.9	2.1	2.1	- - -	734	802	801	- - -	2,404	3,599	3,812	- - -	1,765	2,887	3,055
71–72 years	- - -	1.8	2.0	2.0	- - -	762	827	816	- - -	2,557	3,910	4,183	- - -	1,950	3,235	3,412
73–74 years	- - -	1.7	1.9	2.0	- - -	781	832	842	- - -	2,687	4,287	4,560	- - -	2,099	3,567	3,839
75–79 years	- - -	3.5	3.8	4.0	- - -	802	875	864	- - -	3,032	4,815	5,106	- - -	2,433	4,212	4,414
80–84 years	- - -	2.4	2.8	2.9	- - -	839	900	901	- - -	3,244	5,491	5,980	- - -	2,722	4,943	5,387
85 years and over	- - -	2.2	2.7	2.8	- - -	854	924	925	- - -	3,518	6,168	6,743	- - -	3,004	5,698	6,235
Geographic region[4]																
Northeast	5.7	6.6	7.1	7.1	613	793	866	865	1,426	3,171	5,290	5,503	874	2,513	4,582	4,757
Midwest	6.3	7.4	8.0	8.0	541	756	883	892	1,401	2,969	4,247	4,555	757	2,246	3,751	4,062
South	7.5	9.6	11.1	11.2	556	768	870	869	1,198	2,893	4,842	5,263	666	2,221	4,211	4,576
West	3.8	5.2	6.1	6.2	632	726	692	663	1,341	3,222	4,657	5,036	848	2,339	3,222	3,340

- - - Data not available.

[1]Includes fee-for-service and Health maintenance organization (HMO) enrollees and is as of July 1 each year.
[2]Excludes HMO enrollees.
[3]Excludes amounts for HMO services.
[4]Includes residents of the United States. Excludes unknown residence.

NOTE: Table includes data for Medicare enrollees residing in Puerto Rico, Virgin Islands, Guam, other outlying areas, foreign countries, and unknown residence.

SOURCE: Health Care Financing Administration. Bureau of Data Management and Strategy. Unpublished data.

Table 139. Medicaid recipients and medical vendor payments, according to basis of eligibility: United States, selected fiscal years 1972–96

[Data are compiled by the Health Care Financing Administration]

Basis of eligibility	1972	1975	1980	1985	1990	1993	1994	1995	1996
Recipients					Number in millions				
All recipients	17.6	22.0	21.6	21.8	25.3	33.4	35.1	36.3	36.1
					Percent of recipients[1]				
Aged (65 years and over)	18.8	16.4	15.9	14.0	12.7	11.6	11.5	11.4	11.9
Blind and disabled	9.8	11.2	13.5	13.8	14.7	15.0	15.6	16.1	17.2
Adults in families with dependent children[2] .	17.8	20.6	22.6	25.3	23.8	22.4	21.6	21.0	19.7
Children under age 21[3]	44.5	43.6	43.2	44.7	44.4	48.7	49.0	47.3	46.3
Other Title XIX[4]	9.0	8.2	6.9	5.6	3.9	1.9	1.7	1.7	1.8
Vendor payments[5]					Amount in billions				
All payments	$ 6.3	$ 12.2	$ 23.3	$ 37.5	$ 64.9	$101.8	$107.9	$120.1	$121.7
					Percent distribution				
Total	100.0	100.0	100.0	100.0	100.0	100.0	100.0	100.0	100.0
Aged (65 years and over)	30.6	35.6	37.5	37.6	33.2	31.0	30.9	30.4	30.4
Blind and disabled	22.2	25.7	32.7	35.9	37.6	38.0	39.1	41.1	42.8
Adults in families with dependent children[2] .	15.3	16.8	13.9	12.7	13.2	13.4	12.6	11.2	10.1
Children under age 21[3]	18.1	17.9	13.4	11.8	14.0	16.2	16.0	15.0	14.4
Other Title XIX[4]	13.9	4.0	2.6	2.1	1.6	1.2	1.2	1.2	1.2
Vendor payments per recipient[5]					Amount				
All recipients	$ 358	$ 556	$1,079	$1,719	$2,568	$3,042	$3,080	$3,311	$3,369
Aged (65 years and over)	580	1,206	2,540	4,605	6,717	8,168	8,264	8,868	8,622
Blind and disabled	807	1,276	2,618	4,459	6,564	7,706	7,735	8,435	8,369
Adults in families with dependent children[2] .	307	455	662	860	1,429	1,813	1,791	1,777	1,722
Children under age 21[3]	145	228	335	452	811	1,013	1,007	1,047	1,048
Other Title XIX[4]	555	273	398	657	1,062	1,856	2,165	2,380	2,152

[1]Recipients included in more than one category for 1980 and 1985. From 1990 to 1996 between 0.2 and 2.5 percent of recipients have unknown basis of eligibility.
[2]Includes adults in the Aid to Families with Dependent Children (AFDC) program.
[3]Includes children in the AFDC program.
[4]Includes some participants in the Supplemental Security Income program and other people deemed medically needy in participating States.
[5]Payments exclude disproportionate share hospital payments ($15 billion in 1996) and payments to health maintenance organizations ($14 billion in 1996).

NOTES: 1972 and 1975 data are for fiscal year ending June 30. All other years are for fiscal year ending September 30.

SOURCE: Health Care Financing Administration. Office of Information Services, Enterprise Databases Group, Division of Information Distribution. Unpublished data.

Table 140. Medicaid recipients and medical vendor payments, according to type of service: United States, selected fiscal years 1972–96

[Data are compiled by the Health Care Financing Administration]

Type of service	1972	1975	1980	1985	1990	1993	1994	1995	1996
Recipients					Number in millions				
All recipients.	17.6	22.0	21.6	21.8	25.3	33.4	35.1	36.3	36.1
					Percent of recipients				
Inpatient general hospitals.	16.1	15.6	17.0	15.7	18.2	17.6	16.7	15.3	14.8
Inpatient mental hospitals	0.2	0.3	0.3	0.3	0.4	0.2	0.2	0.2	0.3
Mentally retarded intermediate care facilities . .	- - -	0.3	0.6	0.7	0.6	0.4	0.5	0.4	0.4
Nursing facilities.	- - -	- - -	- - -	- - -	- - -	4.8	4.7	4.6	4.4
Skilled	3.1	2.9	2.8	2.5	2.4	- - -	- - -	- - -	- - -
Intermediate care.	- - -	3.1	3.7	3.8	3.4	- - -	- - -	- - -	- - -
Physician.	69.8	69.1	63.7	66.0	67.6	71.0	69.2	65.6	63.3
Dental	13.6	17.9	21.5	21.4	18.0	18.5	18.1	17.6	17.2
Other practitioner	9.1	12.1	15.0	15.4	15.3	15.6	15.4	15.2	14.8
Outpatient hospital	29.6	33.8	44.9	46.2	49.0	49.2	47.2	46.1	44.0
Clinic.	2.8	4.9	7.1	9.7	11.1	14.5	15.0	14.7	14.0
Laboratory and radiological	20.0	21.5	14.9	29.1	35.5	38.8	38.3	36.0	34.9
Home health.	0.6	1.6	1.8	2.5	2.8	3.2	3.9	4.5	4.8
Prescribed drugs	63.3	64.3	63.4	63.8	68.5	71.5	69.8	65.4	62.5
Family planning	. . .	5.5	5.2	7.5	6.9	7.6	7.3	6.9	6.6
Early and periodic screening	. . .	. . .	. . .	8.7	11.7	17.8	18.4	18.2	18.2
Rural health clinic.	. . .	. . .	. . .	0.4	0.9	2.9	2.7	3.4	3.9
Other care.	14.4	13.2	11.9	15.5	20.3	24.3	28.4	31.5	36.3
Vendor payments[1]					Amount in billions				
All payments	$ 6.3	$ 12.2	$ 23.3	$ 37.5	$ 64.9	$ 101.8	$ 107.9	$ 120.1	$ 121.7
					Percent distribution				
Total	100.0	100.0	100.0	100.0	100.0	100.0	100.0	100.0	100.0
Inpatient general hospitals.	40.6	27.6	27.5	25.2	25.7	25.3	24.2	21.9	20.7
Inpatient mental hospitals	1.8	3.3	3.3	3.2	2.6	2.1	1.9	2.1	1.7
Mentally retarded intermediate care facilities . .	- - -	3.1	8.5	12.6	11.3	8.7	7.7	8.6	7.9
Nursing facilities.	- - -	- - -	- - -	- - -	- - -	25.0	24.9	24.2	24.3
Skilled	23.3	19.9	15.8	13.5	12.4	- - -	- - -	- - -	- - -
Intermediate care.	- - -	15.4	18.0	17.4	14.9	- - -	- - -	- - -	- - -
Physician.	12.6	10.0	8.0	6.3	6.2	6.8	6.7	6.1	5.9
Dental	2.7	2.8	2.0	1.2	0.9	0.9	0.9	0.8	0.8
Other practitioner	0.9	1.0	0.8	0.7	0.6	0.9	1.0	0.8	0.9
Outpatient hospital	5.8	3.0	4.7	4.8	5.1	6.1	5.9	5.5	5.3
Clinic.	0.7	3.2	1.4	1.9	2.6	3.4	3.5	3.6	3.5
Laboratory and radiological	1.3	1.0	0.5	0.9	1.1	1.1	1.1	1.0	1.0
Home health.	0.4	0.6	1.4	3.0	5.2	5.5	6.5	7.8	8.9
Prescribed drugs	8.1	6.7	5.7	6.2	6.8	7.8	8.2	8.1	8.8
Family planning	. . .	0.5	0.3	0.5	0.4	0.5	0.5	0.4	0.4
Early and periodic screening	. . .	. . .	. . .	0.2	0.3	0.8	0.9	1.0	1.1
Rural health clinic.	. . .	. . .	. . .	0.0	0.1	0.2	0.2	0.2	0.2
Other care.	1.8	1.9	1.9	2.5	3.7	4.7	6.0	7.7	8.4
Vendor payments per recipient[1]					Amount				
Total payment per recipient	$ 358	$ 556	$ 1,079	$ 1,719	$ 2,568	$ 3,042	$ 3,080	$ 3,311	$ 3,369
Inpatient general hospitals.	903	983	1,742	2,753	3,630	4,366	4,462	4,735	4,696
Inpatient mental hospitals	2,825	6,045	11,742	19,867	18,548	28,965	24,024	29,847	21,873
Mentally retarded intermediate care facilities . .	- - -	5,507	16,438	32,102	50,048	59,149	52,269	68,613	68,232
Nursing facilities.	- - -	- - -	- - -	- - -	- - -	15,796	16,424	17,424	18,589
Skilled	2,665	3,864	6,081	9,274	13,356	- - -	- - -	- - -	- - -
Intermediate care.	- - -	2,764	5,326	7,882	11,236	- - -	- - -	- - -	- - -
Physician.	65	81	136	163	235	293	296	309	317
Dental	71	86	99	98	130	156	153	160	166
Other practitioner	37	48	61	75	96	179	192	178	205
Outpatient hospital	70	50	113	178	269	378	383	397	409
Clinic.	82	358	209	337	602	714	714	804	833
Laboratory and radiological	23	27	38	53	80	88	88	90	96
Home health.	229	204	847	2,094	4,733	5,249	5,124	5,740	6,293
Prescribed drugs	46	58	96	166	256	333	363	413	474
Family planning	. . .	55	72	119	151	212	201	206	200
Early and periodic screening	. . .	. . .	. . .	45	67	143	152	177	212
Rural health clinic.	. . .	. . .	. . .	81	154	194	199	174	215
Other care.	44	80	172	274	465	584	656	807	782

- - - Data not available.
. . . Category not applicable.

[1]Excludes disproportionate share hospital payments ($15 billion in 1996) and payments to health maintenance organizations ($14 billion in 1996).

NOTES: 1972 and 1975 data are for fiscal year ending June 30. All other years are for fiscal year ending September 30.

SOURCE: Health Care Financing Administration. Office of Information Services, Enterprise Databases Group, Division of Information Distribution. Unpublished data.

Table 141. Department of Veterans Affairs health care expenditures and use, and persons treated according to selected characteristics: United States, selected fiscal years 1970–96

[Data are compiled by Department of Veterans Affairs]

	1970	1980	1990	1991	1992	1993	1994	1995	1996
Health care expenditures					Amount in millions				
All expenditures[1]	$1,689	$ 5,981	$11,500	$12,400	$13,682	$14,612	$15,401	$16,126	$16,373
					Percent distribution				
All services	100.0	100.0	100.0	100.0	100.0	100.0	100.0	100.0	100.0
Inpatient hospital	71.3	64.3	57.5	56.9	55.8	54.8	53.8	49.0	46.3
Outpatient care	14.0	19.1	25.3	25.8	27.1	28.0	28.4	30.2	33.6
Nursing home care	5.5	7.1	9.5	10.0	10.0	10.4	10.5	10.0	10.1
All other[2]	9.1	9.6	7.7	7.3	7.1	6.8	7.3	10.8	10.0
Health care use					Number in thousands				
Inpatient hospital stays[3]	787	1,248	1,029	984	935	920	907	879	807
Outpatient visits	7,312	17,971	22,602	23,035	23,902	24,236	25,158	27,527	29,295
Nursing home care	47	57	75	77	75	78	78	77	79
Inpatients[4]									
Total	- - -	- - -	598	574	564	556	547	527	491
					Percent distribution				
Total	- - -	- - -	100.0	100.0	100.0	100.0	100.0	100.0	100.0
Veterans with service-connected disability	- - -	- - -	38.9	39.1	39.0	39.4	39.1	39.3	39.5
Veterans without service-connected									
disability	- - -	- - -	60.3	60.0	60.1	59.6	60.0	59.9	59.6
Low income	- - -	- - -	54.8	55.4	55.7	55.2	56.6	56.2	55.7
Exempt[5]	- - -	- - -	2.5	2.7	2.7	2.4	0.9	0.8	0.8
Other[6]	- - -	- - -	2.8	1.8	1.6	1.9	2.4	2.8	3.0
Unknown	- - -	- - -	0.2	0.1	0.1	0.1	0.1	0.1	0.1
Nonveterans	- - -	- - -	0.8	0.9	0.9	1.0	0.9	0.8	0.8
Outpatients[4]					Number in thousands				
Total	- - -	- - -	2,564	2,557	2,639	2,684	2,714	2,790	2,846
					Percent distribution				
Total	- - -	- - -	100.0	100.0	100.0	100.0	100.0	100.0	100.0
Veterans with service-connected disability	- - -	- - -	38.3	38.5	37.8	37.4	37.4	37.5	37.8
Veterans without service-connected									
disability	- - -	- - -	49.8	50.1	50.9	50.6	50.5	50.5	50.2
Low income	- - -	- - -	41.1	42.1	42.4	41.5	42.6	42.2	41.9
Exempt[5]	- - -	- - -	2.9	2.9	2.8	2.6	1.0	0.9	0.9
Other[6]	- - -	- - -	3.6	2.6	2.6	2.9	3.6	4.2	4.7
Unknown	- - -	- - -	2.2	2.4	3.1	3.6	3.3	3.2	2.8
Nonveterans	- - -	- - -	11.8	11.4	11.3	12.0	12.1	12.0	12.1

- - - Data not available.

[1]Health care expenditures exclude construction, medical administration, and miscellaneous operating expenses.
[2]Includes miscellaneous benefits and services, contract hospitals, education and training, subsidies to State veterans hospitals, nursing homes, and domiciliaries, and the Civilian Health and Medical Program of the Department of Veterans Affairs.
[3]One-day dialysis patients were included in fiscal year 1980. Interfacility transfers were included beginning in fiscal year 1990.
[4]Individuals.
[5]Prisoner of war, exposed to Agent Orange, and so forth. Prior to fiscal year 1994, veterans who reported exposure to Agent Orange were classified as Exempt. Beginning in fiscal year 1994, those veterans reporting Agent Orange exposure but not treated for it were means tested and placed in the low income or other group depending on income.
[6]Financial means-tested veterans who receive medical care subject to copayments according to income level.

NOTES: Figures may not add to totals due to rounding. In 1970 and 1980, fiscal year ends June 30; for all other years fiscal year ends September 30. The veteran population was estimated at 25.9 million in 1996 with 35 percent age 65 or over, compared with 11 percent in 1980. Twenty-seven percent had served during World War II, 17 percent during the Korean conflict, 32 percent during the Vietnam era, 6 percent during the Persian Gulf War, and 23 percent during peacetime. In fiscal year 1995 categories for health care expenditures and health care use were revised and data may differ from previous editions of Health, United States.

SOURCE: Department of Veterans Affairs, Office of Policy and Planning, National Center for Veteran Analysis and Statistics. Unpublished data.

Table 142. Hospital care expenditures by geographic division and State and average annual percent change: United States, selected years 1980–93

[Data are compiled by the Health Care Financing Administration]

Geographic division and State[1]	Amount in millions						Average annual percent change	
	1980	1985	1990	1991	1992	1993	1980–90	1990–93
United States[2]	$101,510	$166,545	$254,239	$279,820	$303,461	$323,919	9.6	8.4
New England	6,467	10,332	15,540	16,773	17,855	19,056	9.2	7.0
Maine	460	735	1,119	1,207	1,280	1,376	9.3	7.1
New Hampshire	313	590	1,056	1,102	1,233	1,388	12.9	9.5
Vermont	174	290	447	494	532	562	9.9	7.9
Massachusetts	3,646	5,628	8,159	8,826	9,380	10,034	8.4	7.1
Rhode Island	481	760	1,095	1,177	1,237	1,314	8.6	6.3
Connecticut	1,396	2,328	3,664	3,967	4,193	4,380	10.1	6.1
Middle Atlantic	18,361	29,462	45,472	49,673	53,779	57,854	9.5	8.4
New York	9,582	14,585	22,739	24,784	26,387	28,001	9.0	7.2
New Jersey	2,763	4,751	7,857	8,586	9,406	10,312	11.0	9.5
Pennsylvania	6,017	10,126	14,876	16,303	17,987	19,540	9.5	9.5
East North Central	19,590	30,093	42,984	47,026	50,835	54,172	8.2	8.0
Ohio	4,808	8,026	11,419	12,359	13,394	14,305	9.0	7.8
Indiana	2,125	3,399	5,288	5,918	6,473	6,998	9.5	9.8
Illinois	6,217	8,998	12,400	13,560	14,744	15,621	7.1	8.0
Michigan	4,482	6,882	9,500	10,309	11,008	11,711	7.8	7.2
Wisconsin	1,959	2,788	4,377	4,880	5,216	5,537	8.4	8.2
West North Central	7,810	12,261	18,012	19,664	21,116	22,252	8.7	7.3
Minnesota	1,740	2,716	4,094	4,473	4,674	4,796	8.9	5.4
Iowa	1,179	1,733	2,634	2,856	2,996	3,111	8.4	5.7
Missouri	2,532	4,172	5,986	6,527	7,077	7,652	9.0	8.5
North Dakota	313	524	717	786	853	903	8.6	8.0
South Dakota	275	450	694	786	863	920	9.7	9.9
Nebraska	681	1,060	1,587	1,749	1,881	2,003	8.8	8.1
Kansas	1,090	1,607	2,300	2,487	2,771	2,868	7.8	7.6
South Atlantic	15,588	26,925	44,077	48,917	52,971	56,711	11.0	8.8
Delaware	259	434	709	777	854	937	10.6	9.7
Maryland	2,034	2,980	4,655	5,097	5,516	5,926	8.6	8.4
District of Columbia	913	1,469	2,133	2,291	2,437	2,612	8.9	7.0
Virginia	2,077	3,530	5,661	6,240	6,618	7,031	10.5	7.5
West Virginia	831	1,219	1,763	1,977	2,190	2,346	7.8	10.0
North Carolina	1,963	3,250	5,901	6,658	7,311	7,801	11.6	9.8
South Carolina	978	1,753	3,108	3,588	3,962	4,221	12.3	10.7
Georgia	2,148	3,885	6,685	7,398	8,092	8,704	12.0	9.2
Florida	4,385	8,404	13,462	14,890	15,992	17,131	11.9	8.4
East South Central	5,713	9,673	15,149	16,955	18,715	19,921	10.2	9.6
Kentucky	1,230	2,157	3,437	3,900	4,268	4,515	10.8	9.5
Tennessee	2,027	3,483	5,511	6,146	6,761	7,208	10.5	9.4
Alabama	1,590	2,606	4,015	4,511	5,028	5,301	9.7	9.7
Mississippi	867	1,427	2,187	2,398	2,658	2,897	9.7	9.8
West South Central	9,210	16,230	25,344	28,335	31,236	33,601	10.7	9.9
Arkansas	746	1,313	2,109	2,336	2,546	2,723	11.0	8.9
Louisiana	1,744	3,155	4,627	5,164	5,575	5,956	10.2	8.8
Oklahoma	1,177	1,896	2,674	2,938	3,182	3,329	8.6	7.6
Texas	5,543	9,866	15,935	17,897	19,932	21,592	11.1	10.7
Mountain	4,255	7,652	11,748	13,092	14,223	15,095	10.7	8.7
Montana	264	438	679	764	841	894	9.9	9.6
Idaho	243	419	665	752	844	900	10.6	10.6
Wyoming	146	248	353	381	396	417	9.2	5.7
Colorado	1,218	2,087	3,101	3,480	3,776	3,932	9.8	8.2
New Mexico	451	873	1,364	1,538	1,703	1,848	11.7	10.7
Arizona	1,093	2,103	3,218	3,532	3,765	3,999	11.4	7.5
Utah	453	816	1,325	1,483	1,631	1,743	11.3	9.6
Nevada	387	667	1,043	1,162	1,267	1,362	10.4	9.3
Pacific	14,515	23,918	35,912	39,384	42,731	45,259	9.5	8.0
Washington	1,396	2,516	3,961	4,546	5,090	5,305	11.0	10.2
Oregon	928	1,486	2,297	2,403	2,714	2,966	9.5	8.9
California	11,632	18,883	27,949	30,554	32,880	34,827	9.2	7.6
Alaska	199	385	557	631	690	701	10.8	8.0
Hawaii	360	648	1,148	1,250	1,358	1,460	12.3	8.3

[1]States where services were provided.

[2]These estimates differ from National Health Expenditures estimates presented elsewhere in *Health, United States*. See Appendix I, Health Care Financing Administration.

NOTE: Figures may not sum to totals due to rounding.

SOURCE: Health Care Financing Administration, Office of the Actuary. Estimates prepared by the Office of National Health Statistics.

Table 143. Physician service expenditures by geographic division and State and average annual percent change: United States, selected years 1980–93

[Data are compiled by the Health Care Financing Administration]

Geographic division and State[1]	Amount in millions						Average annual percent change	
	1980	1985	1990	1991	1992	1993	1980–90	1990–93
United States[2]	$45,245	$83,636	$140,499	$150,318	$161,783	$171,226	12.0	6.8
New England	2,072	4,010	7,656	8,088	8,678	9,250	14.0	6.5
Maine	142	275	480	520	570	601	13.0	7.8
New Hampshire	130	281	491	583	719	780	14.2	16.7
Vermont	68	131	221	229	248	265	12.5	6.2
Massachusetts	978	1,890	3,766	3,892	4,130	4,442	14.4	5.7
Rhode Island	166	304	514	527	543	575	12.0	3.8
Connecticut	589	1,127	2,185	2,336	2,468	2,587	14.0	5.8
Middle Atlantic	6,636	12,255	20,470	22,035	24,044	25,238	11.9	7.2
New York	3,332	5,822	9,697	10,238	11,287	12,003	11.3	7.4
New Jersey	1,353	2,533	4,519	4,771	5,526	5,776	12.8	8.5
Pennsylvania	1,950	3,901	6,254	7,026	7,230	7,460	12.4	6.1
East North Central	8,078	13,646	21,823	23,280	24,837	26,275	10.4	6.4
Ohio	2,130	3,692	6,048	6,486	6,786	7,118	11.0	5.6
Indiana	891	1,607	2,680	2,821	3,061	3,263	11.6	6.8
Illinois	2,118	3,672	5,864	6,191	6,707	6,970	10.7	5.9
Michigan	2,002	3,080	4,668	5,017	5,224	5,562	8.8	6.0
Wisconsin	938	1,595	2,564	2,765	3,059	3,362	10.6	9.5
West North Central	3,286	5,739	9,125	9,594	10,395	10,987	10.8	6.4
Minnesota	944	1,765	2,957	3,202	3,322	3,617	12.1	6.9
Iowa	488	769	1,142	1,178	1,294	1,376	8.9	6.4
Missouri	877	1,537	2,485	2,581	2,879	2,958	11.0	6.0
North Dakota	139	288	368	371	433	445	10.2	6.5
South Dakota	102	173	274	280	319	342	10.4	7.7
Nebraska	276	433	688	700	785	825	9.6	6.2
Kansas	461	774	1,211	1,280	1,362	1,425	10.1	5.6
South Atlantic	7,141	14,169	25,449	26,853	28,588	30,041	13.6	5.7
Delaware	120	214	377	405	439	466	12.1	7.3
Maryland	835	1,702	2,968	3,249	3,498	3,704	13.5	7.7
District of Columbia	237	362	657	662	651	672	10.7	0.8
Virginia	886	1,772	3,172	3,462	3,565	3,769	13.6	5.9
West Virginia	330	642	856	882	973	988	10.0	4.9
North Carolina	866	1,543	3,005	3,213	3,458	3,717	13.2	7.3
South Carolina	399	734	1,325	1,423	1,552	1,685	12.8	8.3
Georgia	987	1,930	3,645	3,957	4,321	4,543	14.0	7.6
Florida	2,482	5,272	9,444	9,600	10,131	10,498	14.3	3.6
East South Central	2,361	4,188	7,379	8,051	8,418	8,913	12.1	6.5
Kentucky	562	955	1,639	1,762	1,950	2,038	11.3	7.5
Tennessee	841	1,499	2,569	2,822	2,988	3,137	11.8	6.9
Alabama	632	1,167	2,247	2,477	2,466	2,631	13.5	5.4
Mississippi	327	568	925	990	1,015	1,107	11.0	6.2
West South Central	4,649	8,666	13,566	14,280	15,334	15,947	11.3	5.5
Arkansas	374	680	1,134	1,228	1,217	1,244	11.7	3.1
Louisiana	743	1,424	2,129	2,282	2,450	2,537	11.1	6.0
Oklahoma	536	972	1,382	1,431	1,558	1,640	9.9	5.9
Texas	2,996	5,590	8,920	9,340	10,108	10,526	11.5	5.7
Mountain	2,211	4,336	7,347	7,731	8,357	8,897	12.8	6.6
Montana	138	205	311	325	350	392	8.5	8.0
Idaho	140	235	374	410	453	486	10.3	9.1
Wyoming	64	118	146	142	152	160	8.6	3.1
Colorado	600	1,230	1,891	2,032	2,242	2,452	12.2	9.0
New Mexico	182	368	574	590	665	716	12.2	7.6
Arizona	635	1,287	2,500	2,559	2,676	2,799	14.7	3.8
Utah	244	472	739	794	832	864	11.7	5.3
Nevada	207	421	812	879	988	1,029	14.6	8.2
Pacific	8,811	16,627	27,682	30,406	33,132	35,677	12.1	8.8
Washington	909	1,667	2,834	3,155	3,413	3,720	12.0	9.5
Oregon	596	990	1,597	1,626	1,798	1,904	10.4	6.0
California	6,959	13,311	22,365	24,654	26,903	28,981	12.4	9.0
Alaska	97	214	258	265	276	301	10.3	5.3
Hawaii	249	444	629	706	742	771	9.7	7.0

[1]States where services were provided.
[2]These estimates differ from National Health Expenditures estimates presented elsewhere in *Health, United States*. See Appendix I, Health Care Financing Administration.

NOTE: Figures may not sum to totals due to rounding.

SOURCE: Health Care Financing Administration, Office of the Actuary. Estimates prepared by the Office of National Health Statistics.

Table 144. Expenditures for purchases of prescription drugs by geographic division and State and average annual percent change: United States, selected years 1980–93

[Data are compiled by the Health Care Financing Administration]

Geographic division and State[1]	Amount in millions						Average annual percent change	
	1980	1985	1990	1991	1992	1993	1980–90	1990–93
United States	$12,049	$21,405	$38,198	$42,755	$45,730	$48,840	12.2	8.5
New England	625	1,217	2,250	2,463	2,578	2,710	13.7	6.4
Maine	51	93	174	192	202	213	13.1	7.0
New Hampshire	39	77	160	174	185	197	15.2	7.2
Vermont	22	43	86	95	101	108	14.6	7.9
Massachusetts.	290	596	1,113	1,214	1,270	1,337	14.4	6.3
Rhode Island	48	96	174	190	198	206	13.7	5.8
Connecticut	174	312	544	597	622	650	12.1	6.1
Middle Atlantic.	1,817	3,334	5,911	6,513	6,859	7,219	12.5	6.9
New York.	820	1,506	2,665	2,929	3,077	3,232	12.5	6.6
New Jersey	381	723	1,298	1,432	1,515	1,601	13.0	7.2
Pennsylvania	616	1,105	1,948	2,152	2,267	2,386	12.2	7.0
East North Central.	2,219	3,850	6,691	7,437	7,895	8,360	11.7	7.7
Ohio	607	1,010	1,684	1,869	1,982	2,095	10.7	7.6
Indiana	305	508	874	974	1,038	1,106	11.1	8.2
Illinois.	561	1,006	1,771	1,964	2,084	2,206	12.2	7.6
Michigan	527	939	1,654	1,837	1,947	2,054	12.1	7.5
Wisconsin	218	387	708	791	844	899	12.5	8.3
West North Central	887	1,495	2,557	2,835	3,012	3,195	11.2	7.7
Minnesota	191	324	580	648	691	739	11.7	8.4
Iowa	156	255	419	463	490	516	10.4	7.2
Missouri.	274	461	783	868	919	975	11.1	7.6
North Dakota	28	51	86	93	98	103	11.9	6.2
South Dakota.	30	50	82	91	97	104	10.6	8.2
Nebraska.	80	136	235	261	277	293	11.4	7.6
Kansas	128	218	373	412	439	465	11.3	7.6
South Atlantic	1,997	3,694	7,181	8,120	8,746	9,412	13.7	9.4
Delaware	25	49	98	111	120	129	14.6	9.6
Maryland.	226	443	888	998	1,069	1,140	14.7	8.7
District of Columbia	32	57	93	99	101	103	11.3	3.5
Virginia	275	522	1,026	1,154	1,248	1,343	14.1	9.4
West Virginia	116	204	333	369	389	412	11.1	7.4
North Carolina	340	569	1,061	1,199	1,287	1,392	12.1	9.5
South Carolina.	154	268	511	580	622	665	12.7	9.2
Georgia.	294	540	1,035	1,176	1,283	1,397	13.4	10.5
Florida.	536	1,041	2,135	2,435	2,627	2,832	14.8	9.9
East South Central	890	1,537	2,659	2,969	3,175	3,402	11.6	8.6
Kentucky.	225	392	667	741	791	846	11.5	8.2
Tennessee.	288	500	886	996	1,072	1,153	11.9	9.2
Alabama	235	404	707	790	845	904	11.6	8.5
Mississippi.	142	241	399	442	468	499	10.9	7.7
West South Central	1,431	2,440	3,846	4,331	4,671	5,039	10.4	9.4
Arkansas.	153	235	382	425	452	484	9.6	8.2
Louisiana.	254	440	668	740	788	832	10.2	7.6
Oklahoma	175	299	450	500	535	569	9.9	8.1
Texas	848	1,467	2,346	2,666	2,896	3,153	10.7	10.4
Mountain	489	916	1,738	1,998	2,201	2,436	13.5	11.9
Montana	31	54	90	101	110	120	11.2	10.1
Idaho	44	74	129	149	164	182	11.4	12.2
Wyoming.	23	37	49	55	59	64	7.9	9.3
Colorado	127	223	379	434	481	534	11.6	12.1
New Mexico.	52	101	190	216	237	259	13.8	10.9
Arizona	123	250	526	600	659	728	15.6	11.4
Utah	54	110	218	249	274	302	15.0	11.5
Nevada	36	67	158	193	218	246	15.9	15.9
Pacific	1,694	2,921	5,365	6,089	6,593	7,067	12.2	9.6
Washington	212	340	618	711	781	853	11.3	11.3
Oregon	125	187	318	364	396	431	9.8	10.7
California.	1,296	2,274	4,222	4,776	5,155	5,501	12.5	9.2
Alaska.	16	34	58	69	77	85	13.7	13.6
Hawaii.	44	87	148	169	184	197	12.9	10.0

[1]State where prescriptions were provided.

NOTES: Prescription drug expenditures are limited to spending for products purchased in retail outlets. The value of drugs and other products provided by hospitals, nursing homes, or other health professionals is included in estimates of spending for these providers' services. Figures may not sum to totals due to rounding.

SOURCE: Health Care Financing Administration, Office of the Actuary. Estimates prepared by the Office of National Health Statistics.

Table 145. State mental health agency per capita expenditures for mental health services and average annual percent change by geographic division and State: United States, selected fiscal years 1981–93

[Data are based on reporting by State mental health agencies]

Geographic division and State	1981	1983	1985	1987	1990[1]	1993[1,2]	Average annual percent change 1981–93
	Amount per capita						
United States	$ 27	$31	$35	$ 38	$ 48	$ 54	6.0
New England:							
Maine	25	32	36	42	67	70	8.9
New Hampshire	35	39	42	36	63	78	7.0
Vermont	32	40	44	44	54	74	7.2
Massachusetts	32	36	46	62	84	83	8.3
Rhode Island	36	32	35	41	50	61	4.5
Connecticut	32	39	44	56	73	82	8.2
Middle Atlantic:							
New York	67	74	90	99	118	131	5.8
New Jersey	26	31	36	43	57	68	8.2
Pennsylvania	41	47	52	50	57	68	4.4
East North Central:							
Ohio	25	29	30	34	41	47	5.5
Indiana	19	23	27	31	47	39	6.3
Illinois	18	21	24	25	34	36	6.0
Michigan	33	39	49	61	74	75	7.2
Wisconsin	22	27	28	31	37	35	3.8
West North Central:							
Minnesota[3]	17	30	32	42	54	69	8.7
Iowa	8	10	11	12	17	13	4.2
Missouri	24	25	28	32	35	41	4.7
North Dakota	39	42	36	42	40	43	0.9
South Dakota	17	21	22	27	25	47	8.8
Nebraska	17	19	21	21	29	34	6.2
Kansas	18	22	27	28	35	48	8.8
South Atlantic:							
Delaware	44	51	46	41	55	56	2.0
Maryland	33	37	40	49	61	64	5.7
District of Columbia[4]	- - -	23	28	130	268	315	- - -
Virginia	23	29	32	35	45	40	4.8
West Virginia	20	20	22	23	24	22	1.0
North Carolina	24	29	38	41	46	50	6.4
South Carolina	31	33	33	45	51	56	5.1
Georgia	25	26	23	32	51	49	5.7
Florida	20	23	26	25	37	31	3.8
East South Central:							
Kentucky	15	17	19	23	23	25	4.5
Tennessee	18	20	23	24	29	37	6.3
Alabama	20	24	28	29	38	43	6.6
Mississippi	14	16	24	22	34	41	9.6
West South Central:							
Arkansas	17	20	24	24	26	30	5.0
Louisiana	19	23	26	25	28	39	6.2
Oklahoma	22	33	31	30	36	38	4.6
Texas	13	16	17	19	23	31	7.4
Mountain:							
Montana	25	28	29	28	28	34	2.8
Idaho	13	15	15	17	20	26	5.7
Wyoming	23	28	31	30	35	42	5.1
Colorado	24	25	28	30	34	41	4.6
New Mexico	24	25	25	24	23	24	0.1
Arizona	10	10	12	16	27	60	16.1
Utah	13	16	17	19	21	25	5.4
Nevada	22	25	26	28	33	32	3.3
Pacific:							
Washington	18	24	30	37	43	66	11.5
Oregon	21	21	25	28	41	60	9.4
California	28	29	34	30	42	50	4.8
Alaska	38	41	45	50	72	86	7.1
Hawaii	19	22	23	26	38	71	11.7

- - - Data not available.
[1]Puerto Rico is included in U.S. total.
[2]Guam is included in U.S. total.
[3]Data for 1981 not comparable with 1983–93 data for Minnesota. Average annual percent change is for 1983–93.
[4]Transfer of St. Elizabeths Hospital from the National Institute of Mental Health to the District of Columbia Office of Mental Health took place over the years 1985–93.

NOTE: Expenditures for mental illness, excluding mental retardation and substance abuse.

SOURCES: National Association of State Mental Health Program Directors and the National Association of State Mental Health Program Directors Research Institute, Inc.: Final Report: Funding sources and expenditures of State mental health agencies: Revenue/expenditure study results, fiscal year 1990. Nov. 1992; Funding sources and expenditures of State mental health agencies: Supplemental report fiscal year 1993. Mar. 1996.

Table 146. Medicare enrollees, enrollees in managed care, payments per enrollee, and short-stay hospital utilization by geographic division and State: United States, 1990 and 1995

[Data are compiled by the Health Care Financing Administration]

Geographic division and State	Enrollment in thousands 1995	Percent of enrollees in managed care 1990	Percent of enrollees in managed care 1995	Payments per enrollee 1990	Payments per enrollee 1995[1]	Short-stay hospital utilization Discharges per 1,000 enrollees 1990	Short-stay hospital utilization Discharges per 1,000 enrollees 1995[1]	Short-stay hospital utilization Average length of stay in days 1990	Short-stay hospital utilization Average length of stay in days 1995
United States	36,789	5.7	9.5	$3,012	$4,750	316	351	8.8	7.0
New England	2,046	3.4	5.7	3,083	5,134	299	323	10.4	7.0
Maine	202	0.1	0.1	2,410	3,547	301	321	9.3	6.7
New Hampshire	155	0.3	0.6	2,558	3,619	292	277	9.2	7.2
Vermont	83	0.0	0.8	2,297	3,751	281	288	9.7	7.4
Massachusetts	935	5.6	9.4	3,443	6,070	326	354	10.0	6.8
Rhode Island	167	3.7	7.4	2,833	4,644	299	328	10.0	7.2
Connecticut	504	2.1	2.8	3,043	5,034	252	290	10.4	7.3
Middle Atlantic	5,866	4.1	6.5	3,413	5,100	327	361	11.4	9.0
New York	2,623	5.9	7.8	3,525	5,322	299	344	13.1	10.4
New Jersey	1,171	3.2	3.9	3,008	4,815	330	357	11.7	9.3
Pennsylvania	2,072	2.2	6.2	3,496	4,987	361	383	9.5	7.3
East North Central	6,211	2.8	3.1	3,068	4,427	330	348	8.6	6.7
Ohio	1,670	2.2	2.9	3,268	4,320	351	354	8.6	6.6
Indiana	817	2.7	2.6	2,819	4,281	337	342	8.3	6.5
Illinois	1,620	4.8	6.1	3,080	4,693	336	372	8.9	6.8
Michigan	1,347	1.5	0.8	3,290	4,813	307	339	8.9	7.1
Wisconsin	758	2.2	2.0	2,489	3,581	306	311	7.7	6.3
West North Central	2,782	7.0	6.7	2,560	3,889	323	341	7.8	6.2
Minnesota	631	21.9	18.7	2,186	3,731	283	338	6.7	5.5
Iowa	473	3.0	3.3	2,375	3,315	320	332	8.1	6.1
Missouri	827	3.1	4.3	2,966	4,451	346	359	8.6	6.7
North Dakota	102	0.8	0.6	2,534	3,460	338	320	7.2	6.2
South Dakota	116	0.0	0.1	2,264	3,399	344	348	7.2	5.9
Nebraska	250	1.8	2.3	2,319	3,303	300	290	7.6	5.9
Kansas	382	3.4	2.9	2,782	4,274	346	352	7.7	6.2
South Atlantic	6,951	4.7	7.3	2,935	4,753	303	347	8.8	6.9
Delaware	102	0.2	1.3	3,024	4,154	315	315	9.3	7.4
Maryland	606	1.2	2.1	3,665	5,351	345	369	9.4	7.0
District of Columbia	80	2.9	4.8	4,024	5,828	321	360	11.6	8.5
Virginia	824	1.4	2.1	2,726	4,021	343	344	8.9	7.0
West Virginia	330	9.8	7.9	2,648	4,224	370	419	8.2	6.7
North Carolina	1,025	0.4	0.5	2,479	3,943	303	331	9.6	7.3
South Carolina	510	0.1	0.2	2,287	3,944	276	329	9.4	7.4
Georgia	841	0.3	0.5	3,046	4,784	373	377	7.9	6.6
Florida	2,633	10.0	16.6	3,090	5,477	256	333	8.6	6.6
East South Central	2,400	1.1	1.2	2,940	4,676	385	399	8.2	6.7
Kentucky	589	2.9	2.3	2,884	4,141	381	391	8.3	6.6
Tennessee	770	0.4	0.4	2,982	4,859	363	376	8.3	6.6
Alabama	642	0.9	1.9	3,106	4,895	400	413	8.1	6.5
Mississippi	398	0.0	0.1	2,681	4,750	407	432	7.8	7.0
West South Central	3,569	0.9	5.2	3,120	5,249	350	361	8.1	6.7
Arkansas	422	0.3	0.3	2,764	4,026	376	370	8.1	6.6
Louisiana	581	0.0	4.3	3,722	6,119	399	421	7.9	6.8
Oklahoma	487	0.6	3.5	2,812	4,625	361	353	8.0	6.6
Texas	2,079	1.3	6.8	3,099	5,416	328	344	8.2	6.7
Mountain	1,959	8.3	18.4	2,644	4,038	274	303	7.0	5.6
Montana	130	0.3	0.5	2,517	3,532	342	312	6.6	5.5
Idaho	151	0.5	2.7	2,216	3,341	260	273	6.2	5.0
Wyoming	60	0.9	3.2	2,626	3,980	342	327	6.7	5.7
Colorado	425	13.3	20.3	2,524	4,354	264	309	7.3	5.6
New Mexico	211	7.8	14.8	2,512	3,548	298	308	6.8	5.8
Arizona	598	11.7	28.8	2,934	4,269	274	320	7.0	5.5
Utah	187	1.5	9.9	2,370	3,996	236	250	6.3	5.1
Nevada	197	8.2	23.0	2,922	4,440	248	310	8.1	6.4
Pacific	5,004	17.6	30.8	2,873	5,075	258	356	7.2	5.7
Washington	691	10.4	15.4	2,515	3,779	262	275	6.7	5.2
Oregon	475	18.1	31.3	2,047	3,724	244	330	6.2	4.9
California	3,653	18.7	33.9	3,079	5,651	262	384	7.3	5.8
Alaska	34	0.6	0.5	3,223	4,775	260	283	7.7	6.3
Hawaii	151	26.3	30.1	2,044	3,419	208	308	10.1	9.3

[1]These data are not comparable with 1990 data because they do not include Medicare managed care enrollees.

NOTE: Figures may not sum to totals due to rounding.

SOURCE: Health Care Financing Administration, Bureau of Data Management and Strategy. Data for the Medicare Decision Support System; data development by the Office of Research and Demonstrations.

Table 147. Medicaid recipients, recipients in managed care, payments per recipient, and recipients per 100 persons below the poverty level by geographic division and State: United States, selected fiscal years 1980–96

[Data are compiled by the Health Care Financing Administration]

Geographic division and State	Recipients in thousands 1996	Percent of recipients in managed care 1996	Payments per recipient 1980	Payments per recipient 1990	Payments per recipient 1996	Recipients per 100 persons below the poverty level 1989–90	Recipients per 100 persons below the poverty level 1995–96
United States	36,118	40	$1,079	$ 2,568	$3,369	75	99
New England:							
Maine	167	1	903	3,248	4,321	88	117
New Hampshire	100	16	1,603	5,423	5,496	53	148
Vermont	102	–	1,102	2,530	2,954	108	149
Massachusetts[1]	715	70	1,302	4,622	5,285	103	112
Rhode Island	130	63	1,255	[2]3,778	5,280	[2]163	129
Connecticut	329	61	1,615	4,829	6,179	167	100
Middle Atlantic:							
New York.	3,281	23	1,985	5,099	6,811	95	104
New Jersey	714	43	1,119	4,054	5,217	83	112
Pennsylvania	1,168	53	846	2,449	3,993	88	85
East North Central:							
Ohio	1,478	32	1,001	2,566	3,729	98	111
Indiana	594	31	1,726	3,859	4,130	45	119
Illinois	1,454	13	1,137	2,271	3,689	69	104
Michigan	1,172	73	1,101	2,094	2,867	85	104
Wisconsin	434	32	1,619	3,179	4,384	95	98
West North Central:							
Minnesota	455	33	1,814	3,709	5,342	70	105
Iowa	308	41	1,290	2,589	3,534	80	97
Missouri	636	35	918	2,002	3,171	63	135
North Dakota	61	55	1,489	3,955	4,889	58	84
South Dakota.	77	65	1,575	3,368	4,114	51	82
Nebraska.	191	27	1,526	2,595	3,548	61	110
Kansas	251	32	1,319	2,524	3,425	71	90
South Atlantic:							
Delaware.	82	78	920	3,004	3,773	68	117
Maryland.	399	64	1,030	3,300	5,138	74	78
District of Columbia	143	55	1,330	2,629	4,955	86	112
Virginia	623	68	1,125	2,596	2,849	53	90
West Virginia	395	30	520	1,443	2,855	80	126
North Carolina	1,130	37	1,065	2,531	3,255	66	126
South Carolina.	503	1	868	2,343	3,026	52	81
Georgia.	1,185	32	1,075	3,190	2,604	64	118
Florida.	1,638	64	783	2,273	2,851	55	77
East South Central:							
Kentucky	641	53	721	2,089	3,014	81	104
Tennessee.	1,409	100	1,071	1,896	2,049	67	167
Alabama	546	11	812	1,731	2,675	43	73
Mississippi.	510	7	688	1,354	2,633	67	85
West South Central:							
Arkansas.	363	39	1,055	2,267	3,375	55	87
Louisiana.	778	6	1,080	2,247	3,154	58	91
Oklahoma	358	19	1,046	2,516	2,852	56	68
Texas	2,572	4	1,369	1,928	2,672	47	80
Mountain:							
Montana	101	59	1,361	2,793	3,478	47	69
Idaho	119	37	1,182	2,973	3,402	36	76
Wyoming.	51	1	1,300	2,036	3,571	[1]59	87
Colorado.	271	80	1,175	2,705	3,815	45	76
New Mexico.	318	45	800	2,120	2,757	39	65
Arizona[3]	528	86	- - -	- - -	- - -	- - -	- - -
Utah	152	82	1,387	2,279	2,775	72	97
Nevada.	109	41	1,781	3,161	3,361	37	70
Pacific:							
Washington	621	100	1,044	2,128	2,242	98	94
Oregon	450	91	964	2,283	2,915	74	122
California.	5,107	23	798	1,795	2,178	88	94
Alaska.	69	–	1,554	3,562	4,027	70	139
Hawaii.	41	80	1,020	2,252	6,574	73	35

– Quantity zero.
- - - Data not available.
[1]Data for categorically eligible blind Medicaid recipients in 1990 are estimated by the Bureau of Data Management and Strategy, HCFA.
[2]Data are estimated by the Bureau of Data Management and Strategy, Health Care Financing Administration (HCFA).
[3]Arizona has a limited Medicaid program, with care financed largely on a capitated basis.

NOTE: Payments exclude disproportionate share hospital payments ($15 billion in 1996) and payments to health maintenance organizations ($14 billion in 1996).

SOURCES: Health Care Financing Administration, Bureau of Data Management and Strategy, Office of Systems Management, Division of Program Systems and the Office of Managed Care; Department of Commerce, Bureau of the Census, Housing and Household Economic Statistics Division. Data computed by the Centers for Disease Control and Prevention, National Center for Health Statistics, Division of Health and Utilization Analysis.

Table 148. Persons enrolled in health maintenance organizations (HMO's) by geographic division and State: United States, selected years 1980–97

[Data are based on a census of health maintenance organizations]

Geographic division and State	Number in thousands 1997	Percent of population						
		1980	1985	1990	1994	1995	1996	1997
United States[1]	66,801	4.0	7.9	13.5	17.3	19.4	22.3	25.2
New England:								
Maine	198	0.4	0.3	2.6	5.1	7.0	9.5	15.9
New Hampshire	277	1.2	5.6	9.6	14.2	18.5	21.9	23.9
Vermont	–	–	–	6.4	11.2	12.5	13.4	–
Massachusetts	2,716	2.9	13.7	26.5	34.5	39.0	39.0	44.6
Rhode Island	116	3.7	9.1	20.6	26.6	19.6	23.7	11.8
Connecticut	1,138	2.4	7.1	19.9	21.2	21.2	29.8	34.7
Middle Atlantic:								
New York	6,484	5.5	8.0	15.1	23.4	26.6	29.2	35.7
New Jersey	2,193	2.0	5.6	12.3	11.4	14.7	23.0	27.5
Pennsylvania	3,600	1.2	5.0	12.5	18.3	21.5	27.4	29.9
East North Central:								
Ohio	1,965	2.2	6.7	13.3	15.2	16.3	18.5	17.6
Indiana	697	0.5	3.6	6.1	7.4	8.3	9.9	11.9
Illinois	2,029	1.9	7.1	12.6	16.2	17.2	20.0	17.1
Michigan	2,252	2.4	9.9	15.2	18.3	20.5	22.2	23.5
Wisconsin	1,285	8.5	17.8	21.7	22.4	24.0	27.6	24.9
West North Central:								
Minnesota	1,525	9.9	22.2	16.4	25.4	26.5	28.6	32.7
Iowa	131	0.2	4.8	10.1	4.6	4.5	4.9	4.6
Missouri	1,619	2.3	6.0	8.2	15.0	18.5	24.0	30.2
North Dakota	11	0.4	2.5	1.7	0.7	1.2	1.2	1.7
South Dakota	26	–	–	3.3	2.9	2.8	2.8	3.5
Nebraska	254	1.1	1.8	5.1	6.9	8.6	10.8	15.4
Kansas	295	–	3.3	7.9	5.2	4.7	6.3	11.5
South Atlantic:								
Delaware	281	–	3.9	17.5	16.6	18.4	29.3	38.8
Maryland	1,926	2.0	4.8	14.2	24.5	29.5	30.9	38.0
District of Columbia[2]	185	- - -	- - -	- - -	- - -	- - -	- - -	34.1
Virginia	1,049	–	1.1	6.1	7.2	7.7	8.7	15.7
West Virginia	172	0.7	1.7	3.9	4.1	5.8	7.0	9.4
North Carolina	1,070	0.6	1.6	4.8	6.7	8.3	11.1	14.6
South Carolina	312	0.2	1.0	1.9	3.6	5.5	9.0	8.4
Georgia	935	0.1	2.9	4.8	6.7	7.6	9.4	12.7
Florida	4,177	1.5	5.6	10.6	15.7	18.8	23.0	29.0
East South Central:								
Kentucky	1,066	0.9	1.6	5.7	10.6	16.1	15.3	27.4
Tennessee	832	–	1.8	3.7	11.0	12.2	13.9	15.3
Alabama	419	0.3	0.9	5.3	6.2	7.3	7.9	9.8
Mississippi	65	–	–	–	0.1	0.7	1.2	2.4
West South Central:								
Arkansas	219	–	0.1	2.2	5.4	3.8	15.2	8.7
Louisiana	641	0.6	0.9	5.4	7.5	7.2	11.0	14.7
Oklahoma	410	–	2.1	5.5	7.1	7.6	10.3	12.4
Texas	2,930	0.6	3.4	6.9	9.1	12.0	12.3	15.3
Mountain:								
Montana	27	–	–	1.0	1.6	2.4	2.9	3.1
Idaho	51	1.2	–	1.8	1.1	1.4	3.7	4.3
Wyoming	2	–	–	–	–	–	–	0.4
Colorado	1,189	6.9	10.8	20.0	22.2	23.3	25.8	31.1
New Mexico	360	1.4	2.0	12.7	12.7	15.1	15.5	21.0
Arizona	1,275	6.0	10.3	16.2	22.5	25.8	29.0	28.8
Utah	814	0.6	8.8	13.9	23.4	25.1	30.1	40.7
Nevada	334	–	5.8	8.5	11.9	15.9	18.7	20.8
Pacific:								
Washington	1,386	9.4	8.7	14.6	21.0	18.7	23.2	25.1
Oregon	1,511	12.0	14.0	24.7	29.6	40.0	44.8	47.2
California	13,966	16.8	22.5	30.7	33.7	36.0	40.3	43.8
Alaska	–	–	–	–	–	–	–	–
Hawaii	296	15.3	18.1	21.6	21.1	21.0	21.6	25.0

– Quantity zero.

- - - Data not available.

[1]Includes Guam.

[2]Data for the District of Columbia (DC) were not included for 1980–96 because the data were not adjusted for the high proportion of enrollees of DC-based HMO's living in Maryland and Virginia.

NOTES: Data for 1980–90 are for pure HMO enrollment at midyear. Data for 1994–97 are for pure and open-ended enrollment as of January 1. In 1990 open-ended enrollment accounted for 3 percent of HMO enrollment compared with 12 percent in 1997. See Appendix II, Health maintenance organization.

SOURCE: The InterStudy Edge, Managed care: A decade in review 1980–1990. The InterStudy Competitive Edge, vols 4–7, issue 1, 1994–1997. St. Paul, Minnesota (Copyrights 1991, 1994–1997: Used with the permission of InterStudy).

Table 149. Persons without health care coverage by geographic division and State: United States, selected years 1987–96

[Data are based on household interviews of the civilian noninstitutionalized population]

Geographic division and State	Number in thousands 1996	Percent of population							
		1987	1990	1991	1992	1993	1994	1995	1996
United States............................	41,716	12.9	13.9	14.1	15.0	15.3	15.2	15.4	15.6
New England:									
Maine..............................	145	8.4	11.2	11.1	11.1	11.1	13.1	13.5	12.1
New Hampshire......................	110	10.1	9.9	10.1	12.6	12.5	11.9	10.1	9.6
Vermont............................	65	9.8	9.5	12.7	9.5	11.9	8.6	13.0	11.0
Massachusetts......................	766	6.3	9.1	10.9	10.6	11.7	12.5	11.1	12.4
Rhode Island........................	93	6.8	11.1	10.1	9.5	10.3	11.5	12.9	9.9
Connecticut.........................	368	6.4	6.9	7.5	8.2	10.0	10.4	8.8	11.0
Middle Atlantic:									
New York...........................	3,132	11.6	12.1	12.3	13.9	13.9	16.0	15.2	17.0
New Jersey.........................	1,317	7.9	10.0	10.8	13.3	13.7	13.0	14.2	16.8
Pennsylvania.......................	1,133	7.2	10.1	7.8	8.7	10.8	10.6	10.0	9.5
East North Central:									
Ohio...............................	1,292	9.2	10.3	10.3	11.0	11.1	11.0	11.9	11.5
Indiana............................	600	13.4	10.7	13.0	11.0	11.9	10.5	12.6	10.6
Illinois.............................	1,337	9.7	10.9	11.5	13.2	12.6	11.4	11.0	11.3
Michigan...........................	857	8.4	9.4	9.0	10.0	11.2	10.8	9.7	8.9
Wisconsin..........................	438	6.5	6.7	8.0	9.1	8.7	8.9	7.3	8.4
West North Central:									
Minnesota..........................	480	6.6	8.9	9.3	8.1	10.1	9.5	8.0	10.2
Iowa...............................	335	7.3	8.1	8.8	10.3	9.2	9.7	11.3	11.6
Missouri............................	700	10.5	12.7	12.2	14.4	12.2	12.2	14.6	13.2
North Dakota........................	62	7.7	6.3	7.6	8.2	13.4	8.4	8.2	9.8
South Dakota........................	67	13.7	11.6	9.9	15.1	13.0	10.0	9.4	9.5
Nebraska...........................	190	9.6	8.5	8.2	9.4	11.9	10.7	9.0	11.4
Kansas.............................	292	10.3	10.8	11.4	10.9	12.7	12.9	12.4	11.4
South Atlantic:									
Delaware...........................	98	10.5	13.9	13.2	11.2	13.4	13.5	15.8	13.3
Maryland...........................	581	9.8	12.7	13.1	11.3	13.5	12.6	15.3	11.4
District of Columbia.................	80	15.6	19.2	25.7	21.7	20.7	16.4	17.3	14.8
Virginia............................	811	10.4	15.7	16.3	14.6	13.0	12.0	13.5	12.5
West Virginia........................	260	13.5	13.8	15.7	15.4	18.3	16.2	15.3	14.9
North Carolina......................	1,160	13.3	13.8	14.9	13.9	14.0	13.3	14.3	16.0
South Carolina......................	633	11.1	16.2	13.1	17.2	16.9	14.2	14.6	17.1
Georgia............................	1,319	13.0	15.3	14.1	19.1	18.4	16.2	17.9	17.8
Florida.............................	2,723	17.4	18.0	18.6	19.8	19.6	17.2	18.3	18.9
East South Central:									
Kentucky...........................	601	15.2	13.2	13.1	14.6	12.5	15.2	14.6	15.4
Tennessee..........................	841	14.5	13.7	13.4	13.6	13.2	10.2	14.8	15.2
Alabama............................	549	15.8	17.4	17.9	16.8	17.2	19.2	13.5	12.8
Mississippi.........................	518	17.1	19.9	18.9	19.4	17.9	17.8	19.7	18.5
West South Central:									
Arkansas...........................	566	20.7	17.4	15.7	19.9	19.7	17.4	18.0	21.7
Louisiana...........................	890	17.1	19.7	20.7	22.3	23.9	19.2	20.5	20.8
Oklahoma...........................	571	18.1	18.6	18.2	22.0	23.6	17.8	19.2	17.0
Texas..............................	4,680	21.1	21.1	22.1	23.1	21.8	24.2	24.5	24.3
Mountain:									
Montana............................	124	15.5	14.0	12.7	9.4	15.3	13.6	12.7	13.6
Idaho..............................	196	15.3	15.2	17.8	16.5	14.8	14.0	14.0	16.5
Wyoming............................	65	11.4	12.5	11.3	11.7	15.0	15.4	15.9	13.4
Colorado...........................	644	13.8	14.7	10.1	12.7	12.6	12.4	14.1	16.6
New Mexico.........................	412	22.7	22.2	21.5	19.8	22.0	23.1	25.6	22.3
Arizona............................	1,159	18.4	15.5	16.9	15.5	20.2	20.2	20.4	24.1
Utah...............................	240	12.4	9.0	13.8	11.8	11.3	11.5	11.8	12.0
Nevada.............................	255	15.9	16.5	18.7	23.0	18.1	15.7	18.7	15.6
Pacific:									
Washington.........................	761	13.0	11.4	10.4	10.4	12.6	12.7	12.4	13.5
Oregon.............................	497	15.0	12.4	14.2	13.6	14.7	13.1	12.5	15.3
California...........................	6,515	16.8	19.1	18.7	20.0	19.7	21.1	20.6	20.1
Alaska.............................	88	16.2	15.4	13.2	16.8	13.3	13.3	12.5	13.4
Hawaii.............................	101	7.5	7.3	7.0	6.1	11.1	9.2	8.9	8.6

NOTES: These data include revisions and may differ from previous editions of *Health, United States*. New health insurance questions were introduced for a quarter sample for 1993 data and the full sample for 1994 data. Starting with 1993 data, the collection method changed from paper and pencil to computer-assisted interviewing. 1990 census population controls were implemented starting with 1992 data. Estimates of persons lacking health care coverage based on the National Health Interview Survey (NHIS) (table 133) are slightly higher than those based on the March Current Population Survey (CPS). The NHIS questions ask about health insurance coverage over the previous month whereas the CPS asks about coverage over the previous calender year. These differences result in higher estimates of Medicaid and other health insurance coverage and correspondingly lower estimates of persons without health care coverage in the CPS compared with the NHIS.

SOURCES: U.S. Bureau of the Census: Household Economic Studies. Current population reports, series P–60, no 190. Washington: U.S. Government Printing Office. Nov. 1995; and unpublished data from the Current Population Survey provided by the Income Statistics Branch.

Appendixes

I. Sources and Limitations of Data

I. Sources and Limitations of Data _____ 386

Introduction _____ 386
Department of Health and Human Services
  Centers for Disease Control and Prevention
    National Center for Health Statistics
      National Vital Statistics System _____ 387
      National Linked File of Live Births and Infant Deaths _____ 390
      Compressed Mortality File _____ 391
      National Survey of Family Growth _____ 391
      National Health Interview Survey _____ 392
      National Immunization Survey _____ 393
      National Health and Nutrition Examination Survey _____ 393
      National Health Provider Inventory (National Master Facility Inventory) _____ 396
      National Home and Hospice Care Survey _____ 396
      National Hospital Discharge Survey _____ 397
      National Nursing Home Survey _____ 398
      National Ambulatory Medical Care Survey _____ 399
      National Hospital Ambulatory Medical Care Survey _____ 400
    National Center for HIV, STD, and TB Prevention
      AIDS Surveillance _____ 400
    Epidemiology Program Office
      National Notifiable Diseases Surveillance System _____ 401
    National Center for Chronic Disease Prevention and Health Promotion
      Abortion Surveillance _____ 401
    National Institute for Occupational Safety and Health
      National Traumatic Occupational Fatalities Surveillance System _____ 402
  Health Resources and Services Administration
    Bureau of Health Professions
      Physician Supply Projections _____ 402
      Nurse Supply Estimates _____ 403
  Substance Abuse and Mental Health Services Administration
    Office of Applied Studies
      National Household Surveys on Drug Abuse _____ 403
      Drug Abuse Warning Network _____ 404
      Uniform Facility Data Set _____ 404
    Center for Mental Health Services
      Surveys of Mental Health Organizations _____ 405
  National Institutes of Health
    National Cancer Institute
      Surveillance, Epidemiology, and End Results Program _____ 406
    National Institute on Drug Abuse
      Monitoring the Future Study (High School Senior Survey) _____ 406
  Health Care Financing Administration
    Office of the Actuary
      Estimates of National Health Expenditures _____ 407
      Estimates of State Health Expenditures _____ 408
    Medicare National Claims History Files _____ 408
    Medicaid Data System _____ 409
    Online Survey Certification and Reporting Database _____ 410

Appendix Contents

Department of Commerce
  Bureau of the Census
    Census of Population _____ 410
    Current Population Survey _____ 410
    Population Estimates _____ 411
Department of Labor
  Bureau of Labor Statistics
    Annual Survey of Occupational Injuries and Illnesses _____ 411
    Consumer Price Index _____ 412
    Employment and Earnings _____ 413
    Employer Costs for Employee Compensation _____ 413
Department of Veterans Affairs
    The Patient Treatment File _____ 413
    The Patient Census File _____ 414
    The Outpatient Clinic File _____ 414
Environmental Protection Agency
    Aerometric Information Retrieval System (AIRS) _____ 414
United Nations
    Demographic Yearbook _____ 414
    World Health Statistics Annual _____ 415
Alan Guttmacher Institute
    Abortion Survey _____ 415
American Association of Colleges of Osteopathic Medicine _____ 416
American Association of Colleges of Pharmacy _____ 416
American Association of Colleges of Podiatric Medicine _____ 416
American Dental Association _____ 416
American Hospital Association
    Annual Survey of Hospitals _____ 416
American Medical Association
    Physician Masterfile _____ 417
    Annual Census of Hospitals _____ 417
Association of American Medical Colleges _____ 417
Association of Schools and Colleges of Optometry _____ 417
InterStudy
    National Health Maintenance Organization Census _____ 418
National League for Nursing _____ 418

II. Glossary _____ 419

Glossary Tables

  I. Standard million age distribution used to adjust death rates to the U.S. population in 1940 _____ 419
  II. Numbers of live births and mother's age groups used to adjust maternal mortality rates to live births in the United States in 1970 _____ 420
  III. Populations and age groups used to age adjust NCHS survey data _____ 420
  IV. Revision of the *International Classification of Diseases*, according to year of conference by which adopted and years in use in the United States _____ 422
  V. Cause-of-death codes, according to applicable revision of *International Classification of Diseases* _____ 423
  VI. Codes for industries, according to the *Standard Industrial Classification (SIC) Manual* _____ 430
  VII. Codes for diagnostic categories from the *International Classification of Diseases, Ninth Revision, Clinical Modification* _____ 431

VIII. Codes for surgical categories from the *International Classification of Diseases, Ninth Revision, Clinical Modification*_____ 432

IX. Codes for diagnostic and other nonsurgical procedure categories from the *International Classification of Diseases, Ninth Revision, Clinical Modification*_____ 432

X. Mental health codes, according to applicable revision of the *Diagnostic and Statistical Manual of Mental Disorders* and *International Classification of Diseases*_____ 434

Index to Detailed Tables_____ 446

Sources of Data

Introduction

This report consolidates the most current data on the health of the population of the United States, the availability and use of health resources, and health care expenditures. The information was obtained from the data files and/or published reports of many governmental and nongovernmental agencies and organizations. In each case, the sponsoring agency or organization collected data using its own methods and procedures. Therefore, the data in this report vary considerably with respect to source, method of collection, definitions, and reference period.

Much of the data presented in the detailed tables are from the ongoing data collection systems of the National Center for Health Statistics. For an overview of these systems, see: Kovar MG. Data systems of the National Center for Health Statistics. National Center for Health Statistics. Vital Health Stat 1(23). 1989. However, health care personnel data come primarily from the Bureau of Health Professions, Health Resources and Services Administration, and the American Medical Association. National health expenditures data were compiled by the office of the Actuary, Health Care Financing Administration.

Although a detailed description and comprehensive evaluation of each data source is beyond the scope of this appendix, users should be aware of the general strengths and weaknesses of the different data collection systems. For example, population-based surveys obtain socioeconomic data, data on family characteristics, and information on the impact of an illness, such as days lost from work or limitation of activity. They are limited by the amount of information a respondent remembers or is willing to report. Detailed medical information, such as precise diagnoses or the types of operations performed, may not be known and so will not be reported. Health care providers, such as physicians and hospitals, usually have good diagnostic information but little or no information about the socioeconomic characteristics of individuals or the impact of illnesses on individuals.

The populations covered by different data collection systems may not be the same and understanding the differences is critical to interpreting the data. Data on vital statistics and national expenditures cover the entire population. Most data on morbidity and utilization of health resources cover only the civilian noninstitutionalized population. Thus, statistics are not included for military personnel who are usually young; for institutionalized people who may be any age; or for nursing home residents who are usually old.

All data collection systems are subject to error, and records may be incomplete or contain inaccurate information. People may not remember essential information, a question may not mean the same thing to different respondents, and some institutions or individuals may not respond at all. It is not always possible to measure the magnitude of these errors or their impact on the data. Where possible, the tables have notes describing the universe and the method of data collection to enable the user to place his or her own evaluation on the data. In many instances data do not add to totals because of rounding.

Some information is collected in more than one survey and estimates of the same statistic may vary among surveys. For example, cigarette use is measured by the Health Interview Survey, the National Household Survey of Drug Abuse, and the Monitoring the Future Survey. Estimates of cigarette use may differ among surveys because of different survey methodologies, sampling frames, questionnaires, definitions, and tabulation categories.

Overall estimates generally have relatively small sampling errors, but estimates for certain population subgroups may be based on small numbers and have relatively large sampling errors. Numbers of births and deaths from the vital statistics system represent complete counts (except for births in those States where data are based on a 50-percent sample for certain years). Therefore, they are not subject to sampling error. However, when the figures are used for analytical purposes, such as the comparison of rates over a period, the number of events that actually occurred may be considered as one of a large series of possible results that could have arisen under the same circumstances. When the number of events is small and the probability of such an event is small, considerable caution must be observed in interpreting the conditions described by the figures. Estimates that are unreliable because of large sampling errors or small numbers of events have been noted with asterisks in selected tables. The criteria used to designate unreliable estimates are indicated as notes to the applicable tables.

The descriptive summaries that follow provide a general overview of study design, methods of data collection, and reliability and validity of the data. More complete and detailed discussions are found in the publications referenced at the end of each summary. The data set or source is listed under the agency or organization that sponsored the data collection.

Department of Health and Human Services

Centers for Disease Control and Prevention

National Center for Health Statistics

National Vital Statistics System

Through the National Vital Statistics System, the National Center for Health Statistics (NCHS) collects and publishes data on births, deaths, marriages, and divorces in the United States. Fetal deaths are classified and tabulated separately from other deaths. The Division of Vital Statistics obtains information on births and deaths from the registration offices of all States, New York City, the District of Columbia, Puerto Rico, the U.S. Virgin Islands, and Guam. Geographic coverage for births and deaths has been complete since 1933. U.S. data shown in detailed tables in this book are for the 50 States and the District of Columbia, unless otherwise specified.

Until 1972 microfilm copies of all death certificates and a 50-percent sample of birth certificates were received from all registration areas and processed by NCHS. In 1972 some States began sending their data to NCHS through the Cooperative Health

Statistics System (CHSS). States that participated in the CHSS program processed 100 percent of their death and birth records and sent the entire data file to NCHS on computer tapes. Currently, the data are sent to NCHS through the Vital Statistics Cooperative Program (VSCP), following the same procedures as the CHSS. The number of participating States grew from 6 in 1972 to 46 in 1984. Starting in 1985 all 50 States and the District of Columbia participated in VSCP.

In most areas practically all births and deaths are registered. The most recent test of the completeness of birth registration, conducted on a sample of births from 1964 to 1968, showed that 99.3 percent of all births in the United States during that period were registered. No comparable information is available for deaths, but it is generally believed that death registration in the United States is at least as complete as birth registration.

Demographic information on the birth certificate such as race and ethnicity is provided by the mother at the time of birth. Medical and health information is based on hospital records. Demographic information on the death certificate is provided by the funeral director based on information supplied by an informant. Medical certification of cause of death is provided by a physician, medical examiner, or coroner.

U.S. Standard Certificates—U.S. Standard Live Birth and Death Certificates and Fetal Death Reports are revised periodically, allowing careful evaluation of each item and addition, modification, and deletion of items. Beginning with 1989, revised standard certificates replaced the 1978 versions. The 1989 revision of the birth certificate includes items to identify the Hispanic parentage of newborns and to expand information about maternal and infant health characteristics. The 1989 revision of the death certificate includes items on educational attainment and Hispanic origin of decedents as well as changes to improve the medical certification of cause of death. Standard certificates recommended by NCHS are modified in each registration area to serve the area's needs. However, most certificates conform closely in content and arrangement to the standard certificate, and

Sources of Data

all certificates contain a minimum data set specified by NCHS. For selected items, reporting areas expanded during the years spanned by this report. For items on the birth certificate, the number of reporting States increased for mother's education, prenatal care, marital status, Hispanic parentage, and tobacco use; and on the death certificate, for educational attainment and Hispanic origin of the decedent.

Maternal education—Mother's education was reported on the birth certificate by 38 States in 1970. Data were not available from Alabama, Arkansas, California, Connecticut, Delaware, District of Columbia, Georgia, Idaho, Maryland, New Mexico, Pennsylvania, Texas, and Washington. In 1975 these data were available from 4 additional States, Connecticut, Delaware, Georgia, Maryland, and the District of Columbia, increasing the number of States reporting mother's education to 42 and the District of Columbia. Between 1980 and 1988 only three States, California, Texas, and Washington did not report mother's education. In 1988 mother's education was also missing from New York State outside of New York City. In 1989–91 mother's education was missing only from Washington and New York State outside of New York City. Starting in 1992 mother's education was reported by all 50 States and the District of Columbia.

Prenatal care—Prenatal care was reported on the birth certificate by 39 States and the District of Columbia in 1970. Data were not available from Alabama, Alaska, Arkansas, Connecticut, Delaware, Georgia, Idaho, Massachusetts, New Mexico, Pennsylvania, and Virginia. In 1975 these data were available from 3 additional States, Connecticut, Delaware, and Georgia, increasing the number of States reporting prenatal care to 42 and the District of Columbia. Starting in 1980 prenatal care information was available for the entire United States.

Marital status—In 1970 mother's marital status was reported on the birth certificate by 39 States and the District of Columbia, and in 1975, by 38 States and the District of Columbia. In 1970 and 1975 data were not available from California, Connecticut,

Georgia, Idaho, Maryland, Massachusetts, Montana, New Mexico, New York, Ohio, and Vermont; and in 1975 also from Nevada. In 1980 and the following years marital status of mother was reported on the birth certificates of 41–45 States and for the remaining 5–9 States that lacked the item, marital status was inferred from a comparison of the child's and parents' surnames and from other information concerning the father.

Hispanic births—In 1980 and 1981 information on births of Hispanic parentage was reported on the birth certificate by the following 22 States: Arizona, Arkansas, California, Colorado, Florida, Georgia, Hawaii, Illinois, Indiana, Kansas, Maine, Mississippi, Nebraska, Nevada, New Jersey, New Mexico, New York, North Dakota, Ohio, Texas, Utah, and Wyoming. In 1982 Tennessee, and in 1983 the District of Columbia began reporting this information. Between 1983 and 1987 information on births of Hispanic parentage was available for 23 States and the District of Columbia. In 1988 this information became available for Alabama, Connecticut, Kentucky, Massachusetts, Montana, North Carolina, and Washington, increasing the number of States reporting information on births of Hispanic parentage to 30 States and the District of Columbia. In 1989 this information became available from an additional 17 States, increasing the number of Hispanic-reporting States to 47 and the District of Columbia. In 1989 only Louisiana, New Hampshire, and Oklahoma did not report Hispanic parentage on the birth certificate. In 1990 Louisiana began reporting Hispanic parentage. Hispanic origin of the mother was reported on the birth certificates of 49 States and the District of Columbia in 1991 and 1992; only New Hampshire did not provide this information. Starting in 1993 Hispanic origin of mother was reported by all 50 States and the District of Columbia. In 1990, 99 percent of birth records included information on mother's origin.

Tobacco use—Information on tobacco use during pregnancy became available for the first time in 1989 with the revision of the U.S. Standard Birth Certificate. In 1989 data on tobacco use were collected by 43

States and the District of Columbia. The following States did not require the reporting of tobacco use on the birth certificate: California, Indiana, Louisiana, Nebraska, New York, Oklahoma, and South Dakota. In 1990 information on tobacco use became available from Louisiana and Nebraska increasing the number of reporting States to 45 and the District of Columbia. In 1991–93 information on tobacco use was available for 46 States and the District of Columbia with the addition of Oklahoma to the reporting area; and in 1994–96, for 46 States, the District of Columbia, and New York City.

Education of decedent—Information on educational attainment of decedents became available for the first time in 1989 due to the revision of the U.S. Standard Certificate of Death. Mortality data by educational attainment for 1989 was based on data from 20 States and by 1994–96 increased to 45 States and the District of Columbia. In 1994–96 the following States either did not report educational attainment on the death certificate or the information was more than 20 percent incomplete: Georgia, Kentucky, Oklahoma, Rhode Island, and South Dakota. Information on the death certificate about the decedent's educational attainment is reported by the funeral director based on information provided by an informant such as next of kin.

Calculation of unbiased death rates by educational attainment based on the National Vital Statistics System requires that the reporting of education on the death certificate be complete and consistent with the reporting of education on the Current Population Survey, the source of population estimates which form the denominators for death rates. Death records with education not stated have not been included in the calculation of rates. Therefore the levels of the rates shown in this report are underestimated by approximately the percent not stated, which ranged from 3 to 5 percent.

The validity of information about the decedent's education was evaluated by comparing self-reported education obtained in the Current Population Survey with education on the death certificate for decedents in the National Longitudinal Mortality Survey (NLMS). (Sorlie PD, Johnson NJ: Validity of education information on the death certificate, *Epidemiology* 7(4):437–439, 1996.) Another analysis compared self-reported education collected in the first National Health and Nutrition Examination Survey (NHANES I) with education on the death certificate for decedents in the NHANES I Epidemiologic Followup Study. (Makuc DM, Feldman JJ, Mussolino ME: Validity of education and age as reported on death certificates, American Statistical Association 1996 Proceedings of the Social Statistics Section, 102–106, 1997.) Results of both studies indicated that there is a tendency for some people who did not graduate from high school to be reported as high school graduates on the death certificate. This tendency results in overstating the death rate for high school graduates and understating the death rate for the group with less than 12 years of education. The bias was greater among older than younger decedents and somewhat greater among black than white decedents.

In addition, educational gradients in death rates based on the National Vital Statistics System were compared with those based on the NLMS, a prospective study of persons in the Current Population Survey. Results of these comparisons indicate that educational gradients in death rates based on the National Vital Statistics System were reasonably similar to those based on the NLMS for white persons 25–64 years of age and black persons 25–44 years of age. The number of deaths for persons of Hispanic origin in the NLMS was too small to permit comparison for this ethnic group.

Hispanic deaths—In 1985 mortality data by Hispanic origin of decedent were based on deaths to residents of the following 17 States and the District of Columbia whose data on the death certificate were at least 90 percent complete on a place-of-occurrence basis and of comparable format: Arizona, Arkansas, California, Colorado, Georgia, Hawaii, Illinois, Indiana, Kansas, Mississippi, Nebraska, New York, North Dakota, Ohio, Texas, Utah, and Wyoming. In 1986 New Jersey began reporting Hispanic origin of

Sources of Data

decedent, increasing the number of reporting States to 18 and the District of Columbia in 1986 and 1987. In 1988 Alabama, Kentucky, Maine, Montana, North Carolina, Oregon, Rhode Island, and Washington were added to the reporting area, increasing the number of States to 26 and the District of Columbia. In 1989 an additional 18 States were added, increasing the Hispanic reporting area to 44 States and the District of Columbia. In 1989 only Connecticut, Louisiana, Maryland, New Hampshire, Oklahoma, and Virginia were not included in the reporting area. Starting with 1990 data in this book, the criterion was changed to include States whose data were at least 80 percent complete. In 1990 Maryland, Virginia, and Connecticut, in 1991 Louisiana, and in 1993 New Hampshire were added, increasing the reporting area for Hispanic origin of decedent to 47 States and the District of Columbia in 1990, 48 States and the District of Columbia in 1991 and 1992, and 49 States and the District of Columbia in 1993–96. Only Oklahoma did not provide this information in 1993–96. Based on data from the U.S. Bureau of the Census, the 1990 reporting area encompassed 99.6 percent of the U.S. Hispanic population. In 1990 more than 99 percent of death records included information on origin of decedent.

Alaska data—For 1995 the number of deaths occurring in Alaska is in error for selected causes because NCHS did not receive changes resulting from amended records and because of errors in processing the cause of death data. Differences are concentrated among selected causes of death, principally Symptoms, signs, and ill-defined conditions (ICD-9 Nos. 780–799) and external causes.

For more information, see: National Center for Health Statistics, Technical Appendix, *Vital Statistics of the United States, 1992*, Vol. I, Natality, DHHS Pub. No. (PHS)96–1100 and Vol. II, Mortality, Part A, DHHS Pub. No. (PHS) 96–1101, Public Health

Service. Washington. U.S. Government Printing Office, 1996.

National Linked File of Live Births and Infant Deaths

National linked files of live births and infant deaths are data sets for research on infant mortality. To create these data sets, death certificates are linked with corresponding birth certificates for infants who die in the United States before their first birthday. Linked data files include all of the variables on the national natality file, including the more accurate racial and ethnic information, as well as the variables on the national mortality file, including cause of death and age at death. The linkage makes available for the analysis of infant mortality, extensive information from the birth certificate about the pregnancy, maternal risk factors, and infant characteristics and health items at birth. Each year, 97–98 percent of infant death records are linked to their corresponding birth records.

National linked files of live births and infant deaths were first produced for the 1983 birth cohort. Birth cohort linked file data are available for 1983–91 and period linked file data for 1995. While birth cohort linked files have methodological advantages, their production incurs substantial delays in data availability, since it is necessary to wait until the close of a second data year to include all infant deaths to the birth cohort. Starting with data year 1995, more timely linked file data are produced in a period data format, preceding the release of the corresponding birth cohort format. Other changes to the data set in 1995 include the addition of record weights to correct for the 2.5 percent of records that could not be linked and the addition of an imputation for not stated birthweight. For more information, see: Prager K. Infant mortality by birthweight and other characteristics: United States, 1985 birth cohort. National Center for Health Statistics. Vital Health Stat 20(24). 1994; National

Center for Health Statistics, Public Use Data Tape Documentation, Linked Birth/Infant Death Data Set: 1995 Period Data, 1997.

Compressed Mortality File

The Compressed Mortality File (CMF) used to compute death rates by urbanization level is a county level national mortality and population data base. The mortality data base of CMF is derived from the detailed mortality files of the National Vital Statistics System starting with 1968. The population data base of CMF is derived from intercensal and postcensal population estimates and census counts of the resident population of each U.S. county by age, race, and sex. Counties are categorized according to level of urbanization based on an NCHS-modified version of the 1993 rural-urban continuum codes for metropolitan and nonmetropolitan counties developed by the Economic Research Service, U.S. Department of Agriculture. See Appendix II, Urbanization. For more information about the CMF, contact: D. Ingram, Analytic Studies Branch, Division of Health and Utilization Analysis, National Center for Health Statistics, 6525 Belcrest Road, Hyattsville, MD 20782.

National Survey of Family Growth

Data from the National Survey of Family Growth (NSFG) are based on samples of women ages 15–44 years in the civilian noninstitutionalized population of the United States. The first and second cycles, conducted in 1973 and 1976, excluded most women who had never been married. The third, fourth, and fifth cycles, conducted in 1982, 1988, and 1995, included all women ages 15–44 years.

The purpose of the survey is to provide national data on factors affecting birth and pregnancy rates, adoption, and maternal and infant health. These factors include sexual activity, marriage, divorce and remarriage, unmarried cohabitation, contraception and sterilization, infertility, breastfeeding, pregnancy loss, low birthweight, and use of medical care for family planning and infertility.

Interviews are conducted in person by professional female interviewers using a standardized questionnaire. In 1973–88, the average interview length was about 1 hour. In 1995 the average interview lasted about 1 hour and 45 minutes. In all cycles black women were sampled at higher rates than white women, so that detailed statistics for black women could be produced.

Interviewing for Cycle 1 of NSFG was conducted from June 1973 to February 1974. Counties and independent cities of the United States were sampled to form a frame of primary sampling units (PSU's), and 101 PSU's were selected. From these 101 PSU's, 10,879 women 15–44 years of age were selected; 9,797 of these were interviewed. Most never-married women were excluded from the 1973 NSFG.

Interviewing for Cycle 2 of the NSFG was conducted from January to September 1976. From 79 PSU's, 10,202 eligible women were identified; of these, 8,611 were interviewed. Again, most never-married women were excluded from the sample for the 1976 NSFG.

Interviewing for Cycle 3 of NSFG was conducted from August 1982 to February 1983. The sample design was similar to that in Cycle 2: 31,027 households were selected in 79 PSU'S. Household screener interviews were completed in 29,511 households (95.1 percent). Of the 9,964 eligible women identified, 7,969 were interviewed. For the first time in NSFG, Cycle 3 included women of all marital statuses.

Interviewing for Cycle 4 was conducted between January and August 1988. The sample was obtained from households that had been interviewed in the National Health Interview Survey in the 18 months between October 1, 1985, and March 31, 1987. For the first time, women living in Alaska and Hawaii were included so that the survey covered women from the noninstitutionalized population of the entire United States. The sample was drawn from 156 PSU's; 10,566 eligible women ages 15–44 years were sampled. Interviews were completed with 8,450 women.

Between July and November of 1990, 5,686 women were interviewed by telephone in the first

NSFG telephone reinterview. The average length of interview in 1990 was 20 minutes. The response rate for the 1990 telephone reinterview was 68 percent of those responding to the 1988 survey and still eligible for the 1990 survey.

Interviewing for Cycle 5 of NSFG was conducted between January and October of 1995. The sample was obtained from households that had been interviewed in 198 PSU's in the National Health Interview Survey in 1993. Of the 13,795 eligible women in the sample, 10,847 were interviewed. For the first time, Hispanic as well as black women were sampled at a higher rate than other women.

In order to make national estimates from the sample for the millions of women ages 15–44 years in the United States, data for the interviewed sample women were (a) inflated by the reciprocal of the probability of selection at each stage of sampling (for example, if there was a 1 in 5,000 chance that a woman would be selected for the sample, her sampling weight was 5,000), (b) adjusted for nonresponse, and (c) forced to agree with benchmark population values based on data from the Current Population Survey of the U.S. Bureau of the Census (this last step is called "poststratification").

Quality control procedures for selecting and training interviewers, coding, editing, and processing the data, were built into NSFG to minimize nonsampling error.

More information on the methodology of NSFG is available in the following reports: French DK. National Survey of Family Growth, Cycle I: Sample design, estimation procedures, and variance estimation. National Center for Health Statistics. Vital Health Stat 2(76). 1978; Grady WR. National Survey of Family Growth, Cycle II: Sample design, estimation procedures, and variance estimation. National Center for Health Statistics. Vital Health Stat 2(87). 1981; Bachrach CA, Horn MC, Mosher WD, Shimizu I. National Survey of Family Growth, Cycle III: Sample design, weighting, and variance estimation. National Center for Health Statistics. Vital Health Stat 2(98). 1985; Judkins DR, Mosher WD, Botman SL. National Survey of Family Growth: Design, estimation, and inference. National Center for Health Statistics. Vital Health Stat 2(109). 1991; Goksel H, Judkins DR, Mosher WD. Nonresponse adjustments for a telephone follow-up to a National In-Person Survey. Journal of Official Statistics 8(4):417–32. 1992; Kelly JE, Mosher WD, Duffer AP, Kinsey SH. Plan and operation of the 1995 National Survey of Family Growth. Vital Health Stat 1(36). 1997; Potter FJ, Iannacchione VG, Mosher WD, Mason RE, Kavee JD. Sampling weights, imputation, and variance estimation in the 1995 National Survey of Family Growth. Vital Health Stat 2(124). 1998.

National Health Interview Survey

The National Health Interview Survey (NHIS) is a continuing nationwide sample survey in which data are collected through personal household interviews. Information is obtained on personal and demographic characteristics including race and ethnicity by self-reporting or as reported by an informant. Information is also obtained on illnesses, injuries, impairments, chronic conditions, utilization of health resources, and other health topics. The household questionnaire is reviewed each year with special health topics being added or deleted. For most health topics data are collected over an entire calendar year.

The sample design plan of NHIS follows a multistage probability design that permits a continuous sampling of the civilian noninstitutionalized population residing in the United States. The survey is designed in such a way that the sample scheduled for each week is representative of the target population and the weekly samples are additive over time. The response rate for the ongoing portion of the survey (core) has been between 94 and 98 percent over the years. Response rates for special health topics (supplements) have generally been lower. For example the response rate was 80 percent for the 1994 Year 2000 Supplement, which included questions about cigarette smoking and use of such preventive services as mammography.

In 1985 NHIS adopted several new sample design features although, conceptually, the sampling plan remained the same as the previous design. Two major changes included reducing the number of primary sampling locations from 376 to 198 for sampling efficiency and oversampling the black population to improve the precision of the statistics. The sample was designed so that a typical NHIS sample for the data collection years 1985–94 will consist of approximately 7,500 segments containing about 59,000 assigned households. Of these households, an expected 10,000 will be vacant, demolished, or occupied by persons not in the target population of the survey. The expected sample of 49,000 occupied households will yield a probability sample of about 127,000 persons. In 1994 there was a sample of 116,179 persons.

In 1995 the NHIS sample was redesigned again. Major design changes include increasing the number of primary sampling units from 198 to 358 and oversampling the black and Hispanic populations to improve the precision of the statistics. The sample was designed so that a typical NHIS sample for the data collection years 1995–2004 will consist of approximately 7,000 segments. The expected sample of 44,000 occupied respondent households will yield a probability sample of about 106,000 persons. In 1995 there was a sample of 102,467 persons.

A description of the survey design, the methods used in estimation, and the general qualifications of the data obtained from the survey are presented in: Massey JT, Moore TF, Parsons VL, Tadros W. Design and estimation for the National Health Interview Survey, 1985–94. National Center for Health Statistics. Vital Health Stat 2(110). 1989; Kovar MG, Poe GS. The National Health Interview Survey design, 1973–84, and procedures, 1975–83. National Center for Health Statistics. Vital Health Stat 1(18). 1985; Benson V, Marano M. Current estimates from the National Health Interview Survey, 1995. National Center for Health Statistics. Vital Health Stat 10(199). 1998.

National Immunization Survey

The National Immunization Survey (NIS) is a continuing nationwide telephone sample survey among children 19–35 months of age. Estimates of

vaccine-specific coverage are available for national, State, and 28 urban areas considered to be high-risk for under-vaccination.

NIS uses a two-phase sample design. First, a random-digit-dialing (RDD) sample of telephone numbers is drawn. When households with age-eligible children are contacted, the interviewer collects information on the vaccinations received by all age-eligible children. In 1995, 69 percent of households with age-eligible children completed vaccination interviews, yielding data for 31,997 children. In 1996 the response rate was 94 percent, yielding data for 33,305 children. The interviewer also collects information on the vaccination providers. In the second phase, all vaccination providers are contacted by mail. Vaccination information from providers' records was obtained for 52 percent of all children who were eligible for provider followup in 1995 and 64 percent in 1996. Providers' responses are combined with information obtained from the households to provide a more accurate estimate of vaccination coverage levels. Final estimates are adjusted for noncoverage of nontelephone households.

A description of the survey design and the methods used in estimation are presented in: Massey JT. Estimating the response rate in a two stage telephone survey. Proceedings of the Section on Survey Research Methods. Alexandria, Virginia: American Statistical Association. 1995.

National Health and Nutrition Examination Survey

For the first program or cycle of the National Health Examination Survey (NHES I), 1960–62, data were collected on the total prevalence of certain chronic diseases as well as the distributions of various physical and physiological measures, including blood pressure and serum cholesterol levels. For that program, a highly stratified, multistage probability sample of 7,710 adults, of whom 86.5 percent were examined, was selected to represent the 111 million civilian noninstitutionalized adults 18–79 years of age

Sources of Data

in the United States at that time. The sample areas consisted of 42 primary sampling units (PSU's) from the 1,900 geographic units.

NHES II (1963–65) and NHES III (1966–70) examined probability samples of the nation's noninstitutionalized children between the ages of 6 and 11 years (NHES II) and 12 and 17 years (NHES III) focusing on factors related to growth and development. Both cycles were multistage, stratified probability samples of clusters of households in land-based segments and used the same 40 PSU's. NHES II sampled 7,417 children with a response rate of 96 percent. NHES III sampled 7,514 youth with a response rate of 90 percent.

For more information on NHES I, see: Gordon T, Miller HW. Cycle I of the Health Examination Survey: Sample and response, United States, 1960–62. National Center for Health Statistics. Vital Health Stat 11(1). 1974. For more information on NHES II, see: Plan, operation, and response results of a program of children's examinations. National Center for Health Statistics. Vital Health Stat 1(5). 1967. For more information on NHES III, see: Schaible, WL. Quality control in a National Health Examination Survey. National Center for Health Statistics. Vital Health Stat 2(44). 1972.

In 1971 a nutrition surveillance component was added and the survey name was changed to the National Health and Nutrition Examination Survey (NHANES). In NHANES I, conducted from 1971 to 1974, a major purpose was to measure and monitor indicators of the nutrition and health status of the American people through dietary intake data, biochemical tests, physical measurements, and clinical assessments for evidence of nutritional deficiency. Detailed examinations were given by dentists, ophthalmologists, and dermatologists with an assessment of need for treatment. In addition, data were obtained for a subsample of adults on overall health care needs and behavior, and more detailed examination data were collected on cardiovascular, respiratory, arthritic, and hearing conditions.

The NHANES I target population was the civilian noninstitutionalized population 1–74 years of age residing in the coterminous United States, except for people residing on any of the reservation lands set aside for the use of American Indians. The sample design was a multistage, stratified probability sample of clusters of persons in land-based segments. The sample areas consisted of 65 PSU's selected from the 1,900 PSU's in the coterminous United States. A subsample of persons 25–74 years of age was selected to receive the more detailed health examination. Groups at high risk of malnutrition were oversampled at known rates throughout the process. Household interviews were completed for more than 96 percent of the 28,043 persons selected for the NHANES I sample, and about 75 percent (20,749) were examined.

For NHANES II, conducted from 1976 to 1980, the nutrition component was expanded from the one fielded for NHANES I. In the medical area primary emphasis was placed on diabetes, kidney and liver functions, allergy, and speech pathology. The NHANES II target population was the civilian noninstitutionalized population 6 months–74 years of age residing in the United States, including Alaska and Hawaii.

NHANES II utilized a multistage probability design that involved selection of PSU's, segments (clusters of households) within PSU's, households, eligible persons, and finally, sample persons. The sample design provided for oversampling among those persons 6 months–5 years of age, those 60–74 years of age, and those living in poverty areas. A sample of 27,801 persons was selected for NHANES II. Of this sample 20,322 (73.1 percent) were examined. Race information for NHANES I and NHANES II was determined primarily by interviewer observation.

The estimation procedure used to produce national statistics for NHANES I and NHANES II involved inflation by the reciprocal of the probability of selection, adjustment for nonresponse, and poststratified ratio adjustment to population totals. Sampling errors also were estimated to measure the reliability of the statistics.

For more information on NHANES I, see: Miller HW. Plan and operation of the Health and Nutrition Examination Survey, United States, 1971–73. National Center for Health Statistics. Vital Health Stat 1(10a) and 1(10b). 1977 and 1978; and Engel A, Murphy RS, Maurer K, Collins E. Plan and operation of the NHANES I Augmentation Survey of Adults 25–74 years, United States 1974–75. National Center for Health Statistics. Vital Health Stat 1(14). 1978.

For more information on NHANES II, see: McDowell A, Engel A, Massey JT, Maurer K. Plan and operation of the second National Health and Nutrition Examination Survey, 1976–80. National Center for Health Statistics. Vital Health Stat 1(15). 1981. For information on nutritional applications of these surveys, see: Yetley E, Johnson C. 1987. Nutritional applications of the Health and Nutrition Examination Surveys (HANES). Ann Rev Nutr 7:441–63.

The Hispanic Health and Nutrition Examination Survey (HHANES), conducted during 1982–84, was similar in content and design to the previous National Health and Nutrition Examination Surveys. The major difference between HHANES and the previous national surveys is that HHANES employed a probability sample of three special subgroups of the population living in selected areas of the United States rather than a national probability sample. The three HHANES universes included approximately 84, 57, and 59 percent of the respective 1980 Mexican-, Cuban-, and Puerto Rican-origin populations in the continental United States. The Hispanic ethnicity of these populations was determined by self-report.

In the HHANES three geographically and ethnically distinct populations were studied: Mexican Americans in Texas, New Mexico, Arizona, Colorado, and California; Cuban Americans living in Dade County, Florida; and Puerto Ricans living in parts of New York, New Jersey, and Connecticut. In the Southwest 9,894 persons were selected (75 percent or 7,462 were examined), in Dade County 2,244 persons were selected (60 percent or 1,357 were examined),

and in the Northeast 3,786 persons were selected (75 percent or 2,834 were examined).

For more information on HHANES, see: Maurer KR. Plan and operation of the Hispanic Health and Nutrition Examination Survey, 1982–84. National Center for Health Statistics. Vital Health Stat 1(19). 1985.

The third National Health and Nutrition Examination Survey (NHANES III) is a 6-year survey covering the years 1988–94. Over the 6-year period, 39,695 persons were selected for the survey of which 30,818 (77.6 percent) were examined in the mobile examination center.

The NHANES III target population is the civilian noninstitutionalized population 2 months of age and over. The sample design provides for oversampling among children 2–35 months of age, persons 70 years of age and over, black Americans, and Mexican Americans. Race is reported for the household by the respondent.

Although some of the specific health areas have changed from earlier NHANES surveys, the following goals of the NHANES III are similar to those of earlier NHANES surveys:

■ to estimate the national prevalence of selected diseases and risk factors

■ to estimate national population reference distributions of selected health parameters

■ to document and investigate reasons for secular trends in selected diseases and risk factors

Two new additional goals for the NHANES III survey are:

■ to contribute to an understanding of disease etiology

■ to investigate the natural history of selected diseases

For more information on NHANES III, see: Ezzati TM, Massey JT, Waksberg J, et al. Sample design: Third National Health and Nutrition Examination Survey. National Center for Health Statistics. Vital

Health Stat 2(113). 1992; Plan and operation of the Third National Health and Nutrition Examination Survey, 1988–94. National Center for Health Statistics. Vital Health Stat 1(32). 1994.

National Health Provider Inventory (National Master Facility Inventory)

The National Master Facility Inventory (NMFI) is a comprehensive file of inpatient health facilities in the United States. The three broad categories of facilities in NMFI are hospitals, nursing and related care homes, and other custodial or remedial care facilities. To be included in NMFI, hospitals must have at least six inpatient beds; nursing and related care homes and other facilities must have at least three inpatient beds. NMFI is kept current by the periodic addition of names and addresses obtained from State licensing and other agencies for all newly established inpatient facilities. In addition, annual surveys of hospitals and periodic surveys of nursing homes and other facilities are conducted to update name and location, type of business, number of beds, and number of residents or patients in the facilities, and to identify those facilities that have gone out of business.

From 1968 to 1975 the hospital survey was conducted in conjunction with the American Hospital Association (AHA) Annual Survey of Hospitals. AHA performed the data collection for its member hospitals, while NCHS collected the data for the approximately 400 non-AHA registered hospitals. Since 1976, however, all of the data collection has been performed by AHA.

The nursing home and other facilities surveys were conducted by NCHS in 1963, 1967, 1969, 1971, 1973, 1976, 1978, 1980, 1982, 1986, and 1991. Data were collected on facilities and resident characteristics by questionnaires mailed to the facilities.

In 1986 nursing and related care homes and facilities for the mentally retarded were covered and called the Inventory of Long-Term Care Places. In 1991 nursing homes, board and care homes, home health agencies, and hospices were covered, and the survey was called the National Health Provider Inventory.

For more detailed information, see: Sirrocco A. Nursing homes and board and care homes. Advance data from vital and health statistics; no 244. Hyattsville, Maryland: National Center for Health Statistics. 1994.

National Home and Hospice Care Survey

The National Home and Hospice Care Survey (NHHCS) is a sample survey of health agencies and hospices. Initialed in 1992, it was also conducted in 1993, 1994, and 1996. The original sampling frame consisted of all home health care agencies and hospices identified in the 1991 National Health Provider Inventory (NHPI). The 1992 sample contained 1,500 agencies. These agencies were revisited during the 1993 survey (excluding agencies which had been found to be out of scope for the survey). In 1994 in-scope agencies identified in the 1993 survey were revisited, with 100 newly-identified agencies added to the sample. For 1996 the universe was again updated and a new sample of 1,200 agencies was drawn.

The sample design for the 1992–94 NHHCS was a stratified three-stage probability design. Primary sampling units were selected at the first stage, agencies were selected at the second stage, and current patients and discharges were selected at the third stage. The sample design for the 1996 NHHCS has a two-stage probability design in which agencies were selected at the first stage and current patients and discharges were selected at the second stage. Current patients were on the rolls of the agency as of midnight on the day before the survey. Discharges were selected to estimate the number of discharges from the agency during the year prior to the survey.

After the samples had been selected, a patient questionnaire was completed for each current patient and discharge by interviewing the staff member most familiar with the care provided to the patients. The respondent was requested to refer to the medical records for each patient. For additional information see: Haupt BJ. Development of the National Home and Hospice Care Survey. National Center for Health Statistics. Vital Health Stat 1(33). 1994.

National Hospital Discharge Survey

The National Hospital Discharge Survey (NHDS) is a continuing nationwide sample survey of short-stay hospitals in the United States. The scope of NHDS encompasses patients discharged from noninstitutional hospitals, exclusive of military and Department of Veterans Affairs hospitals, located in the 50 States and the District of Columbia. Only hospitals having six or more beds for patient use are included in the survey and before 1988 those in which the average length of stay for all patients was less than 30 days. In 1988 the scope was altered slightly to include all general and children's general hospitals regardless of the length of stay. Although all discharges of patients from these hospitals are within the scope of the survey, discharges of newborn infants from all hospitals are excluded from this report.

The original sample was selected in 1964 from a frame of short-stay hospitals listed in the National Master Facility Inventory. A two-stage stratified sample design was used, and hospitals were stratified according to bed size and geographic region. Sample hospitals were selected with probabilities ranging from certainty for the largest hospitals to 1 in 40 for the smallest hospitals. Within each sample hospital, a systematic random sample of discharges was selected from the daily listing sheet. Initially, the within-hospital sampling rates for selecting discharges varied inversely with the probability of hospital selection so that the overall probability of selecting a discharge was approximately the same across the sample. Those rates were adjusted for individual hospitals in subsequent years to control the reporting burden of those hospitals.

In 1985, for the first time, two data collection procedures were used for the survey. The first was the traditional manual system of sample selection and data abstraction. In the manual system, sample selection

and transcription of information from the hospital records to abstract forms were performed by either the hospital staff or representatives of NCHS or both. The second was an automated method, used in approximately 17 percent of the sample hospitals in 1985, involving the purchase of data tapes from commercial abstracting services. Upon receipt of these tapes they were subject to NCHS sampling, editing, and weighting procedures.

In 1988 NHDS was redesigned. The hospitals with the most beds and/or discharges annually were selected with certainty, but the remaining sample was selected using a three-stage stratified design. The first stage is a sample of PSU's used by the National Health Interview Survey. Within PSU's, hospitals were stratified or arrayed by abstracting status (whether subscribing to a commercial abstracting service) and within abstracting status arrayed by type of service and bed size. Within these strata and arrays, a systematic sampling scheme with probability proportional to the annual number of discharges was used to select hospitals. The rates for systematic sampling of discharges within hospitals vary inversely with probability of hospital selection within PSU. Discharge records from hospitals submitting data via commercial abstracting services and selected State data systems (approximately 34 percent of sample hospitals in 1994) were arrayed by primary diagnoses, patient sex and age group, and date of discharge before sampling. Otherwise, the procedures for sampling discharges within hospitals is the same as that used in the prior design.

In 1994 the hospital sample was updated by continuing the sampling process among hospitals that were NHDS-eligible for the sampling frame in 1994 but not in 1991. The additional hospitals were added at the end of the list for the strata where they belonged, and the systematic sampling was continued as if the additional hospitals had been present during the initial sample selection. Hospitals that were no longer NHDS-eligible were deleted. A similar updating process occurred in 1991.

The basic unit of estimation for NHDS is the sample patient abstract. The estimation procedure involves inflation by the reciprocal of the probability of selection, adjustment for nonresponding hospitals and missing abstracts, and ratio adjustments to fixed totals. In 1994 of the 525 hospitals selected for the survey, 512 were within the scope of the survey, and 478 participated in the survey. Data were abstracted from about 277,000 medical records. In 1995, 525 hospitals were selected, 508 were within scope, 466 participated, and 263,000 medical records were abstracted.

For more detailed information on the design of NHDS and the magnitude of sampling errors associated with the NHDS estimates, see: Graves EJ, Gillum BS. 1994 Summary: and Graves EJ, Owings MF. 1995 Summary: National Hospital Discharge Survey. Advance data from vital and health statistics; no 278 and no 291. Hyattsville, Maryland: National Center for Health Statistics. 1996 and 1997; and Haupt BJ, Kozak LJ. Estimates from two survey designs: National Hospital Discharge Survey. National Center for Health Statistics. Vital Health Stat 13(111). 1992.

National Nursing Home Survey

NCHS has conducted five National Nursing Home Surveys. The first survey was conducted from August 1973 to April 1974; the second survey from May 1977 to December 1977; the third from August 1985 to January 1986; the fourth from July 1995 to December 1995; and the fifth from July 1997 to December 1997.

Much of the background information and experience used to develop the first National Nursing Home Survey was obtained from a series of three ad hoc sample surveys of nursing and personal care homes called the Resident Places Surveys (RPS-1, -2, -3). The three surveys were conducted by the National Center for Health Statistics during April–June 1963, May–June 1964, and June–August 1969. During the first survey, RPS-1, data were collected on nursing homes, chronic disease and geriatric hospitals, nursing home units, and chronic disease wards of general and mental hospitals. RPS-2 concentrated mainly on

nursing homes and geriatric hospitals. During the third survey, RPS-3, nursing and personal care homes in the coterminous United States were sampled.

For the initial National Nursing Home Survey (NNHS) conducted in 1973–74, the universe included only those nursing homes that provided some level of nursing care. Homes providing only personal or domiciliary care were excluded. The sample of 2,118 homes was selected from the 17,685 homes that provided some level of nursing care and were listed in the 1971 National Master Facility Inventory (NMFI) or those that opened for business in 1972. Data were obtained from about 20,600 staff and 19,000 residents. Response rates were 97 percent for facilities, 88 percent for expenditures, 98 percent for residents, and 82 percent for staff.

The scope of the 1977 NNHS encompassed all types of nursing homes, including personal care and domiciliary care homes. The sample of about 1,700 facilities was selected from 23,105 nursing homes in the sampling frame, which consisted of all homes listed in the 1973 NMFI and those opening for business between 1973 and December 1976. Data were obtained from about 13,600 staff, 7,000 residents, and 5,100 discharged residents. Response rates were 95 percent for facilities, 85 percent for expenses, 81 percent for staff, 99 percent for residents, and 97 percent for discharges.

The scope of the 1985 NNHS was similar to the 1977 survey in that it included all types of nursing homes. Excluded were personal or domiciliary care homes. The sample of 1,220 homes was selected from a sampling frame of 20,479 nursing and related care homes. The frame consisted of all homes in the 1982 NMFI; homes identified in the 1982 Complement Survey of NMFI as "missing" from the 1982 NMFI; facilities that opened for business between 1982 and June 1984; and hospital-based nursing homes obtained from the Health Care Financing Administration. Information on the facility was collected through a personal interview with the administrator. Accountants were asked to complete a questionnaire on expenditures or provide a financial statement. Resident data were provided by a nurse familiar with the care provided to the resident. The nurse relied on the medical record and personal knowledge of the resident. In addition to employee data that were collected during the interview with the administrator, a sample of registered nurses completed a self-administered questionnaire. Discharge data were based on information recorded in the medical record. Additional data about the current and discharged residents were obtained in telephone interviews with next of kin. Data were obtained from 1,079 facilities, 2,763 registered nurses, 5,243 current residents, and 6,023 discharges. Response rates were 93 percent for facilities, 68 percent for expenses, 80 percent for registered nurses, 97 percent for residents, 95 percent for discharges, and 90 percent for next of kin.

The scope of the 1995 and 1997 NNHS was similar to the 1985 and the 1973–74 NNHS in that they included only nursing homes that provided some level of nursing care. Homes providing only personal or domiciliary care were excluded. The 1995 sample of 1,500 homes was selected from a sampling frame of 17,500 nursing homes. The frame consisted of an updated version of the 1991 National Health Provider Inventory (NHPI). Data were obtained from about 1,400 nursing homes and 8,000 current residents. Data on current residents were provided by a staff member familiar with the care received by residents and from information contained in resident's medical records.

The 1997 sample of 1,488 nursing homes was the same basic sample used in 1995. Excluded were out-of-scope and out-of-business places identified in the 1995 survey and included were a small number of additions to the sample from a supplemental frame of places not in the 1995 frame. The 1997 NNHS included the discharge component not available in the 1995 survey. Data from this survey should be available in the fall of 1998.

Statistics for all five surveys were derived by a ratio-estimation procedure. Statistics were adjusted for failure of a home to respond, failure to fill out one of the questionnaires, and failure to complete an item on a questionnaire.

For more information on the 1973–74 NNHS, see: Meiners MR. Selected operating and financial characteristics of nursing homes, United States, 1973–74 National Nursing Home Survey. National Center for Health Statistics. Vital Health Stat 13(22). 1975. For more information on the 1977 NNHS, see: Van Nostrand JF, Zappolo A, Hing E, et al. The National Nursing Home Survey, 1977 summary for the United States. National Center for Health Statistics. Vital Health Stat 13(43). 1979. For more information on the 1985 NNHS, see: Hing E, Sekscenski E, Strahan G. The National Nursing Home Survey: 1985 summary for the United States. National Center for Health Statistics. Vital Health Stat 13(97). 1985. For more information on the 1995 NNHS, see: Strahan G. An overview of nursing homes and their current residents: Data from the 1995 National Nursing Home Survey. Advance data from vital and health statistics; no 280. Hyattsville, Maryland: National Center for Health Statistics. 1997.

National Ambulatory Medical Care Survey

The National Ambulatory Medical Care Survey (NAMCS) is a continuing national probability sample of ambulatory medical encounters. The scope of the survey covers physician-patient encounters in the offices of non-Federally employed physicians classified by the American Medical Association or American Osteopathic Association as "office-based, patient care" physicians. Patient encounters with physicians engaged in prepaid practices (health maintenance organizations (HMO's), independent practice organizations (IPA's), and other prepaid practices) are included in NAMCS. Excluded are visits to hospital-based physicians, visits to specialists in anesthesiology, pathology, and radiology, and visits to physicians who are principally engaged in teaching, research, or administration. Telephone contacts and nonoffice visits are excluded, also.

A multistage probability design is employed. The first-stage sample consists of 84 primary sampling units (PSU's) in 1985 and 112 PSU's in 1992 selected from about 1,900 such units into which the United

States has been divided. In each sample PSU, a sample of practicing non-Federal office-based physicians is selected from master files maintained by the American Medical Association and the American Osteopathic Association. The final stage involves systematic random samples of office visits during randomly assigned 7-day reporting periods. In 1985 the survey excluded Alaska and Hawaii. Starting in 1989 the survey included all 50 States.

For the 1996 survey a sample of 3,000 physicians was selected. The physician response rate for 1996 was 70 percent providing data on 29,805 records.

The estimation procedure used in NAMCS basically has three components: inflation by the reciprocal of the probability of selection, adjustment for nonresponse, and ratio adjustment to fixed totals.

For more detailed information on NAMCS, see: Woodwell, DA. National Ambulatory Medical Care Survey: 1996 summary: Advance data from vital and health statistics; no 295. Hyattsville, Maryland: National Center for Health Statistics, 1997.

National Hospital Ambulatory Medical Care Survey

The National Hospital Ambulatory Medical Care Survey (NHAMCS), initiated in 1992, is a continuing annual national probability sample of visits by patients to emergency departments (ED's) and outpatient departments (OPD's) of non-Federal, short-stay, or general hospitals. Telephone contacts are excluded.

A four-stage probability sample design is used in NHAMCS, involving samples of primary sampling units (PSU's), hospitals with ED's and/or OPD's within PSU's, ED's within hospitals and/or clinics within OPD's, and patient visits within ED's and/or clinics. In 1996 the hospital response rate for NHAMCS was 95 percent. Hospital staff were asked to complete Patient Record forms for a systematic random sample of patient visits occurring during a randomly assigned 4-week reporting period. In 1996 the number of Patient Record forms completed for ED's was 21,902 and for OPD's was 29,806.

For more detailed information on NHAMCS, see: McCaig LF, McLemore T. Plan and operation of the National Hospital Ambulatory Medical Care Survey. National Center for Health Statistics. Vital Health Stat 1(34). 1994.

National Center for HIV, STD, and TB Prevention

AIDS Surveillance

Acquired immunodeficiency syndrome (AIDS) surveillance is conducted by health departments in each State, territory, and the District of Columbia. Although surveillance activities range from passive to active, most areas employ multifaceted active surveillance programs, which include four major reporting sources of AIDS information: hospitals and hospital-based physicians, physicians in nonhospital practice, public and private clinics, and medical record systems (death certificates, tumor registries, hospital discharge abstracts, and communicable disease reports). Using a standard confidential case report form, the health departments collect information without personal identifiers, which is coded and computerized either at the Centers for Disease Control and Prevention (CDC) or at health departments from which it is then transmitted electronically to CDC.

AIDS surveillance data are used to detect epidemiologic trends, to identify unusual cases requiring follow up, and for semiannual publication in the *HIV/AIDS Surveillance Report*. Studies to determine the completeness of reporting of AIDS cases meeting the national surveillance definition suggest reporting at greater than or equal to 90 percent.

For more information on AIDS surveillance, see: Centers for Disease Control and Prevention. *HIV/AIDS Surveillance Report*, published semiannually; or contact: Chief, Surveillance Branch, Division of HIV/AIDS, National Center for HIV, STD, and TB Prevention (NCHSTP), Centers for Disease Control and Prevention, Atlanta, GA 30333; or visit the NCHSTP home page at http://www.cdc.gov/nchstp/od/nchstp.html.

Epidemiology Program Office

National Notifiable Diseases Surveillance System

The Epidemiology Program Office (EPO) of CDC, in partnership with the Council of State and Territorial Epidemiologists (CSTE), operates the National Notifiable Diseases Surveillance System. The purpose of this system is primarily to provide weekly provisional information on the occurrence of diseases defined as notifiable by CSTE. In addition, the system also provides summary data on an annual basis. State epidemiologists report cases of notifiable diseases to EPO, and EPO tabulates and publishes these data in the *Morbidity and Mortality Weekly Report* (MMWR) and the *Summary of Notifiable Diseases, United States* (entitled *Annual Summary* before 1985). Notifiable disease surveillance is used by public health practitioners at local, State, and national levels as part of disease prevention and control activities.

Notifiable disease reports are received from 52 areas in the United States and 5 territories. To calculate U.S. rates, data reported by 50 States, New York City, and the District of Columbia, are used. (New York State is reported as Upstate New York, which excludes New York City.)

Completeness of reporting varies because not all cases receive medical care and not all treated conditions are reported. Although State laws and regulations mandate disease reporting, reporting to CDC by States and territories is voluntary. For example, reporting of mumps to CDC is not done by some States in which this disease is not notifiable to local or State authorities. Chlamydia became notifiable starting in 1995.

Estimates of underreporting of some diseases have been made. For example, it is estimated that only 22 percent of cases of congenital rubella syndrome are reported. Only 10–15 percent of all measles cases were reported before the institution of the Measles Elimination Program in 1978. Recent investigations suggest that fewer than 50 percent of measles cases were reported following an outbreak in an inner city and that 40 percent of hospitalized measles cases are

currently reported. Data from a study of pertussis suggest that only one-third of severe cases causing hospitalization or death are reported. Data from a study of tetanus deaths suggest that only 40 percent of tetanus cases are reported to CDC.

For more information, see: Centers for Disease Control and Prevention, Summary of notifiable diseases, United States, 1996. *Morbidity and Mortality Weekly Report*, 45(53), Public Health Service, DHHS, Atlanta, GA, 1997; or write: Director, Division of Public Health Surveillance and Informatics. Epidemiology Program Office, Centers for Disease Control and Prevention, Atlanta, GA 30333; or visit the EPO home page at http://www.cdc.gov/epo.

National Center for Chronic Disease Prevention and Health Promotion

Abortion Surveillance

In 1969 CDC began abortion surveillance to document the number and characteristics of women obtaining legal induced abortions, monitor unintended pregnancy, and assist efforts to identify and reduce preventable causes of morbidity and mortality associated with abortions. For each year since 1969 abortion data have been available from 52 reporting areas: 50 States, the District of Columbia, and New York City. The total number of legal induced abortions is available from all reporting areas; however, not all areas collect information regarding the characteristics of women who obtain abortions. Furthermore the number of States reporting each characteristic and the number of States with complete data for each characteristic varies from year to year. State data with more than 15 percent unknown for a given characteristic are excluded from the analysis of that characteristic.

For 47 reporting areas, data concerning the number and characteristics of women who obtain legal induced abortions are provided by central health agencies such as State health departments and the health departments of New York City and the District of Columbia. For the other five areas, data concerning the number of abortions are provided by hospitals and other medical facilities. In general the procedures are reported by the State in which the procedure is performed. However, two reporting areas (the District of Columbia and Wisconsin) report abortions by State of residence; occurrence data are unavailable for these areas.

The total number of abortions reported to CDC is about 10 percent less than the total estimated independently by the Alan Guttmacher Institute, a not-for-profit organization for reproductive health research, policy analysis, and public education.

For more information, see: Centers for Disease Control and Prevention, CDC Surveillance Summaries, Special Focus: Surveillance for Reproductive Health. *Morbidity and Mortality Weekly Report* 1997; 46(No SS-4), August 1997; or contact: Director, Division of Reproductive Health, National Center for Chronic Disease Prevention and Health Promotion (NCCDPHP), Centers for Disease Control and Prevention Atlanta, GA 30333; or visit the NCCDPHP home page at http://www.cdc.gov.nccdphp.

National Institute for Occupational Safety and Health

National Traumatic Occupational Fatalities Surveillance System

The National Traumatic Occupational Fatalities (NTOF) surveillance system is compiled by the National Institute for Occupational Safety and Health (NIOSH) based on information taken from death certificates. Certificates are collected from 52 vital statistics reporting units (the 50 States, New York City, and the District of Columbia) based on the following criteria: age 16 years or over, an external cause of death (ICD-9, E800-E999), and a positive response to the "Injury at work?" item.

For the period of this analysis there were no standardized guidelines regarding the completion of the "Injury at work?" item on the death certificate, thus, numbers and rates of occupational injury deaths from NTOF should be regarded as the lower bound for the true number of these events. Operational guidelines for

the completion of the "Injury at work?" item have been developed by NIOSH in conjunction with the National Center for Health Statistics, the National Association for Public Health Statistics and Information Systems, and the National Center for Environmental Health and were disseminated in 1992 for implementation in 1993. This should improve death certificate-based surveillance of work-related injuries.

The denominator data for the calculation of rates by industry division were obtained from the U.S. Bureau of Labor Statistics' annual average employment data. All of the rates presented are for the U.S. civilian labor force.

For further information on NTOF, see DHHS (NIOSH). Publication No. 93–108, *Fatal Injuries to Workers in the United States, 1980–1989: A Decade of Surveillance*; or contact: Director, Division of Safety Research, National Institute for Occupational Safety and Health, 1095 Willowdale Road, Mailstop P-1172, Morgantown, WV 26505; or visit the NIOSH home page at http://www.cdc.gov/niosh.

Health Resources and Services Administration

Bureau of Health Professions

Physician Supply Projections

Physician supply projections in this report are based on a model developed by the Bureau of Health Professionals to forecast the supply of physicians by specialty, activity, and State of practice. The 1986 supply of active physicians (M.D.'s) was used as the starting point for the most recent projections of active physicians. The major source of data used to obtain 1986 figures was the American Medical Association (AMA) Physician Masterfile.

In the first stage of the projections, graduates from U.S. schools of allopathic (M.D.) and osteopathic (D.O.) medicine and internationally trained additions were estimated on a year-by-year basis. Estimates of first-year enrollments, student attrition, other medical school-related trends, and a model of net internationally trained medical graduate immigration were used in deriving these annual additions. These year-by-year additions were then combined with the already existing active supply in a given year to produce a preliminary estimate of the active work force in each succeeding year. These estimates were then reduced to account for mortality and retirement. Gender-specific mortality and retirement losses were computed by 5-year age cohorts on an annual basis, using age distributions and mortality and retirement rates based on AMA data.

For more information, see: Bureau of Health Professions, *Health Personnel in the United States Ninth Report to Congress, 1993*, DHHS Pub. No. HRS-P-OD-94–1, Health Resources and Services Administration, Rockville, MD.

Nurse Supply Estimates

Nursing estimates in this report are based on a model developed by the Bureau of Health Professions to meet the requirements of Section 951, P.L. 94–63. The model estimates the following for each State: (a) population of nurses currently licensed to practice; (b) supply of full- and part-time practicing nurses (or available to practice); and (c) full-time equivalent supply of nurses practicing full time plus one-half of those practicing part time (or available on that basis).

The three estimates are divided into three levels of highest educational preparation: associate degree or diploma, baccalaureate, and master's and doctorate.

Among the factors considered are new graduates, changes in educational status, nursing employment rates, age, migration patterns, death rates, and licensure phenomena. The base data for the model are derived from the National Sample Surveys of Registered Nurses, conducted by the Division of Nursing, Bureau of Health Professions, HRSA. Other data sources include National League for Nursing for data on nursing education and National Council of State Boards of Nursing for data on licensure.

Substance Abuse and Mental Health Services Administration

Office of Applied Studies

National Household Surveys on Drug Abuse

Data on trends in use of marijuana, cigarettes, alcohol, and cocaine among persons 12 years of age and over are from the National Household Survey on Drug Abuse (NHSDA). The 1996 survey is the 16th in a series that began in 1971 under the auspices of the National Commission on Marijuana and Drug Abuse. From 1974 to September 1992, the survey was sponsored by the National Institute on Drug Abuse. Since October 1992, the survey has been sponsored by the Substance Abuse and Mental Health Services Administration (SAMHSA).

Since 1991 the National Household Survey on Drug Abuse has covered the civilian noninstitutionalized population 12 years of age and over in the United States. This includes civilians living on military bases and persons living in noninstitutionalized group quarters, such as college dormitories, rooming houses, and shelters. Hawaii and Alaska were included for the first time in 1991.

In 1994 the survey underwent major changes that affect the reporting of substance abuse prevalence rates. New questionnaire and data editing procedures were implemented to improve the measurement of trends in prevalence and to enhance the timeliness and quality of the data. Because it was anticipated that the new methodology would affect the estimates of prevalence, the 1994 NHSDA was designed to generate two sets of estimates. The first set, called the 1994-A estimates, was based on the same questionnaire and editing method that was used in 1993. The second set, called the 1994-B estimates, was based on the new questionnaire and editing methodology. A description of this new methodology can be found in Advance Report 10, available from SAMHSA. Because of the 1994 changes, many of the estimates from the 1994-A and earlier NHSDA's are not comparable with estimates from the 1994-B and later NHSDA's. To be able to describe long-term trends in drug use accurately, an adjustment procedure was developed and applied to the pre-1994 estimates. This adjustment uses the 1994 split sample design to estimate the magnitude of the impact of the new methodology for each drug category. The adjusted estimates are presented in this volume of *Health, United States*. A description of the adjustment method can be found in Advance Report Number 18, Appendix A, available from SAMHSA.

The 1996 survey employed a multistage probability sample design. Young people (age 12–34 years), black Americans, and Hispanics were oversampled. The sample included 18,269 respondents. The screening and interview response rates were 92.7 percent and 78.6 percent, respectively.

For more information on the National Household Survey on Drug Abuse (NHSDA), see: NHSDA Series: H-1 National Household Survey on Drug Abuse Main Findings 1995, H-3 Preliminary Results from the 1996 National Household Survey on Drug Abuse, H-4 National Household Survey on Drug Abuse: Population Estimates 1996; or write: Office of Applied Studies, Substance Abuse and Mental Health Services Administration, Room 16C-06, 5600 Fishers Lane, Rockville, MD 20857; or visit the SAMHSA home page at http://www.samhsa.gov.

Drug Abuse Warning Network

The Drug Abuse Warning Network (DAWN) is a large-scale, ongoing drug abuse data collection system based on information from emergency room and medical examiner facilities. DAWN collects information about those drug abuse occurrences that have resulted in a medical crisis or death. The major objectives of the DAWN data system include the monitoring of drug abuse patterns and trends, the identification of substances associated with drug abuse episodes, and the assessment of drug-related consequences and other health hazards.

Hospitals eligible for DAWN are non-Federal, short-stay general hospitals that have a 24-hour emergency room. Since 1988 the DAWN emergency room data have been collected from a representative sample of these hospitals located throughout the coterminous United States, including 21 oversampled metropolitan areas. Within each facility, a designated DAWN reporter is responsible for identifying drug abuse episodes by reviewing official records and transcribing and submitting data on each case. The data from this sample are used to generate estimates of the total number of emergency room drug abuse episodes and drug mentions in all such hospitals. A response rate of 77 percent was obtained in the 1995 survey.

A methodology for generating comparable estimates for years before 1988 was developed, taking advantage of historical data on the characteristics of the universe of eligible hospitals and the extensive data files compiled over the years by DAWN. After the new probability sample for DAWN was implemented in 1988, old and new DAWN sample data were collected for a period of 1 year. This overlap period was used to evaluate various procedures for weighting the old sample data (from 1978 to 1987). The procedure that consistently produced reliable estimates for a particular metropolitan area was selected as the weighting scheme for that area and used to generate all estimates for that area for years before 1988. These historical estimates are available in Advance Report 16, available from SAMHSA.

For further information, see: The Drug Abuse Warning Network (DAWN), Annual Data, 1994, Series I, Number 14-A; Historical Estimates from the Drug Abuse Warning Network, Advance Report Number 16; DAWN Series D-1: Drug Abuse Warning Network Annual Medical Examiner Data 1995; DAWN Series D-2: Mid-Year Preliminary Estimates from the 1996 Drug Abuse Warning Network or write: Office of Applied Studies, Substance Abuse and Mental Health Services Administration, Room 16C-06, 5600 Fishers Lane, Rockville, MD 20857; or visit the SAMHSA home page at http://www.samhsa.gov.

Uniform Facility Data Set

The Uniform Facility Data Set (UFDS), formerly the National Drug and Alcoholism Treatment Unit Survey (NDATUS), is part of the Drug and Alcohol

Services Information System (DASIS) maintained by the Substance Abuse and Mental Health Services Administration. UFDS is a census of all known drug and alcohol abuse treatment and prevention facilities in the United States and its jurisdictions. It seeks information from all specialized facilities that treat substance abuse. These include facilities that only treat substance abuse, as well as specialty substance abuse units operating within larger mental health (for example, community mental health centers), general health (for example, hospitals), social service (for example, family assistance centers), and criminal justice (for example, probation departments) agencies. UFDS solicits data concerning facility and client characteristics for a specific reference day (on or about October 1) including number of individuals in treatment, substance of abuse (alcohol, drugs, or both), types of services, and source of revenue. Public and private facilities are included.

Treatment facilities contacted through UFDS are identified from the National Facility Register (NFR), which lists providers that are recognized by State substance abuse agencies. Listings of private providers are not complete for all States. The response rates to the survey were 82 percent, 91 percent, and 89 percent, in 1992, 1993, and 1995, respectively. Response rates increased in 1993 and 1995 due to a new policy of conducting a follow-up telephone interview of all nonrespondents to the initial mailed survey.

For further information on UFDS, contact: Office of Applied Studies, Substance Abuse and Mental Health Services Administration, Room 16-105, 5600 Fishers Lane, Rockville, MD 20857; or visit the OAS statistical information section of the SAMHSA home page: http://www.samhsa.gov.

Center for Mental Health Services

Surveys of Mental Health Organizations

The Survey and Analysis Branch of the Division of State and Community Systems Development conducts a biennial inventory of mental health organizations (IMHO) and general hospital mental health services (GHMHS). One version is designed for specialty mental health organizations and another for non-Federal general hospitals with separate psychiatric services. The response rate to most of the items on these inventories is relatively high (90 percent or better) as is the rate for data presented in this report. However, for some inventory items, the response rate may be somewhat lower.

IMHO and GHMHS are the primary sources for Center for Mental Health Services data included in this report. This data system is based on questionnaires mailed every other year to mental health organizations in the United States, including psychiatric hospitals, non-Federal general hospitals with psychiatric services, Department of Veterans Affairs psychiatric services, residential treatment centers for emotionally disturbed children, freestanding outpatient psychiatric clinics, partial care organizations, freestanding day-night organizations, and multiservice mental health organizations, not elsewhere classified.

Federally funded community mental health centers (CMHC's) were included separately through 1980. In 1981, with the advent of block grants, the changes in definition of CMHC's and the discontinuation of CMHC monitoring by the Center for Mental Health Services, organizations formerly classified as CMHC's have been reclassified as other organization types, primarily "multiservice mental health organizations, not elsewhere classified," and "freestanding psychiatric outpatient clinics."

Beginning in 1983 any organization that provides services in any combination of two or more services (for example, outpatient plus partial care, residential treatment plus outpatient plus partial care) and is neither a hospital nor a residential treatment center for emotionally disturbed children is classified as a multiservice mental health organization.

Other surveys conducted by the Survey and Analysis Branch encompass samples of patients admitted to State and county mental hospitals, private mental hospitals, multiservice mental health organizations, the psychiatric services of non-Federal general hospitals and Department of Veterans Affairs medical centers, residential treatment centers for emotionally disturbed children, and freestanding outpatient and partial care programs. The purpose of these surveys is to determine the sociodemographic, clinical, and treatment characteristics of patients served by these facilities.

For more information, write: Survey and Analysis Branch, Division of State and Community Systems Development, Center for Mental Health Services, Room 15C-O4, 5600 Fishers Lane, Rockville, MD 20857. For further information on mental health, see: Center for Mental Health Services, *Mental Health, United States, 1996.* Manderscheid RW, Sonnenschein MA, eds. DHHS Pub. No. (SMA) 96–3098. Washington: Public Health Service. 1996; or visit the Center for Mental Health Services home page at http://www.samhsa.gov/cmhs/cmhs.htm.

National Institutes of Health

National Cancer Institute

Surveillance, Epidemiology, and End Results Program

In the Surveillance, Epidemiology, and End Results (SEER) Program the National Cancer Institute (NCI) contracts with 11 population-based registries throughout the United States to provide data on all residents diagnosed with cancer during the year and to provide current follow-up information on all previously diagnosed patients.

This report covers residents of one of the following geographic areas at the time of their initial diagnosis of cancer: Atlanta, Georgia; Detroit, Michigan; Seattle-Puget Sound, Washington; San Francisco-Oakland, California; Connecticut; Iowa; New Mexico; Utah; and Hawaii.

Population estimates used to calculate incidence rates are obtained from the U.S. Bureau of the Census. NCI uses estimation procedures as needed to obtain estimates for years and races not included in the data provided by the U.S. Bureau of the Census. Rates presented in this report may differ somewhat from previous reports due to revised population estimates and the addition and deletion of small numbers of incidence cases.

Life tables used to determine normal life expectancy when calculating relative survival rates were obtained from NCHS and in-house calculations. Separate life tables are used for each race-sex-specific group included in the SEER Program.

For further information, see: National Cancer Institute, *Cancer Statistics Review, 1973–95* by L.A.G. Ries, et al. Public Health Service. Bethesda, MD, 1998; or visit the SEER home page: http://www-seer.ims.nci.nih.gov.

National Institute on Drug Abuse

Monitoring the Future Study (High School Senior Survey)

Monitoring the Future Study (MTF) is a large-scale epidemiological survey of drug use and related attitudes. It was initiated by the National Institute on Drug Abuse (NIDA) in 1975 and is conducted annually through a NIDA grant awarded to the University of Michigan's Institute for Social Research. MTF is composed of three substudies: (a) annual survey of high school seniors initiated in 1975; (b) ongoing panel studies of representative samples from each graduating class that have been conducted by mail since 1976; and (c) annual surveys of 8th and 10th graders initiated in 1991.

The survey design is a multistage random sample with stage one being the selection of particular geographic areas, stage two the selection of one or more schools in each area, and stage three the selection of students within each school. Data are collected using self-administered questionnaires administered in the classroom by representatives of the Institute for Social Research. Dropouts and students who are absent on the day of the survey are excluded. Recognizing that the dropout population is at higher risk for drug use, this survey was expanded to include similar nationally representative samples of 8th and 10th graders in 1991. Statistics that are published in the Dropout Rates in the United States: 1996 (published by the National Center for Educational Statistics, Pub. No. 98-250) stated that among persons 15 to 16 years of age, 3.5 percent have dropped out of school. Among persons 17 years of age, 3.4 percent have dropped out of school, while the dropout percent increases to 5.9 percent of persons 18 years of age, and to 8.9 percent for persons 19 years of age. Therefore, surveying eighth graders (where drop out rates are much lower than for high school seniors) should be effective for picking up students at higher risk for drug use.

Approximately 50,000 8th, 10th, and 12th graders are surveyed annually. In 1997, the annual senior samples are comprised of roughly 15,400 seniors in 135 public and private high schools nationwide, selected to be representative of all seniors in the continental United States. The 10th grade samples involve about 15,500 students in 125 schools in 1997, and the 1997 eighth grade samples have approximately 18,600 students in 160 schools.

For further information on Monitoring the Future Study, see: National Institute on Drug Abuse, National Survey Results on Drug Use from Monitoring the Future Study, 1975–1995, vol I, secondary students. NIH Pub. No. 96–4139. Washington: Public Health Service. 1996; or visit the NIDA home page at http://www.nida.nih.gov.

Health Care Financing Administration

Office of the Actuary

Estimates of National Health Expenditures

Estimates of expenditures for health (National Health Accounts) are compiled annually by type of expenditure and source of funds.

Estimates of expenditures for health services come from an array of sources. The American Hospital Association (AHA) data on hospital finances are the primary source for estimates relating to hospital care. The salaries of physicians and dentists on the staffs of hospitals, hospital outpatient clinics, hospital-based home health agencies, and nursing home care provided in the hospital setting are considered to be components of hospital care. Expenditures for home health care and for services of health professionals (for example, doctors, chiropractors, private duty nurses, therapists, and podiatrists) are estimated primarily using a combination of data from the U.S. Bureau of the Census' Service Annual Survey and the quinquennial Census of Service Industries.

The estimates of retail spending for prescription drugs are based on results of a HCFA-sponsored study conducted by the Actuarial Research Corporation and on industry data on prescription drug transactions. Expenditures for other medical nondurables and vision products and other medical durables purchased in retail outlets are based on estimates of personal consumption expenditures prepared by the U.S. Department of Commerce's Bureau of Economic Analysis, U.S. Bureau of Labor Statistics' Consumer Expenditure Survey, and the 1987 National Medical Expenditure Survey conducted by the Agency for Health Care Policy and Research. Those durable and nondurable products provided to inpatients in hospitals or nursing homes, and those provided by licensed professionals or through home health agencies are excluded here, but are included with the expenditure estimates of the provider service category.

Nursing home expenditures cover care rendered in establishments providing inpatient nursing and health-related personal care through active treatment programs for medical and health-related conditions. These establishments cover skilled nursing and intermediate care facilities, including those for the mentally retarded. Spending estimates are based upon data from the U.S. Bureau of the Census Services Annual Survey, and the quinequennial Census of Service Industries.

Expenditures for construction include those spent on the erection or renovation of hospitals, nursing homes, medical clinics, and medical research facilities, but not for private office buildings providing office space for private practitioners. Expenditures for noncommercial research (the cost of commercial research by drug companies are assumed to be imbedded in the price charged for the product; to include this item again would result in double counting) are developed from information gathered by the National Institutes of Health.

Source of funding estimates likewise come from a multiplicity of sources. Data on the Federal health programs are taken from administrative records maintained by the servicing agencies. Among the sources used to estimate State and local government spending for health are the U.S. Bureau of the Census' *Government Finances* and Social Security Administration reports on State-operated Workers' Compensation programs. Federal and State-local expenditures for education and training of medical personnel are excluded from these measures where they are separable. For the private financing of health care, data on the financial experience of health insurance organizations come from special Health Care Financing Administration analyses of private health insurers, and from the Bureau of Labor Statistics' survey on the cost of employer-sponsored health insurance and on consumer expenditures. Information on out-of-pocket spending from the U.S. Bureau of the Census' Services Annual Survey, U.S. Bureau of Labor Statistics' Consumer Expenditure Survey, the 1987 National Medical Expenditure Survey conducted by the Agency for Health Care Policy and Research, and from private surveys conducted by the American Hospital Association, American Medical Association, and the American Dental Association are used to develop estimates of direct spending by customers.

For more specific information on definitions, sources and methods used in the National Health Accounts, see: National Health Accounts: Lessons from the U.S. Experience, by Lazenby HC, Levit KR, Waldo DR, et al. Health Care Financing Review, vol 14 no 4. Health Care Financing Administration. Washington: Public Health Service. 1992 and National Health Expenditures, 1994, Levit KR, Lazenby HC, Sivarajan L, et al. Health Care Financing Review, vol

17 no 3. Health Care Financing Administration. Washington: Public Health Service. 1996.

Estimates of State Health Expenditures

Estimates of spending by State are created using the same definitions of health care sectors used in producing the National Health Expenditures (NHE). The same data sources used in creating NHE are also used to create State estimates whenever possible. Frequently, however, surveys that are used to create valid national estimates lack sufficient size to create valid State level estimates. In these cases, alternative data sources that best represent the State-by-State distribution of spending are substituted and the U.S. aggregate expenditures for the specific type of service or source of funds are used to control the level of State-by-State distributions. This procedure implicitly assumes that national spending estimates can be created more accurately than State specific expenditures.

Despite definitional correspondence, NHE differ from the sum of State estimates. NHE include expenditures for persons living in U.S. territories and for military and Federal civilian employees and their families stationed overseas. The sum of the State level expenditures exclude health spending for those groups. For hospital care, exclusion of purchases of services in non-U.S. areas accounts for a 0.9 percent reduction in hospital expenditures from those measured as part of NHE.

For more information, contact: Office of the Actuary, Health Care Financing Administration, 7500 Security Blvd., Baltimore, MD 21244-1850.

Medicare National Claims History Files

The Medicare Common Working File (CWF) is a Medicare Part A and Part B benefit coordination and claims validation system. There are two National Claims History (NCH) files, the NCH 100 percent-Nearline File, and the NCH Beneficiary Program Liability (BPL) File. The NCH files contain claims records and Medicare beneficiary information. The NCH 100 percent Nearline File contains all institutional and physician/supplier claims from the CWF. It provides records of every claim submitted, including all adjustment claims. The NCH BPL file contains Medicare Part A and Part B beneficiary liability information (such as deductible and coinsurance amounts remaining). The records include all Part A and Part B utilization and entitlement data. Records for 1997 were maintained on more than 38 million enrollees and 48,826 institutional providers including 6,246 hospitals, 14,619 skilled nursing facilities, 10,487 home health agencies, 2,239 hospices, 2,689 outpatient physical therapy, 472 comprehensive outpatient rehabilitation facilities, 3,274 end state renal dialysis facilities, 3,447 rural health clinics, 1,175 community mental health centers, 2,406 ambulatory surgical centers, and 1,772 federally qualified health centers. About 708 million claims were processed in fiscal year 1996.

Data from the NCH files provide information about enrollee use of benefits for a point in time or over an extended period. Statistical reports are produced on enrollment, characteristics of participating providers, reimbursement, and services used.

For further information on the NCH files see: Health Care Financing Administration, Office of Information Services, Enterprise Data Base Group, Division of Information Distribution, Data Users Reference Guide or call the Medicare Hotline at 410–786–3689.

For further information on Medicare visit the HCFA home page at http://www.hcfa.gov.

Medicaid Data System

The majority of Medicaid data are compiled from forms submitted annually by State Medicaid agencies to the Health Care Financing Administration (HCFA) for Federal fiscal years ending September 30 on the Form HCFA-2082, *Statistical Report on Medical Care: Eligibles, Recipients, Payments, and Services.*

When using the data keep the following caveats in mind:

■ Counts of recipients and eligibles categorized by

basis of eligibility generally count each person only once based on the person's basis of eligibility as of first appearance on the Medicaid rolls during the Federal fiscal year covered by the report. Note, however, that some States report duplicated counts of recipients; that is, they report an individual in as many categories as the individual had different eligibility statuses during the year. In such cases, the sum of all basis-of-eligibility cells will be greater than the "total recipients" number.

■ Expenditure data include payments for all claims adjudicated or paid during the fiscal year covered by the report. Note that this is not the same as summing payments for services that were rendered during the reporting period.

■ Some States fail to submit the HCFA-2082 for a particular year. When this happens, HCFA estimates the current year's HCFA-2082 data for missing States based upon prior year's submissions and information the State entered on Form HCFA-64 (the form States use to claim reimbursement for Federal matching funds for Medicaid).

■ HCFA-2082's submitted by States frequently contain obvious errors in one or more cells in the form. For cells obviously in error, HCFA estimates values that appear to be more reasonable.

The Medicaid data presented in *Health, United States* are from the Medicaid statistical system (using form HCFA-2082) and may differ from data presented elsewhere using the quarterly financial reports (form HCFA-64) submitted by States for reimbursement. Vendor payments from the Medicaid statistical system exclude disproportionate share hospital payments ($17 billion in 1993) and payments to health maintenance organizations and Medicare ($6 billion in 1993).

For further information on Medicaid data, see: *Health Care Financing Review: Medicare and Medicaid Statistical Supplement, 1995*, HCFA Pub. No. 0374, Health Care Financing Administration, Baltimore, MD. U.S. Government Printing Office, Sept. 1995; or visit the HCFA home page at http://www.hcfa.gov.

Online Survey Certification and Reporting Database

The Online Survey Certification and Reporting (OSCAR) database has been maintained by the Health Care Financing Administration (HCFA) since 1992. OSCAR is an updated version of the Medicare and Medicaid Automated Certification System that has been in existence since 1972. OSCAR is an administrative database containing detailed information on all Medicare and Medicaid health care providers in addition to all currently certified Medicare and Medicaid nursing home facilities in the United States and Territories. (Data for the territories are not shown in this report.) The purpose of the nursing home facility survey certification process is to ensure that nursing facilities meet the current HCFA long-term care requirements and thus can participate in serving Medicare and Medicaid beneficiaries. Included in the OSCAR database are all certified nursing facilities, certified hospital-based nursing homes, and certified units for other types of nursing home facilities (for example, life care communities or board and care homes). Facilities not included in OSCAR are all noncertified facilities (that is, facilities that are only licensed by the State and are limited to private payment sources), and nursing homes that are part of the Department of Veterans Affairs. Also excluded are nursing homes that are intermediate care facilities for the mentally retarded. Approximately 700 nursing homes, which account for about 52,600 beds, are noncertified and not included in OSCAR in 1996. The number of noncertified nursing homes was obtained from the 1995 National Nursing Home Survey; due to the small sample size and/or relative standard error over 30 percent, this figure should not be assumed reliable.

Information on the number of beds, residents, and resident characteristics are collected during an inspection of all certified facilities. All certified nursing homes are inspected by representatives of the State survey agency (generally the Department of Health) at least once every 15 months. The information present on OSCAR is based on each facility's own administrative record system in addition to interviews with key administrative staff members.

For more information, see: HCFA: OSCAR data users reference guide, 1995, available from HCFA, Health Standards and Quality Bureau, HCFA/HSQB S2–11-07, 7500 Security Boulevard, Baltimore, MD 21244; or visit the HCFA home page at http://www.hcfa.gov.

Department of Commerce

Bureau of the Census

Census of Population

The census of population has been taken in the United States every 10 years since 1790. In the 1990 census, data were collected on sex, race, age, and marital status from 100 percent of the enumerated population. More detailed information such as income, education, housing, occupation, and industry were collected from a representative sample of the population. For most of the country, one out of six households (about 17 percent) received the more detailed questionnaire. In places of residence estimated to have less than 2,500 population, 50 percent of households received the long form.

For more information on the 1990 census, see: U.S. Bureau of the Census, *1990 Census of Population, General Population Characteristics*, Series 1990, CP-1; or visit the Census Bureau home page at http://www.census.gov.

Current Population Survey

The Current Population Survey (CPS) is a household sample survey of the civilian noninstitutionalized population conducted monthly by the U.S. Bureau of the Census. CPS provides estimates of employment, unemployment, and other characteristics of the general labor force, the population as a whole, and various other subgroups of the population.

The 1996 CPS sample is located in 754 sample areas, with coverage in every State and the District of

Columbia. In an average month during 1996, the number of housing units or living quarters eligible for interview was about 50,000; of these about 7 percent were, for various reasons, unavailable for interview. In 1994 major changes were introduced, which included a complete redesign of the questionnaire and the introduction of computer-assisted interviewing for the entire survey. In addition, there were revisions to some of the labor force concepts and definitions.

The estimation procedure used involves inflation by the reciprocal of the probability of selection, adjustment for nonresponse, and ratio adjustment. Beginning in 1994 new population controls based on the 1990 census adjusted for the estimated population undercount were utilized.

For more information, see: U.S. Bureau of the Census, *The Current Population Survey, Design and Methodology*, Technical Paper 40, Washington, U.S. Government Printing Office, Jan. 1978; U.S. Department of Labor, Bureau of Labor Statistics, Employment and Earnings, Feb. 1994, vol 41 no 2 and Feb. 1995, vol 42 no 2, Washington: U.S. Government Printing Office, Feb. 1994 and Feb. 1995; or visit the CPS home page at http://www.bls.census.gov.

Population Estimates

National population estimates are derived by using decennial census data as benchmarks and data available from various agencies as follows: births and deaths (National Center for Health Statistics); immigrants (Immigration and Naturalization Service); Armed Forces (Department of Defense); net movement between Puerto Rico and the U.S. mainland (Puerto Rico Planning Board); and Federal employees abroad (Office of Personnel Management and Department of Defense). State estimates are based on similar data and also on a variety of data series, including school statistics from State departments of education and parochial school systems. Current estimates are consistent with official decennial census figures and do not reflect estimated decennial census underenumeration.

After decennial population censuses, intercensal population estimates for the preceding decade are prepared to replace postcensal estimates. Intercensal population estimates are more accurate than postcensal estimates because they take into account the census of population at the beginning and end of the decade. Intercensal estimates have been prepared for the 1960's, 1970's, and 1980's to correct the "error of closure" or difference between the estimated population at the end of the decade and the census count for that date. The error of closure at the national level was quite small during the 1960's (379,000). However, for the 1970's it amounted to almost 5 million and for the 1980's, 1.5 million.

For more information, see: U.S. Bureau of the Census, U.S. population estimated by age, sex, race, and Hispanic origin: 1990–96, release PPL-57, March 1997; or visit the Census Bureau home page: http://www.census.gov.

Department of Labor

Bureau of Labor Statistics

Annual Survey of Occupational Injuries and Illnesses

Since 1971 the Bureau of Labor Statistics (BLS) has conducted an annual survey of establishments in the private sector to collect statistics on occupational injuries and illnesses. The Survey of Occupational Injuries and Illnesses is based on records that employers maintain under the Occupational Safety and Health Act. Excluded from the survey are self-employed individuals; farmers with fewer than 11 employees; employers regulated by other Federal safety and health laws; and Federal, State, and local government agencies.

Data are obtained from a sample of approximately 250,000 establishments, that is, single physical locations where business is conducted or where services of industrial operations are performed. An independent sample is selected for each State and the

District of Columbia that represents industries in that jurisdiction. BLS includes all the State samples in the national sample.

Establishments included in the survey are instructed in a mailed questionnaire to provide summary totals of all entries for the previous calendar year to its Log and Summary of Occupational Injuries and Illnesses (OSHA No. 200 form). Additionally, from the selected establishments, approximately 550,000 injuries and illnesses with days away from work are sampled in order to obtain demographic and detailed case characteristic information. An occupational injury is any injury, such as a cut, fracture, sprain, or amputation, that results from a work-related event or from a single instantaneous exposure in the work environment. An occupational illness is any abnormal condition or disorder, other than one resulting from an occupational injury, caused by exposure to factors associated with employment. It includes acute and chronic illnesses or disease that may be caused by inhalation, absorption, ingestion, or direct contact. Lost workday cases are cases that involve days away from work, or days of restricted work activity, or both. The response rate is about 92 percent.

For more information, see: Bureau of Labor Statistics, Occupational Injuries and Illnesses: Counts, Rates, and Characteristics, 1993. BLS Bulletin 2478, U.S. Department of Labor, Washington, D.C., August 1996; or visit the BLS home page at http://www.bls.gov.

Consumer Price Index

The Consumer Price Index (CPI) is a monthly measure of the average change in the prices paid by urban consumers for a fixed market basket of goods and services. The all-urban index (CPI-U) introduced in 1978 is representative of the buying habits of about 80 percent of the noninstitutionalized population of the United States.

In calculating the index, price changes for the various items in each location were averaged together with weights that represent their importance in the spending of all urban consumers. Local data were then combined to obtain a U.S. city average.

The index measures price changes from a designated reference date, 1982–84, which equals 100. An increase of 22 percent, for example, is shown as 122. This change can also be expressed in dollars as follows: the price of a base period "market basket" of goods and services bought by all urban consumers has risen from $10 in 1982–84 to $11.83 in 1988.

The most recent revision of CPI, completed in 1987, reflected spending patterns based on the Survey of Consumer Expenditures from 1982 to 1984, the 1980 Census of Population, and the ongoing Point-of-Purchase Survey. Using this improved sample design, prices for the goods and services required to calculate the index are collected in 85 urban areas throughout the country and from about 21,000 retail and service establishments. In addition, data on rents are collected from about 40,000 tenants and 20,000 owner-occupied housing units. Food, fuels, and a few other items are priced monthly in all 85 locations. Prices of most other goods and services are collected bimonthly in the remaining areas. All price information is obtained through visits or calls by trained BLS field representatives.

The 1987 revision changed the treatment of health insurance in the cost-weight definitions for medical care items. This change has no effect on the final index result but provides a clearer picture of the role of health insurance in the CPI. As part of the revision, three new indexes have been created by separating previously combined items, for example, eye care from other professional services and inpatient and outpatient treatment from other hospital and medical care services.

Effective January 1997 the hospital index was restructured by combining the three categories room, inpatient services and outpatient services into one category, hospital services. Differentiation between inpatient and outpatient and among service types are under this broad category. In addition new procedures for hospital data collection identify a payor, diagnosis, and the payor's reimbursement arrangement from selected hospital bills.

For more information, see: Bureau of Labor Statistics, *Handbook of Methods*, BLS Bulletin 2490, U.S. Department of Labor, Washington, Apr. 1997; IK Ford and P Sturm. CPI revision provides more accuracy in the medical care services component, *Monthly Labor Review*, U.S. Department of Labor, Bureau of Labor Statistics, Washington, Apr. 1988; or visit the BLS home page at http://www.bls.gov.

Employment and Earnings

The Division of Monthly Industry Employment Statistics and the Division of Employment and Unemployment Analysis of the Bureau of Labor Statistics publish data on employment and earnings. The data are collected by the U.S. Bureau of the Census, State Employment Security Agencies, and State Departments of Labor in cooperation with BLS.

The major data source is the Current Population Survey (CPS), a household interview survey conducted monthly by the U.S. Bureau of the Census to collect labor force data for BLS. CPS is described separately in this appendix. Data based on establishment records are also compiled each month from mail questionnaires by BLS, in cooperation with State agencies.

For more information, see: U.S. Department of Labor, Bureau of Labor Statistics, *Employment and Earnings*, Jan. 1997, vol 44 no 1, Washington: U.S. Government Printing Office. Jan. 1997.

Employer Costs for Employee Compensation

Employer costs for employee compensation cover all occupations in private industry, excluding farms and households and State and local governments. These cost levels are published once a year with the payroll period including March 12th as the reference period.

The cost levels are based on compensation cost data collected for the Bureau of Labor Statistics Employment Cost Index (ECI), released quarterly. Employee Benefits Survey (EBS) data are jointly collected with ECI data. Cost data were collected from

the ECI's March 1993 sample that consisted of about 23,000 occupations within 4,500 sample establishments in private industry and 7,000 occupations within 1,000 establishments in State and local governments. The sample establishments are classified industry categories based on the 1987 Standard Industrial Classification (SIC) system, as defined by the U.S. Office of Management and Budget. Within an establishment, specific job categories are selected to represent broader major occupational groups such as professional specialty and technical occupations. The cost levels are calculated with current employment weights each year.

For more information, see: U.S. Department of Labor, Bureau of Labor Statistics, *Employment Cost Indexes and Levels, 1975–95*, Bulletin 2466, Oct. 1995.

Department of Veterans Affairs

Data are obtained from the Department of Veterans Affairs (VA) administrative data systems. These include budget, patient treatment, patient census, and patient outpatient clinic information. Data from the three patient files are collected locally at each VA medical center and are transmitted to the national databank at the VA Austin Automated Center where they are stored and used to provide nationwide statistics, reports, and comparisons.

The Patient Treatment File

The patient treatment file (PTF) collects data, at the time of the patient's discharge, on each episode of inpatient care provided to patients at VA hospitals, VA nursing homes, VA domiciliaries, community nursing homes, and other non-VA facilities. The PTF record contains the scrambled social security number, dates of inpatient treatment, date of birth, State and county of residence, type of disposition, place of disposition after discharge, as well as the ICD–9–CM diagnostic and procedure or operative codes for each episode of care.

The Patient Census File

The patient census file collects data on each patient remaining in a VA medical facility at midnight on a selected date of each year, normally September 30. This file includes patients admitted to VA hospitals, VA nursing homes, and VA domiciliaries. The census record includes information similar to that reported in the patient treatment file record.

The Outpatient Clinic File

The outpatient clinic file (OPC) collects data on each instance of medical treatment provided to a veteran in an outpatient setting. The OPC record includes the age, scrambled social security number, State and county of residence, VA eligibility code, clinic(s) visited, purpose of visit, and the date of visit for each episode of care.

For more information, write: Department of Veterans Affairs, National Center for Veteran Analysis and Statistics, Biometrics Division 008C12, 810 Vermont Ave., NW, Washington, DC 20420; or visit the VA home page at http://www.va.gov.

Environmental Protection Agency

Aerometric Information Retrieval System (AIRS)

The Environmental Protection Agency's Aerometric Information Retrieval System (AIRS) compiles data on ambient air levels of particulate matter smaller than 10 microns (PM-10), lead, carbon monoxide, sulphur dioxide, nitrogen dioxide, and tropospheric ozone. These pollutants were identified in the Clean Air Act of 1970 and in its 1977 and 1990 amendments because they pose significant threats to public health. The National Ambient Air Quality Standards (NAAQS) define for each pollutant the maximum concentration level (micrograms per cubic meter) that cannot be exceeded during specific time intervals. Data shown in this publication reflect attainment of NAAQS during a 12-month period based

on analysis using county level air monitoring data from AIRS and population data from the Bureau of the Census.

Data are collected at State and local air pollution monitoring sites. Each site provides data for one or more of the six pollutants. The number of sites has varied, but generally increased over the years. In 1993 there were 4,469 sites, 4,668 sites in 1994, and 4,800 sites in 1995. The monitoring sites are located primarily in heavily populated urban areas. Air quality for less populated areas is assessed through a combination of data from supplemental monitors and air pollution models.

For more information, see: Environmental Protection Agency, *National Air Quality and Emissions Trend Report, 1994*, EPA-454/R-95–014, Research Triangle Park, NC, Oct. 1995, or write: Office of Air Quality Planning and Standards, Environmental Protection Agency, Research Triangle Park, NC 27711. For additional information on this measure and similar measures used to track the Healthy People 2000 Objectives and Health Status Indicators, see: National Center for Health Statistics, *Monitoring Air Quality in Healthy People 2000*, Statistical Notes, No. 9. Hyattsville, Maryland: 1995; or visit the EPA AIRS home page at http://www.epa.gov/airs/airs.html.

United Nations

Demographic Yearbook

The Statistical Office of the United Nations prepares the *Demographic Yearbook*, a comprehensive collection of international demographic statistics.

Questionnaires are sent annually and monthly to more than 220 national statistical services and other appropriate government offices. Data forwarded on these questionnaires are supplemented, to the extent possible, by data taken from official national publications and by correspondence with the national statistical services. To ensure comparability, rates, ratios, and percents have been calculated in the statistical office of the United Nations.

Lack of international comparability between estimates arises from differences in concepts, definitions, and time of data collection. The comparability of population data is affected by several factors, including (a) the definitions of the total population, (b) the definitions used to classify the population into its urban and rural components, (c) the difficulties relating to age reporting, (d) the extent of over- or underenumeration, and (e) the quality of population estimates. The completeness and accuracy of vital statistics data also vary from one country to another. Differences in statistical definitions of vital events may also influence comparability.

For more information, see: United Nations, *Demographic Yearbook 1995*, United Nations, New York, NY. 1995; or visit the United Nations home page at http://www.un.org or their website locator at http://www.unsystem.org.

World Health Statistics Annual

The World Health Organization (WHO) prepares the *World Health Statistics Annual*, an annual volume of information on vital statistics and causes of death designed for use by the medical and public health professions. Each volume is the result of a joint effort by the national health and statistical administrations of many countries, the United Nations, and WHO. United Nations estimates of vital rates and population size and composition, where available, are reprinted directly in the *Statistics Annual*. For those countries for which the United Nations does not prepare demographic estimates, primarily smaller populations, the latest available data reported to the United Nations and based on reasonably complete coverage of events are used.

Information published on late fetal and infant mortality is based entirely on official national data either reported directly or made available to WHO.

Selected life table functions are calculated from the application of a uniform methodology to national mortality data provided to WHO, in order to enhance their value for international comparisons. The life table procedure used by WHO may often lead to

discrepancies with national figures published by countries, due to differences in methodology or degree of age detail maintained in calculations.

The international comparability of estimates published in the *World Health Statistics Annual* is affected by the same problems discussed above for the *Demographic Yearbook*. Cross-national differences in statistical definitions of vital events, in the completeness and accuracy of vital statistics data, and in the comparability of population data are the primary factors affecting comparability.

For more information, see: World Health Organization, *World Health Statistics Annual 1995*, World Health Organization, Geneva, Switzerland, 1995; or visit the WHO home page at http://www.who.org.

Alan Guttmacher Institute

Abortion Survey

The Alan Guttmacher Institute (AGI) conducts an annual survey of abortion providers. Data are collected from hospitals, nonhospital clinics, and physicians identified as providers of abortion services. A universal survey of 3,092 hospitals, nonhospital clinics, and individual physicians was compiled. To assess the completeness of the provider and abortion counts, supplemental surveys were conducted of a sample of obstetrician-gynecologists and a sample of hospitals (not in original universe) that were identified as providing abortion services through the American Hospital Association Survey.

The number of abortions estimated by AGI through the mid to late 1980's was about 20 percent more than the number reported to the Centers for Disease Control and Prevention (CDC). Since 1989 the AGI estimates have been about 12 percent higher than those reported by CDC.

For more information, write: The Alan Guttmacher Institute, 120 Wall Street, New York, NY 10005; or visit AGI's home page at http://www.agi-usa.org.

American Association of Colleges of Osteopathic Medicine

The American Association of Colleges of Osteopathic Medicine compiles data on various aspects of osteopathic medical education for distribution to the profession, the government, and the public. Questionnaires are sent annually to all schools of osteopathic medicine requesting information on characteristics of applicants and students, curricula, faculty, grants, contracts, revenues, and expenditures. The response rate is 100 percent.

For more information, see: *Annual Statistical Report, 1996*, American Association of Colleges of Osteopathic Medicine: Rockville, Maryland. 1996; or visit the AACOM home page at http://www.aacom.org.

American Association of Colleges of Pharmacy

The American Association of Colleges of Pharmacy compiles data on the Colleges of Pharmacy, including information on student enrollment, and types of degrees conferred. Data are collected through an annual survey; the response rate is 100 percent.

For further information, see: Profile of Pharmacy Students. The American Association of Colleges of Pharmacy, 1426 Prince Street, Alexandria, VA 22314; or visit the AACP home page at http://www.aacp.org.

American Association of Colleges of Podiatric Medicine

The American Association of Podiatric Medicine compiles data on the Colleges of Podiatric Medicine, including information on the schools and enrollment. Data are collected annually through written questionnaires. The response rate is 100 percent.

For further information, write: The American Association of Colleges of Podiatric Medicine, 1350 Piccard Drive, Suite 322, Rockville, MD 20850–4307; or visit the AACPM home page at http://www.aacpm.org.

American Dental Association

The Division of Educational Measurement of the American Dental Association conducts annual surveys of predoctoral dental educational institutions. The questionnaire, mailed to all dental schools, collects information on student characteristics, financial management, and curricula.

For more information, see: American Dental Association, *1995/96 Survey of predoctoral dental educational institutions*. Chicago, Illinois, 1996; or visit the ADA home page at http://www.ada.org.

American Hospital Association

Annual Survey of Hospitals

Data from the American Hospital Association (AHA) annual survey are based on questionnaires that were sent to all hospitals, AHA-registered and nonregistered, in the United States and its associated areas. U.S. government hospitals located outside the United States were excluded. Questionnaires were mailed to all hospitals on AHA files. For nonreporting hospitals and for the survey questionnaires of reporting hospitals on which some information was missing, estimates were made for all data except those on beds, bassinets, and facilities. Data for beds and bassinets of nonreporting hospitals were based on the most recent information available from those hospitals. Facilities and services and inpatient service area data include only reporting hospitals and, therefore, do not include estimates.

Estimates of other types of missing data were based on data reported the previous year, if available. When unavailable, the estimates were based on data furnished by reporting hospitals similar in size, control, major service provided, length of stay, and geographic and demographic characteristics.

For more information on the AHA Annual Survey of Hospitals, see: American Hospital Association, (Healthcare InfoSource), *Hospital Statistics, 1998 ed.* Chicago. 1998; or visit an AHA page at http://www.aha.org.

American Medical Association

Physician Masterfile

A masterfile of physicians has been maintained by the American Medical Association (AMA) since 1906. The Physician Masterfile contains data on almost every physician in the United States, members and nonmembers of AMA, and on those graduates of American medical schools temporarily practicing overseas. The file also includes graduates of international medical schools who are in the United States and meet education standards for primary recognition as physicians.

A file is initiated on each individual upon entry into medical school or, in the case of international graduates, upon entry into the United States. Between 1969–85 a mail questionnaire survey was conducted every 4 years to update the file information on professional activities, self-designated area of specialization, and present employment status. Since 1985 approximately one-third of all physicians are surveyed each year.

For more information on the AMA Physician Masterfile, see: Division of Survey and Data Resources, American Medical Association, *Physician Characteristics and Distribution in the U.S.*, 1997/98 ed. Chicago. 1997; or visit the AMA home page at http://www.ama-assn.org.

Annual Census of Hospitals

From 1920 to 1953 the Council on Medical Education and Hospitals of the AMA conducted annual censuses of all hospitals registered by AMA.

In each annual census, questionnaires were sent to hospitals asking for the number of beds, bassinets, births, patients admitted, average census of patients, lists of staff doctors and interns, and other information of importance at the particular time. Response rates were always nearly 100 percent.

The community hospital data from 1940 and 1950 presented in this report were calculated using published figures from the AMA Annual Census of Hospitals. Although the hospital classification scheme used by AMA in published reports is not strictly comparable with the definition of community hospitals, methods were employed to achieve the greatest comparability possible.

For more information on the AMA Annual Census of Hospitals, see: American Medical Association, Hospital service in the United States, *Journal of the American Medical Association,* 116(11):1055–1144. 1941; or visit the AMA home page at http://www.ama-assn.org.

Association of American Medical Colleges

The Association of American Medical Colleges (AAMC) collects information on student enrollment in medical schools through the annual Liaison Committee on Medical Education questionnaire, the fall enrollment questionnaire, and the American Medical College Application Service (AMCAS) data system. Other data sources are the institutional profile system, the premedical students questionnaire, the minority student opportunities in medicine questionnaire, the faculty roster system, data from the Medical College Admission Test, and one-time surveys developed for special projects.

For more information, see: Association of American Medical Colleges: *Statistical Information Related to Medical Education*. Washington. 1997; or visit the AAMC home page at http://www.aamc.org.

Association of Schools and Colleges of Optometry

The Association of Schools and Colleges of Optometry compiles data on the various aspects of optometric education including data on schools and enrollment. Questionnaires are sent annually to all the schools and colleges of optometry. The response rate is 100 percent.

For further information, write: Annual Survey of Optometric Educational Institutions, Association of Schools and Colleges of Optometry, 6110 Executive Blvd., Suite 690, Rockville, MD 20852; or visit the ASCO home page at http://www.opted.org.

Sources of Data

InterStudy

National Health Maintenance Organization Census

From 1976 to 1980 the Office of Health Maintenance Organizations conducted a census of health maintenance organizations (HMO's). Since 1981 InterStudy has conducted the census. A questionnaire is sent to all HMO's in the United States asking for updated enrollment, profit status, and Federal qualification status. New HMO's are also asked to provide information on model type. When necessary, information is obtained, supplemented, or clarified by telephone. For nonresponding HMO's State-supplied information or the most current available data are used.

In 1985 a large increase in the number of HMO's and enrollment was partly attributable to a change in the categories of HMO's included in the census: Medicaid-only and Medicare-only HMO's have been added. Also component HMO's, which have their own discrete management, can be listed separately; whereas, previously the oldest HMO reported for all of its component or expansion sites, even when the components had different operational dates or were different model types.

For further information, see: *The InterStudy Competitive Edge,* 1995. InterStudy Publications, St. Paul, MN 55104; or visit the InterStudy home page at http://www.hmodata.com.

National League for Nursing

The division of research of the National League for Nursing (NLN) conducts The Annual Survey of Schools of Nursing in October of each year. Questionnaires are sent to all graduate nursing programs (master's and doctoral), baccalaureate programs designed exclusively for registered nurses, basic registered nursing programs (baccalaureate, associate degree, and diploma), and licensed practical nursing programs. Data on enrollments, first-time admissions, and graduates are complete for all nursing education programs. Response rates of approximately 80 percent are achieved for other areas of inquiry.

For more information, see: National League for Nursing, *Nursing Data Review*, 1996, New York, NY; or visit the NLN home page at http://www.nln.org.

The glossary is an alphabetical listing of terms used in *Health, United States*. It includes cross references to related terms and synonyms. It also contains the standard populations used for age adjustment and *International Classification of Diseases* (ICD) codes for cause of death and diagnostic and procedure categories.

Abortion—The Centers for Disease Control and Prevention's (CDC) surveillance program counts legal abortions only. For surveillance purposes, legal abortion is defined as a procedure performed by a licensed physician or someone acting under the supervision of a licensed physician to induce the termination of a pregnancy.

Acquired immunodeficiency syndrome (AIDS)—All 50 States and the District of Columbia report AIDS cases to CDC using a uniform case definition and case report form. The case reporting definitions were expanded in 1985 *(MMWR 1985; 34:373–5)*; 1987 *(MMWR 1987; 36 (supp. no. 1S): 1S-15S)*; and 1993 *(MMWR 1993; 41 (supp. no. RR-17))*. These data are published semiannually by CDC in HIV/AIDS Surveillance Report. See related *Human immunodeficiency virus (HIV) infection.*

Active physician—See *Physician.*

Addition—An addition to a psychiatric organization is defined by the Center for Mental Health Services as a new admission, a readmission, a return from long-term leave, or a transfer from another service of the same organization or another organization. See related *Mental health disorder; Mental health organization; Mental health service type.*

Admission—The American Hospital Association defines admissions as patients, excluding newborns, accepted for inpatient services during the survey reporting period. See related *Days of care; Discharge; Patient.*

Age—Age is reported as age at last birthday, that is, age in completed years, often calculated by subtracting date of birth from the reference date, with the reference date being the date of the examination, interview, or other contact with an individual.

Age adjustment—Age adjustment, using the direct method, is the application of age-specific rates in a population of interest to a standardized age distribution in order to eliminate differences in observed rates that result from age differences in population composition. This adjustment is usually done when comparing two or more populations at one point in time or one population at two or more points in time.

Age-adjusted death rates are calculated by the direct method as follows:

$$\sum_{i=1}^{n} r_i \times (p_i/P)$$

where r_i = age-specific death rates for the population of interest,

p_i = standard population in age group i,

$P = \sum_{i=1}^{n} p_i$ for the age groups that comprise the age range of the rate being age adjusted,

n = total number of age groups over the age range of the age-adjusted rate.

Mortality data—Death rates are age adjusted to the U.S. standard million population (relative age distribution of 1940 enumerated population of the United States totaling 1,000,000) (table I). Age-adjusted death rates are calculated using

Table I. Standard million age distribution used to adjust death rates to the U.S. population in 1940

Age	Standard million
All ages.	1,000,000
Under 1 year	15,343
1–4 years	64,718
5–14 years.	170,355
15–24 years.	181,677
25–34 years.	162,066
35–44 years.	139,237
45–54 years.	117,811
55–64 years.	80,294
65–74 years.	48,426
75–84 years.	17,303
85 years and over	2,770

age-specific death rates per 100,000 population rounded to 1 decimal place. Adjustment is based on 11 age groups with 2 exceptions. First, age-adjusted death rates for black males and black females in 1950 are based on nine age groups, with under 1 year and 1–4 years of age combined as one group and 75–84 years and 85 years of age and over combined as one group. Second, age-adjusted death rates by educational attainment for the age group 25–64 years are based on four 10-year age groups (25–34 years, 35–44 years, 45–54 years, and 55–64 years).

The rate for years of potential life lost (YPLL) before age 75 years is age adjusted to the U.S. standard million population (table I) and is based on eight age groups (under 1 year, 1–14 years, 15–24 years, and 10-year age groups through 65–74 years).

Maternal mortality rates for Complications of pregnancy, childbirth, and the puerperium are calculated as the number of deaths per 100,000 live births. These rates are age adjusted to the 1970 distribution of live births by mother's age in the United States as shown in table II. See related *Rate: Death and related rates; Years of potential life lost.*

National Health Interview Survey—Data from the National Health Interview Survey (NHIS) are age adjusted to the 1970 civilian noninstitutionalized population shown in table III. The 1970 civilian noninstitutionalized population is derived as follows: Civilian noninstitutionalized population = civilian population on July 1, 1970 – institutionalized population. Institutionalized population = (1 –

proportion of total population not institutionalized on April 1, 1970) × total population on July 1, 1970.

Most of the data from NHIS (except as noted below and in table III) are age adjusted using four age groups: under 15 years, 15–44 years, 45–64 years, and 65 years and over. The NHIS data on health care

Table III. Populations and age groups used to age adjust NCHS survey data

Population, survey, and age	Number in thousands
U.S. civilian noninstitutionalized population in 1970 NHIS, NHDS, NAMCS, and NHAMCS	
All ages.	199,584
Under 15 years	57,745
15–44 years	81,189
45–64 years	41,537
65 years and over	19,113
65–74 years.	12,224
75 years and over	6,889
NHIS smoking data	
18 years and over	130,158
25 years and over	107,694
18–24 years	22,464
25–34 years	24,430
35–44 years	22,614
45–64 years	41,537
65 years and over	19,113
NHIS health care coverage data	
All ages.	199,584
Under 18 years	69,426
18–44 years	69,508
45–64 years	41,537
65–74 years	12,224
75 years and over	6,889
U.S. resident population in 1980 NHES and NHANES	
6–11 years	20,834
6–8 years	9,777
9–11 years	11,057
12–17 years	23,410
12–14 years.	10,945
15–17 years	12,465
20–74 years	144,120
20–34 years	58,401
35–44 years	25,635
45–54 years	22,800
55–64 years	21,703
65–74 years.	15,581

SOURCE: Calculated from U.S. Bureau of Census: Estimates of the Population of the United States by Age, Sex, and Race: 1970 to 1977. Population Estimates and Projections. *Current Population Reports.* Series P–25, No. 721, Washington. U.S. Government Printing Office, April 1978.

Table II. Numbers of live births and mother's age groups used to adjust maternal mortality rates to live births in the United States in 1970

Mother's age	Number
All ages.	3,731,386
Under 20 years	656,460
20–24 years	1,418,874
25–29 years	994,904
30–34 years	427,806
35 years and over	233,342

SOURCE: U.S. Bureau of the Census: Population estimates and projections. *Current Population Reports.* Series P-25, No. 499. Washington. U.S. Government Printing Office, May 1973.

coverage are age adjusted for the population under 65 years of age using three age groups: under 15 years, 15–44 years, and 45–64 years; and for the population 65 years and over using two age groups: 65–74 years and 75 years and over. The NHIS data on smoking in the population 18 years and over are age adjusted using five age groups: 18–24 years, 25–34 years, 35–44 years, 45–64 years, and 65 years and over. The NHIS data on smoking in the population 25 years and over are age adjusted using four age groups: 25–34 years, 35–44 years, 45–64 years, and 65 years and over.

Health Care Surveys—Data from the three health care surveys, the National Hospital Discharge Survey (NHDS), National Ambulatory Medical Care Survey (NAMCS), and National Hospital Ambulatory Medical Care Survey (NHAMCS) are age adjusted to the 1970 civilian noninstitutionalized population using five age groups: under 15 years, 15–44 years, 45–64 years, 65–74 years, and 75 years and over (table III).

National Health and Nutrition Examination Survey— Data from the National Health Examination Survey (NHES) and the National Health and Nutrition Examination Survey (NHANES) are age adjusted to the 1980 U.S. resident population using five age groups for adults: 20–34 years, 35–44 years, 45–54 years, 55–64 years, and 65–74 years (table III). Data for children aged 6–11 years and 12–17 years are age adjusted within each group using two subgroups. 6–8 years and 9–11 years; and 12–14 years and 15–17 years (table III).

AIDS—See *Acquired immunodeficiency syndrome.*

Air quality standards—See *National ambient air quality standards.*

Air pollution—See *Pollutant.* Alcohol abuse treatment clients—See *Substance abuse treatment clients.*

Ambulatory care—Health care provided to persons without their admission to a health facility.

Average annual rate of change (percent change)—In this report average annual rates of change or growth rates are calculated as follows:

$$[(P_n /P_o)^{1/N} - 1] \times 100$$

where P_n = later time period
P_o = earlier time period
N = number of years in interval.

This geometric rate of change assumes that a variable increases or decreases at the same rate during each year between the two time periods.

Average length of stay—In the National Health Interview Survey, the average length of stay per discharged patient is computed by dividing the total number of hospital days for a specified group by the total number of discharges for that group. Similarly, in the National Hospital Discharge Survey, the average length of stay is computed by dividing the total number of days of care, counting the date of admission but not the date of discharge, by the number of patients discharged. The American Hospital Association computes the average length of stay by dividing the number of inpatient days by the number of admissions. See related *Days of care; Discharge; Patient.*

Bed—Any bed that is set up and staffed for use by inpatients is counted as a bed in a facility. In the National Master Facility Inventory, the count is of beds at the end of the reporting period; for the American Hospital Association, it is of the average number of beds, cribs, and pediatric bassinets during the entire reporting period. In the Health Care Financing Administration's Online Survey Certification and Reporting database, all beds in certified facilities are counted on the day of certification inspection. The World Health Organization defines a hospital bed as one regularly maintained and staffed for the accommodation and full-time care of a succession of inpatients and situated in a part of the hospital where continuous medical care for inpatients is provided. The Center for Mental Health Services counts the number of beds set up and staffed for use in inpatient and residential treatment services on the last day of the survey reporting period. See related *Hospital; Mental health organization; Mental health service type; Occupancy rate.*

Birth cohort—A birth cohort consists of all persons born within a given period of time, such as a calendar year.

Birth rate—See *Rate: Birth and related rates.*

Birthweight—The first weight of the newborn obtained after birth. Low birthweight is defined as less than 2,500 grams or 5 pounds 8 ounces. Very low birthweight is defined as less than 1,500 grams or 3 pounds 4 ounces. Before 1979 low birthweight was defined as 2,500 grams or less and very low birthweight as 1,500 grams or less.

Body mass index (BMI)—BMI is a measure that adjusts body weight for height. It is calculated as weight in kilograms divided by height in meters squared. Sex- and age-specific cut points of BMI are used in this book in the definition of overweight.

Cause of death—For the purpose of national mortality statistics, every death is attributed to one underlying condition, based on information reported on the death certificate and utilizing the international rules for selecting the underlying cause of death from the reported conditions. Beginning with 1979 the *International Classification of Diseases, Ninth Revision* (ICD-9) has been used for coding cause of death. Data from earlier time periods were coded using the appropriate revision of the ICD for that time period. (See tables IV and V.) Changes in classification of causes of death in successive revisions of the ICD may introduce discontinuities in cause-of-death statistics over time. For further discussion, see Technical Appendix in National Center for Health Statistics: *Vital Statistics of the United States, 1990, Volume II, Mortality, Part A.* DHHS Pub. No. (PHS) 95–1101, Public Health Service, Washington, U.S. Government Printing Office, 1994. See related *Human immunodeficiency virus infection; International Classification of Diseases, Ninth Revision.*

Table IV. Revision of the *International Classification of Diseases*, according to year of conference by which adopted and years in use in the United States

Revision of the International Classification of Diseases	Year of conference by which adopted	Years in use in United States
First.	1900	1900–1909
Second.	1909	1910–1920
Third	1920	1921–1929
Fourth	1929	1930–1938
Fifth.	1938	1939–1948
Sixth	1948	1949–1957
Seventh	1955	1958–1967
Eighth	1965	1968–1978
Ninth	1975	1979–present

Cause-of-death ranking—Cause-of-death ranking for infants is based on the List of 61 Selected Causes of Infant Death and HIV infection (ICD-9 Nos. *042–*044). Cause-of-death ranking for other ages is based on the List of 72 Selected Causes of Death, HIV infection, and Alzheimer's disease. The List of 72 Selected Causes of Death was adapted from one of the special lists for mortality tabulations recommended by the World Health Organization for use with the *Ninth Revision of the International Classification of Diseases.* Two group titles—Certain conditions originating in the perinatal period and Symptoms, signs, and ill-defined conditions—are not ranked from the List of 61 Selected Causes of Infant Death; and two group titles—Major cardiovascular diseases and Symptoms, signs, and ill-defined conditions—are not ranked from the List of 72 Selected Causes. In addition, category titles that begin with the words "Other" and "All other" are not ranked. The remaining category titles are ranked according to number of deaths to determine the leading causes of death. When one of the titles that represent a subtotal is ranked (for example, unintentional injuries), its component parts are not ranked (in this case, motor vehicle crashes and all other unintentional injuries). See related *International Classification of Diseases, Ninth Revision.*

Civilian noninstitutionalized population; Civilian population—See *Population.*

Table V. Cause-of-death codes, according to applicable revision of *International Classification of Diseases*

Cause of death	Code numbers			
	Sixth Revision	Seventh Revision	Eighth Revision	Ninth Revision
Communicable diseases.................	. . .	. . .	. . .	001–139, 460–466, 480–487
Chronic and other non-communicable diseases.........................	. . .	. . .	. . .	140–459, 467–479, 488–799
Injury and adverse effects.............	. . .	. . .	. . .	E800–E999
Meningococcal infection..............	. . .	. . .	. . .	036
Septicemia........................	. . .	. . .	. . .	038
Human immunodeficiency virus infection[1] . . .	. . .	. . .	. . .	*042–*044
Malignant neoplasms.................	140–205	140–205	140–209	140–208
Colorectal	153–154	153–154	153–154	153, 154
Malignant neoplasm of peritoneum and pleura.........................	. . .	. . .	158, 163.0	158, 163
Respiratory system	160–164	160–164	160–163	160–165
Malignant neoplasm of trachea, bronchus and lung	. . .	. . .	. . .	162
Breast	170	170	174	174–175
Prostate	177	177	185	185
Benign neoplasms	. . .	. . .	. . .	210–239
Diabetes mellitus	260	260	250	250
Anemias	. . .	. . .	. . .	280–285
Meningitis........................	. . .	. . .	. . .	320–322
Alzheimer's disease	. . .	. . .	. . .	331.0
Diseases of heart	410–443	400–402, 410–443	390–398, 402, 404, 410–429	390–398, 402, 404–429
Ischemic heart disease	. . .	. . .	. . .	410–414
Cerebrovascular diseases.............	330–334	330–334	430–438	430–438
Atherosclerosis	. . .	. . .	. . .	440
Pneumonia and influenza	480–483, 490–493	480–483, 490–493	470–474, 480–486	480–487
Chronic obstructive pulmonary diseases	241, 501, 502, 527.1	241, 501, 502, 527.1	490–493, 519.3	490–496
Coalworkers' pneumoconiosis	. . .	. . .	515.1	500
Asbestosis	. . .	. . .	515.2	501
Silicosis	. . .	. . .	515.0	502
Chronic liver disease and cirrhosis	581	581	571	571
Nephritis, nephrotic syndrome, and nephrosis........................	. . .	. . .	. . .	580–589
Complications of pregnancy, childbirth, and the puerperium....................	640–689	640–689	630–678	630–676
Congenital anomalies	. . .	. . .	. . .	740–759
Certain conditions originating in the perinatal period	. . .	. . .	. . .	760–779
Newborn affected by maternal complications of pregnancy	. . .	. . .	. . .	761
Newborn affected by complications of placenta, cord, and membranes........	. . .	. . .	. . .	762
Disorders relating to short gestation and unspecified low birthweight...........	. . .	. . .	. . .	765
Birth trauma....................	. . .	. . .	. . .	767
Intrauterine hypoxia and birth asphyxia ...	. . .	. . .	. . .	768
Respiratory distress syndrome	. . .	. . .	. . .	769
Infections specific to the perinatal period ..	. . .	. . .	. . .	771
Sudden infant death syndrome..........	. . .	. . .	. . .	798.0
Unintentional injuries[2]	E800–E962	E800–E962	E800–E949	E800–E949
Motor vehicle-related injuries[2]	E810–E835	E810–E835	E810–E823	E810–E825
Suicide	E963, E970–E979	E963, E970–E979	E950–E959	E950–E959
Homicide and legal intervention	E964, E980–E985	E964, E980–E985	E960–E978	E960–E978
Firearm-related injuries	. . .	. . .	E922, E955, E965, E970, E985	E922, E955.0–E955.4, E965.0–E965.4, E970, E985.0–E985.4

. . . Category not applicable.

[1]Categories for coding human immunodeficiency virus infection were introduced in 1987. The * indicates codes are not part of the Ninth Revision.

[2]In the public health community, the term "unintentional injuries" is preferred to "accidents and adverse effects" and "motor vehicle-related injuries" to "motor vehicle accidents."

Cocaine-related emergency room episodes—The Drug Abuse Warning Network monitors selected adverse medical consequences of cocaine and other drug abuse episodes by measuring contacts with hospital emergency rooms. Contacts may be for drug overdose, unexpected drug reactions, chronic abuse, detoxification, or other reasons in which drug use is known to have occurred.

Cohort fertility—Cohort fertility refers to the fertility of the same women at successive ages. Women born during a 12-month period comprise a birth cohort. Cohort fertility for birth cohorts of women is measured by central birth rates, which represent the number of births occurring to women of an exact age divided by the number of women of that exact age. Cumulative birth rates by a given exact age represent the total childbearing experience of women in a cohort up to that age. Cumulative birth rates are sums of central birth rates for specified cohorts and show the number of children ever born up to the indicated age. For example, the cumulative birth rate for women exactly 30 years of age as of January 1, 1960, is the sum of the central birth rates for the 1930 birth cohort for the years 1944 (when its members were age 14) through 1959 (when they were age 29). Cumulative birth rates are also calculated for specific birth orders at each exact age of woman. The percent of women who have not had at least one live birth by a certain age is found by subtracting the cumulative first birth rate for women of that age from 1,000 and dividing by 10. For method of calculation, see Heuser RL. *Fertility tables for birth cohorts by color: United States, 1917–73.* Rockville, Maryland. NCHS. 1976. See related *Rate: Birth and related rates.*

Community hospitals—See *Hospital.*

Compensation—See *Employer costs for employee compensation.*

Completed fertility rate—See *Rate: Birth and related rates.*

Condition—A health condition is a departure from a state of physical or mental well-being. An impairment is a health condition that includes chronic or permanent health defects resulting from disease, injury, or congenital malformations. All health conditions, except impairments, are coded according to the *International Classification of Diseases, Ninth Revision, Clinical Modification (ICD-9-CM).*

Based on duration, there are two categories of conditions, acute and chronic. In the National Health Interview Survey, an *acute condition* is a condition that has lasted less than 3 months and has involved either a physician visit (medical attention) or restricted activity. A *chronic condition* refers to any condition lasting 3 months or more or is a condition classified as chronic regardless of its time of onset (for example, diabetes, heart conditions, emphysema, and arthritis). The National Nursing Home Survey uses a specific list of chronic conditions, also disregarding time of onset. See related *International Classification of Diseases, Ninth Revision, Clinical Modification.*

Consumer Price Index (CPI)—CPI is prepared by the U.S. Bureau of Labor Statistics. It is a monthly measure of the average change in the prices paid by urban consumers for a fixed market basket of goods and services. The medical care component of CPI shows trends in medical care prices based on specific indicators of hospital, medical, dental, and drug prices. A revision of the definition of CPI has been in use since January 1988. See related *Gross domestic product; Health expenditures, national.*

Crude birth rate; Crude death rate—See *Rate: Birth and related rates; Rate: Death and related rates.*

Current smoker—In 1992 the definition of current smoker in the National Health Interview Survey (NHIS) was modified to specifically include persons who smoked on "some days." Before 1992 a current smoker was defined by the following questions from the NHIS survey "Have you ever smoked 100 cigarettes in your lifetime?" and "Do you smoke now?" (traditional definition). In 1992 data were collected for half the respondents using the traditional smoking questions and for the other half of respondents using a revised smoking question ("Do you smoke every day, some days, or not at all?"). An unpublished analysis of the 1992 traditional smoking measure revealed that the crude percent of current smokers 18 years of age and over remained the same as 1991. The statistics for 1992 combine data collected using the traditional and the revised questions. For further information on survey methodology and sample sizes pertaining to the NHIS cigarette data for data years 1965 to 1992 and other sources of cigarette smoking data available from the National Center for Health Statistics, see: National Center for Health Statistics, *Biographies and Data Sources, Smoking Data Guide,* No. 1, DHHS Pub. No. (PHS) 91-1308-1, Public Health Service. Washington. U.S. Government Printing Office, 1991.

Starting with 1993 data estimates of cigarette smoking prevalence are based on the revised definition that is considered a more complete estimate of smoking prevalence. In 1993–95 estimates of cigarette smoking prevalence were based on a half-sample.

Days of care—According to the American Hospital Association and National Master Facility Inventory, days, hospital days, or inpatient days are the number of adult and pediatric days of care rendered during the entire reporting period. Days of care for newborns are excluded.

In the National Health Interview Survey, hospital days during the year refer to the total number of hospital days occurring in the 12-month period before the interview week. A hospital day is a night spent in the hospital for persons admitted as inpatients.

In the National Hospital Discharge Survey, days of care refers to the total number of patient days accumulated by patients at the time of discharge from non-Federal short-stay hospitals during a reporting period. All days from and including the date of admission but not including the date of discharge are counted. See related *Admission; Average length of stay; Discharge; Hospital; Patient.*

Death rate—See *Rate: Death and related rates.*

Dental visit—The National Health Interview Survey considers dental visits to be visits to a dentist's office for treatment or advice, including services by a technician or hygienist acting under the dentist's supervision. Services provided to hospital inpatients are not included. Dental visits are based on a 12-month recall period.

Diagnosis—See *First-listed diagnosis.*

Diagnostic and other nonsurgical procedures—See *Procedure.*

Discharge—The National Health Interview Survey defines a hospital discharge as the completion of any continuous period of stay of 1 night or more in a hospital as an inpatient, not including the period of stay of a well newborn infant. According to the National Hospital Discharge Survey, American Hospital Association, and National Master Facility Inventory, discharge is the formal release of an inpatient by a hospital (excluding newborn infants), that is, the termination of a period of hospitalization (including stays of 0 nights) by death or by disposition to a place of residence, nursing home, or another hospital. See related *Admission; Average length of stay; Days of care; Patient.*

Domiciliary care homes—See *Nursing home.*

Drug abuse treatment clients—See *Substance abuse treatment clients.*

Emergency department—According to the National Hospital Ambulatory Medical Care Survey (NHAMCS), an emergency department is a hospital facility for the provision of unscheduled outpatient services to patients whose conditions require immediate care and is staffed 24 hours a day. Off-site emergency departments open less than 24 hours are included if staffed by the hospital's emergency department. An emergency department visit is a direct personal exchange between a patient and a physician or other health care providers working under the physician's supervision, for the purpose of seeking care and receiving personal health services. See related *Hospital; Outpatient department.*

Employer costs for employee compensation—A measure of the average cost per employee hour worked to employers for wages and salaries and benefits. Wages and salaries are defined as the hourly straight-time wage rate, or for workers not paid on an hourly basis, straight-time earnings divided by the corresponding hours. Straight-time wage and salary rates are total earnings before payroll deductions, excluding premium pay for overtime and for work on weekends and holidays, shift differentials, nonproduction bonuses, and lump-sum payments provided in lieu of wage increases. Production bonuses, incentive earnings, commission payments, and cost-of-living adjustments are included in straight-time wage and salary rates. Benefits covered are paid leave—paid vacations, holidays, sick leave, and other leave; supplemental pay—premium pay for overtime and work on weekends and holidays, shift differentials, nonproduction bonuses, and lump-sum payments provided in lieu of wage increases; insurance benefits—life, health, and sickness and accident insurance; retirement and savings benefits—pension and other retirement plans and savings and thrift plans; legally required benefits—social security, railroad retirement and supplemental retirement, railroad unemployment insurance, Federal and State unemployment insurance, workers' compensation, and other benefits required by law, such as State temporary disability insurance; and other benefits—severance pay and supplemental unemployment plans.

Expenditures—See *Health expenditures, national.*

Family income—For purposes of the National Health Interview Survey and National Health and Nutrition Examination Survey, all people within a household related to each other by blood, marriage, or adoption constitute a family. Each member of a family is classified according to the total income of the family. Unrelated individuals are classified according to their own income. Family income is the total income received by the members of a family (or by an unrelated individual) in the 12 months before the interview. Family income includes wages, salaries, rents from property, interest, dividends, profits and fees from their own businesses, pensions, and help from relatives. Family income has generally been categorized into approximate quintiles in the tables.

Federal hospitals—See *Hospital.*

Federal physicians—See *Physician.*

Fertility rate—See *Rate: Birth and related rates.*

Fetal death—In the World Health Organization's definition, also adopted by the United Nations and the National Center for Health Statistics, a fetal death is death before the complete expulsion or extraction from its mother of a product of conception, irrespective of the duration of pregnancy; the death is indicated by the fact that after such separation, the fetus does not breathe or show any other evidence of life, such as beating of the heart, pulsation of the umbilical cord, or definite movement of voluntary muscles. For statistical purposes, fetal deaths are classified according to gestational age. In this report tabulations are shown for fetal deaths with stated or presumed gestation of 20 weeks or more and of 28 weeks or more, the latter gestational age group also known as late fetal deaths. See related *Gestation; Live birth; Rate: Death and related rates.*

First-listed diagnosis—In the National Hospital Discharge Survey this is the first recorded final diagnosis on the medical record face sheet (summary sheet).

General hospitals—See *Hospital.*

General hospitals providing separate psychiatric services—See *Mental health organization.*

Geographic region and division—The 50 States and the District of Columbia are grouped for statistical purposes by the U.S. Bureau of the Census into 4 geographic regions and 9 divisions. The groupings are as follows:

- Northeast
  - New England
    - Maine, New Hampshire, Vermont, Massachusetts, Rhode Island, Connecticut
  - Middle Atlantic
    - New York, New Jersey, Pennsylvania
- Midwest
  - East North Central
    - Ohio, Indiana, Illinois, Michigan, Wisconsin
  - West North Central
    - Minnesota, Iowa, Missouri, North Dakota, South Dakota, Nebraska, Kansas
- South
  - South Atlantic
    - Delaware, Maryland, District of Columbia, Virginia, West Virginia, North Carolina, South Carolina, Georgia, Florida
  - East South Central
    - Kentucky, Tennessee, Alabama, Mississippi
  - West South Central
    - Arkansas, Louisiana, Oklahoma, Texas
- West
  - Mountain
    - Montana, Idaho, Wyoming, Colorado, New Mexico, Arizona, Utah, Nevada
  - Pacific
    - Washington, Oregon, California, Alaska, Hawaii

Gestation—For the National Vital Statistics System and the Centers for Disease Control and Prevention's Abortion Surveillance, the period of gestation is defined as beginning with the first day of the last normal menstrual period and ending with the day of birth or day of termination of pregnancy. See related *Abortion; Fetal death; Live birth.*

Gross domestic product (GDP)—GDP is the market value of the goods and services produced by labor and property located in the United States. As long as the labor and property are located in the

United States, the suppliers (that is, the workers and, for property, the owners) may be either U.S. residents or residents of the rest of the world. See related *Consumer Price Index; Health expenditures, national.*

Health expenditures, national—See related *Consumer Price Index; Gross domestic product.*

Health services and supplies expenditures—These are outlays for goods and services relating directly to patient care plus expenses for administering health insurance programs and government public health activities. This category is equivalent to total national health expenditures minus expenditures for research and construction.

National health expenditures—This measure estimates the amount spent for all health services and supplies and health-related research and construction activities consumed in the United States during the calendar year. Detailed estimates are available by source of expenditures (for example, out-of-pocket payments, private health insurance, and government programs), type of expenditures (for example, hospital care, physician services, and drugs), and are in current dollars for the year of report. Data are compiled from a variety of sources.

Nursing home expenditures—These cover care rendered in skilled nursing and intermediate care facilities, including those for the mentally retarded. The costs of long-term care provided by hospitals are excluded.

Personal health care expenditures—These are outlays for goods and services relating directly to patient care. The expenditures in this category are total national health expenditures minus expenditures for research and construction, expenses for administering health insurance programs, and government public health activities.

Private expenditures—These are outlays for services provided or paid for by nongovernmental sources—consumers, insurance companies, private industry, philanthropic, and other nonpatient care sources.

Public expenditures—These are outlays for services provided or paid for by Federal, State, and local government agencies or expenditures required by governmental mandate (such as, workmen's compensation insurance payments).

Health insurance coverage—National Health Interview Survey (NHIS) respondents are asked about their health insurance coverage at the time of the interview in 1984 and 1989 and in the previous month in 1993 to 1996. They are covered by private health insurance if they indicate private health insurance or they are covered by a single service hospital plan. Private health insurance includes managed care such as health maintenance organizations (HMO's). Persons are covered by Medicaid or other public assistance if they indicate they have either Medicaid or other public assistance, or if they are receiving Aid to Families with Dependent Children (AFDC) or Supplementary Security Income (SSI). Medicare or military health plan coverage is also determined in the interview. If respondents do not indicate coverage under one of the above types of plans and they have unknown coverage on either private health insurance or Medicaid then they are considered to have unknown coverage. The remaining respondents are considered uninsured. See related *Health maintenance organization; Managed care; Medicaid; Medicare.*

Health maintenance organization (HMO)—An HMO is a prepaid health plan delivering comprehensive care to members through designated providers, having a fixed monthly payment for health care services, and requiring members to be in a plan for a specified period of time (usually 1 year). Pure HMO enrollees use only the prepaid capitated health services of the HMO's panel of medical care providers. Open-ended HMO enrollees use the prepaid HMO health services but in addition may receive medical care from providers who are not part of the HMO's panel. There is usually a substantial deductible, copayment, or coinsurance associated with

the use of nonpanel providers. These open-ended products are governed by State HMO regulations. HMO model types are:

Group—An HMO that delivers health services through a physician group that is controlled by the HMO unit or an HMO that contracts with one or more independent group practices to provide health services.

Individual practice association (IPA)—An HMO that contracts directly with physicians in independent practice, and/or contracts with one or more associations of physicians in independent practice, and/or contracts with one or more multispecialty group practices. The plan is predominantly organized around solo-single-specialty practices.

Mixed—An HMO that combines features of group and IPA. This category was introduced in mid-1990 because HMO's are continually changing and many now combine features of group and IPA plans in a single plan.

See related *Managed care.*

Health services and supplies expenditures—See *Health expenditures, national.*

Health status, respondent-assessed—Health status was measured in the National Health Interview Survey by asking the respondent, "Would you say _____'s health is excellent, very good, good, fair, or poor?"

Hispanic origin—Hispanic origin includes persons of Mexican, Puerto Rican, Cuban, Central and South American, and other or unknown Spanish origins. Persons of Hispanic origin may be of any race. See related *Race.*

HIV—See *Human immunodeficiency virus infection.*

Home health care—Home health care as defined by the National Home and Hospice Care Survey is care provided to individuals and families in their place of residence for promoting, maintaining, or restoring health; or for minimizing the effects of disability and illness including terminal illness.

Hospice care—Hospice care as defined by the National Home and Hospice Care Survey is a program of palliative and supportive care services providing physical, psychological, social, and spiritual care for dying persons, their families, and other loved ones. Hospice services are available in home and inpatient settings.

Hospital—According to the American Hospital Association and National Master Facility Inventory, hospitals are licensed institutions with at least six beds whose primary function is to provide diagnostic and therapeutic patient services for medical conditions by an organized physician staff, and have continuous nursing services under the supervision of registered nurses. The World Health Organization considers an establishment to be a hospital if it is permanently staffed by at least one physician, can offer inpatient accommodation, and can provide active medical and nursing care. Hospitals may be classified by type of service, ownership, size in terms of number of beds, and length of stay. In the National Hospital Ambulatory Medical Care Survey (NHAMCS) hospitals include all those with an average length of stay for all patients of less than 30 days (short-stay) or hospitals whose specialty is general (medical or surgical) or children's general. Federal hospitals and hospital units of institutions and hospitals with fewer than six beds staffed for patient use are excluded. See related *Average length of stay; Bed; Days of care; Emergency department; Outpatient department; Patient.*

Community hospitals traditionally included all non-Federal short-stay hospitals except facilities for the mentally retarded. In the revised definition the following additional sites are excluded: hospital units of institutions, and alcoholism and chemical dependency facilities.

Federal hospitals are operated by the Federal Government.

General hospitals provide diagnostic, treatment, and surgical services for patients with a variety of medical conditions. According to the World Health Organization, these hospitals provide medical and nursing care for more than one category of medical discipline (for example, general medicine, specialized medicine, general surgery, specialized surgery, and obstetrics). Excluded are hospitals, usually in rural areas, that provide a more limited range of care.

Nonprofit hospitals are operated by a church or other nonprofit organization.

Proprietary hospitals are operated for profit by individuals, partnerships, or corporations.

Psychiatric hospitals are ones whose major type of service is psychiatric care. See *Mental health organization.*

Registered hospitals are hospitals registered with the American Hospital Association. About 98 percent of hospitals are registered.

Short-stay hospitals in the National Hospital Discharge Survey are those in which the average length of stay is less than 30 days. The National Health Interview Survey defines short-stay hospitals as any hospital or hospital department in which the type of service provided is general; maternity; eye, ear, nose, and throat; children's; or osteopathic.

Specialty hospitals, such as psychiatric, tuberculosis, chronic disease, rehabilitation, maternity, and alcoholic or narcotic, provide a particular type of service to the majority of their patients.

Hospital-based physician—See *Physician.*

Hospital days—See *Days of care.*

Human immunodeficiency virus (HIV) infection—Mortality coding: Beginning with data for 1987, NCHS introduced category numbers *042–*044 for classifying and coding HIV infection as a cause of death. HIV infection was formerly referred to as human T-cell lymphotropic virus-III/lymphadenopathy-associated virus (HTLV-III/LAV) infection. The asterisk before the category numbers indicates that these codes are not part of the *Ninth Revision of the International Classification of Diseases* (ICD-9). Before 1987 deaths involving HIV infection were classified to Deficiency of cell-mediated immunity (ICD-9 No. 279.1) contained in the title All other diseases; to Pneumocystosis (ICD-9 No. 136.3) contained in the title All other infectious and parasitic diseases; to Malignant neoplasms, including neoplasms of lymphatic and hematopoietic tissues; and to a number of other causes. Therefore, beginning with 1987, death statistics for HIV infection are not strictly comparable with data for earlier years.

Morbidity coding: The National Hospital Discharge Survey codes diagnosis data using the *International Classification of Diseases, Ninth Revision, Clinical Modification* (ICD-9-CM). Discharges with diagnosis of HIV as shown in *Health, United States,* have at least one HIV diagnosis listed on the face sheet of the medical record and are not limited to the first-listed diagnosis. During 1984 and 1985 only data for AIDS (ICD-9-CM 279.19) were included. In 1986–94, discharges with the following diagnoses were included: acquired immunodeficiency syndrome (AIDS), human immunodeficiency virus (HIV) infection and associated conditions, and positive serological or viral culture findings for HIV (ICD–9–CM 042–044, 279.19, and 795.8). Beginning in 1995 discharges with the following diagnoses were included: human immunodeficiency virus (HIV) disease and asymptomatic human immunodeficiency virus (HIV) infection status (ICD–9–CM 042 and V08). See related *Acquired immunodeficiency syndrome; Cause of death; International Classification of Diseases, Ninth Revision; International Classification of Diseases, Ninth Revision, Clinical Modification.*

ICD; ICD codes—See *Cause of death; International Classification of Diseases, Ninth Revision.*

Incidence—Incidence is the number of cases of disease having their onset during a prescribed period of time. It is often expressed as a rate (for example, the incidence of measles per 1,000 children 5–15 years of age during a specified year). Incidence is a measure of morbidity or other events that occur within a specified period of time. See related *Prevalence.*

Individual practice association (IPA)—See *Health maintenance organization (HMO).*

Industry of employment—Industries are classified according to the *Standard Industrial Classification (SIC) Manual* of the Office of Management and Budget. Three editions of the SIC are used for coding industry data in *Health, United States*: the 1972 edition; the 1977 supplement to the 1972 edition; and the 1987 edition.

The changes between versions include a few detailed titles created to correct or clarify industries or

Table VI. Codes for Industries, according to the *Standard Industrial Classification (SIC) Manual*

Industry	Code numbers
Agriculture, forestry, and fishing	01–09
Mining	10–14
Construction	15–17
Manufacturing	20–39
Textile mill products	22
Apparel and other finished products made from fabrics and similar materials	23
Lumber and wood products, except furniture	24
Printing, publishing, and allied industries	27
Chemicals and allied products	28
Rubber and miscellaneous plastics products	30
Stone, clay, glass, and concrete products	32
Primary metal industries	33
Fabricated metal products, except machinery and transportation equipment	34
Industrial and commercial machinery and computer equipment	35
Electronic and other electrical equipment and components, except computer equipment	36
Transportation equipment	37
Measuring, analyzing, and controlling instruments; photographic, medical, and optical goods; watches and clocks	38
Miscellaneous manufacturing industries	39
Transportation, communication, and public utilities	40–49
Wholesale trade	50–51
Retail trade	52–59
Finance, insurance, and real estate	60–67
Services	70–89
Public administration	91–97

Table VII. Codes for diagnostic categories from the *International Classification of Diseases, Ninth Revision, Clinical Modification*

Diagnostic category	Code numbers
Females with delivery	V27
Human immunodeficiency virus (HIV) (1984–85)	279.19
(1986–94)	042–044, 279.19, 795.8
(Beginning in 1995)	042, V08
Malignant neoplasms	140–208
Large intestine and rectum	153–154, 197.5
Trachea, bronchus, and lung	162, 197.0, 197.3
Breast	174–175, 198.81
Prostate	185
Diabetes	250
Psychoses	293–299
Diseases of the nervous system and sense organs	320–389
Diseases of the circulatory system	390–459
Diseases of heart	391–392.0, 393–398, 402, 404, 410–416, 420–429
Ischemic heart disease	410–414
Acute myocardial infarction	410
Congestive heart failure	428.0
Cerebrovascular diseases	430–438
Diseases of the respiratory system	460–519
Bronchitis	466.0, 490–491
Pneumonia	466.1, 480–487.0
Asthma	493
Hyperplasia of prostate	600
Decubitus ulcers	707.0
Diseases of the musculoskeletal system and connective tissue	710–739
Osteoarthritis	715
Intervertebral disc disorders	722
Injuries and poisoning	800–999
Fracture, all sites	800–829
Fracture of neck of femur (hip)	820

to recognize changes within the industry. Codes for major industrial divisions (table VI) were not changed between versions.

The category "Private sector" includes all industrial divisions except public administration and military. The category "Civilian sector" includes "Private sector" and the public administration division. The category "Not classified" is comprised of the following entries from the death certificate: housewife, student, or self-employed; information inadequate to code industry; establishments not elsewhere classified.

Infant death—An infant death is the death of a live-born child before his or her first birthday. Deaths in the first year of life may be further classified according to age as neonatal and postneonatal. Neonatal deaths are those that occur before the 28th day of life; postneonatal deaths are those that occur between 28 and 365 days of age. See *Live birth; Rate: Death and related rates.*

Inpatient care—See *Mental health service type.*

Inpatient days—See *Days of care.*

Insured—See *Health insurance coverage.*

Intermediate care facilities—See *Nursing home.*

International Classification of Diseases, Ninth Revision (ICD-9)—The *International Classification of Diseases* (ICD) classifies mortality information for statistical purposes. The ICD was first used in 1900 and has been revised about every 10 years since then. The ICD-9, published in 1977, is used to code U.S. mortality data beginning with data year 1979. (See tables IV and V.) See related *Cause of death; International Classification of Diseases, Ninth Revision, Clinical Modification.*

International Classification of Diseases, Ninth Revision, Clinical Modification (ICD-9-CM)—The ICD-9-CM is based on and is completely compatible with the *International Classification of Diseases, Ninth*

Table VIII. Codes for surgical categories from the *International Classification of Diseases, Ninth Revision, Clinical Modification*

Surgical category	Code numbers
Myringotomy	20.0
Tonsillectomy, with or without adenoidectomy	28.2–28.3
Coronary angioplasty	36.0
Direct heart revascularization (coronary bypass)	36.1
Cardiac catheterization	37.21–37.23
Pacemaker insertion or replacement	37.7–37.8
Carotid endarterectomy	38.12
Appendectomy, excluding incidental	47.0
Cholecystectomy	51.2
Prostatectomy	60.2–60.6
Bilateral destruction or occlusion of fallopian tubes	66.2–66.3
Hysterectomy	68.3–68.7, 68.9
Procedures to assist delivery	72, 73.0–73.3, 73.6–73.8, 73.93–73.99
Cesarean section	74.0–74.2, 74.4, 74.99
Repair of current obstetrical laceration	75.5–75.6
Reduction of fracture (excluding skull and facial)	79.0–79.5
Excision or destruction of intervertebral disc and spinal fusion	80.5, 81.0
Excision of semilunar cartilage of knee	80.6
Arthroplasty and replacement of hip[1] (Prior to 1989)	81.5–81.6
(Beginning in 1990)	81.40, 81.51–81.53
Mastectomy	85.4

[1]The ICD-9-CM codes for arthroplasty and replacement of the hip were substantially revised in October 1989. Arthroplasty data for 1989 are omitted.

Revision. The ICD-9-CM is used to code morbidity data and the ICD-9 is used to code mortality data. Diagnostic groupings and code number inclusions for ICD-9-CM are shown in table VII; surgical groupings and code number inclusions are shown in table VIII; and diagnostic and other nonsurgical procedure groupings and code number inclusions are shown in table IX.

ICD-9 and ICD-9-CM are arranged in 17 main chapters. Most of the diseases are arranged according to their principal anatomical site, with special chapters for infective and parasitic diseases; neoplasms; endocrine, metabolic, and nutritional diseases; mental diseases; complications of pregnancy and childbirth;

certain diseases peculiar to the perinatal period; and ill-defined conditions. In addition, two supplemental classifications are provided: the classification of factors influencing health status and contact with health service and the classification of external causes of injury and poisoning. See related *Condition; International Classification of Diseases, Ninth Revision; Mental health disorder.*

Late fetal death rate—See *Rate: Death and related rates.*

Leading causes of death—See *Cause-of-death ranking.*

Table IX. Codes for diagnostic and other nonsurgical procedure categories from the *International Classification of Diseases, Ninth Revision, Clinical Modification*

Procedure category	Code numbers
Spinal tap	03.31
Endoscopy of large or small intestine without biopsy	45.11–45.13, 45.21–45.24
Cystoscopy	57.31–57.32
Computerized axial tomography (CAT scan)	87.03, 87.41, 87.71, 88.01, 88.38
Arteriography using contrast material	88.4
Angiocardiography using contrast material	88.5
Diagnostic ultrasound	88.7
Magnetic resonance imaging (MRI) (in 1985)	88.99, 89.15, 89.29, 89.39
(Beginning in 1990)	88.91–88.97
Radioisotope scan	92.0–92.1

Length of stay—See *Average length of stay*.

Life expectancy—Life expectancy is the average number of years of life remaining to a person at a particular age and is based on a given set of age-specific death rates, generally the mortality conditions existing in the period mentioned. Life expectancy may be determined by race, sex, or other characteristics using age-specific death rates for the population with that characteristic. See related *Rate: Death and related rates*.

Limitation of activity—In the National Health Interview Survey limitation of activity refers to a long-term reduction in a person's capacity to perform the usual kind or amount of activities associated with his or her age group. Each person is classified according to the extent to which his or her activities are limited, as follows:

■ Persons unable to carry on major activity;

■ Persons limited in the amount or kind of major activity performed;

■ Persons not limited in major activity but otherwise limited; and

■ Persons not limited in activity.

See related *Condition; Major activity*.

Live birth—In the World Health Organization's definition, also adopted by the United Nations and the National Center for Health Statistics, a live birth is the complete expulsion or extraction from its mother of a product of conception, irrespective of the duration of the pregnancy, which, after such separation, breathes or shows any other evidence of life such as heartbeat, umbilical cord pulsation, or definite movement of voluntary muscles, whether the umbilical cord has been cut or the placenta is attached. Each product of such a birth is considered live born. See related *Gestation; Rate: Birth and related rates*.

Live-birth order—In the National Vital Statistics System this item from the birth certificate refers to the total number of live births the mother has had, including the present birth as recorded on the birth certificate. Fetal deaths are excluded. See related *Live birth*.

Low birthweight—See *Birthweight*.

Major activity (or usual activity)—This is the principal activity of a person or of his or her age-sex group. For children 1–5 years of age, the major activity refers to ordinary play with other children; for children 5–17 years of age, the major activity refers to school attendance; for adults 18–69 years of age, the major activity usually refers to a job, housework, or school attendance; for persons 70 years of age and over, the major activity refers to the capacity for independent living (bathe, shop, dress, or eat without needing the help of another person). See related *Limitation of activity*.

Managed care—Managed care is a health care plan that integrates the financing and delivery of health care services by using arrangements with selected health care providers to provide services for covered individuals. Plans are generally financed using capitation fees. There are signifcant financial incentives for members of the plan to use the health care providers associated with the plan. The plan includes formal programs for quality assurance and utilization review. Health maintenance organizations (HMO's), preferred provider organizations (PPO's), and point of service (POS) plans are examples of managed care. See related *Health maintenance organization; Preferred provider organization*.

Marital status—Marital status is classified through self-reporting into the categories married and unmarried. The term married encompasses all married people including those separated from their spouses. Unmarried includes those who are single (never married), divorced, or widowed. The Abortion Surveillance Reports of the Centers for Disease Control and Prevention classified separated people as unmarried before 1978.

Maternal mortality rate—See *Rate: Death and related rates*.

Glossary

Medicaid—This program is State operated and administered but has Federal financial participation. Within certain broad federally determined guidelines, States decide who is eligible; the amount, duration, and scope of services covered; rates of payment for providers; and methods of administering the program. Medicaid provides health care services for certain low-income persons. Medicaid does not provide health services to all poor people in every State. It categorically covers participants in the Aid to Families with Dependent Children program and in the Supplemental Security Income program. In most States it also covers certain other people deemed to be medically needy. The program was authorized in 1965 by Title XIX of the Social Security Act. See related *Health expenditures, national; Health maintenance organization; Medicare.*

Medical specialties—See *Physician specialty.*

Medical vendor payments—Under the Medicaid program, medical vendor payments are payments (expenditures) to medical vendors from the State through a fiscal agent or to a health insurance plan. Adjustments are made for Indian Health Service payments to Medicaid, cost settlements, third party recoupments, refunds, voided checks, and other financial settlements that cannot be related to specific provided claims. Excluded are payments made for medical care under the emergency assistance provisions, payments made from State medical assistance funds that are not federally matchable, disproportionate share hospital payments, cost sharing or enrollment fees collected from recipients or a third party, and administration and training costs.

Medicare—This is a nationwide health insurance program providing health insurance protection to people 65 years of age and over, people entitled to social security disability payments for 2 years or more, and people with end-stage renal disease, regardless of income. The program was enacted July 30, 1965, as Title XVIII, *Health Insurance for the Aged of the Social Security Act,* and became effective on July 1, 1966. It consists of two separate but coordinated programs, hospital insurance (Part A) and supplementary medical insurance (Part B). See related *Health expenditures, national; Health maintenance organization; Medicaid.*

Mental health disorder—The Center for Mental Health Services defines a mental health disorder as any of several disorders listed in the *International Classification of Diseases, Ninth Revision, Clinical Modification* (ICD-9-CM) or *Diagnostic and Statistical Manual of Mental Disorders, Third Edition* (DSM-IIIR). Table X shows diagnostic categories and code numbers for ICD-9-CM/DSM-IIIR and corresponding codes for the *International Classification of Diseases, Adapted for Use in the United States, Eighth Revision* (ICDA-8) and *Diagnostic and Statistical Manual of Mental Disorders, Second Edition* (DSM-II). See related *International Classification of Diseases, Clinical Modification.*

Mental health organization—The Center for Mental Health Services defines a mental health organization as an administratively distinct public or private agency or institution whose primary concern is the provision of direct mental health services to the

Table X. Mental health codes, according to applicable revision of the *Diagnostic and Statistical Manual of Mental Disorders* and *International Classification of Diseases*

Diagnostic category	DSM-II/ICDA-8	DSM-IIIR/ICD-9-CM
Alcohol related	291, 303, 309.13	291, 303, 305.0
Drug related	294.3, 304, 309.14	292, 304, 305.1–305.9, 327, 328
Organic disorders (other than alcoholism and drug) . .	290, 292, 293, 294 (except 294.3), 309.0, 309.2–309.9	290, 293, 294, 310
Affective disorders	296, 298.0, 300.4	296, 298.0, 300.4, 301.11, 301.13
Schizophrenia	295	295

mentally ill or emotionally disturbed. Excluded are private office-based practices of psychiatrists, psychologists, and other mental health providers; psychiatric services of all types of hospitals or outpatient clinics operated by Federal agencies other than the Department of Veterans Affairs (for example, Public Health Service, Indian Health Service, Department of Defense, and Bureau of Prisons); general hospitals that have no separate psychiatric services, but admit psychiatric patients to nonpsychiatric units; and psychiatric services of schools, colleges, halfway houses, community residential organizations, local and county jails, State prisons, and other human service providers. The major types of mental health organizations are described below.

Freestanding psychiatric outpatient clinics provide only outpatient services on either a regular or emergency basis. The medical responsibility for services is generally assumed by a psychiatrist.

General hospitals providing separate psychiatric services are non-Federal general hospitals that provide psychiatric services in either a separate psychiatric inpatient, outpatient, or partial hospitalization service with assigned staff and space.

Multiservice mental health organizations directly provide two or more of the program elements defined under Mental health service type and are not classifiable as a psychiatric hospital, general hospital, or a residential treatment center for emotionally disturbed children. (The classification of a psychiatric or general hospital or a residential treatment center for emotionally disturbed children takes precedence over a multiservice classification, even if two or more services are offered.)

Partial care organizations provide a program of ambulatory mental health services.

Private mental hospitals are operated by a sole proprietor, partnership, limited partnership,

corporation, or nonprofit organization, primarily for the care of persons with mental disorders.

Psychiatric hospitals are hospitals primarily concerned with providing inpatient care and treatment for the mentally ill. Psychiatric inpatient units of Department of Veterans Affairs general hospitals and Department of Veterans Affairs neuropsychiatric hospitals are combined into the category Department of Veterans Affairs psychiatric hospitals because of their similarity in size, operation, and length of stay.

Residential treatment centers for emotionally disturbed children must meet all of the following criteria: (a) Not licensed as a psychiatric hospital and primary purpose is to provide individually planned mental health treatment services in conjunction with residential care; (b) Include a clinical program that is directed by a psychiatrist, psychologist, social worker, or psychiatric nurse with a graduate degree; (c) Serve children and youth primarily under the age of 18; and (d) Primary diagnosis for the majority of admissions is mental illness, classified as other than mental retardation, developmental disability, and substance-related disorders, according to DSM-II/ICDA-8 or DSM-IIIR/ICD-9-CM codes. See related *Table X. Mental health codes.*

State and county mental hospitals are under the auspices of a State or county government or operated jointly by a State and county government.

See related *Addition; Mental health service type.*

Mental health service type—refers to the following kinds of mental health services:

Inpatient care is the provision of 24-hour mental health care in a mental health hospital setting.

Outpatient care is the provision of ambulatory mental health services for less than 3 hours at a single visit on an individual, group, or family basis, usually in a clinic or similar organization. Emergency care on a walk-in basis, as well as care provided by mobile teams who visit patients outside these organizations are included. "Hotline" services are excluded.

Partial care treatment is a planned program of mental health treatment services generally provided in visits of 3 or more hours to groups of patients. Included are treatment programs that emphasize intensive short-term therapy and rehabilitation; programs that focus on recreation, and/or occupational program activities, including sheltered workshops; and education and training programs, including special education classes, therapeutic nursery schools, and vocational training.

Residential treatment care is the provision of overnight mental health care in conjunction with an intensive treatment program in a setting other than a hospital. Facilities may offer care to emotionally disturbed children or mentally ill adults.

See related *Addition; Mental health organization.*

Metropolitan statistical area (MSA)—The definitions and titles of MSA's are established by the U.S. Office of Management and Budget with the advice of the Federal Committee on Metropolitan Statistical Areas. Generally speaking, an MSA consists of a county or group of counties containing at least one city (or twin cities) having a population of 50,000 or more plus adjacent counties that are metropolitan in character and are economically and socially integrated with the central city. In New England, towns and cities rather than counties are the units used in defining MSA's. There is no limit to the number of adjacent counties included in the MSA as long as they are integrated with the central city. Nor is an MSA limited to a single State; boundaries may cross State lines. Metropolitan population, as used in this report in connection with data from the National Health

Interview Survey, is based on MSA's as defined in the 1980 census and does not include any subsequent additions or changes.

Multiservice mental health organizations—See *Mental health organization.*

National ambient air quality standards—The Federal Clean Air Act of 1970, amended in 1977 and 1990, required the Environmental Protection Agency (EPA) to establish National Ambient Air Quality Standards. EPA has set specific standards for each of six major pollutants: carbon monoxide, lead, nitrogen dioxide, ozone, sulfur dioxide, and particulate matter whose aerodynamic size is equal to or less than 10 microns (PM-10). Each pollutant standard represents a maximum concentration level (micrograms per cubic meter) that cannot be exceeded during a specified time interval. A county meets the national ambient air quality standards if none of the six pollutants exceed the standard during a 12-month period. See *related Particulate matter; Pollutant.*

Neonatal mortality rate—See *Rate: Death and related rates.*

Non-Federal physicians—See *Physician.*

Nonpatient revenue—Nonpatient revenues are those revenues received for which no direct patient care services are rendered. The most widely recognized source of nonpatient revenues is philanthropy. Philanthropic support may be direct from individuals or may be obtained through philanthropic fund raising organizations such as the United Way. Support may also be obtained from foundations or corporations. Philanthropic revenues may be designated for direct patient care use or may be contained in an endowment fund where only the current income may be tapped.

Nonprofit hospitals—See *Hospital.*

Notifiable disease—A notifiable disease is one that, when diagnosed, health providers are required, usually by law, to report to State or local public health

.... Appendix II

Glossary

officials. Notifiable diseases are those of public interest by reason of their contagiousness, severity, or frequency.

Nursing care—The following definition of nursing care applies to data collected in National Nursing Home Surveys through 1977. Nursing care is the provision of any of the following services: application of dressings or bandages; bowel and bladder retraining; catheterization; enema; full bed bath; hypodermic, intramuscular, or intravenous injection; irrigation; nasal feeding; oxygen therapy; and temperature-pulse-respiration or blood pressure measurement. See related *Nursing home*.

Nursing care homes—See *Nursing home*.

Nursing home—In the Online Certification and Reporting database, a nursing home is a facility that is certified and meets the Health Care Financing Administration's long-term care requirements for Medicare and Medicaid eligibility. In the National Master Facility Inventory and the National Nursing Home Survey a nursing home is an establishment with three or more beds that provides nursing or personal care services to the aged, infirm, or chronically ill. The following definitions of nursing home types apply to data collected in National Nursing Home Surveys through 1977.

Nursing care homes must employ one or more full-time registered or licensed practical nurses and must provide nursing care to at least one-half the residents.

Personal care homes with nursing have some but fewer than one-half the residents receiving nursing care. In addition, such homes must employ one or more registered or licensed practical nurses or must provide administration of medications and treatments in accordance with physicians' orders, supervision of self-administered medications, or three or more personal services.

Personal care homes without nursing have no residents who are receiving nursing care. These homes provide administration of medications and treatments in accordance with physicians' orders, supervision of self-administered medications, or three or more personal services.

Domiciliary care homes primarily provide supervisory care but also provide one or two personal services.

Nursing homes are certified by the Medicare and/or Medicaid program. The following definitions of certification levels apply to data collected in National Nursing Home Surveys of 1973–74, 1977, and 1985.

Skilled nursing facilities provide the most intensive nursing care available outside of a hospital. Facilities certified by Medicare provide posthospital care to eligible Medicare enrollees. Facilities certified by Medicaid as skilled nursing facilities provide skilled nursing services on a daily basis to individuals eligible for Medicaid benefits.

Intermediate care facilities are certified by the Medicaid program to provide health-related services on a regular basis to Medicaid eligibles who do not require hospital or skilled nursing facility care but do require institutional care above the level of room and board.

Not certified facilities are not certified as providers of care by Medicare or Medicaid.

See related *Nursing care; Resident*.

Nursing home expenditures—See *Health expenditures, national*.

Occupancy rate—The National Master Facility Inventory and American Hospital Association define hospital occupancy rate as the average daily census divided by the average number of hospital beds during a reporting period. Average daily census is defined by the American Hospital Association as the average number of inpatients, excluding newborns, receiving care each day during a reporting period. The occupancy rate for facilities other than hospitals is calculated as the number of residents reported at the time of the interview divided by the number of beds reported. In the Online Survey Certification and Reporting database, occupancy is the total number of residents on the day of certification inspection divided by the total number of beds on the day of certification.

Office—In the National Health Interview Survey, an office refers to the office of any physician in private practice not located in a hospital. In the National Ambulatory Medical Care Survey, an office is any location for a physician's ambulatory practice other than hospitals, nursing homes, other extended care facilities, patients' homes, industrial clinics, college clinics, and family planning clinics. However, private offices in hospitals are included. See related *Office visit; Outpatient visit; Physician; Physician contact.*

Office-based physician—See *Physician.*

Office visit—In the National Ambulatory Medical Care Survey, an office visit is any direct personal exchange between an ambulatory patient and a physician or members of his or her staff for the purposes of seeking care and rendering health services. See related *Outpatient visit; Physician contact.*

Operations—See *Procedure.*

Outpatient department—According to the National Hospital Ambulatory Medical Care Survey (NHAMCS), an outpatient department (OPD) is a hospital facility where nonurgent ambulatory medical care is provided. The following are examples of the types of OPD's excluded from the NHAMCS: ambulatory surgical centers, chemotherapy, employee health services, renal dialysis, methadone maintenance, and radiology. An outpatient department visit is a direct personal exchange between a patient and a physician or other health care provider working under the physician's supervision for the purpose of seeking care and receiving personal health services. See related *Emergency department; Hospital.*

Outpatient visit—The American Hospital Association defines outpatient visits as visits for receipt of medical, dental, or other services by patients who are not lodged in the hospital. Each appearance by an outpatient to each unit of the hospital is counted individually as an outpatient visit. See related *Office visit; Physician contact.*

Partial care organization—See *Mental health organization.*

Partial care treatment—See *Mental health service type.*

Particulate matter—Particulate matter is defined as particles of solid or liquid matter in the air, including nontoxic materials (soot, dust, and dirt) and toxic materials (for example, lead, asbestos, suspended sulfates, and nitrates). See related *National ambient air quality standards; Pollutant.*

Patient—A patient is a person who is formally admitted to the inpatient service of a hospital for observation, care, diagnosis, or treatment. See related *Admission; Average length of stay; Days of care; Discharge; Hospital.*

Percent change—See *Average annual rate of change.*

Perinatal mortality rate, ratio—See *Rate: Death and related rates.*

Personal care homes with or without nursing—See *Nursing home.*

Personal health care expenditures—See *Health expenditures, national.*

Physician—Physicians, through self-reporting, are classified by the American Medical Association and others as licensed doctors of medicine or osteopathy, as follows:

Active (or professionally active) physicians are currently practicing medicine for a minimum of 20 hours per week. Excluded are physicians who are inactive practicing medicine less than 20 hours per week, have unknown addresses, or specialties not classified (when specialty information is presented).

Federal physicians are employed by the Federal Government; non-Federal or civilian physicians are not.

Hospital-based physicians spend the plurality of their time as salaried physicians in hospitals.

Office-based physicians spend the plurality of their time working in practices based in private offices.

Data for physicians are presented by type of education (doctors of medicine and doctors of osteopathy); place of education (U.S. medical graduates and international medical graduates); activity status (professionally active and inactive); employment setting (Federal and non-Federal); area of specialty; and geographic area. See related *Office; Physician specialty*.

Physician contact—In the National Health Interview Survey, a physician contact is defined as a consultation with a physician in person or by telephone, for examination, diagnosis, treatment, or advice. The service may be provided by the physician or by another person working under the physician's supervision. Contacts involving services provided on a mass basis (for example, blood pressure screenings) and contacts for hospital inpatients are not included.

Place of contact includes office, hospital outpatient clinics, emergency room, telephone (advice given by a physician in a telephone call), home (any place in which a person was staying at the time a physician was called there), clinics, HMO's, and other places located outside a hospital.

In the National Health Interview Survey, analyses of the annual number of physician contacts and place of contact are based upon data collected using a 2-week recall period and are adjusted to produce annual estimates. Analyses of children without a physician contact during the past 12-month period are based upon a different question that uses a 12-month recall period. Analyses of the interval since last physician contact are based upon the length of time before the week of interview in which the physician was last consulted. See related *Office; Office visit*.

Physician specialty—A physician specialty is any specific branch of medicine in which a physician may concentrate. Data are based on physician self-reports of their primary area of speciality. Physician data are

broadly categorized into two general areas of practice: generalists and specialists.

Generalist physicians are synonymous with primary care generalists and only include physicians practicing in the general fields of family and general practice, general internal medicine, and general pediatrics. They specifically exclude primary care specialists.

Primary care specialists practice in the subspecialties of general and family practice, internal medicine, and pediatrics. The primary care subspecialties for family practice include geriatric medicine and sports medicine. Primary care subspecialties for internal medicine include diabetes, endocrinology and metabolism, hematology, hepatology, cardiac electrophysiology, infectious diseases, diagnostic laboratory immunology, geriatric medicine, sports medicine, nephrology, nutrition, medical oncology, and rheumatology. Primary care subspecialties for pediatrics include adolescent medicine, critical care pediatrics, neonatal-perinatal medicine, pediatric allergy, pediatric cardiology, pediatric endocrinology, pediatric pulmonology, pediatric emergency medicine, pediatric gastroenterology, pediatric hematology/oncology, diagnostic laboratory immunology, pediatric nephrology, pediatric rheumatology, and sports medicine.

Specialist physicians practice in the primary care specialties, in addition to all other specialist fields not included in the generalist definition. Specialist fields include allergy and immunology, aerospace medicine, anesthesiology, cardiovascular diseases, child and adolescent psychiatry, colon and rectal surgery, dermatology, diagnostic radiology, forensic pathology, gastroenterology, general surgery, medical genetics, neurology, nuclear medicine, neurological surgery, obstetrics and gynecology, occupational medicine, ophthalmology, orthopedic surgery, otolaryngology, psychiatry, public health and general preventive medicine, physical medicine and rehabilitation, plastic surgery, anatomic and clinical pathology, pulmonary diseases, radiation oncology, thoracic surgery, urology, addiction medicine, critical care medicine, legal medicine, and clinical pharmacology.

See related *Physician*.

Pollutant—A pollutant is any substance that renders the atmosphere or water foul or noxious to health. See related *National ambient air quality standards; Particulate matter.*

Population—The U.S. Bureau of the Census collects and publishes data on populations in the United States according to several different definitions. Various statistical systems then use the appropriate population for calculating rates.

Total population is the population of the United States, including all members of the Armed Forces living in foreign countries, Puerto Rico, Guam, and the U.S. Virgin Islands. Other Americans abroad (for example, civilian Federal employees and dependents of members of the Armed Forces or other Federal employees) are not included.

Resident population includes persons whose usual place of residence (that is, the place where one usually lives and sleeps) is in one of the 50 States or the District of Columbia. It includes members of the Armed Forces stationed in the United States and their families. It excludes international military, naval, and diplomatic personnel and their families located here and residing in embassies or similar quarters. Also excluded are international workers and international students in this country and Americans living abroad. The resident population is usually the denominator when calculating birth and death rates and incidence of disease. The resident population is also the denominator for selected population-based rates that use numerator data from the National Health Provider Inventory (National Master Facility Inventory) and National Nursing Home Survey.

Civilian population is the resident population excluding members of the Armed Forces. However, families of members of the Armed Forces are included. This population is the denominator in rates calculated for the NCHS National Hospital Discharge Survey.

Civilian noninstitutionalized population is the civilian population not residing in institutions. Institutions include correctional institutions, detention homes, and training schools for juvenile delinquents; homes for the aged and dependent (for example, nursing homes and convalescent homes); homes for dependent and neglected children; homes and schools for the mentally or physically handicapped; homes for unwed mothers; psychiatric, tuberculosis, and chronic disease hospitals; and residential treatment centers. This population is the denominator in rates calculated for the NCHS National Health Interview Survey; National Health and Nutrition Examination Survey; National Ambulatory Medical Care Survey; and the National Hospital Ambulatory Medical Care Survey.

Postneonatal mortality rate—See *Rate: Death and related rates.*

Poverty level—Poverty statistics are based on definitions originally developed by the Social Security Administration. These include a set of money income thresholds that vary by family size and composition. Families or individuals with income below their appropriate thresholds are classified as below the poverty level. These thresholds are updated annually by the U.S. Bureau of the Census to reflect changes in the Consumer Price Index for all urban consumers (CPI-U). For example, the average poverty threshold for a family of four was $15,569 in 1995 and $13,359 in 1990. See related *Consumer Price Index.*

Preferred provider organization (PPO)—Health plan generally consisting of hospital and physician providers. The PPO provides health care services to plan members usually at discounted rates in return for

Glossary

expedited claims payment. Plan members can use PPO or non-PPO health care providers, however, financial incentives are built into the benefit structure to encourage utilization of PPO providers. See related *Managed care.*

Prevalence—Prevalence is the number of cases of a disease, infected persons, or persons with some other attribute present during a particular interval of time. It is often expressed as a rate (for example, the prevalence of diabetes per 1,000 persons during a year). See related *Incidence.*

Primary admission diagnosis—In the National Home and Hospice Care Survey the primary admission diagnosis is the first-listed diagnosis at admission on the patient's medical record as provided by the agency staff member most familiar with the care provided to the patient.

Primary care specialties—See *Physician specialty.*

Private expenditures—See *Health expenditures, national.*

Procedure—The National Hospital Discharge Survey (NHDS) defines a procedure as a surgical or nonsurgical operation, diagnostic procedure, or special treatment assigned by the physician and recorded on the medical record of patients discharged from the inpatient service of short-stay hospitals. All terms listed on the face sheet of the medical record under captions such as "operation," "operative procedures," and "operations and/or special treatments" are transcribed in the order listed. A maximum of four 4-digit ICD-9-CM codes are assigned per discharge. Tables in *Health, United States* that show operations or diagnostic procedure data include all operations or procedures up to a maximum of four per discharge. In accordance with ICD-9-CM coding, procedures are classified as diagnostic and other nonsurgical procedures or as surgical operations.

Diagnostic and other nonsurgical procedures are procedures generally not considered to be surgery. These include diagnostic endoscopy and

radiography, radiotherapy and related therapies, physical medicine and rehabilitation, and other nonsurgical procedures. Selected diagnostic and other nonsurgical procedures are listed with their ICD-9-CM code numbers in table IX. For a complete listing of nonsurgical procedures, as defined by NHDS, see Graves EJ, Kozak LJ. National Hospital Discharge Survey: Annual summary 1989. National Center for Health Statistics. Vital Health Stat 13(109). 1991.

Surgical operations encompass all ICD-9-CM procedures, except those listed under "Nonsurgical procedures." Selected surgical operations are listed with their ICD-9-CM codes in table VIII. The American Hospital Association defines surgery as a major or minor surgical episode performed in the operating room. During a single episode, multiple surgical procedures may be performed, but the episode is considered only one surgical operation. In contrast the National Hospital Discharge Survey codes up to four ICD-9-CM surgical procedures per surgical episode.

See related *International Classification of Diseases, Ninth Revision, Clinical Modification.*

Proprietary hospitals—See *Hospital.*

Psychiatric hospitals—See *Hospital; Mental health organization.*

Public expenditures—See *Health expenditures, national.*

Race—Beginning in 1976 the Federal Government's data systems classified individuals into the following racial groups: American Indian or Alaskan Native, Asian or Pacific Islander, black, and white. Depending on the data source, the classification by race may be based on self-classification or on observation by an interviewer or other persons filling out the questionnaire. Starting in 1989, data from the National Vital Statistics System for newborn infants and fetal deaths are tabulated according to race of mother, and trend data by race shown in this report have been retabulated by race of mother for all years, beginning with 1980. Before 1980, data were tabulated by race of newborn and fetus according to race of both parents. If the parents were of different races and one parent was white, the child was classified according to the race of the other parent. When neither parent was white, the child was classified according to father's race, with one exception: if either parent was Hawaiian, the child was classified Hawaiian. Before 1964 the National Vital Statistics System classified all births for which race was unknown as white. Beginning in 1964 these births were classified according to information on the previous record.

In *Health, United States*, trends of birth rates, birth characteristics, and infant and maternal mortality rates are calculated according to race of mother unless specified otherwise. In the National Health Interview Survey, children whose parents are of different races are classified according to the race of the mother. Vital event rates for the American Indian or Alaska Native population shown in this book are based on the total U.S. resident population of American Indians and Alaska Natives as enumerated by the U.S. Bureau of Census. In contrast the Indian Health Service calculates vital event rates for this population based on U.S. Bureau of Census county data for American Indians and Alaska Natives who reside on or near reservations. See related *Hispanic origin*.

Rate—A rate is a measure of some event, disease, or condition in relation to a unit of population, along with some specification of time. See related *Age adjustment; Population*.

■ *Birth and related rates*

Birth rate is calculated by dividing the number of live births in a population in a year by the midyear resident population. For census years, rates are based on unrounded census counts of the resident population, as of April 1. For the noncensus years of 1981–89 and 1991, rates are based on national estimates of the resident population, as of July 1, rounded to 1,000's. Population estimates for 5-year age groups are

generated by summing unrounded population estimates before rounding to 1,000's. Starting in 1992 rates are based on unrounded national population estimates. Birth rates are expressed as the number of live births per 1,000 population. The rate may be restricted to births to women of specific age, race, marital status, or geographic location (specific rate), or it may be related to the entire population (crude rate). See related *Cohort fertility; Live birth*.

Fertility rate is the number of live births per 1,000 women of reproductive age, 15–44 years.

■ *Death and related rates*

Death rate is calculated by dividing the number of deaths in a population in a year by the midyear resident population. For census years, rates are based on unrounded census counts of the resident population, as of April 1. For the noncensus years of 1981–89 and 1991, rates are based on national estimates of the resident population, as of July 1, rounded to 1,000's. Population estimates for 10-year age groups are generated by summing unrounded population estimates before rounding to 1,000's. Starting in 1992 rates are based on unrounded national population estimates. Rates for the Hispanic and non-Hispanic white populations in each year are based on unrounded State population estimates for States in the Hispanic reporting area. Death rates are expressed as the number of deaths per 100,000 population. The rate may be restricted to deaths in specific age, race, sex, or geographic groups or from specific causes of death (specific rate) or it may be related to the entire population (crude rate).

Fetal death rate is the number of fetal deaths with stated or presumed gestation of 20 weeks or more divided by the sum of live births plus fetal deaths, stated per 1,000 live births plus fetal deaths. *Late fetal death rate* is the number of fetal deaths with stated or presumed gestation of 28 weeks or more divided by the sum of live births plus late fetal deaths, stated per 1,000 live births plus late fetal deaths. See related *Fetal death; Gestation.*

Infant mortality rate based on period files is calculated by dividing the number of infant deaths during a calendar year by the number of live births reported in the same year. It is expressed as the number of infant deaths per 1,000 live births. *Neonatal mortality rate* is the number of deaths of children under 28 days of age, per 1,000 live births. *Postneonatal mortality rate* is the number of deaths of children that occur between 28 days and 365 days after birth, per 1,000 live births. See related *Infant death.*

Birth cohort infant mortality rates are based on linked birth and infant death files. In contrast to period rates in which the births and infant deaths occur in the same period or calendar year, infant deaths comprising the numerator of a birth cohort rate may have occurred in the same year as, or in the year following the year of birth. The birth cohort infant mortality rate is expressed as the number of infant deaths per 1,000 live births. See related *Birth cohort.*

Perinatal relates to the period surrounding the birth event. Rates and ratios are based on events reported in a calendar year. *Perinatal mortality rate* is the sum of late fetal deaths plus infant deaths within 7 days of birth divided by the sum of live births plus late fetal deaths, stated per 1,000 live births plus late fetal deaths. *Perinatal mortality ratio* is the sum of late fetal deaths plus infant deaths within 7 days of birth divided by the number of live births, stated per 1,000 live births. *Feto-infant mortality rate* is the sum of late fetal deaths plus all infant deaths divided by the sum of live births plus late fetal deaths, stated per 1,000 live births plus late fetal deaths. See related *Fetal death; Gestation; Infant death; Live birth.*

Maternal death is one for which the certifying physician has designated a maternal condition as the underlying cause of death. Maternal conditions are those assigned to Complications of pregnancy, childbirth, and the puerperium. (See related table V.) *Maternal mortality rate* is the number of maternal deaths per 100,000 live births. The maternal mortality rate indicates the likelihood that a pregnant woman will die from maternal causes. The number of live births used in the denominator is an approximation of the population of pregnant women who are at risk of a maternal death.

Region—See *Geographic region and division.*

Registered hospitals—See *Hospital.*

Registered nursing education—Registered nursing data are shown by level of educational preparation. Baccalaureate education requires at least 4 years of college or university; associate degree programs are based in community colleges and are usually 2 years in length; and diploma programs are based in hospitals and are usually 3 years in length.

Registration area—The United States has separate registration areas for birth, death, marriage, and divorce statistics. In general, registration areas correspond to States and include two separate registration areas for the District of Columbia and New York City. All States have adopted laws that require the registration of births and deaths and the reporting of fetal deaths. It is believed that more than 99 percent of the births and deaths occurring in this country are registered.

The *death registration area* was established in 1900 with 10 States and the District of Columbia, and the *birth registration area* was established in 1915, also with 10 States and the District of Columbia. Both areas have covered the entire United States since 1933. Currently, Puerto Rico, U.S. Virgin Islands, and Guam comprise separate registration areas, although their data are not included in statistical tabulations of U.S. resident data. See related *Reporting area.*

Relative survival rate—The relative survival rate is the ratio of the observed survival rate for the patient group to the expected survival rate for persons in the general population similar to the patient group with respect to age, sex, race, and calendar year of observation. The 5-year relative survival rate is used to estimate the proportion of cancer patients potentially curable. Because over one-half of all cancers occur in persons 65 years of age and over, many of these individuals die of other causes with no evidence of recurrence of their cancer. Thus, because it is obtained by adjusting observed survival for the normal life expectancy of the general population of the same age, the relative survival rate is an estimate of the chance of surviving the effects of cancer.

Reporting area—In the National Vital Statistics System, the reporting area for such basic items on the birth and death certificates as age, race, and sex, is based on data from residents of all 50 States in the United States and the District of Columbia. The reporting area for selected items such as Hispanic origin, educational attainment, and marital status, is based on data from those States that require the item to be reported, whose data meet a minimum level of completeness (such as, 80 or 90 percent), and are considered to be sufficiently comparable to be used for analysis. In 1993–96 the reporting area for Hispanic origin of decedent on the death certificate included 49 States and the District of Columbia. See related *Registration area; National Vital Statistics System* in Appendix I.

Resident—In the Online Certification and Reporting database, all residents in certified facilities are counted on the day of certification inspection. In the National Nursing Home Survey, a resident is a person on the roster of the nursing home as of the night before the survey. Included are all residents for whom beds are maintained even though they may be on overnight leave or in a hospital. See related *Nursing home.*

Resident population—See *Population.*

Residential treatment care—See *Mental health service type.*

Residential treatment centers for emotionally disturbed children—See *Mental health organization.*

Self-assessment of health—See *Health status, respondent-assessed.*

Short-stay hospitals—See *Hospital.*

Skilled nursing facilities—See *Nursing home.*

Smoker—See *Current smoker.*

Specialty hospitals—See *Hospital.*

State health agency—The agency or department within State government headed by the State or territorial health official. Generally, the State health agency is responsible for setting statewide public health priorities, carrying out national and State mandates, responding to public health hazards, and assuring access to health care for underserved State residents.

Substance abuse treatment clients—In the Substance Abuse and Mental Health Services Administration's Uniform Facilities Data Set substance abuse treatment clients have been admitted to treatment and have been seen on a scheduled appointment basis at least once in the month before the survey reference date or were inpatients on the survey reference date. Types of treatment include 24-hour detoxification, 24-hour rehabilitation or residential care, and outpatient care.

Surgical operations—See *Procedure.*

Surgical specialties—See *Physician specialty.*

Uninsured—See *Health insurance coverage.*

Urbanization—In this report death rates are presented according to level of urbanization of the decedent's county of residence. Metropolitan and nonmetropolitan counties are categorized into urbanization levels based on an NCHS-modification of the 1993 rural-urban continuum codes. The 1993 rural-urban continuum codes were developed by the Economic Research Service, U.S. Department of Agriculture using the 1993 U.S. Office of Management and Budget definition of metropolitan statistical areas (MSA's). The codes classify metropolitan counties by population size and level of urbanization and nonmetropolitan counties by level of urbanization and proximity to metropolitan areas. NCHS modified the 1993 rural-urban continuum codes to make the definition of core and fringe metropolitan counties comparable to the definitions used for the 1983 codes. For this report, the 10 categories of counties have been collapsed into 5 categories (a) core metropolitan counties contain the primary central city of an MSA with a 1990 population of 1 million or more; (b) fringe metropolitan counties are the noncore counties of an MSA with 1990 population of 1 million or more; (c) medium or small metropolitan counties are in MSA's with 1990 population under 1 million; (d) urban nonmetropolitan counties are not in MSA's and have 2,500 or more urban residents in 1990; and (e) rural counties are not in MSA's and have fewer than 2,500 urban residents in 1990. See related *Metropolitan statistical area (MSA)*.

Usual source of care—Usual source of care was measured in the National Health Interview Survey (NHIS) in 1993 and 1994 by asking the respondent, "Is there a particular person or place that __ usually goes to when ___ is sick or needs advice about __ health?" In the 1995 NHIS, the respondent was asked "Is there one doctor, person, or place that __ usually goes to when __ is sick or needs advice about ___ health?"

Wages and salaries—See *Employer costs for employee compensation*.

Years of potential life lost—Years of potential life lost (YPLL) is a measure of premature mortality. Starting with *Health, United States, 1996–97*, YPLL is presented for persons under 75 years of age because the average life expectancy in the United States is over 75 years. YPLL-75 is caculated using the following eight age groups: under 1 year, 1–14 years, 15–24 years, 25–34 years, 35–44 years, 45–54 years, 55–64 years, 65–74 years. The number of deaths for each age group is multiplied by the years of life lost, calculated as the difference between age 75 years and the midpoint of the age group. For the eight age groups the midpoints are 0.5, 7.5, 19.5, 29.5, 39.5, 49.5, 59.5,

and 69.5. For example, the death of a person 15–24 years of age counts as 55.5 years of life lost. Years of potential life lost is derived by summing years of life lost over all age groups. In *Health, United States, 1995* and earlier editions, YPLL was presented for persons under 65 years of age. For more information, see Centers for Disease Control. *MMWR*. Vol 35 no 25S, suppl. 1986.

Index to Health, United States, 1998 Detailed Tables ....

(Numbers refer to table numbers)

A

Table

Abortion 15, 16, 17
    Abortions per 100 live births 15
    Age. 15
    Deaths, abortion-related. 17
    Gestation 16, 17
    Location of facility 16
    Marital status 15
    Number of abortions 16, 17
    Previous induced abortions 16
    Previous live births 15
    Race 15
    Type of procedure 16
Access to care (see also Physician utilization) 78, 79
    No physician contact in past year. 78
    No usual source of care. 79
Accidents, see Motor vehicle-related injuries; Unintentional injuries.
AIDS, see HIV/AIDS.
Air quality standards 72
Alcohol abuse treatment clients. 84
Alcohol consumption 64, 65, 67
    Age. 64, 67
    Education 65
    Hispanic origin. 64, 67
    Race 64, 65, 67
    Students 65
Alzheimers disease 33, 34
Ambulatory care (see also Access to care; Dental visits; Hospital utilization; Mammography; Mental health care utilization;
  Physician utilization) 81, 82
    Hospital emergency department 81
    Hospital outpatient department 81
    Physician office visits 81, 82
American Indian population
    AIDS cases. 55
    Air quality standards 72
    Birth rates. 3
    Births, number 5
    Birthweight, low 11, 12
    Death rates, all causes. 30, 31, 37
    Death rates, geographic division and State. 30
    Death rates, selected causes 31, 38, 39, 40, 41, 42, 43, 44, 45, 46, 47, 48, 49
    Deaths, number, all causes and leading causes 33
    Dental students. 107
    Education of mother 9, 12, 21
    Infant mortality 20, 21
    Medical students 107, 108
    Nursing students 107
    Optometry students 107
    Pharmacy students. 107
    Podiatry students 107
    Population, resident 1
    Prenatal care. 6
    Smoking status of mother 10
    Teenage childbearing. 7

A—Con.

American Indian population—Con.
Unmarried mothers 8
Years of potential life lost 32
Anemias 34
Asian Population
AIDS cases 55
Air quality standards 72
Birth rates 3
Births, number 5
Birthweight, low 11, 12
Death rates, all causes 30, 31, 37
Death rates, geographic division and State 30
Death rates, selected causes 31, 38, 39, 40, 41, 42, 43, 44, 45, 46, 47, 48, 49
Deaths, number, all causes and leading causes 33
Dental students 107
Education of mother 9, 12, 21
Infant mortality 20, 21
Medical students 107, 108
Nursing students 107
Optometry students 107
Pharmacy students 107
Podiatry students 107
Population, resident 1
Prenatal care 6
Smoking status of mother 10
Teenage childbearing 7
Unmarried mothers 8
Years of potential life lost 32
Asian subgroups (Chinese; Filipino; Hawaiian; Japanese)
Births, number 5
Birthweight, low 11, 12
Education of mother 9, 12, 21
Infant mortality 20, 21
Prenatal care 6
Smoking status of mother 10
Teenage childbearing 7
Unmarried mothers 8
Asthma 90, 91
Atherosclerosis 33, 34

B

Benign neoplasms 34
Birth control, see Contraception.
Birth trauma 34
Births (see also Childless women) 3, 5, 6, 7, 8, 9, 10, 11, 12, 13, 14
Age of mother 3, 8, 10
Birth rates 3, 8
Births, number 5, 8
Birthweight, low 11, 12, 13, 14
Education of mother 9, 10, 12
Geographic division and State 13, 14
Hispanic origin of mother 3, 5, 6, 7, 8, 9, 10, 11, 12
Prenatal care 6
Race 3, 5, 6, 7, 8, 9, 10, 11, 12, 13, 14
Smoking status of mother 10, 11
Teenage childbearing 7
Unmarried mothers 8

Black population
  Abortion 15
  Access to care 78, 79
  AIDS cases 55, 56
  Air quality standards 72
  Alcohol consumption 64, 65, 67
  Birth rates 3, 8
  Births, number 3, 5
  Birthweight, low 11, 12, 13, 14
  Breastfeeding 19
  Cancer incidence rates 58
  Cancer survival, 5-year relative 59
  Cholesterol, serum 69
  Cigarette smoking 62, 63, 64, 65
  Cocaine use 64, 65, 66
  Contraception 18
  Death rates, all causes 30, 31, 37
  Death rates, geographic division and State 30
  Death rates, selected causes 31, 38, 39, 40, 41, 42, 43, 44, 45, 46, 47, 48, 49
  Deaths, number, all causes and leading causes 33
  Dental students 107
  Dental visits 83
  Education of mother 9, 12, 21
  Fetal mortality 23
  Health insurance 133, 134
  Health status, respondent-assessed 61
  Home health care patients 86
  Hospice patients 86
  Hospital utilization, Emergency and Outpatient departments 81
  Hospital utilization, inpatient 87
  Hypertension 68
  Infant mortality 20, 21, 23, 24, 25, 26
  Inhalants 65
  Life expectancy 29
  Limitation of activity 60
  Mammography 80
  Marijuana use 64, 65
  Medical students 107, 108
  Nursing home utilization 95, 96
  Nursing students 107
  Optometry students 107
  Overweight 70, 71
  Pharmacy students 107
  Physician utilization 74, 75, 76, 77, 81, 82
  Podiatry students 107
  Population, resident 1
  Poverty level, persons and families below 2
  Prenatal care 6
  Region, death rates 35
  Smoking status of mother 10
  Teenage childbearing 7
  Unmarried mothers 8
  Urbanization, death rates 35
  Vaccinations 52
  Years of potential life lost 32
Breastfeeding 19
Bronchitis 90, 91

C

Cancer (Malignant neoplasms). 31, 32, 33, 34, 40, 41, 42, 58, 59, 90, 91
    All sites 31, 32, 33, 34, 40, 58, 59, 90, 91
    Breast 31, 32, 42, 58, 59, 90, 91
    Colorectal. 31, 32, 58, 59, 90, 91
    Deaths and death rates. 31, 33, 34, 40
    Hospital utilization. 90, 91
    Incidence rates 58
    Large intestine and rectum 90, 91
    Prostate. 31, 32, 58, 59, 90, 91
    Respiratory system. 31, 32, 41, 90, 91
    Survival, 5-year relative 59
    Trachea, bronchus, lung. 90, 91
    Years of potential life lost. 32
Central and South American population, see Hispanic subgroups.
Cerebrovascular disease (Stroke). 31, 32, 33, 34, 39, 90, 91
    Deaths and death rates. 31, 33, 34, 39
    Hospital utilization. 90, 91
    Years of potential life lost. 32
Certain conditions originating in the perinatal period 33, 34
Chancroid, see Diseases, notifiable
Childless women. 4
Chinese population, see Asian subgroups.
Chiropractors. 99, 106
    Employees, in offices of 99
    Schools. 106
    Students 106
Chlamydia, see Diseases, notifiable.
Cholesterol, serum 69
Chronic liver disease and cirrhosis 31, 32, 33, 34
Chronic obstructive pulmonary diseases (COPD). 31, 32, 33, 34, 43
Cigarette smoking (see also Births, Smoking status of mother) 62, 63, 64, 65
    Age. 62
    Education 63, 65
    Hispanic origin. 64
    Students 65
Cirrhosis, see Chronic liver disease and cirrhosis.
Cocaine use. 64, 65, 66
    Age. 64, 66
    Education 65
    Emergency room episodes. 66
    Hispanic origin. 64, 66
    Students 65
Communicable diseases, see Diseases, notifiable.
Congenital anomalies 33, 34
Consumer Price Index (CPI) 117, 118
    Medical care components 118
    Selected items 118
Contraception 18
Cost, see Employee costs; Employer costs.
Cuban population, see Hispanic subgroups.

D

Deaths, All causes (see also Cause of death titles; Infant mortality; Life expectancy; 30, 31, 32, 33, 34, 35, 36, 37
    Age. 34, 36, 37
    Educational attainment 36
    Hispanic origin. 30, 31, 32, 33, 37

D—Con.

Deaths—Con.
  Race 30, 31, 32, 33, 35, 36, 37
  Sex 31, 32, 33, 35, 36, 37
  State 30
  Urbanization. 35
  Years of potential life lost 32
Dental visits 83
Dentists 99, 103, 106, 107, 108
  Employees, in offices of 99
  Geographic region 103
  Schools. 106
  Students 106, 107, 108
Diabetes mellitus 31, 32, 33, 34, 90, 91
  Deaths and death rates. 31, 33, 34
  Hospital utilization. 90, 91
Diphtheria see Diseases, notifiable; Vaccinations.
Diseases, notifiable. 54
Disorders relating to short gestation and unspecified low birthweight 34
Drug abuse treatment clients 84
Drug use, see Alcohol consumption; Cigarette smoking; Cocaine use; Inhalants; Marijuana use.
DTP (Diphtheria, Tetanus, Pertussis), see Vaccinations.

E

Education
  Alcohol consumption. 65
  Births 9, 10, 12
  Breastfeeding 19
  Cigarette smoking 63, 65
  Cocaine use 65
  Death rates by educational attainment 36
  Dental visits 83
  Infant mortality 21
  Inhalants. 65
  Mammography. 80
  Marijuana use. 65
Elderly population
  AIDS cases. 55
  Alcohol consumption. 67
  Cholesterol, serum 69
  Cigarette smoking 62
  Death rates, all causes. 37
  Deaths, leading causes. 34
  Death rates, selected causes 38, 39, 40, 41, 42, 43, 44, 46, 47, 48, 49, 50
  Dental visits 83
  Health insurance 134
  Health maintenance organizations. 146
  Health status, respondent-assessed 61, 76
  Home health care patients. 86
  Hospice patients. 86
  Hospital utilization, Emergency and Outpatient departments 81
  Hospital utilization, inpatient 87, 88, 90, 91, 92, 93
  Hypertension 68
  Life expectancy at age 65 . . . . 28, 29
  Life expectancy at age 75 29
  Limitation of activity. 60
  Mammography. 80

E—Con.

Elderly population—Con.
Medicaid 134, 139, 140
Medicare 134, 135, 137, 138, 146
Mental health care utilization 97, 98
Nursing home expenditures 120, 125, 127, 128
Nursing home utilization 95, 96, 114, 127, 128
Nursing homes 113, 114
Overweight 70
Physician utilization 74, 75, 76, 77, 81, 82
Population, resident 1
Emergency department, see Hospital utilization, Emergency department.
Employee costs for health insurance 136
Employer costs for employee compensation 122
Employer costs for health insurance 122
Expenditures, national health (see also Consumer Price Index; Health research and development;
    HIV/AIDS, Expenditures by Federal agency; Hospital expenses; Medicaid; Medicare; Mental health
    expenditures; Nursing home expenditures; Physician expenditures; Prescription drug expenditures;
    Public health expenditures; Veterans medical care) 115, 116, 119, 120, 121, 123, 124, 125
Amount in billions 115, 119, 120, 121, 124
Amount per capita 115, 116, 119, 124
Factors affecting growth 123
Federal government 115, 124
International 116
Out-of-pocket payments 121, 124, 125
Percent of Gross Domestic Product 115, 116
Personal health care 123, 124
Source of funds 119, 124, 125
State and local government 115, 124
Type of expenditure 120, 125
Type of payer 121

F

Fertility rates, see Births.
Fetal mortality 23
Filipino population, see Asian subgroups.
Firearm injuries 49
Fractures, see Injuries and poisoning 49

G

Gonorrhea, see Diseases, notifiable.
Gross Domestic Product (GDP) 115, 116
Health expenditures, as percent of 115
International 116

H

Hawaiian population, see Asian subgroups.
Health expenditures, national, see Expenditures, national health.
Health insurance (see also Health maintenance organizations; Medicaid; Medicare) 78, 79, 122, 133, 134, 136, 149
Access to care 78, 79
Employee costs 136
Employer costs 122
Employment 133, 134, 136

H—Con.

Health insurance—Con.

 Family coverage...136
 Occupation...136
 65 years of age and over...134
 Under 65 years of age...133
 Uninsured...133, 149

Health maintenance organizations (HMO) 135, 136, 148

 Employee costs 136
 Geographic division and State 148
 Medicaid and State 147
 Medicare and State 146
 Occupation...136
 Plans and enrollment...135
 Preferred provider organization (PPO)...136

Health research and development (see also HIV/AIDS) 130, 131

 Federal funding, by agency...131
 Source of funds...130

Health status, respondent-assessed...61, 76

 Physician contacts...76
 Selected characteristics...61

Heart disease...31, 32, 33, 34, 38, 90, 91

 Acute myocardial infection...90, 91
 Congestive heart failure...90, 91
 Deaths and death rates...31, 33, 34, 38
 Hospital utilization...90, 91
 Ischemic heart disease...31, 32, 90, 91
 Years of potential life lost...32

Hepatitis, see Diseases, notifiable.

Hib (Haemophilus influenzae type b), see Vaccinations.

Hispanic origin population

 Abortion...15
 Access to care 78, 79
 AIDS cases...55, 56
 Air quality standards 72
 Alcohol consumption...64, 67
 Birth rates...3
 Births, number 5
 Birthweight, low 11, 12
 Breastfeeding...19
 Cigarette smoking 64
 Cocaine use 64, 66
 Death rates, all causes...30, 31, 37
 Death rates, geographic division and State...30
 Death rates, selected causes 31, 38, 39, 40, 41, 42, 43, 44, 45, 46, 47, 48, 49
 Deaths, number, all causes and leading causes 33
 Dental students...107
 Dental visits...83
 Education of mother 9, 12, 21
 Health insurance 133, 134
 Infant mortality 20, 21
 Mammography...80
 Marijuana use...64
 Medical students 107, 108
 Nursing students 107
 Optometry students 107
 Pharmacy students 107
 Podiatry students 107

Hispanic origin population—Con.
Population, resident 1
Poverty level, persons and families below 2
Prenatal care 6
Smoking status of mother 10
Teenage childbearing 7
Unmarried mothers 8
Years of potential life lost 32
Hispanic subgroups (Central and South American; Cuban; Mexican; Puerto Rican)
(see also Mexican; Puerto Rican).
Births, number 5
Birthweight, low 11, 12
Education of mother 9, 12, 21
Health insurance 133, 134
Infant mortality 20, 21
Prenatal care 6
Smoking status of mother 10
Teenage childbearing 7
Unmarried mothers 8
HIV/AIDS 31, 32, 33, 34, 44, 55, 56, 57, 89, 132
Age 34, 44, 55, 89
AIDS cases 55, 56, 57
Death and death rates 31, 33, 34, 44
Expenditures by Federal agency and activity 132
Geographic division and State 57
Hispanic origin 31, 33, 44, 55, 56
Hospital utilization 89
Race 31, 32, 33, 44, 55, 56
Rank as cause of death 33, 34
Sex 32, 33, 44, 55, 56
Transmission category 56
Years of potential life lost 32
Home health care patients (see also Hospice patients) 86
Homicide and legal intervention 31, 32, 33, 34, 47
Hospice patients (see also Home health care patients) 86
Hospital employees (see also Mental health resources) 99, 104, 126
Full-time employees 104, 126
Number employed in hospitals 99
Occupation 104
Hospital expenses (see also Consumer Price Index; Medicaid; Medicare) 125, 126, 142
Amount in billions 125, 126
Employee costs, as percent of 126
Geographic division and State 142
Inpatient care expenses 126
Source of funds 125
Hospital utilization (see also Ambulatory care; Medicaid; Medicare; Physician utilization;
Veterans medical care) 81, 87, 88, 89, 90, 91, 92, 93, 94
Admissions 94
Average length of stay 87, 88, 89, 91, 94
Days of care 87, 88, 89, 90
Diagnoses, selected 89, 90, 91
Diagnostic and other nonsurgical procedures 93
Discharges for inpatients 87, 88, 89, 90, 91
Emergency department 81
Family income 87
Geographic region 87, 88
Outpatient department 81
Outpatient visits 94

H—Con.

Hospital utilization—Con.
Ownership type 94
Race 87
Residence within/outside metropolitan statistical area 87
Sex 87, 88, 90, 91, 92, 93
Size of hospital 94
Surgery, inpatient 92
Surgery, outpatient 94
Hospitals (see also Hospital employees; Mental health resources; Nursing Homes) 94, 109, 111, 112
Beds 109
Beds per 1,000 population 111
Community hospitals 94, 109, 111, 112
Geographic division and State 111, 112
Number of hospitals 109
Occupancy rate 109, 112
Ownership type 94, 109
Size of hospital 94, 109
Hypertension 68

I

Immunizations, see Vaccinations.
Income, family (see also Poverty status)
Health status, respondent-assessed 61
Hospital utilization 87
Limitation of activity 60
Physician utilization 74, 75, 77
Infant mortality (see also Fetal mortality) 20, 21, 22, 23, 24, 25, 26, 27, 34
Birth cohort data 20, 21, 22
Birthweight 22
Cause of death 34
Education of mother 21
Feto-infant mortality 27
Geographic division and State 24, 25, 26
Hispanic origin 20, 21
International 27
Neonatal mortality 20, 23, 25
Perinatal mortality 23
Postneonatal mortality 20, 23, 26, 27
Race 20, 21, 23, 24, 25, 26
Infections specific to the perinatal period 34
Inhalants 65
Injuries, unintentional, see Unintentional injuries.
Injuries and poisoning 90, 91
Fractures 90, 91
Inpatient care, see Hospital utilization; Mental health care utilization; Nursing home utilization.
International health, see Expenditures, International; Infant mortality; Life expectancy.
Intrauterine hypoxia and birth asphyxia 34
Ischemic heart disease, see Heart disease.
Intervertebral disc disorders 90, 91

J

Japanese population, see Asian subgroups.

L

Leading causes of death 33, 34
    Age 34
    Hispanic origin population 33
    Race 33
Life expectancy 28, 29
    International 28
    Race 29
Limitation of activity 60
Liver disease, see Chronic liver disease and cirrhosis.
Low birthweight, see Births, Birthweight, low; Infant mortality, Birthweight.

M

Malignant neoplasms, see Cancer.
Mammography 80
Managed care, see Health maintenance organizations; Preferred provider organizations.
Marijuana use 64, 65
    Age 64
    Education 65
    Hispanic origin 64
    Students 65
Maternal mortality 45
Measles (Rubeola), see Diseases, notifiable; Vaccinations.
Medicaid 125, 133, 134, 139, 140, 147
    Basis of eligibility 139
    Coverage 133, 134
    Expenditures 125
    Geographic division and State 147
    Health maintenance organizations (HMO) 147
    Payments 147
    Recipients 147
    Type of service 140
Medical doctors, see Physicians.
Medicare 125, 134, 137, 138, 146
    Age and sex 138
    Coverage 134
    Enrollment 137, 138, 146
    Expenditures 125, 137
    Geographic division and State 146
    Geographic region 138
    Health maintenance organizations (HMO) 146
    Hospital utilization 138, 146
    Payments 138, 146
    Persons served per 1,000 enrollees 138
    Type of service 137
Meningitis 34
Meningococcal infection 34
Mental health care utilization 85, 97, 98
    Additions 85, 97, 98
    Age 97, 98
    Diagnosis, primary 98
    Race and sex 97
    Type of service 85
Mental health expenditures 129, 145
    Organization type 129
    State mental health agency 145

M—Con.

Mental health resources 105, 110
  Beds 110
  Organizations 110
  Patient care staff 105
Mexican population (see also Hispanic subgroups)
  Cholesterol, serum 69
  Hypertension 68
  Medical students 107, 108
  Overweight 70, 71
  Poverty level, persons and families below 2
MMR (Measles, Mumps, Rubella), see Vaccinations.
Motor vehicle-related injuries 31, 32, 46
Mumps, see Diseases, notifiable; Vaccinations.

N

National health expenditures, see Expenditures, national health.
Neonatal mortality, see Infant mortality.
Nephritis, nephrotic syndrome, nephrosis 33, 34
Newborn affected by complications of placenta, cord, and membranes 34
Newborn affected by maternal complications of pregnancy 34
Nulliparous women 4
Nurses, licensed practical 104, 106
  Full-time employees in community hospitals 104
  Schools 106
  Students 106
Nurses, registered (see also Mental health resources) 103, 104, 106, 107, 108
  Full-time employees in community hospitals 104
  Geographic region 103
  Schools 106
  Students 106, 107, 108
  Type of training 103, 106, 107
Nursing home employees 99
Nursing home expenditures 125, 127, 128
  Age and sex of residents 127
  Amount in billions 125
  Average monthly charges 127, 128
  Facility characteristics 127, 128
  Source of funds 125, 128
Nursing home utilization 95, 96
  Age, sex, and race 95, 96
  Functional status of residents 96
  Geographic region 96
Nursing homes 113, 114
  Beds 113, 114
  Beds per 1,000 population 113
  Number of nursing homes 113, 114
  Occupancy rate 114
  Resident rate 114
Nutrition-related
  Alcohol consumption 64, 65, 67
  Breastfeeding 19
  Cancer death rates 31, 32, 33, 34, 40
  Cancer incidence 58
  Cerebrovascular disease death rates (stroke) 31, 32, 33, 34, 39
  Cholesterol, serum 69
  Diabetes mellitus 31, 32, 33, 34, 91

N—Con.

Nutrition related—Con.
  Hypertension 70
  Infant mortality 20, 21, 22, 23, 24, 25, 26, 27, 34
  Ischemic heart disease. 32, 33
  Low birthweight. 11, 12, 13, 14
  Overweight. 70, 71

O

Occupational diseases. 50
Occupational injuries 51, 73
  Deaths. 51
  With lost workdays 73
Optometrists 103, 106, 107, 108
  Geographic region 103
  Schools. 106
  Students 106, 107, 108
Osteoarthritis. 90, 91
Osteopaths, see Physicians.
Outpatient department, see Hospital utilization, Outpatient department.
Overweight 70, 71
  Adults. 70
  Children 71

P

Perinatal mortality, see Infant mortality.
Personal health care expenditures, see Expenditures, national health.
Pertussis (whooping cough), see Diseases, notifiable; Vaccinations.
Pharmacists 103, 104, 106, 107, 108
  Employed in hospitals 104
  Geographic region 103
  Schools. 106
  Students 106, 107, 108
Physician expenditures (see also Consumer Price Index; Medicaid; Medicare) 125, 143
  Amount in billions. 125
  Geographic division and State 143
  Source of funds 125
Physician utilization (see also Access to care; Ambulatory care; Hospital utilization). 74, 75, 76, 77, 81, 82
  Family income. 74, 75, 77
  Geographic region 74, 75, 77
  Health status, respondent-assessed 76
  Interval since last physician contact 77
  Office visits to physicians 81, 82
  Physician contacts per person 74, 76
  Physician specialty. 82
  Place of physician contact. 75
  Poverty status. 76
  Residence within/outside metropolitan statistical area. 74, 75, 79
Physicians (see also Mental health resources) 99, 100, 101, 102, 103, 106, 107, 108
  Doctors of osteopathy 103, 106, 107, 108
  Employees, in offices of 99
  Geographic division and State 100
  Geographic region 103
  International medical school graduates. 101
  Primary care. 102

Physicians—Con.
  Primary specialty 101, 102
  Schools 106
  Students 106, 107, 108
Pneumonia and influenza 31, 32, 33, 34, 90, 91
  Deaths, Death rates 31, 33, 34
  Hospital utilization 90, 91
  Years of potential life lost 32
Podiatrists 103, 107, 108
  Geographic region 103
  Students 107, 108
Poliomyelitis (Polio), see Diseases, notifiable; Vaccinations.
Population, resident 1
Postneonatal mortality, see Infant mortality
Poverty status (see also Income, family) 2, 52, 76, 78, 79, 80, 83, 133, 134
  Access to care 78, 79
  Dental visits 83
  Health insurance 133, 134
  Mammography 80
  Medicaid 133, 134
  Persons and families below poverty level 2
  Physician contacts 76
  Vaccinations 52
Preferred provider organization (PPO) 136
Prenatal care, see Births.
Prescription drug expenditures (see also Consumer Price Index; Medicaid) 144
Psychoses 90, 91
Puerto Rican population (see also Hispanic subgroups)
  Medical students 107, 108
  Poverty level, persons and families below 2

R

Registered nurses, see Nurses, registered.
Respiratory distress syndrome 34
Rubella (German measles), see Diseases, notifiable; Vaccinations.

S

Salmonellosis, see Diseases, notifiable.
Self-assessment of health, see Health status, respondent-assessed.
Septicemia 33, 34
Shigellosis, see Diseases, notifiable.
Smoking, see Cigarette smoking.
Socioeconomic status, see Education; Income, family; Poverty status.
State data
  AIDS cases 57
  Alcohol abuse treatment clients 84
  Birthweight, low and very low 13, 14
  Death rates 30
  Drug abuse treatment clients 84
  Expenditures, hospital care 142
  Expenditures, physician 143
  Expenditures, prescription drug 144
  Expenditures, State mental health agency 145

S—Con.

State data—Con.
Health maintenance organizations (HMO) 146, 147, 148
Hospital beds 111
Hospital occupancy rates 112
Infant mortality 24, 25, 26
Medicaid 147
Medicare 146
Nursing homes 114
Nursing home beds 113, 114
Nursing home occupancy 114
Nursing home residents 114
Physicians 100
Substance abuse treatment clients 84
Uninsured, health 149
Vaccinations 53
Stroke, see Cerebrovascular disease.
Substance abuse treatment clients 84
Sudden infant death syndrome 34
Suicide 31, 32, 33, 34, 48
Surgery, see Hospital utilization.
Syphilis, see Diseases, notifiable.

T

Tetanus, see Diseases, notifiable; Vaccinations.
Tuberculosis, see Diseases, notifiable.

U

Uninsured, health, see Health insurance, Uninsured.
Unintentional injuries 31, 32, 33, 34
Urbanization, death rates 35

V

Vaccinations 52, 53
Veterans medical care 141

W

Wages and salaries 122
Women's health
Abortion 15, 16, 17
AIDS cases 55, 56
Alcohol consumption 64, 65, 67
Birth rates 3, 8
Births, number 5, 8
Breastfeeding 19
Cancer incidence rates 58
Cancer survival, 5-year relative 59
Childless women 4
Cholesterol, serum 69
Cigarette smoking 62, 63, 65
Cocaine use 64, 65, 66

Women's health—Con.

Contraception 18
Death rates, all causes 31, 35, 37
Death rates, selected causes 31, 38, 39, 40, 41, 42, 43, 44, 45, 46, 47, 48, 49
Deaths, number, leading causes 33
Dental students 108
Dental visits 83
Education of mother 9, 10, 12, 21
Educational attainment, death rates 36
Health insurance 133, 134
Health status, respondent-assessed 61
Home health care patients 86
Hospice patients 86
Hospital utilization, Emergency and Outpatient departments 81
Hospital utilization, inpatient 87, 88, 89, 90, 91, 92, 93
Hypertension 68
Inhalants 65
Life expectancy 28, 29
Limitation of activity 60
Mammography 80
Marijuana use 64, 65
Medical students 108
Medicare 138
Nursing home utilization 95, 96
Nursing students 108
Optometry students 108
Overweight 70
Pharmacy students 108
Physician utilization 74, 75, 76, 77, 81, 82
Population, resident 1
Poverty, families with female householder 2
Prenatal care 6
Region, death rates 35
Smoking status of mother 10, 11
Teenage childbearing 3, 7
Unmarried mothers 8
Urbanization, death rates 35
Years of potential life lost 32

Y

Years of potential life lost 32

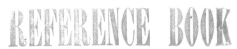

Health, United States, 1998

With Socioeconomic Status and Health Chartbook

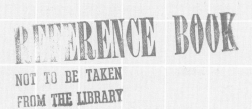

U.S. DEPARTMENT OF HEALTH AND HUMAN SERVICES
Centers for Disease Control and Prevention
National Center for Health Statistics
6525 Belcrest Road
Hyattsville, Maryland 20782

DHHS Publication number (PHS) 98-1232

D1299787

U.S. Department of Health and Human Services

Donna E. Shalala
Secretary

Office of Public Health and Science

David Satcher, M.D., Ph.D.
Assistant Secretary for Health

Centers for Disease Control and Prevention (CDC)

Claire V. Broome, M.D.
Acting Director

National Center for Health Statistics

Edward J. Sondik, Ph.D.
Director

For sale by the U.S. Government Printing Office
Superintendent of Documents, Mail Stop: SSOP, Washington, DC 20402-9328
ISBN 0-16-049631-4

Health, United States, 1998 is the 22d report on the health status of the Nation submitted by the Secretary of Health and Human Services to the President and Congress of the United States in compliance with Section 308 of the Public Health Service Act. This report was compiled by the Centers for Disease Control and Prevention (CDC), National Center for Health Statistics (NCHS). The National Committee on Vital and Health Statistics served in a review capacity.

Health, United States presents national trends in health statistics. Major findings are presented in the Highlights. The report includes a chartbook and detailed tables. In each edition of *Health, United States*, the chartbook focuses on a major health topic. This year socioeconomic status and health was selected as the subject of the chartbook. The chartbook consists of 49 figures and accompanying text divided into sections on the population, children's health, and adults' health. The sections on children's and adults' health include subsections on health status, risk factors, and health care access and utilization.

The chartbook is followed by 149 detailed tables organized around four major subject areas: health status and determinants, utilization of health resources, health care resources, and health care expenditures. A major criterion used in selecting the detailed tables is the availability of comparable national data over a period of several years. The detailed tables report data for selected years to highlight major trends in health statistics. Similar tables appear in each volume of *Health, United States* to enhance the use of this publication as a standard reference source. For tables that show extended trends, earlier editions of *Health, United States* may present data for intervening years that are not included in the current printed report. Where possible, intervening years in an extended trend are retained in the Lotus 1–2–3 spreadsheet files (described below).

Several tables in *Health, United States* present data according to race and Hispanic origin consistent with Department-wide emphasis on expanding racial and ethnic detail in the presentation of health data. The presentation of data on race and ethnicity in the detailed tables is usually in the greatest detail possible, after taking into account the quality of data, the amount of missing data, and the number of observations. The large differences in health status according to race and Hispanic origin that are documented in this report may be explained by several factors including socioeconomic status, health practices, psychosocial stress and resources, environmental exposures, discrimination, and access to health care.

Each year new tables are added to *Health, United States* to reflect emerging topics in public health and new variables are added to existing tables to enhance their usefulness. *Health, United States, 1998* includes the following four new tables. For the first time vaccination rates for children 19–35 months of age are provided for States and selected urban areas (table 53); access to health care according to poverty status and health insurance status is measured by no physican contact in the past year for children under 6 years of age and by no usual source of care for children under 18 years of age (tables 78 and 79); and data on medical care benefits for employees of private companies are presented (table 136). The following enhancements were made to existing tables. Data for racial and ethnic groups were expanded in tables showing years of potential life lost rates (table 32) and maternal mortality rates (table 45). Data by race were added to other tables as follows: the poverty rate in 1990 among the American Indian population (NOTE, table 2); vaccination rates for children by race and poverty status (table 52); and functional status of nursing home residents by race, sex, and age (table 96). Data on health care coverage were expanded to include employer-sponsored private insurance and additional race, age, and poverty status subgroups (tables 133 and 134). To address heightened interest in persons 55–64 years of age approaching Medicare eligibility, data by age were expanded for ambulatory care visits (tables 81 and 82). The percent of Medicare enrollees in managed care and the percent of Medicaid recipients in managed care in each State were added to tables 146 and 147.

To use *Health, United States* most effectively, the reader should become familiar with two appendixes at the end of the report. Appendix I describes each data source used in the report and provides references for further information about the sources. Appendix II is an alphabetical listing of terms used in the report. It also contains standard populations used for age adjustment and *International Classification of Diseases* codes for cause of death and diagnostic and procedure categories.

Health, United States can be accessed electronically in several formats. First, the entire *Health, United States, 1998* is available, along with other NCHS reports, on a CD-ROM entitled "Publications from the National Center for Health Statistics, featuring *Health, United States, 1998*," vol 1 no 4, 1998. These publications can be viewed, searched, printed, and saved using the Adobe Acrobat software on the CD-ROM. The CD-ROM may be purchased from the Government Printing Office or the National Technical Information Service.

Second, the complete *Health, United States, 1998* is available as an Acrobat .pdf file on the Internet through the NCHS home page on the World Wide Web. The direct Uniform Locator Code (URL) address is:

www.cdc.gov/nchswww/products/pubs/pubd/hus/hus.htm.

Third, the 149 detailed tables in *Health, United States, 1998* are available on the FTP server as Lotus 1–2–3 spreadsheet files that can be downloaded. An electronic index is included that enables the user to search the tables by topic. The URL address for the FTP server is:

www.cdc.gov/nchswww/datawh/ftpserv/ftpserv.htm.

The detailed tables and electronic index are also included as Lotus 1–2–3 spreadsheet files on the CD-ROM mentioned above.

Fourth, for users who do not have access to the Internet or to a CD-ROM reader, the 149 detailed tables can be made available on diskette as Lotus 1–2–3 spreadsheet files for use with IBM compatible personal computers. To obtain a copy of the diskette, contact the NCHS Data Dissemination Branch.

For answers to questions about this report, contact:

Data Dissemination Branch
National Center for Health Statistics
Centers for Disease Control and Prevention
6525 Belcrest Road, Room 1064
Hyattsville, Maryland 20782-2003

phone: 301-436-8500

E-mail: nchsquery@cdc.gov

Overall responsibility for planning and coordinating the content of this volume rested with the Office of Analysis, Epidemiology, and Health Promotion, National Center for Health Statistics (NCHS), under the supervision of Kate Prager, Diane M. Makuc, and Jacob J. Feldman. Highlights of the detailed tables were written by Margaret A. Cooke, Virginia M. Freid, Michael E. Mussolino, and Kate Prager. Detailed tables were prepared by Alan J. Cohen, Margaret A. Cooke, Virginia M. Freid, Michael E. Mussolino, Mitchell B. Pierre, Jr., Rebecca A. Placek, and Kate Prager with assistance from La-Tonya Curl, Catherine Duran, Deborah D. Ingram, Patricia A. Knapp, Jaleh Mousavi, Mark F. Pioli, Anita L. Powell, Ronica N. Rooks, Kenneth C. Schoendorf, Fred Seitz, and Jean F. Williams. The appendixes, index to detailed tables, and pocket edition were prepared by Anita L. Powell. Production planning and coordination were managed by Rebecca A. Placek with typing assistance from Carole J. Hunt.

The chartbook was prepared by Elsie R. Pamuk, Diane M. Makuc, Katherine E. Heck, Cynthia Reuben, and Kimberly Lochner in the Office of Analysis, Epidemiology, and Health Promotion under the general direction of Jacob J. Feldman. Data for specific charts were provided by Sylvia A. Ellison (figure 23) and Lois A. Fingerhut (figures 30–31) of NCHS; Joseph Gfroerer of the Substance Abuse and Mental Health Administration (figure 37); and Paul Sorlie of the National Heart, Lung, and Blood Institute (figure 25). Technical help was provided by Alan J. Cohen and Catherine Duran of TRW, Information Services Division; Laura Porter, Joyce Abma, Debra Brody, Catherine W. Burt, Margaret Carroll, Margaret A. Cooke, Virginia M. Freid, Wilbur C. Hadden, Tamy Hickman, Meena Khare, John L. Kiely, Patricia A. Knapp, Lola Jean Kozak, Jeffrey D. Maurer, Laura E. Montgomery, Cynthia Ogden, Linda W. Pickle, Mitchell B. Pierre, Jr., Ronica N. Rooks, Kenneth C. Schoendorf, Richard P. Troiano, Kathleen M. Turczyn, and Clemencia M. Vargas of NCHS; Edmond F. Maes

of the National Immunization Program, CDC; and Deborah Dawson of the National Institute on Alcohol Abuse and Alcoholism.

Dr. Philip R. Lee, former Assistant Secretary for Health and currently at the University of California at San Francisco, was instrumental in the development of the chartbook. Dr. Lee has long been committed to the study of the relationship between socioeconomic status and health and to applying the knowledge gained to improving the health of disadvantaged populations. Advice and encouragement was also graciously provided by the following individuals: Dr. Norman Anderson of the National Institutes of Health; Dr. A. John Fox of the Office for National Statistics, England; Dr. George Kaplan of the University of Michigan; Dr. Roz Lasker of the New York Academy of Medicine; Dr. Paul Newacheck of the University of California at San Francisco; and Dr. David Williams of the University of Michigan.

Publications management and editorial review were provided by Thelma W. Sanders and Rolfe W. Larson. The designer was Sarah M. Hinkle. Graphics were supervised by Stephen L. Sloan. Production was done by Jacqueline M. Davis and Annette F. Holman. Printing was managed by Patricia L. Wilson and Joan D. Burton.

Publication of *Health, United States* would not have been possible without the contributions of numerous staff members throughout the National Center for Health Statistics and several other agencies. These people gave generously of their time and knowledge, providing data from their surveys and programs; their cooperation and assistance are gratefully acknowledged.

Contents

Preface.. iii

Acknowledgments... v

List of Figures on Socioeconomic Status and Health.................................. ix

Geographic Regions and Divisions of the United States............................... xi

Highlights
Socioeconomic Status and Health Chartbook... 3
Detailed Tables.. 9

Socioeconomic Status and Health Chartbook

Introduction... 23

Population... 29
    Income... 32
    Poverty.. 36
    Education.. 40
    Occupation... 44

Children's Health.. 46
    Health Status
        Infant Mortality... 50
        Low Birthweight.. 54
        Activity Limitation.. 56
    Risk Factors
        Teenage Childbearing... 58
        Smoking in Pregnancy... 60
        Blood Lead... 62
        Cigarette Smoking.. 64
        Overweight... 66
        Sedentary Lifestyle.. 68
    Health Care Access and Utilization
        Prenatal Care.. 70
        Health Insurance... 74
        Vaccinations... 76
        No Physician Contact... 78
        Ambulatory Care.. 80
        Asthma Hospitalization... 82

Adults' Health.. 84
    Health Status
        Life Expectancy.. 88
        Cause of Death... 90
        Heart Disease Mortality.. 92
        Lung Cancer Mortality.. 94
        Diabetes Mortality... 96
        Homicide... 98
        Suicide.. 100
        Fair or Poor Health.. 102
        Activity Limitation.. 104
        Activities of Daily Living... 106

Contents ....

Risk Factors
    Cigarette Smoking _____ 108
    Alcohol Use _____ 112
    Overweight _____ 114
    Sedentary Lifestyle _____ 118
    Hypertension _____ 120
    Blood Lead _____ 122
Health Care Access and Utilization
    Health Insurance _____ 124
    No Physician Contact _____ 126
    Mammography _____ 128
    Unmet Need for Care _____ 130
    Avoidable Hospitalization _____ 134
    Dental Care _____ 136

Technical Notes _____ 138
Data Tables for Figures 1–49 _____ 144

Detailed Tables

List of Detailed Tables _____ 163

Health Status and Determinants _____ 169
    Population _____ 169
    Fertility and Natality _____ 172
    Mortality _____ 190
    Determinants and Measures of Health _____ 261
Utilization of Health Resources _____ 287
    Ambulatory Care _____ 287
    Inpatient Care _____ 302
Health Care Resources _____ 321
    Personnel _____ 321
    Facilities _____ 334
Health Care Expenditures _____ 341
    National Health Expenditures _____ 341
    Health Care Coverage and Major Federal Programs _____ 361
    State Health Expenditures _____ 372

Appendixes

Contents _____ 383
I. Sources and Limitations of Data _____ 386
II. Glossary _____ 419

Index to Detailed Tables _____ 446

Population

1. Household income at selected percentiles of the household income distribution: United States, 1970–96__ 33

2. Median household income by race and Hispanic origin: United States, 1980–96_____ 35

3. Percent of persons poor and near poor by race and Hispanic origin: United States, 1996_____ 37

4. Percent of persons in poverty by State: United States, average annual 1994–96_____ 39

5. Educational attainment among persons 25 years of age and over by age, race, and Hispanic origin: United States, 1996_____ 41

6. Median household income among persons 25 years of age and over by education, sex, race, and Hispanic origin: United States, 1996_____ 43

7. Current occupation for persons 25–64 years of age by sex, race, and Hispanic origin: United States, 1996_____ 45

Children's Health

Health Status

8. Infant mortality rates among infants of mothers 20 years of age and over by mother's education and race: United States, 1983–95_____ 51

9. Infant mortality rates among infants of mothers 20 years of age and over by mother's education, race, and Hispanic origin: United States, 1995_____ 53

10. Low-birthweight live births among mothers 20 years of age and over by mother's education, race, and Hispanic origin: United States, 1996_____ 55

11. Activity limitation among children under 18 years of age by family income, race, and Hispanic origin: United States, average annual, 1984–87, 1988–91, and 1992–95_____ 56

Risk Factors

12. Percent of women 20–29 years of age who had a teenage birth, by respondent's mother's education and respondent's race and Hispanic origin: United States, 1995_____ 59

13. Cigarette smoking during pregnancy among mothers 20 years of age and over by mother's education, race, and Hispanic origin: United States, 1996_____ 61

14. Elevated blood lead among children 1–5 years of age by family income, race, and Hispanic origin: United States, average annual 1988–94_____ 62

15. Cigarette smoking among adolescents 12–17 years of age by family income, race, and Hispanic origin: United States, 1992_____ 65

16. Overweight among adolescents 12–17 years of age by family income, race, and Hispanic origin: United States, average annual 1988–94_____ 67

17. Sedentary lifestyle among adolescents 12–17 years of age by family income and sex: United States, 1992__ 69

Health Care Access and Utilization

18. Prenatal care use in the first trimester among mothers 20 years of age and over by mother's education and race: United States, 1980–96_____ 71

19. Prenatal care use in the first trimester among mothers 20 years of age and over by mother's education, race, and Hispanic origin: United States, 1996_____ 73

20. Percent of children under 18 years of age with no health insurance coverage by family income, race, and Hispanic origin: United States, average annual 1994–95_ 75

21. Vaccinations among children 19–35 months of age by poverty status, race, and Hispanic origin: United States, 1996_____ 77

22. Percent of children under 6 years of age with no physician contact during the past year by family income, health insurance status, race, and Hispanic origin: United States, average annual 1994–95_____ 78

23. Ambulatory care visits among children under 18 years of age by median household income in ZIP Code of residence and place of visit: United States, 1995_____ 81

24. Asthma hospitalization rates among children 1–14 years of age by median household income in ZIP Code of residence and race: United States, average annual 1989–91_____ 83

Adults' Health

Health Status

25. Life expectancy among adults 45 and 65 years of age by family income, sex, and race: United States, average annual 1979–89_____ 89

26. Death rates for selected causes for adults 25–64 years of age, by education level and sex: Selected States, 1995_____ 91

27. Heart disease death rates among adults 25–64 years of age and 65 years of age and over by family income, sex, race, and Hispanic origin: United States, average annual 1979–89_____ 92

List of Figures

28. Lung cancer death rates among adults 25–64 years of age and 65 years of age and over by family income and sex: United States, average annual 1979–89 _____ **95**

29. Diabetes death rates among adults 45 years of age and over by family income and sex: United States, average annual 1979–89 _____ **97**

30. Homicide rates among adults 25–44 years of age by education, sex, race, and Hispanic origin: Selected States, average annual 1994–95 _____ **99**

31. Suicide rates among adults 25–64 years of age by education, sex, race and Hispanic origin: Selected States, average annual 1994–95 _____ **101**

32. Fair or poor health among adults 18 years of age and over by family income, sex, race, and Hispanic origin: United States, 1995 _____ **103**

33. Activity limitation among adults 18–64 years of age by family income, race, and Hispanic origin: United States average annual, 1984–87, 1988–91, and 1992–95 _____ **104**

34. Difficulties with one or more activities of daily living among adults 70 years of age and over by family income and sex: United States, 1995 _____ **107**

Risk Factors

35. Cigarette smoking among adults 25 years of age and over by education and sex: United States, 1974–95 _____ **109**

36. Cigarette smoking among adults 18 years of age and over, by family income, sex, race, and Hispanic origin: United States, 1995 _____ **110**

37. Heavy alcohol use during the past month among adults 25–49 years of age by education, sex, race, and Hispanic origin: United States, average annual 1994–96 _____ **112**

38. Overweight among adults 25–74 years of age by sex and education: United States, average annual 1971–74, 1976–80, and 1988–94 _____ **115**

39. Overweight among adults 20 years of age and over by family income, sex, race, and Hispanic origin: United States, average annual 1988–94 _____ **116**

40. Sedentary lifestyle among adults 18 years of age and over by family income, sex, race, and Hispanic origin: United States, 1991 _____ **119**

41. Hypertension among adults 20 years of age and over by family income, sex, race, and Hispanic origin: United States, average annual 1988–94 _____ **120**

42. Elevated blood lead among men 20 years of age and over, by family income, race, and Hispanic origin: United States, average annual 1988–94 _____ **122**

Health Care Access and Utilization

43. No health insurance coverage among adults 18–64 years of age by family income, race, and Hispanic origin, United States, average annual 1994–95 _____ **125**

44. No physician contact within the past year among adults 18–64 years of age with a health problem by family income, race, and Hispanic origin: United States, average annual 1994–95 _____ **127**

45. Mammography within the past 2 years among women 50 years of age and over by family income, race, and Hispanic origin: United States, average annual 1993–94 _____ **128**

46. Unmet need for health care during the past year among adults 18–64 years of age, by family income, age, and sex: United States, average annual 1994–95 _____ **131**

47. Unmet need for health care during the past year among adults 65 years of age and over by family income, race, and Hispanic origin: United States, average annual 1994–95 _____ **132**

48. Avoidable hospitalizations among adults 18–64 years of age by median household income in ZIP Code of residence and race: United States, average annual 1989–91 _____ **135**

49. Dental visit within the past year among adults 18–64 years of age by family income, race, and Hispanic origin: United States, 1993 _____ **136**

Geographic Regions and Divisions of the United States

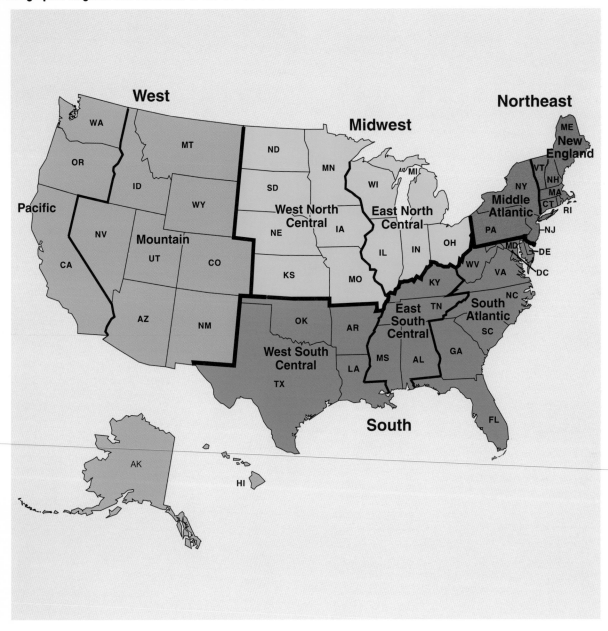

Population

■   **Income inequality** in the United States increased between 1970 and 1996. The growth in inequality was due primarily to larger increases in income among high-income than low-income households. While income increased by 5–7 percent in constant dollars for households in the 20th and the 50th percentiles of income, those at the 80th percentile experienced a 22 percent increase in their earnings, and the income of those in the 95th percentile increased by 36 percent (figure 1).

■   Children under 18 years of age were 40 percent more likely to live in **poverty** than was the population as a whole in 1996 (20 compared with 14 percent). Children in female-headed households were particularly unlikely to have adequate incomes. One-half of children in female-headed households were poor in 1996 and an additional 27 percent were near poor. Black and Hispanic children and adults were more likely than non-Hispanic white or Asian persons to be poor or near poor. On the whole, black persons and Hispanic persons had a poverty rate about 3.3 times that of non-Hispanic white persons (figure 3).

■   State **poverty** rates in 1994–96 varied more than threefold from 7 to 24 percent. Higher rates of poverty tended to be found in Southern and Southwestern States, while lower rates were found among New England and North Central States (figure 4).

■   Between 1980 and 1996 **median household incomes** increased about 5 percent in constant dollars. Non-Hispanic white households saw a 7 percent rise in their median incomes and black households a 14 percent rise, while Hispanic incomes declined by 4 percent. In 1996 Asian or Pacific Islander households had the highest median income, around $43,300, with non-Hispanic white incomes slightly less, at about $38,800; incomes of black and Hispanic households were similar and substantially lower: $23,500 and $24,900, respectively (figure 2).

■   In 1996 median **family incomes** rose with each higher level of **education** for men and women in each race and ethnic group. Among non-Hispanic white, non-Hispanic black, and Hispanic persons the ratio of median family income of college graduates to median income of those with less than a high school education ranged from 2.4–2.7 for men and from 2.9–3.6 for women. This ratio was 1.8–2.0 for Asian women and men (figure 6).

■   Asian or Pacific Islander adults had the most **education** as well as the largest proportion of men whose **occupation** was white collar. Fully 45 percent of Asian or Pacific Islander persons 25–64 years of age had 16 or more years of education in 1996, compared with 29 percent of non-Hispanic white persons, 15 percent of non-Hispanic black persons, and 10 percent of Hispanic persons. Conversely, 44 percent of Hispanic adults 25–64 years of age had less than 12 years of education, compared with 20 percent of non-Hispanic black adults, 14 percent of Asian or Pacific Islander adults, and 10 percent of non-Hispanic white adults. Education levels were lower among adults 65 and over; in each race and ethnic group, 6 to 20 percent of adults in this age group had 16 or more years of education. The distribution of occupational categories by race and ethnicity reflected the educational patterns in race and ethnic groups. A majority of Asian or Pacific Islander and non-Hispanic white men worked in white collar occupations, while a plurality (almost one-half) of non-Hispanic black and Hispanic men were classified as blue collar. A majority (52 to 78 percent) of women in every race and ethnic group were classified as white collar. Non-Hispanic black and Hispanic men and women were about twice as likely as their non-Hispanic white counterparts to be in service occupations. More than one-quarter of Hispanic and black women were in service jobs as were 15–18 percent of non-Hispanic black and Hispanic men (figures 5 and 7).

Children's Health

■ **Infant mortality** declined between 1983 and 1995 for infants of black and white mothers at all educational levels, but substantial socioeconomic disparities remained in 1995. **Low birthweight** and infant mortality were more common among the children of less educated mothers than among children of more educated mothers; for example, in 1995, infants born to non-Hispanic white mothers with less than 12 years of education were 2.4 times as likely to die in the first year of life as those whose mothers had at least 16 years of education. However, not all race and ethnic groups demonstrated identical patterns; a relationship between maternal education and these infant health outcomes was more apparent for non-Hispanic white, non-Hispanic black, and American Indian or Alaska Native infants than for Asian or Pacific Islander and Hispanic infants (figures 8, 9, and 10).

■ Mothers with more education are more likely to have received early **prenatal care** than less educated mothers; in 1996 mothers with 16 or more years of education were 40 percent more likely to obtain first-trimester prenatal care than those with fewer than 12 years of education. Mothers with fewer than 12 years of education were almost 10 times as likely to **smoke during pregnancy** as mothers with 16 or more years of education in 1996. These maternal risk factors are likely contributors to the higher incidence of low birthweight and infant mortality among the infants of less-educated mothers (figures 8–10, 13, 18, and 19).

■ The relationship between maternal education and health differed for **Hispanic** mothers and their infants compared with non-Hispanic mothers and infants. Non-Hispanic white mothers with fewer than 12 years of education were 80 percent more likely to have a low birthweight infant than those with a college degree. However, the incidence of **low birthweight** among Hispanic infants did not vary by mother's education. The relationship between mother's education and both low birthweight and **smoking during pregnancy**

varied according to Hispanic subgroup; for example, Puerto Rican and Cuban American mothers were less likely to smoke during pregnancy if they had higher education levels, but there was no relationship with education for Mexican American and Central and South American mothers, all of whom were unlikely to smoke during pregnancy. Although an inverse educational gradient was found for Hispanic infant mortality, the relationship was weaker for Hispanic infants (40 percent higher mortality in infants of the least educated compared with the most educated mothers) than for non-Hispanic white infants (140 percent higher) (figures 9, 10, and 13).

■ Young children who are exposed to environmental lead may be at risk for a range of mental and physical problems. **Elevated blood lead levels** were more common among poor children and among black children than among children of other groups. Children 1–5 years of age living in poor families in 1988–94 were over seven times as likely to have an elevated blood lead level as children in high-income families. Over one in five non-Hispanic black children who were poor had an elevated level of blood lead, compared with 8 percent of poor non-Hispanic white children and 6 percent of poor Mexican American children (figure 14).

■ Early childbearing is more common among girls from lower socioeconomic-status families. According to a 1995 survey, women in their twenties whose mothers did not finish high school were about five times as likely to have had a **teenage birth** as those whose mothers had 4 years of college education. The adolescent mothers, now in their twenties, had lower family incomes than women the same age who had not had a teenage birth (figure 12).

■ In 1992 non-Hispanic white girls and boys 12–17 years of age from poor families were 45 percent more likely to **smoke** cigarettes than similar adolescents from middle- or high-income families, while poor non-Hispanic black teen boys were almost 3 times as likely to smoke as those from middle- or high-income

families. There was no relationship between family income and smoking for non-Hispanic black girls, while for Hispanic girls the pattern was reversed: those from middle- or high-income families were 60 percent more likely to smoke than those from poor families. However, smoking prevalence tended to differ more by race and ethnicity than by family income: smoking was most common among non-Hispanic white teens, somewhat less common among Hispanic teens, and least common among non-Hispanic black teens. For example, in 1992 among poor adolescents, the proportion who smoked was 33 percent for non-Hispanic white males, 23 percent for Hispanic males, and 12 percent for non-Hispanic black males (figure 15).

■ **Overweight** was inversely related to family income among non-Hispanic white adolescents, but not among Mexican American or non-Hispanic black adolescents. The percent of poor non-Hispanic white adolescents who were overweight during 1988–94 (19 percent) was about 2.6 times that for middle- or high-income adolescents (7 percent). **Sedentary lifestyle** was inversely related to family income among teenage girls and to a lesser extent among teenage boys. Poor female adolescents were more than twice as likely as those with high incomes to be sedentary. Girls were more likely than boys to be sedentary, and this difference was most pronounced among lower income youths. Among the poor and near poor, girls were 70–80 percent more likely than boys to be sedentary (figures 16 and 17).

■ Children from higher income families are more likely to have **health insurance** coverage than those from lower income families. More than one in five poor and near-poor children had no health insurance in 1994–95, while 9 percent of middle-income children and 4 percent of high-income children were uninsured. These differences were reflected in less use of health care for low-income children. During 1994–95, poor and near-poor children under 6 years of age were only about one-half as likely to have seen a physician in the

prior year as middle- or high-income children. Uninsured children were particularly unlikely to have seen a doctor, especially if they were poor: almost one-quarter of poor uninsured young children had not seen a doctor in the past year, compared with about 1 in 12 poor children with health insurance. Poor uninsured children were almost twice as likely to have had **no recent physician contacts** as middle or upper income uninsured children. When children in lower income areas received **ambulatory care** in 1995, it was less likely to be at a physician's office and more likely to be at a hospital emergency room: 22 percent of visits among children living in areas where the median income was less than $20,000 took place in emergency rooms, while only 8 percent of visits were in emergency rooms for children living in areas where the median income was at least $40,000 (figures 20, 22, and 23 and table 78).

■ Children in lower income families are less likely to receive needed health care. In 1996 two-thirds of poor children 19–35 months of age had been fully **vaccinated**, compared with more than three-quarters of those above the poverty level. Children 1–14 years of age living in low-income areas were more than twice as likely to be **hospitalized for asthma** as those in high-income areas during 1989–91, suggesting they may have been unable to receive outpatient care that could prevent such a hospitalization (figures 21 and 24).

Adults' Health

■ **Life expectancy** is related to family income; people with lower family income tend to die at younger ages than those with higher income. During 1979–89 white men who were 45 years of age and who had a family income of at least $25,000 could expect to live 6.6 years longer than men with family income less than $10,000 (33.9 years compared with 27.3 years). Among black men, the difference in life expectancy at age 45 between those with low and high incomes was 7.4 years; among white women, 2.7

years, and among black women, 3.8 years. At age 65, when life expectancy was shorter, the income disparities were somewhat less: the disparity in life expectancy between the lowest and highest income persons was 1.0 to 3.1 years, depending on sex and race (figure 25).

■ Among persons 25–64 years of age **death rates for chronic diseases, communicable diseases, and injuries** are all inversely related to education for men and women. In 1995 the death rate for chronic diseases among men with less than 12 years of education was 2.5 times that for men with more than 12 years education and among women the comparable ratio was 2.1. For men and women non-HIV communicable disease mortality among the least educated was three times that of the most educated. The education gradient in HIV mortality was much stronger among women than men. The ratio of the death rate for injuries for the least educated to the rate for most educated was 3.4 for men and 2.3 for women in 1995 (figure 26).

■ Less educated men and women have higher rates of **homicide** and **suicide** than those with more education. In 1994–95 homicide rates for adults 25–44 years of age were between three (for Hispanic women) and nine (for non-Hispanic white men) times as high among those with less than 12 years of education as among those with 13 or more years of education. In 1994–95 suicide rates for 25–44 year old men and women with less than 13 years of education were generally about twice the rates for those with more education. For non-Hispanic white men, however, suicide rates for the less educated were close to 4 times the rates for those with 13 or more years of education. (figures 30 and 31).

■ Adults with low incomes are far more likely than those with higher incomes to report **fair or poor health** status. In 1995 poor adults 18 years of age and over were about four to seven times as likely (depending on race, ethnicity, and sex) as high-income adults to report that their health status was fair or poor.

Poor persons 18–64 years of age were about three times as likely as middle- or high-income persons to report **limitations in activities** due to chronic conditions (34 percent compared with 11 percent in 1992–95). The gap between poor and middle- or high-income persons widened slightly between 1984–87 and 1992–95, primarily due to a 17 percent increase in the percent reporting limitations among poor non-Hispanic white adults. In addition, adults 70 years of age and over with low incomes were more likely than higher income older persons to report difficulty with **activities of daily living** (the ability to perform routine personal care); in 1995, 36 percent of poor men and 43 percent of poor women reported difficulty with activities of daily living while 20 percent of middle- or high-income men and 28 percent of middle- or high-income women reported such limitations (figures 32, 33, and 34).

■ Cigarette **smoking** among adults 25 years of age and over declined between 1974 and 1995, but rates of decline were steeper among more educated adults. While smoking rates declined 51 percent among men with 16 or more years of education, they declined 24 percent among those with less than a high school education. Declines for women were similar (down 49 percent for the college educated, compared with a drop of 13 percent among those who did not finish high school). In 1995 the least educated men and women were more than twice as likely to smoke as the most educated. Smoking also varies inversely with income. In 1995 poor non-Hispanic white, non-Hispanic black, and Hispanic persons 18 years of age and over were 1.2–2.0 times as likely to smoke as those with middle or high income (figures 35 and 36).

■ Higher prevalence of cigarette smoking among those of lower socioeconomic status was manifested in elevated **lung cancer and heart disease** death rates for lower income adults during 1979–89. Men with family incomes less than $10,000 were more than twice as likely to die of lung cancer as those earning at least $25,000. Among women, whose smoking and

mortality rates were lower, there was no clear income gradient in lung cancer mortality during 1979–89. However, heart disease mortality was higher among those with lower incomes, regardless of sex, age, or race (figures 27 and 28).

■ Between 1971–74 and 1988–94 the prevalence of **overweight** increased by 20 to 80 percent, depending on sex and education level. By 1988–94, overweight prevalence was similar among men with less than 12, 12, or 13 to 15 years of education (37–40 percent), but men with 16 or more years of education were less likely to be overweight (28 percent). There were significant educational differences in the prevalence of overweight for women during 1988–94; each increase in education level was associated with a decline in the percent of women who were overweight, from 46 percent among women with less than 12 years of education, down to 26 percent among women with 16 or more years of education. Prevalence of overweight was similar for men of different income levels but it varied inversely with income among women. Non-Hispanic white and Mexican American (but not non-Hispanic black) women with lower income were more likely to be overweight than their higher income counterparts. **Hypertension** was also more common among lower income women in 1988–94. Poor women were 1.6 times as likely as high-income women to be hypertensive. **Sedentary lifestyle** is more common among lower income persons as well; in 1991 poor persons were 1.6 to 3.1 times as likely to be sedentary as high-income persons, depending on sex, race, and ethnicity. Overweight and sedentary persons are more likely to develop **diabetes**; in 1979–89 the death rate for diabetes among low–income women was three times that for high income women and the income gradient in diabetes mortality was only slightly less steep for men (figures 29, 38, 39, 40, and 41).

■ Heavy and chronic alcohol use can cause cirrhosis, poor pregnancy outcomes, and motor vehicle crashes as well as other health problems. In 1994–96 the percent of men and women 25–49 years of age

reporting **heavy alcohol use** (five or more drinks on at least one occasion in the past month) was 30 percent higher among those with less than a high school education than among college graduates and men were almost three times as likely as women to report heavy drinking during the past month. The percent of heavy alcohol use varied by education and sex from 9 percent among college-educated women to 32 percent among men with less than a high school education (figure 37).

■ Adults under age 65 with low family incomes are less likely to have **health insurance coverage** than higher income adults. In 1994–95 poor men were six to seven times as likely to be uninsured as high-income men, depending on race and ethnicity, while poor women were four to eight times as likely as high-income women to be uninsured. Among the poor and the near poor, coverage for women was somewhat higher than among men, due primarily to higher proportions of women than men with Medicaid coverage. In most income groups, non-Hispanic white and non-Hispanic black adults were more likely to be insured than Hispanic adults (figure 43).

■ The use of sick care, preventive care, and dental care by adults varies with income. Among adults 18–64 years of age who report a health problem there is a strong inverse income gradient in the percent with **no recent physician contact,** and the gradient is similar across race and ethnic groups. In 1994–95 poor women with a health problem were almost three times as likely, and poor men with a health problem almost twice as likely, not to have seen a doctor within the past year as high-income men and women. There is a strong direct relationship between income and use of recent **mammography**. During 1993–94, high-income women 50 years of age and over were about 70 percent more likely than poor women to have received a mammogram in the past 2 years. In 1993 the percent of adults 18–64 years of age with a **dental visit** within the past 12 months rose sharply with income from 41 percent among the poor to 77 percent

among those with high family income (figures 44, 45, and 49).

■ Poor persons were far more likely than middle- or high-income persons to report an **unmet need for health care**. Among adults 18–64 years of age, about one-third of poor persons reported an unmet need for care in 1994–95, compared with about 7 percent of high-income persons; among adults 65 years of age and over, about one-fifth of the poor reported an unmet need, compared with 2 percent of high-income persons. Although the elderly have more health care needs than younger persons, almost universal Medicare coverage among the elderly assisted older adults in obtaining needed care (figures 46 and 47).

■ **Avoidable hospitalizations** are hospital stays for conditions that may be preventable with appropriate outpatient care. In 1989–91 the rate of **avoidable hospitalizations** among adults 18–64 years of age living in areas where median incomes were lowest (less than $20,000) was 2.4 times the rate among those living in areas where incomes were highest ($40,000 or more) (figure 48).

.... Highlights

Tables

Health Status and Determinants

Population

■ In 1996 some 58 million children under the age of 15 years comprised the U.S. population, which totaled 265 million persons. Populations of **Asian or Pacific Islander children and Hispanic children** in the United States are increasing more rapidly than children in the U.S. population as a whole. Between 1990 and 1996 the average annual rate of increase was 4.5 percent for Asian or Pacific Islander children and 4.1 percent for Hispanic children compared with 1.2 percent for all U.S. children (table 1).

Fertility and Natality

■ In 1996 the **birth rate** for teenagers declined for the fifth consecutive year to 54.4 births per 1,000 women aged 15–19 years. Between 1991 and 1996 the teen birth rate declined 12 percent, with larger reductions for 15–17 year-olds than for 18–19 year-olds (13 percent compared with 9 percent) and larger reductions for black than for white teens (21 percent compared with 9 percent). In 1996 the overall fertility rate declined slightly from 65.6 to 65.3 births per 1,000 women 15–44 years of age, after declining at an average annual rate of 1.5 percent between 1990 and 1995 (table 3).

■ Between 1994 and 1996 the percent of **births to unmarried mothers** remained essentially level at about 32–33 percent following a threefold increase between 1970 and 1994. Between 1994 and 1996 the birth rate for unmarried black women declined 9 percent to 74 births per 1,000 unmarried black women aged 15–44 years and the birth rate for unmarried Hispanic women declined 8 percent to 93 per 1,000 while the birth rate for unmarried non-Hispanic white women remained stable at about 28 per 1,000 (table 8).

■ A trend toward **delayed childbearing** in the United States that began in the mid- to late-1960's has been relatively stable since 1985. The percent of women 25–29 years of age who had not had at least

one live birth increased from 20 percent in 1965 to 42 percent in 1985 and 44 percent in 1990–96. Among women 30–34 years of age, the percent who had not had at least one live birth increased from 12 percent in 1970 to 25 percent in 1985 and 26 percent in 1987–96 (table 4).

■ **Low birthweight** is associated with elevated risk of death and disability in infants. In 1996 the incidence of low birthweight (less than 2,500 grams) among live-born infants was 7.4 percent. Between 1991 and 1996 low birthweight increased among white infants from 5.8 to 6.3 percent and decreased among black infants from 13.6 to 13.0 percent. Between 1991 and 1996 the incidence of very low birthweight (less than 1,500 grams) rose slightly for white infants from 1.0 to 1.1 percent and was stable at 3.0 percent for black infants (table 11).

■ In 1995 **mortality for low-birthweight infants** (weighing less than 2,500 grams at birth) was 22 times that for infants of normal weight (2,500 grams or more) (65.3 compared with 3.0 deaths per 1,000 live births). In 1995 mortality for very low birthweight infants (weighing less than 1,500 grams at birth) was 90 times that for infants of normal weight (table 22).

Mortality

■ In 1996 the **infant mortality rate** fell to a record low of 7.3 deaths per 1,000 live births, continuing the longterm downward trend in infant mortality. In 1996 mortality also reached record low rates for black infants (14.7) and white infants (6.1) (table 23).

■ In 1995 **infant mortality** for Puerto Rican and American Indian infants (8.9 and 9.0 deaths per 1,000 live births) was about 40 percent higher than mortality for non-Hispanic white infants. Compared with mortality for non-Hispanic white babies, Puerto Rican neonatal mortality (death before 28 days of age) was about 50 percent higher and postneonatal mortality (death in the 1st through 11th month of life) was nearly 30 percent higher. For American Indian babies the race differential in infant mortality was due entirely

to a postneonatal mortality rate that was more than double that for white postneonates (table 20).

■ In 1996 **life expectancy** at birth reached an all-time high of 76.1 years. Life expectancy for black males increased for the third consecutive year to a record high of 66.1 years in 1996, following a period between 1984 and 1993 generally characterized by year-to-year declines in life expectancy. Life expectancy for white females rose slightly to 79.7 years but was still below the record high attained in 1992. In 1996 the gender gap in life expectancy narrowed to 6.0 years and the race differential between the white and black populations narrowed to 6.6 years (table 29).

■ Substantial **geographic differences** persist in the death rates for States and geographic divisions in the United States. In 1994–96 the age-adjusted death rate for the East South Central Division (575.5 deaths per 100,000 population) was 15 percent higher than for the United States as a whole whereas age-adjusted death rates for the Mountain, Pacific, West North Central, and New England Divisions were 7–10 percent lower than the U.S. average (table 30).

■ **Years of potential life lost** (YPLL) per 100,000 population under 75 years of age is a measure of premature mortality. In 1996 unintentional injuries were the leading cause of YPLL under 75 years of age among Hispanic males and American Indian females and males, accounting for 20–29 percent of all YPLL in each group. Heart disease was the leading cause of YPLL among black males and non–Hispanic white males, accounting for 14–21 percent of all YPLL. Cancer was the leading cause of YPLL among black, Hispanic, Asian American, and non-Hispanic white females, accounting for 18–32 percent of all YPLL in each group (table 32).

■ Although the first three leading causes of death, heart disease, cancer, and stroke, are the same for **males and females** in the United States, other leading causes of death differ for males and females. In 1996 unintentional injuries ranked higher for males (4th)

than for females (7th) and HIV infection and suicide, which ranked 8th and 9th for males, were not among the 10 leading causes for females. For males the age-adjusted death rate for unintentional injuries (43.3 deaths per 100,000 population) was 2.4 times the rate for females and the rates for HIV infection (18.1) and suicide (18.0) were 4–5 times the rates for females (tables 31 and 33).

■ Although the first two leading causes of death, heart disease and cancer, are the same for the **American Indian** and white populations in the United States, other leading causes of death differ for the two populations. In 1996 unintentional injuries and diabetes ranked higher for American Indians (3d and 4th) than for white persons (5th and 7th), and cirrhosis, which ranked 6th for American Indians, ranked 9th for white persons. For American Indians the age-adjusted death rates for unintentional injuries (57.6 deaths per 100,000 population) and diabetes (27.8) were about double the rates for white persons, and the rate for cirrhosis (20.7) was nearly 3 times the rate for white persons (table 31 and 33).

■ In 1996 overall mortality for **Hispanic Americans** was 22 percent lower than for non-Hispanic white Americans. However for males 15–44 years of age death rates were higher for Hispanics than for non-Hispanic white persons, primarily due to elevated death rates for homicide and HIV infection among young Hispanic males. In 1996 homicide rates for Hispanic males 15–24 and 25–44 years of age were 8 times and 4 times the rates for non-Hispanic white males of similar ages and the death rate for HIV infection for Hispanic males 25–44 years of age was about double the rate for non-Hispanic white males (tables 31, 37, 44, and 47).

■ In 1996 the age-adjusted death rate for **black Americans** declined 4 percent to 738 deaths per 100,000 population. Between 1995 and 1996 mortality due to HIV infection, the fourth leading cause of death among black persons, declined 20 percent, following an average increase of 15 percent per year between

1990 and 1995. Mortality among black persons continued to decline for heart disease and injuries. In 1996 age-adjusted death rates declined 4 percent for heart disease, 2 percent for unintentional injuries, and 8 percent for homicide, and homicide dropped from sixth to seventh in the ranking of leading causes of death for black persons (tables 31 and 33).

■   Between 1992 and 1996 the age-adjusted death rate for **stroke,** the third leading cause of death overall, was stable following a long downward trend. Between 1980 and 1992 stroke mortality declined at an average rate of 3.6 percent per year. Stroke mortality is higher for the black population than for other racial groups. In 1996 the age-adjusted death rate for stroke for the black population was 80 percent higher than for the white population (tables 31, 33, and 39).

■   In 1996 age-adjusted death rates for cancer and heart disease for the **Asian-American** population were 39 percent and 45 percent lower than the rates for the white population, while death rates for stroke were similar for the two populations. Death rates for stroke for Asian-American males 55–64 and 65–74 years of age were 14–28 percent higher than for white males of those ages, while death rates for Asian males age 75 years and over were 12–14 percent lower than for elderly white males (tables 31 and 39).

■   Between 1990 and 1996 the age-adjusted death rate for **cancer,** the second leading cause of death, decreased 5 percent, after increasing slowly but steadily over the 20-year period, 1970 to 1990 (tables 31 and 33).

■   In 1996 the age-adjusted death rate for **chronic obstructive pulmonary diseases (COPD),** the fourth leading cause of death overall, was 47 percent higher for males than females (25.9 and 17.6 deaths per 100,000 population). Between 1980 and 1996 age-adjusted death rates for males were relatively stable while death rates for females nearly doubled. COPD death rates are highest for the elderly and have been increasing most rapidly among females age 75 years and over (tables 33 and 43).

■   In 1996 the age-adjusted death rate for **HIV infection** declined 29 percent to 11.1 deaths per 100,000 population. Between 1994 and 1995 HIV mortality increased by only 1 percent following a period between 1987 and 1994 in which mortality had increased at an average rate of 16 percent per year. In 1996 the death rate for HIV infection for persons 25–44 years of age declined 30 percent and HIV infection dropped from first to third in the ranking of leading causes of death for this age group (tables 31, 34, and 44).

■   Between 1980 and 1996 the age-adjusted **maternal mortality** rate declined by nearly one-third, to 6.4 maternal deaths per 100,000 live births. In 1996, 294 women died of maternal causes compared with 334 women in 1980. In 1996 age-adjusted maternal mortality for black women (19.9 per 100,000 live births) was 5 times the rate for non-Hispanic white women. Maternal mortality for Hispanic women (4.8) was 23 percent higher than the rate for non-Hispanic white women (table 45).

■   Between 1993 and 1996 the age-adjusted death rate for **firearm-related injuries** declined by about 6 percent annually on average to 12.9 deaths per 100,000 population, after increasing almost every year since the late 1980's. Two-thirds of the decline in the firearm-related death rate resulted from the decline in the homicide rate associated with firearms. Between 1993 and 1996 the firearm-related death rate for young black males 15–24 years of age declined at an average annual rate of nearly 10 percent to 131.6 deaths per 100,000. Despite the decline, the firearm-related death rate for young black males was still 6.5 times the rate for young non-Hispanic white males (table 49).

■   In general the workplace is safer today than it was over a decade ago. Between 1980 and 1993 the overall **occupational injury death rate** declined 45 percent to 4.2 deaths per 100,000 workers and decreases occurred in all industries. Of the industries with the highest occupational injury mortality, declines of 52 percent occurred in transportation, communication, and public

Tables

utilities; 45 percent in construction; 42 percent in mining; and 24 percent in agriculture, forestry, and fishing. Although occupational injury mortality in 1993 for wholesale and retail trade was lower than in 1980, rates have increased since 1989. In 1993 the occupational injury death rate was 3.6 deaths per 100,000 workers for wholesale trade and 2.9 for retail trade (table 51).

Determinants and Measures of Health

■ In 1996, 77 percent of children 19–35 months of age received the combined **vaccination** series of 4 doses of DTP (diphtheria-tetanus-pertussis) vaccine, 3 doses of polio vaccine, 1 dose of measles-containing vaccine, and 3 doses of Hib (Haemophilus influenzae type b) vaccine, up from 69 percent in 1994. Substantial differences exist among the States in the percent of children 19–35 months of age who received the combined vaccination series, ranging from a high of 87 percent in Connecticut to a low of 63 percent in Utah (tables 52 and 53).

■ In 1996 **tuberculosis** incidence declined to 8 cases per 100,000 population. This, the fourth consecutive year of decline, is the lowest rate ever reported and reflects improvements in TB-prevention and TB-control programs. Between 1990 and 1996 the case rate for primary and secondary syphilis declined nearly 80 percent to 4 cases per 100,000 and gonorrhea incidence declined 55 percent to 124 per 100,000 (table 54).

■ Between 1995 and 1996 the number of reported **AIDS cases** decreased 6 percent overall. However the decrease was not observed for all population groups. In contrast to other groups, incident AIDS cases for non-Hispanic black females 13 years of age and over increased 6 percent. In 1996 incident AIDS cases decreased for all exposure categories except for the undetermined category, which increased 24 percent overall, and for persons infected through heterosexual contact, which increased 14 percent for non-Hispanic black persons (tables 55 and 56).

■ In 1997 the first leveling off of drug use was found in eighth graders since 1992, with **marijuana** use in the past month declining to 10 percent. The percent of eighth graders who drank alcohol (25) or smoked cigarettes (19) also decreased slightly in 1997. Among high school seniors, 37 percent reported smoking cigarettes in the past month; 1997 marked the fifth consecutive year of increase. Marijuana use among high school seniors in 1997 was 24 percent, double that in 1992 (table 65).

■ In 1996, 51 percent of the population 12 years of age and over reported using **alcohol** in the past month and 15 percent reported having five or more drinks on at least one occasion in the past month. Young people 18–25 years of age were more likely to drink heavily than were other age groups. Among 18–25 year olds, heavy drinking was more than twice as likely for males as females (44 and 21 percent) and about twice as likely for non-Hispanic white persons as for non-Hispanic black persons (37 and 19 percent) (table 64).

■ In 1994 and 1995 there were more than 142,000 **cocaine-related emergency room episodes** per year, the highest number ever reported since these events were tracked starting in 1978. Between 1988 and 1995 cocaine-related episodes among persons 35 years of age and over have almost tripled, reflecting an aging population of drug abusers being treated in emergency departments (table 66).

■ An **environmental health** objective for the year 2000 is that at least 85 percent of the U.S. population should be living in counties that meet the Environmental Protection Agency's National Ambient Air Quality Standards (NAAQS). In 1996, 81 percent of Americans lived in counties that met the NAAQS for all pollutants, up from 68 percent in 1995. In 1995, one of the hottest summers on record, a 7-percentage point decline in compliance with air quality standards occurred, following 3 years of higher levels of compliance (table 72).

■ Between 1990 and 1996 the **injuries with lost workdays** rate decreased 21 percent to 3.1 per 100 full-time equivalents (FTE's) in the private sector. The industries reporting the largest declines during this period (33–35 percent) were mining; agriculture, fishing, and forestry; and construction. The 1996 rate for the manufacturing industry (4.3 per 100 FTE's) was 19 percent lower than in 1990 and the rate for the transportation, communication, and public utilities industry (5.0 per 100 FTE's) was 7 percent lower than in 1990 (table 73).

Utilization of Health Resources

Ambulatory Care

■ In 1994–95, 4 percent of children under 6 years of age had no **usual source of health care**. Being without a usual source of care was more likely for Hispanic children than for non-Hispanic white and non-Hispanic black children (8 percent compared with 3–4 percent); more likely for poor and near poor children (in families whose income was below 200 percent of the poverty threshhold) than for nonpoor children (6 percent compared with 2 percent); and more likely for children without health insurance than for children with insurance (16 percent compared with 2 percent). Among poor children under 6 years of age, 21 percent of uninsured children had no usual source of care compared with 4 percent of insured children (table 79).

■ In 1996 there were 892 million **ambulatory care visits,** 82 percent occurring in physician offices, 8 percent in hospital outpatient departments, and 10 percent in hospital emergency departments. Compared with older persons, a larger proportion of the ambulatory care visits by younger persons are to hospital emergency departments. In 1996 hospital emergency department visits accounted for 12–14 percent of ambulatory care visits among persons under 45 years of age and 8 percent of visits among persons 75 years of age and over (table 81).

■ In 1996, 60 percent of all **surgical operations** in community hospitals were performed on an outpatient basis, almost 4 times the percent in 1980. The upward trend in the proportion of surgery performed on outpatients is slowing. During the 1980's the proportion of surgery that was outpatient increased 12 percent per year on the average whereas by the 1990's that growth had slowed to 3 percent per year (table 94).

■ In 1995 there were 457 **clients in specialty substance abuse treatment** per 100,000 population 12 years of age and over, 5 percent higher than in 1992. Nearly one-half (46 percent) of the clients were enrolled in simultaneous treatment for alcohol and drug abuse in 1995, up from 38 percent in 1992. In 1995 30 percent of clients were enrolled in alcohol-only treatment and 23 percent in drug abuse-only treatment. The total number of substance abuse clients in all specialty treatment units per 100,000 population was lowest in the West South Central (258) and West North Central divisions (279) and highest in the Pacific (618) and Middle Atlantic divisions (596) (table 84).

■ In 1996 **home health agencies** provided care to about 2.4 million persons on an average day. Two-thirds of users of home health services were female. Home health services are provided mainly to the elderly. In 1996 one-third of those being served were 75–84 years of age at the time of admission and one-sixth were 85 years of age and over. In 1996 the most common primary admission diagnoses were heart disease (11 percent of patients), diseases of the musculoskeletal system and diabetes (9 percent each), and cerebrovascular diseases and diseases of the respiratory system (8 percent each) (table 86).

Inpatient Care

■ Utilization of **inpatient short-stay hospital care** is greater for persons with low family income (less than $15,000) than for persons with high family income ($50,000 or more). In 1995 the age-adjusted

Highlights ....

Tables

days of care rate for low income persons was almost 3 times the rate for high income persons (880 and 300 days of care per 1,000 population) (table 87).

■ Between 1988 and 1995 the age-adjusted **hospital discharge rate** for non-Federal short-stay hospitals declined 11 percent to 105 discharges per 1,000 population. The decline was greater for persons under 64 years of age (14–17 percent) than for persons 65–74 years of age (3 percent). By contrast the hospital discharge rate increased 5 percent for persons 75 years of age and over. Between 1988 and 1995 the **average length of stay** decreased for persons of all ages with larger declines for elderly than for younger persons. The average length of stay declined by more than 2 days for persons 65 years of age and over, 1.3 days for persons 45–64 years of age, and by less than 1 day for persons under 45 years of age (table 88).

■ In 1995 among elderly persons with a first-listed diagnosis of **ischemic heart disease**, the hospital discharge rate for non-Federal short-stay hospitals was higher for men than for women, but the difference diminished with increasing age. In 1995 among persons 65–74 years of age the rate of ischemic heart disease discharges for men was 1.8 times the rate for women (43.7 and 24.0 per 1,000 population). Among persons 75 years of age and over, the rate for men was 1.4 times the rate for women (51.6 and 36.8) (table 90).

■ In 1995 for persons 65 years of age and over, the hospital discharge rate for **coronary bypass surgery** for men was 3 times the rate for women and this difference did not diminish with increasing age. For persons 65–74 years of age, the discharge rate for men was 11.2 per 1,000 population compared with 3.8 for women. For persons 75 years of age and over, the rate for men was 8.9 compared with 3.0 for women (table 92).

■ Between 1990 and 1994, overall **additions to mental health inpatient and residential treatment organizations** (admissions and readmissions) remained stable at 830–840 per 100,000 civilian population.

However, trends differed for different types of mental health organizations. Additions declined 19–24 percent in State and county mental health organizations and the Department of Veterans Affairs while additions increased 5–11 percent in non-Federal general hospitals and private psychiatric hospitals (table 85).

■ Between 1985 and 1995 the number of **nursing home residents** 85 years of age and over per 1,000 population decreased 10 percent to 199. During this 10-year period the number of nursing home residents 85 years of age and over increased 21 percent while this age group in the population increased 36 percent. In 1995 the nursing home residency rate among persons 85 years and over was about 70 percent higher for women than men and 20 percent higher for white persons than for black persons (tables 1 and 95).

■ Functional dependencies most commonly afflicting **nursing home residents** are in mobility, incontinence, and eating. In 1995, 79 percent of nursing home residents 65 years of age and over were dependent in mobility, 64 percent were incontinent, 45 percent were dependent in eating, and 37 percent were dependent in all three functionalities. Compared with 1985 a larger proportion of nursing home residents were functionally dependent in 1995. In 1995 a larger proportion of black than white residents had functional dependencies (table 96).

Health Care Resources

Personnel

■ In 1996 the number of active **doctors of medicine in patient care** per 10,000 civilian population was 22 for the United States as a whole, an increase of 61 percent since 1975. In 1996 the divisions with the highest ratios were New England and Middle Atlantic (28–29) and the divisions with the lowest ratios were East South Central, West South Central, and Mountain (18), a pattern similar to that in 1975 (table 100).

■ Between 1980 and 1995 the **supply of active registered nurses** increased 42 percent to 798 per

100,000 population. Registered nurses are generally more educated today than they were 15 years ago. In 1995, 58 percent of active registered nurses were prepared at the associate and diploma level, 32 percent at the baccalaureate level, and 10 percent at the masters and doctoral level. By contrast in 1980, the mix was 71 percent associate and diploma, 23 percent baccalaureate, and 5 percent masters and doctoral nurses (table 103).

■ In 1993 through 1996 the annual number of **graduates from dentistry school** was stable at 3,700–3,800 after declining steadily from 5,400 in 1985. Between 1985 and 1996 the number of professional schools of dentistry declined from 60 to 53 (table 106).

■ In academic year 1995–96, women comprised 42 percent of total student enrollment in **allopathic schools of medicine** compared with 27 percent in academic year 1980–81. In academic year 1995–96 women comprised 40–45 percent of the non-Hispanic white, Asian, Hispanic, and American Indian students compared with 60 percent of the non-Hispanic black students (table 108).

Facilities

■ In 1996 **occupancy rates in community hospitals** averaged 62 percent. Community hospital occupancy varied inversely by bed size ranging from 33 percent for hospitals with 6–24 beds to 70 percent for hospitals with 500 beds or more (table 109).

■ Between 1990 and 1994 the number of **mental health inpatient and residential treatment beds** per 100,000 population declined 13 percent to 98 after remaining relatively stable between 1984 and 1990. Between 1990 and 1994, the bed to population ratio declined 24 percent for State and county mental hospitals to 31 per 100,000 and declined 14 percent for private psychiatric hospitals to 16. By contrast, the mental health bed to population ratio remained relatively stable for non-Federal general hospitals, Department of Veterans Affairs hospitals, and

residential treatment centers for emotionally disturbed children (table 110).

■ Between 1992 and 1996 the number of **nursing home beds** in the United States increased by 9 percent to 1.8 million beds. During the same period, occupancy rates in nursing homes declined by 3 percentage points from 86 percent to 83 percent. In 1996 occupancy rates varied among the geographic divisions from a low of 72 percent in the West South Central division to a high of 90–93 percent in the East South Central, New England, and Middle Atlantic divisions (table 114).

Health Care Expenditures

National Health Expenditures

■ In 1996 **national health care expenditures** in the United States totaled $1,035 billion, an average of $3,759 per person. In 1996 the 4-percent increase in national health expenditures continued the steady slowdown in growth of the 1990's. During the 1980's national health expenditures grew at an average annual rate of 11 percent compared with 7 percent between 1990 and 1995 (tables 115 and 119).

■ **Health expenditures as a percent of the gross domestic product** remained stable at 13.6 percent between 1993 and 1996, after increasing steadily from 8.9 percent in 1980 (table 115).

■ In 1995 health spending in the United States continued to account for a larger **share of gross domestic product** (GDP) than in any other major industrialized country. The United States devoted 13.6 percent of GDP to health in 1995. The countries with the next highest share of GDP devoted to health in 1995 were Germany with 10.4 percent and Canada, Switzerland, and France with 9.7 to 9.9 percent each. In the United Kingdom the percent of GDP devoted to health care has been stable at 6.9 percent during 1992–95 while in Japan the percent has been steadily rising during the 1990's to 7.2 percent in 1995 (table 116).

■ During the 1990's the rate of increase in the medical care component of the **Consumer Price Index** (CPI) has declined every year from 9.0 percent in 1990 to 2.8 percent in 1997. From 1990 to 1995 the inflation rate for the medical care component of CPI (6.3 percent) averaged more than double the overall inflation rate of 3.1 percent. However for the last two years medical care inflation averaged 20 percent higher than the overall rate of inflation. In 1997 inflation for dental services (4.7 percent) and outpatient services (4.6 percent) outpaced inflation for all other types of medical care services and commodities (tables 117 and 118).

■ During the 1990's the percent of **national health expenditures that were publicly funded** increased steadily to 47 percent in 1996. Between 1990 and 1996 public funds for national health expenditures grew at an average annual rate of 9.2 percent compared with 4.9 percent for private funds (table 119).

■ Expenditures for hospital care continued to decline as a percent of **national health expenditures** from 42 percent in 1980 to 35 percent in 1996. Physician services accounted for 20 percent of the total in 1996 and drugs and nursing home care each for 8–9 percent (table 120).

■ In 1995, 34 percent of **expenditures for health services and supplies** was paid by households, 26 percent by private business, and 38 percent by the Federal and State and local governments. Between 1990 and 1995 the share of expenditures from out-of-pocket health spending by individuals declined from 22 percent to 19 percent and the share of expenditures paid by private business declined from 28 percent to 26 percent (table 121).

■ Between 1994 and 1997 **private employers' health insurance costs** per employee-hour worked declined from $1.14 to $.99 per hour after increasing by 24 percent between 1991 and 1994. In 1997 private employers with 500 or more employees paid 2.2 times as much for health insurance per employee-hour worked ($1.57) as did the employers with fewer than

100 employees ($.72), and 2.4 times as much for health insurance per employee-hour worked for union workers ($2.01) as for nonunion workers ($.85). Among private employers the share of total compensation devoted to health insurance declined from 6.7 percent in 1994 to 5.5 percent in 1997 (table 122).

■ In 1996, 19 percent of **personal health care expenditures** were paid out-of-pocket; private health insurance paid 32 percent, the Federal Government paid 36 percent, and State and local government paid 10 percent. Between 1990 and 1996 the share paid by the Federal Government increased nearly 7 percentage points, while the share paid out-of-pocket decreased by nearly 5 percentage points (table 124).

■ In 1996 the major **sources of funds** for hospital care were Medicare (33 percent) and private health insurance (32 percent). In 1996 physician services were also primarily funded by private health insurance (50 percent) and Medicare (21 percent). In contrast, in 1996 nursing home care was financed primarily by Medicaid (48 percent) and out-of-pocket payments (31 percent). In 1996 out-of-pocket payments financed only 3 percent of hospital care and 15 percent of physician services (table 125).

■ Between 1990 and 1996 the proportion of **health expenditures** paid by Medicaid increased from 12 to 15 percent for hospital care and from 5 to 8 percent for physician services. Over the same period Medicare funding for hospital care increased from 27 to 33 percent and for nursing home care increased from 3 to 11 percent (table 125).

■ Between 1993 and 1996 the average annual increase in **total expenses in community hospitals** was 3.4 percent, following a period of higher growth that averaged 9.3 percent per year from 1985 to 1993. Between 1993 and 1996 expenses per inpatient day increased by 5.1 percent per year in nonprofit hospitals and by 1.1 percent per year in proprietary hospitals, while expenses per inpatient stay increased by 0.9 percent per year in nonprofit community hospitals

and decreased by 2.6 percent per year in proprietary hospitals. In 1996 employee costs accounted for 53 percent of total hospital costs in nonprofit community hospitals compared with 48 percent in proprietary hospitals (table 126).

■ In 1995 the **average monthly charge in a nursing home** was $3,135 per resident. The monthly charge varied widely by geographic region from about $2,700 in the Midwest and South to $3,700 and $3,900 in the West and Northeast. In 1995 nearly one-half of the nursing home residents were 85 years of age or older and nearly three-quarters were women (table 127).

■ The **average monthly nursing home charge** varies according to the primary source of payment. In 1995 the average monthly charge for patients funded by Medicaid (60 percent of residents) was $2,769 per resident, one-half of the charge of $5,546 for Medicare patients (10 percent of residents). Medicare funds nursing home patients who have been discharged directly from the hospital to the nursing home and who are likely to be sicker than nursing home patients funded by Medicaid. Residents paying for nursing home care with their own income, family support, or private health insurance paid $3,081 per month (28 percent of residents) (table 128).

■ **Expenditures by mental health organizations** increased between 1990 and 1994 from $28 to $33 billion. Spending on mental health was $128 per capita in 1994, up from $117 per capita in 1990 and 1992. Private psychiatric hospitals continued to account for about one-fifth of the mental health dollar. State and county mental hospitals continued to decrease their share of mental health expenditures from 27 percent in 1990 to 24 percent in 1994 (table 129).

■ In 1995 **funding for health research and development** increased by 7 percent to $36 billion. The average annual rate of increase in health research funding during 1992–95 (7 percent) was less rapid than during 1990–92 (12.5 percent). Between 1990 and 1995 industry's share of funding for health research

increased from 46 to 52 percent while the Federal Government's share decreased from 42 to 37 percent (table 130).

■ Between 1995 and 1997 **Federal expenditures for HIV-related activities** increased at an average annual rate of 11 percent to $8.5 billion compared with an average annual increase of 17 percent between 1990 and 1995. Of the total Federal spending in 1997, 56 percent was for medical care, 21 percent for research, 15 percent for cash assistance (Disability Insurance, Supplemental Security Income, and Housing and Urban Development assistance), and 8 percent for education and prevention. Between 1996 and 1997 expenditures for medical care increased by 17 percent, cash assistance by 10 percent, education and prevention expenditures by 7 percent, and research by 5 percent (table 132).

Health Care Coverage and Major Federal Programs

■ Between 1993 and 1996 the age-adjusted proportion of the population under 65 years of age with **private health insurance** has remained stable at 70–71 percent after declining from 76 percent in 1989. More than 90 percent of private coverage was obtained through the workplace (a current or former employer or union) in 1996. Compared with persons living in the South, those living in the Northeast and Midwest geographic regions were about 14–19 percent more likely to have private health insurance in 1996. Persons living in the South and West were about equally likely to have private health insurance (table 133).

■ Expansions in the **Medicaid** program have resulted in an increase in the percentage of poor children under 18 years of age with Medicaid or other public assistance from 48 percent in 1989 to 66 percent in 1996. During this period the percentage of near poor children with Medicaid doubled from 12 to 25 percent for children at 100–149 percent of the poverty threshold and from 6 to 11 percent for children at 150–199 percent of the poverty threshold (table 133).

■ Nearly all persons 65 years of age or older are eligible for **Medicare**, the Federal health program for the elderly, but most of the elderly have additional health care coverage. In 1996, 72 percent of the elderly had private health insurance and 38 percent had private health insurance obtained through the workplace (a current or former employer or union). In 1996, 9 percent of the elderly had Medicaid or other public assistance and 18 percent had Medicare only, with no other health plan (table 134).

■ In 1997, one-quarter of the U.S. population was enrolled in **health maintenance organizations (HMO's)**, ranging from only 18 percent in the South to 36 percent in the West. HMO enrollment is steadily increasing. Enrollment in 1997 was 67 million persons, double the enrollment in 1991. The distribution of enrollees among model types is also changing. Between 1991 and 1997 the percent of HMO members enrolled in group HMO's declined from 50 to 17 percent while the percent enrolled in mixed HMO's increased from 10 to 43 percent. During the same period the percent of HMO members enrolled in individual practice associations was relatively unchanged at about 40 percent (table 135).

■ Employee participation in **medical care benefits** is related to the size of the company. In 1995, 77 percent of full-time and 19 percent of part-time employees in medium and large private establishments (100 or more employees) participated in the medical care benefits offered by their company. In 1994, 66 percent of full-time and only 7 percent of part-time employees in small private establishments (less than 100 employees) participated in the company's medical care benefits (table 136).

■ In private companies with 100 or more employees the percent of full-time **employees participating in health care benefits** declined between 1991 and 1995 from 83 to 77 percent. The decline among blue collar and service employees was 9 percentage points compared with a 5-percentage point decline among employees in other occupational groups (table 136).

■ During the 1990's the use of **traditional fee-for-service** medical care benefits by employees in private companies declined sharply. In 1994 in small companies, 55 percent of full-time employees who participated in medical care benefits were in traditional fee-for-service medical care, down from 74 percent in 1990. In 1995 in medium and large companies, only 37 percent of participating full-time employees were in traditional fee-for-service medical care, down from 67 percent in 1991 (table 136).

■ During the 1990's **full financing of medical care coverage** became less common. In 1994, 47 percent of full-time participating employees in small companies received full financing of individual medical coverage compared with 58 percent in 1990. In 1995, 33 percent of full-time participating employees in larger companies received full financing of individual medical coverage compared with 49 percent in 1991. Similar declines in full financing of family medical coverage were also seen in small and larger companies (table 136).

■ The average **monthly contribution** by full-time employees for family **medical care benefits** was 36 percent higher in small companies ($160 in 1994) than in medium and large companies ($118 in 1995). Average monthly contributions by full-time employees for individual medical care benefits were more than 20 percent higher in small than in medium and large companies ($41 in 1994 compared with $34 in 1995). Average employee contributions for HMO medical care benefits were higher than for non-HMO fee arrangements, regardless of company size (table 136).

■ In 1996 the **Medicare** program had 38.1 million enrollees and expenditures of $200 billion. The total number of enrollees increased less than 2 percent over the previous year while expenditures increased nearly 9 percent. In 1996 supplementary medical insurance (SMI) accounted for 35 percent of Medicare expenditures. Expenditures for home health agency care increased to 13.5 percent of hospital insurance (HI) expenditures in 1996 up from 5.5 percent in 1990.

Expenditures for skilled nursing facilities more than doubled to 9 percent of the HI expenditures over the same period. Group practice prepayment increased from 6 percent of the SMI expenditures in 1990 to 13 percent in 1996 (table 137).

■ Of the 33.1 million elderly **Medicare** enrollees in 1995, 11 percent were 85 years of age and over. In 1995 the average payment per Medicare enrollee for those 85 years of age and over ($6,356) was 2.5 times that for those aged 65–66 years ($2,546). In every age group for those 65 years of age and over, Medicare payments per person served and payments per enrollee were higher for men than for women. In 1995 in the West there were 663 persons served per 1,000 enrollees compared with 865 or more in the other three regions of the country (table 138).

■ In 1996 **Medicaid** vendor payments totaled $122 billion for 36.1 million recipients, showing little change from the previous year. Between 1993 and 1995 the average annual increase slowed to 9 percent for payments and 4 percent for recipients, about one-half the growth during the period 1990 to 1993. In 1996 children under the age of 21 years comprised 46 percent of recipients but accounted for only 14 percent of expenditures. The aged, blind, and disabled accounted for 29 percent of recipients and 73 percent of expenditures (table 139).

■ In 1996 nearly one-quarter of **Medicaid** payments went to nursing facilities and 21 percent to general hospitals. Home health care accounted for 9 percent of Medicaid payments in 1996, up from 1 percent in 1980. In 1996, 5 percent of Medicaid recipients received home health care at a cost averaging $6,293 per recipient. Early and periodic screening, rural health clinics, and family planning services combined received less than 2 percent of Medicaid funds in 1996, with the cost per recipient averaging between $200 and $215 (table 140).

■ Between 1995 and 1996 spending on health care by the **Department of Veterans Affairs** increased by less than 2 percent to $16.4 billion. In 1996, 46 percent

of the total was for inpatient hospital care, down from 58 percent in 1990, one-third for outpatient care, up from one-quarter in 1990, and 10 percent for nursing home care. The number of inpatient stays decreased by 8 percent between 1995 and 1996 and the number of outpatient visits increased by 6 percent. In 1996 veterans with service-connected disabilities accounted for 40 percent of inpatients and 38 percent of outpatients. Low-income veterans with no service-connected disability were the largest group served accounting for 56 percent of inpatients and 42 percent of outpatients (table 141).

State Health Expenditures

■ In 1995 **Medicare payments per enrollee** averaged $4,750 in the United States, ranging from $3,300 in Nebraska, Iowa, and Idaho to more than $6,000 in Massachusetts and Louisiana. In 1995 utilization of short-stay hospitals by Medicare enrollees varied among the States from 250 discharges per 1,000 enrollees in Utah to 432 in Mississippi. The length of stay in short-stay hospitals by Medicare enrollees averaged 5.6 and 5.7 days in the Mountain and Pacific geographic divisions compared with 9.0 days in the Middle Atlantic division in 1995 (table 146).

■ In 1996 **Medicaid payments per recipient** averaged $3,369 and ranged from $2,049 in Tennessee to $6,811 in New York. For the United States as a whole, the ratio of Medicaid recipients to persons below the poverty level increased from 75 per 100 in 1989–90 to 99 per 100 in 1995–96. For 1995–96 the ratio of Medicaid recipients to persons below the poverty level was above the average in all States in the New England geographic division and below the average in all States in the West South Central and Mountain divisions (table 147).

■ In 1997 the percent of the population enrolled in a **health maintenance organization (HMO)** varied among the States from 0 in Alaska and Vermont to 47 percent in Oregon. In seven other States more than one-third of the population was enrolled in an HMO in

Tables

1997 including Massachusetts (45 percent), New York (36 percent), Connecticut (35 percent), Maryland and Delaware (38–39 percent), Utah (41 percent), and California (44 percent) (table 148).

■   In 1996 the proportion of the population without **health care coverage** was 15.6 percent, compared with 15.4 percent the previous year and 12.9 percent in 1987. In 1996 the proportion of the population without health care coverage varied from less than 9 percent in Wisconsin, Michigan, and Hawaii to more than 20 percent in Arkansas, Louisiana, Texas, New Mexico, Arizona, and California (table 149).

Socioeconomic Status and Health Chartbook

One of the three overarching goals of *Healthy People 2000*, the Public Health Service's national health objectives for the year 2000, is to reduce health disparities among Americans (1). *Healthy People 2000*, the Nation's prevention agenda, seeks to reduce such disparities by encouraging preventive efforts targeted for "special population" groups: low-income persons, racial and ethnic minorities, and persons with disabilities. In the United States health disparities among racial and ethnic subgroups of the population, especially between white persons and black persons, have received much of the attention. However, individuals' access to social and economic resources, as indicated by income, level of education, or type of occupation, is a major source of disparities in health in this country, and many others (2–4). *Healthy People 2000* implicitly recognizes the strength and persistence of disparities in health outcomes and access to health services by setting separate targets for special population groups that represent a more rapid rate of improvement and thus a narrowing of the gap. In 1997, goals for *Healthy People 2010* were proposed that seek to eliminate, rather than reduce, health disparities.

The first section of this chartbook documents the strong relationship between race, ethnicity, and various measures of socioeconomic status: household or family income (figures 2 and 6), poverty status (figure 3), level of education (figure 5), and type of occupation (figure 7). Racial and ethnic minorities are disproportionately represented among the poor in the United States. In 1996 African Americans comprised 13 percent of the overall U.S. population and 26 percent of the poor population; persons of Hispanic origin comprised 11 percent of the overall population and 22 percent of the poor; while non-Hispanic white persons made up 72 percent of the overall population and 45 percent of the poor. By contrast, the high-income population was considerably more homogeneous with respect to race and Hispanic origin; 87 percent of individuals with incomes of $50,000 or more in 1996 were non-Hispanic white persons. This chartbook addresses the overlap between race, ethnicity, and socioeconomic status by documenting

health disparities across levels of socioeconomic status for as many race and ethnic subgroups as possible, given the limitations of the data.

The chartbook includes separate sections on the health of children under 18 years of age (figures 8–24) and adults 18 years of age and over (figures 25–49). Each of these sections is divided into subsections on health status, health risk factors, and health care access and utilization. Many of the charts in each section present data by gender where appropriate and feasible. The charts are followed by Technical Notes that describe data sources, definitions, and methods and a Data Table that includes data points presented in the charts and standard errors. Appendixes I and II present additional information on data sources and definitions.

Data Issues

With the exception of data derived from the Census and from the vital registration system (birth and death certificates), the existing sources of health data do not permit examination of socioeconomic differences for any but the three largest race and ethnic categories: non-Hispanic white persons, non-Hispanic black persons, and persons of Hispanic or Mexican origin. Much of the data used in this chartbook was collected by surveys that may provide reliable estimates for entire race and ethnic subgroups, but usually have insufficient numbers to make good estimates for detailed subcategories within these populations. This problem is particularly acute when the subcategories reflect socioeconomic levels, because of the tendency for race and ethnic groups to be disproportionately concentrated at either the low or high ends of the socioeconomic distribution (as shown in the Population section). The reader will notice that, even for the three largest race and ethnic groups, sample sizes often require collapsing socioeconomic variables into fewer categories than reported for the population as a whole.

Combining into larger groups is an expedient solution to problems of small numbers, but it is not without cost. Readers should be aware that the broad groupings presented in this chartbook may mask

differences among subgroups. For example, "Asian or Pacific Islander" includes persons with ancestry in such countries as China, Vietnam, the Phillippines, Japan, and Samoa, while "Hispanic" combines persons whose origins were in Cuba, Puerto Rico, Mexico, or any of the countries of Central or South America. These subgroups often have very diverse socioeconomic profiles and may also have very different health status and risk behaviors.

This problem of hidden heterogeneity also affects the socioeconomic categories. For example, in many of the charts that follow, "high income" persons may have a family income for the year ranging from $50,000 to $500,000 or more; the category of 16 or more years of education combines persons with baccalaureate degrees with those with graduate and professional degrees, such as lawyers and doctors. There are likely to be differences within each of these categories that are not discernable in the charts. In addition, race and ethnic groups are likely to have different "mixes" of persons within a uniformly named category. In 1996, in an income category labeled "$50,000 or more," 25 percent of the non-Hispanic white households in this group would have incomes of $100,000 or more, compared with only 17 percent of Hispanic households and 14 percent of black households (5). The reader should also bear in mind that race and ethnic groups are distributed very differently across socioeconomic strata, although the categories are depicted equally in the charts. Thus, in the charts for children under the age of 18, the category "poor" usually represents around 11 percent of non-Hispanic white children, but 40 percent or more of Hispanic or black children (figure 3).

Another difficulty in presenting health data by socioeconomic status is that each indicator used to stratify the population into levels of SES has certain conceptual and practical limitations.

Income is the most common measure of socioeconomic status, and is probably the most relevant to health policy formulation. Current income provides a direct measure of the quality of food, housing, leisure-time amenities, and health care an

individual is able to acquire, as well as reflecting their relative position in society. However, income may fluctuate over time so that income received in a given year may not accurately reflect one's lifetime income stream, the measure of resources more relevant to health. Among the elderly, persons who have low incomes may also have accumulated assets that offset their need for a high annual income. Of particular importance in considering the relationship between income and health is the fact that income may be low because illness has limited the amount of income earned or prevented earning income entirely.

The use of income as a measure of SES also involves more practical difficulties. A fairly high percent of persons either do not know or refuse to report their incomes. In the income-based charts shown in this report, the proportion of the population excluded because of missing data on family income generally varied between 10 and 16 percent, although it was as high as 24 percent for persons 70 years of age and older (figure 34). To reduce nonresponse, income is most often collected in categories. The categorization of income, however, introduces a certain amount of error into calculation of poverty status (family income as a percent of the Federal poverty level), although the error is likely to be small when the number of categories is large. Since low-income populations are of particular interest to health researchers, income data has traditionally been collected at a finer level of detail at the lower end of the income distribution. In most of the surveys used in this report, less detailed income categories were collected at higher income levels; in particular, all persons with family incomes of $50,000 or more were grouped together (see Technical Notes).

Converting family income into percent of the Federal poverty level is generally desirable because family size is taken into account and poverty definitions are adjusted each year to account for inflation (See Technical Notes and Appendix II). Since the calculation of poverty status was not feasible for the full range of incomes, trend data are generally presented by level of education. Education is

frequently used as the measure of SES in presentations of health data. There are several reasons for this preference. Education is generally better reported than income; usually 95 percent or more of respondents report their attained level of education. Unlike occupation, all adults may be characterized by their education level. Education, unlike income, remains fixed for most people after the age of 25 and usually is not influenced by health. In addition, education is highly related to income as shown in figure 6. However, education cannot be used to characterize the socioeconomic position of children (except through parental education), and the average education level of the U.S. population has increased dramatically over time, complicating comparisons across age groups.

This chartbook relies most heavily on poverty, income, and education as measures of socioeconomic status. We have included average income level in the individual's area of residence as a measure of SES where an individual-level indicator was not available (figures 23, 24, and 48). Occupation is another indicator of SES that reflects education and income. However, occupation as usually collected is not relevant to children, retired persons, or women not currently employed, which characterizes a significant portion of women during childbearing. Since these stages of the life cycle are of great interest to health researchers and policymakers, we have not included in this report charts showing health variables by occupation.

Socioeconomic Disparities in Health

This chartbook is intended to document the extent to which socioeconomic disparities continue to exist in indicators of health status, health behaviors and other risk factors, and health care access and utilization within the United States. This demonstration provides a cautionary note when examining progress toward the *Healthy People 2000* objectives for the population as a whole. Although progress is occurring toward most targets, data presented in this chartbook demonstrate that, for many objectives, only the higher socioeconomic groups have achieved or are close to achieving the target, while lower socioeconomic

groups lag farther behind. For a broad cross section of indicators where substantial progress toward the year 2000 objectives has already occurred—mortality from heart disease (figure 27) and lung cancer (figure 28), infant mortality (figures 8 and 9), cigarette smoking (figures 35 and 36) and smoking during pregnancy (figure 13), receipt of early prenatal care (figure 19), and having regular mammograms (figure 45)—further improvement clearly depends on achieving greater gains among persons of lower socioeconomic status. This chartbook does not attempt to present a complete examination of differential progress toward all of the Year 2000 objectives since this is routinely presented in the *Healthy People 2000 Progress Reviews* (6). We have however tried to include a broad cross-section of indicators reflecting different aspects of health and health care and applicable to several age groups, that demonstrate both the magnitude and complexity of the effects of socioeconomic status.

Often examinations of the relationship between SES and health have focused on the lowest end of the SES distribution, comparing poor persons to those above the poverty threshold or persons with less than a high school education to everyone else (7). Although poverty is a powerful determinant and consequence of ill health, focus on the extreme end of the SES distribution implies uniformity among persons above the thresholds of poverty or high school graduation. Evidence from previous studies in Europe and the United States have indicated that the association between SES and health generally takes the form of a gradient; that is, while persons of lowest SES have the worst health outcomes, persons of middle SES have worse health than persons of high SES (8,9).

The data presented in this chartbook support the existence of a socioeconomic gradient in most of the health indicators examined; each increase in social position, measured either by income or education, improves the likelihood of being in good health. For most of the health indicators, this SES gradient was observed for persons in every race and ethnic group examined. In general, the SES gradient was strongest for non-Hispanic white persons and weakest for Mexican American or all Hispanic persons or, in the few instances where data were available, for Asians

and Pacific Islanders. In addition, lower SES Hispanic persons tend to have better health status than non-Hispanic persons at a similar social position. The different pattern of SES and health among persons of Hispanic origin characterizes Mexican Americans, who make up the largest share of the U.S. Hispanic population. Evidence suggests that this pattern may be due, in part, to protective effects of traditional culture, which is likely to be more prevalent among recent immigrants who are also most likely to have lower incomes and educational attainment (10–12).

Although documenting socioeconomic disparities in health is not new, identifying and understanding the causes still remain a challenge. The sections of this chartbook on risk factors and health care access demonstrate the likely contributions of these two broad areas toward disparities seen in health outcomes. The socioeconomic differences apparent in risk factors, such as smoking (figures 13, 15, 35, and 36), overweight (figures 16, 38, and 39), elevated blood lead (figures 14 and 42), and sedentary lifestyle (figures 17 and 40), as well as differential access to and utilization of health care, such as seen in health insurance coverage (figures 20 and 43), physician visits (figures 22, 23, 44, 46, and 47), and avoidable hospitalizations (figures 24 and 48), influence the rates of health outcomes such as low birthweight (figure 10), heart disease mortality (figure 27), fair or poor health (figure 32), diabetes mortality (figure 29), and activity limitation (figures 11 and 33).

Given the ubiquity of SES differences in health risk factors, we need to address the question of why these behaviors are disproportionately concentrated among persons with fewer socioeconomic resources. Differences in the life circumstances of high- and low-SES persons in the United States are substantial. Higher socioeconomic position may directly influence health through income- and education-related differences including having knowledge and time to pursue healthy behaviors, having sufficient income to assure access to comfortable housing, healthy food, and appropriate health care, access to safe and

affordable locations to exercise and relax, and living and working in a safe, healthy environment (13,14). In addition, a more direct connection may exist in that persons whose attention and energy are focused on attaining economic security, or dealing with the lack of it, may have few resources, financial and emotional, for pursuing healthy lifestyles and obtaining preventive health care. It has also been suggested that simply being at a lower position on the economic distribution exacts an emotional or psychological cost that translates into poorer health practices, or simply poorer health (15,16). This latter explanation may also apply to the effects of racial and ethnic discrimination, proposed by some as a contributor to the poorer health outcomes experienced by many minorities even after adjusting for differences in their socioeconomic profile (17,18).

References

1. U.S. Department of Health and Human Services. Healthy people 2000: National health promotion and disease prevention objectives. Washington: Public Health Service. 1990.

2. Department of Health (U.K.). Variations in health: What can the Department of Health and the N.H.S. do? London. 1996.

3. Williams DR. Socioeconomic differentials in health: A review and redirection. Social Psychology Quarterly 53:81–99. 1990.

4. Townsend P, Davidson N. Inequalities in health: The Black report. Penguin: London. 1982.

5. U.S. Bureau of the Census. Current Population Survey, 1996.

6. Department of Health and Human Services. Office of Disease Prevention and Health Promotion. <http://odphp.osophs.dhhs.gov/pubs/hp2000>.

7. Haan MN, Kaplan GA, Syme SL. Socioeconomic status and health: Old observations and new thoughts, in Bunker DS, Gomby DS, Kehrer BH (eds.) Pathways to health: The role of social factors. Menlo Park, CA: Henry Kaiser Family Foundation. 1989.

8. Marmot M, Smith GD, Stansfeld S et al. Health inequalities among British civil servants: The Whitehall Study II. Lancet 337:1387–93. 1991.

9. Adler N, Boyce T, Chesney M, et al. Socioeconomic status and health: The challenge of the gradient. Am Psychol 49:15–24. 1994.

10. Marin G, Perez-Stable EJ, Marin BV. Cigarette smoking among San Francisco Hispanics: The role of acculturation and gender. Am J Public Health 79:196–8. 1989.

11. Council on Scientific Affairs. Hispanic health in the United States. JAMA 265:248–52. 1991.

12. Molina CW, Aguirre-Molina M (eds.). Latino Health in the US: A growing challenge. American Public Health Association. 1994.

13. Lundberg O. Causal explanations for class inequality in health an empirical analysis. Soc Sci Med 32:385–93. 1991.

14. Link BG, Phelan J. Social conditions as fundamental causes of disease. J Health Soc Behav (extra issue):80–94. 1995.

15. Wilkinson RG. The epidemiologic transition: From material scarcity to social disadvantage. Daedalus 123:61–77. 1994.

16. Wilkinson RG. Health inequalities: Relative or absolute material standards? BMJ 314:1427–28. 1997.

17. Krieger N, Rowley D, Herman AA, et al. Racism, sexism, and social class: Implications for studies of health disease and well-being. Am J Prev Med 9:82–122. 1993.

18. Williams DR. Racism and health: A research agenda. Ethn Dis 6:1–6. 1996.

This section presents current patterns and recent trends in measures of socioeconomic status (SES) in the United States population. To the extent possible, distributions and trends in measures of SES are shown for major race and ethnic subgroups of the population, and for gender and age groups where appropriate.

Figure 1 shows household income at selected percentiles of the household income distribution for the years 1970 to 1996 and demonstrates increasing income inequality in recent years in the United States. In 1996 the bottom 20 percent of U.S. households had incomes below $14,770; adjusted for inflation, this represents an increase of less than $800 since 1970. In contrast, the top 20 percent of households had incomes above $68,000 in 1996, $12,300 more than in 1970. A major contributor to the increase in income inequality has been increasing inequality in wages. The increase in earnings inequality over the last 25 years was primarily produced by technological change that increased returns to highly skilled labor at the same time that less skilled workers saw their real wages stagnate or decline. This trend was exacerbated to some degree by "globalization" of the economy, declines in the real minimum wage and in unionization, and an increase in immigration. Household income, however, is also a product of household composition and income from sources other than earnings. A significant part of the increase in income inequality can be attributed to changes in family composition and an increase in female labor-force participation. Because individuals tend to marry individuals with similar earnings profiles, increasing the number of families with both husband and wife working increases income inequality. In addition, an increase in families headed by women (from 10 percent of families in 1970 to 18 percent in 1996) has acted to increase income inequality since these households generally have lower incomes (1–5).

Income may be related to health because it increases access to medical care, enables one to live in better neighborhoods and afford better housing, and increases the opportunity to engage in health-promoting behaviors. Income may also be affected by poor health, by restricting type or amount of employment, or preventing an individual from working entirely. Figure 2 shows median household income by race and Hispanic origin for the years 1980 to 1996. Throughout this period, the median income of non-Hispanic white households has been much higher than that of black or Hispanic households, but the income gap between white and Hispanic households widened, whereas the gap between white and black households narrowed slightly. In 1996 Asian or Pacific Islander households had the highest median income, with the median income of these households showing no significant change between 1991 and 1996. Trends in median income for Hispanic and Asian or Pacific Islander households are likely to have been affected by increasing immigration into the United States in recent years since recent immigrants have a lower median income than natives or longer term residents (6).

As mentioned above, household income is affected by household composition. The poverty index takes household size and composition into account (see Technical Notes). Figure 3 shows the proportion of persons poor and near poor by race and Hispanic origin for 1996. Overall, almost 14 percent of the population lived in poverty in 1996 and 20 percent more had incomes that were near poverty.

There are distinct demographic differences in poverty by age, race, ethnicity and household composition. In accordance with differences in median household income, black persons and persons of Hispanic origin are disproportionately represented among the poor and near poor. Poverty rates also vary across age groups. In 1996 over one-fifth of all children lived in poverty. Between 1970 and 1980 the poverty rate among children rose from around 15 percent to more than 20 percent and it has remained at or above 20 percent for the last 16 years. In contrast, nearly one-quarter of persons 65 years of age and over were poor in 1970, but by 1980 the proportion in poverty had decreased to 16 percent. Between 1980 and 1996 poverty among the elderly continued to decline to 10.8 percent, slightly below the rate for working-age adults (18–64 years of age) (7).

Race and ethnic differences in the poverty rate are as pronounced among children as among adults; in 1996, 11 percent of non-Hispanic white children were poor compared with 40 percent of black and Hispanic

children. Children in female-headed households had the highest rates of poverty; nearly one-half of the children living in female-headed households in 1996 were below the poverty line. Even among female-headed households, however, poverty rates for children were higher in black and Hispanic households than white households.

Figure 4 demonstrates that there are substantial geographic differences in poverty rates in the United States. The average State poverty levels for the years 1994–96 ranged from 7–8 percent in New Hampshire and Utah to 22 percent and more in New Mexico, the District of Columbia, and Louisiana with the South and West having disproportionately larger shares of the Nation's poor population. Geographic differences in health outcomes may be related to these variations in poverty.

Education is a widely used indicator of socioeconomic status in the United States. Educational attainment is a major determinant of earnings. In addition, education is also likely to influence health through a variety of cultural, social, and psychological mechanisms (8). For example, higher levels of education may increase exposure to health-related information as well as equip individuals with the skills to adopt health promoting behaviors. Education may also influence health-related values such as a belief in prevention.

Figure 5 shows the distribution of educational attainment for persons 25 years and over by age, race, and Hispanic origin in 1996. Educational attainment is presented for persons 25–64 years and 65 years or over because educational attainment varies by age cohort, with persons 65 years and over much less likely to have completed high school. Educational attainment also differs substantially by race and ethnicity. The race and ethnic patterns in household income (figure 2) are mirrored in the educational distributions of these groups. Among persons 25 to 64 years of age in 1996, 45 percent of Asian or Pacific Islanders and nearly 30 percent of non-Hispanic white persons have college degrees, compared with 15 percent of non-Hispanic black persons and 10 percent of Hispanic persons. This pattern is essentially reversed at the low end of educational

attainment; 10 percent of non-Hispanic white persons and 14 percent of Asian or Pacific Islander persons have not completed high school, compared with 20 percent of non-Hispanic black persons and 44 percent of Hispanic persons.

Figures 2 and 5 show that income and education vary by race and ethnicity, but even within the same category of educational attainment, median family income varies by race and ethnicity and also gender (figure 6). For men and women across all race and ethnic groups, the higher the level of education, the higher the median family income. However, within education level categories, men have higher median family incomes than women, and median family incomes of Asian or Pacific Islander and white persons were higher than median family incomes of black or Hispanic men and women. Some of these differences, especially differences between men and women, may be attributed to the number of family members who are employed and to whether employed family members work full-time or part-time.

Type of occupation can also significantly impact health, largely because occupation and income are intrinsically connected. However, occupation may additionally influence health directly by determining exposure to hazards in the work environment, as well as exposure to job-associated stress (9). Figure 7 shows the distribution of men and women by racial and ethnic groups across occupational categories (see Technical Notes for a description of each occupational category). The majority of persons 25–64 years of age are employed in white collar occupations. However, a greater proportion of Asian or Pacific Islander and non-Hispanic white men are employed in white collar jobs while more black and Hispanic men are employed in blue collar jobs. Women were twice as likely to be employed in service occupations than men, with black and Hispanic women more likely to be employed in service occupations than Asian or Pacific Islander or white women.

As these charts briefly demonstrate, the most common measures of socioeconomic status (income, education, and occupation) can vary substantially by race, ethnicity, and sex. The two following sections of the chartbook will demonstrate how measures of

socioeconomic status—particularly income and education—are strongly associated with health outcomes, health-related behaviors and other risk factors, and measures of health care access and utilization.

References

1. Ryscavage P, Henle P. Earnings inequality accelerates in the 1980's. Monthly Labor Review 113:3–16. 1990.

2. Danziger S, Gottschalk (eds.). Uneven tides: Rising inequality in America. New York: Russell Sage Foundation. 1993.

3. Karoly LA, Burtless G. Demographic change, rising earnings inequality, and the distribution of personal well-being, 1959–89. Demography 32(3):379–405. 1995.

4. U.S. Council of Economic Advisors. Economic report of the President. Washington: U.S. Government Printing Office. Chapter 4. 1992.

5. U.S. Council of Economic Advisors. Economic report of the President Washington: U.S. Government Printing Office. Chapter 5. 1995.

6. Hansen KA, Faber CS. The foreign-born population, 1996. U.S. Bureau of the Census. Current Population Survey, P20–494. 1997.

7. U.S. Council of Economic Advisors. Economic report of the President. Washington: U.S. Government Printing Office. Chapter 5. 1997.

8. Liberatos P. Link BG. Kelsey JL. The measurement of social class in epidemiology. Epidemiologic Reviews.10:87–121. 1988.

9. Karasek R, Theorell T. Healthy work: Stress, productivity, and the reconstruction of working life. New York: Basic Books. 1990.

Income

■ In 1996, 20 percent of U.S. households had incomes above $68,015 and 20 percent had incomes below $14,768, so that household income at the 80th percentile of the household income distribution was 4.6 times household income at the 20th percentile.

■ The ratio of income at the 80th percentile to that at the 20th percentile increased over the past 26 years; in 1970 this ratio was 4.0. The increase in the ratio of income at the 95th percentile to that at the 20th percentile has been even greater, from 6.3 in 1970 to 8.1 in 1996. By contrast, income at the 50th percentile remained approximately 2.4 times income at the 20th percentile over the 26 year period.

■ Measured in 1996 dollars, household income at the 20th and 50th percentiles changed little between 1970 and 1996. Between 1970 and 1990, income at the 20th percentile increased slightly, then fell by a small amount between 1990 and 1996, yielding an average annual increase of 0.20 percent over the 26-year period. Income at the 50th percentile followed a similar pattern with an average annual increase of 0.26 percent between 1970 and 1996. Income at the 80th percentile increased consistently over the period at an average annual rate of 0.77 percent, while the top 5 percent of the income distribution showed the greatest increase at 1.18 percent per year.

Figure 1. Household income at selected percentiles of the household income distribution: United States, 1970–96

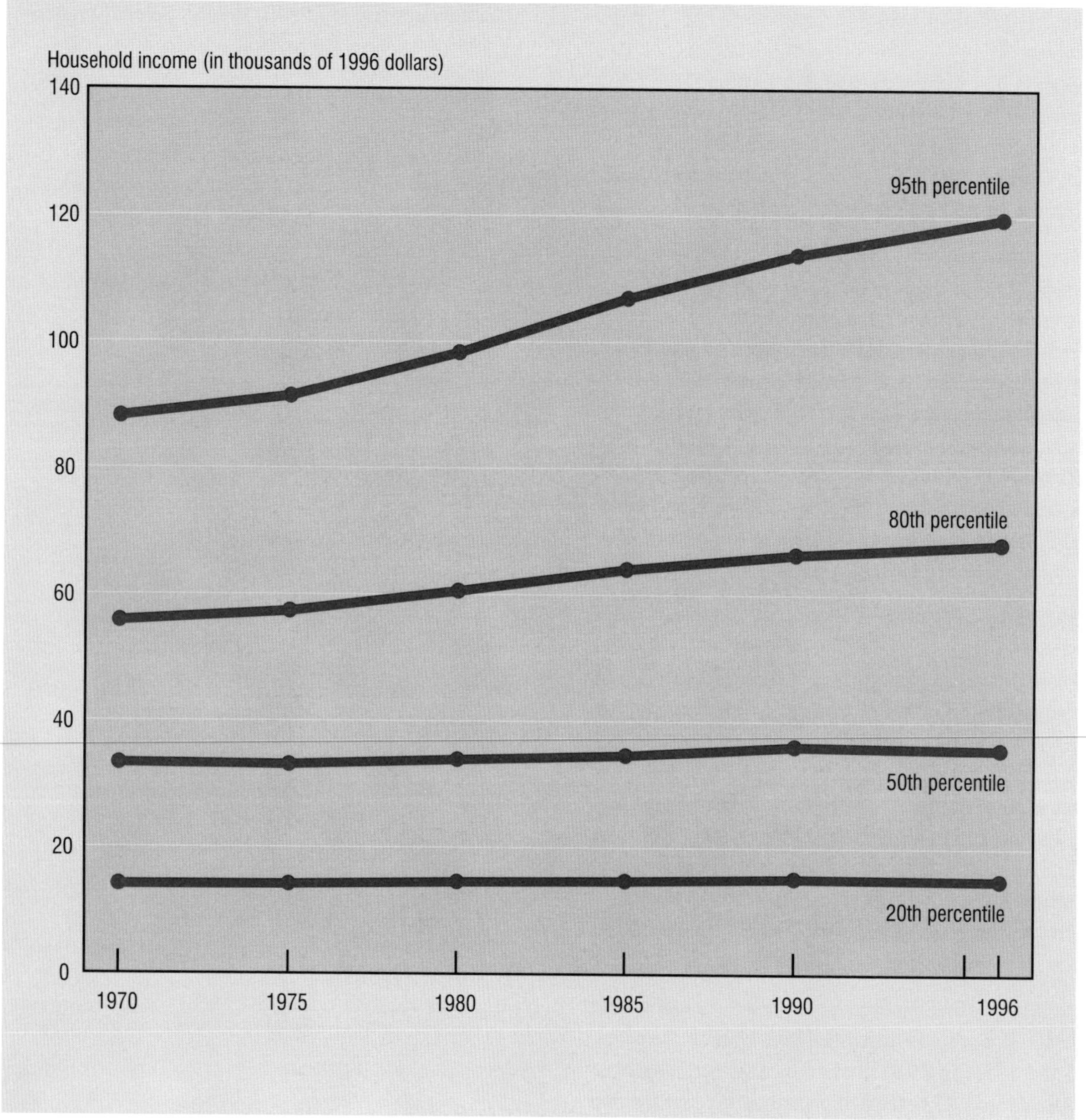

Household income (in thousands of 1996 dollars)

95th percentile

80th percentile

50th percentile

20th percentile

NOTES: See Technical Notes for the definition of income. In 1995, the 1990 Census adjusted population controls and sample redesign were implemented: there was a change in data collection method from paper-pencil to computer-assisted interviewing, and income reporting limits changed. In 1980, the 1980 Census population controls were implemented. In 1975, the 1970 population controls were implemented.

SOURCE: U.S. Census Bureau. Money Income in the United States: 1996. Current Population Reports, Series P60-197, Washington: U.S. Government Printing Office. September 1997.

Income

■ In 1996 median household income in the United States was $35,492. Asian or Pacific Islander households had the highest median income ($43,276), followed by non-Hispanic white households ($38,787). Median incomes for black and Hispanic households ($23,482 and $24,906) were less than 65 percent of the median for non-Hispanic white households.

■ Between 1982 and 1989, median income increased for black, non-Hispanic white, and Hispanic households (by 17 percent, 12 percent and 11 percent, respectively), then declined for all race and ethnic groups between 1989 and 1992. Between 1992 and 1996 median incomes rose for black, Asian or Pacific Islander, and non-Hispanic white households, but not for Hispanic households. In 1996 median income for black households was slightly higher than it had been in 1989, but median income for white households was still slightly lower than in 1989.

■ Between 1980 and 1996 the difference in income between non-Hispanic white households and black households decreased slightly, but the difference between Hispanic households and non-Hispanic white households widened. In 1980 the median income for white households was 39 percent higher than for Hispanic households; in 1990, 43 percent higher; and in 1996, 56 percent higher. In contrast, median income for non-Hispanic white households in 1980 was 77 percent higher than for black households; it was 71 percent higher in 1990, and 65 percent higher in 1996.

■ Similarly, the income difference between Hispanic and black households decreased considerably between 1980 and 1996. In 1980 median income for Hispanic households was 27 percent higher than median income

for black households; in 1990 it was 20 percent higher, but by 1996 it was only 6 percent higher.

■ Household income is influenced by number of earners per household and comparison across race and ethnic groups is affected by differences in average household size. In 1996, the total money income per household member was $20,216 for non-Hispanic white persons, $17,928 for persons of Asian or Pacific Islander origin, $11,543 for black persons, and $9,545 for persons of Hispanic origin (1).

Reference

1. U.S. Census Bureau. "Historical Income Tables, Household Table H-15. Total Money Income Per Household Member, by Race and Hispanic Origin of Householder: 1980 to 1996." Published 29 September, 1997.<www.census.gov/hhes/income/histinc/h15.html>

Figure 2. Median household income by race and Hispanic origin: United States, 1980–96

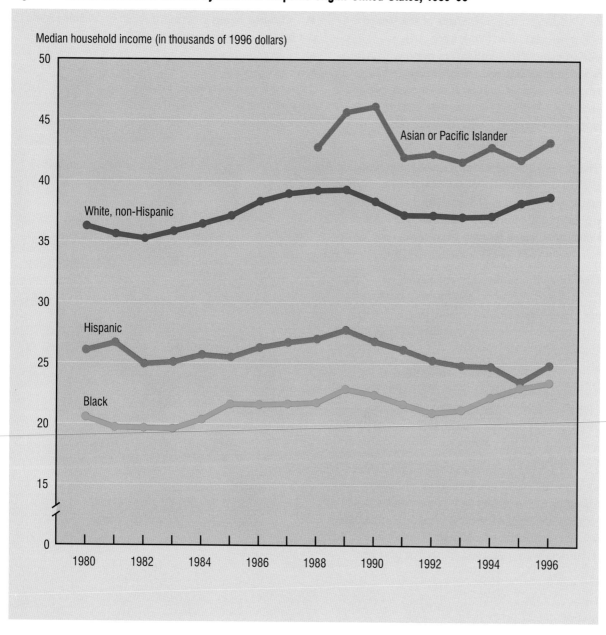

Median household income (in thousands of 1996 dollars)

NOTES: See Technical Notes for the definition of income. In 1995 the 1990 census adjusted population controls and sample redesign were implemented; there was a change in data collection method from paper-pencil to computer-assisted interviewing, and income reporting limits changed. In 1980, the 1980 Census population controls were implemented. In 1975, the 1970 population controls were implemented.

SOURCE: U.S. Census Bureau. "Historical Income Tables, Household Table H-5. Race and Hispanic Origin of Householder—Households by Median and Mean Income: 1967 to 1996." Published 29 September 1997. <www.census.gov/hhes/income/histic/h05.html>

Poverty

■ In 1996, 36.5 million residents of the United States (14 percent) were living in poverty. Forty-five percent (16.5 million) of persons living below the poverty line were non-Hispanic white persons, 27 percent (9.7 million) were black persons, 24 percent (8.7 million) were persons of Hispanic origin, and 4 percent (1.5 million) were persons of Asian or Pacific Islander origin.

■ The poverty rate was lowest among non-Hispanic white persons (9 percent) followed by persons of Asian or Pacific Islander origin (15 percent). Poverty rates for black persons and persons of Hispanic origin were more than three times the rate for non-Hispanic white persons.

■ Over one-third of the U.S. population was living in or near poverty in 1996. The majority of black persons (55 percent) and persons of Hispanic origin (60 percent) lived in families classified as poor or near poor.

■ In 1996, one out of every five children in the United States (14.5 million) lived in poverty. Poverty rates for black and Hispanic children were much higher (40 percent in each group) than the overall rate, and almost 4 times the poverty rate for non-Hispanic white children.

■ Over two-thirds of black children and nearly three-quarters of Hispanic children were living in or near poverty in 1996; 31 percent of non-Hispanic white children and 36 percent of children of Asian or Pacific Islander origin were classified as poor or near poor.

■ Children living in female-headed households had the highest rates of poverty. In 1996 nearly one-half of all children in female-headed households (8 million) were living below the poverty line and another 27 percent were near poor. Poverty rates for black and Hispanic children in female-headed households were considerably higher than the rates for non-Hispanic white children or children of Asian or Pacific Islander origin.

Figure 3. Percent of persons poor and near poor by race and Hispanic origin: United States, 1996

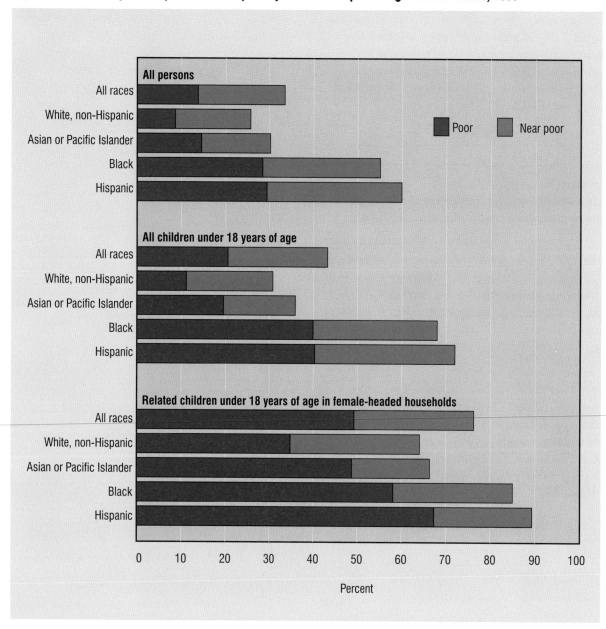

NOTES: All figures refer to persons. "All children under 18 years of age" includes unrelated children. "Female-headed households" above are families with female householder and no spouse present. See Technical Notes for a description of poverty status.

SOURCE: U.S. Census Bureau. "Detailed Poverty Tables, Table 2. Age, Sex, Household Relationship, Race and Hispanic origin, and Selected Statuses-Ratio of Income to Poverty level in 1996." Last revised: October 3, 1997. <http://ferret.bls.census.gov/macro/031997/pov/2_001-3.htm>. See related *Health, United States, 1998*, table 2.

Poverty

■ Across States the average annual poverty rates for the years 1994–96 varied over threefold from 7 to 24 percent. Poverty rates were lowest in New Hampshire and Utah (7–8 percent) and highest in Louisiana, New Mexico, and the District of Columbia (22–24 percent).

■ The South has a disproportionately large share of the Nation's poor population. In 1996, 35 percent of the U.S. population, but 38 percent of persons below the poverty line, lived in the South. One-quarter of poor persons lived in the West, while the Midwest and Northeast each contained 18 percent of the Nation's poor.

■ Before 1994 the South had the highest poverty rate of any region. In 1996 the poverty rate in the West was not significantly different from that in the South; both were 15 percent. Thirteen percent of persons living in the Northeast were poor in 1996, as were 11 percent of persons living in the Midwest.

■ Within the West, the States with the highest poverty rates during 1994–96 include New Mexico (24 percent), Arizona (18 percent), and California (17 percent). Within the South the following eight States had poverty rates of 16 percent or higher during 1994–96: Louisiana, the District of Columbia, Mississippi, West Virginia, Alabama, Texas, Oklahoma, and Kentucky.

Figure 4. Percent of persons in poverty by State: United States, average annual 1994–96

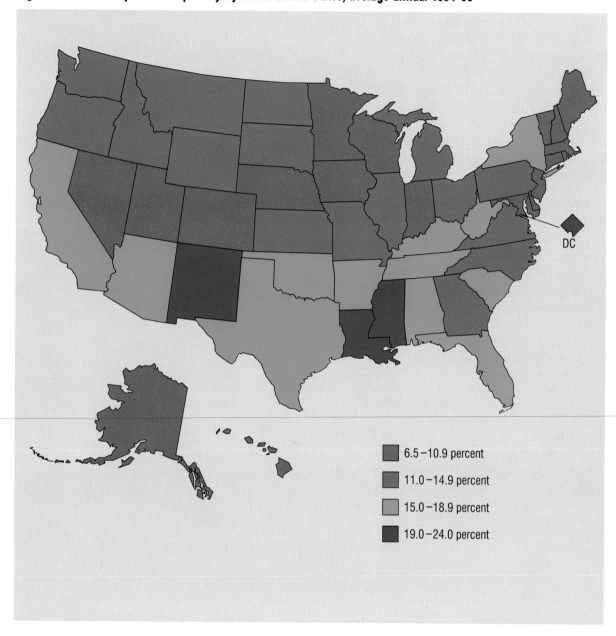

■	6.5–10.9 percent
■	11.0–14.9 percent
■	15.0–18.9 percent
■	19.0–24.0 percent

NOTE: See Technical Notes for a description of poverty status.

SOURCE: U.S. Bureau of the Census. Poverty in the United States: 1996. Current Population Reports, Series P60-194. Washington: U.S. Government Printing Office. September 1997.

Education

■ The average level of education in the U.S. population has increased steadily since this information was first collected by the Current Population Survey in 1947. In 1996, 35 percent of persons 65 years of age and over, but only 14 percent of persons ages 25–64 years, had not completed high school. In contrast, more than one-half of persons 25–64 years of age had some education beyond high school, whereas only 31 percent of persons 65 years of age and over had more than a high school diploma.

■ Educational levels vary considerably among race and ethnic subgroups. Among persons 25–64 years of age, the proportion who had not completed high school in 1996 ranged from 10 percent for white persons to 44 percent for Hispanic persons. In this age group, one out of every five black persons and one out of every eight Asian or Pacific Islander persons had less than a high school education. The percent with a college degree or higher level of education ranged from 10 percent for Hispanic persons to 45 percent for Asian or Pacific Islander persons.

■ Among persons 65 years of age and older, the percent who did not complete high school ranged from 31 percent for white persons to 70 percent for Hispanic persons. In this age group, one-third of white persons and 35 percent of Asian or Pacific Islander persons had some education beyond high school, compared with 18 percent of black persons and 14 percent of Hispanic persons.

Figure 5. Educational attainment among persons 25 years and over by age, race, and Hispanic origin: United States, 1996

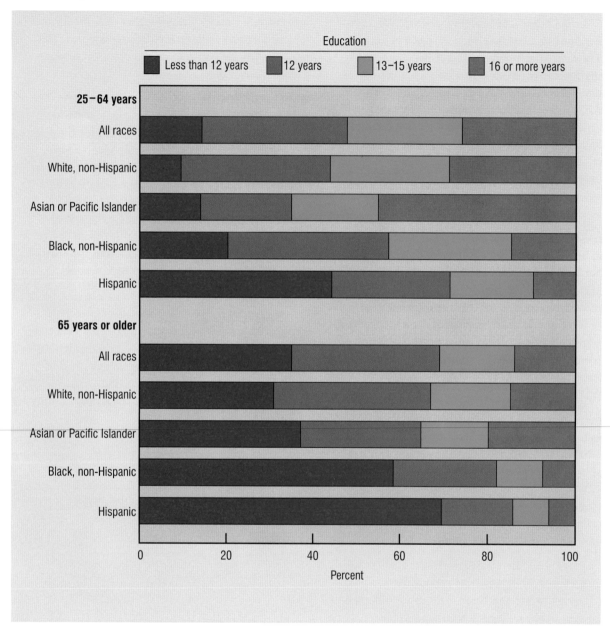

NOTES: Less than 12 years includes persons with 12 years of schooling but no high school diploma. Twelve years includes persons with a high school diploma or G.E.D. Thirteen to fifteen years includes persons without a degree and persons with associate's degrees. Sixteen years or more includes all persons with a baccalaurate degree or higher.

SOURCE: U.S. Bureau of the Census. Current Population Survey, March 1996.

Education

■ Median household income increases with each higher level of education. Men 25 years of age and over with at least a college degree had a median family income of $66,690 in 1996, 2.7 times the median for men who did not complete high school ($24,386). The income gradient with increasing education was similar for women; median family income for women with a college degree or higher level of education was 3.4 times as high as the median for women without a high school diploma ($62,050 compared with $18,200).

■ At each level of attained education, women generally lived in households with less income than men, but the gender disparity tended to decrease at higher levels of education. Median household income for men who had not finished high school was 34 percent higher than the median for women with the same level of education; median household income for men with at least a college degree was 7 percent higher than the median for women at the same education level.

■ The disparity between the median household incomes of men and women at the same level of education was greatest for black persons; median income for men exceeded that for women by 52 percent for persons with less than a high school education, and by 16 percent for college graduates. Among Asian or Pacific Islander persons, there was essentially no gender disparity in median household income within levels of education.

■ Among men, the education-related gradient in median household income was greatest for non-Hispanic white and black men; in 1996 black and white men with a college degree had median household incomes 2.7 times higher than the median income for those with no high school diploma. This ratio was 2.4 for Hispanic men and 2.0 for Asian or Pacific Islander men.

■ The education-related gradient in median household income was similar for black and white women; those with at least a college degree lived in households where the median family income was approximately 3.5 times greater than that for women who had not finished high school. Among Hispanic women, this ratio was 2.9. There was less of an education-related gradient in income for Asian or Pacific Islander women; those with a college degree or higher lived in households with a median income less than twice that of women with no high school diploma.

■ At each level of education, median household incomes for women varied more across the race and ethnic subgroups than did those for men. Within each education level, median household income in 1996 was similar for Hispanic and black men, but the median for black women was lower than that for Hispanic women.

Figure 6. Median household income among persons 25 years of age and over by education, sex, race, and Hispanic origin: United States, 1996

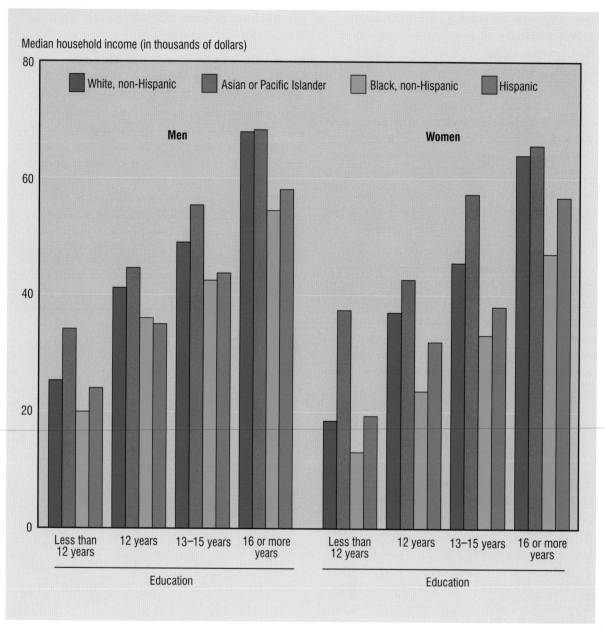

NOTES: Median income is based on total household income (earnings and other income) and is not adjusted for work status or number of hours worked by household members. Median is calculated using actual reported household income, not grouped data. Educational attainment is as of March 1997. Less than 12 years includes persons with 12 years of schooling but no high school diploma. Twelve years includes persons with a high school diploma or G.E.D. Thirteen to fifteen years includes persons without a degree and persons with Associate's degrees. Sixteen years or more includes all persons with a baccalaurate degree or higher.

SOURCE: U.S. Bureau of the Census. Current Population Survey: March 1997.

Occupation

■ The U.S. labor force has become increasingly concentrated in white collar occupations: executive, professional, managerial, administrative, technical, clerical, and sales positions. In 1996, among civilians 25–64 years of age reporting a current occupation, 48 percent of men and 73 percent of women held white collar positions. Thirty–nine percent of civilian men in this age range held blue collar jobs, compared with only 10 percent of women. By contrast, women were nearly twice as likely as men to be employed in service occupations (16 percent compared with 9 percent). Only 4 percent of men and just 1 percent of women reported their major occupation as farm related.

■ Asian or Pacific Islander men and non-Hispanic white men were much more likely to hold white collar positions than black or Hispanic men; three out of every five Asian or Pacific Islander men and over one-half of white men were employed in white collar occupations, compared with one out of every three black men and about one-quarter of Hispanic men. For each race and ethnic group examined, the majority of employed civilian women between 25 and 64 years of age held white collar positions, from 52 percent of Hispanic women to over three-quarters of white women.

■ In 1996 average compensation for persons holding blue-collar jobs was 81 percent of that for white collar workers (see *Health, United States, 1998*, table 122). Nearly one-half of employed civilian Hispanic and black men were working in blue collar jobs in 1996, but only 28 percent of Asian or Pacific Islander men were in blue collar employment. Only 8 percent of currently employed white women held blue collar jobs,

compared with between 15 and 18 percent of women in other race and ethnic groups.

■ In 1996 average compensation for service workers was 41 percent of that for persons in white collar employment (see *Health, United States, 1998*, table 122). Black and Hispanic women were nearly twice as likely as white and Asian or Pacific Islander women to be employed in service occupations (26 and 27 percent compared with 13 and 15 percent, respectively) in 1996. White and Asian or Pacific Islander men were least likely to be employed in service occupations, 7 and 9 percent compared with 15 and 18 percent for Hispanic and black men, respectively.

■ Hispanic men and women were more likely to be employed in farm occupations than those in other race and ethnic groups. In 1996, 9 percent of Hispanic men and 3 percent of Hispanic women reported farm-related work as their major occupation.

Figure 7. Current occupation for persons 25–64 years of age by sex, race, and Hispanic origin: United States, 1996

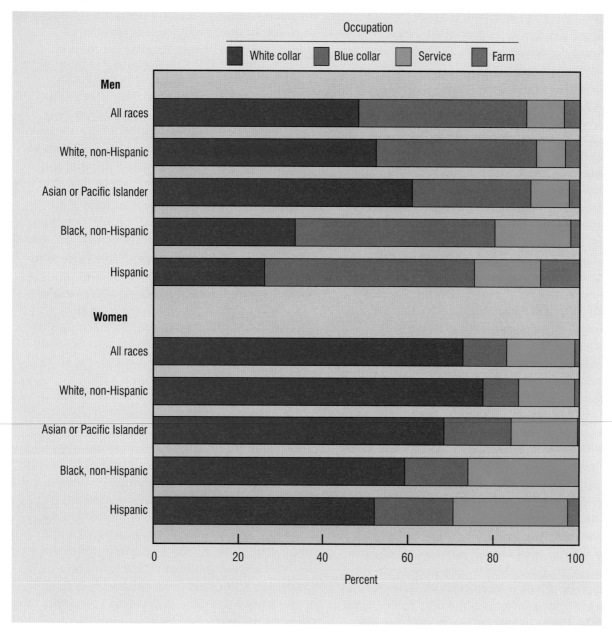

NOTES: Within the occupational categories there is a great deal of occupational diversity. See Technical Notes for description of each occupational category. Persons in the military are excluded.

SOURCE: U.S. Bureau of the Census. Current Population Survey: March 1996.

Children's Health

A healthy childhood is a foundation of success and health in later life. This section of the chartbook shows the relationship between socioeconomic status (SES) of a child's family and indicators of health status in childhood, risk factors for poor health during pregnancy through adolescence, and health care access and utilization for children.

Receiving prenatal care and maintaining good health behaviors during pregnancy are the first steps toward having a healthy child. Early and consistent prenatal care reduces the risk of poor birth outcomes. Figures 18 and 19 present data on prenatal care utilization. During the 1990's early initiation of prenatal care increased for mothers at every level of education. This improvement may have been due partly to expansions in Medicaid coverage for pregnant women (1). However, data indicated that in 1996 more educated mothers were still more likely than less educated mothers to obtain prenatal care in the first trimester, regardless of race or ethnicity. The *Healthy People 2000* goal for prenatal care is for 90 percent of live births to have received prenatal care in the first trimester. While mothers with 16 or more years of education were close to the goal or achieved it in most race and ethnic groups, fewer than three-quarters of mothers who had not completed high school obtained early prenatal care in any race and ethnic group; in some groups the percent with early prenatal care was closer to one-half. In addition to lack of insurance or other financial problems, other factors, such as lack of transportation, scheduling difficulties, or lack of knowledge about the pregnancy, may act as barriers to receiving early care (2,3).

Maternal behaviors also influence the health of the infant at birth. Infants whose mothers smoked during pregnancy are more likely to experience health problems, such as low birthweight, abruptio placentae (4), intrauterine growth retardation (5), Sudden Infant Death Syndrome (6), and asthma in childhood (7). Figure 13 demonstrates that in 1996 less educated women were more likely to smoke during pregnancy, but there were significant differences by race and ethnicity; less educated non-Hispanic white women were far more likely to smoke than women of other backgrounds. Almost one-half of non-Hispanic white women without a high school diploma smoked during pregnancy, compared with less than one-third of women in any other group. Hispanic and Asian or Pacific Islander women were particularly unlikely to smoke, yet even in these groups, an education-related gradient was apparent.

Adolescent childbearing, another risk factor for poor health in childhood, was more common among mothers of lower socioeconomic status (figure 12). Women whose own mothers were less educated were more likely to become teenage parents. The low education levels of the respondents' mothers likely reflected lower household incomes, on average, when the teenage mothers were young, and perhaps different expectations for educational attainment or childbearing than were found among the daughters of more educated women (8). Early childbearing is associated with a wide range of poor health and economic outcomes (9), and the teenage mothers in this data set had much lower incomes in adulthood than those who delayed their first birth. Lower socioeconomic status was a predictor and a consequence of early childbearing.

Infants born to mothers of lower socioeconomic status tended to have poorer health, as measured by their rates of low birthweight and infant mortality. In addition to the importance of infant survival in its own right, the infant mortality rate is correlated strongly with a variety of other health measures, and is considered to be a good measure of overall community health (10). Low birthweight is associated with an increased risk of health and developmental problems during infancy and childhood (11). Infants whose mothers had fewer years of education were more likely to have a low weight at birth (less than 5.5 pounds) and to die before reaching their first birthday (figures 8, 9, and 10). These two measures are closely associated as low birthweight is a frequent antecedent to infant mortality. Among white and black infants,

each increase in maternal education was associated with a decline in low birthweight and infant mortality rates. This pattern was evident among Hispanic children for infant mortality but not for low birthweight. Neither infant mortality nor low birthweight was clearly associated with maternal education among American Indian or Alaska Native children or among Asian or Pacific Islander children, although the infants of the least educated American Indian or Alaska Native women had higher rates of both measures. Analysis of data for Hispanic and Asian or Pacific Islander subgroups found the association with socioeconomic status to be evident among some groups and less so among others. Analysis of trends in infant mortality (figure 8) indicated that the health gaps between children of higher and lower socioeconomic status have been fairly wide throughout the 1980's and early 1990's, and that declines in infant mortality during 1983–95 were fairly consistent across maternal education groups.

Health insurance may be a contributing factor in health disparities. Children without health insurance coverage are likely to have difficulties obtaining medical care (12,13). The parents of children with public (usually Medicaid) coverage may also have trouble finding a physician since many do not accept Medicaid patients, often because Medicaid reimburses at a lower rate than does private insurance (14). Children who have no insurance may be forced to bypass well-child and preventive visits. Those without adequate access may procure services at an emergency room as a last-resort location for health care (13).

Children from low-income families were much less likely to be insured (figure 20), although there were few differences between poor and near-poor children. Among black and Hispanic children, the near-poor had lower coverage rates, probably because many of the poor were insured through the Medicaid program, for which most of the near-poor children were not eligible. Very few children in high-income families were uninsured (from 4 to 7 percent), while

up to one-third of children in low-income families had no health insurance.

Several measures of health status and health care utilization indicated that children from lower SES families had worse health status and more risk factors for poor health while having less adequate access to and utilization of health services. Health care utilization reflected the disparities evident in insurance coverage. Children under age 6 who were from poor and near-poor families were less likely than those from middle- or high-income families to have seen a physician in the past year, and uninsured children from every income group were substantially less likely than insured children to have seen a doctor (figure 22). Children living in lower income areas had lower rates of outpatient visits than those living in higher income areas, and were more likely to have received care in hospital emergency or outpatient departments than at a physician's office (figure 23).

Children from poor families were less likely to be fully vaccinated on schedule than children from higher income families (figure 21). Prompt vaccination is important to protect children's health, and may be a marker of the quality of children's health care early in life. Insufficient vaccine levels may indicate that the child has not had timely use of well-child visits.

Another indicator of adequacy of preventive care is hospitalization for asthma. Asthma is one of the most common chronic diseases in childhood, and is generally managed via outpatient care and, occasionally, emergency room visits. Hospitalization for asthma indicates severe disease and may suggest that the child has not had adequate care from a physician who can help them control their asthma (15). Children who lived in poorer neighborhoods had higher rates of hospitalization for asthma (figure 24) and black children had higher rates than those of white children at every level of neighborhood socioeconomic status during 1989–91.

Disparity in environmental quality is another factor contributing to the influence of socioeconomic

status on health. Figure 14 shows that children in lower income households were more likely to have elevated levels of blood lead, which is associated with less than optimal developmental outcome, such as lower intelligence (16). Poorer children may be more subject to environmental degradation, such as substandard housing, putting them at greater risk of lead intake (17).

Activity limitation due to a chronic health condition is a broad measure of health and functioning. In contrast to the declines in infant mortality, rates of reported activity limitation among children increased slightly between 1984–87 and 1992–95. This increase appeared to be greater among children in lower income than higher income families, resulting in a slight widening of the disparity by income (figure 11). Hispanic children had lower rates of reported activity limitation in each income group and a less marked income gradient than white or black children. The increase in reported rates of activity limitation may have been a result of a true increase in limitation, but also may have been influenced if there was an increase in diagnosis of existing limitations (such as the diagnosis of learning disability) or a change in awareness of such limitations.

Many risk factors for poor health in later life develop in adolescence. Smoking is most frequently begun in adolescence (18), and obesity in youth may remain into adulthood (19). Although smoking rates among pregnant women were inversely related to level of education, there was no clear gradient in smoking rates for adolescents by family income group overall (figures 13 and 15). However, when adolescent smoking data were broken down by race and ethnic group, results appeared more similar to those of childbearing women: the proportion smoking was highest and the income gradient strongest among white adolescents. However, smoking was more common among Hispanic adolescents and less common among black adolescents than among pregnant women of the same race or ethnicity.

Overall, adolescents from lower income families were more likely to be overweight than those from higher income families. However, within the race and ethnic subgroups examined, the negative relationship of income and overweight was true only for non-Hispanic white adolescents (figure 16). Black adolescents had no clear pattern of overweight in relation to family socioeconomic status, while Mexican American teenagers from higher income families were more likely to be overweight. Since sedentary behavior is a strong risk factor for overweight, one might expect the two to have a similar socioeconomic profile, and sedentariness was associated with socioeconomic status (figure 17), with the association more marked for girls than for boys. The overall relationship between income and sedentary behavior may obscure substantial differences among race and ethnic groups, which could not be examined here due to insufficient sample size.

Data suggested that health status of children has improved in some areas since the early 1980's and worsened in others. However, the health gap between children of higher and lower socioeconomic status parents was constant through the time period and remained in the mid-1990's. Children who had well-educated or high-income parents had a better chance of being born healthy and continuing to remain healthy throughout childhood. Access to appropriate health care, health behaviors of parents and children, and exposure to environmental risks are among the factors contributing to the socioeconomic disparities in children's health.

References

1. Ray WA, Mitchel EF, Piper JM. Effect of Medicaid expansions on preterm birth. Am J Prev Med 13(4): 292–7. 1997.

2. Lewis CT, Mathews TJ, Heuser RL. Prenatal care in the United States, 1980–94. Vital Health Stat 21(54):1–17. 1996.

3. Rogers C, Schiff M. Early versus late prenatal care in New Mexico: Barriers and motivators. Birth 23(1):26–30. 1996.

4. Kramer MS, Usher RH, Pollack R, Boyd M, Usher S. Etiologic determinants of abruptio placentae. Obstet Gynecol 89:221–6. 1997.

5. Nordentoft M, Lou HC, Hansen D, et al. Intrauterine growth retardation and premature delivery: The influence of maternal smoking and psychosocial factors. Am J Public Health 86: 1996.

6. Hoffman HJ, Damus K, Hillman L, Krongrad E. Risk factors for SIDS: Results of the National Institute of Child Health and Human Development SIDS Cooperative Epidemiological Study. Ann NY Acad Sci1 8: 113–20. 1988.

7. Ehrlich RI, Du-Toit D, Jordaan E, et al. Risk factors for childhood asthma and wheezing: Importance of maternal and household smoking. Am J Respir Crit Care Med 154: 681–8. 1996.

8. Nord CW, Moore KA, Morrison DR, et al. Consequences of teenage parenting. J School Health 62:310–8. 1992.

9. Hoffman SD, Foster EM, Furstenberg FF Jr. Reevaluating the costs of teenage childbearing. Demography 30(1):1–13. 1993.

10. Freedman MA. Health status indicators for the year 2000. Healthy People 2000 Statistical Notes 1(1): 1–4. National Center for Health Statistics. 1991.

11. Hack M, Klein NK, Taylor HG. Long-term developmental outcomes of low birth weight infants. In: The Future of Children. Low Birth Weight. Shiano PH and Berhman RE, eds. David and Lucille Packard Foundation. 176–96. 1995.

12. Newacheck PW, Hughes DC, Stoddard JJ. Children's access to primary care: Differences by race, income, and insurance status. Pediatrics 97(1):26–32. 1996.

13. Weissman JS, Epstein AM. Falling through the safety net. Baltimore, Maryland: The Johns Hopkins University Press. 1994.

14. Cykert S, Kissling G, Layson R, Hansen C. Health insurance does not guarantee access to primary care: A national study of physicians' acceptance of publicly insured patients. J Gen Intern Med 10(6):345–8. 1995.

15. Lieu TA, Quesenberry CP Jr, Capra AM, et al. Outpatient management practices associated with reduced risk of pediatric asthma hospitalization and emergency department visits. Pediatrics 100(3 Pt 1): 334–41. 1997.

16. Pocock SJ, Smith M, Baghurst P. Environmental lead and children's intelligence: A systematic review of the epidemiological evidence. BMJ 309:1189–97. 1994.

17. Lanphear BP, Weitzman M, Eberly S. Racial differences in urban children's environmental exposures to lead. Am J Public Health 86:1460–63. 1996.

18. Centers for Disease Control and Prevention. Trends in smoking initiation among adolescents and young adults - United States, 1980–1989. MMWR 44(28): 521–5. 1995.

19. Serdula MK, Ivery D, Coates RJ, et al. Do obese children become obese adults? A review of the literature. Prev Med 22:167–77. 1993.

Infant Mortality

■ Infant mortality is comprised of deaths that occur before an infant's first birthday. Infant mortality is an important indicator of the health of infants and pregnant women because it is closely related to factors such as maternal health, quality of and access to medical care, socioeconomic conditions, and public health practices. About two-thirds of infant deaths are associated with problems of the infant or the pregnancy, while one-third result from conditions arising after the delivery, often reflecting social or environmental factors (1). The *Healthy People 2000* target is for no more than 7 deaths per 1,000 infants in the United States as a whole, and no more than 11 deaths per 1,000 black infants.

■ Between 1983 and 1995, the infant mortality rate in the United States among infants born to mothers 20 years of age and over declined from 10.3 to 7.1 deaths per 1,000 live births. Reductions in infant mortality were seen in all race and education groups examined, though the decline occurred more steadily in some groups than in others.

■ The infant mortality gap across education levels remained approximately constant during the time period among white and black infants. In every year, infants born to less educated mothers had higher rates of mortality than infants born to more educated mothers, but the disparity was constant or decreased slightly over time. Between 1983 and 1995, among infants born to white mothers, the relative decline in infant mortality was greatest among infants born to women with less than 12 years of education (39 percent) and least among infants of mothers with 12 years of education (26 percent). Among infants born to black women the relative decline in infant mortality ranged from 16 percent among those born to the most

educated mothers to 27 percent among those born to the least educated mothers.

■ In every year black infants remained at higher risk of dying than white infants at every level of mother's education. By 1995 rates among infants born to more educated black mothers were approaching rates seen in the mid-1980's among infants of less educated white mothers.

■ White infants' mortality rates declined more rapidly than those of black infants at each level of mother's education. In 1983, the ratio of black to white infant mortality rates ranged from 1.9 for infants born to the least educated mothers to 2.1 among infants born to the most educated mothers. In 1995 the black-white infant mortality ratio increased to 2.2 for infants born to the least educated mothers to 2.7 among infants born to the most educated mothers.

Reference

1. Centers for Disease Control and Prevention. Poverty and infant mortality. United States, 1988. MMWR 44(49): 922–27. 1995.

Figure 8. Infant mortality rates among infants of mothers 20 years of age and over by mother's education and race: United States, 1983–95

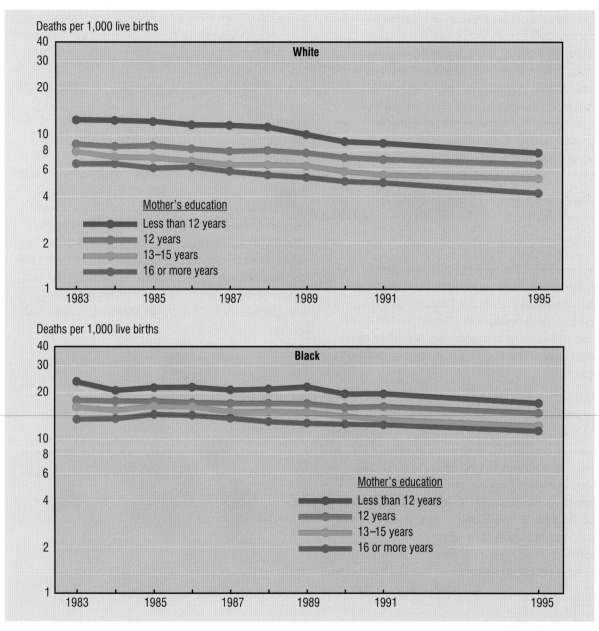

NOTES: 1995 data were calculated on a period basis, while prior years were calculated on a cohort basis; 1995 data used weighting for the first time. See *Health, United States, 1998* Appendix I for an explanation of the differences in the methods.

SOURCE: Centers for Disease Control and Prevention, National Center for Health Statistics, National Linked Files of Live Births and Infant Deaths. See related *Health, United States, 1998*, table 21.

Infant Mortality

■ During 1995 about seven in every thousand infants died before their first birthday. The likelihood of death in infancy was related to the mother's education; each higher level of maternal education was associated with an improvement in the infant mortality rate. Among live births to mothers 20 years of age and over in 1995, babies born to mothers who did not finish high school were almost 1.9 times as likely to die as those whose mothers graduated from college.

■ Infant mortality rates varied significantly among racial and ethnic groups. Hispanic and Asian or Pacific Islander infants tended to have similar infant mortality rates. Black infants had higher rates. Non-Hispanic white and American Indian or Alaska Native infants had intermediate rates at lower education levels, but rates among non-Hispanic white infants approached Hispanic and Asian or Pacific Islander rates at the highest education levels. The *Healthy People 2000* goal for American Indian or Alaska Native infants is 8.5 deaths per 1,000.

■ Although apparent for all race and ethnic groups, the educational gradient in infant mortality was stronger for white and American Indian or Alaska Native infants than for black, Asian or Pacific Islander, or Hispanic infants. White infants had the steepest gradient; infants born to mothers with fewer than 12 years of education were 2.4 times as likely to die as those born to mothers with 16 or more years of education. Among both Hispanic and Asian or Pacific Islander infants, babies born to the least educated mothers were 1.4 times as likely to die as those born to the most educated mothers.

■ There was diversity in the educational disparities among Hispanic and Asian or Pacific Islander subgroups. When Hispanic subgroups were examined separately for the 3-year period 1989–91, Cuban and Puerto Rican infants had stronger maternal educational gradients in mortality (the infants of the least educated women were 1.8 or 1.9 times as likely to die as infants of the most educated women) than did Mexican or Central and South American infants (where the disparity was 1.1–1.3). *Healthy People 2000* sets a target for Puerto Rican infants of 8 deaths per 1,000 by the year 2000. During the same time period, among Asian or Pacific Islander infants, Filipino American and Chinese American infants had a relatively lower gradient (infants born to the least educated women were 1.2 to 1.4 times as likely to die as infants of the most educated), while Japanese American (infants of the least educated were 1.7 times as likely to die) and Hawaiian infants (infants of the least educated were over three times as likely to die) had steeper maternal educational gradients.

Figure 9. Infant mortality rates among infants of mothers 20 years of age and over by mother's education, race, and Hispanic origin: United States, 1995

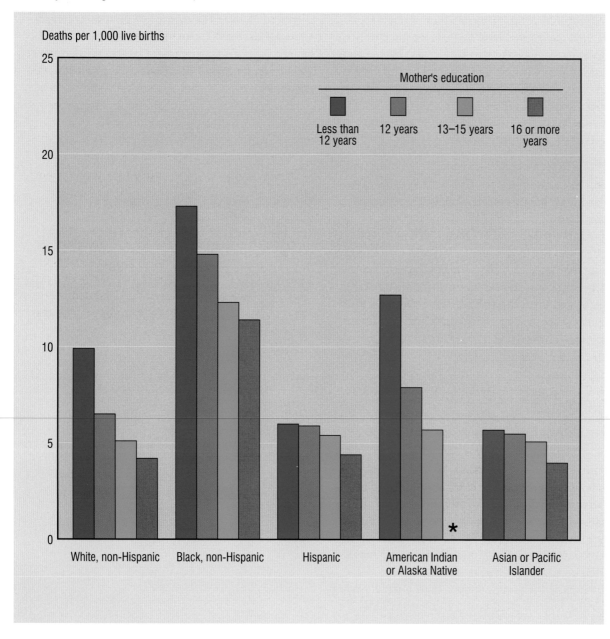

*The number of infant deaths among American Indian or Alaska Native mothers with 16 or more years of education was too small for stable rate calculation.

SOURCE: Centers for Disease Control and Prevention, National Center for Health Statistics, National Linked File of Live Births and Infant Deaths. See related *Health, United States, 1998*, table 21.

Low Birthweight

■ Low-birthweight infants are born weighing less than 2,500 grams, or about 5.5 pounds. Infants of low birthweight are less likely to survive and have a higher risk of disability if they live. Low birthweight may result from premature birth and/or from insufficient growth for the gestational age. *Healthy People 2000* sets a low-birthweight goal of 5 percent overall, and 9 percent for black infants.

■ Among births to non-Hispanic white, black, and American Indian or Alaska Native mothers 20 years of age and over, greater maternal education was associated with a decreased likelihood of low birthweight. In 1996 the prevalence of low birthweight among births to white mothers with less than 12 years of education was 1.8 times as high as among mothers with at least 16 years of education; among black mothers, the least educated had low birthweight rates 1.5 times those of their counterparts who had 16 or more years of education. For American Indian or Alaska Native infants, low birthweight was 1.2 times as high among births to mothers with less than a high school education as among births to mothers who had at least some college.

■ Overall, births to Hispanic and Asian or Pacific Islander mothers did not show the same kind of trend; no matter what the mother's education level, the infants were equally likely to be low birthweight, and the rates were uniformly low (on average, 6 percent of Hispanic infants and 7 percent of Asian or Pacific Islander infants). When Asian or Pacific Islander subgroups were examined, only Hawaiian mothers had a strong relationship between education and birthweight; other groups did not show a trend. Among Hispanics, less educated Puerto Rican and Cuban

American mothers had higher low birthweight rates, while Mexican and Central and South American mothers had no such gradient. The *Healthy People 2000* target for Puerto Rican infants is 6 percent with low birthweight.

■ There was a greater disparity in low birthweight across race and ethnic groups than by maternal education. Black women were much more likely to have a low-birthweight infant than women of any other background. Over 13 percent of black infants were low birthweight, compared with between 6 and 7 percent of infants for the four other groups. The reasons for this disparity are unclear, but socioeconomic status could not fully account for it; the most educated black women were more likely to have a low-birthweight infant than the least educated women of any other race or ethnic group.

Figure 10. Low-birthweight live births among mothers 20 years of age and over by mother's education, race, and Hispanic origin: United States, 1996

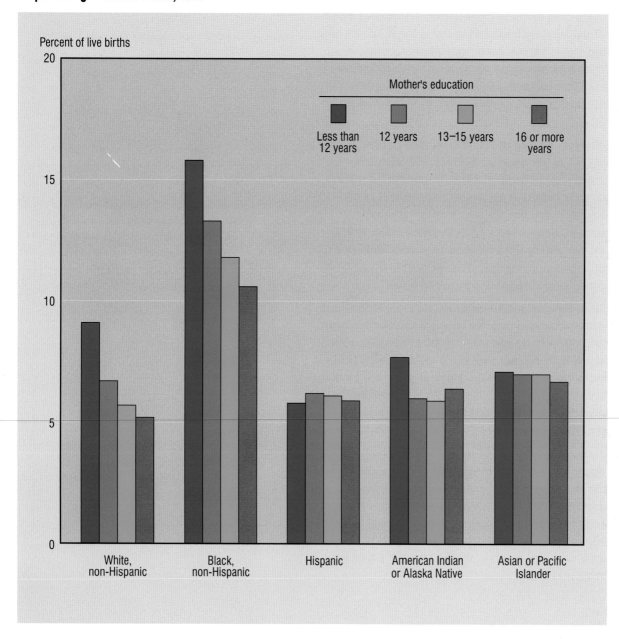

NOTE: Low birthweight refers to an infant weighing less than 2,500 grams at birth.

SOURCES: Centers for Disease Control and Prevention, National Center for Health Statistics, National Vital Statistics System. See related *Health, United States, 1998*, table 12.

Activity Limitation

■ This chart refers to the proportion of children whose usual activities, such as playing and going to school, are limited due to chronic health conditions. Conditions included here have persisted at least 3 months and may include illnesses, such as asthma or diabetes, injuries, or impairments affecting abilities such as vision, hearing, or speech.

■ Overall, the rate of children who are reported to have some kind of limitation in their everyday activities increased slightly between 1984–87 and 1992–95. There was a clear pattern of socioeconomic disparity in each time period, such that children from lower income families were more likely to have some kind of activity limitation. During 1992–95 children in poor families were about 1.9 times as likely to have an activity limitation as children living in higher income households.

■ In every race and ethnic group for every time period, limitation of activity rates increased as income declined. In 1992–95, poor non-Hispanic white children were about 2.2 times as likely, and poor black children twice as likely, to have an activity limitation as white and black children in higher income households. Hispanic children, however, had less of a gradient; the lower income children were only 1.4 times as likely as upper income children to have a limitation.

■ Data suggested that the disparity between the lowest and highest income groups may have increased over time. During 1984–87 children living in poor families were 1.7 times as likely to have a limitation of activity as those in the highest income families, while in 1992–95 poor children were almost twice as likely to have a limitation as wealthier children.

Figure 11. Activity limitation among children under 18 years of age by family income, race, and Hispanic origin: United States, average annual, 1984–87, 1988–91, and 1992–95

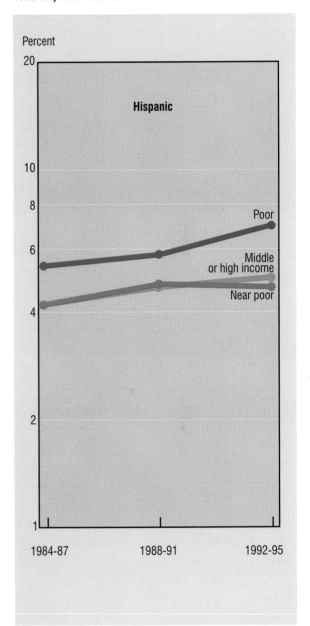

Figure 11. Activity limitation among children under 18 years of age by family income, race, and Hispanic origin: United States, average annual, 1984–87, 1988–91, and 1992–95—Continued

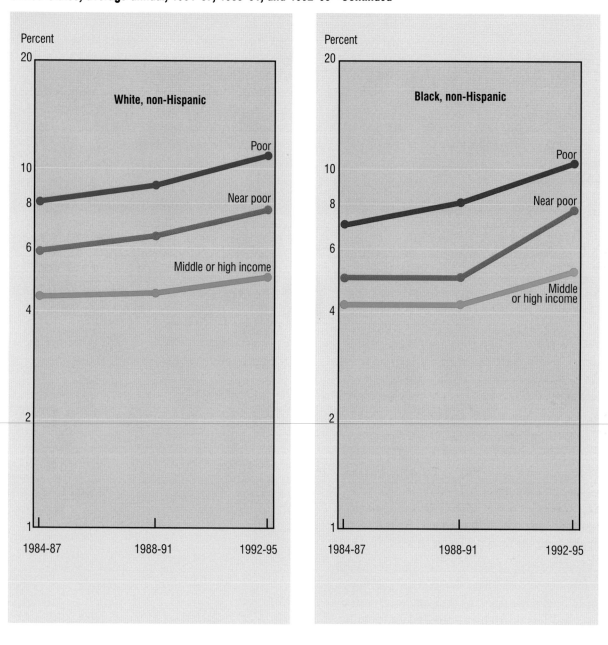

NOTE: See Technical Notes for definitions of activity limitation and family income categories.

SOURCE: Centers for Disease Control and Prevention, National Center for Health Statistics, National Health Interview Survey. See related *Health, United States, 1998*, table 60.

Teenage Childbearing

■ Teenage childbearing often leads to poor economic and social outcomes for teenage parents and their children. Adolescent mothers are unlikely to attain a high level of education, their relationships with the father are highly unstable, and they are far more likely than other women to live in poverty. Children born to teenagers have higher infant mortality rates, and sequelae continue throughout childhood, including higher rates of abuse and neglect and poorer rates of high school completion.

■ Almost one out of five women aged 20–29 in 1995 had a first birth before the age of 20. The likelihood of having had a child as a teenager was much higher among women whose own mothers were less educated. Nearly one out of every three women whose mothers had not completed high school began childbearing as an adolescent. The proportion dropped to fewer than one in five among those whose mothers had completed only high school, to 13 percent of women whose mothers had some college, and to 7 percent of women whose mothers had completed college.

■ In every race and ethnic group analyzed, there was an inverse relationship between the respondent's mother's education level and the proportion of women who had a teenage birth. Women whose mothers had more education were less likely to have become a teenage parent, no matter what their race or ethnic background, although the magnitude of this disparity differed among the race and ethnic groups.

■ The proportion of non-Hispanic white women in their twenties who had their first birth as a teenager declined from more than 1 in 4 among those whose mothers had less than a high school education to less than 1 in 20 among those whose mothers completed college. Among black women, almost one-half of women with the least educated mothers had a teenage birth while about one in seven of those with college-educated mothers had a teenage birth. Hispanic women showed the least disparity; about one-third of women whose mothers were the least educated had a teen birth while one in five daughters of college-educated mothers were teen parents.

■ The family income of women in their twenties at the time of the survey suggested that those who had been teen mothers were much worse off economically than those who were not (data not shown). Forty-three percent of women who began childbearing in adolescence were poor in their twenties, while only 16 percent had high incomes in their twenties. Among women in their twenties who had not been teenage mothers, these figures were almost reversed; 13 percent were below the poverty line at the time of the survey and 40 percent were in high-income families.

Figure 12. Percent of women 20–29 years of age who had a teenage birth, by respondent's mother's education and respondent's race and Hispanic origin: United States, 1995

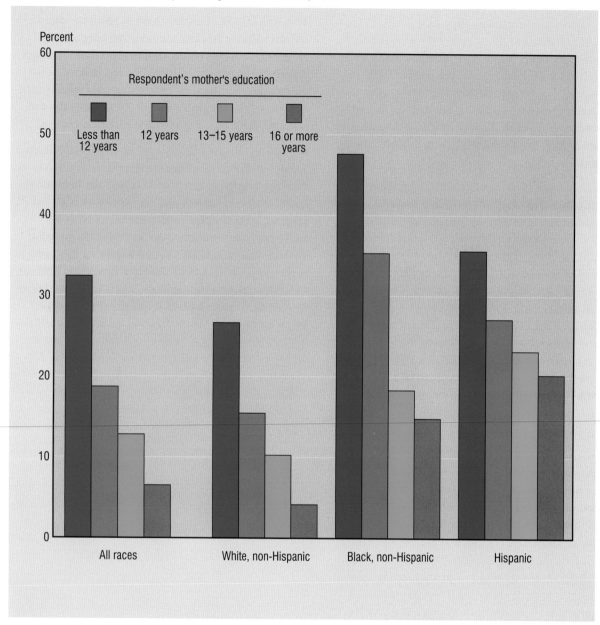

NOTES: Education level is for the infant's maternal grandmother. See Technical Notes for further information.

SOURCE: Centers for Disease Control and Prevention, National Center for Health Statistics, 1995 National Survey of Family Growth.

Risk Factors

Smoking in Pregnancy

■ Infants whose mothers smoke cigarettes during pregnancy are more likely to be born with low birthweight. Other health outcomes associated with maternal smoking include Sudden Infant Death Syndrome (1), pregnancy complications such as placenta previa and abruptio placentae (2), and asthma in childhood (3). The *Healthy People 2000* goal is for no more than 10 percent of mothers to smoke during pregnancy.

■ Data from 1996 birth certificates for mothers 20 years of age and older indicated that smoking cigarettes during pregnancy was strongly associated with socioeconomic status among all racial and ethnic groups. In every race and ethnic group, the more education women had, the less likely they were to report smoking during their pregnancy. Overall, non-Hispanic white mothers (16 percent) and American Indian or Alaska Native mothers (21 percent) were most likely to report smoking during their pregnancies, while black mothers had a somewhat lower rate (12 percent), and Hispanic (4 percent) and Asian or Pacific Islander mothers (3 percent) had the lowest rates of smoking.

■ Non-Hispanic white mothers with less than a high school education were the most likely of any group to smoke during pregnancy. In 1996 nearly one-half of these women reported smoking during pregnancy, compared with only 3 percent of white mothers with 16 or more years of education. Among American Indian or Alaska Native mothers, the percent who smoked during pregnancy decreased from 32 percent among the least educated to 7 percent among those at the highest level of education. Over one-quarter of black mothers with less than 12 years of education smoked, compared with 3 percent among those with 16

or more years of education. Among Hispanic and Asian or Pacific Islander mothers, smoking during pregnancy was rare but an education gradient was still apparent. The proportion varied from 5 percent at the lowest education level to 1 percent at the highest education level for both Asian or Pacific Islander and Hispanic mothers.

■ Among Hispanic subgroups, more educated Puerto Rican and Cuban American mothers were less likely to smoke during pregnancy, but Mexican and Central and South American mothers did not show a strong gradient; their smoking rates were very low at all levels of education. Among Asian or Pacific Islander mothers, data suggested a strong negative relationship between education and smoking for Hawaiian, Filipino, and Japanese American mothers, but Chinese American mothers were very unlikely to smoke at all levels of education.

References

1. Golding J. Sudden infant death syndrome and parental smoking—a literature review. Paediatr Perinat Epidemiol 11(1): 67–77. 1997.

2. Andres RL. The association of cigarette smoking with placenta previa and abruptio placentae. Semin Perinatol 20(2): 154–159. 1996.

3. Oliveti JF. Pre- and perinatal risk factors for asthma in inner city African-American children. Am J Epidemiol 143(6): 570–577. 1996.

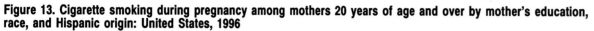

Figure 13. Cigarette smoking during pregnancy among mothers 20 years of age and over by mother's education, race, and Hispanic origin: United States, 1996

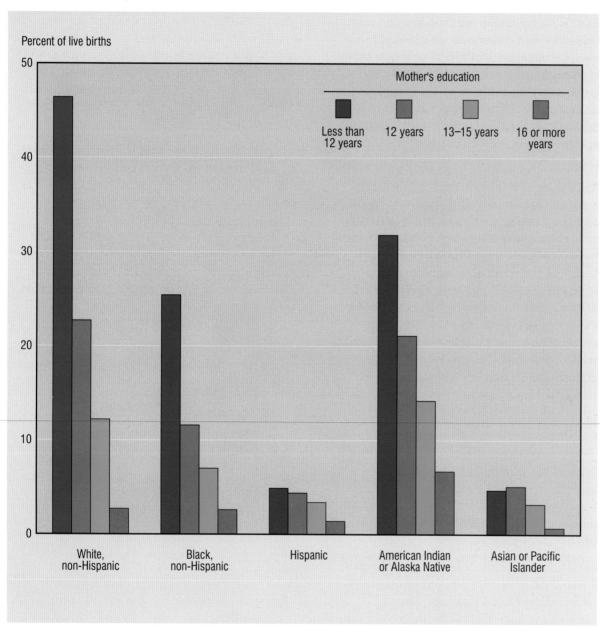

SOURCE: Centers for Disease Control and Prevention, National Center for Health Statistics, National Vital Statistics System. See related *Health, United States, 1998*, table 10.

Risk Factors

Blood Lead

■   Lead is dangerous for small children because it can lead to lowered intelligence (1). Elevated blood lead among children in the United States most often results from residence in an older house that has lead paint, which may flake or peel, causing lead dust to be distributed in the house. Young children may eat paint chips or inadvertently take in lead by tasting dusty objects.

■   Data presented here are drawn from the Third National Health and Nutrition Examination Survey. In general, children 1 to 5 years of age who lived in families with lower socioeconomic status had a greater likelihood of having a high blood lead level (defined as a level of blood lead at or above 10 μg/dL). About 12 percent of children living in poor families had an elevated lead level, compared with about 2 percent of children in high-income families. There was a clear income-related gradient in the prevalence of high blood lead levels; each increase in family income level was associated with a decline in the proportion of children with elevated blood lead.

■   The income-associated gradient in the prevalence of high blood lead levels was seen in each of the race and ethnic groups examined. The gradient was strongest for non-Hispanic black children; 22 percent of black children in families below poverty had an elevated blood lead level, compared with only 6 percent in high-income families.

■   In each income group, black children were more likely than children of other race and ethnic groups to have an elevated blood lead level. Among children living in households below the poverty line, black children were 2.7 times as likely as non-Hispanic white children and 3.4 times as likely as Mexican American children to have an elevated blood lead level.

Reference

1. Pocock SJ, Smith M, Baghurst P. Environmental lead and children's intelligence: A systematic review of the epidemiological evidence. BMJ 309:1189–97. 1994.

Figure 14. Elevated blood lead among children 1–5 years of age by family income, race, and Hispanic origin: United States, average annual 1988–94

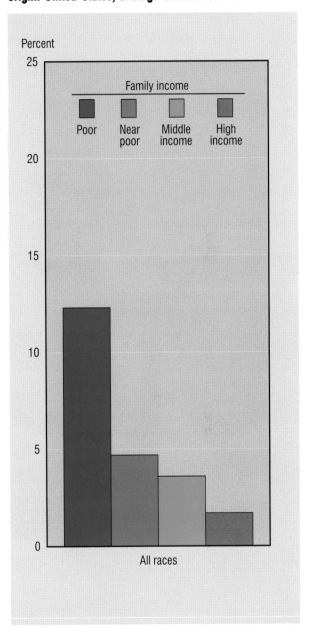

Figure 14. Elevated blood lead among children 1–5 years of age by family income, race, and Hispanic origin: United States, average annual 1988–94—Continued

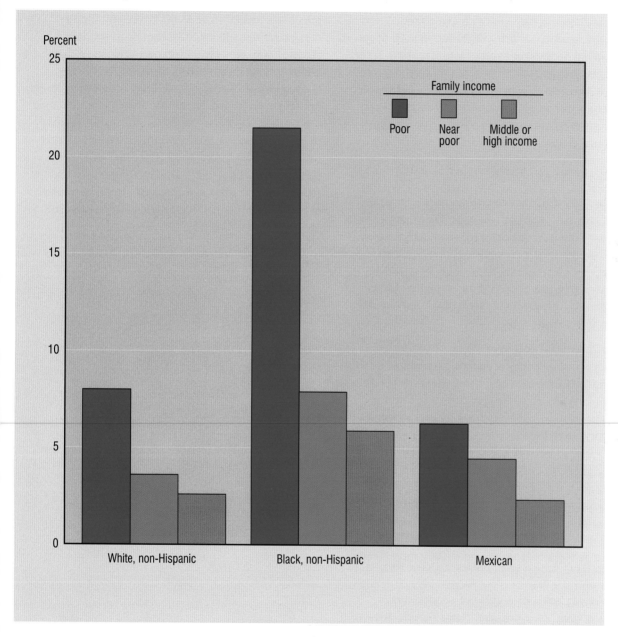

NOTES: Elevated blood lead was defined as having at least 10 micrograms of lead per deciliter of blood. See Technical Notes for definition of family income categories.

SOURCE: Centers for Disease Control and Prevention, National Center for Health Statistics, Third National Health and Nutrition Examination Survey.

Cigarette Smoking

■ Adolescence is the most common time to take up cigarette smoking, which kills about 400,000 people in the United States every year. Each day, about 3,000 teenagers become daily smokers (1). Smoking may lead to heart disease, lung or other forms of cancer, bronchitis and emphysema (also known as chronic obstructive pulmonary disease), and other health problems. The *Healthy People 2000* goal is for no more than 6 percent of adolescents 12–17 to have smoked in the past month.

■ In 1992 about one in five adolescents age 12–17 years said they were current cigarette smokers. When all race and ethnic groups were examined together, there was no clear socioeconomic trend in smoking: teenagers in low-income households were about equally likely to smoke as those in higher income households. Boys and girls were also about equally likely to smoke.

■ However, a breakdown by race and ethnicity demonstrated that socioeconomic gradients in smoking did exist. In each race and ethnic group, the prevalence of smoking among adolescent boys was lower in households with higher incomes. In every income category, non-Hispanic white boys had higher rates of smoking than boys of any other race or ethnic background. Among teenagers in poor families, white teen boys were 2.8 times as likely as black teen boys to smoke and 1.5 times as likely as Hispanic teen boys. Among adolescents in higher income households, white teen males were over five times as likely to smoke as black teen males and slightly more likely than Hispanic teen males.

■ Among adolescent girls the socioeconomic patterns were less consistent. Non-Hispanic white teen girls had a similar trend to the boys, with higher income girls less likely to smoke. However, in Hispanic teen girls the pattern was reversed with higher income girls more likely to smoke. Among black teen girls there appeared to be little difference in smoking rates by income group. Smoking rates among black adolescents were uniformly lower than the rates in any other race or ethnic group. Almost 1 in 3 poor white, but fewer than 1 in 12 poor black adolescent girls, was a smoker in 1992. About one in five middle- or high-income white and Hispanic teen girls smoked, but only 8 percent of black teen girls in this income group smoked.

Reference

1. Centers for Disease Control and Prevention. The great American smokeout–November 21, 1996. MMWR 45(44): 961. 1996.

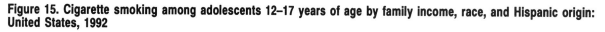

Figure 15. Cigarette smoking among adolescents 12–17 years of age by family income, race, and Hispanic origin: United States, 1992

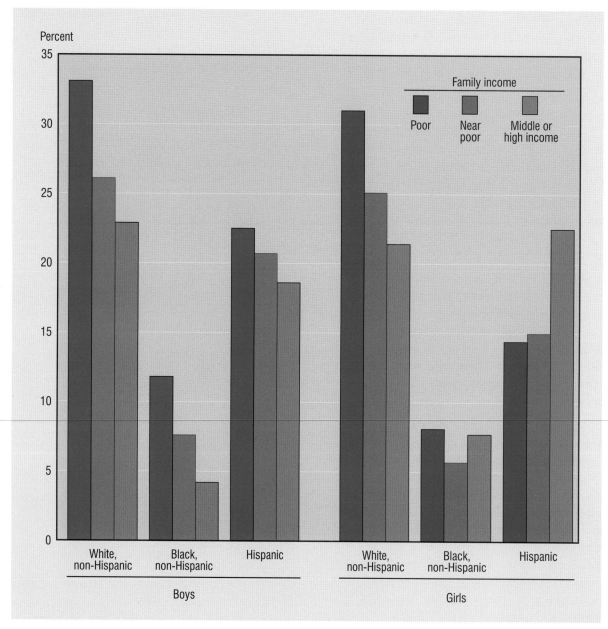

NOTES: Smoking is defined as any smoking in the past month. Percents are age adjusted. See Technical notes for definition of family income categories and age adjustment procedure.

SOURCE: Centers for Disease Control and Prevention, National Center for Health Statistics, National Health Interview Survey, Youth Risk Behavior Survey, 1992.

Overweight

■   Overweight in adolescence is associated with overweight in adulthood. Excessive weight for height is a risk factor for heart disease, several forms of cancer, diabetes, and other health problems (1).

■   Data from the third National Health and Nutrition Examination Survey suggested that among adolescents 12–17 years of age during 1988–94, socioeconomic status was closely related to the prevalence of overweight in some race and ethnic groups. Overall, adolescents in higher income households were less likely to be overweight than those in poorer households. Among adolescents in middle- or high-income households, 9 percent were overweight, compared with 17 percent in poor households.

■   Despite the apparent socioeconomic gradient in overweight, only non-Hispanic white adolescents exhibited an association between overweight and socioeconomic status. Poor white adolescents were about 2.6 times as likely to be overweight as those in middle- or high-income families, and adolescents with near-poor family income had an intermediate prevalence.

■   Among black and Mexican-origin adolescents, there was no such trend. Adolescents in these groups had lower rates of overweight if they were poor than if they were in middle- or high-income households. The highest rates of overweight were found among Mexican American adolescents whose families were middle- or high-income; about one in five of these teens were overweight. The lowest rates were in middle- or high-income white teens, 7 percent of whom were overweight.

Reference

1. Troiano RP, Flegal KM, Kuczmarski RJ, Campbell SM, Johnson CL. Overweight prevalence and trends for children and adolescents. The National Health and Nutrition Examination Surveys, 1963 to 1991. Arch Pediatr Adolesc Med 149(10):1085–91. 1995.

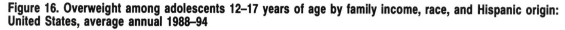

Figure 16. Overweight among adolescents 12–17 years of age by family income, race, and Hispanic origin: United States, average annual 1988–94

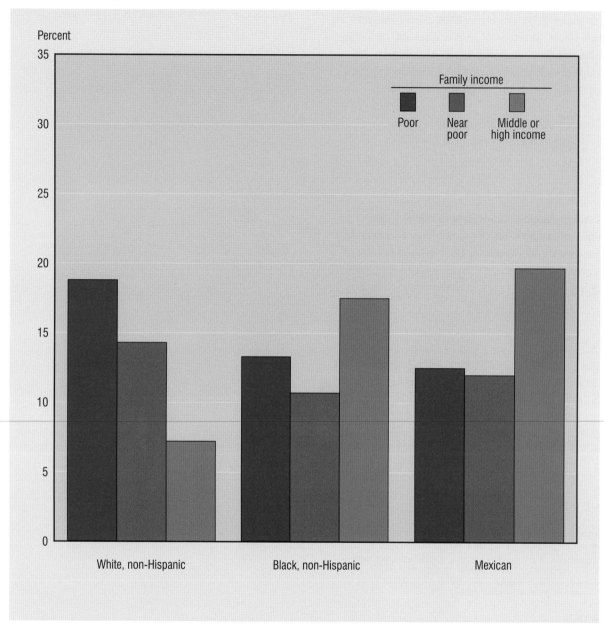

NOTES: Overweight was defined for adolescents by the sex-specific 95th percentile of weight for height and age in the National Health Examination Survey, 1966–70. Percents are age adjusted. See Technical Notes for definition of family income categories, age adjustment, and for more information on classifying overweight.

SOURCE: Centers for Disease Control and Prevention, National Center for Health Statistics, Third National Health and Nutrition Examination Survey. See related *Health, United States, 1998*, table 71.

Risk Factors

Sedentary Lifestyle

■ Sedentary lifestyle, or the lack of physical activity, is a risk factor for several chronic diseases, including heart disease, stroke, diabetes, and certain forms of cancer. Physical activity has been shown to improve mental health and is important for the health of muscles, bones and joints. Lack of physical activity contributes to obesity. Participation in all forms of physical activity declines dramatically during adolescence (1). *Healthy People 2000* sets a goal of no more than 15 percent of individuals 6 years of age and over to have a sedentary lifestyle.

■ Data from the Youth Risk Behavioral Survey showed that females 12–17 years of age in lower income households were more likely to be sedentary than those in higher-income households. Among male adolescents, there was less socioeconomic variation. Poor females were over twice as likely as high-income females to be sedentary, while poor males were 1.4 times as likely as high-income males to be sedentary.

■ In every income group, girls were more likely than boys to say they were sedentary during the past week. However, the differences between boys and girls also varied with socioeconomic status. The sex differential appeared primarily among lower income youth; poor and near-poor girls were 1.7–1.8 times as likely to be sedentary as poor or near-poor boys, while girls and boys in high-income families had nearly equal rates of inactivity.

Reference

1. U.S. Department of Health and Human Services. Physical activity and health: A report of the Surgeon General. Atlanta, Georgia: U.S. Department of Health and Human Services, Centers for Disease Control and Prevention, National Center for Chronic Disease Prevention and Health Promotion. 1996.

Figure 17. Sedentary lifestyle among adolescents 12–17 years of age by family income and sex: United States, 1992

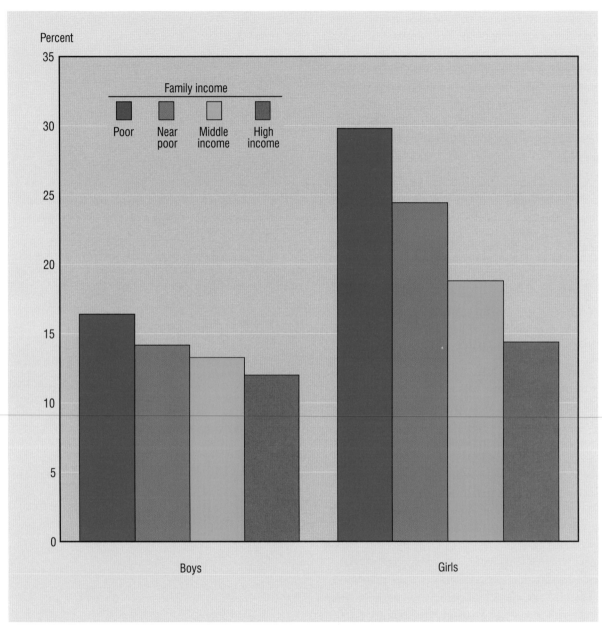

NOTES: Percents are age adjusted. See Technical Notes for definition of family income categories, sedentary lifestyle, and age adjustment procedure.

SOURCE: Centers for Disease Control and Prevention, National Center for Health Statistics, National Health Interview Survey, Youth Risk Behavior Survey, 1992.

Prenatal Care

■ Pregnant women are encouraged to obtain regular prenatal care beginning in the first trimester of pregnancy to help ensure a healthy pregnancy and birth. The *Healthy People 2000* goal is for 90 percent of pregnant women to obtain first-trimester prenatal care. Expansion of the Medicaid program to cover pregnant women with incomes up to 185 percent of poverty improved access to prenatal care in some States (1).

■ After declining slightly during the 1980's, prenatal care attendance rates increased steadily if slowly during the 1990's.

■ Prenatal care utilization is directly associated with education level. Pregnant women who have more education are more likely to start prenatal care early and to have more visits. Throughout the period 1980–96, rates of early prenatal care use among mothers at least 20 years of age were higher among those with more education.

■ Among white mothers, there was little change in rates of prenatal care use between 1980 and 1996 except among mothers with fewer than 13 years of education; prenatal care use among white mothers who had not finished high school declined until 1990, when it began to rise again and in 1994 attained the level achieved in 1980. White mothers with 12 years of education evidenced a similar though more moderate pattern. Those with 16 or more years of education had rates that rose throughout the period, resulting in a 3-percent increase in prenatal care use by 1995; among mothers with some college, rates changed relatively little during the time period with less than a 2 percent increase in usage overall. In both 1980 and 1996 white mothers with at least 16 years of education were 1.4

times as likely to have early prenatal care as those with fewer than 12 years of education.

■ Black mothers' rates in each education group tended to be lower than the rates among white mothers, but their early prenatal attendance rates increased more rapidly in the 1990's than white mothers' rates. Particularly among those without any college education, rates declined until 1990 and then increased again to surpass the 1980 levels. By 1989 only about one-half of black mothers with fewer than 12 years of education received first-trimester prenatal care. However, between 1990 and 1996 these mothers' rates rose rapidly, so that about 61 percent received early prenatal care in 1996. Similar changes were seen among mothers with 12 years of education, while those with 13–15 and 16 or more years of education experienced slower increases. In 1996 black mothers with 16 or more years of education were about 1.4 times as likely to receive early prenatal care as those with fewer than 12 years of education.

Reference

1. Ray WA. Effect of Medicaid expansions on preterm birth. Am J Prev Med 13(4): 292–7. 1997.

Figure 18. Prenatal care use in the first trimester among mothers 20 years of age and over by mother's education and race: United States, 1980–96

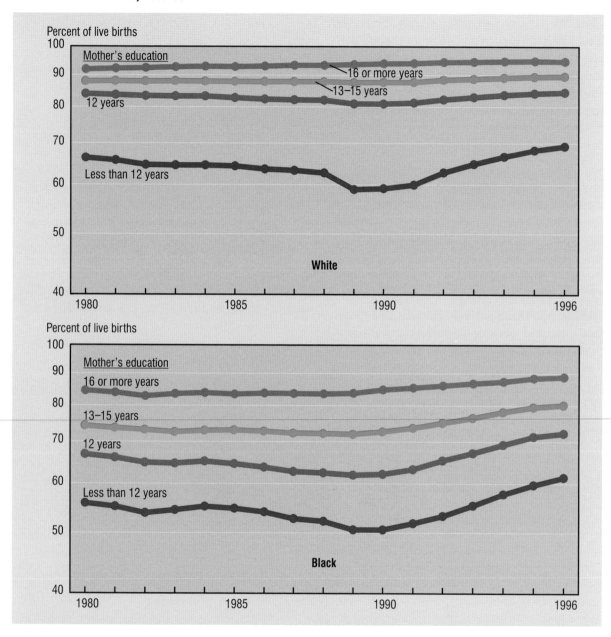

SOURCES: Centers for Disease Control and Prevention, National Center for Health Statistics, National Vital Statistics System. See related *Health, United States, 1998*, table 6.

Prenatal Care

■ In 1996, 82 percent of mothers received early (first trimester) prenatal care, though there was substantial variation among racial and ethnic groups. Japanese and Cuban American mothers were the most likely to obtain early prenatal care in 1996 (89 percent), while American Indian or Alaska Native mothers were the least likely (68 percent).

■ In 1996 there was a clear socioeconomic gradient among mothers 20 years of age and over in use of early prenatal care. In every race and ethnic group, mothers with more education were more likely to receive early prenatal care; overall, the most educated mothers (those with at least 16 years of education) were 1.4 times as likely to receive early prenatal care as the least educated mothers (those with fewer than 12 years of education).

■ Among non-Hispanic white, Hispanic, and Asian or Pacific Islander mothers, the most educated were 1.3 times as likely to have early prenatal care as the least educated. The most educated black and American Indian or Alaska Native mothers were 1.5 times as likely to receive early care as the least educated. White mothers with at least 13 years of education have achieved the *Healthy People 2000* goal of 90 percent or more first trimester prenatal care attendance; rates were above 87 percent among the most educated mothers of all other racial and ethnic groups, but substantially lower among less educated mothers.

Figure 19. Prenatal care use in the first trimester among mothers 20 years of age and over by mother's education, race, and Hispanic origin: United States, 1996

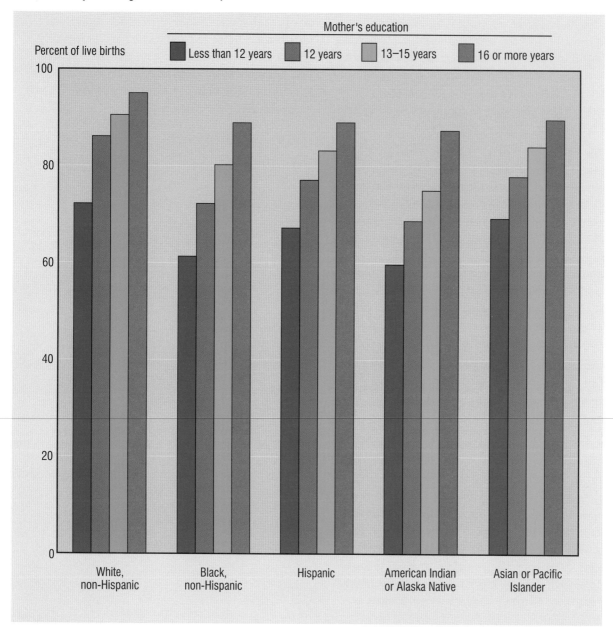

SOURCE: Centers for Disease Control and Prevention, National Center for Health Statistics, National Vital Statistics System. See related *Health, United States, 1998*, table 6.

Health Care

Health Insurance

■ Health insurance coverage is an important component of financial access to health care. Children without health insurance coverage are less likely to have a usual source of health care and are more likely to delay or not receive care when it is needed (1). The *Healthy People 2000* goal is for no one to be without health insurance.

■ In 1995, 14 percent of children under age 18 had no health insurance coverage during the month prior to interview in the National Health Interview Survey, while 21 percent had Medicaid or public assistance coverage, and 66 percent had private coverage (see *Health, United States, 1998*, table 133). Between 1989 and 1995 the proportion of children covered by Medicaid increased by more than 60 percent, primarily due to State expansions in Medicaid eligibility for children, while the proportion of children with private coverage declined by 8 percent, and the percent with no coverage remained fairly stable.

■ The percent of children who are uninsured is strongly associated with family income. Overall, in 1994–95 poor and near-poor children were more than five times as likely as those with high family income to be uninsured.

■ Family income is a strong predictor of insurance coverage, regardless of race and ethnicity. Poor white children were six times as likely as those with high incomes to be uninsured. Among black and Hispanic children those with near-poor family income were somewhat more likely to be uninsured than poor children. Near-poor black children were 3.2 times as likely as high- income black children to be uninsured and near-poor Hispanic children were 4.5 times as likely as high-income Hispanic children to be uninsured.

■ Poor Hispanic children were twice as likely as poor black children to be uninsured and near-poor Hispanic children were almost 80 percent more likely than near-poor black children to be uninsured, due in large part to lower rates of Medicaid coverage among Hispanic than black children.

Reference

1. Simpson G, Bloom B, Cohen RA, Parsons PE. Access to health care. Part 1: Children. National Center for Health Statistics. Vital Health Stat 10(196). 1997.

Figure 20. Percent of children under 18 years of age with no health insurance coverage by family income, race, and Hispanic origin: United States, average annual 1994–95

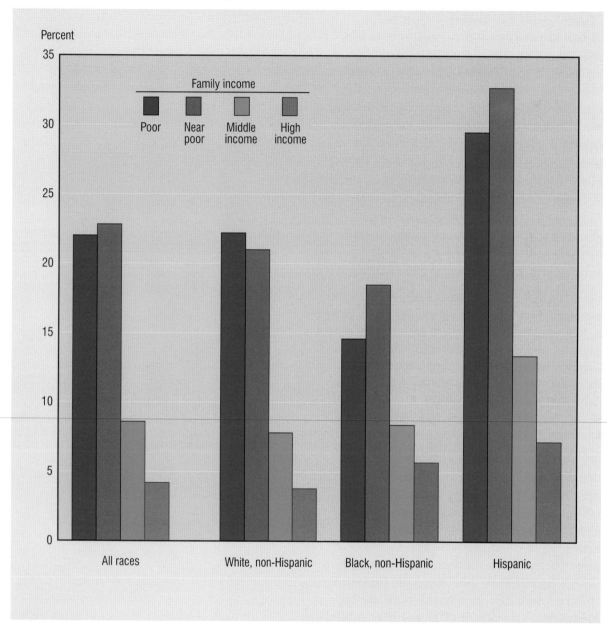

NOTE: See Technical Notes for definitions of the uninsured and family income categories.

SOURCE: Centers for Disease Control and Prevention, National Center for Health Statistics, National Health Interview Survey. See related *Health, United States, 1998*, table 133.

Vaccinations

■ Timely vaccination protects children from life-threatening and disabling diseases. In 1996 over three-quarters (77 percent) of children ages 19–35 months received the combined series of recommended vaccines consisting of 4 doses of diphtheria, tetanus, and pertussis (DTP) vaccine, 3 doses of polio vaccine, 1 dose of measles-containing vaccine, and 3 doses of *Haemophilus influenzae* type b (Hib) vaccine. The *Healthy People 2000* goal is for 90 percent of children under 2 years of age to have received the recommended immunization series.

■ Children with family incomes below the poverty level were less likely to receive the combined series than children with family incomes at or above the poverty level (69 percent compared with 80 percent).

■ Non-Hispanic white, black, and Hispanic children whose families were not poor were slightly more likely to be fully vaccinated than those in poor families. Poor white, black, and Hispanic children had similar levels of vaccine coverage, with 68–70 percent having a full series of vaccines. Among those in families above the poverty line, non-Hispanic white children were slightly more likely to be fully vaccinated than Hispanic children; black children had an intermediate level of vaccination.

■ In 1996 about 92 percent of children living in families at or above the poverty level were fully vaccinated with polio, Hib, and a measles-containing vaccine (data not shown). About 88 percent of poor children were vaccinated for these diseases. About 84 percent of children in nonpoor families were fully vaccinated for DTP (4 or more doses) and Hepatitis B (3 or more doses). Among children in poor families, 73 percent were vaccinated for DTP and 78 percent for Hepatitis B.

Figure 21. Vaccinations among children 19–35 months of age by poverty status, race, and Hispanic origin: United States, 1996

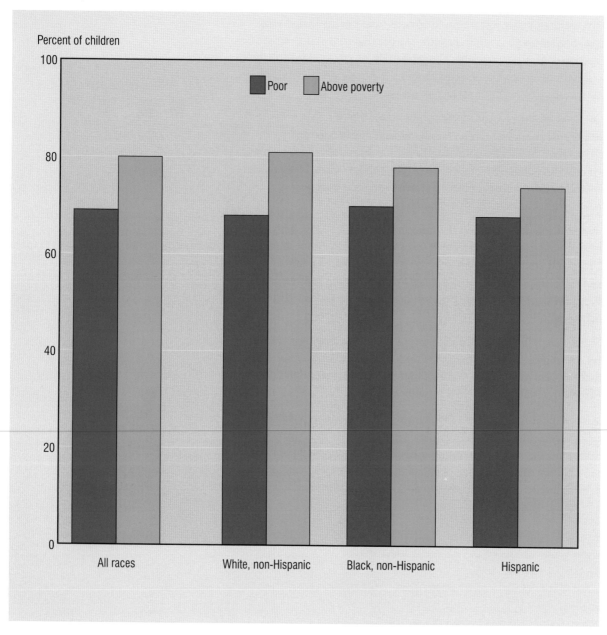

NOTES: Vaccinations included in the full series are 4 doses of diphtheria-tetanus-pertussis (DTP) vaccine, 3 doses of polio vaccine, 1 dose of a measles-containing vaccine, and 3 doses of *Haemophilus influenzae* type b (Hib) vaccine. See Technical Notes for definition of poverty status.

SOURCE: Centers for Disease Control and Prevention, National Center for Health Statistics and National Immunization Program, National Immunization Survey. See related *Health, United States, 1998*, table 52.

No Physician Contact

■ All children under age 6 should have at least one physician visit each year to assess the child's growth and development and to ensure that vaccinations are up to date. The proportion of young children who have visited a physician at least once in the previous year varies with family income and health insurance coverage.

■ In 1994–95 the percent of young children without a recent physician visit declined with increasing income. Near poor and poor children were 2.5–2.7 times as likely to lack a recent physician visit as high-income children. Eleven percent of poor children and 10 percent of near-poor children lacked a physician visit within the past year compared with 4 percent of high-income children.

■ Within each income group the percent of young children without a recent physician visit did not vary by race and ethnicity. In each of the three race and ethnic groups shown, the percent of young children without a recent physician visit declined with increasing income and 11 percent of poor children within each group did not have a recent physician visit.

■ Within each income group the percent without a recent visit was greater for uninsured than insured children. Poor children without health insurance coverage were 2.8 times as likely to lack a recent physician visit as poor children with health insurance.

■ Among uninsured children the percent without a recent visit ranged from 12 percent for those with middle or high incomes to 23 percent for poor children. Lacking a recent physician visit was less common among insured children at each income level and ranged from 5 percent of those with middle or high incomes to 8–9 percent of the poor and near poor.

Figure 22. Percent of children under 6 years of age with no physician contact during the past year by family income, health insurance status, race, and Hispanic origin: United States, average annual 1994–95

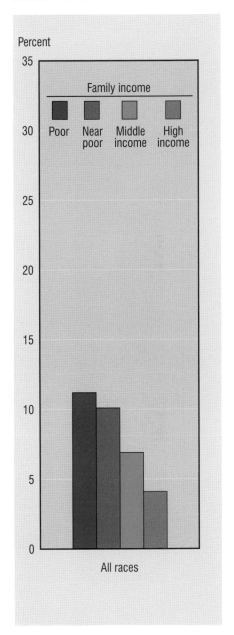

Figure 22. Percent of children under 6 years of age with no physician contact during the past year by family income, health insurance status, race, and Hispanic origin: United States, average annual 1994–95—Continued

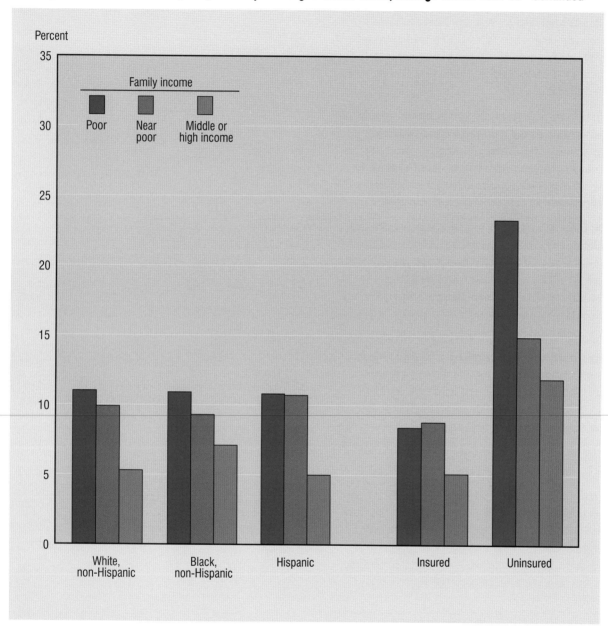

NOTES: See Technical Notes for definitions of the uninsured and family income categories.
SOURCE: Centers for Disease Control and Prevention, National Center for Health Statistics, National Health Interview Survey. See related *Health, United States, 1998*, table 78.

Ambulatory Care

■ In 1995 ambulatory care utilization among children who resided in areas with a median income of $40,000 or more was 65–75 percent higher than for children who resided in areas with a median income below $30,000.

■ There was a particularly strong income gradient in the use of ambulatory care in physician offices. Children who resided in the highest-income areas had more than twice as many visits as those residing in areas with a median income of less than $20,000 (339 and 145 visits per 100 children, respectively).

■ In contrast to physician offices, the use of ambulatory care in hospital settings (emergency departments and outpatient departments) was almost 50 percent higher for children residing in the lowest-income areas (median income below $20,000) than for those in the highest income areas (79 and 54 visits per 100 children, respectively).

■ The distribution of the place of ambulatory care visits for children varies substantially by median income of the patient's area of residence. In 1995, 22 percent of visits by children residing in the lowest income areas were to hospital emergency departments, compared with only 8 percent of visits by children in the highest income areas. Hospital outpatient departments accounted for 13 percent of visits by children residing in the lowest income areas and only 6 percent of visits by children in the highest income areas. In contrast, 86 percent of visits by children in the highest income areas took place in physician offices while 65 percent of visits by children residing in the lowest income areas occurred in physician offices.

Figure 23. Ambulatory care visits among children under 18 years of age by median household income in ZIP Code of residence and place of visit: United States, 1995

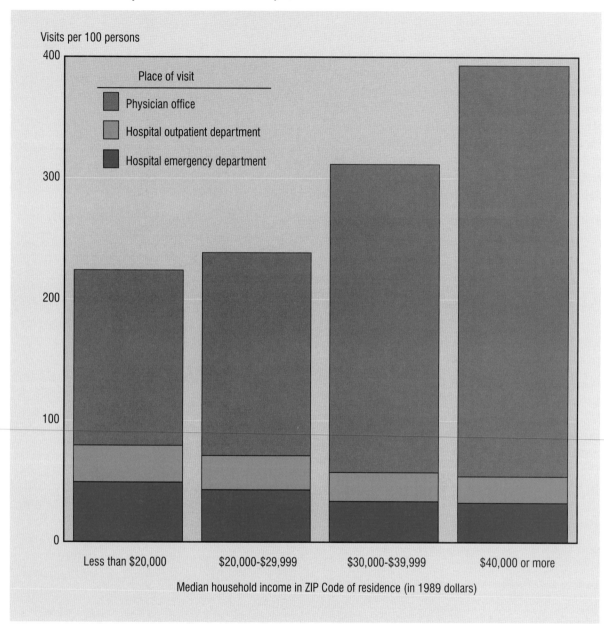

Visits per 100 persons

Place of visit
- Physician office
- Hospital outpatient department
- Hospital emergency department

Less than $20,000 $20,000-$29,999 $30,000-$39,999 $40,000 or more

Median household income in ZIP Code of residence (in 1989 dollars)

NOTES: Median income is for persons who resided in the ZIP Code area in 1990. See Technical Notes for methods.

SOURCE: Centers for Disease Control and Prevention, National Center for Health Statistics, 1995 National Ambulatory Medical Care Survey and 1995 National Hospital Ambulatory Medical Care Survey. Bureau of the Census, 1990 decennial Census.

Asthma Hospitalization

■ Access to and utilization of appropriate medical care can prevent severe episodes of asthma in many cases. Hospitalization for asthma may indicate that the child has not had adequate outpatient management for the disease. Research suggests that asthma, which is the most common chronic disease in childhood, may be increasing in the United States (1,2). The *Healthy People 2000* goal is for no more than 2.25 asthma hospitalizations per 1,000 population for children 0–14 years of age. White, but not black, children in each socioeconomic group attained the goal by 1989–91.

■ Data presented here were for hospitalizations in 1989–91 and were categorized by the median family income in the child's ZIP Code in 1990. There was an inverse relationship between median income and hospital admission rates for asthma among children 1–14 years of age. Children living in communities with a median family income below $20,000 were 2.4 times as likely to be hospitalized with asthma as those living in neighborhoods with an income of at least $40,000.

■ Asthma hospitalization rates were higher among black children than among white children. Black children had a rate 3.3 times that of white children, and the hospitalization rates of black children were higher than those of white children in each neighborhood income group. Racial disparities were similar within neighborhood income groups.

References

1. Farber HJ. Trends in asthma prevalence: The Bogalusa heart study. Ann Allergy Asthma Immunol 78(3): 265–69. 1997.

2. Centers for Disease Control and Prevention. Asthma mortality and hospitalization among children and young adults—United States, 1980–1993. MMWR 45(17): 350–3. 1996.

Figure 24. Asthma hospitalization rates among children 1–14 years of age by median household income in ZIP Code of residence and race: United States, average annual 1989–91

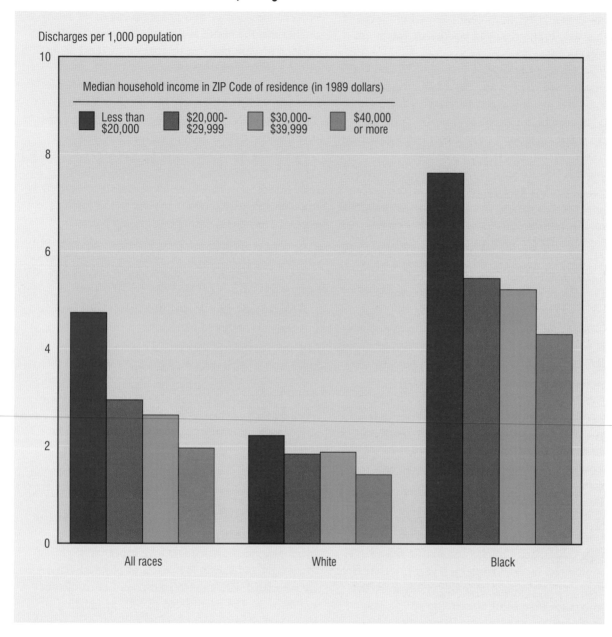

Discharges per 1,000 population

Median household income in ZIP Code of residence (in 1989 dollars)

■ Less than $20,000   ■ $20,000-$29,999   ■ $30,000-$39,999   ■ $40,000 or more

All races   White   Black

NOTE: See Technical Notes for methods.

SOURCE: Centers for Disease Control and Prevention, National Center for Health Statistics, National Hospital Discharge Survey; Bureau of the Census, 1990 decennial Census.

This section describes the relationship between socioeconomic status (SES) and adult health. Using national data from several sources, the figures in this section show this relationship for several indicators of health status, health risk, and health care access and utilization.

The negative relationship between SES and health is perhaps made most evident by examining differences in death rates and life expectancy. As far back as the mid-19th century, vital records from Great Britain indicated that death rates were higher and average age at death lower for men in trade and laboring occupations than for men in the professional class (1). Several of the factors, such as grossly inadequate housing, poor sanitation, and insufficient nutrition, that contributed to SES differences in health a century ago no longer contribute substantially to mortality today; and yet, persons of lower SES still experience higher death rates and lower life expectancy. Furthermore, there is evidence that socioeconomic disparities in death rates have widened since 1960 (2).

Throughout this century, average life expectancy for all persons in the United States has been increasing (*Health, United States, 1998*, table 29), but data show that during 1979–89, 45-year-olds with the highest incomes could expect to live 3 to 7 years longer than those with the lowest incomes (figure 25). Figure 26 shows that the advantage experienced by those with higher social position is evident in death rates for the major categories of natural causes (chronic and communicable diseases) and injuries.

Deaths due to chronic disease now account for nearly three-fourths of all deaths to persons 25–64 years of age. Considered together, cardiovascular diseases, cancer, and diabetes account for over $300 billion in direct medical costs each year (3). Data from the National Longitudinal Mortality Study show that mortality rates from heart disease (figure 27), lung cancer (figure 28), and diabetes (figure 29) increased as family income decreased, indicating that much of the burden of chronic disease is disproportionately concentrated among persons with fewer resources.

These discrepancies tended to be larger for young and middle-aged adults than for the elderly.

The consistency of the inverse relationship between measures of SES and most causes of death implies that the health of persons of lower social position is more likely to be affected by these same diseases or injuries while they remain alive. In addition, the greater susceptibility associated with lower SES implies a greater likelihood of having multiple health conditions adversely affecting overall health status. Global health assessments, such as a person rating his or her health as "poor," "fair," "good," or "excellent," have been shown to be reliable indicators of a person's health status as well as being an independent risk factor for mortality (4,5). Figure 32 shows the strong relationship between self-reported health and family income; regardless of gender, race, or ethnicity, the percent reporting their health as only "fair" or "poor" increases as family income decreases.

Chronically poor health often results in a decline in a person's ability to perform their usual activities; it may prevent them from holding a job or limit the kinds of work they can do, affect their ability to do routine chores inside or outside the home, or, when health impairment is severe, render them incapable of handling their personal care needs (6,7). Figure 33 shows a strong inverse association between income level and health-related activity limitation among working-age adults, while figure 34 demonstrates a similar association for difficulty performing personal care activities among the elderly.

Many chronic diseases have common risk factors. For example, smoking increases a person's risk of developing heart disease and lung cancer while being overweight and having low levels of physical activity are associated with an increased risk of heart disease and diabetes. The relationship of SES to smoking, prevalence of overweight, and lack of physical activity are described in figures 35–36 and 38–40. The decline in cigarette smoking among U.S. adults since the publication of the first Surgeon General's report on

smoking in 1964 has been one of the major success stories of public health (8). However, figure 35 shows that the decline in smoking has been disproportionately concentrated among the more educated, and figure 36 shows the prevalence of smoking among lower income persons remains higher than among middle- and high-income persons regardless of gender, race, or ethnicity.

In contrast to smoking, the prevalence of overweight in the United States is increasing among adults and children (9,10). A consistent inverse relationship between overweight and SES exists for women, but not for men, and the gradient is strongest for non-Hispanic white women (figures 38–39). Overweight contributes to diabetes (11) and to hypertension (12), health conditions that are also major risk factors for heart disease and stroke. Like overweight, hypertension is strongly related to SES among women, but not men (figure 41). Lack of physical activity, however, increases sharply as family income decreases within each sex, race, and ethnic group examined (figure 40).

The reasons why lower SES groups experience higher morbidity and mortality are complex. Established risk factors for chronic diseases, such as smoking, being overweight, and low physical activity levels that tend to increase as SES declines account for part of the observed relationship between SES and health. However, many studies have found that an elevated risk of heart disease among lower SES groups remains even after adjustment for the known major behavioral risk factors, such as smoking, obesity, and hypertension (13). This suggests that the relationship between SES and chronic disease mortality may not be fully explained by the differential distribution of health-related behaviors. In addition, as figure 26 demonstrates, the SES gradients in mortality from communicable diseases and injuries are larger, relatively, than that for chronic disease mortality, indicating that environmental and social exposures may be even more unequally distributed than the behavioral risk factors for chronic diseases. For example,

figure 42 shows a strong income gradient in elevated blood lead level among adult men that likely results from differential occupational and environmental exposures.

The association between socioeconomic status and the health status of adults may also be explained in part by reduced access to health care among those with lower socioeconomic status. Figures 43–48 provide national data on the relationship between income and a selected set of indicators of access to health care and health care utilization. Access to health care may be defined as "the attainment of timely, sufficient, and appropriate health care of adequate quality such that health outcomes are maximized" (14). Having adequate health insurance coverage is key to assuring access to health care. However, nonfinancial factors such as race, ethnicity, language, culture, education, geographic isolation, and provider availability also have been shown to affect access to care (14).

Almost all U.S. adults age 65 and over have Medicare coverage. About three-quarters of adults 18–64 years of age have private health insurance coverage, most commonly through an employer-sponsored health insurance plan. However, in 1994–95 almost one-fifth of adults under age 65 lacked coverage and the proportion uninsured rose sharply as income declined (figure 43). Reasons for lacking employer-sponsored coverage include not being offered health insurance through work or not being able to afford the coverage offered, losing a job or changing employers, or losing coverage through divorce or the death of a spouse. Persons employed in small firms are less likely to be offered coverage than those in large firms and part-time workers are less likely to be offered coverage than full-time workers. Establishments with predominantly low-wage workers are also less likely to offer coverage than establishments where a majority of employees earn at least $10,000 per year (15). Even those with health insurance may have problems accessing health care for financial reasons. Insurance plans may exclude

coverage for certain types of care or require substantial out-of-pocket spending through deductibles and copayments.

Medicaid provides coverage to eligible needy persons, but eligibility varies from State to State and is undergoing major changes with the implementation of welfare reform. Those eligible for Medicaid have included families with children receiving Aid to Families with Dependent Children (AFDC), pregnant women and young children in low-income families, the aged, blind, and disabled receiving assistance under Supplemental Security Income (SSI), and the medically needy (persons who become poor due to illness). The Medicaid eligibility criteria have resulted in greater Medicaid coverage and lower proportions uninsured among poor women than poor men (figure 43). In addition to meeting Medicaid eligibility requirements, individuals must know about the program, complete necessary forms, and provide required documentation to gain access to benefits. These requirements may present difficult barriers to some persons who are eligible for Medicaid. Among the poor and near poor, Hispanic adults are more likely to be uninsured than non-Hispanic white or black adults (figure 43). Immigration status and language and cultural barriers as well as their greater likelihood of employment in service and farm occupations may contribute to the lower proportions with coverage among the Hispanic population.

Low-income adults are more likely to experience financial barriers to health care use than those with higher incomes. They are less able to afford out-of-pocket expenses for health care, but are also more likely to lack health insurance coverage and incur high out-of-pocket expenses when they use health care. Results from the RAND Health Insurance Experiment indicate that cost sharing reduces the use of appropriate and inappropriate services (16). Cost sharing also reduces the use of preventive care (16). While financial barriers may discourage the use of health care among the low-income population, adults with low incomes are more likely to be sick than those

with higher incomes and therefore could be expected to need more health care (figures 32–33).

The use of sick care, preventive care, and dental care by adults varies with income. Among adults 18–64 years of age who report a health problem there is a strong inverse income gradient in the percent without a recent physician contact (figure 44), and the gradient is similar across race and ethnic groups. Similarly, the percent of adults 18–64 years of age with a recent dental visit rises sharply with income (figure 49). Women 50 years of age and older from higher income families are more likely to have recently used mammography (figure 45). This relationship is particularly pronounced among non-Hispanic white women. Poor and near-poor black women were more likely than poor and near-poor non-Hispanic white women to have received recent mammography, perhaps as a result of targeted screening programs (17).

Perceived unmet need for health care provides another indicator of access to health care (18,19). Data from the National Health Interview Survey show a strong inverse income gradient in the percent of adults who perceive that they have unmet needs for health care (figures 46–47). This measure incorporates needs for services that may not be covered by health insurance plans (prescription drugs, mental health care, and dental care) as well as delaying or not receiving needed medical care. Although the percent who report unmet need for care is lower among the elderly (who have Medicare coverage) than among those 18–64 years of age, there was a strong inverse relationship between income and unmet need for the elderly as well as for younger adults.

Persons who delay or do not receive needed ambulatory care may become more seriously ill and require hospitalization. Avoidable hospitalizations have been defined as those that could potentially be avoided in the presence of appropriate and timely ambulatory care (20,21). Among adults 18–64 years of age the rate of avoidable hospitalizations during 1989–91 was inversely associated with the median household income

of ZIP Code of residence (figure 48). In addition, among residents of low-income areas the avoidable hospitalization rate for black persons was substantially greater than that for white persons. The higher rate of avoidable hospitalizations among black persons than white persons in low income-areas could be due in part to lower family income among black persons than white persons who reside in low income ZIP Code areas.

The direct provision and financing of personal health care services is an area where government has played an important role in the United States (22). Programs such as Medicaid, community health centers, and the National Health Service Corps have had an important effect on improving access to health care for disadvantaged groups. Recent legislative efforts to further extend health insurance coverage to the uninsured have focused on expanding coverage for uninsured children. However, the data in figures 43–48 as well as other published literature demonstrate that low-income adults also clearly face difficulties in accessing the health care system (23).

References

1. Macintyre S. The Black report and beyond: What are the issues? Soc Sci Med 44(6):723–45. 1997.

2. Feldman JJ, Makuc DM, Kleinman JC, Cornoni-Huntley J. National trends in educational differentials in mortality. AJE 129: 919–33. 1989.

3. Institute of Medicine. Disability in America. 1991.

4. Tissue T. Another look at self-rated health among the elderly. J Geront 27:91–4. 1972.

5. Idler EL, Benyamini Y. Self-rated health and mortality: A review of twenty-seven community studies. J Hlth Soc Beh 38:21–37. 1997.

6. Centers for Disease Control and Prevention. Prevalence of work disability—United States, 1990. MMWR 42:757—9. 1993.

7. Centers for Disease Control and Prevention. Prevalence of mobility and self-care disability—United States, 1990. MMWR 42:760–7. 1993.

8. Centers for Disease Control and Prevention. Reducing the health consequences of smoking: 25 years of progress—a report of the Surgeon General. Rockville, Maryland: Department of Health and Human Services. Public Health Service. 1989.

9. Kuczmarski RJ, Flegal KM, Campbell SM, Johnson CL. Increasing prevalence of overweight among U.S. adults: The National Health and Nutrition Examination surveys, 1960 to 1991. JAMA 272:205–11. 1994.

10. Centers for Disease Control and Prevention. Update: Prevalence of overweight among children, adolescents, and adults—United States, 1988–94. MMWR 46:199—202. 1997.

11. Pi-Sunyer FX. Medical hazards of obesity. Ann Intern Med 119:655–60. 1993.

12. Joint National Committee on Detection, Evaluation, and Treatment of High Blood Pressure. The fifth report on the Joint National Committee on Detection, Evaluation, and Treatment of High Blood Pressure. Arch Intern Med 153:154–83. 1993.

13. Davey Smith G, Shipley R, Rose G. Magnitude and causes of socioeconomic differentials in mortality: Further evidence from the Whitehall Study. J Epid Comm Hlth 44:265–70. 1990.

14. Weissman JS, Epstein AM. Falling through the safety net. Insurance and access to health care. The Johns Hopkins University Press: Baltimore. 1994.

15. National Center for Health Statistics. Employer-sponsored health insurance: State and national estimates. Hyattsville, Maryland. 1997.

16. Newhouse JP and the Insurance Experiment Group. Free for all? Lessons from the RAND Health Insurance Experiment. Harvard University Press: Cambridge. 1993.

17. Henson RM, Wyatt SW, Lee NC. The National Breast and Cervical Cancer Early Detection Program: a comprehensive public health response to two major health issues for women. J Public Health Management Practice 2(2): 36–47. 1996.

18. Bloom B, Simpson G, Cohen RA, Parsons PE. Access to health care. Part 2: Working-age adults. National Center for Health Statistics. Vital Health Stat 10(197). 1997.

19. Cohen RA, Bloom B, Simpson G. Parsons PE. Access to heath care. Part 3: Older adults. National Center for Health Statistics. Vital Health Stat 10(198). 1997.

20. Weissman JS, Gatsonis C, Epstein AM. Rates of avoidable hospitalization by insurance status in Massachusetts and Maryland. JAMA 268: 2388–94. 1992.

21. Pappas G, Hadden WC, Kozak LF, Fisher GF. Potentially avoidable hospitalizations: Inequalities in rates between U.S. socioeconomic groups. AJPH 87(5):811–16. 1997.

22. Shonick W. Government and health services. Oxford University Press: New York. 1995.

23. Schoen C, Lyons B, Rowland D, et al.. Insurance matters for low income adults: results from a five-State survey. Health Affairs 16 (5), 163–71. 1997.

Health Status

Life Expectancy

■ U.S. vital statistics data show that average life expectancy of all persons in the United States has been increasing. Life expectancy from birth has increased from 70.8 years in 1970 to 75.8 years in 1995. Life expectancy varies by race and sex. Women have a longer life expectancy than men and black persons have a shorter life expectancy than white persons (see *Health, United States, 1998*, table 29). Data from the National Longitudinal Mortality Study for 1979–89 indicate that, among the noninstitutionalized population of the United States, life expectancy also varies by family income level.

■ During 1979–89 life expectancy at age 45 increased with each increase in family income, regardless of sex or race. Black men 45 years of age in families earning at least $25,000 could expect to live 7.4 years longer than black men in families earning less than $10,000; among white men the difference was 6.6 years. The differences between the highest and the lowest income groups tended to be smaller for women than for men. At 45 years of age, black women in the highest income group could expect to live 3.8 years longer than those in the lowest income group; among white women the difference was 2.7 years.

■ At age 65, white men in the highest income families could expect to live 3.1 years longer than white men in the lowest income families; the difference was 2.5 years for black men, 1.3 years for black women, and 1 year for white women.

■ Race differences in life expectancy were larger at age 45 than at age 65. The life expectancy of white persons at age 45 exceeded that of black persons at every income level. Differences between black and white persons in life expectancy at age 45 were larger for women than for men, and larger for persons with family incomes below $15,000 than for persons with higher incomes.

Figure 25. Life expectancy among adults 45 and 65 years of age by family income, sex, and race: United States, average annual 1979–89

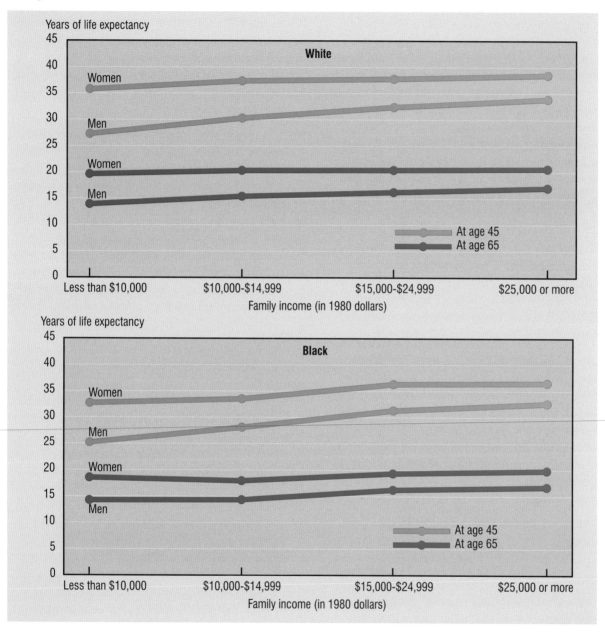

NOTE: See Appendix II for definition of life expectancy.

SOURCE: U.S. Bureau of the Census and National Institutes of Health, National Heart, Lung, and Blood Institute, National Longitudinal Mortality Study.

Health Status

Cause of Death

■ Although socioeconomic (SES) differences in mortality have been persistent over time, the nature of the SES relationship for specific causes of death has changed. In earlier times when communicable diseases were the primary causes of death, the higher death rate among persons of lower SES was due to their poor nutrition and unsanitary living conditions. Today chronic diseases, such as heart disease, are the major contributors to death, and although heart disease currently fits the pattern of higher rates among lower SES, this represents a change from the pattern in the past. As recently as the 1950's, heart disease mortality rates were greater among higher SES groups (1). As the factors that influence chronic diseases, such as smoking, high-fat diet, and preventive care, have diffused throughout society, there has been a shift to lower SES groups being more adversely affected, presumably because higher SES groups more quickly adopt practices to reduce their risk of chronic diseases.

■ In 1995 nearly three out of every four deaths to persons 25–64 years of age was due to a chronic disease, intentional and unintentional injuries accounted for 15 percent of deaths in this age range, and communicable diseases accounted for 11 percent. Communicable diseases and injuries were responsible for a larger proportion of deaths to men (13 and 18 percent, respectively) than to women (7 and 10 percent, respectively).

■ Men and women with more than a high school education had lower age-adjusted death rates than their less educated counterparts within each of these major cause groupings.

■ Education gradients in mortality attributed to chronic diseases were similar for men and women

25–64 years of age. In 1995 the chronic disease death rate for men with a high school education or less was 2.3–2.5 times that for men with more than a high school education; less educated women had death rates 1.9–2.2 times the rate of women with education beyond high school.

■ The overall death rate and the education gradient for injuries was higher for men than women. In 1995 the death rate from injuries for men was over three times that for women. Men with 12 years of education or less had age-adjusted injury death rates approximately three times that for men with more than 12 years of education. Among women, the education gradient in injury mortality was similar to that for mortality from chronic diseases; less educated women had injury mortality rates approximately twice that of women with more than a high school education.

■ At ages 25–64 years, mortality from communicable diseases was 3.5 times higher for men than women, and the education gradient was much stronger for women than for men. The discrepancy between men and women in the education gradient for communicable diseases was due entirely to mortality from HIV infection (see data table). For men and women, non-HIV communicable disease mortality among the least educated was three times that of the most educated, and those with 12 years of education had mortality rates twice as high as persons with more than 12 years. In contrast, mortality from HIV infection among men with 12 or fewer years of education was 60–70 percent higher than among those with more than 12 years. By contrast, women with less than 12 years of education were almost six times as likely to die from HIV infection as those with more than 12 years.

Reference

1. Marmot MG, Shipley MJ, Rose G. Inequalities in death: Specific explanations of a general pattern? Lancet 1:1003–6. 1984.

Figure 26. Death rates for selected causes for adults 25–64 years of age, by education level, and sex: selected States, 1995

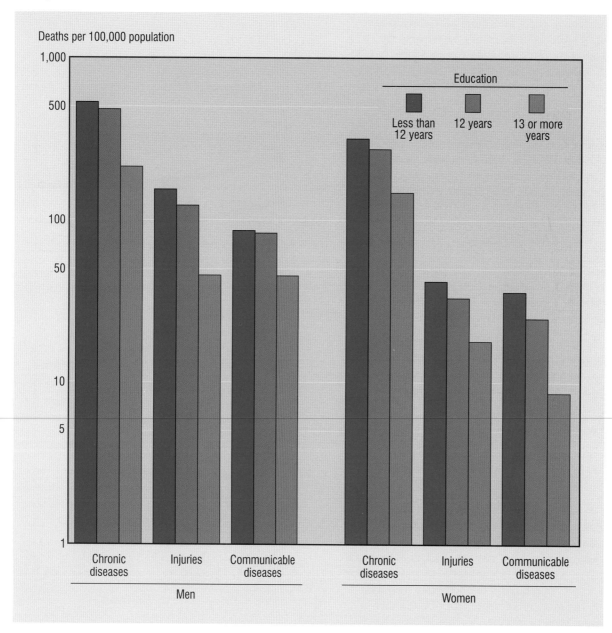

Deaths per 100,000 population

NOTES: Death rates are age adjusted; see Technical Notes. For a description of International Classification of Diseases code numbers for causes of death, see Appendix II. "Injuries" includes homicide, suicide, unintentional injuries, and deaths from adverse effects of medical procedures. See Appendix I, National Vital Statistics System, for a discussion of reporting of education of decedent on death certificates. Rates are plotted on a log scale.

SOURCE: Centers for Disease Control and Prevention, National Center for Health Statistics, National Vital Statistics System.

Health Status

Heart Disease Mortality

■ Although death rates from heart disease have dropped since 1970, heart disease remains the leading cause of death in the United States. In 1995 heart disease accounted for an estimated $79 billion in direct medical expenditures (1). Risk factors for heart disease include diabetes, hypertension, high serum cholesterol, smoking, obesity, and lack of physical activity (2).

■ During 1979–89 death rates from heart disease declined as family income increased. Among men 25–64 years of age, heart disease mortality for those with incomes less than $10,000 was 2.5 times that for those with incomes of $25,000 or more. The poorest women in this age range were 3.4 times as likely to die from heart disease as those with the highest incomes. For persons 65 years of age and over, the income gradient in heart disease mortality was similar for men and women and flatter than at younger ages.

■ At ages 25–64, income-related gradients in heart disease mortality were similar across sex, race, and ethnic groups; persons with incomes under $10,000 were 2.4–2.9 times as likely to die from heart disease as those with incomes of $15,000 or more. Among persons 65 years of age and older, income gradients were less steep. Ratios of the heart disease death rate in the lowest income group to that in the highest income group ranged from 1.3 for black women to 1.7 for black men.

■ Within each income level, non-Hispanic black women had higher mortality from heart disease than non-Hispanic white women. At 25–64 years of age the death rate for heart disease was higher for black men than white men, regardless of income; at older ages, however, the death rate for white men was nearly the same or exceeded that of black men at the same level of income.

■ Heart disease mortality varied by sex. The poorest women had death rates similar to those of the highest income men.

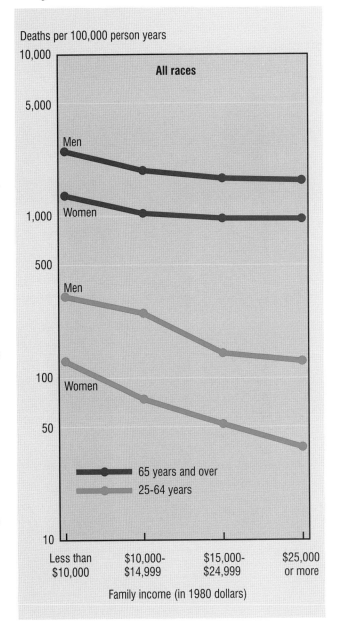

Figure 27. Heart disease death rates among adults 25–64 years of age and 65 years of age and over by family income, sex, race, and Hispanic origin: United States, average annual 1979–89

References

1. Hodgson TA. National Center for Health Statistics, Centers for Disease Control and Prevention. Unpublished estimates. 1997.

2. White CC, Tolsma DD, Haynes SG, McGee D. Cardiovascular disease. In: Amler RW, Dull HB, eds. Closing the gap: The burden of unnecessary illness. New York: Oxford University Press. 1987.

Figure 27. Heart disease death rates among adults 25–64 years of age and 65 years of age and over by family income, sex, race, and Hispanic origin: United States, average annual 1979–89—Continued

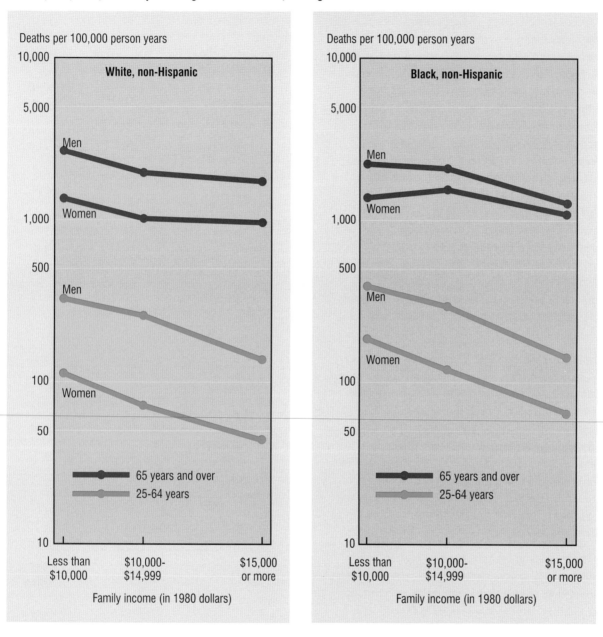

NOTES: Death rates are age adjusted; see Technical Notes. For a description of International Classification of Diseases code numbers for causes of death, see Appendix II. Rates are plotted on a log scale.

SOURCE: U.S. Bureau of the Census and National Institutes of Health, National Heart, Lung, and Blood Institute, National Longitudinal Mortality Study.

Lung Cancer Mortality

■ Cancer is the second leading cause of death in the United States, and lung cancer accounted for approximately 28 percent of all cancer deaths in 1996 (1,2). Since 1987 lung cancer has been the leading cause of cancer deaths for men and women. Death rates for lung cancer have been consistently higher for men than women. Between 1950 and 1990 the overall age-adjusted death rate for lung cancer increased. However, among men, the rate of increase began to slow during the early 1980's while the rate for women continued to increase sharply. Between 1990 and 1995 the age-adjusted death rate for lung cancer for males decreased 9 percent while the corresponding rate for females increased 5 percent. In 1995 medical expenditures for lung cancer were estimated to be nearly $4 billion (3). Tobacco is the leading contributor to lung cancer incidence, and the majority of lung cancer cases could be prevented by refraining from smoking (4).

■ Data from the National Longitudinal Mortality Study for 1979–89 show that, among men, lung cancer mortality rates declined as family income increased. The relationship between family income and lung cancer mortality was somewhat stronger for younger than for older men. Men 25–64 years of age in families earning less than $10,000 had a mortality rate 2.4 times the rate among men in families with an income of at least $25,000. Among men 65 years and over, the lowest income group had a rate twice as high as that of the highest.

■ Among women the relationship between family income and lung cancer mortality was weaker and less consistent than among men. Women 25–64 years of age in families earning less than $15,000 had lung cancer death rates 40–60 percent higher than the rates for women with incomes of $15,000 and more. For women ages 65 years and over, there was some indication that mortality from lung cancer increased with income, although differences were small. Lung cancer mortality among elderly women with incomes of $25,000 and more was 25–30 percent higher than among those with incomes below $15,000.

References

1. Ventura SJ, Peters KD, Martin JA, Maurer JD. Births and deaths: United States, 1996. Monthly vital statistics report; vol 46 no 1, supp 2. Hyattsville, Maryland: National Center for Health Statistics. 1997.

2. Ries LAG, Miller BA, Hankey BF, eds. SEER Cancer Statistics Review, 1973–1993. National Cancer Institute. NIH Pub. No. 94–2789. 1996.

3. Hodgson TA. National Center for Health Statistics, Centers for Disease Control and Prevention. Unpublished estimates. 1997.

4. National Cancer Institute. Cancer control objectives for the nation: 1985–2000. National Cancer Institute Monographs 2. Bethesda, Maryland: U.S. Department of Health and Human Services. 1986.

Figure 28. Lung cancer death rates among adults 25–64 years of age and 65 years of age and over by family income and sex: United States, average annual 1979–89

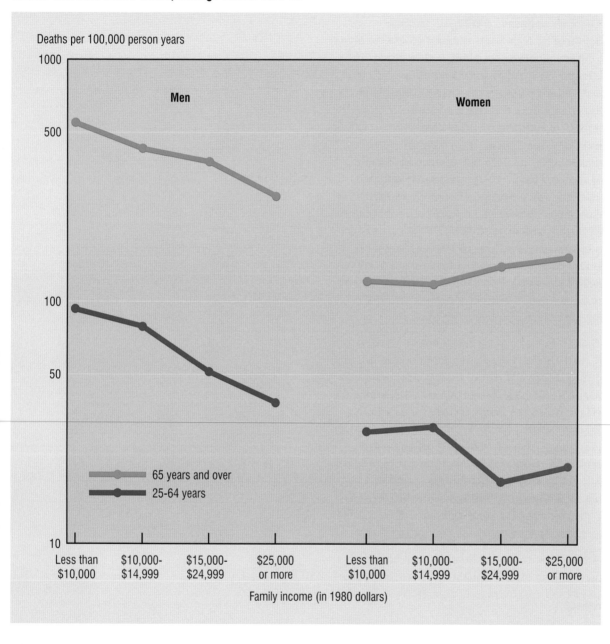

NOTES: Death rates are age adjusted; see Technical Notes. For a description of International Classification of Diseases code numbers for causes of death, see Appendix II. Rates are plotted on a log scale.

SOURCE: U.S. Bureau of the Census and National Institutes of Health, National Heart, Lung, and Blood Institute, National Longitudinal Mortality Study.

Diabetes Mortality

■   Diabetes mellitus is a group of diseases characterized by high levels of blood glucose resulting from defects in insulin secretion, insulin action, or both. In 1995 diabetes was the seventh leading cause of death for all persons in the United States. In recent years mortality from diabetes has been increasing; between 1990 and 1995, the age-adjusted death rate for diabetes increased 17 percent for men and 12 percent for women. Diabetes death rates vary considerably across race and ethnic groups; compared with non-Hispanic white persons, diabetes death rates were 2.5 times higher among black persons, 2.4 times higher among American Indians or Alaska Natives, and 1.7 times higher among persons of Hispanic origin in 1995. Diabetes was responsible for nearly $48 billion in medical expenditures in 1995 (1). The primary risk factor for noninsulin dependent diabetes mellitus is obesity (2).

■   Data from the National Longitudinal Mortality Study for 1979–89 show a strong relationship between diabetes mortality and family income. For persons 45 years of age and over, the age-adjusted death rate from diabetes decreased as family income increased. The relationship between family income and death from diabetes was similar for men and women; for both sexes mortality from diabetes decreased at each higher level of family income. The diabetes death rate for women in families with incomes below $10,000 was 3 times the death rate for those with incomes of $25,000 or more; among men, the death rate for the lowest income group was 2.6 times that of the highest income group.

References

1. Hodgson TA. National Center for Health Statistics, Centers for Disease Control and Prevention. Unpublished estimates. 1997.

2. Herman WH, Teutsch SM, Geiss LS. Diabetes mellitus. In: Amler RW, Dull HB, eds. Closing the gap: The burden of unnecessary illness. New York: Oxford University Press. 1987.

Figure 29. Diabetes death rates among adults 45 years of age and over by family income and sex: United States, average annual 1979–89

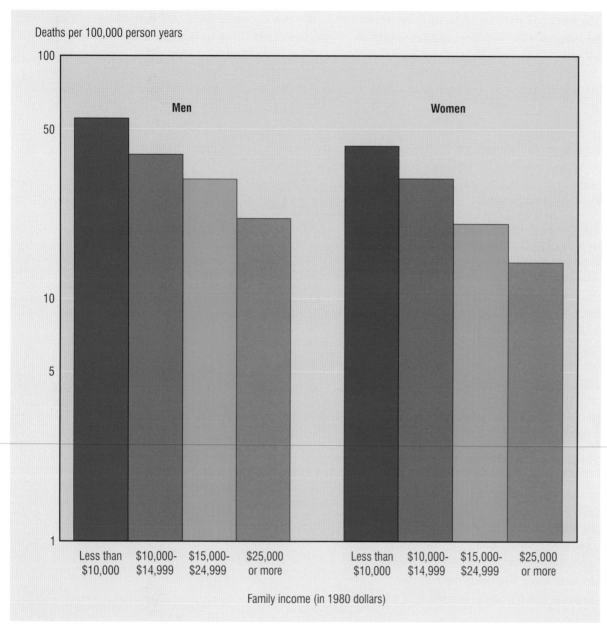

Deaths per 100,000 person years

Family income (in 1980 dollars)

NOTES: Death rates are age adjusted; See Technical Notes. For a description of International Classification of Diseases code numbers for causes of death, see Appendix II. Rates are plotted on a log scale.

SOURCE: U.S. Bureau of the Census and National Institutes of Health, National Heart, Lung, and Blood Institute, National Longitudinal Mortality Study.

Homicide

■ The homicide rate in the United States increased sharply between 1985 and 1991 and then began to decline in 1992 (1). In 1995 homicide ranked as the 11th leading cause of death in the United States overall and the 6th leading cause among persons 25–44 years of age.

■ In 1994–95 homicide rates decreased as years of education increased for persons 25–44 years of age. For those with less than 12 years of education, the rate was more than 7 times the rate for persons who had 13 or more years of education.

■ The education gradient in homicide rates was strongest for non-Hispanic white men. The homicide rate for white men with less than 12 years of education was 8.6 times the rate for those with 13 or more years; for black and Hispanic men, those with the least education were about 5 times as likely to be the victim of homicide as those with the most education. Among women the education gradient for homicide was also strongest for non-Hispanic whites; the rate of the least educated women was 6.4 times the rate for the most educated. Homicide rates for Hispanic and black women with less than 12 years of education were 3–4 times that of those with 13 or more years.

■ For all levels of education combined, the homicide rates for black and Hispanic men were 12 and 4 times the rate for non-Hispanic white men. For those with less than a high school education, the relative difference in homicide rates among the race and ethnic groups was much smaller than for those with more education. By contrast, homicide rates for black women were about 4–6 times the rates for non-Hispanic white women, regardless of educational attainment.

■ Among white, black, and Hispanic men 25–44 years of age, firearms were the cause of about 70–80 percent of homicides; among women 50–60 percent of homicides were caused by firearms. The proportion of homicides caused by firearms did not vary by education level for any sex, race, or ethnic group.

Reference

1. Centers for Disease Control and Prevention. Trends in rates of homicide-United States, 1985–94. MMWR 45:460–64. 1996.

Figure 30. Homicide rates among adults 25–44 years of age by education, sex, race, and Hispanic origin: Selected States, average annual 1994–95

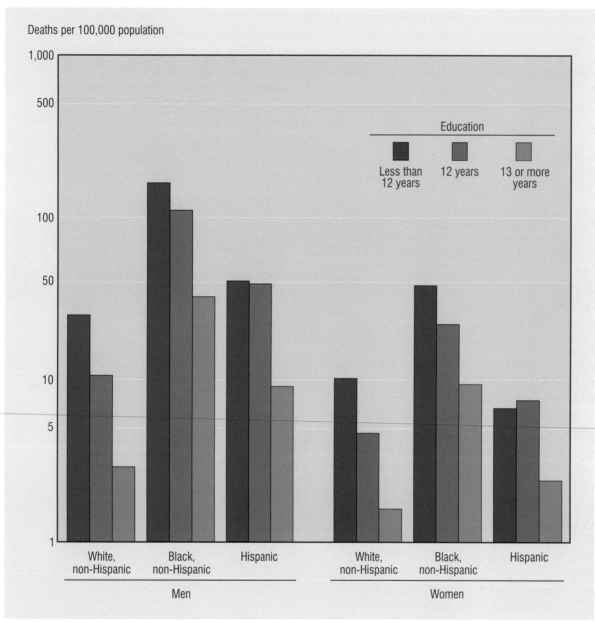

NOTES: Death rates are age adjusted; see Technical Notes. For a description of International Classification of Diseases code numbers for causes of death, see Appendix II. See Appendix I, National Vital Statistics System, for a discussion of reporting of education of decedent on death certificates. Rates are plotted on a log scale.

SOURCE: Centers for Disease Control and Prevention, National Center for Health Statistics, National Vital Statistics System.

Suicide

■ In 1994–95 suicide was the ninth leading cause of death in the United States. Suicide rates tend to be higher for men than women, higher for the elderly than for younger persons, and higher among American Indian or Alaska Native and non-Hispanic white persons than other race and ethnic groups (see *Health, United States, 1998*, table 48). Suicide rates vary by geographic region; for 1990–94, suicide rates were higher in the West and lower in the Northeast, after adjustment for differences in the age, sex, race, and ethnic distributions of regional populations(1).

■ In 1994–95 suicide rates at ages 25–44 were highest for non-Hispanic white persons, and slightly higher for non-Hispanic black persons than for persons of Hispanic origin. In this age group, suicide rates among men were 4–6 times higher than among women for each race and ethnic group examined.

■ For 1994–95, the relationship between education and suicide at ages 25–44 differed by race and ethnicity. The strongest education-related gradient in suicide rates was observed for non-Hispanic white men; the rate for those with less than a high school education was 3.7 times the rate for men with at least some college. Suicide rates for black men who had not gone to college were twice that of those who had, but there was little evidence of a gradient among Hispanic men. Among women 25–44 years of age, the education-related patterns in suicide were similar to those of men in the same race and ethnic group, although not as pronounced. Non-Hispanic white women who had not completed high school had a suicide rate 2.2 times that of those with some college; among non-Hispanic black women this ratio was 1.8. Similar to Hispanic men, there appeared to be no education-related gradient in suicide for Hispanic women.

■ Firearms caused about 55 percent of suicides among men and 40 percent among women. Firearm use in suicide did not vary by education among men, but was more common among less educated women than among more-educated women. Poisoning as a method was more common among those of higher education, while suffocation was more common among less educated persons.

Reference

1. Centers for Disease Control and Prevention. Regional variations in suicide rates, United States, 1990–94. MMWR 46:789–93. 1997.

Figure 31. Suicide rates among adults 25–44 years of age by education, sex, race, and Hispanic origin: Selected States, average annual 1994–95

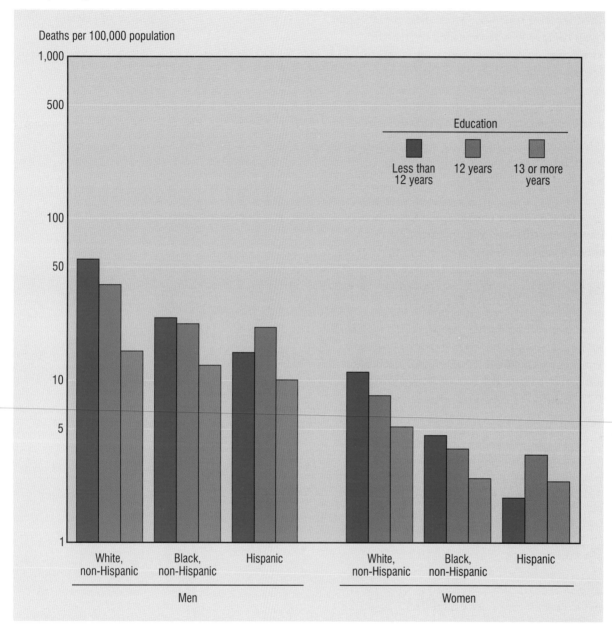

NOTES: Death rates are age adjusted; see Technical Notes. For a description of International Classification of Diseases code numbers for causes of death, see Appendix II. See Appendix I, National Vital Statistics System, for a discussion of reporting of education of decedent on death certificates. Rates are plotted on a log scale.

SOURCE: Centers for Disease Control and Prevention, National Center for Health Statistics, National Vital Statistics System.

Health Status

Fair or Poor Health

■ Self-assessed health is a broad indicator of health and well being, which incorporates a variety of physical, emotional, and personal components of health. Several studies have shown self-assessed health to be a valid and reliable indicator of a person's overall health status (1) and a powerful predictor of mortality (2) and changes in physical functioning (3).

■ In 1995, one in eight persons 18 years of age and over classified themselves as being in fair or poor health, while seven in eight said they were in good to excellent health. Black and Hispanic persons were more likely to consider themselves in fair or poor health than non-Hispanic white persons. However, within each race and gender group there was a strong income gradient in self-assessed health.

■ Men in poor households were 1.5 times as likely to be in fair or poor health as men near the poverty line, and over 7 times as likely to report their health as fair or poor as men in the highest-income households. Only 4–5 percent of high-income white, black, and Hispanic men were in fair or poor health, compared with 27–37 percent of those below the poverty line.

■ Similar to men, poor women were 1.6 times as likely to say their health was fair or poor as women near the poverty line and over 5 times as likely as high-income women to report their health as less than good. Income disparities in self-assessed health were similar across race and ethnic groups; poor women were four to five times as likely to be in fair or poor health as high-income women.

References

1. Tissue T. Another look at self-rated health among the elderly. J Gerontol (27):91–4. 1972.

2. Idler EL, Benyamini Y. Self-rated health and mortality: A review of twenty-seven community studies. J Health Soc Behav (38):21–37. 1997.

3. Idler EL, Kasl SV. Self-ratings of health: Do they also predict change in functional ability? J Gerontol 50B(6):S344–53. 1995.

Figure 32. Fair or poor health among adults 18 years of age and over by family income, sex, race, and Hispanic origin: United States, 1995

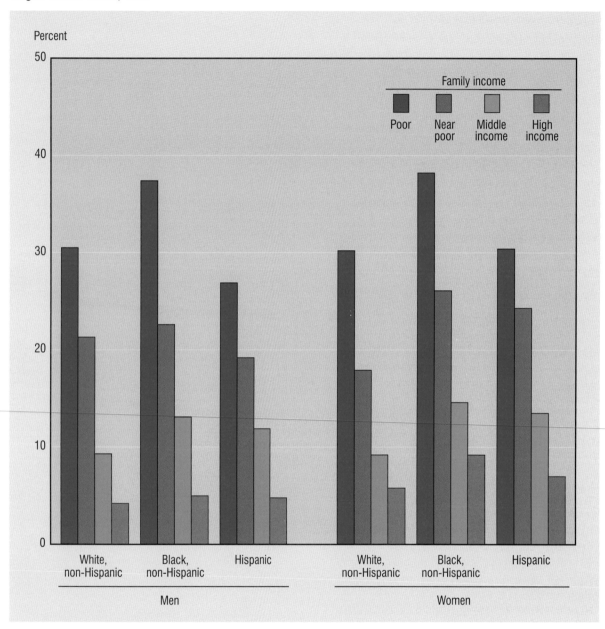

NOTE: Percents are age adjusted. See Technical Notes for definition of family income categories and age adjustment procedure.

SOURCE: Centers for Disease Control and Prevention, National Center for Health Statistics, National Health Interview Survey. See related *Health, United States, 1998*, table 61.

Health Status

Activity Limitation

■   Chronic conditions and injuries can have long term health consequences, sometimes resulting in limiting individuals in the performance of their usual activities, such as work, household tasks, or other routine activities. In 1995, 22.5 million Americans 18 to 64 years of age experienced some limitation in normal activities because of a chronic health problem. The conditions responsible for most activity limitation in nonelderly adults include back, spine, and lower extremity injuries and impairments, heart disease, arthritis, and visual problems (1,2).

■   In 1992–95 the age-adjusted percent reporting activity limitation was slightly higher among black persons (19 percent) than among white or Hispanic persons (14 percent). However, at each level of income, white persons had the highest rates of activity limitation.

■   At each period and within each race and ethnic group, a larger proportion of poor persons reported activity limitation. In 1992–95 one-third of poor persons, 22 percent of near-poor persons, and 11 percent of middle- and high-income persons had activity limitation.

■   In 1992–95 the income gradient was larger for non-Hispanic black and non-Hispanic white persons than for Hispanic persons; white and black persons in poor families were nearly 3.5 times as likely to be limited as their middle- and high-income counterparts. Poor Hispanic persons were 2.6 times as likely to be limited as those with middle or high incomes.

■   Between 1984–87 and 1992–95 the prevalence of activity limitations among poor white persons increased by 17 percent while the prevalence among those with middle and high incomes increased by only 3 percent. Among black persons increases in the percent with a limitation were similar across income levels (11–15 percent), while among Hispanic persons there was some evidence of an increase in activity limitation for those with incomes above poverty (9–11 percent), but there was no change for those below poverty.

References

1. Verbrugge LM, Patrick DL. Seven chronic conditions and their impact on U.S. adult activity levels and use of medical services. Am J Public Health 85(2):173–82. 1995.

2. Stoto MA, Durch JS. National health objectives for the year 2000: The demographic impact of health promotion and disease prevention. Am J Public Health 1991 81(11):1456–65. 1995.

Figure 33. Activity limitation among adults 18–64 years of age by family income, race, and Hispanic origin: United States, average annual, 1984–87, 1988–91, and 1992–95

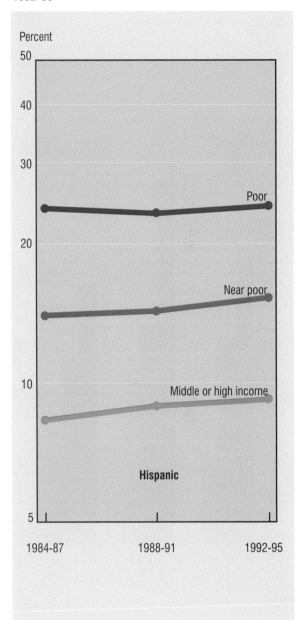

Figure 33. Activity limitation among adults 18–64 years of age by family income, race, and Hispanic origin: United States, average annual, 1984–87, 1988–91, and 1992–95—Continued

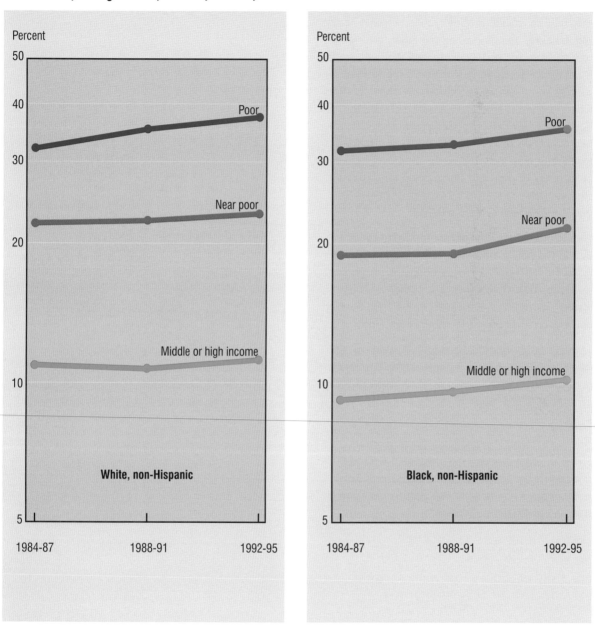

NOTES: Percents are age adjusted and plotted on a log scale. See Technical Notes for definition of family income categories and age adjustment procedure.

SOURCE: Centers for Disease Control and Prevention, National Center for Health Statistics, National Health Interview Survey. See related *Health, United States, 1998*, table 60.

Activities of Daily Living

■　The ability to take care of routine personal needs (eating, bathing, dressing, using the toilet, getting in and out of chairs or bed, walking, and getting outside), is an important aspect of health status, particularly for the elderly population. Needing the assistance of other persons to perform these activities of daily living (ADL) constitutes a physical and psychological burden to the individual affected. The inability to function independently may also impose an additional burden, either in terms of time and foregone opportunities to family members, or a financial burden, if help is obtained from a paid service provider.

■　In 1995, 24 percent of men and 32 percent of women in the noninstitutionalized population 70 years of age and over reported having difficulty performing one or more ADL. Twelve percent of men and 15 percent of women received assistance from another person with at least one of these daily activities.

■　Among noninstitutionalized men 70 years of age and over, poor men were 1.8 times as likely to report having difficulty and 2.5 times as likely to receive help as were middle- and high-income men.

■　Among noninstitutionalized women 70 years of age and over, income gradients in the proportions experiencing difficulty and receiving help were similar. Poor women were about 1.5 times as likely to have difficulty and to receive help with routine care as were middle- and high-income women.

Figure 34. Difficulty with one or more activities of daily living among adults 70 years of age and over by family income and sex: United States, 1995

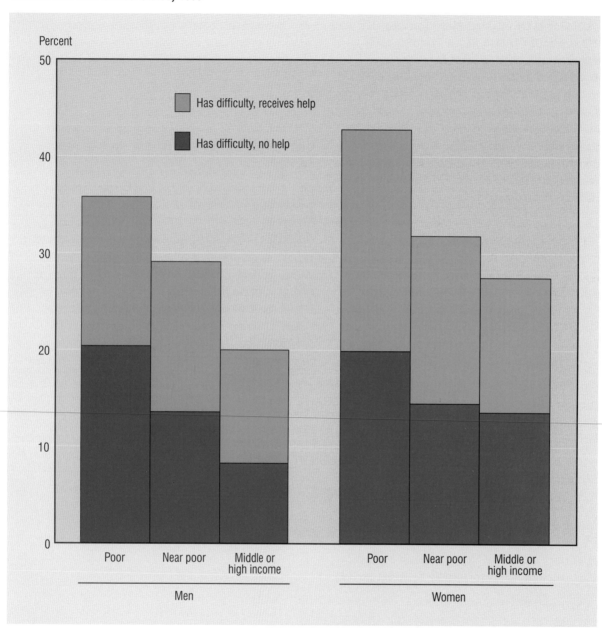

NOTES: Based on interviews conducted between October 1994 and March 1996 with noninstitutionalized persons. Percents are age adjusted. See Technical Notes for definitions of activities of daily living, family income categories, and age adjustment procedure.

SOURCE: Centers for Disease Control and Prevention, National Center for Health Statistics, National Health Interview Survey.

Risk Factors

Cigarette Smoking

■ Smoking is the leading cause of preventable death and disease in the United States. Smoking leads to an increased risk for heart disease, lung cancer, emphysema, and other respiratory diseases. Each year approximately 400,000 deaths in the United States are attributed to smoking (1) and smoking results annually in more than $50 billion in direct medical costs (1). Although there have been recent declines in the prevalence of smoking, the public health burden of smoking-related illness is expected to continue over the next several decades.

■ Between 1974 and 1990, cigarette smoking in the United States declined substantially for persons 25 years of age and over. Among men, the age adjusted prevalence of smoking decreased from 43 percent in 1974 to 28 percent in 1990; among women, smoking declined from 32 percent to 23 percent over the same period. Between 1990 and 1995, however, there was little change in smoking prevalence; in 1995, the age adjusted smoking prevalence was 26 percent for men and 23 percent for women.

■ Between 1974 and 1990, cigarette smoking declined at all levels of education for both men and women. The rate of decline, however, was greater among persons with more education. Among men, smoking declined at an average annual rate of about 1.5 percent among those with a high school diploma or less education and 2.9 percent per year among those with some college. Average annual declines ranged from 0.9 to 2.2 percent for women with less than a college degree. Among college graduates, cigarette smoking declined by approximately 4 percent per year for men and women.

■ Between 1990 and 1995, the rate of decline in smoking prevalence was considerably less than occurred during 1974 to 1990. In addition, declines showed no education-related gradient, ranging from 0.4 percent per year among high school graduates to 1.5 percent per year among men with some college. For women at all levels of education, the age-adjusted prevalence of smoking in 1995 was nearly the same as in 1990.

■ Differential declines across education groups have produced a widening in the socioeconomic gradient in smoking prevalence. In 1974, men with less than a high school education were nearly twice as likely to smoke as those with a college degree or more; by 1995, the least educated men were nearly 3 times as likely to smoke as the most educated. Likewise, in 1974, the least educated women were 1.4 times as likely to smoke as women with 16 or more years of education; by 1995 they were 2.4 times as likely to smoke.

Reference

1. Centers for Disease Control and Prevention. Cigarette smoking-attributable mortality and years of potential life lost—United States, 1990. MMWR 42:654–9. 1993.

Figure 35. Cigarette smoking among adults 25 years of age and over by education and sex: United States, 1974–95

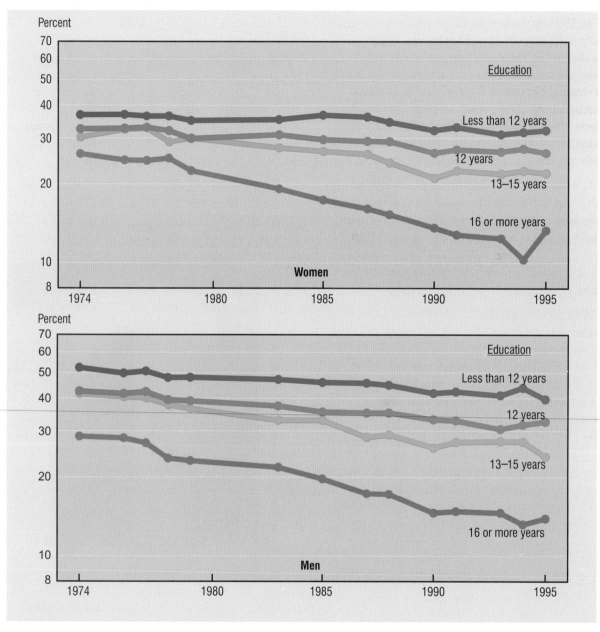

NOTES: Percents are age adjusted (see Technical Notes) and plotted on a log scale. The definition of current smoker was revised in 1992 and 1993. See Appendix II for definition of "current smoker."

SOURCE: Centers for Disease Control and Prevention, National Center for Health Statistics, National Health Interview Survey. See related *Health, United States, 1998*, table 63.

Cigarette Smoking

■ In 1995 approximately one out of every four U.S. residents 18 years of age and over was a current cigarette smoker. However, the percent currently smoking decreased as family income increased. For men and women, cigarette smoking was about twice as common among poor persons as among high-income persons. The *Healthy People 2000* goal is to reduce smoking prevalence to no more than 15 percent among persons 18 years of age and older.

■ Non-Hispanic white and black persons living below poverty were more likely to smoke than persons with higher incomes. Poor black men and women were twice as likely to smoke as those with middle and high incomes; for white men and women the ratio was 1.7. There appeared to be less of an income gradient in smoking prevalence among Hispanic persons.

■ At all income levels, the prevalence of cigarette smoking was similar for non-Hispanic white and black men, whereas non-Hispanic white women were more likely to smoke than black women regardless of income Hispanic men and women in or near poverty were less likely to smoke than their non-Hispanic white or black counterparts.

Figure 36. Cigarette smoking among adults 18 years of age and over, by family income, sex, race, and Hispanic origin: United States, 1995

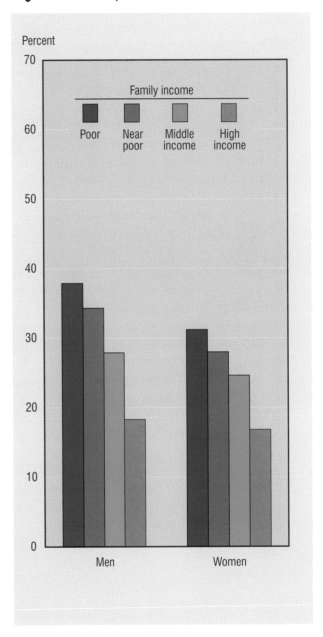

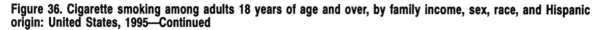

Figure 36. Cigarette smoking among adults 18 years of age and over, by family income, sex, race, and Hispanic origin: United States, 1995—Continued

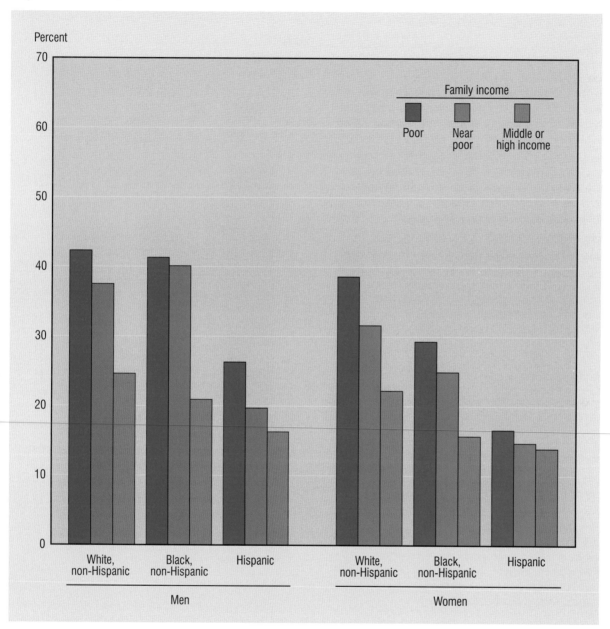

NOTES: Percents are age adjusted. See Technical Notes for definition of family income categories and age adjustment procedure. See Appendix II for definition of "current smoker."

SOURCE: Centers for Disease Control and Prevention, National Center for Health Statistics, National Health Interview Survey.

Alcohol Use

■ Heavy and chronic alcohol use has numerous harmful effects on the body (1). For example, alcohol use and abuse can cause cirrhosis, poor pregnancy outcomes, and motor vehicle crashes (1). The relationship between socioeconomic status and alcohol differs for moderate and heavy use of alcohol. Heavy drinking decreases with more education, whereas moderate alcohol use increases with educational level (2).

■ In 1994–96, 19 percent of persons 25–49 years of age reported heavy alcohol use, defined as having five or more drinks on at least one occasion in the past month. Men were 2.8 times as likely as women to report heavy drinking during the past month.

■ The relationship between education and heavy drinking in the past month differed by race, ethnicity, and gender. In 1994–96 black men and women with less than a high school education were almost twice as likely to report heavy alcohol use in the past month as those with more than a high school education. White men with a high school degree were 20 percent more likely to report heavy alcohol use than those with more education and white women with less than a high school degree were 40 percent more likely to report heavy drinking than women with more education. Heavy drinking in the past month did not differ by education among Hispanic women.

■ Another measure of heavy alcohol use, drinking five or more drinks on five or more occasions in the past month, shows an even stronger inverse relationship with educational attainment (see data table for figure 37). In 1994–96, 7 percent of persons 25–49 years reported this measure of heavy alcohol use. Those with less than a high school education were 2.7 times as likely to report frequent heavy alcohol use during the past month as college graduates. Except for Hispanic women, all race, ethnicity, and gender groups showed a strong inverse relationship between education and frequent heavy alcohol use.

References

1. U.S. Department of Health and Human Services. Eighth special report to Congress on alcohol and health. National Institutes of Health, National Institute on Alcohol Abuse and Alcoholism. Public Health Service. 1993.

2. Substance Abuse and Mental Health Services Administration. Race/ethnicity, socioeconomic status, and drug abuse. U.S. Department of Health and Human Services. No. (SMA) 93–2062. 1993.

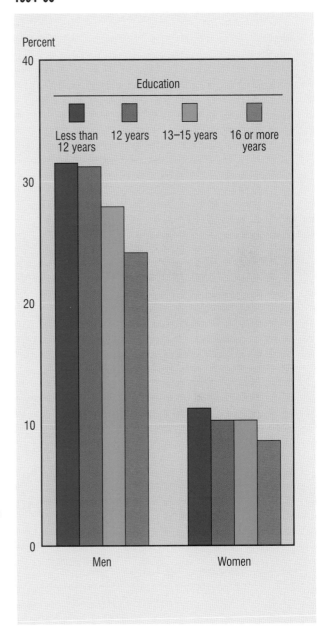

Figure 37. Heavy alcohol use during the past month among adults 25–49 years of age by education, sex, race, and Hispanic origin: United States, average annual 1994–96

Figure 37. Heavy alcohol use during the past month among adults 25–49 years of age by education, sex, race, and Hispanic origin: United States, average annual 1994–96—Continued

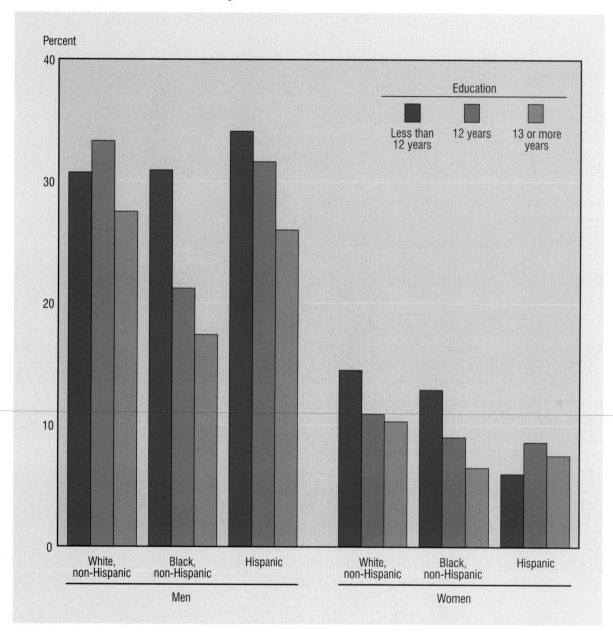

NOTE: Heavy alcohol use during the past month is defined as drinking five or more drinks on the same occasion at least once in the past month.

SOURCE: Substance Abuse and Mental Health Services Administration, Office of Applied Studies, National Household Survey on Drug Abuse, 1994B–96.

Overweight

■ Overweight adults are at increased risk for hypertension, heart disease, diabetes and some types of cancer (1). A healthy diet and engaging in regular physical activity are important for maintaining a healthy weight.

■ Between 1971–1974 and 1976–80 the prevalence of overweight among U.S. adults 25–74 years of age remained nearly constant at around 26 percent for men and 29 percent for women. By 1988–94, however, 36 percent of men and 39 percent of women in this age range were overweight, an increase of 38 and 33 percent, respectively.

■ Over the three time periods, the prevalence of overweight among men has risen continuously only for those with less than 12 years of education, increasing from 25 percent in 1971–74 to 40 percent in 1988–94. For men at all higher levels of education, the prevalence of overweight remained stable between 1971–74 and 1976–80 and then increased between 1976–80 and 1988–94. Among women the trends were different. Between 1971–74 and 1976–80 the prevalence of overweight was stable for women with less than 12 years of education and increased most among women with higher levels of education. Between 1976–80 and 1988–94 overweight increased among women at all levels of education. The increases were greatest for women with 13–15 years of education.

■ Among men the greatest educational differences in prevalence of overweight are between men with 16 or more years of education and men with fewer than 16 years. Overweight prevalences among men with less than a college degree were similar at each time period and 1.3–1.5 times as high as those of college

graduates. However, among women, overweight prevalence declined as education increased. In 1971–74, overweight prevalence among women with less than 12 years of education was nearly 2.5 times the prevalence among those with 16 or more years. By 1988–94 overweight prevalence among women with less than 12 years of education was only 1.7 times as high as the prevalence among college graduates, due to increases in overweight among college graduates between 1971–74 and 1988–94.

Reference

1. Pi-Sunyer FX. Medical hazards of obesity. Annals of Internal Medicine 119:655–60. 1993.

Figure 38. Overweight among adults 25–74 years of age by sex and education: United States, average annual 1971–74, 1976–80, and 1988–94

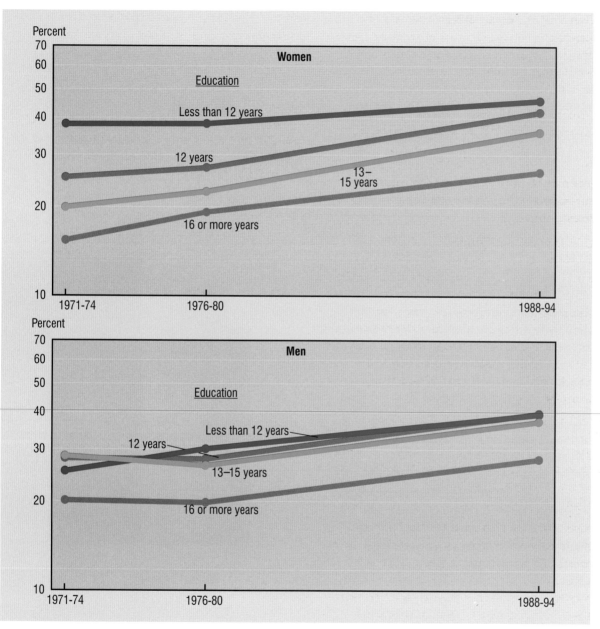

NOTES: Percents are age adjusted and plotted on a log scale. See Technical Notes for definition of overweight and age adjustment procedure.

SOURCE: Centers for Disease Control and Prevention, National Center for Health Statistics, National Health and Nutrition Examination Surveys. See related *Health, United States, 1998*, table 70.

Overweight

■ The *Healthy People 2000* goal is for no more than 20 percent of adults 20–74 years of age to be overweight; the target for low-income women is 25 percent. During 1988–94, approximately one-third of adults in the United States were overweight. The prevalence of overweight was similar for men and women, except for persons living below the poverty line. Among the poor, 46 percent of women and 31 percent of men were overweight.

■ For men of all races there was little evidence of an income-related gradient in the prevalence of overweight. In contrast, there was a clear income gradient in overweight prevalence among women, with overweight prevalence for poor women 1.4 times that of women with middle incomes and 1.6 times that for women with high incomes.

■ The prevalence of overweight was 58 percent higher for black women than for black men. Mexican American women were also more likely than Mexican American men to be overweight, while the prevalence of overweight was the same for white women and men.

■ For Mexican American and non-Hispanic white women, there was an income-related gradient in the prevalence of overweight. In 1988–94, 42 percent of poor white women were overweight, 1.4 times the proportion overweight among middle- or high-income white women. Among Mexican American women, overweight prevalence for those in poverty was 1.2 times that for those with middle or high incomes. Among black women, however, the prevalence of overweight did not vary much across the income categories.

Figure 39. Overweight among adults 20 years of age and over by family income, sex, race, and Hispanic origin: United States, average annual 1988–94

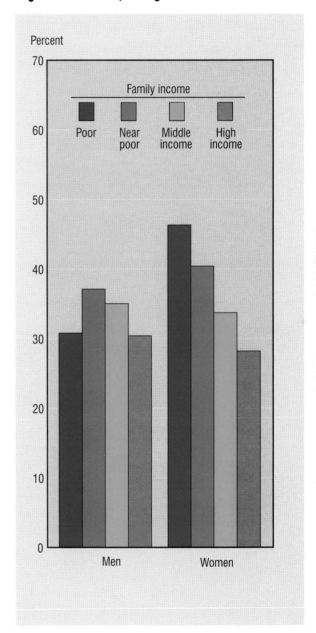

Figure 39. Overweight among adults 20 years of age and over by family income, sex, race, and Hispanic origin: United States, average annual 1988–94—Continued

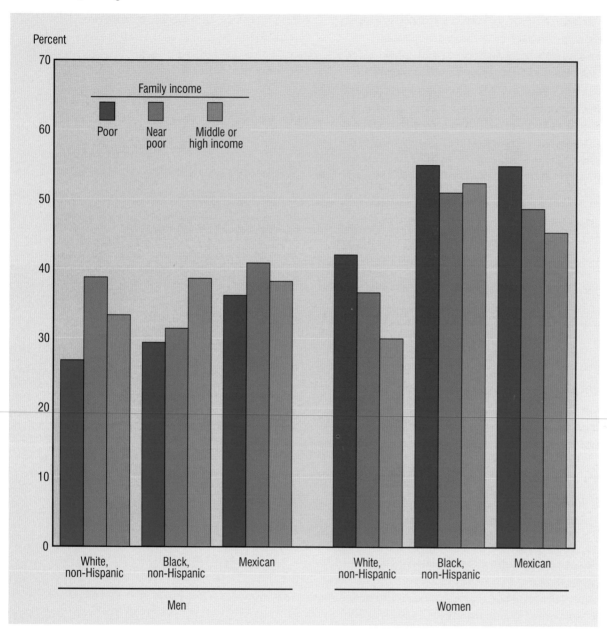

NOTES: Percents are age adjusted. See Technical Notes for definition of family income categories, overweight, and age adjustment procedure.

SOURCE: Centers for Disease Control and Prevention, National Center for Health Statistics, National Health and Nutrition Examination Survey. See related *Health, United States, 1998*, table 70.

Sedentary Lifestyle

■   Regular physical activity can reduce the risk of developing coronary heart disease, noninsulin-dependent diabetes, hypertension, and colon cancer, and thus lower the risk of premature death and disability. Physical activity also helps to control and maintain weight as well as reduce anxiety and depression. Recent research has shown that adults and children do not have to engage in strenuous physical activity to gain health benefits, but rather Americans can improve their health and quality of life by incorporating moderate amounts of physical activity (for example, walking, dancing, or yard work) in their daily lives (1). No more than 15 percent of adults 18 years of age and over should lead a sedentary lifestyle, according to the *Healthy People 2000* goal.

■   In 1991 one out of every five men and one out of every four women 18 years of age and over were not physically active during their leisure time. Although sedentary lifestyle was more common for Hispanic and black persons than for white persons, sedentary lifestyle showed a strong relationship to income in every sex, race, and ethnic group. The percent who were sedentary in their leisure time declined at each higher income level.

■   Black men living in poverty were three times as likely to have a sedentary lifestyle as those with high family incomes. For Hispanic and non-Hispanic white men, the prevalence of sedentary lifestyle for the poor was around 2.5 times the prevalence among those with high family incomes.

■   Women had similar income-related gradients in sedentary lifestyle, with higher income groups having lower prevalences. Poor Hispanic women and poor white women were more than twice as likely to be sedentary as their high income counterparts. The percent sedentary among poor black women was 1.6 times the percent sedentary among black women with high incomes.

Reference

1. U.S. Department of Health and Human Services. Physical activity and health: A report of the Surgeon General. Atlanta, Georgia: Public Health Service. Centers for Disease Control and Prevention, National Center for Chronic Disease Prevention and Health Promotion. 1996.

Figure 40. Sedentary lifestyle among adults 18 years of age and over by family income, sex, race, and Hispanic origin: United States, 1991

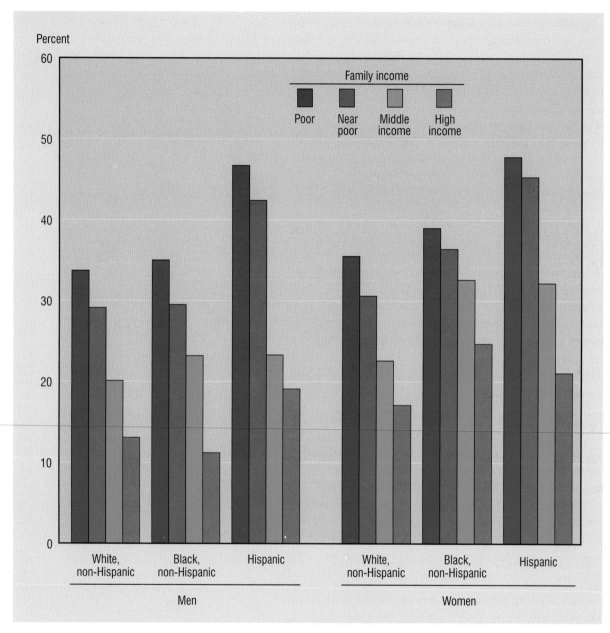

NOTES: Percents are age adjusted. See Technical Notes for definitions of sedentary lifestyle, family income categories, and age adjustment procedure.

SOURCE: Centers for Disease Control and Prevention, National Center for Health Statistics, National Health Interview Survey.

Hypertension

■ Hypertension is a risk factor for heart disease and stroke, the first and third leading causes of death in the United States. During 1988–94 hypertension affected nearly one in four U.S. adults 20 years of age and over, 25 percent of men and 23 percent of women. Twenty percent of men and 17 percent of women had uncontrolled high blood pressure while 18 percent of hypertensive men and 28 percent of hypertensive women were controlling their blood pressure with medication. The *Healthy People 2000* goal is for 50 percent of hypertensives (40 percent of hypertensive men) to be controlling their hypertension.

■ For men of all races, there was little evidence of an income-related gradient in hypertension prevalence in 1988–94. The prevalence of hypertension was 26–27 percent for poor, near poor, and middle income men. Men with high family incomes, however, had a somewhat lower prevalence of hypertension (22 percent). In contrast, there was a clear income-related gradient in hypertension prevalence among women. The prevalence of hypertension ranged from 31 percent for poor women to 19 percent for high-income women and poor women were 1.8 times as likely as high-income women to have uncontrolled hypertension.

■ The income-associated prevalences of hypertension for all men and women mask considerable differences across race and ethnic groups. Among non-Hispanic white men, hypertension prevalence was similar across income groups. Hypertension prevalence was higher for black men than for white and Mexican American men, and also varied little across income categories (33–34 percent). However, poor black men were less likely than those with higher incomes to control their hypertension with medication. Among Mexican American men, uncontrolled hypertension increased at higher levels of income.

■ In 1988–94 total hypertension prevalence and uncontrolled hypertension declined as income increased for white and black women. Forty percent of poor black women had hypertension, compared with 30 percent of middle- and high-income women. Among white women the prevalence of hypertension ranged from 30 percent for those in poverty to 20 percent for those with middle or high incomes. Among Mexican American women there was no association between income and hypertension.

Figure 41. Hypertension among adults 20 years of age and over by family income, sex, race, and Hispanic origin: United States, average annual 1988–94

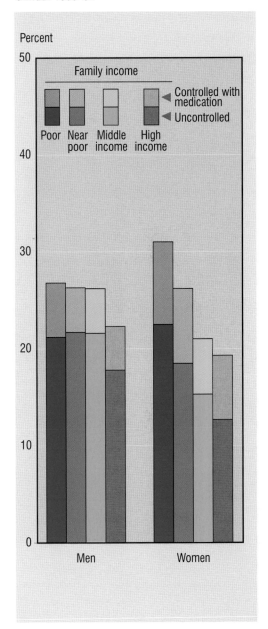

Figure 41. Hypertension among adults 20 years of age and over by family income, sex, race, and Hispanic origin: United States, average annual 1988–94—Continued

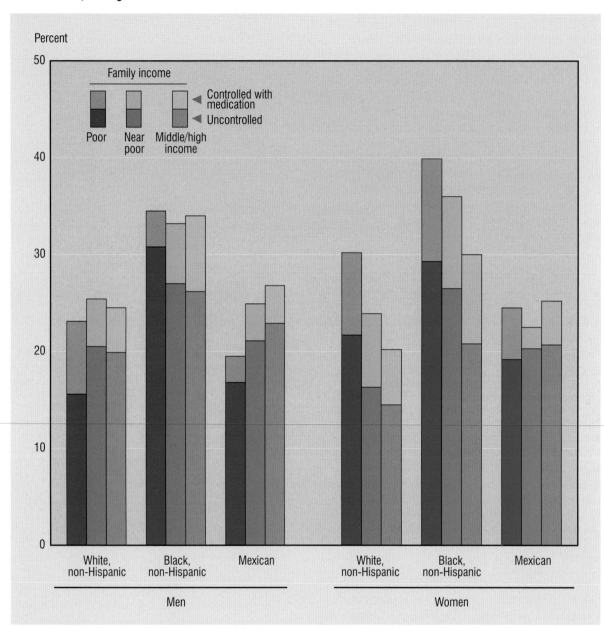

NOTES: Percents are age adjusted. See Technical Notes for definition of family income categories and age adjustment procedure. A person with hypertension is defined as either having elevated blood pressure (systolic pressure of at least 140 mmHg or diastolic pressure of at least 90 mmHg) or taking antihypertensive medication. Percents are based on an average of up to six measurements of blood pressure.

SOURCE: Centers for Disease Control and Prevention, National Center for Health Statistics, Third National Health and Nutrition Examination Survey. See related *Health, United States, 1998*, table 68.

Blood Lead

■ Lead can be absorbed by breathing air that is contaminated with lead particles, drinking water that comes from lead pipes or lead-soldered fittings, or eating foods that have been grown in soil containing lead. Adults may be exposed to lead in the environment, but the most common high-dose exposures for men come from the workplace. There are a wide variety of occupations in which a worker may be exposed to lead including smelting and refining industries, battery manufacturing plants, gasoline stations, construction, and residential painting. Elevated levels of lead in adults may have a variety of adverse effects on health including decreased reaction time, possible memory loss, anemia, kidney damage, as well as damaging male and female reproductive functions (1).

■ There is a clear gradient between income and prevalence of high blood lead in men. (Rates for women were very low and are not presented here.) In 1988–94 poor men had a greater likelihood of having high levels of lead in their blood (defined as blood lead at or above 10 μg/dL) than men with higher incomes. Over 13 percent of poor men had an elevated blood lead level, a prevalence that was 1.8 times that for near-poor men, 2.8 times that for middle-income men, and almost six times that for men with high incomes.

■ Across all race and ethnic groups, poor men had higher prevalences of elevated blood lead than men with high incomes. Non-Hispanic white men living in poverty were over three times as likely to have high blood lead as white men with middle and high incomes. Poor black and Mexican American men had a prevalence of elevated blood lead that was over twice as high as those of black and Mexican American men with middle and high incomes.

■ Non-Hispanic white and Mexican American men had similar prevalences of high blood lead levels at each income category; however, the data suggest that black men were more likely to have high blood lead levels than white or Mexican American men at each income level.

Reference

1. U.S. Department of Health and Human Services. Toxicological profile for lead. Atlanta, Georgia: Agency for Toxic Substances and Disease Registry (ATSDR). Public Health Service.1993.

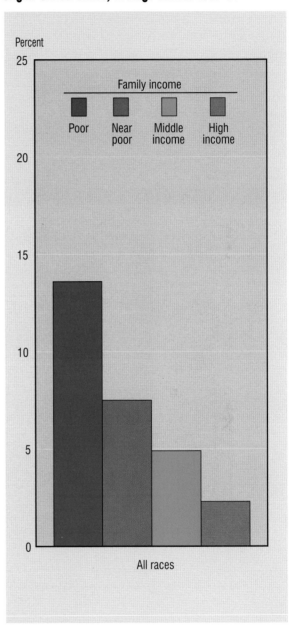

Figure 42. Elevated blood lead among men 20 years of age and over, by family income, race, and Hispanic origin: United States, average annual 1988–94

Figure 42. Elevated blood lead among men 20 years of age and over, by family income, race, and Hispanic origin: United States, average annual 1988–94—Continued

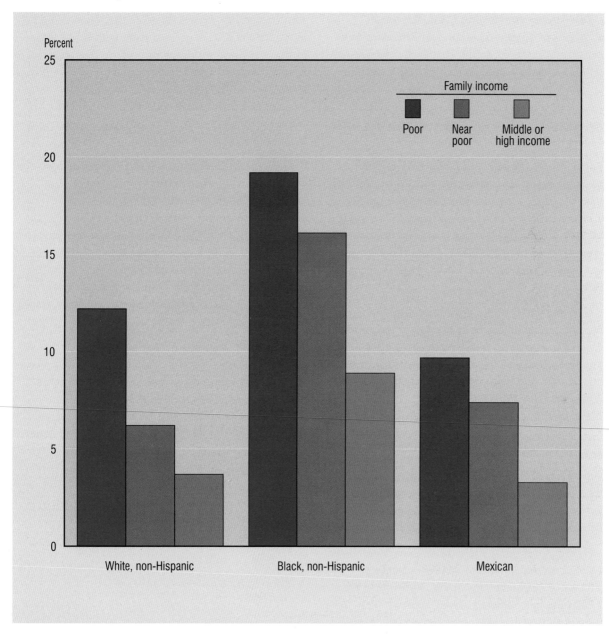

NOTES: Percents are age adjusted. See Technical Notes for definition of family income categories and age adjustment procedure. An elevated blood lead level is defined as blood lead at or above 10 μg/dL.

SOURCE: Centers for Disease Control and Prevention, National Center for Health Statistics, Third National Health and Nutrition Examination Survey.

Health Insurance

■ Health insurance coverage is an important determinant of access to health care. Persons without either private or public health insurance coverage are less likely to have a usual source of health care, are more likely to report an unmet need for health care, and are less likely to receive preventive health care services (1,2). The *Healthy People 2000* goal is for no one to be without health insurance.

■ In 1994–95, 18 percent of adults 18–64 years of age had no health insurance coverage, 73 percent had private coverage, 7 percent had Medicaid or public assistance coverage, and 2 percent had other coverage (Medicare or military). Among adults age 65 and over, the proportion who were uninsured was very low (less than 1 percent) due to Medicare coverage of older persons.

■ Hispanic adults under age 65 are substantially more likely to be uninsured than white or black adults. In 1994–95, 34 percent of Hispanic adults 18–64 years of age lacked health care coverage, more than twice the percent of non-Hispanic white persons without coverage and about 60 percent more than the percent of black persons without coverage.

■ The percent of adults under 65 years of age who are uninsured is strongly associated with family income. Overall, in 1994–95 poor adults were seven times as likely to be uninsured as those with high incomes and near-poor adults were six times as likely to be uninsured.

■ Poor and near-poor adults were much more likely to be uninsured than those with high incomes regardless of race, ethnicity, or sex. Poor white, black, and Hispanic men were six–seven times as likely to be uninsured as their high-income counterparts. Among white women the poor were more than eight times as likely and the near poor were more than seven times as likely as those with high incomes to be uninsured. Among Hispanic women the poor and near poor were about five-six times as likely as those with high incomes to be uninsured; poor and near-poor black women were about four times as likely as those with high incomes to be uninsured.

■ At each level of income Hispanic men and women were more likely to be uninsured than either their black or white counterparts. Within most income groups the percent of black men and women without coverage was somewhat higher or similar to the percent of white men and women without coverage. However, poor and near-poor black women were less likely to be uninsured than white women at those income levels due to greater Medicaid coverage among black women.

■ Men were more likely than women to be uninsured and the difference was greatest among black adults. Poor black men were about 70 percent more likely than poor black women to be uninsured, primarily due to the fact that poor black women were more than twice as likely as poor black men to have Medicaid coverage (55 percent compared with 27 percent).

References

1. Bloom B, Simpson G, Cohen RA, Parsons PE. Access to health care. Part 2: Working-age adults. National Center for Health Statistics. Vital Heath Stat 10(197). 1997.

2. Makuc DM, Freid VM, Parsons PE. Health insurance and cancer screening among women. Advance data from vital and health statistics; no 254. National Center for Health Statistics. 1994.

Figure 43. No health insurance coverage among persons 18–64 years of age by family income, race, and Hispanic origin: United States, average annual 1994–95

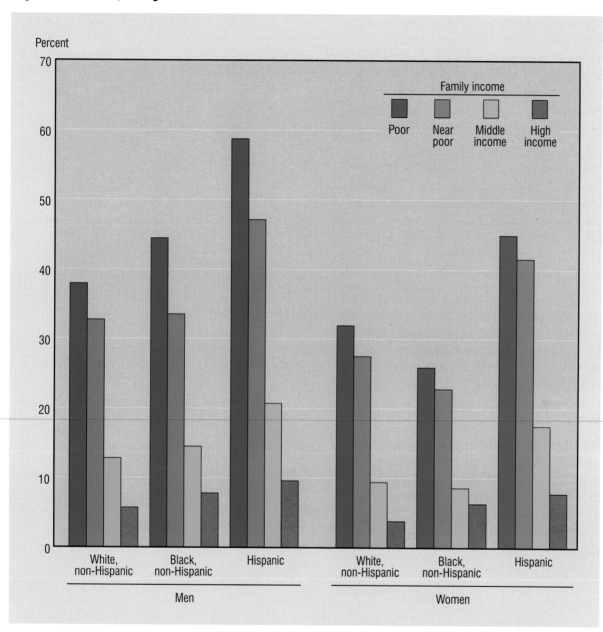

NOTES: Percents are age adjusted. See Technical Notes for definitions of the uninsured, family income categories, and age adjustment procedure.

SOURCE: Centers for Disease Control and Prevention, National Center for Health Statistics, National Health Interview Survey. See related *Health, United States, 1998,* table 133.

No Physician Contact

■   Those who do not receive timely and appropriate ambulatory care when ill may suffer adverse health consequences that require more intensive care in the future. The proportion of adults without a physician visit within the past year among those with health problems is one measure of access to care for those who are ill and may have a need for health care.

■   In 1993–95, 22 percent of persons 18–64 years of age reported a health problem, defined as reporting any one of the following: fair or poor health, a limitation in activity due to a chronic condition, or 10 or more bed-days in the past year. The percent of persons who had not visited a physician in the past year was 12 percent among those with a health problem and 31 percent among those without a health problem.

■   Among adults with a health problem the percent who had not visited a physician in the past year was inversely related to family income, regardless of race, ethnicity, or sex. Poor women were almost three times as likely to be without a recent physician visit as women with high incomes and poor men were almost two times as likely to lack a recent physician visit as men with high incomes.

■   Men with a health problem were more likely than women with a health problem to lack a recent physician contact, regardless of income, race, and ethnicity. Among the poor and near-poor, men were almost twice as likely as women to lack a recent physician contact, and among middle- and high-income persons men were about 2.5 times as likely as women to lack a recent physician contact.

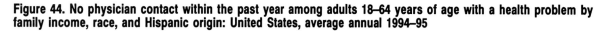

Figure 44. No physician contact within the past year among adults 18–64 years of age with a health problem by family income, race, and Hispanic origin: United States, average annual 1994–95

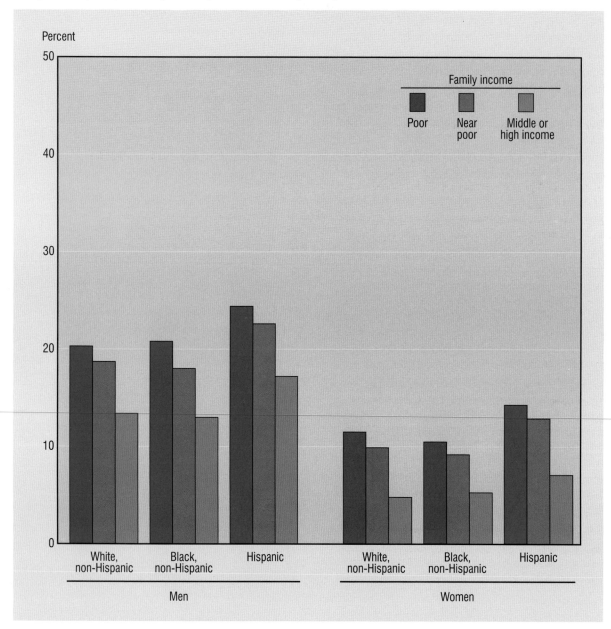

NOTES: Percents are age adjusted. See Technical Notes for definitions of persons with a health problem, family income categories, and age adjustment procedure.

SOURCES: Centers for Disease Control and Prevention, National Center for Health Statistics, National Health Interview Survey. See related *Health, United States, 1998*, table 77.

Mammography

■ Breast cancer is the most common site of new cancers among women and second to lung cancer as a leading cause of cancer deaths among women. Regular mammography screening has been shown to be effective in reducing breast cancer mortality. For women ages 50 years and over the National Cancer Institute recommends screening with mammography every 1 to 2 years. The *Healthy People 2000* goal is for 60 percent of women 50 years and older to have received a breast examination and mammogram within the past 2 years.

■ Overall in 1993–94, 60 percent of women 50 years of age and over reported having a mammogram in the last 2 years. Women with high incomes were about 60–70 percent more likely than poor or near-poor women to have had a recent mammogram. The income gradient in the percent with recent mammography holds for middle-aged women 50–64 years of age as well as for older women 65 years of age and over (data not shown).

■ Within each race and ethnic group women with middle and high incomes were more likely than poor or near-poor women to have recent mammography. This relationship was strongest among white women; the proportion of middle- and high-income white women with a recent mammogram was almost twice that for poor white women.

■ After controlling for income, black women were as likely or more likely than white women to report having a recent mammogram. Among the poor, black women were about 60 percent more likely than white women to have a recent mammogram. Among near-poor women, Hispanic women were less likely than either white women or black women to have recent mammography screening.

Figure 45. Mammography within the past 2 years among women 50 years of age and over by family income, race, and Hispanic origin: United States, average annual 1993–94

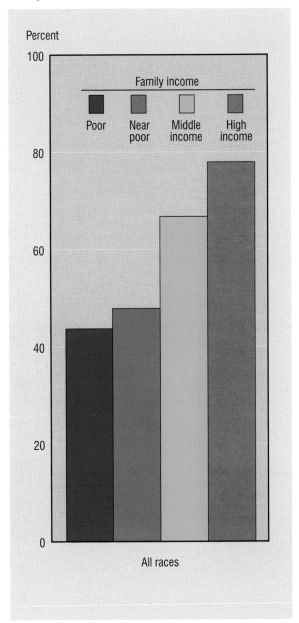

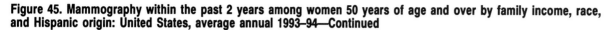

Figure 45. Mammography within the past 2 years among women 50 years of age and over by family income, race, and Hispanic origin: United States, average annual 1993–94—Continued

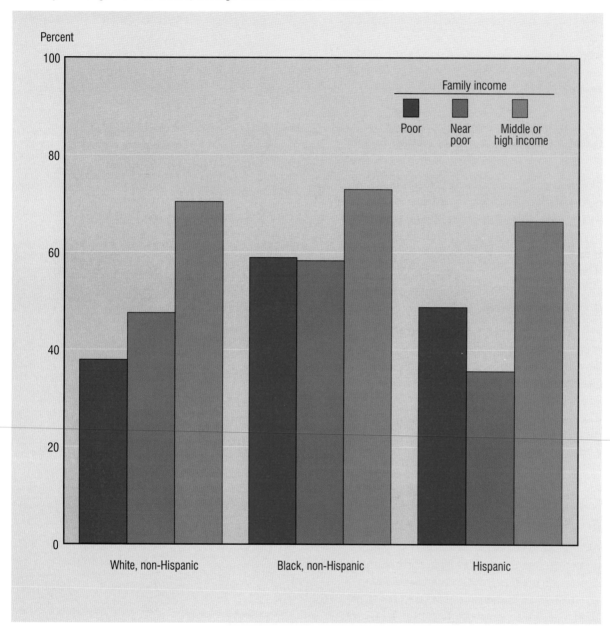

NOTES: Percents are age adjusted. See Technical Notes for definition of family income categories and age adjustment procedure.

SOURCE: Centers for Disease Control and Prevention, National Center for Health Statistics, National Health Interview Survey. See related *Health, United States, 1998*, table 80.

Unmet Need for Care

■ Delaying or not receiving needed health care can have adverse health consequences and may eventually result in the need for more intensive care if health status worsens. One approach to measuring the extent of unmet need for health care is to ask respondents whether they delayed or received care that they needed. This approach relies on the ability of respondents to accurately determine whether care was needed.

■ The proportion of persons who report unmet need for health care increases sharply as income declines. In 1994–95 the age-adjusted percent of poor persons 18–64 years of age who reported unmet need for health care was almost five times that for adults with high family income, and near-poor persons were four times as likely as those with high incomes to report unmet need for health care.

■ The inverse relationship between unmet need for health care and family income held true for young and middle-aged adults and for men and women. The relationship between income and having an unmet need was even stronger for middle-aged persons 45–64 years of age than for younger adults 18–44 years. Poor middle-aged men and women were almost seven times as likely as high-income men and women to report unmet need for care. Poor and near-poor men and women 18–44 years of age were almost four times as likely as their high-income counterparts to report unmet need for care.

■ Among the poor the percent of persons with unmet need for health care was higher among those 45–64 years of age than younger adults, whereas among middle- and high-income persons the percent with unmet need was somewhat lower for 45–64 year

olds than for younger adults. Poor men 45–64 years of age were 40 percent more likely than poor men 18–44 years of age to report unmet need for health care. Poor women 45–64 years of age were about one–third more likely than younger adult women to report unmet need for health care.

■ The proportion of adult women who report unmet need for health care tended to be somewhat higher than for adult men, regardless of income or age.

Figure 46. Unmet need for health care during the past year among adults 18–64 years of age, by family income, age, and sex: United States, average annual 1994–95

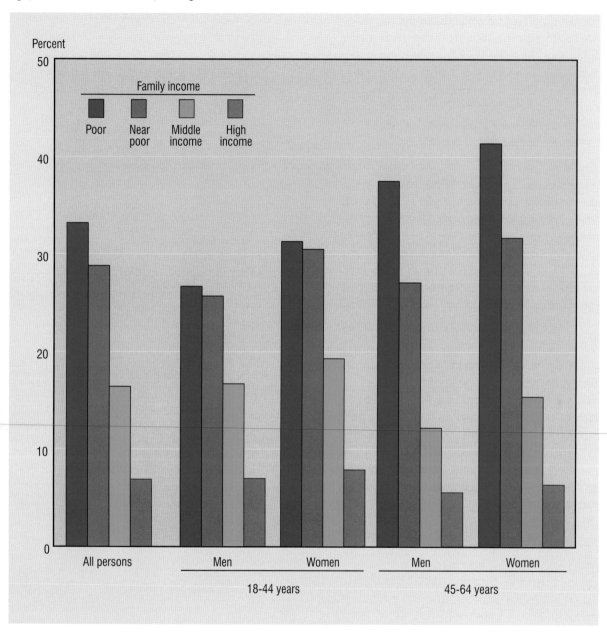

NOTE: See Technical Notes for definitions of unmet need for health care and family income categories.

SOURCE: Centers for Disease Control and Prevention, National Center for Health Statistics, National Health Interview Survey.

Unmet Need for Care

■ Unmet need for health care increases sharply as income declines among the elderly as well as among younger adults. In 1994–95, 22 percent of persons 65 years and over who were poor reported unmet need for health care, 10 times the percent for older persons with high incomes. Twelve percent of near-poor older persons reported unmet need for health care, five times the percent for those with high incomes.

■ Compared with middle-aged persons 45–64 years of age, older persons are substantially less likely to report unmet need for care, due in large part to the fact that Medicare coverage comes into effect at age 65. The drop in unmet need between middle-aged and older persons occurs in every income group. Poor persons 45–64 years of age were 1.8 times as likely to report unmet need for care as poor persons 65 years and over. Among the near-poor the percent of those 65 years and over reporting unmet need was less than one–half that for middle-aged persons.

■ Among poor elderly persons and among near-poor elderly persons the percent with unmet need for health care did not differ significantly by race and Hispanic origin. However, in the middle- or high-income group, black and Hispanic older persons were about twice as likely to report unmet need as non-Hispanic white older persons. As a result the income gradient in unmet need was greater for white older persons than for black or Hispanic older persons.

Figure 47. Unmet need for health care during the past year among adults 65 years of age and over by family income, race, and Hispanic origin: United States, average annual 1994–95

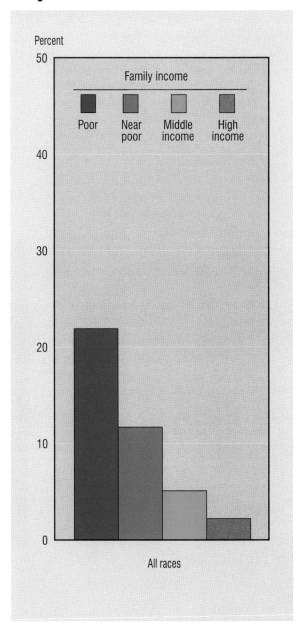

Figure 47. Unmet need for health care during the past year among adults 65 years of age and over by family income, race, and Hispanic origin: United States, average annual 1994–95—Continued

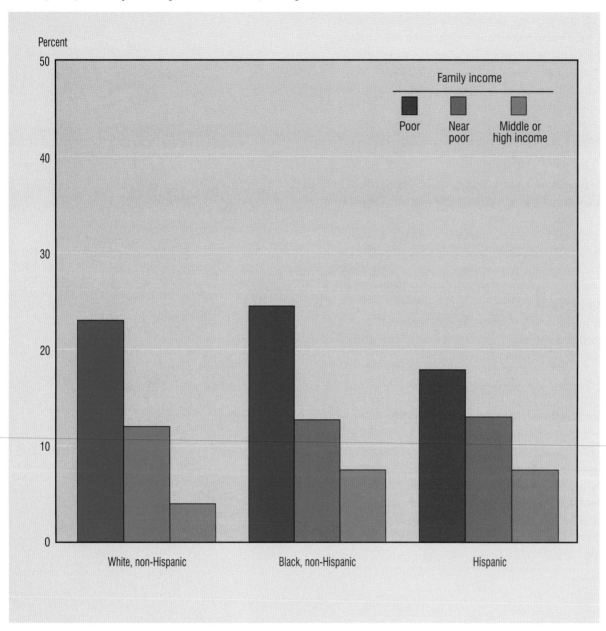

NOTE: See Technical Notes for definitions of unmet need for health care and family income categories.

SOURCE: Centers for Disease Control and Prevention, National Center for Health Statistics, National Health Interview Survey.

Avoidable Hospitalization

■ Delaying or not receiving timely and appropriate care for chronic conditions and other health problems may lead to the development of more serious health conditions that require hospitalization. Hospital stays for specific conditions have been identified as potentially avoidable in the presence of appropriate and timely ambulatory care. Hospitalization rates for these conditions provide a measure of access to ambulatory medical care.

■ The rate of avoidable hospitalizations is inversely associated with the median income of the patient's area of residence. In 1989–91 the avoidable hospitalization rate among residents of low-income areas with median household income less than $20,000 was 2.4 times that for residents of high-income areas with median income $40,000 and over. There was an income gradient in avoidable hospitalization rates for white persons and black persons. The ratio of low-income to high-income rates was 1.7 for white persons and 2.2 for black persons.

■ At each level of median area income, the avoidable hospitalization rate for black persons was higher than for white persons. This racial difference was largest for residents of the lowest income areas. The rate of avoidable hospitalizations for black persons living in the lowest income areas was 2.7 times that of white persons residing in areas with the lowest median income. In areas with higher median incomes black persons had about twice the rate of avoidable hospitalizations as white persons.

Figure 48. Avoidable hospitalizations among adults 18–64 years of age by median household income in ZIP Code of residence and race: United States, average annual 1989–91

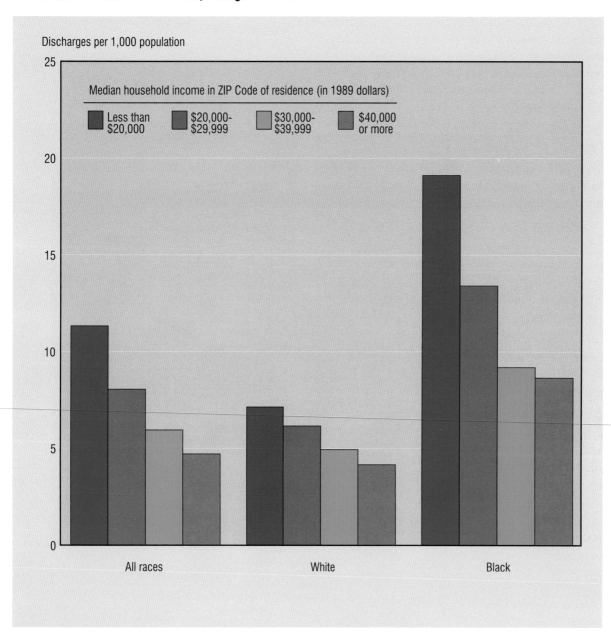

Discharges per 1,000 population

Median household income in ZIP Code of residence (in 1989 dollars)

- Less than $20,000
- $20,000–$29,999
- $30,000–$39,999
- $40,000 or more

All races   White   Black

NOTES: Rates are age adjusted. See Technical Notes for definition of avoidable hospitalizations and methods.

SOURCE: Centers for Disease Control and Prevention, National Center for Health Statistics, National Hospital Discharge Survey. U.S. Bureau of the Census, 1990 decennial Census.

Dental Care

■ Regular dental visits are important for preventing and treating oral diseases. Having at least one dental visit per year is an indicator of appropriate use of dental care services. The *Healthy People 2000* objective is for 70 percent of adults 35 years and over to use the oral health care system during each year.

■ In 1993, 63 percent of adults 18–64 years of age had a dental visit during the previous 12 months. The percent of adults with a recent dental visit rose sharply with income from 41 percent among the poor to 77 percent among those with high family income.

■ The strength of the association between family income and dental care utilization was similar for white, black, and Hispanic persons. The percent of middle- or high-income adults with a dental visit during the past 12 months was 60–65 percent higher than the percent of poor adults with a recent dental visit within each of these three race and ethnic groups.

■ Among poor adults non-Hispanic white persons were more likely to have had a dental visit in the past 12 months than black or Hispanic persons (45 percent compared with 38 and 36 percent). Among middle or high income adults a similar pattern was found with non-Hispanic white persons more likely than black or Hispanic persons to have had a recent dental visit.

Figure 49. Dental visit within the past year among adults 18–64 years of age by family income, race, and Hispanic origin: United States, 1993

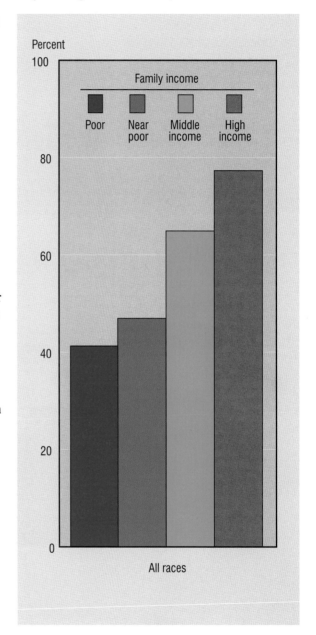

Figure 49. Dental visit within the past year among adults 18–64 years of age by family income, race, and Hispanic origin: United States, 1993—Continued

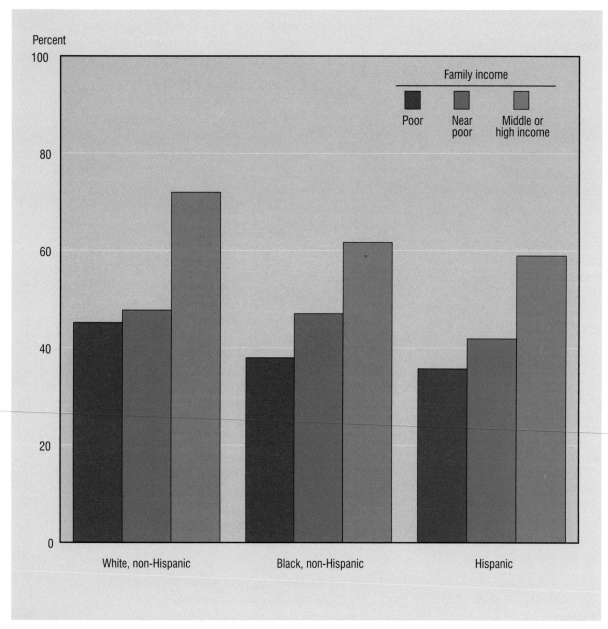

NOTES: Percents are age adjusted. See Technical Notes for definition of family income categories and age adjustment procedure.

SOURCE: Centers for Disease Control and Prevention, National Center for Health Statistics, National Health Interview Survey. See related *Health, United States, 1998*, table 83.

Technical Notes ....

Data Sources

Appendix I describes the data sources used in the chartbook except for the two surveys described below.

National Longitudinal Mortality Study (figures 25 and 27–29)

The National Longitudinal Mortality Study (NLMS) is a long-term prospective study of mortality in the United States. The study is funded and directed by the National Heart, Lung, and Blood Institute and is carried out with the help of the Census Bureau and the National Center for Health Statistics.

The study population for NLMS consists of samples drawn from the Current Population Survey (CPS). The primary purpose of CPS is to provide estimates of employment, unemployment, and other characteristics of the labor force, but it also includes data needed for the record linkage with the National Death Index.

The CPS sample includes persons of all ages, both sexes, and all races. Each sample is designated as a "cohort" for mortality follow up; that is, the persons in the sample were known to be alive on the survey date, and therefore are eligible for follow up for survivorship from that date forward. The CPS surveys used for the full NLMS were conducted in February 1978, March 1979, April 1980, August 1980, December 1980, March 1981, March 1982, March 1983, and March 1985. Data for figures 27–29 were obtained from the NLMS Public Use File, Release 2, which includes 9 years of follow up for the five CPS surveys conducted over the period 1979–81 (1).

Youth Risk Behavior Survey (figures 15 and 17)

The 1992 Youth Risk Behavior Survey is a followback survey of children 12–21 years of age, drawn from families who were interviewed in the 1992 National Health Interview Survey (NHIS). Interviews were completed for 10,645 children. The questionnaire focused on selected types of health behaviors that could lead to a greater risk for disease and injuries among youths.

Measures of Socioeconomic Status

Income refers solely to money income before taxes and does not include the value of noncash benefits such as food stamps, Medicare, Medicaid, public housing, and employer-provided fringe benefits.

Poverty status (figures 3, 4, 21) is based on family income and family size using the poverty thresholds developed by the U.S. Bureau of the Census (see Appendix II). Poor persons are defined as having incomes below the poverty threshold. Near poor persons have incomes of 100 percent to 199 percent of the poverty threshold.

Poverty rates by State (figure 4) are grouped into the following intervals according to the percent below the poverty threshold: 6.5–10.9 percent (19 States); 11.0–14.9 percent (16 States); 15.0–18.9 percent (12 States); and 19.0–24.0 (3 States and the District of Columbia).

Occupational category (figure 7) is based on current occupation and excludes persons on full-time active duty in the military. The category "white collar" includes executive, administrative, and managerial occupations, professional specialty occupations, technicians and related support occupations, sales occupations, and administrative support occupations. The category "blue collar" includes precision production, craft and repair occupations, machine operators, assemblers and inspectors, transportation and material moving occupations, handlers, equipment cleaners, helpers, and laborers. The category "service" includes private household occupations, protective and other service occupations. The category "farm" includes farming, forestry, and fishing occupations.

Family income categories (figures 11, 14–17, 20, 22, 32–34, 36, 39–47, and 49) were defined as follows:

■ **Poor** persons have family incomes below the Federal poverty level (See Appendix II). For a family of four, the Federal poverty level was $15,569 in 1995.

■ **Near poor** persons have family incomes between 100 and 199 percent of the Federal poverty level.

■ **Middle income** persons have family incomes at least 200 percent of the Federal poverty level but less than $50,000.

■ **High income** persons have family incomes at least 200 percent of the Federal poverty level and at least $50,000.

■ **Middle or high income** persons have family income at least 200 percent of the Federal poverty level.

Three or four family income categories were used in each chart, depending on whether there were sufficient numbers of observations to subdivide those persons with family incomes above twice the poverty level into two groups. Limitations in data collection required the subdivision of the group with incomes at least 200 percent of poverty to be based on family income rather than on percent of poverty level (the National Health Interview Survey and National Health and Nutrition Examination Survey had an upper income category of $50,000 or more for the survey years analyzed).

Median household income in ZIP Code of residence (figures 23, 24, and 48) based on the 1990 decennial Census was used as a measure of socioeconomic status for charts based on data sources that did not include a measure of socioeconomic status at the individual level. Four categories of median household income were used: under $20,000 (13 percent of the U.S. population), $20,000–$29,999 (39 percent of the U.S. population), $30,000–$39,999 (27 percent of the U.S. population), $40,000 and over (21 percent of the U.S. population) (2).

Race and Ethnicity

This chartbook presents data by race and ethnicity as well as socioeconomic status. In many charts, data are presented by both race and ethnicity (e.g., presenting information for Hispanic as well as non-Hispanic white and non-Hispanic black persons).

The chart labels provide a complete description of the data that are presented. In the text that accompanies the charts, in some places, shorthand terms ("white" and "black") were used for the sake of brevity. For example, where a chart presents data for black, non-Hispanic persons, the term "black" in the text refers to only non-Hispanic black persons.

Data throughout the chartbook were generally presented for each race and ethnic subgroup where data were available and numbers were sufficient to allow calculation of reliable estimates. Many charts present data only for the largest race and ethnic groups: non-Hispanic white, non-Hispanic black, and Hispanic (or Mexican-American) persons. National health data sources that permit tabulation by socioeconomic status are limited for smaller groups such as American Indians or Alaska Natives and Asians or Pacific Islanders. Figures 8 and 18 do not present trends for Hispanic births because the number of states reporting Hispanic origin on birth certificates has changed over the time period 1980–95 (See Appendix I, National Vital Statistics System). Figures 14, 16, 39, 41, and 42 present data for Mexican Americans, rather than all Hispanic persons, because Mexican Americans were oversampled in the National Health and Nutrition Examination Survey III. Figures 24 and 48, based on the National Hospital Discharge Survey, do not present data by Hispanic origin because ethnicity is not well reported in that survey.

Data are generally presented by both race and ethnicity so that data are shown for non-Hispanic white and non-Hispanic black persons rather than all white persons and all black persons. However, figures 2 and 3 present data for non-Hispanic white persons and all black persons because the data sources for these figures did not include tabulations for non-Hispanic black persons. Failing to separate black Hispanics from all black persons should not have a large effect on results for black persons, however. While 12.4 percent of the white population is Hispanic, only 2.4 percent of the black population is Hispanic.

Technical Notes ....

The proportion of the black population that is of Hispanic origin by sex and age is shown in the following table.

Percent of black persons who are of Hispanic origin, United States, 1996

Age	Male	Female
0–17 years.	2.7	2.6
18–64 years.	2.4	2.4
65 years and over	0.8	1.7

SOURCE: Current Population Survey, 1996.

The method of collection of race or ethnicity varies with the data source. Most of the data sources used in the chartbook collect race and ethnicity through self-report or the report of a household member. However, in medical records-based data sources such as the National Hospital Discharge Survey these data may be obtained through some self-reports and some observer reports. Race and ethnicity on death certificates are reported by the funeral director based on information provided by an informant such as next of kin, while birth certificates may combine some self-reports and some observer reports.

Age Adjustment

The age adjustment section of Appendix II explains age adjustment procedures and defines standard populations. The standard populations used in the chartbook are consistent with those used in the detailed tables section of Health, United States and vary with the data source.

- Figures 15, 16, and 17: data were age adjusted to the 1980 U.S. resident population using two age groups: 12–14 years and 15–17 years (see Appendix II, table III).

- Figures 26–31: data were age adjusted to the 1940 U.S. standard million age distribution (see Appendix II, table I) using 10-year age groups.

- Figures 32–36, 40, 44, 45, 46, 48: data were age adjusted to the 1970 U.S. civilian noninstitutionalized population (see Appendix II, table III) using the following age groups: 18–44, 45–64, 65–74, 75 and over (figure 32); 18–24, 25–34, 35–44, 45–64, and 65 and over (figures 36, 40); 18–24, 25–34, 35–44, 45–64 (figure 33); 70–74, 75–84, 85 and over (figure 34); 25–34, 35–44, 45–64, 65 and over (figure 35); 18–44, 45–64 (figures 44, 46); 50–64, 65 and over (figure 45); 18–24, 25–34, 35–44, 45–54, 55–64 (figure 48).

- Figures 38, 39, 41, and 42: data were age-adjusted to the 1980 U.S. resident population using the following age groups: 25–34, 35–44, 45–54, 55–64, 65–74 (figure 38); 20–34, 35–44, 45–54, 55–64, 65–74, 75 and over (figures 39, 41, 42).

Other Measures and Methods

Activity limitation among children (figure 11) refers to limitation in ability to perform activities usual for children of the same age. For children under 5 years of age, the National Health Interview Survey (NHIS) asked about "the usual kinds of play activities done by most children his/her age." For children ages 5 to 17, the NHIS asked whether "any impairment or health problem" limits school attendance, or requires the child "to attend a special school or special classes." In addition, respondents are asked whether the child is "limited in any way in any activities because of an impairment or health problem."

Teenage childbearing (figure 12) estimates are based on the 1995 National Survey of Family Growth (NSFG). Women were asked their age at first birth and some information about their family of origin. The education level shown is education of the respondent's mother, to provide information about the socioeconomic status of the respondent's family of origin. This chart included only women 20–29 years of age at the time of the survey in order to reduce recall bias and reduce age-related variability in respondents' current income.

Blood lead (figures 14 and 42) levels are based on data from the third National Health and Nutrition Examination Survey. Blood was drawn from most survey participants and the level of lead in the blood was assessed. These charts present the proportion of the population who were determined to have a high level of blood lead. An elevated blood lead level was defined as having at least 10 micrograms of lead per deciliter of blood. Data for adults are shown only for men; values for women were very low in every socioeconomic category.

Overweight among adolescents (figure 16) is measured by the body mass index (BMI), a measure of weight for height (kg/m^2). The lower boundaries for overweight in adolescents were defined by the sex-specific 95th percentile of BMI for every 6 months of age among respondents 12–17 years of age in the 1966–70 National Health Examination Survey (NHES). Adolescents in NHANES III (the third National Health and Nutrition Examination Survey) whose BMI's were greater than the 95th percentiles for NHES were defined as being overweight. Pregnant girls were excluded.

Sedentary lifestyle among adolescents (figure 17) is defined as having no heavy physical activity that resulted in sweating or heavy breathing during the past week.

Health insurance coverage (figures 20, 22, and 43) is defined as coverage during the month prior to interview in the National Health Interview Survey. The uninsured are defined as those who reported that they did not have the following types of health insurance coverage: private coverage, Medicaid, public assistance, Medicare, and military coverage. Persons who reported that they had any of these types of coverage during the month prior to interview are categorized as insured in figure 22. In the data table for figures 20 and 43 persons who had Medicaid and private coverage are classified as having Medicaid coverage.

Ambulatory care visits among children (figure 23) by median household income of ZIP Code of residence were estimated by linking records from the 1995 National Ambulatory Medical Care Survey (NAMCS) and the National Hospital Ambulatory Medical Care Survey (NHAMCS) with 1990 Census data on median household income of ZIP Code of residence. Ratios of the number of ambulatory care visits during 1995 to Census population estimates in 1990 by median household income of ZIP Code of residence were estimated. The 1995 data on numbers of visits were used because 1995 was the first year with ZIP Code of residence available on NAMCS and NHAMCS. The only year for which information on median household income by ZIP Code is readily available from the Bureau of the Census is 1990.

Asthma hospitalizations among children (figure 24) include inpatient hospital stays; emergency room visits that did not result in a hospital stay are excluded. The data are based on the National Hospital Discharge Survey (NHDS). ZIP Code of the patient's place of residence from NHDS was linked with 1990 Census data on median household income by ZIP Code to produce hospitalization rates by median household income in the ZIP Code of residence. Census population estimates in 1990 by median household income of ZIP Code of residence, age, and race were used as the denominators of rates. These estimates were based on data for 1989–91 because 1990 is the only year for which information on median household income by ZIP Code is readily available from the Bureau of the Census.

Activity limitation among adults (figure 33) refers to a long-term reduction in a person's capacity to perform the usual kind or amount of activities associated with his or her age group.

Activities of daily living among persons 70 years and over (figure 34) are based on the activities of daily living scale (ADL) that is used to measure functional limitation, primarily in community dwelling populations. The ADL scale is comprised of a set of self-maintenance activities specifically designed to measure the ability to perform routine personal care functions. The activities included in the measure are:

Technical Notes

bathing or showering, dressing, eating, getting in and out of bed or chairs, walking, using the toilet, and getting outside. Questions about these activities ask whether, because of a health or physical problem, an individual has any difficulty performing the activity without personal assistance or the assistance of special equipment. If the individual has difficulty then the degree of difficulty is obtained, including whether he or she receives help from another person.

Overweight among adults (figures 38 and 39) is measured by the body mass index (BMI), a measure of weight for height (kg/m^2). Overweight is defined for men as a BMI greater than or equal to 27.8 kg/m^2, and for women as a BMI greater than or equal to 27.3 kg/m^2. These cut points were used because they represent the sex-specific 85th percentiles for persons 20–29 years of age in the 1976–80 National Health and Nutrition Examination Survey. Height was measured without shoes. Pregnant women were excluded.

Sedentary lifestyle among adults (figure 40) is defined as no self-reported leisure time physical activity during the past 2 weeks. Individuals with disabilities were asked if they had done any exercises, sports, or physically active hobbies in the past 2 weeks. All other persons were asked about the following specific activities: walking for exercise, gardening or yard work, stretching exercises, lifting weights, jogging or running, aerobics or aerobic dancing, bicycle riding, stair climbing, swimming for exercise, bowling, golfing, or playing the following sports: softball, baseball, tennis, handball/racquetball/squash, basketball, volleyball, soccer, or football. A final question was asked about doing any other sport, exercise, or physically active hobbies.

Physician contacts among adults (figure 44) are based on data from the 1993, 1994, and 1995 National Health Interview Survey. This figure presents the average annual age-adjusted proportion of adults 18–64 years of age who have not had a physician visit during the past 12 months among those who reported a health problem. Persons with a health problem are defined as those who met at least one of the following criteria: (a) respondent reported fair or poor health status, (b) a limitation in activity due to a chronic condition, or (c) 10 or more bed days within the past 12 months where a bed day is defined as staying in bed for at least half a day due to a health condition.

Mammography (figure 45) estimates are based on data from the 1993 and 1994 Healthy People Year 2000 Supplements to the National Health Interview Survey. These 1993 and 1994 supplements asked about selected topic areas related to the Department of Health and Human Service's year 2000 health objectives. These supplements were administered to one adult per family in one-half of the sampled households each year. During the 2-year period 1993–94 about 9,400 women age 50 and over responded to questions on mammography.

Unmet need for health care (figures 46 and 47) is based on data from the 1994 and 1995 Access to Care Supplements of the National Health Interview Survey. Persons who responded "yes" to at least one of the following series of questions on unmet need for care during the 12 months prior to being interviewed were categorized as having unmet need for health care: needed medical care or surgery, but did not get it; delayed medical care because of the cost; needed dental care, prescription medicine, eyeglasses, or mental health care but could not get it.

Avoidable hospitalizations (figure 48) were defined as hospital stays with a principal or first-listed diagnosis for which hospitalization may potentially be avoided if ambulatory care is provided in a timely and effective manner. Avoidable hospitalizations were defined as those with the following first-listed diagnoses based on *International Classification of Diseases, 9th Revision, Clinical Modifications* (ICD–9–CM) codes: pneumonia (481–483, 485–486); congestive heart failure (402.01, 402.11, 402.91, 428); asthma (493); cellulitis (681, 682); perforated or bleeding ulcer (531.0, 531.2, 531.4, 531.6, 532.0, 532.2, 532.4, 532.6, 533.0–533.2, 533.4–533.6);

pyelonephritis (590.0, 590.1, 590.8); diabetes with ketoacidosis or coma (250.1–250.3, 251.0); ruptured appendix (540.0–540.1), malignant hypertension (401.0, 402.0, 403.0, 404.0, 405.0, 437.2); hypokalemia (276.8); immunizable conditions (032, 033, 037, 045, 055, 072); and gangrene (785.4) (2, 3). ZIP Code of the patient's place of residence from NHDS was linked with 1990 Census data on median family income by ZIP Code to produce avoidable hospitalization rates by median family income in the ZIP Code of residence. Population estimates for denominators were based on the 1990 Census.

Dental visit estimates (figure 49) are based on data from the 1993 Healthy People 2000 Supplement to the National Health Interview Survey. This supplement was administered to one adult sample person per family during the last half of 1993. Adults defined as having a dental visit within the past year responded that they had one or more dental visits when asked the number of visits that they had made to a dentist during the past 12 months.

References

1. Rogot E, Sorlie PD, Johnson NJ, Schmitt C. NIH Publication No 92–3297. National Institutes of Health, PHS, DHHS. 1992.

2. Pappas G, Hadden WG, Kozak LJ, Fisher G. Potentially avoidable hospitalizations: Inequalities in rates between U.S. socioeconomic groups. AJPH 87(5), 811–6. 1997.

3. Weissman JS, Gatsonis C, Epstein AM. Rates of avoidable hospitalization by insurance status in Massachusetts and Maryland. JAMA 268:2388–94. 1992.

Data Tables for Figures 1–49

Figure 1. Household income at selected percentiles of the household income distribution

Year	Percentiles of income distribution			
	20th percentile	50th percentile	80th percentile	95th percentile
1970	$14,007	$33,181	$55,698	$ 88,054
1975	14,029	32,943	57,221	91,239
1980	14,405	33,763	60,434	98,182
1985	14,582	34,439	63,881	106,830
1990	15,006	35,945	66,271	113,741
1996	14,768	35,492	68,015	119,540

Figure 2. Median household income

Year	All races	White, non-Hispanic	Black[1]	Hispanic	Asian or Pacific Islander
1980	$33,763	$36,251	$20,521	$26,025	– – –
1981	33,215	35,601	19,693	26,643	– – –
1982	33,105	35,238	19,642	24,910	– – –
1983	32,900	– – –	19,579	25,057	– – –
1984	33,849	36,451	20,343	25,660	– – –
1985	34,439	37,137	21,609	25,467	– – –
1986	35,642	38,323	21,588	26,272	– – –
1987	35,994	38,967	21,646	26,706	– – –
1988	36,108	39,224	21,760	27,002	$42,795
1989	36,575	39,301	22,881	27,737	45,681
1990	35,945	38,349	22,420	26,806	46,158
1991	34,705	37,236	21,665	26,140	41,989
1992	34,261	37,229	20,974	25,271	42,274
1993	33,922	37,105	21,209	24,850	41,638
1994	34,158	37,188	22,261	24,796	42,858
1995	35,082	38,276	23,054	23,535	41,813
1996	35,492	38,787	23,482	24,906	43,276

– – – Data not available.
[1]Includes persons of Hispanic origin.

Figure 3. Percent of persons poor and near poor

Race and Hispanic origin	All persons		Children under 18 in families		Related children under 18 in female-headed households	
	Poor	Near poor	Poor	Near poor	Poor	Near poor
All races	13.7	19.8	20.5	22.7	49.3	27.0
White, non-Hispanic	8.6	17.0	11.1	19.7	34.9	29.2
Asian or Pacific Islander	14.5	15.7	19.5	16.4	48.8	17.6
Black[1]	28.4	26.7	39.9	28.1	58.2	26.8
Hispanic	29.4	30.5	40.3	31.7	67.4	21.9

[1]Includes persons of Hispanic origin.

Figure 4. Percent of persons in poverty

State	Percent	SE	State	Percent	SE	State	Percent	SE
Alabama	16.8	1.4	Kentucky	16.7	1.4	North Dakota	11.1	1.2
Alaska	8.5	1.0	Louisiana	22.0	1.5	Ohio	12.8	0.7
Arizona	17.5	1.3	Maine	10.6	1.3	Oklahoma	16.8	1.3
Arkansas	15.8	1.3	Maryland	10.4	1.2	Oregon	11.6	1.2
California	17.2	0.6	Massachusetts	10.3	0.8	Pennsylvania	12.1	0.7
Colorado	9.5	1.1	Michigan	12.5	0.7	Rhode Island	10.6	1.3
Connecticut	10.7	1.3	Minnesota	10.2	1.1	South Carolina	15.6	1.4
Delaware	9.1	1.2	Mississippi	21.3	1.5	South Dakota	13.6	1.2
District of Columbia . . .	22.5	1.7	Missouri	11.5	1.2	Tennessee	15.3	1.3
Florida	15.1	0.7	Montana	14.6	1.3	Texas	17.7	0.7
Georgia	13.6	1.1	Nebraska	9.5	1.1	Utah	8.0	0.9
Hawaii	10.4	1.2	Nevada	10.1	1.1	Vermont	10.2	1.2
Idaho	12.8	1.2	New Hampshire	6.5	1.1	Virginia	11.1	1.1
Illinois	12.3	0.7	New Jersey	8.7	0.6	Washington	12.0	1.2
Indiana	10.3	1.1	New Mexico	24.0	1.5	West Virginia	17.9	1.4
Iowa	10.8	1.2	New York	16.7	0.6	Wisconsin	8.8	1.0
Kansas	12.3	1.2	North Carolina	13.0	0.8	Wyoming	11.1	1.2

SE Standard error.

Figure 5. Educational attainment among persons 25 years of age and over

	Education			
Age, race, and Hispanic origin	Less than 12 years	12 years	13–15 years	16 or more years
25–64 years				
All races	14.3	33.5	26.3	25.8
White, non-Hispanic	9.5	34.4	27.3	28.8
Asian or Pacific Islander	14.0	21.0	20.0	45.1
Black, non-Hispanic	20.3	37.1	27.9	14.8
Hispanic	44.3	27.1	18.9	9.7
65 years and over				
All races	35.1	34.0	17.0	13.9
White, non-Hispanic	31.0	36.1	18.1	14.8
Asian or Pacific Islander	37.2	27.7	15.3	19.8
Black, non-Hispanic	58.6	23.5	10.5	7.4
Hispanic	69.6	16.2	8.2	6.0

Data Tables for Figures 1–49

Figure 6. Median family income among persons 25 years of age and over

Sex, race, and Hispanic origin	Education			
	Less than 12 years	12 years	13–15 years	16 or more years
Men				
All races	$24,386	$40,000	$47,944	$66,690
White, non-Hispanic	$25,274	$41,200	$49,000	$67,952
Asian or Pacific Islander	$34,146	$44,612	$55,392	$68,327
Black, non-Hispanic	$19,957	$36,020	$42,500	$54,500
Hispanic	$24,000	$35,000	$43,734	$58,079
Women				
All races	$18,200	$35,300	$43,628	$62,050
White, non-Hispanic	$18,471	$37,000	$45,510	$64,007
Asian or Pacific Islander	$37,420	$42,658	$57,300	$65,675
Black, non-Hispanic	$13,100	$23,556	$33,162	$47,100
Hispanic	$19,310	$32,000	$38,000	$56,765

Figure 7. Current occupation for persons 25–64 years of age

Race and Hispanic origin	Men				Women			
	White collar	Blue collar	Service	Farm	White collar	Blue collar	Service	Farm
All races	48.4	39.2	8.7	3.8	72.9	10.2	15.8	1.1
White, non-Hispanic	52.6	37.4	6.7	3.4	77.6	8.3	13.0	1.1
Asian or Pacific Islander	60.9	27.7	8.9	2.5	68.5	15.7	15.4	0.4
Black, non-Hispanic	33.5	46.9	17.6	2.0	59.3	14.8	25.7	0.1
Hispanic	26.1	49.4	15.4	9.0	52.3	18.4	26.7	2.7

Figure 8. Infant mortality rates among infants of mothers 20 years of age and over

Maternal education and race	1983	1984	1985	1986	1987	1988	1989	1990	1991	1995
White[1]										
Less than 12 years	12.5	12.4	12.2	11.6	11.5	11.2	10.0	9.0	8.8	7.6
12 years	8.7	8.4	8.5	8.1	7.8	7.9	7.6	7.1	6.9	6.4
13–15 years	7.8	7.2	7.1	6.8	6.4	6.4	6.3	5.8	5.5	5.2
16 or more years	6.5	6.5	6.1	6.2	5.8	5.5	5.3	5.0	4.9	4.2
Black[1]										
Less than 12 years	23.4	20.6	21.5	21.6	20.7	21.0	21.7	19.5	19.6	17.0
12 years	17.8	17.6	17.6	17.2	17.0	17.0	16.9	16.0	16.2	14.7
13–15 years	16.1	15.4	16.4	16.2	15.0	15.1	14.9	14.1	13.4	12.2
16 or more years	13.5	13.6	14.5	14.3	13.7	13.0	12.7	12.5	12.4	11.3

[1]Includes persons of Hispanic origin. Method of rate calculation changed in 1995. See Technical Notes.

Figure 9. Infant mortality rates among infants of mothers 20 years of age and over

Maternal education	White, non-Hispanic	Black, non-Hispanic	Hispanic	American Indian or Alaska Native	Asian or Pacific Islander
Less than 12 years.	9.9	17.3	6.0	12.7	5.7
12 years	6.5	14.8	5.9	7.9	5.5
13–15 years.	5.1	12.3	5.4	5.7	5.1
16 or more years	4.2	11.4	4.4	*	4.0

* Number in this category is too small for stable rate calculation.

Figure 10. Low birthweight live births among mothers 20 years of age and over

Maternal education	All races	White, non-Hispanic	Black, non-Hispanic	Hispanic	American Indian or Alaska Native	Asian or Pacific Islander
Less than 12 years.	8.4	9.1	15.8	5.8	7.7	7.1
12 years	7.7	6.7	13.3	6.2	6.0	7.0
13–15 years.	6.7	5.7	11.8	6.1	5.9	7.0
16 or more years	5.7	5.2	10.6	5.9	6.4	6.7

Figure 11. Activity limitation among children under 18 years of age

Race, Hispanic origin, and family income	1984–87		1988–91		1992–95	
	Percent	SE	Percent	SE	Percent	SE
All races						
Poor	7.1	0.2	7.8	0.3	9.4	0.2
Near poor	5.5	0.2	5.9	0.2	7.1	0.2
Middle/high income.	4.3	0.1	4.4	0.1	5.0	0.1
White, non-Hispanic						
Poor	8.1	0.4	9.0	0.5	10.9	0.4
Near poor	5.9	0.2	6.5	0.3	7.7	0.2
Middle/high income.	4.4	0.1	4.5	0.1	5.0	0.1
Black, non-Hispanic						
Poor	7.0	0.3	8.1	0.4	10.4	0.5
Near poor	5.0	0.4	5.0	0.4	7.7	0.5
Middle/high income.	4.2	0.3	4.2	0.3	5.2	0.4
Hispanic						
Poor	5.4	0.5	5.8	0.4	7.0	0.4
Near poor	4.2	0.4	4.8	0.4	4.7	0.3
Middle/high income.	4.2	0.4	4.7	0.3	5.0	0.3

SE Standard error.

Figure 12. Percent of women 20–29 years of age who had a teenage birth

Respondent's mother's education	All races		White, non-Hispanic		Black, non-Hispanic		Hispanic	
	Percent	SE	Percent	SE	Percent	SE	Percent	SE
Less than 12 years.	32.4	1.6	26.7	2.6	47.6	3.5	35.6	2.8
12 years	18.7	1.2	15.5	1.3	35.3	3.2	27.1	4.1
13–15 years.	12.8	1.6	10.3	1.8	18.4	4.2	23.2	5.5
16 or more years	6.5	1.1	4.2	1.1	14.9	3.5	20.3	8.0

SE Standard error.

Data Tables for Figures 1–49

Figure 13. Cigarette smoking during pregnancy among mothers 20 years of age and over

Maternal education	All races	White, non-Hispanic	Black, non-Hispanic	Hispanic	American Indian or Alaska Native	Asian or Pacific Islander
Less than 12 years..............	25.3	46.4	25.4	4.9	31.8	4.7
12 years	18.0	22.7	11.6	4.4	21.1	5.1
13–15 years..................	10.4	12.2	7.0	3.4	14.2	3.2
16 or more years	2.6	2.7	2.6	1.4	6.7	0.7

Figure 14. Elevated blood lead among children 1–5 years of age

Family income	All races		White, non-Hispanic		Black, non-Hispanic		Mexican	
	Percent	SE	Percent	SE	Percent	SE	Percent	SE
Poor	12.3	1.7	8.0	1.7	21.5	3.2	6.3	1.6
Near poor	4.7	1.3	3.6	1.5	7.9	2.2	4.5	1.3
Middle income	3.6	0.9 }	2.6	0.8	5.9	1.5	2.4	1.3
High income..........	1.7	0.8 }						

SE Standard error.

Figure 15. Cigarette smoking among adolescents 12–17 years of age

Family income	Total		Boys		Girls	
	Percent	SE	Percent	SE	Percent	SE
Poor	20.3	1.7	22.0	2.1	18.5	2.4
Near poor	21.5	1.4	22.5	2.0	20.4	1.9
Middle income	21.0	1.2	19.5	1.7	22.6	1.8
High income.............................	20.3	1.1	22.6	1.8	18.0	1.3

Sex and family income	White, non-Hispanic		Black, non-Hispanic		Hispanic	
	Percent	SE	Percent	SE	Percent	SE
Boys						
Poor	33.1	4.0	11.8	3.2	22.5	3.0
Near poor	26.1	2.5	7.6	2.7	20.7	4.3
Middle/high income.......................	22.9	1.6	4.2	1.6	18.6	3.6
Girls						
Poor	31.0	4.3	8.1	2.8	14.4	3.4
Near poor	25.1	2.6	5.7	1.9	15.0	2.9
Middle/high income.......................	21.4	1.3	7.7	3.4	22.5	4.2

SE Standard error.

Figure 16. Overweight among adolescents 12–17 years of age

Family income	All races		White, non-Hispanic		Black, non-Hispanic		Mexican	
	Percent	SE	Percent	SE	Percent	SE	Percent	SE
Poor	16.6	3.0	18.8	5.1	13.3	2.0	12.5	2.7
Near poor	12.6	2.0	14.3	3.0	10.7	2.1	12.0	2.4
Middle/high income.....	8.5	1.4	7.2	1.6	17.5	3.4	19.7	5.3

SE Standard error.

Figure 17. Sedentary lifestyle among adolescents 12–17 years of age

Family income	Boys		Girls	
	Percent	SE	Percent	SE
Poor	16.4	1.8	29.8	2.3
Near poor	14.2	1.8	24.4	2.0
Middle income	13.3	1.5	18.8	1.6
High income.	12.0	1.5	14.4	1.4

SE Standard error.

Figure 18. Prenatal care use in the first trimester among mothers 20 years of age and over

Year	Race and maternal education							
	White[1]				Black[1]			
	Less than 12 years	12 years	13–15 years	16 or more years	Less than 12 years	12 years	13–15 years	16 or more years
1980	66.3	83.9	87.9	91.9	55.8	66.8	74.2	84.5
1981	65.7	83.6	88.0	92.2	55.1	66.0	73.6	83.9
1982	64.6	83.3	87.9	92.4	53.8	64.8	73.1	82.8
1983	64.5	83.2	88.0	92.7	54.4	64.6	72.5	83.5
1984	64.5	83.2	87.9	92.9	55.1	65.1	72.9	83.8
1985	64.3	82.7	87.8	92.8	54.7	64.5	73.0	83.4
1986	63.6	82.3	87.8	93.0	54.0	63.7	72.7	83.7
1987	63.3	82.1	87.8	93.3	52.7	62.7	72.2	83.6
1988	62.7	82.0	87.8	93.3	52.2	62.4	72.1	83.5
1989	59.0	80.9	87.5	93.6	50.6	61.9	71.9	83.7
1990	59.2	80.9	87.6	93.9	50.6	62.1	72.6	84.8
1991	60.0	81.2	87.6	94.0	51.8	63.2	73.6	85.4
1992	62.8	82.2	88.4	94.4	53.2	65.3	75.0	86.1
1993	64.8	82.9	88.7	94.5	55.3	67.1	76.4	86.8
1994	66.6	83.6	89.1	94.7	57.7	69.2	78.1	87.4
1995	68.2	84.1	89.4	94.8	59.7	71.3	79.5	88.5
1996	69.2	84.4	89.6	94.7	61.4	72.2	80.1	88.9

[1]Includes persons of Hispanic origin.

Figure 19. Prenatal care use in the first trimester among mothers 20 years of age and over

Maternal education	All races	White, non-Hispanic	Black, non-Hispanic	Hispanic	American Indian or Alaska Native	Asian or Pacific Islander
Less than 12 years.	68.0	72.2	61.3	67.2	59.7	69.3
12 years	82.0	86.1	72.2	77.1	68.7	77.9
13–15 years.	87.8	90.5	80.2	83.2	75.0	84.1
16 or more years	93.9	95.0	88.9	89.0	87.4	89.7

Data Tables for Figures 1–49

Figure 20. Percent of children under 18 years of age with no health insurance coverage

Race, Hispanic origin, and family income	Type of health insurance coverage					
	Uninsured		Medicaid		Private	
	Percent	SE	Percent	SE	Percent	SE
All races						
Poor	22.0	0.7	64.5	0.8	12.7	0.6
Near poor	22.8	0.6	18.1	0.5	55.5	0.8
Middle income	8.6	0.4	3.5	0.2	85.4	0.5
High income	4.2	0.2	1.4	0.2	93.4	0.3
White, non-Hispanic						
Poor	22.2	1.2	60.0	1.4	16.5	1.0
Near poor	21.0	0.7	14.5	0.6	60.8	1.0
Middle income	7.8	0.4	2.8	0.2	87.2	0.6
High income	3.8	0.3	1.1	0.2	94.3	0.3
Black, non-Hispanic						
Poor	14.6	1.1	74.3	1.3	10.5	1.0
Near poor	18.5	1.4	30.7	1.6	46.4	1.8
Middle income	8.4	1.0	7.7	1.0	79.2	1.6
High income	5.7	1.1	4.9	1.0	88.6	1.5
Hispanic						
Poor	29.5	1.3	60.4	1.4	9.7	0.8
Near poor	32.7	1.4	21.6	1.2	43.4	1.5
Middle income	13.4	1.3	5.8	0.8	78.3	1.6
High income	7.2	1.0	3.0	0.7	88.2	1.3

SE Standard error.

Figure 21. Vaccinations among children 19–35 months of age

Race and Hispanic origin	Poor		Above poverty level	
	Percent	SE	Percent	SE
All races	69	1.5	80	0.7
White, non-Hispanic	68	2.4	81	0.8
Black, non-Hispanic	70	2.7	78	2.3
Hispanic	68	2.9	74	2.6

SE Standard error.

Figure 22. Percent of children under 6 years of age with no physician contact during the past year

Family income	All races		White, non-Hispanic		Black non-Hispanic		Hispanic		Insured		Uninsured	
	Percent	SE	Percent	SE	Percent	SE	Percent	SE	Percent	SE	Percent	SE
Poor	11.2	0.6	11.0	1.1	10.9	1.0	10.8	0.9	8.4	0.6	23.3	1.9
Near poor	10.1	0.5	9.9	0.6	9.3	1.3	10.7	1.0	8.7	0.6	14.9	1.3
Middle income	6.9	0.5 }	5.3	0.3	7.1	1.2	5.0	0.7	5.1	0.3	11.8	1.6
High income.	4.1	0.4										

SE Standard error.

Figure 23. Ambulatory care visits among children under 18 years of age

Median income in ZIP Code of residence	Place of visit							
	All places		Emergency department		Outpatient department		Physician office	
	Ratio	SE	Ratio	SE	Ratio	SE	Ratio	SE
Less than $20,000	224.1	29.0	49.3	6.2	30.2	5.5	144.6	26.9
$20,000–29,999	238.5	19.1	43.1	3.2	28.1	5.1	167.3	16.3
$30,000–39,999	311.7	25.8	33.7	2.4	23.8	3.4	254.2	24.1
$40,000 or more.	393.0	40.8	32.6	3.0	21.7	4.6	338.8	39.9

SE Standard error.

Figure 24. Asthma hospitalization rates among children 1–14 years of age

Race	Median income in ZIP Code of residence									
	All incomes		Less than $20,000		$20,000–29,999		$30,000–39,999		$40,000 or more	
	Rate	SE	Rate	SE	Rate	SE	Rate	SE	Rate	SE
All races	3.1	0.4	4.7	1.0	3.0	0.4	2.6	0.5	2.0	0.2
White[1]	1.9	0.3	2.2	0.6	1.8	0.3	1.9	0.4	1.4	0.2
Black[1]	6.3	1.0	7.6	1.6	5.5	0.8	5.2	1.1	4.3	1.0

SE Standard error.
[1]Includes persons of Hispanic origin.

Data Tables for Figures 1–49

Figure 25. Life expectancy among adults 45 and 65 years of age

Family income	White men[1]		Black men[1]		White women[1]		Black women[1]	
	45 years	65 years	45 years	65 years	45 years	65 years	45 years	65 years
Less than $10,000	27.3	14.0	25.2	14.3	35.8	19.7	32.7	18.6
$10,000–14,999	30.3	15.5	28.1	14.4	37.4	20.4	33.5	18.0
$15,000–24,999	32.4	16.3	31.3	16.3	37.8	20.5	36.3	19.4
$25,000 or more.	33.9	17.1	32.6	16.8	38.5	20.7	36.5	19.9

[1]Includes persons of Hispanic origin.

Figure 26. Death rates for selected causes among adults 25–64 years of age

Education	Chronic diseases	Injuries	Communicable diseases		
			Total	HIV	Other
Men					
Less than 12 years.	530.8	154.0	85.7	58.9	26.8
12 years	479.2	122.7	82.8	63.5	19.3
13 years or more	212.3	45.6	45.3	36.9	8.4
Women					
Less than 12 years.	317.9	41.9	36.0	19.8	16.2
12 years	273.8	33.1	24.8	13.8	11.0
13 years or more	147.6	17.9	8.6	3.4	5.2

HIV Human immunodeficiency virus.

Figure 27. Heart disease death rates among adults 25–64 years of age and 65 years of age and over

Race, Hispanic origin, and family income	Men		Women	
	25–64 years	65 or more years	25–64 years	65 or more years
All races				
Less than $10,000	318.7	2524.6	126.9	1346.0
$10,000–$14,999	251.4	1920.6	74.1	1043.6
$15,000–$24,999	142.3	1715.3	51.9	969.7
$25,000 or more.	126.8	1666.6	37.3	963.4
White, non-Hispanic				
Less than $10,000	324.1	2658.3	112.2	1352.6
$10,000-$14,999	255.4	1951.1	71.3	1016.2
$15,000 or more.	136.9	1723.1	43.7	961.4
Black, non-Hispanic				
Less than $10,000	390.8	2216.2	184.7	1374.2
$10,000-$14,999	292.8	2079.8	119.2	1542.0
$15,000 or more.	142.2	1272.5	64.8	1088.1

Figure 28. Lung cancer death rates among adults 25–64 years of age and 65 years of age and over

	Men		Women	
Family income	25–64 years	65 or more years	25–64 years	65 or more years
Less than $10,000	93.3	547.9	29.1	122.1
$10,000–$14,999	79.3	428.9	30.6	118.8
$15,000–$24,999	51.5	379.0	18.1	140.7
$25,000 or more.	38.5	273.6	20.9	153.4

Figure 29. Diabetes death rates among adults 45 years of age and over

Family income	Men	Women
Less than $10,000	55.3	42.6
$10,000–$14,999	39.3	31.3
$15,000–$24,999	31.1	20.3
$25,000 or more.	21.4	14.1

Figure 30. Homicide rates among adults 25–44 years of age

	Education		
Sex, race and Hispanic origin	Less than 12 years	12 years	13 or more years
Men			
White, non-Hispanic	25.0	10.6	2.9
Black, non-Hispanic	163.3	110.7	32.4
Hispanic	40.6	39.0	9.1
Women			
White, non-Hispanic	10.2	4.7	1.6
Black, non-Hispanic	38.2	22.0	9.4
Hispanic	6.7	7.5	2.4

Figure 31. Suicide rates among adults 25–44 years of age

	Education		
Sex, race, and Hispanic origin	Less than 12 years	12 years	13 or more years
Men			
White, non-Hispanic	56.0	38.9	15.2
Black, non-Hispanic	24.4	22.4	12.4
Hispanic	14.9	21.3	10.1
Women			
White, non-Hispanic	11.3	8.1	5.2
Black, non-Hispanic	4.6	3.8	2.5
Hispanic	1.9	3.5	2.4

Figure 32. Fair or poor health among adults 18 years of age and over

Sex and family income	All races		White, non-Hispanic		Black, non-Hispanic		Hispanic	
	Percent	SE	Percent	SE	Percent	SE	Percent	SE
Men								
Poor	31.1	1.1	30.5	1.5	37.4	2.3	26.9	2.0
Near poor	21.1	0.7	21.3	0.8	22.6	1.7	19.2	1.3
Middle income	9.8	0.3	9.3	0.3	13.1	1.1	11.9	1.2
High income.	4.3	0.3	4.2	0.3	5.0	1.0	4.8	1.4
Women								
Poor	32.4	0.8	30.2	1.2	38.2	1.6	30.4	1.4
Near poor	19.8	0.6	17.9	0.7	26.1	1.6	24.3	1.4
Middle income	9.9	0.3	9.2	0.3	14.6	1.1	13.5	1.2
High income.	6.0	0.3	5.8	0.3	9.2	1.7	7.0	1.2

SE Standard error.

Figure 33. Activity limitation among adults 18–64 years of age

Race and Hispanic origin, and year	Poor		Near poor		Middle/high income	
	Percent	SE	Percent	SE	Percent	SE
All races						
1984–87	30.4	0.4	20.6	0.3	10.5	0.2
1988–91	31.9	0.4	20.7	0.3	10.4	0.1
1992–95	33.6	0.4	21.5	0.3	10.9	0.1
White, non-Hispanic						
1984–87	32.1	0.6	22.1	0.4	10.9	0.2
1988–91	35.3	0.5	22.4	0.4	10.7	0.1
1992–95	37.5	0.5	23.2	0.3	11.2	0.1
Black, non-Hispanic						
1984–87	31.8	0.7	18.9	0.6	9.2	0.4
1988–91	32.8	0.7	19.1	0.6	9.6	0.3
1992–95	35.5	0.7	21.7	0.6	10.2	0.3
Hispanic						
1984–87	23.9	1.1	14.0	0.8	8.3	0.5
1988–91	23.3	0.7	14.3	0.6	8.9	0.3
1992–95	24.2	0.8	15.3	0.6	9.2	0.3

SE Standard error.

Figure 34. Difficulty with one or more activities of daily living among adults 70 years of age and over

Family income	Men						Women					
	Any difficulty		Receives help		No help		Any difficulty		Receives help		No help	
	Percent	SE	Percent	SE	Percent	SE	Percent	SE	Percent	SE	Percent	SE
Poor	35.8	2.8	20.4	2.7	15.4	2.3	42.8	1.9	19.9	1.5	22.9	1.7
Near poor	29.1	1.6	13.6	1.2	15.5	1.4	31.8	1.3	14.5	1.1	17.3	1.1
Middle/high income.	20.0	1.1	8.3	0.7	11.7	0.9	27.5	1.1	13.6	0.9	13.9	0.9

SE Standard error.

Figure 35. Cigarette smoking among adults 25 years of age and over

	Education							
	Less than 12 years		12 years		13–15 years		16 or more years	
Sex and year	Percent	SE	Percent	SE	Percent	SE	Percent	SE
Men								
1974	52.4	0.9	42.6	1.9	41.6	1.4	28.6	1.3
1976	49.9	1.0	41.7	1.0	40.5	1.6	28.2	1.3
1977	50.8	1.1	42.4	1.2	40.1	1.6	27.0	1.2
1978	48.0	1.6	39.5	1.4	37.8	2.2	23.6	1.5
1979	48.1	1.0	39.1	0.9	36.5	1.3	23.1	1.1
1983	47.2	1.3	37.4	0.9	33.0	1.4	21.8	1.1
1985	46.0	1.2	35.5	0.9	33.0	1.2	19.7	0.9
1987	45.7	1.1	35.2	0.8	28.4	1.0	17.3	0.7
1988	44.9	0.8	35.2	0.7	29.0	1.0	17.2	0.7
1990	41.8	1.2	33.2	0.7	25.9	0.8	14.6	0.6
1991	42.4	1.1	32.9	0.7	27.2	1.0	14.8	0.7
1993	41.0	1.6	30.5	1.1	27.4	1.4	14.6	0.9
1994	43.9	1.5	31.7	1.1	27.3	1.3	13.2	0.8
1995	39.7	1.7	32.6	1.1	24.0	1.3	13.9	0.9
Women								
1974	36.8	0.8	32.5	0.8	30.2	1.4	26.1	1.4
1976	36.9	0.9	32.7	0.7	32.4	1.3	24.7	1.3
1977	36.4	0.9	33.0	0.7	32.7	1.2	24.6	1.4
1978	36.4	1.3	32.0	0.9	29.0	1.9	25.1	2.0
1979	35.0	0.9	29.9	0.7	30.0	1.2	22.5	1.1
1983	35.3	1.1	30.9	0.7	27.5	1.2	19.2	1.1
1985	36.7	1.0	29.6	0.6	26.7	1.0	17.4	1.0
1987	36.1	0.9	29.2	0.6	26.0	0.8	16.1	0.8
1988	34.5	0.9	29.1	0.6	24.1	0.7	15.3	0.8
1990	32.1	1.0	26.3	0.5	21.1	0.8	13.6	0.8
1991	33.0	0.9	27.1	0.6	22.5	0.8	12.8	0.7
1993	31.0	1.5	26.6	0.7	21.9	1.0	12.4	0.9
1994	31.6	1.4	27.3	0.9	22.5	1.1	10.3	0.7
1995	32.1	1.4	26.3	0.9	22.0	1.1	13.3	0.9

SE Standard error.

Figure 36. Cigarette smoking among adults 18 years of age and over

	All races				White, non-Hispanic				Black, non-Hispanic				Hispanic			
	Men		Women		Men		Women		Men		Women		Men		Women	
Family income	Percent	SE	Percent	SE	Percent	SE	Percent	SE	Percent	SE	Percent	SE	Percent	SE	Percent	SE
Poor	37.9	2.3	31.2	1.7	42.3	3.5	38.6	2.5	41.3	4.4	29.3	2.7	26.3	3.3	16.6	2.4
Near poor	34.3	1.6	28.0	1.3	37.5	2.0	31.6	1.7	40.1	4.5	24.9	3.0	19.7	2.5	14.7	1.9
Middle income	27.9	1.1	24.6	1.0	} 24.6	0.9	22.2	0.8	20.9	2.6	15.7	2.0	16.3	2.0	13.9	1.8
High income.	18.3	1.2	16.8	1.2												

SE Standard error.

Figure 37. Heavy alcohol use during the past month among adults 25–49 years of age

	Heavy alcohol use during the past month							
	On 1 or more occasions				On 5 or more occasions			
	Men		Women		Men		Women	
Race, Hispanic origin, and education	Percent	SE	Percent	SE	Percent	SE	Percent	SE
All races								
Less than 12 years.....................	31.5	1.5	11.3	0.8	16.3	1.1	3.9	0.5
12 years	31.2	1.2	10.3	0.7	14.0	0.8	2.6	0.3
13–15 years..........................	27.9	1.4	10.3	0.6	9.0	0.7	2.4	0.3
16 or more years	24.1	1.2	8.6	0.6	6.1	06	1.4	0.3
White, non-Hispanic								
Less than 12 years.....................	30.7	2.5	14.5	1.6	17.7	1.9	4.9	0.9
12 years	33.3	1.6	10.9	0.8	14.8	1.0	2.7	0.4
13 or more years	27.5	1.2	10.3	0.6	7.7	0.5	2.0	0.2
Black, non-Hispanic								
Less than 12 years.....................	30.9	3.1	12.9	1.4	17.6	2.6	5.0	0.8
12 years	21.2	1.7	9.0	0.9	10.6	1.3	2.9	0.4
13 or more years	17.4	1.5	6.5	0.9	5.7	0.8	1.9	0.5
Hispanic								
Less than 12 years.....................	34.1	1.9	6.0	0.7	13.6	1.3	1.8	0.4
12 years	31.6	1.9	8.6	1.1	13.5	1.6	3.2	0.9
13 or more years	26.0	1.9	7.5	1.1	8.4	1.3	1.7	0.5

SE Standard error.

Figure 38. Overweight among adults 25–74 years of age

| | Men | | | | | | Women | | | | | |
| | 1971–74 | | 1976–80 | | 1988–94 | | 1971–74 | | 1976–80 | | 1988–94 | |
Education	Percent	SE	Percent	SE	Percent	SE	Percent	SE	Percent	SE	Percent	SE
Less than 12 years....	25.2	1.3	30.0	1.5	39.5	1.7	38.0	1.4	38.1	1.3	45.8	1.8
12 years	27.9	2.0	27.7	1.3	39.8	1.8	25.1	1.0	27.1	1.4	41.8	1.6
13–15 years.........	28.4	2.7	26.4	1.9	37.3	2.3	19.9	2.2	22.5	1.3	35.9	2.0
16 or more years	20.1	2.2	19.8	1.5	27.9	2.3	15.4	2.1	19.2	1.8	26.3	2.1

SE Standard error.

Figure 39. Overweight among adults 20 years of age and over

| | All races | | | | White, non-Hispanic | | | | Black, non-Hispanic | | | | Mexican | | | |
| | Men | | Women | | Men | | Women | | Men | | Women | | Men | | Women | |
Family income	Percent	SE	Percent	SE	Percent	SE	Percent	SE	Percent	SE	Percent	SE	Percent	SE	Percent	SE
Poor	30.8	2.4	46.3	1.9	26.8	3.2	42.0	3.2	29.4	1.8	55.0	2.3	36.2	1.8	54.9	2.4
Near poor	37.1	1.8	40.4	1.8	38.7	2.7	36.6	2.4	31.4	2.1	51.0	1.9	40.8	2.0	48.7	2.2
Middle	35.0	1.5	33.7	1.3 }	33.3	1.3	30.0	1.2	38.6	1.7	52.4	2.4	38.2	2.2	45.3	2.2
High	30.4	2.3	28.2	1.7 }												

SE Standard error.

Figure 40. Sedentary lifestyle among adults 18 years of age and over

Sex, race, and Hispanic origin	Poor		Near poor		Middle income		High income	
	Percent	SE	Percent	SE	Percent	SE	Percent	SE
Men								
White, non-Hispanic	33.7	2.1	29.1	1.7	20.1	0.8	13.1	0.9
Black, non-Hispanic	35.0	3.4	29.5	3.2	23.2	2.3	11.2	3.0
Hispanic	46.7	5.0	42.4	3.9	23.3	3.2	19.1	5.3
Women								
White, non-Hispanic	35.5	1.7	30.6	1.2	22.6	0.8	17.1	1.0
Black, non-Hispanic	39.0	2.5	36.4	2.6	32.6	2.1	24.7	4.0
Hispanic	47.8	2.8	45.3	4.5	32.2	3.0	21.1	4.3

SE Standard error.

Figure 41. Hypertension among adults 20 years of age and over

Race, Hispanic origin, and family income	Men						Women					
	Hypertension		Uncontrolled		Controlled with medication		Hypertension		Uncontrolled		Controlled with medication	
	Percent	SE	Percent	SE	Percent	SE	Percent	SE	Percent	SE	Percent	SE
All races												
Poor	26.7	1.6	21.2	1.7	5.6	1.1	31.0	1.8	22.5	1.7	8.5	1.2
Near poor	26.3	1.7	21.7	1.5	4.6	1.5	26.1	1.3	18.5	1.2	7.7	0.7
Middle income	26.2	1.2	21.6	1.2	4.6	0.5	21.0	0.7	15.3	0.6	5.7	0.5
High income.	22.4	1.7	17.8	1.7	4.5	0.8	19.3	1.1	12.7	1.0	6.6	1.1
White, non-Hispanic												
Poor	23.2	2.6	15.6	2.5	7.5	1.7	30.2	3.1	21.7	2.6	8.5	2.2
Near poor	25.3	2.3	20.5	2.1	4.9	0.8	23.9	1.7	16.3	1.6	7.6	0.9
Middle/high income. . . .	24.5	1.1	19.9	1.1	4.6	0.5	20.2	0.7	14.5	0.5	4.6	0.5
Black, non-Hispanic												
Poor	34.4	1.6	30.8	1.6	3.7	0.7	39.9	1.6	29.3	2.5	10.6	1.8
Near poor	33.3	1.6	27.0	1.8	6.2	1.0	35.9	2.2	26.5	2.1	9.5	1.0
Middle/high income. . . .	34.0	1.7	26.2	1.4	7.8	0.9	30.0	1.5	20.8	1.4	9.2	1.3
Mexican												
Poor	19.5	1.6	16.8	1.4	2.7	0.6	24.5	1.4	19.2	1.3	5.3	0.8
Near poor	24.9	2.1	21.1	1.9	2.8	0.9	22.4	1.4	20.3	1.1	2.2	0.5
Middle/high income. . . .	26.8	1.1	22.9	1.1	3.9	0.8	25.2	2.1	20.7	2.3	4.5	1.2

SE Standard error.

Figure 42. Elevated blood lead among men 18 years of age and over

Family income	All races		White, non-Hispanic		Black, non-Hispanic		Mexican	
	Percent	SE	Percent	SE	Percent	SE	Percent	SE
Poor	13.6	1.6	12.2	2.7	19.2	2.2	9.7	1.5
Near poor	7.5	0.7	6.2	1.1	16.1	1.9	7.4	1.1
Middle income	4.9	0.7 }	3.7	0.7	8.9	1.2	3.3	0.7
High income.	2.3	0.7						

SE Standard error.

Figure 43. *Health insurance coverage among adults 18–64 years of age*

Race, Hispanic origin, and family income	Men						Women					
	Uninsured		Medicaid		Private		Uninsured		Medicaid		Private	
	Percent	SE	Percent	SE	Percent	SE	Percent	SE	Percent	SE	Percent	SE
All races												
Poor	44.1	1.0	23.0	0.8	26.9	1.0	33.3	0.7	42.6	0.8	21.6	0.8
Near Poor	35.3	0.6	5.8	0.3	52.9	0.6	28.6	0.5	11.2	0.4	56.4	0.6
Middle income	13.8	0.3	0.9	0.1	83.1	0.3	10.2	0.2	1.6	0.1	86.2	0.3
High income.	6.1	0.2	0.3	0.1	92.7	0.2	4.4	0.2	0.6	0.1	93.9	0.2
White, non-Hispanic												
Poor	37.9	1.4	22.3	1.0	32.7	1.6	31.9	1.0	37.1	1.1	28.2	1.3
Near poor	32.7	0.7	5.3	0.4	55.5	0.8	27.5	0.6	9.2	0.4	59.6	0.7
Middle income	12.8	0.3	0.8	0.1	84.3	0.3	9.4	0.3	1.3	0.1	87.4	0.3
High income.	5.7	0.2	0.3	0.1	93.2	0.3	3.8	0.2	0.5	0.1	94.7	0.2
Black, non-Hispanic												
Poor	44.4	2.0	26.5	1.7	22.4	1.9	25.9	1.2	55.4	1.4	16.4	1.0
Near poor	33.5	1.6	8.6	1.1	50.6	1.8	22.8	1.2	18.8	1.1	54.2	1.4
Middle income	14.5	0.9	1.7	0.3	80.1	1.1	8.6	0.7	2.4	0.4	86.4	0.9
High income.	7.8	1.0	1.1	0.4	90.0	1.1	6.3	0.9	1.4	0.4	91.4	1.0
Hispanic												
Poor	58.7	1.6	22.0	1.6	16.6	1.1	44.9	1.5	41.9	1.7	12.0	0.9
Near poor	47.1	1.4	5.6	0.7	44.6	1.4	41.5	1.3	12.3	0.9	43.4	1.3
Middle income	20.7	1.2	1.1	0.3	76.5	1.2	17.5	1.1	3.3	0.5	77.1	1.2
High income.	9.6	1.0	–	. . .	89.6	1.1	7.8	0.9	1.3	0.4	89.7	1.0

– Quantity zero.
. . . Not applicable
SE Standard error.

Figure 44. *No physician contact within the past year among adults 18–64 years of age with a health problem*

Race, Hispanic origin, and family income	Men		Women	
	Percent	SE	Percent	SE
All races				
Poor	21.2	0.8	11.7	0.5
Near poor	19.1	0.7	10.3	0.5
Middle income	14.9	0.6	5.7	0.3
High income.	11.4	0.7	4.0	0.3
White, non-Hispanic				
Poor	20.3	1.1	11.5	0.8
Near poor	18.7	0.8	9.9	0.5
Middle/high income.	13.4	0.5	4.8	0.2
Black, non-Hispanic				
Poor	20.8	1.6	10.5	0.8
Near poor	18.0	2.0	9.2	1.2
Middle/high income.	13.0	1.5	5.3	0.7
Hispanic				
Poor	24.4	1.8	14.3	1.2
Near poor	22.6	1.8	12.9	1.3
Middle/high income.	17.2	1.9	7.1	1.0

SE Standard error.

Figure 45. Mammography within the past 2 years among women 50 years of age and over

Family income	All races		White, non-Hispanic		Black, non-Hispanic		Hispanic	
	Percent	SE	Percent	SE	Percent	SE	Percent	SE
Poor	44.7	2.2	37.5	2.5	60.0	3.7	49.3	6.8
Near poor	48.2	1.5	47.9	1.8	57.4	3.7	38.2	5.1
Middle income	67.2	1.0 }	70.4	0.9	72.2	3.4	64.7	4.8
High income.	76.3	1.8						

SE Standard error.

Figure 46. Unmet need for health care during the past year among adults 18–64 years of age

Family income	18–64 years		18–44 years				45–64 years			
	Percent	SE	Percent	SE	Percent	SE	Percent	SE	Percent	SE
Poor	33.2	0.6	26.7	0.9	31.3	0.7	37.5	1.6	41.4	1.3
Near poor	28.8	0.	25.7	0.6	30.5	0.6	27.1	1.0	31.7	0.9
Middle income	16.4	0.3	16.7	0.4	19.3	0.4	12.2	0.4	15.4	0.5
High income.	6.9	0.2	7.0	0.3	7.9	0.3	5.6	0.3	6.4	0.3

SE Standard error.

Figure 47. Unmet need for health care during the past year among adults 65 years of age and over

Family income	All races		White, non-Hispanic		Black, non-Hispanic		Hispanic	
	Percent	SE	Percent	SE	Percent	SE	Percent	SE
Poor	21.9	0.9	22.6	1.2	24.5	1.8	17.9	2.2
Near poor	11.7	0.5	11.6	0.6	12.7	1.5	13.0	2.1
Middle income	5.1	0.3 }	4.2	0.2	7.9	1.5	7.5	1.5
High income.	2.2	0.4						

SE Standard error.

Figure 48. Avoidable hospitalizations among adults 18–64 years of age

Median income in ZIP code of residence	All races		White[1]		Black[1]	
	Rate	SE	Rate	SE	Rate	SE
Less than $20,000	11.3	1.0	7.1	0.8	19.1	2.4
$20,000–29,999	8.1	0.4	6.2	0.4	13.4	1.0
$30,000–39,999	5.9	0.3	4.9	0.4	9.2	0.8
$40,000 or more.	4.7	0.3	4.2	0.2	8.6	0.9

SE Standard error.
[1]Includes persons of Hispanic origin.

Figure 49. Dental visit within the past year among adults 18–64 years of age

Family income	All races		White, non-Hispanic		Black, non-Hispanic		Hispanic	
	Percent	SE	Percent	SE	Percent	SE	Percent	SE
Poor	41.3	1.4	45.2	2.0	38.0	2.4	35.7	3.3
Near poor	46.9	1.1	47.7	1.3	47.0	3.1	41.9	3.2
Middle income	64.9	0.8 }	72.0	0.7	61.7	2.3	58.9	2.4
High income.	77.3	1.1						

SE Standard error.

Detailed Tables

Health Status and Determinants

Population

1. **Resident population,** according to age, sex, detailed race, and Hispanic origin: United States, selected years 1950–96_____ 169

2. Persons and families below **poverty** level, according to selected characteristics, race, and Hispanic origin: United States, selected years 1973–96_____ 171

Fertility and Natality

3. Crude birth rates, **fertility rates, and birth rates** by age of mother, according to detailed race and Hispanic origin: United States, selected years 1950–96_____ 172

4. **Women 15–44 years of age who have not had at least one live birth,** by age: United States, selected years 1960–96_____ 174

5. **Live births,** according to detailed race of mother and Hispanic origin of mother: United States, selected years 1970–96_____ 175

6. **Prenatal care** for live births, according to detailed race of mother and Hispanic origin of mother: United States, selected years 1970–96_____ 176

7. **Teenage childbearing,** according to detailed race of mother and Hispanic origin of mother: United States, selected years 1970–96_____ 177

8. **Nonmarital childbearing** according to detailed race of mother, Hispanic origin of mother, and maternal age and birth rates for unmarried women by race of mother and Hispanic origin of mother: United States, selected years 1970–96_____ 178

9. **Maternal education** for live births, according to detailed race of mother and Hispanic origin of mother: United States, selected years 1970–96_____ 179

10. **Mothers who smoked cigarettes** during pregnancy, according to mother's detailed race, Hispanic origin, age, and educational attainment: Selected States, 1989–96_____ 180

11. **Low-birthweight** live births, according to mother's detailed race, Hispanic origin, and smoking status: United States, selected years 1970–96_____ 181

12. **Low-birthweight** live births among mothers 20 years of age and over, by mother's detailed race, Hispanic origin, and educational attainment: Selected States, 1989–96_____ 182

13. **Low-birthweight** live births, according to race of mother, geographic division, and State: United States, average annual 1984–86, 1989–91, and 1994–96_____ 183

14. **Very low-birthweight** live births, according to race of mother, geographic division, and State: United States, average annual 1984–86, 1989–91, and 1994–96_____ 184

15. Legal **abortion ratios,** according to selected patient characteristics: United States, selected years 1973–95_____ 185

16. Legal **abortions,** according to selected characteristics: United States, selected years 1973–95_____ 186

17. Legal abortions, **abortion-related deaths,** and abortion-related death rates, according to period of gestation: United States, 1974–76 through 1989–91_____ 187

18. Methods of **contraception** for women 15–44 years of age, according to race and age: United States, 1982, 1988, and 1995_____ 188

19. **Breastfeeding** by mothers 15–44 years of age by year of baby's birth, according to selected characteristics of mother: United States, 1972–74 to 1993–94_____ 189

Mortality

20. **Infant, neonatal, and postneonatal mortality rates,** according to detailed race of mother and Hispanic origin of mother: United States, selected birth cohorts 1983–95_____ 190

21. **Infant mortality rates** for mothers 20 years of age and over, according to educational attainment, detailed race of mother, and Hispanic origin of mother: United States, selected birth cohorts 1983–95_____ 191

22. **Infant mortality rates** according to birthweight: United States, selected birth cohorts 1983–95_____ 192

23. **Infant mortality rates,** fetal mortality rates, and perinatal mortality rates, according to race: United States, selected years 1950–96_____ 193

24. **Infant mortality rates,** according to race, geographic division, and State: United States, average annual 1984–86, 1989–91, and 1994–96_____ 194

25. **Neonatal mortality rates,** according to race, geographic division, and State: United States, average annual 1984–86, 1989–91, and 1994–96_____ 195

26. **Postneonatal mortality rates,** according to race, geographic division, and State: United States, average annual 1984–86, 1989–91, and 1994–96_____ 196

27. **Infant mortality rates,** feto-infant mortality rates, and postneonatal mortality rates, and average annual percent change: Selected countries, 1989 and 1994_____ 197

List of Detailed Tables ....

28. **Life expectancy** at birth and at 65 years of age, according to sex: Selected countries, 1989 and 1994_____ 198

29. **Life expectancy** at birth, at 65 years of age, and at 75 years of age, according to race and sex: United States, selected years 1900–96_____ 200

30. **Age-adjusted death rates,** according to detailed race, Hispanic origin, geographic division, and State: United States, average annual 1984–86, 1989–91, and 1994–96_____ 201

31. **Age-adjusted death rates** for selected causes of death, according to sex, detailed race, and Hispanic origin: United States, selected years 1950–96_____ 203

32. **Years of potential life lost** before age 75 for selected causes of death, according to sex, detailed race, and Hispanic origin: United States, selected years 1980–96_____ 207

33. **Leading causes of death** and numbers of deaths, according to sex, detailed race, and Hispanic origin: United States, 1980 and 1996_____ 212

34. **Leading causes of death** and numbers of deaths, according to age: United States, 1980 and 1996_____ 216

35. Age-adjusted death rates, according to race, sex, region, and **urbanization:** United States, average annual 1984–86, 1989–91, and 1993–95_____ 218

36. Death rates for persons 25–64 years of age, for all races and the white population, according to sex, age, and **educational attainment:** Selected States, 1994–96_____ 220

37. **Death rates** for all causes, according to sex, detailed race, Hispanic origin, and age: United States, selected years 1950–96_____ 221

38. Death rates for **diseases of heart,** according to sex, detailed race, Hispanic origin, and age: United States, selected years 1950–96_____ 225

39. Death rates for **cerebrovascular diseases,** according to sex, detailed race, Hispanic origin, and age: United States, selected years 1950–96_____ 228

40. Death rates for **malignant neoplasms,** according to sex, detailed race, Hispanic origin, and age: United States, selected years 1950–96_____ 231

41. Death rates for **malignant neoplasms of respiratory system,** according to sex, detailed race, Hispanic origin, and age: United States, selected years 1950–96_____ 235

42. Death rates for **malignant neoplasm of breast** for females, according to detailed race, Hispanic origin, and age: United States, selected years 1950–96_____ 238

43. Death rates for **chronic obstructive pulmonary diseases,** according to sex, detailed race, Hispanic origin, and age: United States, selected years 1980–96_____ 240

44. Death rates for **human immunodeficiency virus (HIV) infection,** according to sex, detailed race, Hispanic origin, and age: United States, 1987–96_____ 243

45. **Maternal mortality** for complications of pregnancy, childbirth, and the puerperium, according to race, Hispanic origin, and age: United States, selected years 1950–96_____ 245

46. Death rates for **motor vehicle-related injuries,** according to sex, detailed race, Hispanic origin, and age: United States, selected years 1950–96_____ 246

47. Death rates for **homicide** and legal intervention, according to sex, detailed race, Hispanic origin, and age: United States, selected years 1950–96_____ 250

48. Death rates for **suicide,** according to sex, detailed race, Hispanic origin, and age: United States, selected years 1950–96_____ 253

49. Death rates for **firearm-related injuries,** according to sex, detailed race, Hispanic origin, and age: United States, selected years 1970–96_____ 256

50. Deaths from selected **occupational diseases** for males, according to age: United States, selected years 1970–96_____ 259

51. **Occupational injury deaths,** according to industry: United States, selected years 1980–93_____ 260

Determinants and Measures of Health

52. **Vaccinations** of children 19–35 months of age for selected diseases, according to race, Hispanic origin, poverty status, and residence in metropolitan statistical area (MSA): United States, 1994–96_____ 261

53. **Vaccination coverage** among children 19–35 months of age according to geographic division, State, and selected urban areas: United States, 1994–96_____ 262

54. Selected **notifiable disease rates,** according to disease: United States, selected years 1950–96_____ 264

55. Acquired immunodeficiency syndrome **(AIDS)** cases, according to age at diagnosis, sex, detailed race, and Hispanic origin: United States, selected years 1985–97_____ 265

56. Acquired immunodeficiency syndrome (**AIDS**) cases, according to race, Hispanic origin, sex, and transmission category for persons 13 years of age and over at diagnosis: United States, selected years 1985–97_____ **266**

57. Acquired immunodeficiency syndrome (**AIDS**) cases, according to geographic division and State: United States, selected years 1985–97_____ **268**

58. Age-adjusted **cancer incidence rates** for selected cancer sites, according to sex and race: Selected geographic areas, selected years 1973–95__ **269**

59. Five-year relative **cancer survival rates** for selected cancer sites, according to race and sex: Selected geographic areas, 1974–79, 1980–82, 1983–85, 1986–88, and 1989–94_____ **270**

60. **Limitation of activity** caused by chronic conditions, according to selected characteristics: United States, 1990 and 1995_____ **271**

61. **Respondent-assessed health status,** according to selected characteristics: United States, 1987–95__ **272**

62. Current **cigarette smoking** by persons 18 years of age and over, according to sex, race, and age: United States, selected years 1965–95_____ **273**

63. Age-adjusted prevalence of current **cigarette smoking** by persons 25 years of age and over, according to sex, race, and education: United States, selected years 1974–95_____ **274**

64. **Use of selected substances** in the past month by persons 12 years of age and over, according to age, sex, race, and Hispanic origin: United States, selected years 1979–96_____ **275**

65. **Use of selected substances** in the past month and heavy alcohol use in the past 2 weeks by high school seniors and eighth-graders, according to sex and race: United States, selected years 1980–97____ **277**

66. **Cocaine-related emergency room episodes,** according to age, sex, race, and Hispanic origin: United States, selected years 1985–95_____ **279**

67. **Alcohol consumption** by persons 18 years of age and over, according to sex, race, Hispanic origin, and age: United States, 1985 and 1990_____ **280**

68. **Hypertension** among persons 20 years of age and over, according to sex, age, race, and Hispanic origin: United States, 1960–62, 1971–74, 1976–80, and 1988–94_____ **281**

69. **Serum cholesterol levels** among persons 20 years of age and over, according to sex, age, race,

and Hispanic origin: United States, 1960–62, 1971–74, 1976–80, and 1988–94_____ **282**

70. **Overweight persons** 20 years of age and over, according to sex, age, race, and Hispanic origin: United States, 1960–62, 1971–74, 1976–80, and 1988–94_____ **283**

71. **Overweight children** and adolescents 6–17 years of age, according to sex, age, race, and Hispanic origin: United States, selected years 1963–65 through 1988–94_____ **284**

72. Persons residing in counties that met **national ambient air quality standards** throughout the year, by race and Hispanic origin: United States, selected years 1988–96_____ **285**

73. **Occupational injuries** with lost workdays in the private sector, according to industry: United States, selected years 1980–96_____ **286**

Utilization of Health Resources

Ambulatory Care

74. **Physician contacts,** according to selected patient characteristics: United States, 1987–95_____ **287**

75. **Physician contacts,** according to place of contact and selected patient characteristics: United States, 1990 and 1995_____ **288**

76. **Physician contacts,** according to respondent-assessed health status, age, sex, and poverty status: United States, 1987–89 and 1993–95_____ **289**

77. **Interval since last physician contact,** according to selected patient characteristics: United States, 1964, 1990, and 1995_____ **290**

78. **No physician contact** within the past 12 months among children under 6 years of age according to selected characteristics: United States, average annual 1993–94 and 1994–95_____ **291**

79. **No usual source of health care** among children under 18 years of age according to selected characteristics: United States, average annual 1993–94 and 1994–95_____ **292**

80. Use of **mammography** for women 40 years of age and over according to selected characteristics: United States, selected years 1987–94_____ **293**

81. **Ambulatory care visits** to physician offices and hospital outpatient and emergency departments by selected patient characteristics: United States, 1993–96_____ **295**

List of Detailed Tables

82. **Ambulatory care visits** to physician offices, percent distribution according to selected patient characteristics and physician specialty: United States, 1975, 1985, and 1996___ 297

83. Persons with a **dental visit** within the past year among persons 25 years of age and over, according to selected patient characteristics: United States, selected years 1983–93___ 298

84. **Substance abuse clients** in specialty treatment units according to substance abused, geographic division, and State: United States, 1992 and 1995___ 299

85. **Additions to mental health organizations** according to type of service and organization: United States, selected years 1983–94___ 300

86. **Home health care and hospice patients,** according to selected characteristics: United States, 1992–96___ 301

Inpatient Care

87. **Discharges,** days of care, and average length of stay in short-stay hospitals, according to selected characteristics: United States, 1964, 1990, and 1995___ 302

88. **Discharges,** days of care, and average length of stay in non-Federal short-stay hospitals, according to selected characteristics: United States, selected years 1980–95___ 303

89. **Discharges,** days of care, and average length of stay in non-Federal short-stay hospitals for discharges with the diagnosis of human immunodeficiency virus (HIV) and for all discharges: United States, 1986–95___ 304

90. **Rates of discharges** and days of care in non-Federal short-stay hospitals, according to sex, age, and selected first-listed diagnosis: United States, 1985, 1990, 1994, and 1995___ 305

91. **Discharges** and average length of stay in non-Federal short-stay hospitals, according to sex, age, and selected first-listed diagnosis: United States, 1985, 1990, 1994, and 1995___ 308

92. **Operations** for inpatients discharged from non-Federal short-stay hospitals, according to sex, age, and surgical category: United States, 1985, 1990, 1994, and 1995___ 311

93. Diagnostic and other **nonsurgical procedures** for inpatients discharged from non-Federal short-stay hospitals, according to sex, age, and procedure category: United States, 1985, 1990, 1994, and 1995___ 314

94. Hospital admissions, average length of stay, and outpatient visits, according to type of ownership and size of hospital, and percent **outpatient surgery:** United States, selected years 1975–96___ 316

95. **Nursing home** and personal care home residents 65 years of age and over according to age, sex, and race: United States, 1963, 1973–74, 1985, and 1995___ 317

96. **Nursing home residents** 65 years of age and over, according to selected functional status and age, sex, and race: United States, 1985 and 1995___ 318

97. **Additions** to selected inpatient **psychiatric organizations** according to sex, age, and race: United States, 1975, 1980, and 1986___ 319

98. **Additions** to selected inpatient **psychiatric organizations,** according to selected primary diagnoses and age: United States, 1975, 1980, and 1986___ 320

Health Care Resources

Personnel

99. **Persons employed** in health service sites: United States, selected years 1970–96___ 321

100. Active non-Federal **physicians** and doctors of medicine in patient care, according to geographic division and State: United States, 1975, 1985, 1990, and 1996___ 322

101. **Physicians,** according to activity and place of medical education: United States and outlying U.S. areas, selected years 1975–96___ 324

102. **Primary care doctors of medicine,** according to specialty: United States and outlying U.S. areas, selected years 1949–96___ 325

103. Active **health personnel** according to occupation and geographic region: United States, 1980, 1990, and 1995___ 326

104. Full-time equivalent **employment in** selected occupations for **community hospitals:** United States, selected years 1983–93___ 327

105. Full-time equivalent patient care **staff in mental health organizations,** according to type of organization and staff discipline: United States, selected years 1984–94___ 328

106. First-year enrollment and **graduates of health professions schools** and number of schools, according to profession: United States, selected years 1950–96 and projections for year 2000___ 330

107. Total **enrollment of minorities** in schools for selected health occupations, according to detailed race and Hispanic origin: United States, academic years 1970–71, 1980–81, 1990–91, and 1995–96___ 331

108. First-year and total **enrollment of women** in schools for selected health occupations, according to detailed race and Hispanic origin: United States, academic years 1971–72, 1980–81, 1990–91, and 1995–96___ 333

Facilities

109. **Hospitals,** beds, and occupancy rates, according to type of ownership and size of hospital: United States, selected years 1975–96___ 334

110. Inpatient and residential **mental health organizations** and beds, according to type of organization: United States, selected years 1984–94_ 335

111. **Community hospital beds** and average annual percent change, according to geographic division and State: United States, selected years 1940–96___ 336

112. **Occupancy rates** in community hospitals and average annual percent change, according to geographic division and State: United States, selected years 1940–96___ 337

113. **Nursing homes** with 3 or more beds, beds, and bed rates, according to geographic division and State: United States, 1976, 1986, and 1991___ 338

114. **Nursing homes,** beds, occupancy, and residents, according to geographic division and State: United States, 1992 and 1996___ 339

Health Care Expenditures

National Health Expenditures

115. Gross domestic product, **national health expenditures,** and Federal and State and local government expenditures and average annual percent change: United States, selected years 1960–96___ 341

116. **Total health expenditures** as a percent of gross domestic product and per capita health expenditures in dollars: Selected countries and years 1960–95___ 342

117. **Consumer Price Index** and average annual percent change for all items and selected items: United States, selected years 1960–97___ 343

118. **Consumer Price Index** and average annual percent change for all items and medical care components: United States, selected years 1960–97___ 344

119. **National health expenditures** and average annual percent change, according to source of funds: United States, selected years 1929–96___ 345

120. **National health expenditures,** percent distribution, and average annual percent change, according to type of expenditure: United States, selected years 1960–96___ 346

121. **Expenditures for health services** and supplies and percent distribution, by type of payer: United States, selected calendar years 1965–95___ 348

122. **Employers' costs** per employee hour worked for total compensation, wages and salaries, and **health insurance,** according to selected characteristics: United States, selected years 1991–97___ 350

123. **Personal health care expenditures** average annual percent increase and percent distribution of factors affecting growth: United States, 1960–96___ 351

124. **Personal health care expenditures** and percent distribution, according to source of funds: United States, selected years 1929–96___ 352

125. **Expenditures on hospital care,** nursing home care, physician services, and all other personal health care expenditures and percent distribution, according to source of funds: United States, selected years 1960–96___ 353

126. **Hospital expenses,** according to type of ownership and size of hospital: United States, selected years 1975–96___ 354

127. **Nursing home average monthly charges** per resident and percent of residents, according to selected facility and resident characteristics: United States, 1964, 1973–74, 1977, and 1985___ 355

128. **Nursing home average monthly charges** per resident and percent of residents, according to primary source of payments and selected facility characteristics: United States, 1977 and 1985___ 356

129. **Mental health expenditures,** percent distribution, and per capita expenditures, according to type of mental health organization: United States, selected years 1975–94___ 357

130. National **funding for health research** and development and average annual percent change, according to source of funds: United States, selected years 1960–95___ 358

List of Detailed Tables ....

131. Federal **funding for health research** and development and percent distribution, according to agency: United States, selected fiscal years 1970–95_____ **359**

132. Federal **spending for human immunodeficiency virus (HIV)-related activities,** according to agency and type of activity: United States, selected fiscal years 1985–97_____ **360**

Health Care Coverage and Major Federal Programs

133. **Health care coverage** for persons under 65 years of age, according to type of coverage and selected characteristics: United States, selected years 1984–96_____ **361**

134. **Health care coverage** for persons 65 years of age and over, according to type of coverage and selected characteristics: United States, selected years 1984–96_____ **363**

135. **Health maintenance organizations** (HMO's) and enrollment, according to model type, geographic region, and Federal program: United States, selected years 1976–97_____ **365**

136. **Medical care benefits** for employees of private establishments by size of establishment and occupation: United States, selected years 1990–95_ **366**

137. **Medicare** enrollees and expenditures and percent distribution, according to type of service: United States and other areas, selected years 1967–96_____ **367**

138. **Medicare** enrollment, persons served, and payments for Medicare enrollees 65 years of age and over, according to selected characteristics: United States and other areas, selected years 1977–95_____ **368**

139. **Medicaid** recipients and medical vendor payments, according to basis of eligibility: United States, selected fiscal years 1972–96_____ **369**

140. **Medicaid** recipients and medical vendor payments, according to type of service: United States, selected fiscal years 1972–96_____ **370**

141. **Department of Veterans Affairs** health care expenditures and use, and persons treated according to selected characteristics: United States, selected fiscal years 1970–96_____ **371**

State Health Expenditures

142. **Hospital care expenditures** by geographic division and State and average annual percent change: United States, selected years 1980–93_____ **372**

143. **Physician service expenditures** by geographic division and State and average annual percent change: United States, selected years 1980–93_____ **373**

144. **Expenditures for purchases of prescription drugs** by geographic division and State and average annual percent change: United States, selected years 1980–93_____ **374**

145. State mental health agency per capita **expenditures for mental health services** and average annual percent change by geographic division and State: United States, selected fiscal years 1981–93_____ **375**

146. **Medicare** enrollees, enrollees in managed care, payments per enrollee, and short-stay hospital utilization by geographic division and State: United States, 1990 and 1995_____ **376**

147. **Medicaid** recipients, recipients in managed care, payments per recipient, and recipients per 100 persons below the poverty level by geographic division and State: United States, selected fiscal years 1980–96_____ **377**

148. Persons enrolled in **health maintenance organizations** (HMO's) by geographic division and State: United States, selected years 1980–97_____ **378**

149. **Persons without health care coverage** by geographic division and State: United States, selected years 1987–96_____ **379**

Table 1 (page 1 of 2). Resident population, according to age, sex, detailed race, and Hispanic origin: United States, selected years 1950–96

[Data are based on decennial census updated by data from multiple sources]

Sex, race, Hispanic origin, and year	Total resident population	Under 1 year	1–4 years	5–14 years	15–24 years	25–34 years	35–44 years	45–54 years	55–64 years	65–74 years	75–84 years	85 years and over
All persons						Number in thousands						
1950	150,697	3,147	13,017	24,319	22,098	23,759	21,450	17,343	13,370	8,340	3,278	577
1960	179,323	4,112	16,209	35,465	24,020	22,818	24,081	20,485	15,572	10,997	4,633	929
1970	203,212	3,485	13,669	40,746	35,441	24,907	23,088	23,220	18,590	12,435	6,119	1,511
1980	226,546	3,534	12,815	34,942	42,487	37,082	25,634	22,800	21,703	15,580	7,729	2,240
1990	248,710	3,946	14,812	35,095	37,013	43,161	37,435	25,057	21,113	18,045	10,012	3,021
1995	262,755	3,848	15,743	38,134	35,947	40,873	42,468	31,079	21,131	18,759	11,145	3,628
1996	265,284	3,769	15,516	38,422	36,221	40,368	43,393	32,370	21,361	18,669	11,430	3,762
Male												
1950	74,833	1,602	6,634	12,375	10,918	11,597	10,588	8,655	6,697	4,024	1,507	237
1960	88,331	2,090	8,240	18,029	11,906	11,179	11,755	10,093	7,537	5,116	2,025	362
1970	98,912	1,778	6,968	20,759	17,551	12,217	11,231	11,199	8,793	5,437	2,436	542
1980	110,053	1,806	6,556	17,855	21,418	18,382	12,570	11,009	10,152	6,757	2,867	682
1990	121,239	2,018	7,581	17,971	18,915	21,564	18,510	12,232	9,955	7,907	3,745	841
1995	128,314	1,970	8,055	19,529	18,352	20,432	21,062	15,182	10,044	8,342	4,330	1,017
1996	129,810	1,928	7,940	19,681	18,618	20,191	21,569	15,837	10,166	8,325	4,486	1,070
Female												
1950	75,864	1,545	6,383	11,944	11,181	12,162	10,863	8,688	6,672	4,316	1,771	340
1960	90,992	2,022	7,969	17,437	12,114	11,639	12,326	10,393	8,036	5,881	2,609	567
1970	104,300	1,707	6,701	19,986	17,890	12,690	11,857	12,021	9,797	6,998	3,683	969
1980	116,493	1,727	6,259	17,087	21,068	18,700	13,065	11,791	11,551	8,825	4,862	1,559
1990	127,471	1,928	7,231	17,124	18,098	21,596	18,925	12,824	11,158	10,139	6,267	2,180
1995	134,441	1,878	7,688	18,606	17,595	20,441	21,406	15,897	11,087	10,417	6,815	2,611
1996	135,474	1,841	7,577	18,741	17,604	20,177	21,825	16,533	11,195	10,345	6,944	2,692
White male												
1950	67,129	1,400	5,845	10,860	9,689	10,430	9,529	7,836	6,180	3,736	1,406	218
1960	78,367	1,784	7,065	15,659	10,483	9,940	10,564	9,114	6,850	4,702	1,875	331
1970	86,721	1,501	5,873	17,667	15,232	10,775	9,979	10,090	7,958	4,916	2,243	487
1980	94,924	1,485	5,397	14,764	18,110	15,928	11,005	9,771	9,149	6,095	2,600	621
1990	102,143	1,604	6,071	14,467	15,389	18,071	15,819	10,624	8,813	7,127	3,397	760
1995	106,994	1,547	6,377	15,539	14,714	16,858	17,743	13,125	8,778	7,455	3,940	919
1996	108,052	1,546	6,294	15,622	14,910	16,587	18,128	13,649	8,864	7,419	4,076	959
White female												
1950	67,813	1,341	5,599	10,431	9,821	10,851	9,719	7,868	6,168	4,031	1,669	314
1960	80,465	1,714	6,795	15,068	10,596	10,204	11,000	9,364	7,327	5,428	2,441	527
1970	91,028	1,434	5,615	16,912	15,420	11,004	10,349	10,756	8,853	6,366	3,429	890
1980	99,788	1,410	5,121	14,048	17,643	15,887	11,227	10,282	10,324	7,950	4,457	1,440
1990	106,561	1,524	5,762	13,706	14,599	17,757	15,834	10,946	9,698	9,048	5,687	2,001
1995	111,092	1,467	6,060	14,737	13,965	16,529	17,645	13,459	9,487	9,189	6,168	2,385
1996	111,696	1,469	5,980	14,816	13,937	16,230	17,953	13,946	9,551	9,093	6,273	2,447
Black male												
1950	7,300	- - -	- - -	1,442	1,162	1,105	1,003	772	460	299	- - -	- - -
1960	9,114	281	1,082	2,185	1,305	1,120	1,086	891	617	382	137	29
1970	10,748	245	975	2,784	2,041	1,226	1,084	979	739	461	169	46
1980	12,612	270	970	2,618	2,813	1,974	1,238	1,026	855	568	228	53
1990	14,420	322	1,164	2,700	2,669	2,592	1,962	1,175	878	614	277	66
1995	15,721	314	1,256	2,994	2,730	2,565	2,416	1,466	925	674	302	79
1996	15,903	277	1,218	3,044	2,756	2,565	2,485	1,545	937	682	311	83
Black female												
1950	7,745	- - -	- - -	1,446	1,300	1,260	1,112	796	443	322	- - -	- - -
1960	9,758	283	1,085	2,191	1,404	1,300	1,229	974	663	430	160	38
1970	11,832	243	970	2,773	2,196	1,456	1,309	1,134	868	582	230	71
1980	14,071	267	953	2,583	2,942	2,272	1,490	1,260	1,061	777	360	106
1990	16,063	316	1,137	2,641	2,700	2,905	2,279	1,416	1,135	884	495	156
1995	17,420	307	1,223	2,908	2,730	2,855	2,762	1,770	1,201	943	526	195
1996	17,600	270	1,185	2,953	2,741	2,847	2,830	1,864	1,221	951	535	203

See notes at end of table.

Table 1 (page 2 of 2). Resident population, according to age, sex, detailed race, and Hispanic origin: United States, selected years 1950–96

[Data are based on decennial census updated by data from multiple sources]

Sex, race, Hispanic origin, and year	Total resident population	Under 1 year	1–4 years	5–14 years	15–24 years	25–34 years	35–44 years	45–54 years	55–64 years	65–74 years	75–84 years	85 years and over
American Indian or Alaska Native male						Number in thousands						
1980	702	17	60	153	164	114	75	53	37	22	9	2
1990	1,024	24	88	206	192	183	140	86	55	32	13	3
1995	1,110	21	84	234	196	186	163	106	61	38	17	5
1996	1,136	20	82	236	203	192	168	110	63	39	18	5
American Indian or Alaska Native female												
1980	718	16	57	149	158	118	79	57	41	26	12	4
1990	1,041	24	85	200	178	186	148	92	61	41	21	6
1995	1,132	21	82	227	190	180	170	113	69	46	25	10
1996	1,152	20	80	228	195	182	174	118	71	47	26	11
Asian or Pacific Islander male												
1980	1,814	35	129	321	334	367	252	159	110	72	29	6
1990	3,652	68	258	598	665	718	588	347	208	133	57	12
1995	4,489	87	340	761	713	823	740	485	280	176	72	14
1996	4,719	86	346	779	749	849	788	532	302	185	82	22
Asian or Pacific Islander female												
1980	1,915	34	127	307	325	423	269	193	126	70	33	9
1990	3,805	65	247	578	621	749	664	371	264	166	65	17
1995	4,797	83	323	734	710	877	828	556	330	238	96	22
1996	5,024	83	332	743	731	918	867	605	352	254	110	31
Hispanic male												
1980	7,280	187	661	1,530	1,646	1,255	761	570	364	201	86	19
1990	11,388	279	980	2,128	2,376	2,310	1,471	818	551	312	131	32
1995	13,676	338	1,306	2,600	2,397	2,674	1,978	1,105	652	419	164	43
1996	14,519	343	1,334	2,658	2,677	2,779	2,164	1,212	683	439	179	51
Hispanic female												
1980	7,329	181	634	1,482	1,547	1,249	805	615	411	257	116	30
1990	10,966	268	939	2,039	2,028	2,073	1,448	868	632	403	209	59
1995	13,318	321	1,246	2,488	2,214	2,359	1,903	1,167	744	528	260	87
1996	13,750	326	1,269	2,534	2,298	2,373	2,016	1,242	769	549	275	99
Non-Hispanic White male												
1980	88,035	1,308	4,773	13,318	16,555	14,739	10,285	9,229	8,802	5,906	2,519	603
1990	91,743	1,351	5,181	12,525	13,219	15,967	14,481	9,875	8,303	6,837	3,275	729
1995	94,540	1,239	5,184	13,186	12,529	14,426	15,949	12,117	8,179	7,067	3,786	878
1996	94,799	1,232	5,075	13,216	12,455	14,049	16,160	12,542	8,237	7,012	3,909	911
Non-Hispanic White female												
1980	92,872	1,240	4,522	12,647	16,185	14,711	10,468	9,700	9,935	7,708	4,345	1,411
1990	96,557	1,280	4,909	11,846	12,749	15,872	14,520	10,153	9,116	8,674	5,491	1,945
1995	98,983	1,174	4,921	12,485	11,955	14,393	15,921	12,397	8,806	8,703	5,926	2,302
1996	99,179	1,171	4,821	12,521	11,843	14,075	16,125	12,817	8,848	8,587	6,017	2,353

- - - Data not available.

NOTES: The race groups, white, black, American Indian or Alaska Native, and Asian or Pacific Islander, include persons of Hispanic and non-Hispanic origin. Conversely, persons of Hispanic origin may be of any race. Population figures are census counts as of April 1 for 1950, 1960, 1970, 1980, and 1990 and estimates as of July 1 for other years. See Appendix I, Department of Commerce. Populations for age groups may not sum to the total due to rounding. Although population figures are shown rounded to the nearest 1,000, calculations of birth rates and death rates shown in this volume are based on unrounded population figures for decennial years and starting with data year 1992. See Appendix II, Rate. Some numbers have been revised and differ from the previous edition of *Health, United States*.

SOURCES: U.S. Bureau of the Census: 1950 Nonwhite Population by Race. Special Report P-E, No. 3B. Washington. U.S. Government Printing Office, 1951; U.S. Census of Population: 1960, Number of Inhabitants, PC(1)-A1, United States Summary, 1964; 1970, Number of Inhabitants, Final Report PC(1)-A1, United States Summary, 1971; U.S. population estimates, by age, sex, race, and Hispanic origin: 1980 to 1991. Current Population Reports. Series P-25, No. 1095. Washington. U.S. Government Printing Office, Feb. 1993; U.S. resident population—estimates by age, sex, race, and Hispanic origin (consistent with the 1990 Census, as enumerated): 1992. Census files RESP0792 in PPL-21, series 1294. 1993; July 1, 1993. RES0793. 1994; July 1, 1994. RESD0794. 1995; July 1, 1995. RESD0795. 1996; July 1, 1996. NESTV96 in PPL-S7. 1997.

Table 2. Persons and families below poverty level, according to selected characteristics, race, and Hispanic origin: United States, selected years 1973–96

[Data are based on household interviews of the civilian noninstitutionalized population]

Selected characteristics	1973	1980	1985	1989	1990	1991	1992	1993	1994	1995	1996
All persons					Percent below poverty						
All races	11.1	13.0	14.0	12.8	13.5	14.2	14.8	15.1	14.5	13.8	13.7
White	8.4	10.2	11.4	10.0	10.7	11.3	11.9	12.2	11.7	11.2	11.2
Black	31.4	32.5	31.3	30.7	31.9	32.7	33.4	33.1	30.6	29.3	28.4
Asian or Pacific Islander	- - -	- - -	- - -	14.1	12.2	13.8	12.7	15.3	14.6	14.6	14.5
Hispanic origin	21.9	25.7	29.0	26.2	28.1	28.7	29.6	30.6	30.7	30.3	29.4
Mexican	- - -	- - -	28.8	28.4	28.1	29.5	30.1	31.6	32.3	31.2	31.0
Puerto Rican	- - -	- - -	43.3	33.0	40.6	39.4	36.5	38.4	36.0	38.1	35.7
White, non-Hispanic	- - -	- - -	- - -	8.3	8.8	9.4	9.6	9.9	9.4	8.5	8.6
Related children under 18 years of age in families											
All races	14.2	17.9	20.1	19.0	19.9	21.1	21.6	22.0	21.2	20.2	19.8
White	9.7	13.4	15.6	14.1	15.1	16.1	16.5	17.0	16.3	15.5	15.5
Black	40.6	42.1	43.1	43.2	44.2	45.6	46.3	45.9	43.3	41.5	39.5
Asian or Pacific Islander	- - -	- - -	- - -	18.9	17.0	17.1	16.0	17.6	17.9	18.6	19.1
Hispanic origin	27.8	33.0	39.6	35.5	37.7	39.8	39.0	39.9	41.1	39.3	39.9
Mexican	- - -	- - -	37.4	36.3	35.5	38.9	38.2	39.5	41.8	39.3	40.7
Puerto Rican	- - -	- - -	58.6	48.0	56.7	57.7	52.2	53.8	50.5	53.2	49.4
White, non-Hispanic	- - -	- - -	- - -	10.9	11.6	12.4	12.4	12.8	11.8	10.6	10.4
Related children under 18 years of age in families with female householder and no spouse present											
All races	- - -	50.8	53.6	51.1	53.4	55.5	54.3	53.7	52.9	50.3	49.3
White	- - -	41.6	45.2	42.5	45.9	47.1	45.3	45.6	45.7	42.5	43.1
Black	- - -	64.8	66.9	63.1	64.7	68.2	67.1	65.9	63.2	61.6	58.2
Asian or Pacific Islander	- - -	- - -	- - -	63.7	32.2	31.9	43.5	32.2	36.8	42.4	48.8
Hispanic origin	- - -	65.0	72.4	64.3	68.4	68.6	65.7	66.1	68.3	65.7	67.4
Mexican	- - -	- - -	64.4	64.5	62.4	66.6	63.5	64.6	69.5	65.9	68.1
Puerto Rican	- - -	- - -	85.4	74.4	82.7	83.3	74.1	73.4	73.6	79.6	76.6
White, non-Hispanic	- - -	- - -	- - -	36.2	39.6	41.0	39.6	39.0	38.0	33.5	34.9
All persons					Number below poverty in thousands						
All races	22,973	29,272	33,064	31,528	33,585	35,708	38,014	39,265	38,059	36,425	36,529
White	15,142	19,699	22,860	20,785	22,326	23,747	25,259	26,226	25,379	24,423	24,650
Black	7,388	8,579	8,926	9,302	9,837	10,242	10,827	10,877	10,196	9,872	9,694
Asian or Pacific Islander	- - -	- - -	- - -	939	858	996	985	1,134	974	1,411	1,454
Hispanic origin	2,366	3,491	5,236	5,430	6,006	6,339	7,592	8,126	8,416	8,574	8,697
Mexican	- - -	- - -	3,220	3,777	3,764	4,149	4,404	5,373	5,781	5,608	5,815
Puerto Rican	- - -	- - -	1,011	720	966	924	874	1,061	981	1,183	1,116
White, non-Hispanic	- - -	- - -	- - -	15,599	16,622	17,741	18,202	18,882	18,110	16,267	16,462
Related children under 18 years of age in families											
All races	9,453	11,114	12,483	12,001	12,715	13,658	14,521	14,961	14,610	13,999	13,764
White	5,462	6,817	7,838	7,164	7,696	8,316	8,752	9,123	8,826	8,474	8,488
Black	3,822	3,906	4,057	4,257	4,412	4,637	5,015	5,030	4,787	4,644	4,411
Asian or Pacific Islander	- - -	- - -	- - -	368	356	348	352	358	308	532	553
Hispanic origin	1,364	1,718	2,512	2,496	2,750	2,977	3,440	3,666	3,956	3,938	4,090
Mexican	- - -	- - -	1,589	1,785	1,733	2,004	2,019	2,520	2,805	2,655	2,853
Puerto Rican	- - -	- - -	535	354	490	475	457	537	485	610	545
White, non-Hispanic	- - -	- - -	- - -	4,779	5,106	5,497	5,558	5,819	5,404	4,745	4,656
Related children under 18 years of age in families with female householder and no spouse present											
All races	- - -	5,866	6,716	6,808	7,363	8,065	8,032	8,503	8,427	8,364	7,990
White	- - -	2,813	3,372	3,255	3,597	3,941	3,783	4,102	4,099	4,051	4,029
Black	- - -	2,944	3,181	3,326	3,543	3,853	3,967	4,104	3,935	3,954	3,619
Asian or Pacific Islander	- - -	- - -	- - -	115	80	81	103	72	59	145	167
Hispanic origin	- - -	809	1,247	1,158	1,314	1,398	1,289	1,673	1,804	1,872	1,779
Mexican	- - -	- - -	553	677	615	785	679	890	1,054	1,056	948
Puerto Rican	- - -	- - -	449	281	382	369	363	430	394	459	444
White, non-Hispanic	- - -	- - -	- - -	2,160	2,411	2,661	2,588	2,636	2,563	2,299	2,419

- - - Data not available.

NOTES: The race groups, white and black, include persons of both Hispanic and non-Hispanic origin. Conversely, persons of Hispanic origin may be of any race. Poverty status is based on family income and family size using Bureau of the Census poverty thresholds. See Appendix II. In 1989, 31.2 percent of the American Indian population in the United States, or 585,000 persons, were below the poverty threshhold, based on 1989 income data from the 1990 decennial census (U.S. Bureau of the Census, 1990 Census of Population, *Characteristics of American Indians by Tribe and Language*, 1990 CP–3–7).

SOURCE: U.S. Bureau of the Census. Lamison-White L. Poverty in the United States: 1996. Current population reports, series P–60, no 198. Washington: U.S. Government Printing Office. 1997; unpublished data.

Table 3 (page 1 of 2). Crude birth rates, fertility rates, and birth rates by age of mother, according to detailed race and Hispanic origin: United States, selected years 1950–96

[Data are based on the National Vital Statistics System]

Race of mother, Hispanic origin of mother, and year	Crude birth rate[1]	Fertility rate[2]	10–14 years	15–19 years Total	15–17 years	18–19 years	20–24 years	25–29 years	30–34 years	35–39 years	40–44 years	45–49 years
All races						Live births per 1,000 women						
1950	24.1	106.2	1.0	81.6	40.7	132.7	196.6	166.1	103.7	52.9	15.1	1.2
1960	23.7	118.0	0.8	89.1	43.9	166.7	258.1	197.4	112.7	56.2	15.5	0.9
1970	18.4	87.9	1.2	68.3	38.8	114.7	167.8	145.1	73.3	31.7	8.1	0.5
1980	15.9	68.4	1.1	53.0	32.5	82.1	115.1	112.9	61.9	19.8	3.9	0.2
1985	15.8	66.3	1.2	51.0	31.0	79.6	108.3	111.0	69.1	24.0	4.0	0.2
1990	16.7	70.9	1.4	59.9	37.5	88.6	116.5	120.2	80.8	31.7	5.5	0.2
1991	16.3	69.6	1.4	62.1	38.7	94.4	115.7	118.2	79.5	32.0	5.5	0.2
1992	15.9	68.9	1.4	60.7	37.8	94.5	114.6	117.4	80.2	32.5	5.9	0.3
1993	15.5	67.6	1.4	59.6	37.8	92.1	112.6	115.5	80.8	32.9	6.1	0.3
1994	15.2	66.7	1.4	58.9	37.6	91.5	111.1	113.9	81.5	33.7	6.4	0.3
1995	14.8	65.6	1.3	56.8	36.0	89.1	109.8	112.2	82.5	34.3	6.6	0.3
1996	14.7	65.3	1.2	54.4	33.8	86.0	110.4	113.1	83.9	35.3	6.8	0.3
Race of child:[3] White												
1950	23.0	102.3	0.4	70.0	31.3	120.5	190.4	165.1	102.6	51.4	14.5	1.0
1960	22.7	113.2	0.4	79.4	35.5	154.6	252.8	194.9	109.6	54.0	14.7	0.8
1970	17.4	84.1	0.5	57.4	29.2	101.5	163.4	145.9	71.9	30.0	7.5	0.4
1980	14.9	64.7	0.6	44.7	25.2	72.1	109.5	112.4	60.4	18.5	3.4	0.2
Race of mother:[4] White												
1980	15.1	65.6	0.6	45.4	25.5	73.2	111.1	113.8	61.2	18.8	3.5	0.2
1985	15.0	64.1	0.6	43.3	24.4	70.4	104.1	112.3	69.9	23.3	3.7	0.2
1990	15.8	68.3	0.7	50.8	29.5	78.0	109.8	120.7	81.7	31.5	5.2	0.2
1991	15.4	67.0	0.8	52.8	30.7	83.5	109.0	118.8	80.5	31.8	5.2	0.2
1992	15.0	66.5	0.8	51.8	30.1	83.8	108.2	118.4	81.4	32.2	5.7	0.2
1993	14.7	65.4	0.8	51.1	30.3	82.1	106.9	116.6	82.1	32.7	5.9	0.3
1994	14.4	64.9	0.8	51.1	30.7	82.1	106.2	115.5	83.2	33.7	6.2	0.3
1995	14.2	64.4	0.8	50.1	30.0	81.2	106.3	114.8	84.6	34.5	6.4	0.3
1996	14.1	64.3	0.8	48.1	28.4	78.4	107.2	116.1	86.3	35.6	6.7	0.3
Race of child:[3] Black												
1960	31.9	153.5	4.3	156.1	- - -	- - -	295.4	218.6	137.1	73.9	21.9	1.1
1970	25.3	115.4	5.2	140.7	101.4	204.9	202.7	136.3	79.6	41.9	12.5	1.0
1980	22.1	88.1	4.3	100.0	73.6	138.8	146.3	109.1	62.9	24.5	5.8	0.3
Race of mother:[4] Black												
1980	21.3	84.9	4.3	97.8	72.5	135.1	140.0	103.9	59.9	23.5	5.6	0.3
1985	20.4	78.8	4.5	95.4	69.3	132.4	135.0	100.2	57.9	23.9	4.6	0.3
1990	22.4	86.8	4.9	112.8	82.3	152.9	160.2	115.5	68.7	28.1	5.5	0.3
1991	21.9	85.2	4.8	115.5	84.1	158.6	160.9	113.1	67.7	28.3	5.5	0.2
1992	21.3	83.2	4.7	112.4	81.3	157.9	158.0	111.2	67.5	28.8	5.6	0.2
1993	20.5	80.5	4.6	108.6	79.8	151.9	152.6	108.4	67.3	29.2	5.9	0.3
1994	19.5	76.9	4.6	104.5	76.3	148.3	146.0	104.0	65.8	28.9	5.9	0.3
1995	18.2	72.3	4.2	96.1	69.7	137.1	137.1	98.6	64.0	28.7	6.0	0.3
1996	17.8	70.7	3.6	91.4	64.7	132.5	136.8	98.2	63.3	29.1	6.1	0.3
American Indian or Alaska Native mothers[4]												
1980	20.7	82.7	1.9	82.2	51.5	129.5	143.7	106.6	61.8	28.1	8.2	*
1985	19.8	78.6	1.7	79.2	47.7	124.1	139.1	109.6	62.6	27.4	6.0	*
1990	18.9	76.2	1.6	81.1	48.5	129.3	148.7	110.3	61.5	27.5	5.9	*
1991	18.3	75.1	1.6	85.0	52.7	134.3	144.9	106.9	61.9	27.2	5.9	0.4
1992	18.4	75.4	1.6	84.4	53.8	132.6	145.5	109.4	63.0	28.0	6.1	*
1993	17.8	73.4	1.4	83.1	53.7	130.7	139.8	107.6	62.8	27.6	5.9	*
1994	17.1	70.9	1.9	80.8	51.3	130.3	134.2	104.1	61.2	27.5	5.9	0.4
1995	16.6	69.1	1.8	78.0	47.8	130.7	132.5	98.4	62.2	27.7	6.1	*
1996	16.6	68.7	1.7	73.9	46.4	122.3	133.9	98.5	63.2	28.5	6.3	*

See footnotes at end of table.